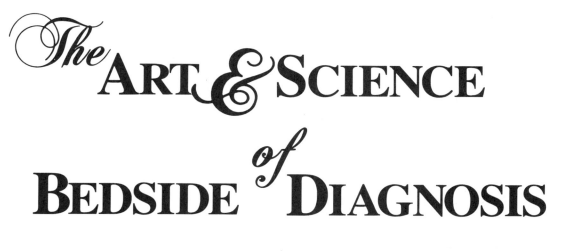

The ART & SCIENCE
of
BEDSIDE DIAGNOSIS

by

D0100854

Joseph D. Sapira, M.D.
Professor of Medicine
St. Louis University School of Medicine

Edited by Jane M. Orient, M.D.

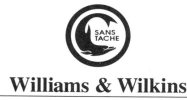

Williams & Wilkins
BALTIMORE • PHILADELPHIA • HONG KONG
LONDON • MUNICH • SYDNEY • TOKYO
A WAVERLY COMPANY

Editor: Charles W. Mitchell
Production Service: Stony Run Publishing Services, Baltimore, MD

Accurate indications, adverse reactions, and dosage schedules for drugs are provided in this book, but it is possible that they may change. The reader is urged to review the package information data of the manufacturers of the medications mentioned.

Printed in the United States of America

First Edition 1990

Library of Congress Cataloging-in-Publication Data

Sapira, Joseph D., 1936–
   The art and science of bedside diagnosis / by Joseph D. Sapira.
      p.   cm.
   Includes bibliographical references.
   ISBN 0-8067-1791-2
   1.   Physical diagnosis.   I.   Title.
   [DNLM: 1. Medical History Taking.   2. Physical Examination.
   WB 200 S241a]
RC76.S25   1989
616.07′54—dc19
DNLM/DLC   89-16654
for Library of Congress   CIP

95   96   97   98
   7   8   9   10

Contents

Preface

"As the decay of the Chou Dynasty grew worse, studies were neglected and the scribes became more and more ignorant. When they did not remember the genuine character, they blunderingly invented a false one. These non-genuine characters, copied out again by other ignorant writers, became usual."

L. Wieger, SJ, *Chinese Characters*

The goal of this book is to help the reader achieve the correct personal, metaphysical, and epistemologic perspectives on the artful science of clinical examination. This is not a textbook of medicine. In analogy to football, a textbook of medicine is the playbook. This book is about learning the skills of blocking, tackling, punting, passing, and so forth, so that one may execute the plays with diligence and facility.

The style is intentionally unusual, attempting to capture the excitement of actual rounds with diversions along the way. This should help to hold the attention of today's students and residents, who are often caught up in pointless memorizing and unproductive errand-running at the expense of scholastic preparation for the lifelong task of self-teaching.

This book is written with a sense of great sadness about American academic medicine, and from a prerevolutionary point of view (the revolution in academic medicine having occurred about 1968,* when the intellectual approach to diagnosis and its attendant techniques of clinical examination fell into disrespect, superseded by an inappropriately exclusive reliance on dogma and modern technologic devices). If the current civilization preserves even more trivial records of its behavior than did the Sumerian culture, then the present text may be of interest to historians of future ages. Some may think this book will be held in the same regard as the work of the 19th century translator of Galen, who believed that medicine could be greatly improved if only the ignorant physicians of his day had access to Galen's work. After devoting his life to translating Galen into modern languages, he found that his task had immediately become an exercise in obsolescence, due to the beginning of the scientific era of medicine. Yet, one daily observes patients for whom the history and physical examination could lead one to the correct diagnosis hours, days, and even weeks before it can be achieved by those who rely solely on modern technology. And for some diagnoses (vascular headache, depression, irritable colon, for example) there is no substitutive technology.

Plowing through this tome, learning what you can and noting other passages for future use, is hopefully part of your initiation into a very special and elite club. This club collects no dues and has no scheduled meetings (although you can attend a meeting any time you wish by picking up a book). It is founded on a certain value hierarchy, irrespective of dramatic changes in technology, and exists in the dimension of time, mostly irrespective of place.

The tradition of clinical examination dates back 2500 years or longer. The author of this book, who is attempting to help train you, was trained by Dr. Jack Myers, who was trained

---

*Chargaff, working independently from completely different observations, also selects 1968 as the year of revolution. (See E. Chargaff, *Heraclitean Fire: Sketches from a Life Before Nature,* Rockefeller University Press, New York, 1978.)

by Dr. Soma Weiss. With sufficient scholarly effort, it would be possible to trace a lineage from any reader back to Laennec, or even to Hippocrates.

We owe a great debt to those who taught us. The only way to repay the debt is to transmit the knowledge to the next generation, in so far as it is possible. In every hospital and every school that I visit, I meet young persons of the prerevolutionary type. This book is for them.

Acknowledgments

Dr. Jane M. Orient, of Tucson, Arizona, edited this book. She also wrote the first draft of the breast examination chapter (15) and the pelvic examination chapter (22) and contributed other significant original writing. She literally read every word in the original manuscript, removed many passages and illustrations, and provided other illustrations and written material. Additionally, she did many experiments with the internal arrangement of the chapters, sections, and even paragraphs, all to make the work more accessible to the reader. In addition to bringing the critical skills of one trained in physical science and mathematics to bear on such problems as the Phillips equation, she also brought the perspective of the literate practitioner to bear on the writing of the author, forcing the text to be not only correct and entertaining, but as referenced and perspicacious as the facts would permit. Without such an editor, this would have been a far different work.

This manuscript was reviewed by Dr. David Rosen of Minnesota (Chapters 1 through 17), Dr. Bill Mootz of Missouri (material on diagnostic decision making in Chapters 1 and 27), Dr. Dennis Patton of Arizona (Chapter 1), Dr. Joe Ojile of Missouri (Chapter 2), Dr. Herbert Weiner of California (Chapter 2), Dr. Bernie Davis of Missouri (Chapters 2 and 3), Dr. Gert Muelheims of Missouri (blood pressure section of Chapter 6), Dr. Don Kennedy of Missouri (temperature section of Chapter 6), Dr. John Bass of Alabama (respiratory section of Chapter 6, and Chapter 16), Dr. Alvin Shapiro of Pennsylvania (blood pressure section of Chapter 6), Dr. H. J. Roberts of Florida (Chapter 7), Dr. David Clarkson of Alabama (Chapter 8), Dr. Rene Wegria of Missouri (Chapter 9), Dr. Eugene de Juan of North Carolina (Chapter 10), Dr. William G. Troyer of Illinois (Chapters 12 and 13), Dr. Fouad Abbas of Maryland (Chapters 15 and 22), Dr. Ben Friedman of Alabama (percussion sections of Chapters 16 and 17), and Dr. Simon Horenstein of Missouri (Chapter 26).

For instruction in library science, I am indebted to Beverly MacVaugh, Debbie Gustin, Alfrieda Keeling, Ann Repetto, and Nancy Besselsen.

Dr. R. A. Fiscella of Baltimore helped translate Rondot. The Spanish-English data base was reviewed by Teresa Federico, Pamela Potter, Dr. M. Lenore Fines, and Dr. Joseph Knapp of Arizona.

Permission to quote from pages 268 to 269 of his book *The Healing Hand* was granted by Dr. Guido Majno. The translations of Herodotus are reproduced by courtesy of Penquin Books. Henry Miller is quoted with permission of Grove Press, publisher of *Sexus,* and New Directions Publishing Company, publisher of *Sunday After the War.* The *Hippocratic Writings*, translated by Iain M. Lonie, are quoted courtesy of Penguin Books and Iain M. Lonie. Permission to quote from Philip Wayne's translation of *Faust* was granted by Penguin Books. An excerpt from Ernest Hemingway's *Death in the Afternoon* (copyright 1932 Charles Scribner's Sons, 1960 Ernest Hemingway) is reprinted with permission of Charles Scribner's Sons, an imprint of Macmillan Publishing Company. Some of the tables and illustrations in Chapter 10 originally appeared in the November 1984 issue of *Disease-a-Month* and are reproduced through the courtesy of Year Book Medical Publishers. Permission to quote Albert Jay Nock was granted by Frank Chodorov, who first printed the speech on Pantagruelism in the August 1946 issue of *Analysis*, and by the Nockian Society.

Dr. David Spodick of Massachusetts contributed to the section on further considerations on the second heart sound, Chapter 17.

I thank Dr. Harold N. Segall for the copy of his privately printed book *Experiments for Determining the Efficiency of Arterial Collaterals* by N. S. Korotkoff, with notes and translation by Dr. Harold N. Segall.

Much of the material on clinical reasoning is reprinted with permission from *Southern Medical Journal*, edited by Dr. John Thomison.

The manuscript was inspired by teachers at the University of Pittsburgh (1957–1971), who taught by diligent example and vigorous expectation, including Doctors Jack Myers, Eugene Robin, T. Danowski, Campbell Moses, W. Jensen, A. I. Braude, T. Benedek, Herbert Heineman, James Leonard, Frank Kroetz, P. Bromberg, Alvin P. Shapiro, J. Field, Jessica Lewis, William Earley, Henry Brosin, James McLaughlin, and Arthur Mirsky. Thanks to Doctors Stewart Wolf, Ben Friedman, Wladimir Wertilecki, and so many others in the South. There are no truly single-authored texts.

In memory of Gerry Rodnan, M.D., and Joan Rodnan, M.D., and for all the other wonderful teachers and students who taught me by diligent example and vigorous expectation to listen compassionately and examine thoughtfully, and who encouraged me to "pass it on."

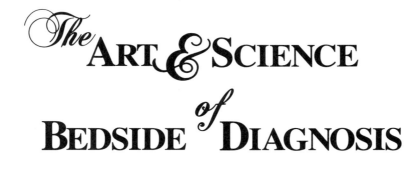

1
Introduction

"If you would converse with me, you must first define your terms."

Voltaire

How to Use This Book

This book is written for clinicians of differing levels of experience, from medical students in their first class in physical diagnosis to attending physicians of long experience. Therefore, a layered style of writing is employed, with sections intended for the more advanced reader set in this typeface. The presence of this type should suggest to the beginning student that there is more to physical diagnosis than that tiny piece he* is able to assimilate at the beginning of his studies. Physical diagnosis, and clinical diagnosis, cannot be learned in a week, a month, or even a year.

How long does it take to learn clinical diagnosis? I am still learning after 30 years. According to Tinsley Harrison, Ben Friedman of Alabama was the best diagnostician he knew, and Ben Friedman was still learning (and teaching) pearls when he was more than 70 years old. The best diagnostician I ever knew, Jack Myers of Pennsylvania, was at the age of 70 entering his second decade of trying to teach a computer to think the way he did. On the other hand, I have had to tell some 24-year-old medical students that they were too old to become physicians because they had already lost their curiosity.

This textbook is intended for physicians, not for subspecialist technicians. Thus, the interviewing chapter is meant to apply to medical patients, not psychiatric patients. It is necessary to emphasize this point because of the present tendency, derived from the evolution of specialty medicine, to teach an abbreviated form of interviewing. And beneath the specialist stands the subspecialist, who may only need to diagnose four or five diseases, and so does not require much of a data base from which to construct his history. Furthermore, an interview may not be considered necessary for building a relationship if the contact with the patient is to be episodic or even singular. In this increasingly prevalent situation, the whole patient has become less than the sum of his parts.

The early chapters on physical diagnosis introduce concepts in clinical reasoning that are reinforced throughout the book;

---

*Use of the masculine pronouns throughout this book is meant to include the feminine counterparts when not referring to a specific person. This is done for simplicity and is not intended to be discriminatory or exclusionary.

they are not intended to be exhaustively descriptive. The scientific method is implicitly reviewed in the section on vital signs, wherein some small group self-experiments are described. By the time one has reached the examination of the heart, one will be reading long passages of physiology, pathophysiology, and hortative instruction.

Many of the advanced maneuvers would not belong in a routine physical examination. However, in order to learn "how to do it" the student needs to perform a certain number of such special examinations in normal subjects. Just what constitutes an acceptable number as well as which special maneuvers ought to become routine in a given population are questions whose answers are left to the discretion of a wise preceptor.

In many sections, I describe "a method" that I have used and taught and found to be successful. These methods are not necessarily encyclopedic. For instance, I once wrote a paper on physical examination of the spleen (Sapira, 1981a), which included a review of the world's literature and more different methods than any reasonable person could possibly be interested in. Although the paper was published in an obscure state journal, within 2 months I was instructed at the lunch table by three different persons, each of whom preferred a favorite but unique method, all of which had been left out of my paper.

Throughout this work, certain "pearls" are marked with a ○ in the margin. Their selection is based upon the author's decades of clinical teaching. Some of them may not be pearls for you, whereas other statements might be so. You are encouraged to mark your own pearls.

In addition to the pearls, there are also marginal **$$**. These symbols mark equipment that you may want to buy for your black bag (also see p. 2).

Finally, there are marginal flags ⚑ to indicate certain situations indicative of a real or impending emergency, wherein the beginner should immediately seek experienced aid for the patient.

To afford some respite from the prose, and to give the reader a chance to entertain one's speculative powers amidst so much concrete instruction, some *objets d'art* are interspersed. These figures (some of which have been doctored) serve as illustrations of phenomena that were not photographed when I encountered them clinically. In addition, they illustrate the points that one is always a physician, even at the art museum, and that medicine is a learned profession that exists within the context of Western civilization.

The beginning student should not attempt to master everything on the first reading. The text is designed to permit you to reread the introductory passages, and, when you have mastered those, to go on to the complex material. In this way, the book and your experience can be concordant. Do not expect to understand much of the material until you have seen it demonstrated in real patients (e.g., if you are seeing many patients with pulmonary disease, but no orthopedic patients, initially concentrate your attention on the chest examination and merely skim the sections having to do with the bones and the joints).

Dr. Rene Wegria of Missouri offers an interesting study technique especially suitable for passages that do not have numbers or statements to be memorized, but rather interconnected ideas. Read a paragraph and then close the text and repeat the paragraph back to yourself in your own words, not those of the author. Then reread the paragraph to be sure you understood it. If you cannot paraphrase the passage correctly, read it again and repeat the procedure. Do not go on to the next paragraph until you have mastered the first one.

It is important for you to be an active, not a passive, reader. To help in this regard, there are various quizzes throughout the book, or sometimes simply questions. As soon as you come to a question, attempt to answer it, and write down your answer. Too many students and "educators" alike act as if learning were a passive act. It is not like getting a suntan. You cannot simply show up and wait for it to happen! On the rare occasion when an answer to the quiz is not given, the author means to imply that just attempting to solve the problem should make the answer apparent.

For the junior student.   The mind grows slowly, one skill or fact at a time. Therefore, you are encouraged to read about each patient seen every day, and try to learn at least one new fact about that patient and his disease. Similarly, you may wish to introduce one new maneuver a day from this book.

The greatest library known to the ancients, and possibly the greatest library of all time, was the one at Alexandria. It was built by requiring that no ship could dock in the harbor unless it brought payment of a book. Thus, the library was built one book at a time.

Unfortunately, the library at Alexandria was burnt in a tumult. The one at Constantinople was also burnt, but only so that the manuscripts could be used to heat the water for the public baths. It is said to have taken weeks to consume that library.

The mark of degenerate societies is that they foolishly consume the accumulated wisdom of their predecessors. So too is the accumulated wisdom of the clinician consumed by time and senility. Like the library at Constantinople, the only evidence of a former vigor may be the length of time it takes to burn out.

For the attending.   One curriculum is to have the students begin the interviewing course by taking the chief complaint the first week. The physical diagnosis course begins concurrently, with the students determining the vital signs of the same patient. The first case record consists only of the chief complaint and the vital signs, and whatever differential diagnosis that the students can develop. Each week a portion of the history and the physical are added. For instance, the second week the students are asked to compose a history of the present illness (in addition to the chief complaint), and to record the general appearance as well as the vital signs. The next week, the integument is added, and the following week, the lymph nodes. By then, the students may be comfortable with the concepts involved in the history of the present illness, and they may begin adding the other portions of the history.

This system slows down the bright students, and the class does not get to the examination of the heart until half the course has passed. Also, the course is very expensive in terms of faculty time. The advantage is that any student of reasonable intelligence can be taught to do a thorough history and physical and to construct a differential diagnosis.

$$ Diagnostic Equipment to Purchase

The Sphygmomanometer

Be sure that the blood pressure cuff that you purchase is sufficiently long; alternately you could purchase an extra wide one (see Ch. 6, p. 88). For instance, when I recently needed a new sphygmomanometer cuff, I purchased a thigh cuff, as I no longer see children but do see a lot of people with big arms. If you purchase an anaeroid pressure gauge, which is less expensive than a mercury manometer, be sure that it does not have a pin stop. Calibrate it according to the method in Chapter 6 (p. 86).

The Ophthalmoscope

These are the minimum *requirements* for a satisfactory ophthalmoscope:

1.   An on-off switch (a rheostat is unnecessary)
2.   A circle of light (you don't *need* the other apertures, although they are fun and may sometimes be helpful)
3.   A focusing wheel

Additionally, you may be wise to purchase an instrument whose handle will also take the otoscope head to avoid buying two separate power sources.

If you have astigmatism, you may prefer to examine patients while wearing your spectacles. If so, purchase an ophthalmoscope with a rubber cushion on the facing, so that it won't scratch your lenses.

See Chapter 10 (pp. 173–174) for a discussion of the optional features on ophthalmoscopes.

Tuning Forks

I prefer to use a 1024 Hz or 512 Hz tuning fork for the Rinne and Weber tests (see Ch. 11, p. 211), since high frequency sounds are often the first ones lost in sensorineural defects, which are the hardest to detect. For testing vibratory sensation, the 256 Hz tuning fork is suggested (see Ch. 26, p. 507).

Any tuning fork needs to have a sturdy handle with a base broad enough to ensure good contact with the bony prominences, and tines that are weighted or sufficiently supple to vibrate for a reasonable period of time. Many of the free tuning forks that medical students receive from drug companies are worth what the students pay for them.

The Stethoscope

I was consulted in 1816 by a young woman who presented some general symptoms of disease of the heart, in whose case the application of the hand and percussion gave but slight indications, on account of her corpulency. On account of the age and sex of the patient, the common modes of exploration being inapplicable, I was led to recollect a well known acoustic phenomenon, namely, if the ear is applied to one extremity of a beam, a person can, very distinctly, hear the scratching of a pin at the other end. I imagined this property of bodies might be made use of in the present case. I took a quire of paper which I rolled together as closely as possible, and applied one end to the precordial region; by placing my ear at the other end, I was agreeably surprised at hearing the pulsation of the heart much more clearly and distinctly than I had ever been able to do by the immediate application of the ear. (RTH Laennec, *The Treatise on Mediated Auscultation*, vol. 1, 1821)

The student should purchase a stethoscope with two different heads: a flat diaphragm, useful for picking up high-pitched sounds, and a bell, which when softly applied is better for detecting low-pitched sounds. Some bells have a rubber rim, which helps to prevent the examiner from pressing so hard as to convert the bell into a diaphragm by tightening the skin beneath it. It is also useful for ausculting skinny, bony chests, being capable of forming a seal that cannot be achieved with a metal-rimmed bell. You should be able to switch from one head to the other quickly and easily.

The length of the tubing is usually 12 inches or more. It has been scientifically proved that the shorter the tubing the better (Rappaport & Sprague, 1941), but for tubing less than 12 inches, what one loses in comfort (and consequently in ability to concentrate) offsets the gain in proximity. The very long-tubed stethoscopes (rarely seen nowadays) date from an era when the physician wished to keep as great a distance as possible between himself and a potentially infectious tubercular patient.

The most important criterion for the earpieces is that they be comfortable in your ears. Under no circumstances should you ever purchase a stethoscope with uncomfortable earpieces. Most surgical supply houses will have sets of interchangeable earpieces so that one can get a comfortable set. (You might also find that you can hear much better with one style of earpiece.) Also check to be sure that the earpieces are slanted forward in approximately the same vectors as your external ear canals; some are slanted more than others. Since you will keep your first stethoscope for about 20 years, choose it with care, and do not buy it with the expectation that you will "adjust to it."

If you wish to compare the acoustic properties of two stethoscopes, the following method will detect gross differences without the use of fancy equipment: Place an earpiece of one stethoscope into your left ear and an earpiece of the second stethoscope into your right ear. Place the (connected) diaphragms of both stethoscopes in front of you, equidistant from a point 2 or 3 feet away on a solid surface. Tap on the point, and in the manner of someone adjusting stereo speakers, notice whether the sound is louder in one ear than the other. To control for the possibility that your hearing is better in one ear, switch the earpieces and repeat the experiment. If the louder sound is now in the opposite ear, you have identified the stethoscope that is better for you. If you have an extra pair of hands, you might want to try this experiment with the unattached earpiece of each stethoscope occluded by a finger.

Question: *What is the most important part of the stethoscope?* (See Appendix 1-1, p. 8.)

Clean the earpiece of your stethoscope from time to time with a Q-tip soaked in alcohol. A pipe cleaner might help to clean out earwax that has migrated beyond the part that fits in the ear. Persons who produce copious quantities of earwax have on occasion noted it to be appearing at the chest piece. In former days, cardiologists regularly used compressed air to clean their stethoscopes.

Reflex Hammers

Purchase any kind of reflex hammer that you wish. The most popular type at the present time is the Taylor hammer whose head is a rubber triangle (see Fig. 26-26). This is a good hammer for beginners because it has both a point (which is optimal for circumstances in which even the beginner knows the exact spot to be struck, such as the biceps tendon) and a broad surface (which can bolster one's confidence when examining the ankle jerk). The head is usually mounted on a steel handle that ends in a point that may be used for producing a noxious stimulus (e.g., for the Babinski reflex) (see Ch. 26).

The Queen's Square hammer (see Fig. 26-27) is popular in England. It has a round rubber ring for striking, mounted on a long wooden handle whose sharpened end can be used for producing noxious stimuli (e.g., for waking medical students during lectures).

My original reflex hammer from medical school was simply a round rubber ball about the diameter of a nickel, mounted on a handle. This illustrates the point that *any* hammer is satisfactory if the examiner knows where to strike the tendon. I have even used the diaphragm of a Sprague stethoscope, and a former resident, a Vanderbilt graduate, used her knuckle.

Other Equipment

It is helpful to have a spring-loaded tape measure, calibrated in both inches and centimeters. It is cheaper to buy one from a fabric store than from a medical supply store.

Do not buy a single pin to use for sensory testing. Chopsticks and a pencil sharpener or a fresh safety pin for each patient may be used for this purpose (see Ch. 26, p. 509).

Calipers for measuring lymph nodes and other swellings are described in Chapter 8 (p. 139).

The Science of Clinical Examination

Clinical diagnosis is currently the most neglected of the bases for the scientific practice of medicine. Yet unlike the secondhand information with which the clinician often works, the clinical examination provides information obtained firsthand from the patient. Working with the primary source introduces in an almost effortless fashion the issues of level of certainty, normal variability, interrater reliability, intrarater reliability, and that unique, almost unconscious type of factor analysis used by the expert diagnostician. Experience with the clinical examination thus refines the techniques for handling information in general, and develops the faculty for critical analysis that marks the scientist.

Unfortunately, the teaching of clinical examination is often marred by Olympian pronouncements sans references for specific statements. Providing references in areas that should be controversial is one of the unique features of this book. Specific articles may be cited in the text where appropriate, and listed at the end of a section or chapter. Where no article is mentioned, I have sometimes named the individual who first taught me the sign. Unreferenced statements are usually based on my own clinical experience (for a caveat about clinical experience, see Ch. 24, p. 424). General references are critically reviewed in the annotated bibliography in the last chapter. Though not without faults, these books, which might be called "golden oldies," have been helpful to me over the past 30 years, and the statements that I quote have been personally tested by me.

•

At bedside rounds at the University of Pittsburgh in the 1960s, Dr. Eugene D. Robin always asked for the evidence, for the data. His retinue of students and house officers felt that these carefully knotted strings of questions were but a requisite evil to be endured in passage to the Nirvana of his 13 nostrums for the treatment of patients with chronic obstructive lung disease. Since there was a reason for each of the treatment orders (tea, supersaturated potassium iodide solution, ephedrine, etc.), it was clear to us that they were engraved on stone and would never change.

None of these nostrums is now used in the treatment of chronic obstructive pulmonary disease, and atropine (which was then forbidden) is enjoying a renewed popularity. But the habit of asking, "What is the evidence?" remains current.

•

The Art of Clinical Examination

Because clinical examination remains a personal activity, historical and anecdotal approaches have a place, and many items in this text are based on experiences that actually occurred during bedside rounds. The occasional use of the first person singular pronoun may be disturbing to some readers who are accustomed to the impersonal tone of most contemporary texts. The impersonal tone is an implication of universality, implying that the author, like the physicist, has embarked on the discovery of truly universal truths. Alas, there are not many universal truths in medicine, and when there are—when something becomes 100% perfect—that something usually moves into the field of public health or is assigned to a physician extender. On the other hand, the personal pronoun is a statement of limitation, nonuniversality, probability, and conditionality. This is not egotism, but the exact opposite: the plaint of Hippocrates about the difficulty of learning the art, the perils of secure prognosis in our *techne* (a Greek word meaning science, art, profession, and career, all wrapped up into one).

The use of the personal pronoun is also an exhortation to the student. A student who has made carefully controlled observations in an area where no others have done so makes not only a contribution to the body of knowledge, but shows that he has learned, at an early stage, the levers by which corrigible minds are moved. Such a student has learned the intellectual ground rules of science, the laws of scientific evidence, by which he can stand on the shoulders of his elders. But his observations are still quite personal. They are limited by the environment and circumstances in which they were collected. Another time and place might yield different results to some other person. Thus, the personal pronoun is meant as a reminder of limitation, not a banner of grandiosity.

Definitions

Semantics has a profound effect on our thinking (Sapira 1980a, 1981a, 1982). Conversely, the way in which I will use certain terms reflects the philosophy that underlies the approach to interviewing and diagnosis that will be taught in this book. The terms

are listed alphabetically to facilitate future reference, but should be skimmed now for purposes of orientation.

Academic medicine: that practice of medicine in which the practitioner is mainly concerned with the development of new knowledge.

Basic science: the parochially impractical but clinically useful sciences concerned with discipline-bound language and the general rules of scientific evidence.

Compliance: 1) change in volume per unit change in pressure (dV/dP)—a measure of the ease with which a structure may be deformed; 2) a tendency to give in to others; 3) obedience to a dictate given by an authority; 4) (vulgar medical parlance) doing what the doctor wants.

I have never had a patient who was completely noncompliant. As a rule, the bones are noncompliant, but the muscles and subcutaneous tissues are almost always compliant (myositis ossificans and calcinosis being the exceptions that prove the rule). I have had a number of patients who chose not to follow my advice. It is quite likely that the problem was with me, not with the patient. I had failed to spend enough time to persuade the patient of the presumed wisdom of my advice; or perhaps I had not gotten to know the patient well enough to understand why the advice would not be attractive. That failure on my part does not justify appropriating a word from the physical sciences to hide behind while blaming the patient.

Conversion: 1) to turn all together: as in, "the patient with atrial fibrillation and a high degree of atrioventricular dissociation underwent DC conversion to normal sinus rhythm"; 2) certain neurologic events of psychogenic origin such as paralyses and somatosensory impairments. The Freudian belief is that the unconscious conflict would be unbearable if it became conscious, so instead it manifests itself symbolically in a conversion reaction. (This is a glib summary of a very large body of work that I find quite convincing.)

Diagnosis: 1) the process of identifying the patient's disease; 2) a thorough understanding.

Disease: a member of a set of verbal symbols used by physicians to communicate with each other in reference to individual human events. See *Illness*.

Education: teaching the selection of contexts within which acts are performed. See *Training*.

Empiric: reliably based upon experience, even if not yet scientific in terms of being connected to a substrate of knowledge or concepts sufficient to permit the observation to be understood within the framework of a general scientific theory. Contrast with expectant.

Expectant: often confused with empiric, this adjective applied to a therapeutic endeavor is synonymous with "hopeful" or "anticipatory." However, there is no reliably predictable outcome based upon past experience.

Falsifiable hypothesis: a hypothesis susceptible to being proved wrong. (The "best" diagnoses are falsifiable, a principle derived from Popper's statement about scientific hypotheses (Sapira, 1980b), which was anticipated by Nietzsche in *Beyond Good and Evil*, I, 18: "It is certainly not the least charm of a theory that it is refutable."*) For further discussion, see Chapter 27, page 529.

---

*Nietzsche may thus be fulfilled in his own stated "ambition to say in ten sentences what everyone else says in a whole book."

Functional: a word used to cover the physician's ignorance. Like "stress" (vide infra), this word should preferably not be used.

Historian: the person who composes a history of events that have happened to someone else.

History: the physician's abstraction of certain facts developed in the course of the interview and arranged in a manner that facilitates diagnosis.

Illness: the totality of effects, predicaments, and repercussions of the disease, deformity, or circumstances produced (directly or indirectly) in the patient.

Internal medicine: 1) (*obsolete*) that nonsurgical medical specialty concerned with clinical diagnosis and scientific therapy. Previously a secondary care consultant specialty, it experienced crisis by lysis in the late 1960s. 2) (*contemporary*) a biopolitical consortium of balkanized tertiary nonsurgical subspecialties, which, oxymoronically, claim it to be a "*primary care specialty.*"

Interview: the process of talking with the patient. See *History*.

Malingering: pretending to signs and symptoms that do not in fact exist. This is always a tenuous and sometimes a tendentious concept. It implies that the physician can know the thoughts of a patient who has chosen not to articulate those thoughts. Since the physician is not a mind reader, he must make an inference about what the patient is consciously thinking, based upon the physician's knowledge of medicine and the signs and symptoms that are found.

Management: the art of keeping the patient alive without furthering one's understanding of why the patient came into the hospital in the first place (*contemporary definition*).

Mutatis mutandis: (*Latin*) "changing with change" (i.e., everything else changed accordingly).

Neurologic: referring to all aspects of the nervous system and its examination except those having to do with affect, motivation, behavior, and the reporting of mental phenomena.

Objective: 1) (*non-Cartesian*) capable of providing sufficient replicability to be used with a high degree of confidence; 2) (*Cartesian*) observable by more than one reporter.

Organic: one of the languages in which patients can be described (Graham, 1967). It is hardly ever used correctly, and should be dropped from our vocabulary.

Practical: capable of being perceived by the speaker as of immediate use in the solution of whatever problems can be identified by the speaker at that point in his intellectual development (*parochial*).

Provisional diagnosis: same as a conditional diagnosis, that is, a diagnosis suggested and favored but not yet proved. Provisional diagnoses are most useful when one has a simple test to refute them (disprove the hypothesis), but they are often diagnoses of common conditions for which no perfectly specific and sensitive laboratory test has yet been developed (e.g., essential hypertension). The provisional diagnosis is often elevated to "the" diagnosis by a process of elimination.

Psychiatric disease: 1) (*concrete*) a disease capable of afflicting psychiatrists; 2) (*relativistic*) a disease which at some time and place may be studied, diagnosed, or treated by a psychiatrist. (Notice that this definition tells you about nothing inherent in the ultimate nature of the disease.)

Psychogenic: *in strictu sensu*, caused by the psyche. This term should be used only on those rare occasions in which this mechanism has been clearly demonstrated. It should not be used as a synonym for "imaginary," "functional," or any other adjective used to cover the physician's own ignorance or un-

certainty. A good test for the strict, rare use of this word would be to see whether one could reasonably and certainly substitute the word "cerebral."

Psychosomatic: 1) referring to the interaction between mental and physical levels of understanding; 2) used to imply linearity or causality, especially on those occasions when it is used with the word "somatopsychic," as in: "the personality and behavior of some patients with hemophilia may be considered somatopsychic in origin and mechanism. But the explanation of certain of the episodes of activation of duodenal ulcer are more likely to be psychosomatic." This word is often used incorrectly by the ignorant as a fancy synonym for "imaginary." In fact, there are no imaginary diseases except those afflicting imaginary animals. Persons who diagnose and treat imaginary illnesses and their host (imaginary) animals must be delusional. The term is also used incorrectly as a pejorative synonym for "psychogenic," especially when no positive evidence supports this putative mechanism.

Semiophysiology: the study of the physiologic basis by which signs are produced (Sapira, 1981b); from the Greek *semeion*, meaning sign or signal.

Specialty: a practice that is restricted in some way.

Stress: The concept of stress was developed by Hans Selye, who defined it as the sum of all nonspecific biologic responses. Several aspects of this definition are noteworthy. First, as a clinician and diagnostician one is most interested in specific responses, rather than nonspecific ones. Second, stress was originally defined as a response, not a stimulus. At present, stress is colloquially referred to as if it were a stimulus, or what Selye called a "stressor." (A stressor was defined as any stimulus that would produce the stress response.) Lumping the stimulus and the response together has occasionally been a useful construct in medicine. For example, antigens and antibodies were once a tautology. Now it is possible to isolate antigens and antibodies and to determine their chemical structure. However, it is not possible to determine the specific structure of a concept such as stress. The third difficulty with the term stress is that the nonspecific biologic responses, summed, may actually be so variable as to make the word semantically useless. For instance, in an experiment in which swine were exsanguinated, the cortisol and epinephrine secretory rates increased in swine bled over 30 minutes, but not in swine bled over 80 minutes (Carey et al., 1976; Sapira, 1975). Should we conclude that bleeding to death slowly is not a stress, a stressor, or stressful? Finally, the best reason for not using the word stress comes from a semantic analysis of its use on medical services and in the medical literature. As currently used, the word obfuscates meaning, aborts communication, confounds data, distracts intelligence, and generally muddies the diagnostic water. Since the word is unnecessary and inconsistently used, since it has no positive value that I have been able to determine, and since its many drawbacks are not balanced by any good feature, I feel it should be deleted—*stress delendam esse* (apologies to Cato).

Subjective: 1) (*non-Cartesian*) incapable of consistently providing sufficient replication; 2) (*Cartesian*) observable by only one observer; 3) (*current misusage*) unconvincing and less true than "objective."

Test: a historical fact, a physical sign, or a laboratory procedure that has diagnostic value.

Training: teaching the performance of specific acts irrespective of their logical context. See *Education*.

In this section, we have referred to Freud and to some of his influences on American psychosomatic medicine. In this view, problems began with conflicts in the psyche that mysteriously "leaped" into the soma. If one could but resolve the nuclear conflict, one could prevent the pathogenetic "leap" to the soma, and the disease would get better. (Of course, this leap turned out to be more like a leap between parallel trails than like a leap across a chasm in one trail. Or to be specific, following Graham, it was a leap between two different languages used to describe two different aspects of the same patient (Graham, 1967). Nevertheless, this philosophical point is not requisite to understanding the previous era's emphasis on interviewing medical patients about their inner (mental) lives and attempting to make some judgments based upon the premise that behavior is to a large extent determined by prior experiences.) In the course of spending time with the patient, as opposed to his laboratory tests and consultant reports, doctors did indeed note that patients improved. Some physicians were even able to perceive patterns that were not universally useful in a diagnostic sense, but that seemed to be statistically associated with diseases, and thus to tantalize with the promise of heuristic value. Although this approach required a great investment of time initially, the material developed was of more or less permanent value in understanding the patient. Unfortunately, the tendency in recent decades has been to emphasize activities with a guaranteed payoff and very little front-end loading. As a result, we have wondrous ways to image the patient's organs, but no commonly used way to understand why the patient with a high pepsinogen II trait does or does not manifest peptic ulcer disease at any particular time.

Evaluation of Diagnostic Signs: More Definitions

Since modern medicine is becoming more and more a quantitative science, it is increasingly important for physicians to become comfortable with quantitative reasoning. Furthermore, the physician who is not overawed by the mystique of objectivity that emanates from data expressed in three significant figures will not be betrayed by an uncritical dependence upon them. Finally, if one understands certain definitions, one can avoid some common errors of inference.

Incidence and Prevalence

Many physicians use the word incidence when they mean prevalence. *Incidence* refers to events that occur during some period of time. For instance, "on a certain island, there are 10 new cases of disease X each year." Incidence may also include the population denominator (e.g., 0.1 new cases per thousand per year). *Prevalence* is the prevailing rate of cases extant at any given point in time. For instance, "on the second anniversary of the arrival of the first case of disease X on the island, the prevalence of the disease was 20 per 100,000."

Question: *If all of the above statements came from the same source, and disease X is neither fatal nor curable, what was the population of the island in question?* (See Appendix 1-2, p. 8.)

Sensitivity and Specificity

The *sensitivity* of a test is the fraction of people with disease that have a positive test (see Table 1-1). Formally, it is defined as the

ratio: true positives/ (true positives + false negatives). (This is also called the true positive rate.)

A test with high sensitivity is not necessarily a useful test. The sign "10 fingers" would be extremely sensitive for almost any disease, since most patients with the disease will have 10 fingers. Very few patients with the disease will have a different number of fingers. Thus, the ratio of true positives (number of patients with disease who have 10 fingers) to the sum of true positives plus false negatives (where false negatives are people who have the disease and do not have 10 fingers) will usually be greater than 0.99 (except in a sanitarium for Hansen's disease). Yet common sense tells us that the possession of 10 fingers, however sensitive on paper, is not of great use to the diagnostician. Why not? The reason is that most of the people in the world have 10 fingers, but do not have the disease.

As a rule, tests with low sensitivity are useful only if they have a very high specificity. Such tests would never be used for screening, but can help separate the true from the false positive results after a prior, more sensitive test.

Specificity is mathematically defined as the true negative rate, or true negatives/(true negatives + false positives) (i.e., the proportion of people who do *not* have disease that will *not* have a positive test) (see Table 1-1).

A Self-Study Question

Test A has a sensitivity of 100%, but a specificity of only 20% for disease X. Test B, which is very expensive, has a specificity of about 100%, but a sensitivity of 50%. How should one go about finding cases of disease X? Write down your solution. Take your time; this is a critical issue. (See Appendix 1-3, p. 8.)

A Caveat

When many clinicians use the term specificity, they have in mind the ratio: true positives/(true positives + false positives) (i.e., the probability that a person with a positive test will have the disease, or the predictive value of a positive test) (see Table 1-1). In fact, specificity once was understood in that way. (*Stedman's Medical Dictionary*, 21st edition, 1966, defined specificity as "the state of having a fixed relationship to a single cause or to a definite result.") Note that *if* a test has a very high positive predictive value (i.e., very few false positives), it will also have a high specificity. But the converse of this statement is not necessarily true.

The clinician's tendency to translate mathematical specificity into a sense of the significance of a positive test is a hazardous pitfall. A mathematical specificity of 90% sounds very good, and the clinician might think that a positive result is very reliable. But in reality, the likelihood of a false positive might be

Table 1-1. Definitions

Disease Present		Yes (D+)	No (D−)
Test Positive	Yes (T+)	TP	FP
	No (T−)	FN	TN

Sensitivity (true positive rate)	= TP/(TP + FN)
Specificity (true negative rate)	= TN/(TN + FP)
Predictive value of positive test	= TP/(TP + FP)
Predictive value of negative test	= TN/(TN + FN)

TP = true positives; FP = false positives; TN = true negatives; FN = false negatives.

quite high, as the next example shows, because the predictive value of a test is highly dependent upon the prevalence of disease.

To avoid misunderstanding, in this text the term *pathognomonic* is used to refer to a sign with a very high positive predictive value, although other texts or journal articles might call such a sign "highly specific." The word is derived from the Greek *pathos*, meaning disease, and the Greek *gnomonikos*, meaning capable of making a judgment. The term *diagnosticity* is generally used in this text to mean the predictive value of a positive test.

Example

To understand the definitions in Table 1-1, you must work an example, and fill in a 2 × 2 table like Table 1-1 yourself. Consider a sign that is 100% sensitive and 90% specific. (The 90% specificity means that there are only 10% false positives—that sounds good, wouldn't you agree?) The sensitivity and specificity were derived from filling in a 2 × 2 table for a test population, which is probably very different from the general population, having been selected to include a lot of patients with the disease being tested for. You now want to apply the results to the real world, to a population of say 100 patients, to judge whether the presence of the sign is of diagnostic value.

At this point, you do not know enough to write any numbers in your table. You only know that (TP + FN + FP + TN) = 100. The missing piece of information is prevalence. In your population, the prevalence of disease is estimated to be 9%. In that case, 9 patients will have the disease and 91 will not. Since the sensitivity of the test is conveniently 100%, all 9 of the patients with disease will have a positive test, so you can write a "9" in the TP box, and a "0" in the FN box. Since the test is 90% specific, 90% of the 91 patients who do not have the disease, or 81.9, will have a negative test, and 9.1 will have a positive test. Thus, you can fill in the remaining boxes, and check that the numbers add to 100.

Now look at the patients who have a positive sign: 9 of them have the disease and a true positive test and 9.1 of them do not have the disease but have a false positive test, giving a total of 18.1 patients with a positive sign, out of the original population of 100. But only 9 of these 18.1 cases (49.7%) actually have a true positive. This is the predictive value of a positive test, here quite weak, despite the high specificity.

For the neophyte.   Master clinicians know all of the above at an unconscious level, and hence seldom explicate it. Most students find these points difficult to understand at first. These crucial definitions will be reemphasized throughout this text in terms of illustrative findings. By the end of the book, you should be able to use these concepts with confidence. They are brought to your attention now, because some of the findings described in this book are very important whenever you find them (because there are few false positives), whereas others become important only when they are absent (because they are highly sensitive, and their absence thus nearly excludes the disease). Obviously, if you are to have confidence in the application of these powerful concepts, you must become very accurate in your detection of the findings, and equally confident of not "finding" them when they are not present.

In the example given above (a test of 100% sensitivity and 90% specificity applied to a population with 9% prevalence), the predic-

tive value of the positive test was so low that you would be slightly better off guessing that a patient with a positive test did not have the disease, a conclusion that may seem to be contrary to common sense. However, a positive test raises the probability of disease from 9% (*prior probability*) to 49.7% (*posterior probability*, i.e., the probability *after* the test). Unfortunately, this is the kind of result that makes skeptics laugh and exclaim that the test is about as good as flipping a coin. This last statement is not true because the majority of patients without disease will have a negative test. The 49.7% is a *conditional* probability: *if* the result is positive, the probability of disease is 49.7%. Furthermore, there is a chain of reasoning in clinical problem solving. The figure of 49.7% may now become the input (the *prior probability*) for the next test ordered. Sequential positive tests with a positive predictive value of about 50% would make the sequential probabilities 50%, 75%, 87.5%, 93.75%, and so forth, tending asymptotically towards 100%. Since questions can be asked quickly, and physical maneuvers done quickly in sequence, many skillful physicians can thus come to a rapid diagnosis, even though the individual maneuvers may be likened to flipping a coin.

There is an even more important consideration. In the example above, the predictive value of a *negative* test is excellent. In fact, it is an incredible 100% (because of the 100% sensitivity). In other words, the absence of the sign is a virtual guarantee of the absence of the disease (also see Ch. 27).

By way of a clinical example, consider heart murmurs in making or excluding a diagnosis of valvular heart disease. The absence of a systolic murmur is more important than its presence because systolic murmurs tend to have a high sensitivity (few false negatives) and a lower mathematical specificity (many false positives). On the other hand, the presence of a diastolic murmur is very helpful because there are few, if any, "innocent" (false positive) diastolic murmurs. Thus, the predictive value (and also the specificity) of diastolic murmurs is high.

For the experienced clinician.   The tendency to confuse specificity with the predictive value of a positive test may result from the fact that the clinician is considering signs and symptoms (as opposed to laboratory tests) in search of positive leads to the existence of disease. In contrast, laboratory tests, for which the concept of specificity was developed, have traditionally been used to exclude entities in the differential diagnosis. It is true that laboratory tests are more commonly used today to search for positive leads (or misused by the clinically inept). However, if one keeps the original use of laboratory tests as definitive excluders in mind, the conceptual relationship of mathematical specificity (in a laboratory test) to the predictive value of a positive sign or symptom (in clinical examination) should be clear.

Although sensitivity and specificity have definite numerical values determined from a sample population, they are not constants. They are, in a sense, a trade-off. By changing the cutoff points for a "positive" and "negative" test, the sensitivity could be increased at the cost of a lower specificity, and vice versa. (See Ch. 10, p. 188 for a discussion of alpha and beta errors, which have a reciprocal relationship, and depend upon the chosen cutoff points.)

For the guru.   Specialists in disease Y study their *patients* to learn the sensitivities of tests C and D. An insurance company studies the specificities of tests C and D in insurance applicants (presumably healthy *controls* shown not to have the disease). If the prevalence of the disease is 50%, will the positive and negative predictive values of the tests be any different than if the prevalence of the disease is only 5%? (When data appear in the literature, people often do not notice that they come from widely disparate populations, which will greatly affect predictive value.)

False Positives

In this text, the term *false positives* generally means the percentage of patients whose positive test was a false positive (i.e., FP/(TP + FP)). However, the student should note that this term seems to be undergoing an evolution similar to that of *specificity*. In the decision analysis literature (Weinstein & Fineberg, 1980), the false positive rate is defined as the frequency of positive test results in those without disease (i.e., FP/(TN + FP), cf. the definition of specificity).

Normal

Sometimes normal can be defined dichotomously as the presence or absence of a sign. (Dichotomous means "cut in two.") However, many measurements are in terms of units that are numerically continuous, such as pounds, inches, milligrams per deciliter, and so forth. Often, if one plots a frequency distribution of these measures (for weight, height, serum uric acid, etc.), one obtains the famous bell-shaped curve of Gauss. This curve is unimodal; it has one hump (see the unimodal camel in Ch. 16, p. 277). Doctors would prefer a bimodal distribution, so that one hump could be labeled "normal" and the other "abnormal." With the unimodal distribution, we are often faced with the problem of determining "how far is up?" At what point does the patient become too short, too tall, too fat, too skinny, or hyperuricemic? Whatever dichotomizing point we propose, the question could be asked: Why is 20 units abnormal, whereas 19.5 units is normal?

When a mortal argues with God about the number of just men required to spare a city (Rabbenu, 1200 B.C.), God can arbitrarily choose 10 (and so instantly dichotomize the universe of cities). Scientists sometimes choose two standard deviations above or below the mean as the cutoff point for normality, but to take these points too seriously would be to engage in arbitrarily God-like behavior.

In these days of multichannel machines for determining blood chemistries, it is especially important to remember the definition of "normal." The "greater than 1.96 standard deviations from the mean" criterion arbitrarily designates 5% of a normal population as "abnormal" (2.5% as "abnormally high" and 2.5% as "abnormally low)". This means that each test will be normal in only 19 out of 20 healthy subjects. Many people think that this means the chance of an abnormality on a 20-channel machine is only 1 in 20. But by the binomial expansion, the probability of having 20 normal test results is actually 0.95 to the 20th power (0.358), and the probability of one or more abnormal results is 0.64. (Actually, tests on the chemistry screen are not independent; the liver enzymes are correlated with each other, as are the BUN and creatinine, to name just two examples. Therefore, the situation is more complicated than this paragraph indicates.)

Appendix 1-1. Answer to the Question on Page 3

The most important part of the stethoscope is the part that goes between the ears.

Appendix 1-2. Answer to the Question on Page 6

If the incidence is 10 cases per year and the disease is neither curable nor lethal, then by the end of the second year after the appearance of the disease there should have been 10 new cases plus the 10 old cases, or 20 cases on the island. If the prevalence is 20 per 100,000, then the population of the island must (conveniently) have been about 100,000, assuming the birth rate and death rate to be equal and quite small and further assuming that no special perturbations have occurred.

Appendix 1-3. Analysis of Example Given on Page 6

Test A will find all the cases of the disease, but it will also falsely diagnose four patients as having the disease for every patient who is correctly identified as healthy. (Look at the definition of specificity again, especially the denominator.) So test A alone would have too much "noise" in its signal detection.

Test B will not erroneously label so many healthy persons as diseased. But it will only find half of the persons who actually have the disease. Alone, it would not be a good screening test.

The correct answer is test A followed by test B. All the patients who are positive on test A, and only those persons, should subsequently be given test B. In this way, all diseased persons, and only such persons, will be identified.

The reverse sequence is not correct. First, one does not like to use the more expensive test first. What is the other reason?

References

Carey LC, Curtin R, Sapira JD: Influence of hemorrhage on adrenal secretion, blood glucose, and serum insulin in the awake pig. *Ann Surg* 183:185–191, 1976.

Graham DT: Health, disease, and the mind-body problem: Linguistic parallelism. *Psychosom Med* 29:52–70, 1967.

Rabbenu M: In the beginning. In: Rabbenu M (ed), *Five Books*. Sforim Books, Mount Nebo, 1200 B.C. [Also known as Moses. *Genesis* 18:32.]

Rappaport MB, Sprague HB: Physiologic and physical laws that govern auscultation, and their clinical application. *Am Heart J* 21:258–381, 1941.

Sapira JD: Letter to the editor. *J Human Stress* 1:28, 1975.

Sapira JD: Semantics of general medicine. *South Med J* 73:227–230, 1980a.

Sapira JD: Logical handling of clinical data. *South Med J* 73:1437–1438, 1980b.

Sapira JD: . . . And how big is the spleen? *South Med J* 74:53–59, 1981a.

Sapira JD: Quincke, De Musset, Duroziez and Hill: Some aortic regurgitations. *South Med J* 74:459–467, 1981b.

Sapira JD: Words. *South Med J* 75:1108–1109, 1982.

Weinstein MC, Fineberg HV: *Clinical Decision Analysis*. WB Saunders, Philadelphia, 1980.

2
The Interview

"It began to dawn on me that the healing art was not at all what people imagined it to be, that it was something very simple, too simple, in fact, for the ordinary mind to grasp. To put it in the simple way that it came to my mind I would say that it was like this: Everybody becomes a healer the moment he forgets about himself."

Henry Miller, *The Rosy Crucifixion*
Book One: Sexus, Vol. 4, Ch. 14

First Principles of the Interview

1. The most important person in the room is the patient—any patient, any room.
2. Anything that the patient tells the interviewer must be held in strictest confidence. No medical person should ever say anything about any patient in a public place where laity are present (such as a hospital elevator.)

The sign once posted in the Medical Records Department of the Falk Outpatient Clinic at the University of Pittsburgh should be reproduced in all medical institutions:

What you see here,
What you hear here,
When you leave here,
Let it stay here.

Interviewing Style

Winning the Patient's Confidence

My father devoted a number of lectures before the fourth-year medical students at the Philadelphia General Hospital to the nonscientific aspects of medicine. . . . He believed that confidence in a physician was of the utmost importance both for the well-being of the patient and for the doctor's success. Confidence, he explained, was first gained through the impression created by the doctor during the interview and physical examination.

He thought a physician should appear to be pleased to see the patient; to think of nothing but the complaint; to be sympathetic and understanding; to be confident of affecting a cure, and if not, to take a cheerful note and inspire hope; to feel privileged to treat the patient; to be courteous and considerate; and be glad to take the time to hear the patient's problems.

He made other suggestions about the ways the interview should be conducted. When extraneous matters came up, he said, the conversation should be gently and tactfully directed

to the illness. He warned against talking about oneself, no matter how trivial or innocent it might seem. (Schnabel, 1983)

○ Forget about yourself during the interview. Just permit yourself to get lost in the patient's story of his illness.

The Process of the Interview

The history is the story that the physician composes to help himself and others understand the patient's disease(s) as well as the patient's illness(es). The interview is the interpersonal process during which the raw material of such a narrative is evoked. The process is interactional, involving both verbal and nonverbal events. As the physician is evaluating the patient, the patient is evaluating the physician. Both patient and physician tell each other what they want to discuss and what they prefer not to discuss. Sometimes the physician tells the patient exactly what answer is desired, and sometimes the patient may also let the physician know what he is ready to hear.

All of this information is conveyed as the patient is describing numbers, colors, dates, and events, and as the physician is recording these facts. Yet both are recording, almost effortlessly, impressions of each other that will govern the relationship more or less in perpetuity.

The Czech poet Milan Kundera says that much of what occurs between a man and a woman devolves from the implied rules that they agreed to in the first few weeks of their relationship. Similarly, I would say that much of what occurs between a physician and a patient derives from the first 10 minutes of their first interview.

Most sophomore medical students are acutely aware that they are being scrutinized during the interview, just as they are scrutinizing the patient. In some cases, the attendant anxiety becomes disabling to the student. In other cases, the intensity of this new situation prompts the student to say and to do that which he can immediately recognize as ineffective and revealing of his or her own neurosis. Yet in other cases, just the fear of looking foolish in itself produces ineffective behavior. All of these problems resolve with experience, although some students secretly doubt that they will ever be comfortable in the interviewing situation.

It is important for the student to remember his feelings of weakness and inadequacy so that he will always be able to recognize the same feelings in his patient, and thus respond in an empathetic manner.

I have found from auditing sophomore medical students in their initial clinical encounters that they usually acquit themselves very well in spite of the feelings described above. A sense of mastery comes with practice. Feelings of the most severe apprehension generally subside when the student simply jumps into the situation and starts to work.

For the senior student.   By now you have seen so many patients that you no longer have stage fright. The hospital has become a familiar workplace, and you have developed good techniques for getting things done. Perhaps now is a good time for you to reflect upon the way you felt the first few times that you introduced yourself to a patient. Your sense of novelty and strangeness has been replaced by confidence. But the hospital is still a strange and possibly frightening place to your patient. You need to respond appropriately to the patient's signs of anxiety or fear or discomfort, rather than ignoring them because they are not germane to the piece of information you are trying to evoke at the moment. Although you should feel confident, you should not allow yourself to relax too much. Remember that the patient is observing your response to him, and deciding whether he will confide in you, what he will tell his family and visitors about the hospital or clinic, and to some extent whether he will agree to undergo the surgery or take the medication that you recommend.

The physician should be neatly dressed and groomed. If the (male) interviewer is not wearing scrubs or other medical costume, he should wear a collared shirt and tie. Interviewers of either sex should dress in a professional style; the patient should be able to tell at a glance the difference between a medical interviewer and the television repairman. Shoes should be of a type suitable for serious employment, rather than for a day at the beach. There are a few rare situations in which certain types of transference can be facilitated by wearing informal clothing. However, many older patients are offended by physicians who dress informally, as can be easily learned by asking them (providing that the interviewer really wants to find out the answer, and is wearing a tie at the time).

Remember that the patient evaluates the doctor as the doctor is evaluating the patient.

Before Beginning the Formal Interview

First introduce yourself to the patient and shake the patient's hand. The handshaking puts the patient at ease and is a sign of cordiality and respect. Diagnoses that can be made from handshaking are discussed in Chapter 25 (p. 438).

It is wise, after introducing yourself, to turn off all radios, television sets, tape recorders, record players, and other distractions. The door should be closed and the curtains pulled. If the patient's friends or relatives are present, they should be courteously asked to leave, with an estimate of how long you expect to be there. If close relatives are there, you should tell them, in the patient's presence, that you will not discuss anything substantive about the patient's care unless the patient is present, and that they should ask the patient whatever questions they have. If

there is a roommate, try to get the roommate to leave the room. Don't forget to close the door when everyone is gone.

Next, make sure that the patient is comfortable. You may need to plump up the pillows, or to fetch the patient a glass of water. I have even been known to feed a patient soup or cereal, much to the amusement of house staff who believe that such tasks are suited only for nurses and female medical students, or other persons below the stature of a full professor. Such acts win the patient's confidence, and convince him of your interest in him. The patient may subsequently tell you things that the other doctors didn't learn.

Occasionally, the patient's family will not want to leave the room, and it is useful to find out why. On rare occasions, the interviewer may change his mind about allowing them to stay, at least for a portion of the interview, particularly if the patient is for some reason unable to tell his own story. With outpatients, the family may be most concerned about understanding the instructions for treatment, so that they may help a forgetful patient to cooperate. In that case, they will usually leave cheerfully if you promise to invite them back at the end, when you are explaining your instructions. (You should also write them down clearly and in large letters that a presbyopic patient can see.)

The patient usually does not want his family to be present, even though you may not be able to determine that fact until the family has departed. **The most important person in the room is the patient.**

Just as relatives should be physically excluded from participation in the patient's personal interview, so should we also subtly diminish their roles as diagnosticians of the patient. Many patients are so dependent upon significant others that the physician's reasonable recommendations are ignored because of the counter-recommendations of a relative. The physician should not defer to a relative's opinion early in the interview. Although this attitude seems to be authoritarian in an egalitarian age, students who are to be taught to seize responsibility with one hand must also be given the opportunity to grasp authority with the other.

This advice is not meant to provoke confrontations with relatives. Mature physicians exert their authority subtly, kindly, gently, and unconsciously. If you smile at the relatives when you ask them to leave the room, they will usually not be offended.

Occasionally, a family member will insist on speaking to you—often by telephone—without the patient being present. The reason is frequently to confide information that they think the patient will not tell you, such as the amount of alcohol consumption. This information can be extremely helpful, and might not be obtainable in any other way. (The same family member might deny the alcohol consumption if asked about it in the patient's presence.) However, it should not be accepted without skepticism; it may actually be a ploy to obtain information about the patient from you. A patient's wife once told the housestaff that the patient was abusing amphetamines, but the patient denied it. When all the laboratory tests for the drug returned negative, and she was so informed, she said, "Oh, I guess he isn't taking them then."

One way in which persons other than the patient can help in obtaining historical information in cases of poisoning is in performing the *box test* (Fig. 2-1). Give the relative, or whoever found the patient, an empty box and ask him to collect all the empty and partially empty containers in the place where the patient was found, including those in the wastebaskets, under the bed, in the night table, and so forth.

Methods to Facilitate the Interview

Sit in a chair close to the head of the bed so that your head is down at the level of the patient's head, or as close to that level as you can comfortably get. It helps to raise the bed; this will also

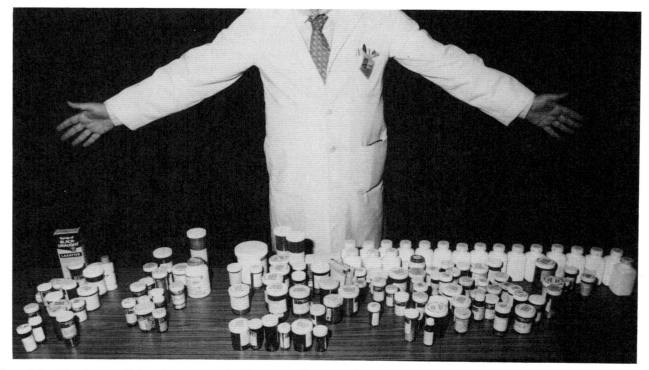

Figure 2-1. *The "box test." A patient presented with an unusual picture of impaired consciousness, so a "box test" was requested. It was initially reported as "negative" for any drugs. In fact, the family member who had been sent home with the box was intoxicated and had returned with three onions! When the test was repeated the next day by a sober family member, the above medications were found in the apartment occupied solely by the patient. Six replicate benzodiazepine prescriptions in the front row were the major psychoactive material eventually identified in his blood. Not surprisingly, a large number of the medications were indigestion remedies.*

facilitate your movements during the subsequent physical exam, and reduce your own low back strain.

Lean toward the patient. Make eye contact. Ask an open-ended question and just maintain eye contact until something in the patient's narrative particularly draws your attention. Forget about anyone else at the bedside. There should be no one in the universe but you and the patient.

Allow no interruptions. Do not allow anyone to break into the interview. This is a rule that is very difficult to put into practice, but that best teaches us its value when it is violated.

If at all possible, touch the patient during the interview. I find it useful to take the patient's pulse during the interview.

●

An illustrative story. There is an old story about the Arabic physician Ibn-Sinna, who was consulted to see the king's only son. The son had fallen into a severe melancholia, and was so withdrawn that he would not even speak to the physician. While the wise physician took the patient's pulse, he asked him, "Are you thinking about something happening here in the palace, or something in the city?" The prince said nothing, but the physician noticed that the pulse rate increased just after the words "or in the city."

"Are you thinking about something on this side of the river or across the river?" asked the wise physician. Again, the young prince said nothing, but his pulse increased at the words "across the river." In this manner, the wise physician continued to examine the young man, learning that the young man had been smitten in love by a young woman he had seen in the town. The physician was even able to determine the exact location of the woman's house, although the young man had given not a single verbal answer.

Upon hearing the physician's report, the king had his guards send for the young woman. The king's son experienced a miraculous recovery as soon as she was brought into his bedroom. The wise physician was rewarded handsomely.

Question: *What does this teach us about medical practice?* (Write your answer before reading on.)

Answer: *First, the story teaches us that all reactions are important, including nonverbal communication. Also, we learn that it is very difficult to maintain confidentiality, especially when powerful third-party payers are involved. It also teaches that dealing with third-party payers is sometimes financially rewarding to the physician. And, of course, it teaches us to stay in tune with the patient throughout the interview—the answer that you should have written down.*

●

Ask an Open-Ended Question

The best way to begin the interview is with an open-ended question. Skill at asking such questions probably determines one's success as a physician more than any other factor.

Two requisites must be satisfied, in the given order. First, *the patient must know who you are.* The introduction may be performed by one of the patient's physicians:

1. "Mr. Smith, these are the two medical students I told you about. They are going to spend about 2 hours with you this afternoon, if that's still all right with you." Or:
2. "Mr. Smith, this is Dr. Blue. He is our attending physician. I mentioned to you earlier that we would be bringing him around to meet you." Or one may introduce oneself:

3. "Mr. Smith, I'm medical student Jones, and this is my partner, Mr. Black." Or:
4. "Mr. Smith, I'm Dr. White. I'm a consultant in endocrinology. Your doctor, Dr. Green, asked me to come by and see you about your diabetes, your sugar problem."

After the introduction, pause to give the patient a chance to ask a question if he has one ready. If not, as is usually the case, proceed with the interview.

The second requirement for success is that *the patient must know what you are doing.* With a brand new patient, I like to explain: "I am going to take the story of your life. I'm going to ask you an awful lot of questions. Then from your answers I am going to have some general idea of what the problem may be. Then when I've finished asking you most of the questions, I am going to examine you. When I finish that examination of your body, I'll have a much better idea of what the problem may be. At that time, I'll also have an idea of what laboratory tests and/or X rays we'll need to solve your problem. Do you have any questions now about how I'm going to proceed?"

Continuing the four dialogues begun above, this second stage might be accomplished by the following statements:

1. "We're Jones and Black. We're sophomore medical students, and we won't be participating in your medical care after today. We're only student doctors, and we're your doctors just for this afternoon. Before we get started, is there anything you need to make you comfortable?"
2. "Hello, Mr. Smith. We've been discussing you in the conference this morning, and I felt it very important that I actually meet you and go over the details of your story. I also want to examine your heart to double check a few things."
3. "We are going to talk with you and go over the details of your medical history, and then we are going to examine you just as your other doctors did."
4. "Dr. Green is a bit puzzled as to why your sugar has been swinging up and down so much, and I am going to try to help him and you, if I can."

Each of these statements is followed by a pause and a check to see that the patient understands what has been said.

Finally, the stage is set for the first of many open-ended questions. To continue the four dialogues, these might be:

1. *"Can you tell us what brought you to the hospital?"*
   "Yes. It was my nephew's Ford." (This patient has examined many sophomore students.)
   "No. I mean, what was bothering you? What were your symptoms? (A double question. See p. 000.)
   "What was bothering me? My mother-in-law."
   "No, we meant why did you come to the hospital?"
   "Well, I'm a Korean War veteran. And this is the Veteran's Hospital, isn't it?"
   "No, we meant why come to the hospital at all? In what way did you feel sick?" (Another double question.)
   "I always feel this way when I'm sick."
   "Well, when did you last feel well?" (An excellent open-ended question.)
2. "Could you begin by telling me *when was the very first time you noticed anything* that might be related to your heart trouble in any way?"
3. *"When was the last time you felt in perfect health?"*
4. *"When was the very first time you were aware that there was anything different* about your sugar?"

Notice that the second and fourth questions would not be open-ended for an initial evaluation, but in reality are open-ended for an interviewer who has already heard a complete history secondhand. To see what I mean, consider the following counterexamples of unhelpful "closed" questions:

1. "When did a doctor first tell you what was wrong?"
2. "Did you have orthopnea before last January?"
3. "Have you ever been in the hospital before for the same problem you are having now?"
4. "When did Dr. Green first tell you your sugar was too high?"

For the neophyte. Much of the material in this chapter may seem quite formal and rigid to the thoughtful reader. However, those students who initially learn to be very obsessive, rigid, compulsive, and thorough will develop excellent interviewing skills; later, they can discard any excrescences. On the other hand, individuals who initially use a sloppy interviewing technique tend later to have a smaller repertoire of adjustments for the individuality of patients.

To illustrate the value of the rules, I like to tell the following story to my students.

●

There was an extremely busy physician who had a large and ever-increasing general practice, which included many families. One night he was running late as usual. After his office nurse had helped him an hour past her quitting time, he asked if there was anyone left in the waiting room.

"Just Mrs. Smith," she said.

"Well, you can go home," said the doctor. "I can gown her and put her on the examining table as well as you, and you have worked long enough."

The doctor finished what he was doing, put away the previous patient's chart, and went to the waiting room, where he saw a man and a woman sitting together.

"Come in," he said, holding the door open as they walked in and sat in the two chairs opposite the doctor's desk.

He seated himself and asked, "What seems to be the problem?"

"Well, doctor," said the man, "to tell you the truth it's a little bit embarrassing." The man then launched into a description of a skin lesion that seemed related to some sexual difficulties. The patient explained in great detail the highly unusual things he had done in the course of acquiring his lesion.

"Well," said the doctor, "just go into the examining room, take off all your clothes, and lie down on the table. I will come in and examine you."

When the man had left the consulting room, the physician turned toward Mrs. Smith, whom he had never imagined would engage in such unusual practices. "Is all this true?"

"I don't know, doctor," said the woman. "I've never seen that man before."

●

This apocryphal story demonstrates that if you violate too many of the rules given in this book, you will sooner or later get into trouble. It also demonstrates the enormous authority afforded a physician in his area of expertise, as well as the physician's ability to sanction social behavior.

The patient-centered principles underlying this style of interviewing will serve one well in other circumstances, including seemingly unrelated cases. For example, consider this story in which the student had to decide what to do when the patient's biopsy was positive for disseminated carcinoma.

Self-Study

A woman was admitted to the hospital for a diagnostic evaluation. Both she and her husband were aware that the doctors might find a terminal form of cancer. The husband, a patriarchal Sicilian, took the doctors aside and said that if the biopsy was positive, the patient was to learn of the diagnosis only from him, the husband. The woman separately told the doctors that she wanted them to tell her the biopsy result if it was positive for malignancy.

The biopsy was positive, and the medical student told the patient the results, as she had requested. When the husband learned that the information had not been "filtered" through him, he became furious with the medical student. The student was castigated by the house officer for not considering the cultural traditions of the patient and her husband.

What would you have done?

Discussion

While the house officer is to be commended for his consideration of cultural factors in the management of patients (if not his delegation of such a responsibility to a third-year medical student), we must return to the patient's wishes. Obviously, in this situation, the patient herself was not willing to maintain total dependency in her relationship with her husband; thus, she may be considered to have abrogated any obligation of the physician's to adhere to any (putative) culturally determined sequencing of the presentation of information. In other words, she was better aware of her own culture than anyone else and yet had clearly stated whom she wished to be informed first of the diagnosis—herself.

Interviewing Versus Interrogation

Thirteen Rue Madeleine, a World War II motion picture formerly popular on late night television, is named for the address of Gestapo headquarters in Paris. In the final scene, an American spy (played by James Cagney) is interrogated by the head of the Gestapo (played by Richard Conte). Cagney has called in a bomber strike on Thirteen Rue Madeleine that will destroy the Gestapo operations in occupied France, but will just as surely destroy the patriotic Cagney. Conte is torturing Cagney to find out what radio message he had sent back to the Allied Forces.

I use this scene in teaching because there is a certain style and rhythm to that interview as it becomes an interrogation. Conte's voice and attitude are those of a superior figure addressing one who is in a dependent position. Furthermore, the superior figure is obviously indifferent to Cagney's suffering, and is hostile and wantonly cruel.

Except in the movies, I have heard that interviewing style only in hospitals when I have been thrust into the role of unintended eavesdropper on medical house staff, and sad to say, some medical students. This style is not suitable for physicians. It is certainly not the way to elicit sensitive information. Students should choose to identify with a more desirable mode of behavior and to overcome any latent tendency to become brusque with patients.

Avoid "Leading the Witness"

Interviewing is a two way-street. The patient responds to the doctor's wishes, and sometimes doctors with poor interviewing style insist on being told what they want to hear, as the following story illustrates.

●

A patient was transferred to the medical service of a tertiary care hospital, instead of the neurologic service, despite the fact that he was suffering from a stroke. At the referring hospital, no one had been interested in his paralysis, but they had been interested in chest pain. In fact, the patient had experienced no chest pain, but after vigorous and repetitive questioning about this symptom, "They talked me into having chest pain." Since the doctors at the tertiary hospital were also concerned about the paralysis, it again became permissible for him not to "have" chest pain.

●

Choice of Language

Always use words that the patient understands. Never use technical or medical terms in the interview. This seems like good common sense, but you need to be aware that because you are just beginning your own mastery of these words, they will slip into the clinical interview, and the patient may not tell you that he doesn't understand. If you are sure that you would never make such a mistake, audit tape recordings of your own interviews. Sooner or later, you too will use a medical term the patient does not understand. As in so much of medicine, awareness of the problem is an obligatory first step toward its solution.

On the other hand, try not to go overboard in the opposite direction. When interviewing a patient who belongs to a subculture with its own jargon (such as a drug abuser or a prisoner), one should not enter into the patient's argot (see p. 25). First of all, language serves important ego defensive functions. Second, the physician should never interview in an unnatural style any more than he should attempt to perform surgery from an unnatural posture.

Of course, the problem of misunderstanding the terminology can go in the other direction as well. Certain obscure slang terms and abstruse euphemisms are used by patients, especially when the disease may have social significance. For example, "bad blood" was a term used to denote syphilis, and later, by augmentation, any venereal disease. (At other times "a hair cut" had the same meaning.) But "bad blood" had to be distinguished from "low blood," which could be either anemia or psychasthenia in a patient with a normal blood pressure. Worse, in different parts of the country, the same phenomenon may have different names. Lymph nodes have been variously referred to as "knots," "lungs," "kernels," and "risings" (the last may also be an abscess). Even within one locality, the names may change from time to time. For instance, when I started work at the hospital for drug addicts then in Lexington, Kentucky, I found a glossary of terms that someone had compiled a few years earlier, apparently to distribute to new medical officers. However, half of the terms were arcane or forgotten, and many had been replaced by new ones.

"Can You Tell Me What Bothers You the Most?"

Some patients will come in with lists of problems, written or otherwise. They may jump from problem to disease to event to syndrome to hospitalization to symptom, without ever finishing the description of any of them. For the neophyte intent on eliciting all the dimensions (see pp. 26–27), getting the correct chronology, or simply developing a clear understanding of what the patient is trying to say, this can be very annoying. The title of this section is a useful response. This question helps the patient focus on whatever he or she really feels is important. In some patients it also makes it clear that they do not need a particular problem to serve as the "ticket for admission"; you are interested in whatever is making them ill with life, if not nominally diseased.

Why do patients need a "ticket of admission"? Many patients would like to talk to a sympathetic doctor about personal problems not parochially thought of as "medical problems." In fact, the urgency to talk about such problems and to take up the physician's time has led to the creation, in some institutions, of whole departments (psychiatry, psychology, social work, behavioral medicine, ombudsmen) devoted to listening to patients talk about what really bothers them, while the physician obliviously orders more non-diagnostic tests. The truly thoughtful physician will want to know about these concerns. However, some patients can only come to see the physician if they have something that will get the receptionist to give them an appointment, or, in larger institutions, that will satisfy some bureaucratic, algorithmic guideline. Once the patients get into your office or the hospital there will be a natural tendency to talk about the true subject of their discomfort—as soon as they believe they can safely bring it up. The question that is the title of this section can help the patient to bring up the problem. Some professors may object to this use of their time, but if they will recall the number of patients who have tried to rekindle a conversation while being shoved out of the office, they may reconsider and use the question to initiate the discussion at the beginning of the hour or quarter hour. (See the section on the "organ recital," p. 27.) Because we insist, properly, on the patient having a chief complaint, we should not be surprised that the patient wants to satisfy us.

For a number of years, I abandoned the teaching of this question because of its misuse. Instead of using it to encourage the patient to talk, some were using it defensively to get the patient to stop talking about problems that did not interest the doctors. Further, if challenged on having missed an important diagnosis, the resident might respond, "Well, I asked her what bothered her the most, and that's what she told me."

An important principle in medicine is that even the best teachings can be subverted. The corollary is that the thoughtful physician will choose his company wisely, associating with those who are wiser than himself, if possible. As the *Talmud* instructs, "If you wish to be a scholar, you must seek out the company of other scholars."

"Tell Me More . . ."

In the initial open-ended portion of the interview, the patient will usually stop talking before he has told you all the details of some important event (such as the dimensions discussed in Ch. 3, p. 34). He may previously have been interrogated, not interviewed; or he may previously have had so many bad doctors that he is puzzled that anyone should want to spend so much time listening to him; he may simply be taciturn; or he may simply not be aware of the importance of certain details. You want to keep the patient talking, but how do you do it?

Just say to the patient, "Tell me more." A few of these phrases sprinkled into the interview act like yeast in bread dough. Some patients will ask, "About what?" The answer is, "About what you were just telling me." Others will ask, "What do you want to know about it?" Your answer is, "How you felt about it," if you cannot think of a specific aspect in which you are interested.

Once the patient senses that you are truly interested in him, he will respond positively to, "Tell me more."

Of course, later on in the more staccato portion of the interview, there will be events or symptoms about which you may wish to have more detail. Here too, it is a good idea to say, "Tell me more." If you have already used the phrase effectively in the initial part of the interview, it will begin to function like a conditioned reflex.

The student must master the open-ended interview before proceeding to the decorticated checklists being promulgated by some supposed medical educators.

Assessing and Improving Your Interviewing Skills

If medicine is truly a science humanely practiced (Eichna, 1980), we must note that science inevitably depends upon measurement. In order to make measurements, one must have a method of recording events and data. One should not expect an electrocardiographer to teach a neophyte if the latter could only describe an arrhythmia as a "little wiggle, then a pause followed by a big wiggle." But if the neophyte brought an electrocardiographic tracing, the electrocardiographer could measure, diagnose, and teach; and the neophyte could learn in a meaningful way. The same is true for interviewing; one learns best from a recording that can be played back and examined.

Videotaping is discussed later. For the time being, let us consider audiotape recorders because these are cheap, ubiquitous, and familiar to most medical students.

Making a Recording

Immediately after you have introduced yourself (if not before), turn on your tape recorder and place it where it will not interfere with eye contact between you and the patient. Stretch the microphone out away from the body of the tape recorder and place it near the patient's mouth, or clip it to his pillow. Remember, the patient is the most important person in the room. Most of the interview content comes from the patient, not the interviewer.

It should be obvious that recorders with built-in microphones are usually not very good for our purposes. In order to obtain good quality recordings, one must place the microphone very close to the patient's mouth. Using a recorder with a built-in microphone may thus result in sticking a large machine near the patient's head. Also, as the patient turns his head, he can quickly get out of range of the built-in microphone. Furthermore, when turned up to high gain, machines with built-in microphones tend also to amplify their own motor hum. It is to avoid such an annoyance that one is advised to stretch the microphone cable as far away from the motor of the portable tape recorder as possible.

Tell the patient, "I'm going to record what you tell me so that I am certain to get everything correct," or words to that effect. If you are recording only for technique (form) and not for content (vide infra), the statement is not strictly true. Since we do nothing with the patient *sub rosa*, you might simply say, "I want to record what you say" or "I want to record our conversation," or "I want to have a record of what we say to each other so that I can review it later."

No matter what explanation you give for recording the interview, be sure to assure the patient of confidentiality. You might say, "I am going to review this alone, using an earpiece, so no one else will hear," or "I am going to go over our interview with a more senior doctor who is teaching me about talking with patients," or "No one will hear the tape recording but me," or whatever is true. Be sure to add that the tape will be permanently erased, and that no one who knows the patient will ever hear it.

Needless to say, your promise of confidentiality must be honored. Listen to the tape privately, only with concerned parties. If you share lodging with a nonprofessional, you should use an earpiece. And, of course, if you promise the patient to erase the tape, you must do so.

I have never had a patient decline to be recorded. Those situations in which students claim the patient refused to give permission to record the interview were themselves always unrecorded. If you are truly concerned about legal issues, you may say at the end of your introductory comments, "Do you mind if I record us," or "May I have your permission to make a recording?" If you are afraid of listening to your own interview, you will ask the question in a manner that guarantees many patients will oblige you by refusing to give permission.

During many years of interviewing medical patients in front of small groups, I have found that, recorded or not, most patients have little hesitancy about speaking openly, with absolutely no embarrassment, if they sense that the listeners are really interested in them. The patients realize that the situation is a well defined professional one, not a social one. If you carry yourself as a professional, and treat the patient in a professional manner, the patient will treat you as a professional, and give you an amazingly sensitive and accurate account of his experiences.

Reviewing the Recording

After you have made the recording, listen to it in the quiet of your own room. You can review the content of the history of the present illness, although if that were the main purpose, I would have placed this section in the chapter on history, not in the one on interviewing. The most important purpose of the recording is to improve your skills in interacting with the patient.

Studies of medical students interviewing patients have found that there are four different objectively measurable phenomena that are highly correlated with experienced clinicians' global ratings of the quality of the interviews: interruptions, percentage of time that the interviewer speaks, pregnant pauses, and double questions.

These four criteria permit you to score your own tape recordings. However, even within one interview, different portions of the interview have somewhat different structures. Thus, to be perfectly scientific, one should randomly select samples from different portions of the entire interview. With each criterion to be discussed we will also discuss its major variations among different portions of the interview.

Criterion 1: Interruptions

On the average, there should be no more than 1.5 interruptions per minute of interview. This is especially critical in the portion of the interview that comes at the beginning and produces content usually found in the history of present illness portion of the case record.

An interruption should be scored whenever the interviewer interrupts the patient while the patient is speaking.

Example of an interruption:
    Patient: ". . . You know doctor, I have always wondered if that shortness of breath had anything to do with the time—"
    Interviewer: "When did you say your ankles first swelled up?"

A distinction can be made between flagrant interruptions and the skillful interviewer's *shaping comments*. A shaping comment gets the patient back to where the interviewer wishes to be by recounting something that the patient has already said.

Example of a shaping comment:
    Patient: ". . . and the following spring, regular as clockwork, I got another one of the asthmatic attacks. It was the same thing as last time, starting with coughing and spitting and getting me up at night just like the first two . . . there was that coughing and spitting. It seemed like every night I would get up just like the past year. Regular as clockwork at 1:00 a.m. there was that coughing and spitting—"
    Interviewer: "Was that spring the first time you noticed the blood?"

Criterion 2: Percentage of Time the Interviewer Speaks

On the average, the interviewer should speak no more than 50% of the time, and no less than 10% of the time. With a young, healthy person who has a completely negative review of systems, it is not uncommon for the interviewer to be speaking from 45% to 50% of the time during that portion of the interview. However, in the history of the present illness portion, the interviewer should be speaking closer to 10% of the time.

The reason for the 10% lower limit is that in certain interviews the interviewer loses control to a loquacious patient. It is true that an excellent interviewer with good nonverbal cuing can let the patient speak more than 90% of the time during fruitful portions of the interview that will produce material for the history of the present illness. But on the average, over the course of the entire interview, no skillful medical interviewer will speak less than 10% of the time.

Criterion 3: Pregnant Pauses

This is the hardest portion of the interview to learn. One must be aware of the technique and use it deliberately. A really good interviewer should be able to produce a pregnant pause, 4 or 5 seconds in length, several times during the interview.

A pregnant pause is defined as the silent interval between the apparent end of a patient's response to the question and a thoughtful continuation, not interrupted by any comment or next question from the interviewer. The pregnant pause is terminated by the patient himself resuming a more detailed description of whatever he was discussing, usually with an enriched context.

Four or five seconds may not seem like a very long pause, but it is long enough to make the naive interviewer very uncomfortable. It is suggested that the novice develop a nonverbal cue such as smiling, leaning forward, motioning with the hand, or taking off one's spectacles and motioning with them in a "continue, please" manner. Extremely skilled interviewers can leave up to 20-second pauses when asking about prior imprisonment, sexual matters, or other taboos for that particular patient. Pregnant pauses are usually found in the portions of the interview having to do with such potentially sensitive subject matter.

Criterion 4: Double Questions

Always ask one question at a time. Although this dictum seems rather obvious, you will almost inevitably violate it. If you carefully audit the recordings of your interviews, you will find instances in which you have asked a second question without waiting for a response to the first.

Example:
   Interviewer: "During any of this time did you cough up any blood—did you say you once worked in shipbuilding? Were you ever exposed to asbestos?" Or:
   Interviewer: "Have you noticed any change in the frequency of your bowel movements since the operation? What about the color? Did it change?

   A study of paired tape recordings and case records reveals that the answer to the first question is always omitted from the case record, and for very good reason. The patient always answers the second question, never the first. Worse, the interviewer never goes back and reasks the first unanswered question.

   If one interviews the interviewer and asks about the omitted information, the inevitable response is frustration, as he remembers asking the question, but is not able to remember the patient's answer—because, of course, it was never given.

Other Criteria

Any good physician who has been in practice for a long time has a number of interview criteria of which he is not consciously aware. You might wish to play an interview for a private physician who is willing to serve as a tutor. Physicians of experience can immediately point out technical errors even though they may never have specifically thought about the right and wrong ways to conduct an interview.

Nonverbal Communication

There are three aspects of nonverbal communication to be considered: tone of voice, body position, and facial expression. The latter two are best taught by means of a videotape.

Tone of Voice

While the importance of this factor is rather obvious, persons who do not use tape recorders often do not realize that their tone of voice is sometimes not what they believe it to be. Many students, upon hearing themselves interview a patient for the first time, remember the patient's voice, but wonder who is the person asking the questions! Again, the simple use of the recorder will solve this problem, given a student of intelligence and sensitivity.

Body Position

The interviewer's body position with respect to the patient determines much about the content of the interview. Physicians who always stand above a supine patient are perhaps unconsciously reinforcing the patient's dependent position and the authoritarian position of the physician. While some physicians know how to utilize this discrepancy to the ultimate advantage of the patient, others may abuse it. In later years, I have always attempted to spend at least some time sitting by the bedside at eye level with the patient. My having the chair at the bedside, while the rest of the team is standing, is often misinterpreted by the junior members of the team. But it makes better eye contact possible, and it shows the patient that I plan to sit and listen to him. Patients also perceive that physicians who sit at the bedside are spending

more time with them than physicians who stand, whether or not that is true by objective measurements.

   The physician's body position can be consciously used to control certain aspects of the interview. Conversely, body movements of which you may be unaware can be counterproductive. For example, breaking eye contact, turning your body away from the patient, looking at your wristwatch, or staring into the corner will decrease communication, both quantitatively and qualitatively. Conversely, if you wish to get a reticent patient to talk, kinesic encouragements could include the following: holding your body so that your line of vision is in line with that of the patient; leaning forward slightly but comfortably; and using skillfully placed signs or motions of encouragement when the patient stops talking. The last include, but are not limited to, a "come here" motion with the hands; taking off one's spectacles and using them in a "hooking the patient in like a fish" movement, with or without accompanying head movement; nonverbally saying, "Yes, go ahead" by smiling; head nodding, which also indicates approval; and a rotary mixing-in motion of pen or pencil with the fast component moving from the patient to the interviewer.

Suggested Teaching Exercise

Videotape an interview, but with the camera pointing at the interviewer rather than the patient. Play it back first with sound, but no picture. Then play back the picture with no sound. Finally, play the sound and picture together.

   When listening to sound only, note what unexplained pauses occur. When looking at the picture only, analyze the body signals. Do you see any negative ones? When listening to the sound with picture, do you see any correlations or contradictions between the patient's verbal behaviors and the interviewer's physical behavior? What other obvious mismatches could you detect with sound and picture that were not apparent viewing just one?

Facial Expressions

Frowning at the patient will decrease communication. Smiling at the patient will encourage the patient to talk. Salesmen of all types use this technique.

An Experiment

If you would like to see the power of the three aspects of nonverbal communication, there is a very simple experiment that you can perform. The time spent analyzing the data is well worthwhile; it is certain to convince the neophyte to utilize these techniques.

   The experiment involves asking any individual who is naive to the experiment, usually a class member, to speak about anything that comes to mind. An interviewer sits opposite the subject and gives positive reinforcement whenever the subject uses a noun (or a verb, an adjective, or other selected part of speech). Positive reinforcement consists of leaning toward the subject, smiling, making positive motions, and the other items suggested above. It is particularly easy to smile whenever the subject uses a verb. This is done for a 5- or 10-minute experimental sampling time.

   The dependent variable is the chosen part of speech, as a percentage of all the words used. The second half of the experimental interview is compared with the first half.

   Don't forget to elicit the subject's observations before you explain the experimental design to him. Most subjects who exhibit good responses (large increases in the use of the chosen part of speech) will not be aware of what they have done. Many of them, on hearing the tape recordings played back, will be aware that they "sound funny."

I have lost the reference for this exercise, and suggest that you do not believe me until you have tried it yourself.

Autognosis

Autognosis is a combination word from auto (meaning self) and diagnosis. It refers to diagnosis through awareness of the feelings that the patient engenders in one's self. While it may be formally taught as part of the specialty known as psychiatry, its application need not be limited to psychiatrists, any more than the interpretation of chest films need be left to radiologists.

Autognosis is useful in certain specific disorders (see Ch. 26, p. 521). Some depressed patients tend to make the physician feel depressed by the end of the encounter; similarly, some manic patients tend to be amusing, making the physician smile or laugh. Patients with less well defined psychiatric disorders (or no psychiatric disorder at all) may evoke in the physician feelings similar to those they evoke in their employers, employees, associates, parents, children, siblings, or spouses.

Again, I emphasize that interviewing is an interactive process. The physician can learn to take advantage of a spontaneous, free, and noninvasive diagnostic aid: his own emotional response.

Last Question in the Interview

As you move from the open-ended questions at the beginning of the interview to the more specific kinds of questions that are covered in the next chapter, you will be formulating differential diagnoses in your head. Then you will move on to the physical examination. When you finish the physical examination, you will be considering which laboratory tests you wish to order. I would suggest interrupting the sequence by inserting, just before the physical examination, the following question: "Is there anything else you want to tell me?"

Some British-trained physicians say, "What do you think is wrong with you, Mr. Smith?" in order to get the patient to think of more diagnostically related material, and to learn the patient's as yet unspoken fears, but this is not really the same question. The "anything else" question is not limited to diagnosis, but includes prognosis, therapeutics, fears, worries, terrors, and even trivia (from the physician's standpoint) such as information concerning restrooms, visiting hours, or parking near the office. The question does not guarantee the quality of the diagnostic content of the response, but it does facilitate the doctor-patient relationship.

This closes the interview in an open-ended style. It also prepares the patient to begin the next interview in an open-ended fashion.

One difference between psychoanalysis and the interview is that the interview never terminates, for the life of the doctor-patient relationship. (See Freud's essay on the subject of psychoanalysis, terminable or interminable [Freud, 1937]).

The Psychodynamic Termination of the Physical Examination

This section is not out of sequence. There is a portion of the interview, or potential portion of the interview, that actually occurs at the very end of the doctor-patient contact. Of course, everyone realizes that we continue to talk to the patient (to perform an interview) even as we perform the physical examination. However, most people do not understand that the termination of the physical examination is also the termination of the interview and is psychologically very important.

Patients often say very important things to you as you are leaving the room. As an aid, I suggest that you leave your tape recorder running as you exit, since you may be inattentive to the patient's comments after you have said goodbye. You may not want to leave your tape recorder running all through the physical examination for logistic reasons. In that case, turn it back on just before you leave, and study the last part of the recording carefully.

From a psychodynamic standpoint, a most important part of the interview occurs as the physician and patient part company. The phenomenon is much easier to observe in an office setting such as your clinic.

There are several reasons why patients give psychologically important material as they are leaving. You are distracted, unguarded, and not really concentrating on the patient. You may have put away his chart and pulled out the chart of the next patient, to whom you are, appropriately, switching your attention. The patient, for his part, is in a relatively safe position. He is no longer recumbent, dependent, prone, or under your gaze. He can throw out a comment and observe your response. If he does not like your look, gesture, or tone of voice, he already has his hand on the doorknob and will soon be safely outside. His remark may be a new symptom (see "Organ Recital," p. 26).

What can be done about this situation? First, use a tape recorder in the outpatient department to convince yourself that the above is true. Second, awareness in itself is helpful, as in so much of medicine. One way to handle the situation is to look up at the patient and say, "That would be a good place for us to start next time," assuming of course that there is to be a next time, and that you will start there.

To understand the nuances of the patient's parting remarks requires some training in psychodynamics. The lack of availability of such training in most medical residencies is a serious deficiency.

For the attending (a rounding ploy).   As the rounding group leaves the bedside, turn your back to the patient and begin washing your hands. (Those who believe in the germ theory think this is a good idea in any case.) This will permit you to eavesdrop upon the rest of the group as they leave the patient's bedside. Listen to the patient's last words to the group.

After you have left the patient's room, ask if anyone can remember the last thing the patient said. If no one can, remind them of what it was, and possibly also comment on why some people cannot remember. It will probably not be difficult to interpret the patient's comments, if they did have some especially significant meaning. Experienced attending physicians know far more about human behavior and patient-doctor interactions than they realize. These insights should be shared with younger colleagues, since one of the purposes of civilization is to spare the young of the species from having to learn everything the hard way.

Interviewing Patients with an Organic Brain Syndrome

Recognizing the Presence of an Organic Brain Syndrome

The most common cause of forgetfulness is cerebral insufficiency (*organic mental syndrome* or *organic brain syndrome* in modern terminology), either the acute form (delirium) or the chronic form (dementia). Organic brain syndrome (an unfortunate term; see the definition of *organic* in Ch. 1) is further manifested during the interview by the patient's contradicting himself, having difficulty recalling details, or in some cases evading the questions. The patient may seem to do well on open-ended questions but develops difficulty when asked more specific ones.

The word *history* comes from the Greek *historia*, meaning inquiry, which was the title of the earliest extant historical work, written by Herodotus. The practical point is that the *historian* does not live the history, but records it (as Herodotus did; see the quotation in Ch. 9, p. 145). When we read in a case record of a *poor historian*, this refers to the same person as would the term *poor auscultator* or *poor ophthalmoscopist*. If *poor historian* refers to the patient, it would mean that he is an impecunious student of the past, a piece of information that belongs in the social history, not following the statement of reliability (see Ch. 4, p. 48). In other words, *the physician is the historian*.

What the historian might have meant to say by his phrase *poor historian* was that the patient has difficulty remembering. Such a memory problem is a biologic event, like fever or tachycardia, and is equally deserving of an explanation. To note the patient's difficulty in recounting his story the same way on any two sequential attempts, or his inability to remember material of the type that most patients would be expected (by us) to remember, should be the beginning of an evaluation, not its termination. These observations should suggest to the physician that the patient may be suffering from an organic brain syndrome. Suspicion should also be aroused if the patient's performance is variable or fluctuating, or if he is disorganized, shows lapses in concentration, or confabulates, often to the annoyance of the physician. The physician is obligated to determine whether the forgetfulness is in fact due to such a syndrome, then to find out the etiology of the syndrome, so any potentially reversible problems can be treated.

Accordingly, when one is eliciting the history from such a patient and one even barely suspects that the patient may be suffering from an organic brain syndrome, one must stop the interview per se and evaluate this problem.

It should be noted that the brief cognitive portion of the mental status examination about to be described is actually part of the neurologic examination (see p. 516). However, the neurologic examination is not described until the end of this book (as is true of most other textbooks and courses). Because between 10% and 40% of the patients on a medical or surgical service will have an organic brain syndrome at some time during their stay, and because such patients will give a very confusing history, it is important that the cognitive portion of the mental status be assessed as soon as possible, if for no other reason than to avoid wasting the physician's time gathering confabulated data. Thus, this is one portion of the physical examination that must, in many cases, be performed near the beginning of the interview.

Acute Organic Brain Syndrome, or Delirium

This term is not specific enough, because only the cerebrum is affected, not the whole brain. In a classic paper, the name *cerebral insufficiency* is suggested as a better synonym for delirium (Engel & Romano, 1959). Nevertheless, the term delirium is still incorrectly used by some to refer to an agitated patient, a patient who is hallucinating, or even a stuporous or comatose patient. To avoid confusion, it is probably best to avoid using the term delirium, except among the cognoscenti.

The terms *toxic psychosis* and *metabolic encephalopathy* actually describe subsets of the organic brain syndrome; they are not synonyms. A patient with severe cerebral insufficiency due to a febrile condition such as meningitis, or a poison (such as bromides, now a rarity), is said to be both toxic and psychotic, and hence to have a toxic psychosis. "Nontoxic" patients may have a cerebral milieu metabolically hostile to the normal function of the cerebral cortex as in hypoxia, hypoglycemia, and so on; thus, they are said to have a metabolic encephalopathy. Sometimes an electroencephalogram (EEG) from such a patient will have the characteristic diffuse slowing of the background rhythm and will be diagnosed as metabolic encephalopathy, or metabolic dysrhythmia.

If the acute form of the syndrome (for example, due to hypoglycemia) is not recognized and treated, the patient may develop the chronic form of the disease, although many persons with the chronic form have etiologies (discussed later) that may never show an acute phase, nor be reversible (e.g., Alzheimer's disease).

Chronic Organic Brain Syndrome

The chronic form of cerebral insufficiency has been variously called chronic brain syndrome, chronic organic brain syndrome, chronic organic mental syndrome, or dementia. I prefer the last term although it has been tainted by some authors who maintain that dementia is by definition irreversible. Actually, a good percentage of the dementias are reversible, as discussed further in Chapter 26 (p. 518). (Please note that both the acute and chronic syndrome imply the loss of function previously available. If a patient is mentally retarded from birth, his examination findings may be similar to those of a patient with the organic brain syndrome, but the term is not applied in this case. Conversely, one should be very careful not to diagnose mental retardation in a patient suffering from a reversible acute brain syndrome.)

Examination for the Syndrome of Cerebral Insufficiency (i.e., Organic Brain Syndrome)

Again, this examination is actually the cognitive portion of the mental status examination, which is performed out of sequence, and possibly written up out of sequence for those whose case records forms contain a statement of "patient reliability" on the first page.

Examination for Disorientation

Types of disorientation.   There are three spheres of orientation: time, place, and person. Some authorities recommend a fourth dimension, called situation, which I do not find useful. Also, it is difficult to teach in that it requires the physician to make some rather sophisticated judgments about the patient's ego defenses. For example, if a patient could not tell the doctor the specific medical circumstances of his hospitalization, it might be because the patient is disoriented to the situation. On the other hand, it might be because previous doctors neglected to inform the patient, or because the details are so dismal that the patient is utilizing the ego defense of denial. Or, the patient might not understand the question.

Disorientation develops in a stereotyped sequence. Orientation to time is lost first, followed by orientation to place, and finally to person. When the patient is successfully diagnosed and treated, the orientation returns in the same order: first the patient remembers who he is, then he can remember (or be taught) where he is, and finally he can be reoriented to time.

When the patient is disoriented to person, that is, when he does not know who he is and cannot even tell the doctor his own name, he is probably in a nearly stuporous condition. Diseases that can cause this state (e.g., severe diffuse lupus cerebritis, multiple staphylococcal brain abscesses) usually have many other findings and do not constitute a diagnostic problem. Thus, I shall say no more about disorientation to person.

We refer to teaching the patient where he is and to reorienting him in the dimension of time because if the patient is found unconscious in the streets and revived in the hospital, it is unreasonable to expect him to know where he is or how many days have elapsed unless someone tells him. For this reason, every patient who is disoriented should be reoriented to the correct place and date, which should be noted in the case record. Patients who are slowly recovering from their cerebral insufficiency may pass through a phase of intermittent disorientation.

Checking for orientation in time. Simply ask the patient to tell you the day of the month, the name of the month, and the year.

This is easy to say, but sometimes difficult to perform. But remember, this is part of the physical examination. Although one is "only" talking to the patient, one is checking a very specific point and must be as tenacious as one is in the search for an important diastolic murmur. This is not an open-ended interview question, a historical review-of-systems question, or a social chat. It is a critical part of the physical examination.

Students sometimes feel awkward about this point, but then they also feel awkward about doing rectal examinations. The student should consider the consequence of missing a possibly reversible brain syndrome. The patient whose feelings were supposedly being spared might remain undiagnosed and untreated, and live out his days in a state mental institution in a vegetative state. Those who believe that this does not happen should peruse Chapter 26 (p. 518).

Some persons like to look up at the patient when they are recording this material and ask the patient the date as if they, the historians, do not know the correct date. This sometimes works, but an evasive patient might turn to a patient in another bed and ask him. And there are many other questions in the cognitive examination, so I tend to explain what I am doing: "I am going to ask you a lot of questions now. Some you will know the answer to, and some you won't. Just answer the ones you can." It is better to be straightforward. Even the patient with an organic brain syndrome might be able to perceive a subterfuge.

Some persons only ask the patient his birth date and then compare it with his stated age. This device gives a few false positives and many false negatives. Because we desire screening tests to have some false positives, but no false negatives, this technique is not recommended.

I have heard a skillful attending physician ask patients directly, "You've been having a little trouble with your memory lately, haven't you?" with an accepting smile and in a tone of voice that gives patients permission to report the problem. The less confident neophyte has difficulty with this approach.

I require that the patient know the year, the month, and the exact day, in order to be called oriented. Now many persons, including me, pay no attention to the day of the month, and so are technically disoriented to time. This does not mean that they necessarily have organic brain syndrome, but they have failed the screen, and the examiner must proceed to further testing (vide infra). The point to be emphasized is that one can accept false positives with a screening test, but no false negatives. Thus, the patient must give the correct year (even on January 1), the correct name of the month (not "Christmas" month because the patient has noticed the hallway decorations) and the exact correct day of the month (not weekday name), not even missing by a single day.

False positives for disorientation in time. In addition to normal persons who simply do not attend to the date, there are other patients who commonly do not know the exact date. First, there are very severe schizophrenics. While most schizophrenics are oriented to time, some are either disoriented or so disturbed that they cannot cooperate with the testing. Some patients with very severe depression are likewise unable to give the date, but it is not always clear whether they are truly disoriented or simply unable to cooperate. A severely excited manic patient may have so much tangentiality* and pressure of speech that he cannot answer the question. Patients suffering from any of the Freudian dissociative states may be unable to answer. This category includes Ganser's syndrome, which is seen in prisoners and inmates of other institutions. Whatever the cause, patients with Ganser's syndrome always answer incorrectly, and thus appear disoriented. However, they would also answer "four" to the question "How many legs on a three-legged stool?" (Thus, they are easy to diagnose, if not to treat.) I have also seen patients who were either malingering or suffering from a hysterical conversion reaction who appeared disoriented on direct questioning. Finally, patients suffering from sensory deprivation will be disoriented to time, regardless of whether the deprivation is experimental, political, or nosocomial (as in patients who are immobilized without vision after retinal surgery, or who are placed in intensive care units without light, time, or calendar cues). All of these false positives can be easily diagnosed on affirmative grounds by a competent clinician.

False negatives for disorientation in time. If the patient with an organic brain syndrome notices that his physicians have taken a very strong interest in his ability to recall the date, he may take some steps to satisfy what he perceives as their wish. For instance, some disoriented patients who have been repeatedly asked about temporal orientation learn to read the date from the physician's calendar watch. Others will keep a newspaper or hospital menu at their bedside table so that they can glance at the date when asked.

Tangentiality refers to the habit of changing the subject of speech by moving gradually away from it, at a tangent, and never coming back to it. It may be distinguished from *circumstantiality*, which is used to mean either (1) dealing with the subject in great detail or (2) circling around the subject and eventually returning to it.

One patient who was described as completely oriented put the date 3 days in the future when I examined him. (Most disoriented patients put the date in the past.) When I examined the examiners, I was told that his answer was always exactly three days in the future, leading someone to conclude (erroneously) that he really was oriented and did not need to be reoriented. Further investigation revealed that the patient realized that his doctors were interested in the date. Accordingly, he daily removed his milk container from his breakfast tray and placed it on his nightstand. Each time he was checked for orientation in time, he read the milk's expiration date from the container. As is so often true in medicine, awareness of the problem may be the solution.

•

In only one patient have I made the diagnosis of benign forgetfulness of senescence, a diagnosis that is ordinarily to be eschewed. This patient complained of failing memory and was disoriented to time, always being off by 1 day. However, she passed every other test (vide infra).

•

Summary.   If the patient is oriented to time, I may not do any more of the cognitive portion of the mental status examination at this point in the interview, unless there is reason to suspect one of the rare false negatives. But if the test is positive, I proceed to the rest of the cognitive examination, until I am convinced one way or the other.

Checking for orientation in place.   This test is useful when the patient is obviously disoriented and thinks he is at home or in an airplane. But it is not a very good screening test. Many false positives occur if one is very rigid and requires a perfect answer for the name of the hospital. (Some patients may know it is a Veterans Hospital, but are unable to give the specific name. Or they may know the name of the city, which is often a partly correct answer for certain hospitals, but in the case of the Veterans Hospital, an incomplete one. If the name of the hospital has changed, the patient may only know the former name.) Worse, there are false negatives. Some patients with organic brain syndrome still know the name of the hospital. Accordingly, I do not use this question often, usually proceeding directly to a test of calculation.

Examination for Ability to Calculate

Performing the serial sevens test.   The standard test is called "serial sevens" because the patient is asked to serially subtract seven from the residual of each operation. It is traditional to begin with the number 100. It goes like this:

MD: "Can you take 7 from 100?"
Patient: "Yes, I guess so."
MD: "Go ahead."
Patient: "You mean 100 minus 7?"
MD: "Yes."
Patient: ". . . That's 93."
MD: "And 7 from that?"
Patient: ". . . 86."
MD: "Minus 7?"
Patient: ". . . 79."
MD: "Minus 7?"

Patient: "Uh, . . . 72."
MD: "Keep going. Seven from that?" (Note that you should *not* help the patient by reminding him of the last number. The ability to remember that number is part of the test.)
Patient: "Uh, 65, . . . uh 58 . . . 51 . . . " etc.

Such a patient is said to be able to do serial sevens.

Validation studies done during World War II in California revealed that sixth grade school children could go all the way down from 100, with correction of their mistakes, in under 2 minutes (Hayman, 1941). This suggests that timed daily serial sevens could be used to follow the progress of a given patient. However, if you do that, remember to start from a different number each day, because the practice effect can permit a cognitively impaired patient to learn the right answers just as a visually impaired patient can learn the letters on the eye chart. For example, the second day start with 102, the third day with 105, and so on.

A teaching trick.   If you doubt that a patient can "learn" serial sevens, do the following experiment: Test the patient twice daily, once with different starting numbers, and once from the same starting number (usually 100). Make the same measurements— number of errors and seconds required to complete the test. If you use the same prompting rules (no correction of errors and no encouragement to "go ahead and try"), there will eventually be a divergence in the results, even with testing only twice a day, unless the patient is recovering rapidly.

In contemporary use, the mistakes are not corrected, to allow us the opportunity to observe perseveration (e.g., "93, 90, 83, 80, 73, 70," etc.) on the part of some patients with the organic brain syndrome. However, many patients with the organic brain syndrome will not perseverate.

Most normal subjects will do serial sevens without a mistake or with only one mistake in the first six subtractions. Two mistakes out of the first six is indeterminate, although it almost always implies a mild degree of cerebral impairment. But three or more mistakes out of the first six, or an inability to continue, is a reliable sign of organic brain syndrome.

Some patients are unable to finish the serial sevens, even with errors. The neophyte may feel embarrassed for the patient. The situation is best handled by smiling at the patient even when he fails the task. Your attitude should be, "Maybe you can't do that test right now, but you were a good chap for showing me that you couldn't do it, and now that I have that piece of information, I will be more able to help you. I am your friend." You might actually say something reassuring to the patient, such as, "I don't really expect anyone to be able to do all these tasks, but I want to see how many of them you can do."

If you think in your own mind that none of these tests are very important in measuring the worth of the patient as a human being, you will find that your instructions convey your acceptance of the patient no matter how well he performs. It will also help you to feel less upset, so that you are not inhibited from doing the test specifically in those situations in which it will be most helpful (i.e. when the patient is most likely to fail).

False positives.   A retarded person or one who left school in the second grade in order to chop cotton may never have had the ability to perform serial sevens. Because the test is intended to detect loss of function, and one cannot lose what one never had, the test is invalid in such a person, who should be identified by the social history. Do not try to compensate by making the test easier, say by asking the patient to perform serial threes, because the normal results have not been determined. Serial fives are worse than useless because the correct answer sounds the same as a perseverating one (95 . . . 90 . . . 85 . . . 80 . . . etc.).

False negatives.   There should not be any false negatives with a properly performed test.

Examination for Impaired Memory

There are a large number of tests for memory. One can ask the patient to repeat six digits forward or to repeat the last four of the six, going backward. The individual digits should be given slowly, one per second, so that the patient does not make compound numbers out of them.

An alternate method is to give the subject three words to remember and see if he can recall them later in the examination. Or one can ask the subject to remember three numbers. He should be able to recall them after counting aloud slowly from 1 to 10.

Persons who have never been to school pose special problems, and special psychometric tests are available for them. A good test is to ask the patient to say the days of the week backward. Patients without an organic brain syndrome can always do this, regardless of level of schooling.

At this point, you should be able to tell whether or not a person who is disoriented to time has an organic brain syndrome. If you are still having difficulty, you may wish to consider the following additional features of organic brain syndromes, both acute and chronic.

Testing for Impaired Judgment and Abstracting Ability

Examples of questions that test for judgment are these: "What would you do if you found an addressed envelope on the sidewalk and it had an uncancelled stamp on it?" Or, "What would you do if you were in a theater and you noticed a fire?"

To test for abstracting ability, one can ask for the interpretation of proverbs such as "a stitch in time saves nine" or "a rolling stone gathers no moss." Alternately, one can ask how things are alike, such as an apple and a pear, or a penny and a dime. Or, one can ask which item doesn't fit in a group, for example, an orange, a nickel, and a banana.

(These questions are also good for examining the examiners. Some people have accepted "banana" as the correct response to the last question, reasoning that the other two are round, an example of a concrete response. Similarly, a patient who gave an abnormal concrete interpretation of the proverb ["a rolling stone will never get green"] was judged cognitively normal by one examiner.)

Other Tests

The affect of a patient with an organic brain syndrome may be labile and shallow, but it is usually not. I would never make the diagnosis only on affect. Furthermore, it is difficult to teach skills such as the evaluation of affect to a large group without using videotape.

Some patients with an organic brain syndrome may hallucinate, but most do not. There are many other causes of hallucinations (see Ch. 26, p. 518). Accordingly, this symptom is not helpful in diagnosing or excluding an organic brain syndrome.

There are a large number of structured, scorable evaluations of the cognitive portion of the mental status examination. Of these, I recommend the Jacobs test, which was developed for use with medically ill patients (Jacobs et al., 1977), or the "Mini-

Mental State," which has been extensively validated (Folstein et al., 1975). The test I use, which is similar, is found in Appendix 2-1. This screening instrument will probably fare no better than any of the established ones, all of which are imperfect in certain circumstances (Nelson et al., 1986).

The EEG, actually a laboratory test, may be of value. In the acute organic brain syndrome, the EEG will show a slowing of the background rhythm compared with the premorbid tracing. Unfortunately, it is of little use if there is no premorbid tracing available. Furthermore, in some patients with a chronic organic brain syndrome, the abnormal cells that generate the slowed rhythm may die, so that this diagnostic sign will no longer be present.

A number of psychologic tests may be available to the examiner, including the Benton Visual Motor Test. A 10-point disparity between the verbal and performance subscales of the IQ test (in favor of the verbal) can also be a clue to organic brain syndrome. The Bender Gestalt test, for which scoring systems are available, is excellent. In the past, I carried the last card of the Bender Gestalt test in my bag, because the inability to draw the two superimposed polyhedra after viewing them was an efficient (positive) test for organic brain syndrome. (The test is also sensitive; the ability to copy the design accurately from memory is good evidence against organic brain syndrome.) Since some certified psychologists objected to this, on the grounds that I lacked the proper wall hangings, I discontinued the practice on the advice of my lawyer.

An alternate test is to draw two intersecting pentagons at least one inch on a side, and ask the patient to copy it. All 10 angles must be present and at least two must intersect to be counted correct, but rotation and tremor are to be ignored (Folstein et al., 1975). The drawings may be placed in the case record for making future comparisons.

Self-Test

Write down three reasons why you want to identify the patient with organic brain syndrome as soon as possible. (See Appendix 2-2, p. 30.)

For the attending.   One of the major problems in teaching the approach described above is the high opinion that the jejune (of all ages) have of their own diagnostic ability. They are all convinced that if there were any cognitive impairment in the patients, they would surely pick it up without specifically testing for orientation. Unfortunately, the only guaranteed way to dissuade them is to interview some of their own organic brain syndrome patients whom they thought "seemed okay to me." Even this doesn't always work the first time, since the illegitimately secure will always rebut, "He must have gotten this way in the last 24 hours." I have even tried playing a tape-recorded genuine (unstaged) interview of such a putatively "oriented" patient, who on direct questioning was disoriented by 20 years (see Ch. 26, p. 517), only to find on follow-up members of that laughing audience making the same mistakes a year or two later. Ben Hecht's description of John Barrymore's "last performance" is probably the most dramatic example of how a person with a known severe organic brain syndrome can deceive keen but uneducated observers (Hecht, 1985).

Approach to the Elderly Patient

The most important thing to remember about elderly people is that patients over the age of 79 years may still "see" themselves as 39. I am not speaking of demented patients, but of normal people. In my experience, this is probably even an understatement. A 79-year-old may see himself as 59, or 39, or 19, or sometimes all three in the course of one interview. The problem is that the interviewer has difficulty seeing the 79 year old patient as a 19-year-old. And whereas the physician has experience with many 79-year-olds, the patient has only recently become 79, and that for the very first time. Thus, it is a novel experience for him, and he must fall back on prior experiences in order to cope, just as you will fall back on critical educational experiences from your youth in times of medical crisis.

For the attending. A unique question to have a medical student or young resident ask the older patient is this: "Mr. Smith, when you were the age that I am now, what did you think your life would be like when you got to be the age you are now?" The young interviewer should be instructed to remain silent for 30 seconds after any verbal interaction required to clarify the question for the patient.

The main purpose of this exercise is to promote empathy, as well as to broaden the education of the young physician. For example, a patient whose present socioeconomic situation is different from that of the resident will often surprise the resident by revealing that his own aspirations and hopes were at one time the same as those presently cherished by the resident. Also, some young persons are detached from the old and impoverished whom they must care for as house officers; the younger may feel that the older arrived at their present decrepitude through some basic moral fault, poor planning, or absence of youthful ambition. To learn that things are otherwise may provide the young with a vicarious shared experience and the basis for better patient understanding.

Many patients over the age of 50 are secretly worried about having cancer. If you keep that idea at the back of your mind while doing the initial history and physical, you will be able to listen perceptively to the patient's fears. You can test this belief by asking a direct (but not a leading) question about what the patient is afraid you will discover, reassuring the patient, when appropriate (Sapira, 1972), and observing what happens. Sometimes, when you wish to reassure patients about what appears to be free-floating anxiety, you can ask about their fears; sometimes the anxiety is not as free-floating as initially believed. The patients will be impressed that such a jejune-appearing person could have perceived their innermost thoughts, and may attribute to you great qualities of intellect and sensitivity, as a result of using this simple technique.

This reasonable and ubiquitous, albeit unspoken, concern about cancer is to be distinguished from *cancerophobia*, which is an unusual psychiatric disorder encountered more commonly in the offices of internists than of psychiatrists. It is characterized by a conviction on the part of the patient that he has or shortly will develop a noxious cancer. Further, this cancer is either producing no symptoms (and must therefore be vigorously sought before it gets bigger) or it is producing symptoms whose significance the patient feels is unappreciated by his doctors. Either the doctor isn't taking the symptoms as seriously as the patient feels he should, or his searching techniques are in some way defective since the cancer remains undetected. Some patients seem to think that the cancers come and go, so that the search may be extended for several years.

The Patient Who Seems to Be Changing His Story

When the patient seems to be changing his story, there are several possible explanations:

1. The interviewer-historian may not be very good.
2. If there are several mediocre interviewer-historians, they may be spending more time conversing with each other than with the patient.
3. The patient may be retarded or have an organic brain syndrome, and simply be unable to remember, while attempting to be cooperative. Or he may not speak the language well.
4. The patient may be overly cooperative because he does not understand that the history is intended to generate information that will determine the specifics of his treatment. He may believe (especially in county, city, and other governmental hospitals) that the interview is for the purpose of determining whether he will receive any medical care at all. Such patients will gladly change their account as often as they believe the doctors want them to do so, in order to demonstrate how compliant they are.
5. The patient may be changing his story because of a motivation that no one can figure out. This rarely happens, and is a diagnosis of exclusion.
6. The patient is simply inattentive and cannot remember his account without a great deal of review and repetition.
7. The patient is developing a relationship with his doctor that is permitting him to remember previously unconscious events that were not accessible to him during earlier interviews.

The Patient Who Is Vague

Bracketing and Other Forms of Forced Choice

In attempting to determine the duration or the frequency of a symptom in a patient who is vague, a useful technique is to "bracket" the correct answer by giving the patient extremes to choose from, then reducing the size of the bracket. For instance, if the patient could not tell you the duration of his symptom, you could begin as follows:

Physician: "Was it about a day long or a year long?"
Patient: "Oh it didn't last a year . . ."
Physician: "Well was it a day long or a month long?"
Patient: "Oh I've had it for more than a month . . . ?"
Physician: "Well, can you remember if you had it around Christmas time?"
Patient: ". . . now that you mention it, I remember I did have it at Christmas."

In this way, you can eventually narrow the estimate of duration within a range of one or two units of time, say months or days. Even this limited information will often be useful.

Patients frequently have difficulty recounting frequency, especially when suffering symptoms whose frequency varies in a phasic manner in the course of time. Thus:

Physician: "Do you get it once a day or once a month?"
Patient: "Well, some days I don't get it at all, but when I get it, it's more than once a day."
Physician: "When you do get it, would it be twice a day or 20 times a day?" (Focusing on frequency per day.)
Patient: "Oh, never 20 times a day."
Physician: "How about 10 times a day?"
Patient: "On no, just two or three times a day, but a lot of days I don't get it at all."
Physician: "In an average week, how many days will you be

free of the symptom?" (Focusing on asymptomatic periods per unit of time.)

Patient: "Well, last March I would sometimes go several weeks without it. But beginning here lately, I noticed it started coming at least once a week . . ."

Here, the physician has accomplished the following:

1. Determined how many times a day the patient will have the symptom when he is symptomatic.
2. Approximated the frequency of symptomatic days.
3. Elicited the fact that there has been an increase in the frequency of symptomatic days.

To determine exactly when this last change in frequency occurred, the physician could now proceed as follows:

Physician: "You say that you are having more days with [the symptom]. When did you start having more days with [the symptom]?"
Patient: "I'm not sure exactly."
Physician: "Well, did this happen a week ago or a year ago?"
Patient: "Oh, it hasn't been a year. But it has been more than a week . . ."

The interview continues in a similar manner.

Being Persistent

Some patients are vague in ways that are not susceptible to bracketing or other forms of forced choice. For example:

Physician: "Can you remember how you felt when your mother died?"
Patient: ". . . I guess I can . . ."
Physician: ". . . Well, what did you feel then?"
Patient: ". . . Oh, I don't know, I guess I don't know."

When confronted with such a frustrating response, it is tempting to change the line of inquiry. This tactic is recommended by many experts, but I disagree. In the desire to get some information, any information, the physician may rapidly slide from one of the seven dimensions to another, never getting a complete data base. It is better to persist, and to give the patient at least three tries at answering the question. At that time, you can change the subject to the difficulty the patient has with answering the question:

Physician: ". . . I notice that you are having a lot of difficulty talking about how you felt at that time. Why do you suppose that might be?"
Patient: ". . . Now . . . maybe . . . uh . . . you know, I've started wondering lately, well actually how much did I really like my mother?"

Although one doesn't often get such a revealing answer, one will never get a revealing answer by sliding off to another dimension or another question, without giving the patient a full opportunity to respond.

The Patient Who Is Addicted to Drugs or Behaviors

It is a good idea to determine, as soon as possible, whether the drug abuse, alcohol use, gambling, philandering, or other prob-

lem is ego-syntonic or ego-alien (ego-dystonic). If the behavior is ego-syntonic (that is, the patient accepts it and does not perceive it as wrong or damaging to himself), one will not expect to bring about a permanent change. If the habit itself (not just its secondary consequences) is ego-alien, one may be more hopeful about change.

To make this determination, simply ask the patient, "Why do you want to stop this?" Most intake interviews do not do this but rather assume that if the patient shows up, he will be "compliant" (see definitions in Ch. 1, p. 4, for a discussion of this word).

The patient whose behavior is ego-syntonic will give a reason that is contingent upon a specific time, place, situation, noxious outcome, or other temporary factor, for example:

"I don't want to be like that for my daughter's wedding."
"If they catch you doing that in that state, they are very hard on you."
"I told her that if she would, I would too."
"Because now I have to stop until . . ."

While each of these may be a good reason to change behavior, they will only apply for a period of time. To test the impression that the behavior is ego-syntonic, one could counter each of these reasons with an appropriate rebuttal:

"But what are you going to do after the wedding?"
"What are you planning to do after you pass through there?"
"I guess then if she doesn't, you won't have to either."
"But then when that's over, I guess you can start all over."

This probing is not cruel to the patient because it is in his best interest to arrive at an understanding of his true motivation. A covert game involving the patient and the organization offering care wastes the patient's opportunity to change while making the staff cynical. In the long run, it is best for the patient to know his motive, and to know that the staff also knows. When he is ready for a genuine change, there will be a responsive facility available to help him.

Certain habituees are manipulative, and will learn to tell each member of the staff what that individual wishes to hear. One drug abuser gave each interviewer a different, highly convincing reason for quitting. He told the student nurse that he wanted to marry a fine girl, after telling the medical student that he wanted to go back to school. The social worker heard that he wanted to take care of his aging parents. The senior resident was told that he wanted to take better care of his health. When an experienced attending interviewed the patient, it became obvious that the drug abuse was ego-syntonic. It should be noted that all of the interviewers who believed the drug abuse to be ego-alien wanted to believe that because the patient was very personable and likeable (Sapira & Cherubin, 1975).

The Patient Who May Be Involved in Illegal Activities

Although one can sometimes omit the introductory explanation about why doctors take histories and ask so many questions (once one can tell which patients are familiar with the procedure), one must always explain the reasons to any patients who might be involved in illegal activities.

Such patients may be met with in jail, or at the hospital prior to being sent to jail, or simply in the hospital after having engaged in an activity that could lead to a jail sentence. Such persons have learned to be very suspicious of those in fiduciary positions, such as lawyers, and those in positions of authority, such as judges and policemen. A doctor may be perceived to be in both categories. To all such patients, I say, "I may ask you about things you do not want to discuss. If I do, then just tell me you don't want to talk about it, and we'll go on to something else. It is more important to have good information to work with, even if it is incomplete, than to have wrong information and make mistakes in your evaluation."

Even this introduction does not guarantee that the interviewer will learn the whole truth. Patients have later approached me (especially when they have been seen in jail), to tell me things they had at first denied.

Whenever I think that a patient, especially one in a private hospital, is seeking sanctuary or is getting "straight" for court appearances, I ask, in the middle of an interview, "When is your court date set?" As I say this, I look at the patient as if I am certain that there is a court appearance approaching, and I am only uncertain about the date. The patient will inevitably look puzzled and inquire further as to my meaning. I simply repeat the original statement, up to three times.

If the patient does not tell me about the court date, or denies having one, I may tell him that I had the feeling that there was one in the offing, since his expectations for care were unusual, given his chief complaint. Sometimes, this produces the desired information. Sometimes, I am simply wrong. Over the years, I have been surprised at how often my intuition has been correct.

If you decide to use this question, drop it unexpectedly into the middle of the interview. Try to restrict it to those in whom the answer is likely to be positive. That judgment is based on intuition; I do not know how to teach it.

The Patient Who May Have Other Legal Involvements

Physicians are increasingly consulted in cases in which the patient's primary motive is not to obtain medical advice but to gain compensation through the legal system, for example, to collect disability payments, or an award in a personal injury case. It is helpful for the physician to know this, because the court schedule has a profound influence on the prognosis. The patient cannot expect to collect benefits if he improves too much. This knowledge can save the physician considerable frustration.

If you suspect that the record of the visit is likely to be subpoenaed, you must be particularly circumspect about writing down information that should be kept confidential. In addition, you will want to be especially precise about chronology related to the incident that sparked the litigation.

The Patient Who Might Have a Factitious Disease

Autogenic illness (e.g., Munchausen's syndrome) is sometimes the final diagnosis in a patient with a complex and puzzling story. The interviewer whose mental status examination goes beyond "oriented times three," and who does more than a perfunctory "coffee, tea, or milk" social history, may suspect this diagnosis during the first interview.

An interactional style characterized by "truculence and evasiveness" has been described in patients with Munchausen's

syndrome (Ireland et al., 1967). The patient's affect may not be immediately appropriate to the verbal content of the interview. There may be self-contradictions within the historic material, and the patient may try to avoid discussing any one aspect of the past medical history in depth. The failure of all attempts to locate family members at the given addresses and telephone numbers is a "positive" diagnostic sign, said to be highly sensitive for the pseudologia phantastica variant of Munchausen's syndrome (Sapira, 1981).

When the diagnosis of any autogenic illness has been established, it has been suggested that the patient should be gently confronted by the internist in the presence of the psychiatrist, who can then initiate a relationship in a supportive nonjudgmental manner. My approach has been to initiate psychiatric consultation from the beginning, regardless of the issue of confrontation. First of all, not all physicians are capable of participating in direct confrontation in a gentle manner, especially after they have been through a diagnostic wild goose chase. Furthermore, if one views the patient's total behavior as a biologic event, one can quickly formulate a hypothesis (usually affirmed later) that this specific pathologic behavior is, for the time, the patient's only way of communicating an intense distress. If so, it may be impossible for the patient to "confess" when confronted, and usually such patients do not "confess." Even if they do, that is no guarantee that the behavior will cease. There is always another doctor and another hospital. Therefore, one would wish to initiate the patient-psychiatrist therapeutic alliance independent of the presenting illness and before any confrontations. The psychotherapeutic process would presumably broaden the patient's repertoire of coping responses beyond the production of autogenic disease.

Almost all "medical" patients have some underlying psychopathology, at the very least, life's everyday unhappiness and problems, about which they will gladly unburden themselves if given the opportunity. A psychiatric consultation can be presented as an "opportunity" to assess the consultant's ability to help resolve the patient's personal problems, independent of the internist's diagnostic evaluation, which will proceed *parri passu*. After diagnostic closure, the internist now has a number of options. He may confront the patient, or he may simply tell the patient, in a nonaccusatory manner, as in the case of a warfarin eater, "We have found some warfarin in your blood on admission, but its effects are all gone now. This condition should not recur." Finally, even if an angry internist confronts the patient in an accusatory manner, there is a preestablished patient relationship with another physician, not related to the subject of the diagnostic physician's anger (Sapira, 1981).

Sexual Orientation

It is important to determine not only the patient's sexual orientation(s), but also his sexual behavior with various types of partners. I simply ask, "With whom do you like to have sex?" and wait for an answer. Some patients become confused by this question, to which they believe the answer should be obvious, so one can add, "Do you prefer men or women as sexual partners, or both?" Watch the patient's eyes during this question. Some distrustful patients will break eye contact or flick their glance down at your pen and up again, if you have not earned their confidence. Patients who are worried about their sexual orientation, but who are not yet active, may also respond in this way. (Of course, generalizations such as the correlation between good eye contact and trustfulness are not perfect, but are simply reminders of the importance of observing nonverbal behavior, and the potential effect of social forces on historical responses.)

Next I ask how active they are sexually at the present time, and possibly when they were last sexually active. Then I inquire about the specific descriptions of behavior if this is important.

Recording this information in a manner that preserves confidentiality is covered in Chapter 4 (p. 67).

The Patient Who Is a Member of a Subculture with Its Own Jargon

The single principle to be observed with a patient of this description is not to use the individual's language unless it is completely natural to you. This is especially true for the language of the criminal, drug-abusing, or juvenile subcultures. Remember that language serves a protective function. Permit the patient to maintain that protection, or he will have to achieve it in some other way.

Many recognize the protective function of language, but assume that if they show themselves to be cognoscenti, or even if they show their interest by trying to "get into" the language, the patient's natural cautions will disappear. In fact, the contrary is the case.

Once the patient has sufficiently assessed you and decided to accept you as a physician, he will not need to hide behind the mask of his argot.

There are certain obvious situations in which it may be in everyone's interest to violate the rule. For example, the physician who sees a patient in the emergency room for a stab wound needs to know whether the patient has been "juked" or "stobbed," to help assess which internal organs are likely to be involved. (The assailant's knife points up in "juking" and down in "stobbing.") If the patient uses unfamiliar terminology, the physician must ask its meaning if he is not sure he understands it.

The Non-English-Speaking Patient

For interviewing the patient who does not speak English, the student should collect articles from the better throw-away journals, such as *Resident and Staff Physician*, which formerly printed bilingual clinical examination synopses, including phonetic pronunciation guides. These should be kept in view of the patient and the interviewer should point to the phrase as he phonetically pronounces it. This permits a literate patient to understand, even if the interviewer is not an excellent phonetic mime. I tear such pages from the journals as they appear, or as someone tells me about them. Occasionally, several will be reprinted together. For a nominal price, they are available from *Resident and Staff Physician*, 80 Shore Road, Port Washington, NY 11050. Blue Cross also publishes a similar text, oriented to the traveling patient and less useful for the physician. A data-base form for the Spanish-speaking patient is given in Appendix 4-1. *Southwestern Medical Dictionary: Spanish-English, English-Spanish* by Margarita Artschwager Kay (University of Arizona Press, Tucson, 1977) is especially good because it includes idiomatic expressions.

In some hospitals, the social service department keeps a list of translators available. When using a translator, especially a member of the patient's family, special care must be taken to preserve the patient's privacy, by swearing the translator to secrecy. The translator is never to reveal anything that he hears to anyone, and is never to speak of it again. He may be asked to lift his hand as in taking an oath, and to translate the exchange for the patient. By watching the patient, especially his eyes, during the translation, you can often perceive whether the patient has completely accepted the translator or not.

You should address your remarks to the patient, not to the translator, because sometimes the patient will understand part of what you say, and you will be better able to read the patient's nonverbal messages if you are looking at him directly.

The biggest problem in my personal experience has been the patient who speaks a little English, enough to carry on a conversation, but who does not have sufficient vocabulary to get through a review of systems. In this instance, the patient may agree to statements that he does not fully understand, in order to please the physician. As always, it is better to have incomplete information than wrong information. Stating the same question in several different ways at different points in the interview (in order to be sure you have consistent answers) may be helpful. (This technique is also good for English-speaking patients, since it is surprising how often the patient has not understood a question, but has answered it anyway.)

The Patient Who Cannot Hear Well

The patient may be able to hear better if you place your stethoscope's earpieces in his ears and speak through the bell. This method was invented by Laennec.

Your tape recording equipment can be useful here, if the patient does not have an adequate hearing aid but can benefit from amplification. Place the earpiece in the patient's ear, or better still, use stereo earphones, since these also help block the ambient noise. Speak into the microphone yourself. With the machine set on "record," its amplifier will serve as a hearing aid for the patient. It is easier to speak in a civil tone when you do not have to speak loudly to enable the patient to hear. If there is not a tape in the machine, it can still be used in this manner by pushing "eject," then depressing the "record" lever.

In any situation involving hearing impairment, it is useful to attempt not to raise the pitch of your voice as you increase the volume. Many persons have a greater loss for high-frequency tones than for middle- and low-frequency tones. If one follows the natural instinct to shout at a higher frequency, the gain in volume may be offset by the move into a frequency range at which the patient's hearing is more severely impaired.

If the patient is completely deaf, I take the history with a typewriter, letting the patient also type in his answers if he prefers. This lengthens the interview, but not as much as you might think, providing that the patient is not also visually or cognitively impaired. Admittedly, the review of systems portion of the interview can be quite boring, and this is one of the few situations in which I would gladly use a printed form.

The Hostile Patient

Quite often, one will become aware at the beginning of the interview that the patient is very hostile. Sometimes, the patient seems specifically angry with the interviewer. One method of handling this situation is simply to say to the patient: "Gosh, Mr. Smith, you seem awfully angry, yet you can't be angry with me because we have never met before. What has upset you?"

It may develop that the patient is upset because his lunch tray was late. Or he may have been treated in a demeaning manner in the admitting area. Or he may be reacting to some other frustration that preceded your entrance into the room. Of course, if the patient starts out in a good mood, but becomes angry in mid-interview, it may well be that you have induced the hostility in some manner. In that case, it is a good idea to stop the interview and ask the question above. By finding out what you did that was offensive, and dealing with it in a considerate manner, you can reestablish rapport in the interview.

The Patient Who Refers to Himself as a "Guinea Pig"

Patients often refer to themselves as "guinea pigs," especially when they are in a teaching hospital. In dealing with this perception, one must first determine what the term *guinea pig* means to the patient. Probably the best way to do that is to ask the patient. (The concept of ego-syntonicity can be applied here.)

If the patient feels that he is the object of experimentation, with no benefit to him (as in a drug study), or that he is being used for education of students and house staff, again with no personal benefit, then the use of the phrase is clearly pejorative. In that case, one must dispel the patient's fantasies; or if the perceptions are accurate, one must help free the patient from the situation.

On the other hand, some patients who were the first in their city or the first in a given hospital to have a certain experience are very proud of this. In this case, the term *guinea pig* is not pejorative, but complimentary, or at least indicative of a psychologic situation wherein the patient may gain some sense of mastery of an otherwise noxious circumstance.

In fact, most of the time the phrase *guinea pig* has both connotations; in other words, the patient feels ambivalent. Here one should, as best one can, "align oneself with the patient's ego" and support the positive meaning of the word while dealing (as above) with the negative.

The Patient Who Will Only Be Examined by a "Real Doctor"

It is tempting for the resident to show solidarity with the team and to reject in turn the patient's rejection of the student or the intern. However, it is better to defer making any kind of response until one has assessed exactly what is conditioning the patient's behavior, which is in no way concerned with the specifics of his care, but rather with the age of those who will provide his care. Sometimes, it is the patient's way of distracting his own attention from more frightening problems. At other times, it is a reflection of prior feelings, which he was unable to express (or perhaps even to experience at a conscious level) while he was in the situation that elicited them. (For example, they might have been feelings such as anger, resentment, or envy, which were unacceptable to that particular patient's makeup). Sometimes the patient is angry at a specialist upon whom he feels very dependent. Since he cannot express his anger at the specialist, he may displace them onto more acceptable targets—like house staff who

are like such a specialist but not in a preexisting dominant relationship to the patient.

The above is an example of the set of transference relationships, which are ubiquitous in clinical medicine, although generally discussed only in the context of psychiatric interviews (e.g., MacKinnon & Michels, 1971). In the example the transference is negative, in terms of its predominant affective tone. Often, the physician is inclined to respond with a countertransference, a relationship that flows from physician to patient. For instance, if a patient who refused to let the intern examine him reminded the supervising resident of one of the resident's past relationships, and if the resident reacted to the patient noxiously but within the rules of that prior relationship (as if the patient were the other person in that relationship), then we would say that the resident had a negative countertransference to the patient.

Positive countertransference (where "positive" again refers to the affective tone) can be just as neurotic and destructive as the negative type. For instance, if a patient experiences a positive transference to the physician and attempts to seduce him, the physician might allow her to succeed, if he is having a positive countertransference. Yet the outcome for the doctor–patient relationship might ultimately not be "positive," either in terms of predominant mood tone or the achievement of therapeutic goals.

The Patient Who Asks Personal Questions

Questions about the interviewer's personal life may involve several different types of transference, or they simply may reveal concern about the interviewer's ability to understand or help the patient. Experienced interviewers generally recognize the meaning of the question, and know when it is best simply to answer it directly, but beginners are generally advised to inquire of the patient, "What did you have in mind?" or "What leads to your question?" Sometimes the interviewer may want to try to interpret the meaning of the question for the patient: "Perhaps you ask about my age because you're not sure if I'll be competent to help you?"

Patients who attempt to socialize should be tactfully discouraged, by saying something like this: "I'm your doctor. If we had a social relationship, my objectivity would be lost."

The Organ Recital (or "By the Way, Doctor . . .")

Quite often in the outpatient practice of chronic disease medicine, the patient asks you about an organ other than the one you had been attending to, just as he has his hand on the door to leave, and just as you are getting the chart ready for the next patient.

For example:
Physician: ". . . and I will give you an appointment for 3 months, so that we can be sure that your blood pressure is under good control."
Patient (rising to leave): "Thank you, doctor."
Physician (signing his note and filing the chart): "Any time."
Patient (reaching the door): ". . . What about my shortness of breath?"
Physician (looking up, startled): "What shortness of breath?"
Patient: "I get shortness of breath."
Physician (flustered): "Shortness of breath! You never told me about that."

Although patients may switch from organ to organ (hence the name "organ recital"), some patients stay within one organ system, alternating symptoms. Some describe the syndrome in this way: "As soon as one thing is fixed, something else goes wrong."

Like most syndromes, this one has multiple etiologies. One of the most common is a failure of the physician to attend to the patient as a person because of an exclusive concern with the patient's various organs. Therefore, in order to deal with this treatable cause, one must return to paying attention to the patient.

One method is to stop near the end of the interview and ask, "Is there anything else you wanted to tell me about or ask me about?" Then wait and let the patient talk for as long as he wants, even if he is talking about psychosocial concerns.

Of course there are some situations in which that method will not work. It is well worth remembering that the ticket of admission to seeing the doctor is a "complaint." We ourselves speak of the medical skill required to determine the patient's "chief complaint." Most patients would feel very strange about telling a doctor, "I really don't feel too bad, but I am worried about something going on (at home or work) and want somebody I trust to talk it over with." Furthermore, some physicians would be startled by such a request, because they have effectively, but unconsciously, trained their patients not to say such things to them. In that situation, the patient has no recourse other than to pause, with his hand on the door (a safe position from which he may escape if he does not get the answer he wants), and try to titillate the doctor back into paying attention to him by offering the doctor something he knows the doctor will respond to: complaints referable to organs.

The Aphasic Patient

For an aphasic patient, one "without speech," the history might have to be constructed from data gathered from old charts and from interviews with the patient's family and friends. The main problem arises when one does not realize that the patient is aphasic and keeps trying to interview the patient when one should give up.

Aphasia is discussed more fully under the neurologic exam, but two "pearls" are worth mentioning at this time.

○ Don't diagnose aphasia too quickly in the absence of other neurologic findings.

○ Do not confuse aphasia with an organic brain syndrome, schizophrenia, retarded depression, or dysarthria (the inability to articulate sounds clearly, see Ch. 26, p. 466).

The Evasive Patient

If an oriented, otherwise cooperative patient withholds information in selected areas of the interview, you should proceed as described below.

Step 1

Ask the patient why he did not tell you what you asked (whether about sexual matters, suicidal ideation, hospitals where he has been, etc.). You must make clear to the patient that you are not simply repeating the query, but rather you are asking a new question, namely why he will not answer the original query.

Patients will usually make one of three types of response:

A. There may be a logical reason based on fear of what you might do with the information. If their fears are specific but incorrect, you can reassure them. Alternately, their reluctance may be diffuse and nonspecific. For instance, they may wish that you do not make a written or electronic recording of what they say. In that case, you should turn off the tape recorder or put down your pen.

B. The patient may have come to a conclusion based on the assumptions inherent in a delusional system. For instance, the patient may refuse to give you information about sexual activities because of his fear that you might report it to the FBI or the CIA. You should gently undercut any statements that are fantastic; you might assure the patient that you don't work for those organizations, but rather that you work for the patient. Then you should pursue his system of thought, particularly if he persists in irrational beliefs.

C. The patient may not even be willing to discuss his refusal to answer. In that case, proceed directly to the next step.

Step 2

Ask the patient, "Why have you come here?" This returns the interview to the subject of the original doctor-patient relationship, because the patient will usually say the visit was for an evaluation or treatment or relief of a symptom. If the patient is one of the few who gives a reason that is inappropriate and/or discordant to the original chief complaint, this discrepancy should immediately be pointed out and pursued. Most patients, however, will refer to their original reason for coming, which falls into the general category of "I-want-you-to-help-me-with-something-doctor." For these patients, proceed to the next step.

Step 3

Tell the patient, "I want to help you, but in order for me to make correct decisions, we have to have correct information on which to base those decisions," or words to that effect. Whatever the other words, the sentence should begin with, "I want to help you, but . . ." and the second half of the sentence should use the first person plural, which is grammatically incorrect but psychologically sound. This sentence helps to prevent the consultation from becoming a doctor-versus-patient battle. It reminds the patient that you want to help, but that your assistance derives from a mutual, joint, team effort.

(At this point, most patients will give you the requested data and also the real reason for their withholding it in the first place. These reasons should be dealt with at this time as described in step 1, parts A and B, if appropriate.)

Step 4

A very few patients will still withhold the information. If the specific information does not seem to be critical at this point, you should proceed with the historytaking. Upon discovering that they have not been rejected, some patients will later disclose the requested information. However, if the withheld information is critical to the diagnosis and treatment, the patient should be apprised of your opinion in this regard. Then instruct the patient to return to the office in a week to resume the consultation, giving the patient the option of canceling the appointment if he still feels that he cannot trust you. It is essential that this step be carried out tactfully and considerately so that it will not be viewed by the patient as punishment or rejection. For instance, one might explain to the patient, "I can't proceed without this information. I certainly respect your privacy, but I want to do right by you, and in order to do that, I need to have this information. Why don't you come back in a week, and we can continue the consultation at that time. If I were to try to make a decision for you at this point, I am afraid that I would be wasting your time and money, and worse, we might erroneously come to judgments that might not be in your best interest."

Some critics have argued that this technique is not suitable for situations in which there may not be a "next week" (as in the emergency room). What to do then? Part of the medical art is deciding which problems are solvable and which are not; I have no solution for this interviewing problem in "no next week" situations. However, those who insist on solutions for every problem, or who believe that they can somehow make a correct diagnosis without obtaining the necessary information, must also believe in miracles. For them, I suggest they visit the tomb of the Voodoo Queen Marie of New Orleans, located in the Basin Street Cemetery. A century after her death, the upkeep on this tomb is still maintained by donations from her grateful followers, to whom she has granted miracles.

The Uncooperative ("Noncompliant") Patient

Is the Patient Taking the Medication?

Numerous studies have shown that outpatient "compliance" with the physician's prescription ranges from 70% to as low as 30% (e.g. Blackwell, 1972). It is essential for the physician to determine whether or not a patient is truly taking his medication. If not, this (biologic) event may give useful information about the patient's interaction with his physician, but is not to be taken as evidence for any enduring character trait of the patient.

There are a number of strategies that may be employed. It is an unfortunate paradox that they all work best for those physicians who need them least. Before beginning your inquiries, you must seriously and honestly consider how you will react if the patient states that he is not taking his medications. What will you do, say, and feel? Will you view the patient's behavior as an event with past determinants in the patient's life, or as a personal affront with past determinants in your own life?

One way to find out how you really feel about such things is to ask yourself what you did the last time you felt, but did not know, that the patient who said that he was taking his medicines as prescribed was in fact not doing so? Did you simply order drug levels, or did you share your feeling with the patient in a way that opened communications? If the latter, did you come to believe the patient when he stated that he was taking his medications as prescribed, or did you then order a drug level as an opening gambit in cops and robbers (rather than as, possibly, evidence of a problem with the patient's metabolism of the drug)? Remember, if you entered clinical medicine to become a detective, the patient should be your client, not your chief suspect. Nor should you be deceived by those with more experience than you who claim to be able to predict which patients are "compliant." When the issue has been scientifically studied, and the results analyzed for statistical significance, physicians have not been able to predict "compliance," and their ability does not improve with increasing experience. In one study, the physicians' prediction that the patient was not taking his medicine as instructed proved to be erroneous 75% of the time (Mushlin & Appel, 1977)!

Here are the techniques:

1. Acknowledgment

"I know how terribly hard it is to remember to take all those pills every day. How many times a week do you think you have trouble taking all your pills?"

Or: "I know how hard it is to keep taking those pills for your blood pressure when you feel perfectly well. Which of them do you think you skip most often?"

Or: "When you went to visit the family on the Coast last month, I guess you went off your pills. How long after you came back did you start taking the medications again?"

Or: "How can you remember to take your medicine on the weekend?"

Or: "What happened the last time you told one of our doctors that you were not taking every single one of those pills?"

Remember that the purpose of the question is to facilitate communication, not to replicate the tone of a Gestapo interrogation (see p. 000.)

Quite often, none of these questions seems to work at the time. The patient may convince you that he has taken all of his medicines, but later will tell you that he has not. Or he may "try you out" by telling about a time with another doctor that he did not take all his medications but could not tell that doctor. In that case, try to learn the patient's fantasies about what the other doctor would have done. This is the patient's chance to tell you about his feelings toward all doctors, including you. The time invested here will pay good dividends later.

2. A Diary

Many clever physicians who have their patients keep diaries for diagnostic purposes do not realize that the diary may also be used therapeutically. Ask the patient to keep a diary of all the times that he forgets to take his medicines and bring it in on the next visit. This accomplishes several purposes. First, it makes it legitimate for the patient to tell you that he has not taken his medications. Second, it may decrease the number of skipped doses by requiring the patient to attend to the issue more closely. It is often easier to take a pill than to find the diary and a pencil. Third, it makes the patient a more active participant in his medical care. Finally, it is an expression of trust between doctor and patient.

3. Sharing the Decision Making

To empower the patient while using a preventive technique, give the patient a choice of the medications to be prescribed. Give a brief description of their differences, and allow him a choice where possible. Most patients will turn the choice over to you again, but at least they will not feel trapped into a particular drug. Eliminating this sense of being trapped seems to be very important for some patients.

None of the above are definitive methods comparable to the tricks we use to elicit a subtle heart murmur. All of them can be ruined by the physician's tone of voice or subsequent behavior. They are simply facilitators. How you react to the patient's admission of skipping medications is the most important factor.

The Counterphobic Patient

One type of noncompliant patient of special interest is the one who is engaged in counterphobic behavior. The patient wishes to deny the disease, the illness, the doctor's prognosis, and its significance to him. One way to do this is to stop taking the prescribed medications. When nothing disastrous happens immediately, the behavior works well in helping the patient to deny his illness. However, as in a patient with congestive heart failure, the continued omission of the medication eventually, perhaps 2 weeks later, may result in a hospital admission for what the doctor sees as the same condition. But the counterphobic patient has had 2 solid weeks of reinforcement for his belief that the original illness is gone and that the doctors were wrong. The new symptoms, therefore, are seen as evidence of a new disease, about whose prognosis the doctors may once again be in error. Obviously, such patients should not be scolded, and threats of a bad prognosis may not frighten them, since they have already proved the physician wrong.

Sometimes a counterphobic tendency will be spontaneously manifested in the interview; the patient will appear to be proud of not taking his medications. But most of the time, the physician must be aware of this possibility, and actively look for evidence of this type of behavior.

Dealing with Fantasies

A fantasy is a private, imaginary scenario. If it is conscious, the fantasizer knows that it is imaginary. The fantasy embodies some belief. It is set in the dimension of time, and may be in the past, present, or future. Those set in the future are the most important for medicine.

We all have fantasies; a daydream is one type. But the fantasies of patients that concern us are different from daydreams in several important ways. Daydreams usually have a positive affective tone (e.g., the "day I won the Nobel Prize"). Patients' fantasies often have a negative tone (e.g., "If I let them do a lumbar puncture, I will become paralyzed from the waist down"). Even those with a positive tone may interfere in the doctor-patient relationship by bringing in a degree of unreality. (e.g., "If I let the doctor do this biopsy, then maybe he will like me enough to give me a special medicine that only he can obtain and that is the only medicine that will keep me alive"). Often we do not learn of patients' fantasies unless we are particularly good interviewers, or unless they prohibit us from doing something important that we wish to do.

Psychiatrists and others comfortable with projective tests are good at learning of patients' fantasies. Sometimes, as with Rorschach cards, they ask the patient to create a fantasy or they may ask the patient to make three wishes. Many doctors seem uncomfortable with such methods, and for them the simplest way to learn the fantasy is to ask about it. For example:

> "I know that you don't want us to do the lumbar puncture, and I understand that you feel strongly about it. And I know you understand how important it is. I was wondering if you could tell me just what you think a lumbar puncture is?"
> or: ". . . tell me what you think a lumbar puncture means?"
> or: ". . . tell me what you think of when you hear the words 'lumbar puncture.'"
> or: "What have you heard about lumbar punctures?" In a patient who was reluctant to have a biopsy, you might say, "What kind of thoughts come to mind when you hear about a biopsy like yours?"
> or: ". . . what do you think is going to happen after the biopsy is done?"
> or: "You were dead set against the biopsy yesterday. What made you change your thinking?"

The important thing is to ask the provocative question, and get the patient to start talking. Eventually, the fantasy will be produced. Now, you will understand the belief system upon which the patient's conclusion was based, and can deal with it openly, in some cases by undercutting it. For example:

> "I have never had a patient become paralyzed from the waist down, or any other place for that matter, after a lumbar puncture. In fact, if I thought that could happen to you, I would not have suggested it."
> or: "There are neurologic procedures in which something like that can happen, but this is not one of them. It is true that some people get a temporary headache afterwards, but there is no paralysis."

In this example, the imbedded belief system is: "Doctors can hurt you as well as help you; this one might hurt me." While one may not be successful at overcoming the belief and altering the patient's behavior, without getting the fantasy out into the open, one will only be skirmishing at the border.

Physicians have fantasies too. If you find yourself getting angry while interviewing a patient, you might ask yourself which of your fantasies the patient has interfered with. Many times, he has challenged what has been called the Omnipotence Fantasy. Physicians wish to believe that they have powers much greater that those they really do possess, particularly over life and death. (In-

deed, these fantasies receive powerful cultural reinforcement.) The patient who dies, or who fails to respond to treatment, may undercut the physician's fantasy of omnipotence, producing a very negative affect, usually in direct proportion to the power of the fantasy's positive affect. Often these fantasies are not completely conscious, but are still powerful motivators of behavior.

The Patient Who Begins to Cry

If the patient begins to cry, this is a signal that indicates that the interview technique was successful in eliciting emotion laden material, and in a manner that permitted the patient to express it. Give the patient a tissue, and permit him to finish crying. Do not abandon the patient either directly by leaving the room, or indirectly by letting the crying patient leave while the physician remains in the room.

The Patient Who Is Undiagnosable

Certain patients who are not suffering from hysteria or conversion come to the physician with objective complaints that have eluded diagnosis. (By objective, it is meant that the patient reports an event that occurred at a clearly stated time, and which the physician can record.) I wish to indicate clearly that patients do not have imaginary symptoms. (I can do this in the current intellectual climate only by rejecting the Cartesian duality of objective versus subjective.)

With clinical experience, one can often discern at the beginning whether these patients are undiagnosed or undiagnosable. An example of the former is a patient who is suffering from acute intermittent porphyria, a diagnosis that no physician has thought of and confirmed with appropriate laboratory tests. An undiagnosable patient, however, is one whose symptoms are not yet part of any syndrome or disease described in the scientific medical literature. Such patients remind us of the imperfections of science and humble us with the inutility of scientific medicine in their cases. Sometimes, we become angry and call them names, but these names are not collectively or individually a diagnosis, as scientists understand that term.

A Method

1. If, at the end of my history and physical I am concerned that the patient may be undiagnosable, I say, "I must tell you that of the patients I see in consultation, I am only able to make a diagnosis in about half of them. We doctors are very good at diagnosing bad diseases, that is, diseases that need urgent surgery or strong medicines. But there are many other patients who have symptoms that come and go, in whom we never make a diagnosis."

Sometimes, with a sophisticated, relaxed, and intelligent patient I might add, "Diagnostic medicine originated in the 19th century from the autopsy table. So, most of the diseases we know about are diseases that are very bad and killed people. But there are many other diseases that don't kill people that we don't know about. Half of the patients I see are in the latter group."

2. I then state, "I am going to order a few laboratory tests and X rays, but there is a very good possibility that all of these tests will be negative. We can then be sure that you don't have a bad disease that requires surgery or strong medicines. However, if you have one of the mild diseases that doesn't kill people, we may not yet have a test for it, and all the tests may come back negative."

3. I then ask, "How do you think you will feel if all of your tests are negative?"

Patients' responses to this question are quite revealing and can usually be easily dichotomized. One group of patients will say, "I will be so relieved." Or, "I don't think there is anything wrong; I only came because my (significant other) wanted me to come in." Or, "I won't be surprised, I figured I was just getting old."

But another type of patient will say verbally and/or visually, "Well, I *know* there is something wrong; why can't you find out?" Or, "Do you have to find out the name of the disease?" Or, "Can't you just give me something?" Or, "How can you be sure it isn't my (organ or disease important to the patient)?"

Although this problem may seem to be beyond the bounds of a clinical diagnosis chrestomathy, it is important to know what you are going to say at the end of the workup, or else one's clinical examination of such patients can become desultory. Since these patients eventually will contract a disease, at least the one that finally kills them (no one lives forever), one wishes to continue practicing good diagnostic medicine with such patients.

Question: *What do you put on the insurance form?*

Answer: *I put down one of the acceptable nondiagnoses such as psychophysiologic nervous system reaction. I tell the patient that I am going to put such a diagnosis down. If the patient asks what disease they have, I say something like, "Mrs. Smith, you have Smith's disease; you are the only one who has it." This is not said flippantly, but in a manner that indicates that the patient does not fit into a pigeonhole and is recognized to be an individual. It can also be a useful statement to make for those patients in whom one is continuing the use of insight therapy.*

The Demanding Patient

Some patients pressure the physician with an insistent demand for rapid treatment or laboratory procedures. The physician who has grown in his diagnostic skill and has confidence in his method will usually communicate this to most patients who simply want relief. Other patients, who want to "master" the doctor-patient relationship will not be comforted by the competent physician's communication of security in his diagnostic method, but will attack it. The sequence of diagnostic maneuvers (history, physical examination, laboratory tests) should be explained patiently once. If the request for intervention becomes repetitive, the physician may choose to interpret it as a symptom: "Mr. Smith, you keep asking me for a prescription, but I haven't yet figured out what your diagnosis is. Don't you think I'll be able to find out what is wrong with you?"

The Patient Who Denies the Relevance of Psychologic Factors

Some patients, just like some physicians, are psychologically inept. These patients will deny psychologic factors or simply not see their relevance, even though they may be apparent to others (family members, physicians, nurses). Since the patient (or his organization) is paying for the physician's services, he is entitled to accept or reject any diagnosis made at any level, and such patient-rejected diagnoses (or connections between life events and illnesses) should not be chronically harped upon by the doctor in a contentious manner.

Further Reading

Other ways to handle the inherent difficulties in working with patients have been discussed elsewhere (Bird, 1973; Coulehan, 1987; Lipkin, 1987; Stevenson, 1971).

Appendix 2-1. Abbreviated Cognitive Examination

Orientation (8 points maximum)

1. Ask the patient for the date. Whatever scorable items are initially omitted should be specifically sought by prompting for the category but not the answer. Score 1 point for each correct answer: year, month, day, weekday.

2. Ask the patient for his location, as above. Score 1 point for each correct answer: state, county, town, hospital.

Memory and Calculation (16 points maximum)

3. (Registration). Name three objects (e.g., hat, orange, watch), taking about 1 second to say each. Have the patient repeat, giving one point for each correct. After recording the score, repeat until he learns all three.

4. Ask the patient to do serial sevens, starting with 103. Score the first five, 1 point for each correct answer.

5. (Recall). Ask the patients for the three objects learned in #3. One point for each correct.

6. Ask the patient to spell "earth" backward. (One point for each letter in correct position.)

Language (6 points maximum)

7. Point to two objects (e.g., a shoe and a pen) and have the patient name them. (One point for each correct.)

8. Ask the patient to repeat the sentence, "No ifs, ands, or buts." (One point if completely correct.)

9. Ask the patient to follow a three stage command: "Pick up this paper, fold it in half, and place it on the nightstand." (One point for each part done correctly.)

Interpretation

Normal persons should be able to get 20 or more out of the 30 possible points. Fewer than 20 points implies that the patient is significantly impaired, either cognitively, linguistically, and/or culturally.

Appendix 2-2. Reasons for Identifying the Patient with Organic Brain Syndrome

1) If you fail to make this diagnosis, you will waste time seeking historical details that the patient simply cannot recall; 2) If the syndrome is acute, prompt treatment may be necessary to reverse it; and 3) The syndrome is of high prevalence (from 10% to 40% of medical patients have it at some time during their hospital stay) and is one of the most underdiagnosed conditions in

medicine. If the primary doctor misses the diagnosis, it is unlikely to be discovered by an infraspecialist.

References

Bird B: *Talking with Patients*, ed 2. JB Lippincott, Philadelphia, 1973.

Blackwell B: The drug defaulter. *Clin Pharmacol Ther* 13:841–848, 1972.

Coulehan JL: *The Medical Interview: A Primer for Students of the Art.* Davis, Philadelphia, 1987.

Eichna LW: Medical-school education, 1975–1979. *N Engl J Med* 303:727–734, 1980.

Engel GL, Romano J: Delirium, a syndrome of cerebral insufficiency. *J Chronic Dis* 9:260–277, 1959.

Folstein MF, Folstein SE, McHugh PR: "Mini-Mental State": A practical method for grading the cognitive state of patients for the clinician. *J Psychiatr Res* 12:189–198, 1975.

Freud S. Analysis terminable and interminable. In: *Collected Papers,* vol 5, p 316 (Standard edition, vol 23), London, Hogarth Press, 1937.

Hayman M: The use of serial sevens in psychiatric examination. *Am J Orthopsychiatry* 11:341–355, 1941.

Hecht B: *A Child of the Century.* Donald I. Fine, New York, 1985.

Ireland P, Sapira JD, Templeton, B: Munchausen's syndrome. Review and report of an additional case. *Am J Med* 43:579–592, 1967.

Jacobs JW, Bernhard MR, Delgado A, Strain, JJ: Screening for organic mental syndromes in the medically ill. *Ann Intern Med.* 86:40–46, 1977.

Lipkin M Jr: The medical interview and related skills. In: Branch WT (ed), *Office Practice of Medicine*, ed 1. WB Saunders, Philadelphia, 1987.

MacKinnon RA, Michels R: *The Psychiatric Interview in Clinical Practice.* WB Saunders, Philadelphia, 1971.

Mushlin AI, Appel FA: Diagnosing potential noncompliance: Physicians' ability in a behavioral dimension of medical care. *Arch Intern Med* 137:318–321, 1977.

Nelson A, Fogel BS, Faust D: Bedside cognitive screening instruments: A critical assessment. *J Nerv Ment Dis* 174:73–83, 1986.

Sapira JD: Reassurance therapy: What to say to symptomatic patients with benign disease. *Ann Intern Med* 77:603–604, 1972.

Sapira JD: Munchausen's syndrome and the technologic imperative. *South Med J* 74:193–196, 1981.

Sapira JD, Cherubin CE: *Drug Abuse.* American Elsevier, New York, 1975.

Schnabel TG: Is medicine still an art? *N Engl J Med* 309:1258–1261, 1983.

Stevenson I: *The Diagnostic Interview*, ed 2. Harper & Row, New York, 1971.

3
The History

"To consider the sense of a question, consider what an answer to it would look like."
Ludwig Wittgenstein

Importance of the History

For decades, medical students beginning the course in clinical examination were told that 90% of all diagnoses are suggested or made by the history, 90% of the remainder (9% of the total) by the physical examination, and only 1% of the total by the laboratory tests. (The purpose of laboratory tests is to confirm diagnoses already hypothesized on the basis of the history and physical.)

A careful study of competent clinicians (Hampton et al., 1975) reveals that 82% of diagnoses are still made by the history, 9% by the physical examination, and 9% by the laboratory.

The importance of the history is best illustrated by a recent research project from the Mayo Clinic (Beart & O'Connell, 1983). One hundred sixty-eight patients with carcinoma of the colon were entered into a prospective study comparing the history, physical, and a variety of laboratory tests in detecting recurrent carcinoma. The patients were seen at least every 15 weeks. The most sensitive sign of recurrence turned out to be the history. Of the 48 patients who developed a recurrence, 85% had coughing, abdominal or pelvic pain, a change in bowel habit, rectal bleeding, or malaise, before signs of disease appeared on physical examination, radiologic examination, or serial determinations of the carcinoembryonic antigen level.

The fact remains that anyone can order laboratory tests; only a physician can make a diagnosis. The acquisition of the requisite clinical skills cannot be completed in a week, a month, a year, or probably much less than a decade. To achieve the results shown by the British and the Mayo Clinic studies, one must be quite skillful in eliciting and composing the history. The leading symptom must be described in as many dimensions as possible, and the story must be composed in a chronologically organized manner.

The Difference Between Facts and Information

Facts are true statements. Information consists of facts arranged in a useful manner.

A history is not simply a collection of facts. It must also contain information, although a good history even goes beyond that. Simply to write down or to recite a gaggle of true statements is not to compose a history. The facts must be placed in a form that makes them informative.

Many medical schools "teach" by having the students memorize a large number of facts. But these schools do not teach the students how to decide what a fact is, or how to collect facts in a useful and informative manner. This method is like teaching a neophyte cab driver to work in a new city by having him memorize all the names and addresses in the telephone book, instead of by showing him how to read a map.

Overview of History of Present Illness (HPI)

As an aid in composing the HPI, the student needs to have in mind a structure. Figure 3-1 is a handout used for over 15 years to help students initiate an adequate bedside presentation of the HPI.

Example: An Unacceptable Presentation

"John is an unemployed veteran who is back again for his hypertension. His doctor said that he needs a different medicine. He had something like this once before, but he isn't certain whether it was when he was a little boy or not."

Example: A Satisfactory Presentation

"Mr. Smith is a 42-year-old black man who enters our hospital for the second time with a chief complaint of a "nosebleed" of about 6 hours duration. The history of the present illness begins 5 years ago when a blood pressure of 180/120 was recorded by a plant physician at the time of a routine preemployment examination.

"He sought no medical advice for this and remained asymptomatic until 4 years ago when he noted the gradual onset of headaches, usually but not always pounding, occurring on the average twice a week. There were no aggravating or alleviating factors (other than aspirin), nor any associated symptoms, until 2 years ago, when the headaches became more severe and blurred vision supervened. For this latter reason, he visited our ER, and was admitted. At that time, he was also told for the first time that he had blood in his urine, although he himself recalls no change in its color . . . (etc.)."

Mr./Mrs./Miss _____ (name of patient) is a _____-year-old _____ (race, ethnic group, and/or occupation), who enters the hospital for the _____ th time with a chief complaint _____ (a symptom, not a sign or a diagnosis) of _____ (a number followed by a unit of time) duration. The history of the present illness begins _____ ago when the patient first noted the (gradual/sudden/other) onset of _____ .

Figure 3-1.   Form used by students to compose the history of the present illness.

Chief Complaint

The chief complaint is a statement in the patient's own words of the index symptom that you have selected from the interview material as being chief or principal. Because it is a direct (albeit edited) quotation, it is placed in quotation marks. It is followed by a statement of duration: a number followed by a unit of time (e.g., 1 hour, 2 days, 3 weeks, 4 months, 5 years, etc.). Placing the chief complaint in the patient's words is a device that prevents the inexperienced as well as the senile from placing their own diagnostic conclusions in the data base. For instance, a patient who had actually complained of "spitting up blood" was presented as a case of hematemesis. After a protracted and fruitless workup, a consultant quickly discovered the fact that the patient was actually suffering from hemoptysis (see p. 39).

The statement of time is a modifier that helps the reader, or listener, select which computer program his brain will run to solve the patient's problem (e.g., chronic diarrhea, acute shortness of breath, acute chest pain, etc.).

In psychiatry, the axiom is that the chief complaint "tells it all." Although at first one does not have enough information about the patient to understand the true, deep meaning of the stated chief complaint, it is a key datum to the psychiatrist.

For the attending.   In a recent study of four house officers presenting cases to senior clinicians at morning report (and unaware that they were being studied), no chief complaint was ever stated in 17%. In the remaining 83%, there was an average wait of 36 seconds (range: 5 seconds to 3 minutes 20 seconds) before the chief complaint was announced. This is simply too long a wait for "selecting a program," since unassimilable facts are meanwhile being presented with no framework upon which they could be arranged.

Dimensions of a Symptom

In order to analyze any symptom, including the leading symptom of the present illness, one must fully describe the symptom in all its dimensions. (If you have already learned the PQRST method of describing a symptom, or the "seven dimensions" listed in Morgan and Engel [1969], you may elect to skip this section and continue with the good habits already formed. If you have not already learned a set of dimensions, this one is offered. A list of the dimensions [whichever one you choose] is probably the only list in all of clinical examination worth memorizing. Everything else can be learned by repetition, and kept on an index card or a notebook in the interim.)

The dimensions I use are these:

1. Time
2. Quantity
3. Location
4. Aggravating factors
5. Alleviating factors
6. Quality
7. Setting
8. Associated symptoms
9. Inconstant dimensions (color, clarity, consistency, etc.)

Time

Time may actually be several dimensions, as we shall shortly see. At first glance, it might seem that the dimension of time has already been presented for the symptom of the chief complaint, because the duration is a statement in this dimension. And for some symptoms this is true (e.g., "cyanosis since birth" in cases of congenital heart disease with right-to-left shunting). But in other cases, the issue is much more complicated than a simple issue of duration.

For instance, consider this account of crescendo angina:

"At first that squeezing pain just lasted about 10 or 20 seconds. It started to go away as soon as I stopped walking up the hill; but later, around that Christmas, when that aching became more frequent I mean I started getting attacks almost every day by then, and just stopping didn't do anything for me. I had to get the nitro under my tongue, and then I had to wait for it to work, oh maybe 2, 3 minutes, but I was still doing okay, going to work every day. Well, Sunday morning when we were getting ready for the birthday party, I noticed all of a sudden . . .

Here the patient is describing the duration of the individual attack, the duration of the relief of symptoms, and the frequency of the attacks, all of which are expressed in units of time and each of which must also be described in the record within the chronologic dimension. If one had only the duration of the symptom, one could not make the diagnosis of crescendo angina.

With further questioning, one could add still another time measure: how long the patient could walk up that hill before the "squeezing-aching" would appear.

It will become obvious that there are many other important symptoms existing in time that we have not discussed here. To give one additional example, students are taught to ask whether there is an "aura" or warning in evaluating the complaint of syncope. But even more useful is the time dimension of the aura, since patients with vasovagal syncope tend to have a long aura (about 2.5 minutes), while those with cardiac syncope usually have a very brief aura (less than 3 seconds) rather than none at all (Martin et al., 1983).

When the onset of the illness is vague or the description seems somewhat sparse, a useful question to ask the patient is this: "When is the last time you can remember feeling perfectly healthy?" Use exactly those words.

The purpose of this question is to get the patient talking. It is not intended to determine when the history of the present illness began, although sometimes it will do that. The idea is to increase the number of historical facts at your disposal. After you get all the facts, you will be able to determine the beginning of the present illness. In addition to sharpening up the early history of the present illness by giving the patient a chance to reflect and recall, this question often stimulates patients to talk about other symptoms that they had momentarily pushed out of consciousness, or that the listener had not attended to at first.

It is important to understand that this question is not the same as, "When did you first get sick?" or even, "When is the last time you did not have (the given symptom)?" Those are not really open-ended questions. The question as stated in the first paragraph is open-ended, providing that you listen to the answer without interrupting.

Quantity

Some examples of quantity are these: "three tablespoons of sputum each morning," "two-pillow orthopnea," "about one half cup of bloody emesis," or "claudication that had formerly appeared after four or five level blocks, now occurring regularly at one block."

Some symptoms, such as pain, have no international units but can still be expressed on an analogue scale from 0 to 10, where 0 is the absence of the symptom and 10 is an extreme, such as "so bad you would have killed yourself."

Other symptoms cannot be described in cardinal numbers, but still require a salient, concrete description. Adjectives (such as "terrible") are much less useful than the answer to the question: "What could you do in the past, that you cannot do now, because of (this symptom)?" The patient might respond that he can no longer walk across the room to the toilet because of shortness of breath.

Location

Although location might well have been covered in the chief complaint, if the chief complaint is the leading symptom of the present illness, the use of the patient's own words might preclude a precise description at that point. The pain in the "tummy" might be in the epigastrium, hypochondrium, periumbilical area, suprapubic area, or even the colon and rectum. A misinterpretation of the term "tummy" by the physician will, at best, delay the diagnosis. Similarly, the "hip" can be the buttock, the rectum, the actual hip joint, the iliac crest, the skin on the lateral surface of the buttock, or nodes in the inguinal or femoral areas. Sometimes it is the doctor who is imprecise; he might change the patient's "thigh," "knee," "calf," "ankle," or "instep" into the "left lower extremity," homogenizing, instead of refining these terms.

Some symptoms, such as weakness, do not always have a location. This is also important to establish and to note in the record. The differential diagnosis of weakness in the right hand is completely different from that of generalized weakness that is not focal.

For certain symptoms, particularly pain, the dimension of location also includes radiation, which is where the symptoms move. Symptoms related to the skin may also have radiation, whereas some symptoms, such as dyspnea, characteristically do not change location.

Aggravating and Alleviating Factors

The patient should be asked about aggravating factors in an open-ended manner: "What kinds of things might make it worse?" Although aggravating factors are usually analyzed in conjunction with alleviating factors, a separate question should be used for the latter. If you ask the patient, "What kinds of things make this better or worse?" most patients will answer only the second part of the question, and will never return to the alleviating factors. The physician who asks this question may then remember "no data" as the alleviating factor. (This, of course, is one form of the dreaded double question, see pp. 15–16. If you audit your tape recordings carefully, you will be amazed by how often you use double questions. Eschewing them is a learned skill.)

To illustrate the utility of the aggravating and alleviating factors, consider two patients with left-sided anterior chest pain. One patient's pain is induced by exercise and strong emotions, but consistently relieved by rest and sublingual nitroglycerin; this is characteristic of angina pectoris. The other patient's pain is aggravated by sneezing, coughing, and respiration, but alleviated by shallow breathing and splinting of the left side of the chest; this patient has pleurisy. Although the patient may not always have such a classic history, the physician will never learn of these diagnostic clues, even when readily available, if he does not ask the proper questions.

Aggravating and alleviating factors are very useful in evaluating back pain. If back pain is made worse by holding or carrying a weight in the arms, one should think of disease of the vertebral column or the paraspinal muscles and other such soft tissues, rather than of the intraperitoneal or retroperitoneal organs. The weight may seem trivial, such as a book or an empty briefcase, or it may be considerable, such as bags of groceries. The diagnosis may be a relatively benign "low back strain" or a significant disease of the vertebral bodies or disk space.

Quality

The quality of the symptom is most important for the very symptoms that at first glance seem to be least susceptible to a qualitative description. For instance, Samuel Levine used to tell his students that if the patient's chest pain was glibly and clearly communicated, it was probably not myocardial in origin. The difficulty that the patient experienced in describing the pain was in itself a diagnostic clue.

When a patient complains of "spells," "falling out," "risings" (or "kernels"), weakness, back pain, or fatigue, a good opening question is, "Could you tell me more about what that was like?"

Not all the information obtained in response to that question will necessarily be in the dimension of quality. In fact, some patients will proceed to describe almost everything else except the quality: where he was when the symptom occurred, the time of day, statements of other persons, opinions of other physicians, and accounts of the symptoms of other family members. Ask such patients, "Could you tell me more about what it felt like to you?" If the patient truly seems to display alexithymia (the inability to describe mood and feelings) try, "What might I have had that would feel most like what you are describing?"

Setting

Determination of the setting in which a symptom began is useful in direct proportion to the breadth of the interviewer's view of the word "setting." A narrow interviewer may only inquire, and episodically at that, as to the patient's position (as in syncope), or time of day (as for ulcer pain), or recent ingestion of alcoholic beverages (for determining the etiology of pancreatitis), and so forth. This restricted view leads to a number of problems.

Narrow inquiries into "setting" are not open-ended information-gathering devices, but branch-point signs at best, or more usually, a means of confirming diagnoses already suggested to the interviewer. The answers to "setting" questions generated in this fashion cannot be used for research purposes because they are not asked of all patients. They cannot be used for learning purposes for a related reason (i.e., their unknown specificity). They are not useful in patient care, because they are post facto to diagnoses considered for some other reason, or are simply window dressing, as in the following example.

•

One morning, I was presented a 28-year-old black man who had been admitted with crushing chest pain, precordial Q waves, huge ST segment elevations, T wave inversions, and increased levels of the cardiac enzymes. The diagnosis of myocardial infarction was evident to everyone.

Most of the history of the present illness was a recitation of the following facts:

1. The patient was not sedentary, being a basketball player.
2. He was not overweight.
3. He had never smoked.
4. He did not have diabetes mellitus; his blood sugar was normal on a recent preemployment physical.
5. The cholesterol and triglyceride levels were known to be normal.
6. There was no family history of heart disease.
7. He was not hypertensive.

When I inquired why I was being given this information, I was told that the patient had been diagnosed (correctly) as suffering from a myocardial infarction, and that these were the risk factors for atherosclerotic coronary artery disease. Although the patient did not have any of these risk factors, the cardiology consultant had nonetheless suggested atherosclerosis as the etiology of the disease. Because of the narrowness of focus in contemporary medicine (engendered, in part, by such post facto lists), unusual diagnoses, such as coronary artery arteritis, a coronary embolus, or a congenital anomaly of the coronary circulation, were not considered. Once the patient was labeled as having atherosclerosis, despite the absence of risk factors, all investigations were stopped cold. (Actually, the team had not checked for the risk factor of "type A" personality, which an abundance of evidence has implicated in the pathogenesis of coronary artery disease [Friedman et al., 1984; Nunes et al., 1987; Rosenman et al., 1975], or for anger and hostility, the "type A" features with the strongest correlation to this disease [Williams, 1986].)

•

Open-ended setting questions will often provide important clues to a correct diagnosis that will be missed by the Procrusteans (i.e., those who insist that the patient's story must fit their preconceived notions, just as travelers had to fit the mythical innkeeper's bed.) The patient might start talking about something he had not told anyone before, for example, recent recurring spells of despondency, leading to further questions and possibly to a diagnosis of anxiety or depression on a positive basis, rather than the always treacherous exclusionary one. Also, open-ended questions help the interviewer understand the patient as a person.

Another error of the Procrusteans is to insist that the setting must be the one expected on a post facto basis, regardless of what the patient says. If the patient has told you that his symptoms do not occur in a setting of strong emotional arousal, you should not insist that they do. I have seen this error made in more than one patient suffering with (undiagnosed) acute intermittent porphyria, whose symptoms had been attributed to "nerves" by several physicians.

A broad interpretation of setting may lead to the discovery of new diseases, as in the story of Soma Weiss's streetcar conductor (see Ch. 18, p. 340). An interest in the setting is also important to the mental hygiene of the physician. If you do not have this basic curiosity about your patients and their illnesses, you will soon be practicing apple-sorter medicine. After a few years of seeing the apples only in the single dimension of size, and ignoring their colors, tastes, smells, bumps, bruises, and curious travels, your medical practice will become one-dimensional, causing boredom and burnout in your life's work.

Finally, a broad understanding of the onset-setting may be useful in management as well as diagnosis. The physician should be particularly sensitive to absences and partings. If the onset of the illness was in the setting of the loss of a significant other, then a similar loss of the physician (who may be quite significant to the patient) may be expected to produce perturbations both in the patient and in the doctor-patient relationship. Loss can be permanent (death or abandonment), temporary (vacation or illness on the part of the physician), or anticipated (either based in reality or the fantasy of the patient).

For the junior student.   If you do attempt to elicit the history in the manner described here, you may find yourself in conflict with some of the medical residents with whom you must work. They will want you to "get in and get out" and "just get the facts" as they perceive them. While their approach may yield certain short-term benefits, it will deprive you of the opportunity to learn certain enduring skills, which are not easily acquired later. You must decide whether you want to learn a difficult but valuable technique from the patients assigned to you, or whether you would prefer to be a donut-and-cup bearer to the tin gods of the buffed chart.

For the attending.   The patient's culture and language are extremely important parts of the setting, both for the interviewing process and the composition of the history. Unfortunately, this is very difficult to teach to the beginning student who is going through an acculturation process himself. By the time the young physician can appreciate these issues fully, he no longer needs to be reminded of them by the written word. The only effective method of instruction is at the bedside with a live patient.

Associated Symptoms

Associated symptoms are those that appear in some regular relationship to the symptom under analysis. This dimension often increases the diagnostic significance of the symptom several fold. For instance, while polydipsia, polyphagia, and polyuria are each individually nonspecific, when combined they are so characteristic of new-onset diabetes mellitus as to be considered a diagnostic triad. Weight loss, fatigue, and anorexia might suggest an occult neoplasm, but weight loss, fatigue, and perspiration could be symptoms of hyperthyroidism or tuberculosis. If paroxysms of perspiration and headaches were accompanied by palpitations, one would think of pheochromocytoma, but if they were temporally associated with bed-shaking chills, one would suspect an infectious process. The associated symptoms of dolor pectoris (chest pain) and angor animi (impending doom, vide infra) from myocardial infarction are an example of concurrent symptoms that may occur only once. Associated symptoms of a chronic complaint may not always be exactly concurrent; but they should be more or less consistent.

In infection, bed shaking occurs during the "chill" part of the temperature curve. Unfortunately, some patients may not notice the phases of their febrile illness, and may report bed-shaking chills concurrent with or even preceding the fever. The association of symptoms is useful, even if the sequence is imprecisely remembered.

Associated symptoms do not lend themselves to easy listing like some of the other dimensions. Inquiring about them requires some knowledge of medicine. Otherwise, who would think to ask about itching when trying to evaluate jaundice? Yet this symptom can help to distinguish hepatic obstruction (in which itching due to bile salt retention can occur before the individual becomes overtly jaundiced) from hemolytic jaundice. Factors that facilitate the appearance of bile salt pruritis are hot baths and aging, dry skin. Again, who would think to ask about hot baths if he had not seen or read much medicine?

Inconstant Dimensions

Inconstant dimensions are those that do not apply to all symptoms but that are nevertheless very important for some, such as color, clarity, consistency, and so forth.

Color Card

Color must be described for urine, sputum, feces, skin lesions, and the skin overlying an arthralgia. Sometimes it is of great importance to know the exact color. To be sure that you and the patient are thinking of the same colors, prepare a color card consisting of patches of various colors, particularly blood red, currant jelly purple, robin's egg blue, tar black, very dark brown (almost but not quite black), cola brown, medium brown (umber or sienna), light brown, clay white, biliverdin green, bilirubin orange, lemon yellow, and several shades of gray. These can be mixed from oil paints or composed of paint store sample chips. More simply, cut the appropriate colors from magazine illustrations, paste them on a card, and for permanence laminate in plastic.

Clarity, Consistency, and So Forth

Body fluids may be clear, opalescent, translucent, opaque, transparent, turbid, like "gold paint," and so forth. Each of these adjectives might be of diagnostic value when applied to a pleural effusion, if one is so fortunate as to have a patient who remembered what his pleural fluid looked like the last time it was tapped.

A description of the consistency of materials may be very helpful. For example, the term *diarrhea* may mean many different things, referring either to the frequency or to the volume of bowel movements. However, a statement of consistency (i.e., whether the stool would assume the shape of its container) is clearly understandable.

Similarly, pain, which does not have the properties of color or consistency, may have the property of being "colicky," especially when it is abdominal (see p. 39).

Although precise descriptions are important, one must also avoid becoming dogmatic about the meaning of certain findings.

An example. Pseudomonas was formerly known as *Bacillus pyocyaneus. Pyocyaneus* means bluish pus, although sometimes the pus from *Pseudomonas* infections is actually green from the fluorescein produced by the organism. However, the idea that green pus is diagnostic for *Pseudomonas* is not correct. Any pus can be green if it contains sufficient white cells and their verdoperoxidase, a copper-containing myeloperoxidase.

Abbreviated History in Trauma Patients

In trauma patients, especially those with suspected head injury, an expedited history (and complete if rapid physical examination) must be obtained because the patient might lose consciousness after an initial lucid interval. In the context of an emergency in which surgery may be necessary, obtain at least the "AMPLE" history recommended by the Advanced Trauma Life Support Course of the American College of Surgeons: allergies, medications, past illnesses, last meal, and events preceding the injury.

Elaboration of Selected Symptoms

The symptoms discussed in this section might occur either in the review of systems or in the history of the present illness. The treatment is not encyclopedic, but rather illustrative of how useful the history can be, and how detailed the history may *need* to be in order to arrive at a diagnosis. The actual inventory discussed here is quite small compared with the entire inventory of questions available to the clinician; it is even small compared with the short inventory of questions given in Chapter 4.

Angina and Other Chest Discomfort Syndromes

If you want to experience severe anginal pain yourself, place a blood pressure cuff on your upper arm, pump it up to 300 mm Hg, and occlude the tubing with a towel clip so there is no slippage. After 5 minutes, work your fist. The feeling in your forearm is the same as the feeling in your chest in severe angina.

Angina is a peculiar disorder in that its timing in some patients is absolutely predictable, coming on at certain times of day, or with taking a certain number of steps (Swartout, 1987).

Angina pectoris may be associated with *angor animi*, which literally means anguish of the soul. Since modern man has shed his soul, we now call this a sense of impending doom, which may often accompany myocardial infarction, dissecting aneurysm, or massive pulmonary embolism. The visceral sensation that accompanies the catecholamine discharge can be confused with nausea.

•

An illustrative case. A patient with retrosternal pain and what was reported as nausea was sent to the gastroenterology unit for evaluation.

Patient: ". . . and with the pain I had this feeling in my stomach . . ."

Attending: "Nausea?" (the word the resident had used)

Patient: "Yeah, I guess it was nausea. You could call it that. The pain was terrible."

Attending: "Did you want to throw up, vomit, with the pain and nausea?

Patient: "No, not at all. I just wanted to be still."

Attending: "You had nausea but you didn't want to throw up."

Patient: "No. If I was sick like that I would ordinarily want to vomit to feel better, but this wasn't the same thing."

Attending: (Motions "tell me more" with his hand.)

Patient: ". . . This was a bad feeling all over and also in the pit of my stomach. When that pain came on and stayed and would not go away, I got this feeling that the end of the world was coming . . . I didn't think I was going to make it . . ."

Attending: "And the nausea? The feeling? . . . Was it really nausea? . . ."

Patient: "No, it was a bad feeling, it was worse than what I call nausea. It was this clutching feeling you get when you are very excited. Like in sports, when you are in sporting events, and you are about to go out there, . . . go on the playing field, . . . you get before a football game. I used to play football. Well that was the feeling I got in my stomach when this pain came on. I thought, my God, this is it. I was terrified. I thought maybe if I did nothing it would go away. I thought this is it, and that is when I got the stomach, the nausea feeling you [*sic*] call it. But I didn't want to vomit, I didn't want to do nothing, I just wanted to live. That was the worst part of the pain, knowing that there was something about that pain that could . . . you know, it could do you in."

•

This patient was subsequently found to have had a myocardial infarction and was transferred from the gastroenterology unit to the coronary care unit.

In a description of angina pectoris and other chest pains based on personal experience (Swartout, 1987), it is noted that the substernal pressure caused by severe asthma and the pain of acute cholecystitis, which may be just as severe as angina, are not associated with angor animi.

The pain of pericarditis is boring and continuous, but it is also positional.

Arrhythmias

The diagnosis of arrhythmias from the history requires a knowledge of the physiology (see Ch. 6, p. 94).

Sternbach Pain Thermometer

In situations involving chronic pain, it is often helpful for the interviewer to have an understanding both of the quantitative aspect of the patient's pain as well as the patient's reporting of the pain. Sternbach has developed just such a technique, which he calls the "pain thermometer" (Sternbach, 1974).

A Method

The patient is first asked to quantitate the intensity (not the character) of his pain, on a scale from 0 to 10, wherein 0 is absolutely no pain and 10 is a pain so terrible that it would cause one to commit suicide.

A blood pressure cuff is then placed in the usual position and inflated to far above the systolic so as to produce ischemic pain. At the same time, a stopwatch is started. The patient is instructed to report the time at which the ischemic pain is of the same intensity as the pain reported in the history.

When the patient reports this experience, record the number of elapsed seconds, but do not deflate the cuff. This will be the numerator. The end point or denominator of the pain thermometer ratio is reached when the patient either rips off the cuff or demands that it be removed.

Interpretation

For a hypothetical situation in which a patient reported his naturally occurring pain to be a 5 on a scale from 0 to 10, there are three possible results with the pain tourniquet test.

1. The patient hypothetically experienced the same intensity of pain after 50 seconds of tourniquet pressure and ripped off the cuff at 100 seconds, yielding a fraction exactly equal to that predicted from his subjective estimation of 5 out of 10. We would say that this patient is an excellent "reporter" of pain. That is, he is precise and accurate.

2. Overreporting would be suggested if the tourniquet test yielded, say, a fraction of 20 seconds over 200 seconds. This result would have been the equivalent of a 1 out of 10 on the patient's subjective rating scale. This would suggest that the patient is sensitive to naturally occurring pain, and tends to overrate or overreport it, or that the patient could have a superior tolerance for experimental pain superior even to his own estimation!

3. The patient might report the tourniquet pain to equal the naturally occurring pain at 90 seconds, and rip the tourniquet off at 100 seconds, yielding a ratio of 0.9, rather than the expected 0.5. This patient could either be underreporting the naturally occurring pain, or demonstrating a low tolerance for the experimental pain.

Note that the pain thermometer, in itself, tells you nothing about the etiology of the pain, although occasionally it may be helpful in suggesting a more aggressive diagnostic effort. A malingerer might be expected to have widely varying tourniquet ratio scores from trial to trial, or response 2, described above. One woman with a subjective rating of 5 out of 10 was thought to be a malingerer, especially after a completely negative radiologic evaluation of her epigastric pain. She still had not reported even the numerator for the pain thermometer after 9 minutes of ischemia. This was so startling that she was subjected to endoscopy, revealing a large gastric ulcer that had been missed by the contrast studies.

Chills and Night Sweats

Patients who report chills should be asked whether the bed actually shook or moved on the floor. A true shaking chill also tends to last a definite period of time, on the order of $1/2$ hour. Shaking chills, as opposed to a sensation of chilliness, have diagnostic implications, and are always high on the list of findings that must be explained by the primary diagnosis. They also imply that the fever was high, even though the patient may not have measured it.

Night sweats should be described in quantitative, practical terms. For example, "Were the sweats so bad that you had to change your pajamas?" Or, "Did you have to change the pillowcase to get back to sleep?" Or, "Did your wife change the sheets?" Note that patients who sleep in warm weather in nonair-conditioned rooms do not soak the sheets as highly febrile patients do. They simply cast the sheets off and roll away from any dampness; and, of course, they are never awakened by a chill.

The old teaching that viral diseases did not cause bed-shaking chills is probably incorrect; patients with dengue fever, for instance, shake the bed.

Itching

Itching is usually a manifestation of cutaneous disease, but may also result from a systemic condition (Bernhard, 1987). A drug history is most important. Phenothiazines, tolbutamide, erythromycin, anabolic hormones, estrogen, progesterone, and testosterone may cause itching by inducing cholestasis; narcotics through histamine release; and aspirin through prostaglandin effects. Any drug may cause pruritis through an idiosyncratic effect, even if the patient has been taking it for years.

Inquire about exposures to fiberglass, dusts, and chemicals. In addition, veterinary examination may identify exposure to ectoparasites from pets in many patients with unexplained pruritis.

Itching severe enough to waken the patient at night should arouse suspicion of scabies or dermatitis herpetiformis. If these conditions are ruled out in a patient with severe itching, consider a systemic cause.

Systemic diseases associated with itching include renal failure (due to secondary hyperparathyroidism); endocrine conditions (thyroid dysfunction, diabetes mellitus, and carcinoid syndrome); and hepatobiliary disease, especially with biliary obstruction (as in primary biliary cirrhosis or carcinoma causing extrahepatic obstruction—note that itching due to the retention of bile salts may precede the appearance of jaundice). Itching produced by bathing (aquagenic pruritis) may be a symptom of polycythemia vera. Nearly 30% of patients with Hodgkin's disease have severe burning pruritis (Bernhard, 1987). Other malignant causes include visceral cancers, mycosis fungoides, multiple myeloma, and central nervous system tumors.

Hemoptysis Versus Hematemesis

The first term literally means "to spit up blood," and the second term means "to vomit up blood." As actually used, hemoptysis refers to the experience of coughing up blood and by extension refers to any blood produced through the mouth but originating in the pulmonary system.

The four main causes of hemoptysis used to be bronchogenic carcinoma, bronchiectasis, rheumatic mitral valve disease (especially mitral stenosis), and tuberculosis. While this remains a useful mnemonic for the previously asymptomatic patient who presents with a sudden hemoptysis, it is probably less accurate today. The prevalence of bronchiectasis, tuberculosis, and rheumatic heart disease has decreased substantially. In the areas of the world where tuberculosis is still a problem, more specific etiologies of hemoptysis need to be considered, including Rasmussen's aneurysm or secondary aspergillosis. (Taking one item out of a differential diagnosis, and performing a more sophisticated differential of that condition, as was just done, is called "going up to the next level of complexity.")

Of course, hematemesis is caused by an entirely different set of diagnostic possibilities. It usually implies a source of blood proximal to the ligament of Treitz and therefore includes gastric ulcer, gastric carcinoma, Osler-Weber-Rendu syndrome, esophageal varices, and so forth. Conceivably, it could be caused by

epistaxis, assuming the patient swallowed the blood and vomited it later.

The physician is responsible for making the distinction if the patient reports, "I spit up blood." A good rule of thumb is to require that the patient actually have gagged and regurgitated the bolus of blood in order to qualify it as hematemesis. On the other hand, patients with hemoptysis usually can recall a clear episode of coughing. Often, they can point to the side of the thorax from which the blood came. Unfortunately, even excellent interviewers may not be able to make the distinction 100% of the time. However, one becomes more skilled by interviewing many patients with this complaint prior to knowing the anatomically determined source of the bleeding.

Abdominal Pain

The differential diagnosis of abdominal pain in various locations is discussed in Chapter 20 (p. 375).

Is the Pain Colicky?

To determine whether an abdominal pain is colicky, I prefer to get a description of temporal waves of pain, whose peak comes and goes with some regularity, like labor pains. Do not use the nonspecific descriptor "crampy." To some patients, especially men, a cramp is a continuous muscle pain that does not have waves of intensity.

Colicky pain originates from a hollow viscus.   If the pain is colicky, one knows that it is not coming from the liver, spleen, or kidney, but could come from the bowel or the ureters. (Ureteral pain is easy to recognize because of its location in the flank. The distal ureters refer pain to the testicles.) However, a steady pain could also come from a hollow viscus, such as the gallbladder. Pain caused by pancreatitis (an inflammation of a solid organ) might be colicky because of associated small bowel ileus, or a stone in the pancreatic ducts (although the latter, like a common bile duct obstruction, could also be steady).

If the pain is colicky, one should try to determine its periodicity. Women patients who have experienced childbirth are particularly good informants. The periodicity of the colic in pain from the upper ileum is stated to be 3 to 5 minutes, as opposed to 6 to 10 minutes for the lower ileum (see Cope's classic work [Silen, 1979], reviewed in Ch. 29, p. 557).

This contention seems contrary to current gastrointestinal physiology, which leads one to expect pacemakers lower in the gut to have shorter periods. Cope (Silen, 1979) does not offer any data, but cites a reference that states:

There is support for the thesis that the waves of propulsive activity in the intestine come with somewhat greater frequency high in the ileum than lower down. In practice, an obstruction high in the ileum appears to be characterized oftener by a period of three to five minutes between peaks of crampy pain, and obstruction in the terminal ileum by intervals between the pains that are as much as twice as long. (Dennis, 1954)

Sometimes the periodicity of abdominal pain exists in a much longer time framework than we are used to thinking about when we describe the periodicity of colic. Abdominal pain due to allergic eosinophilic gastrointestinal disease has a periodicity of days; pain due to lead poisoning, a periodicity of days to weeks; pain due to porphyria, a periodicity of weeks; and pain due to familial Mediterranean fever, a periodicity of weeks to months.

Epigastric Pain

If the patient is over 50 years of age, with his first attack of epigastric pain, and is also experiencing weight loss not clearly related to significant vomiting, one should suspect gastric carcinoma.

On the other hand, peptic ulcer, especially of the duodenum, is more likely to be associated with night pain, relief from food or antacids, a family history of ulcer disease, and a gesture of pointing to the epigastrium. Peptic ulcer is confusing because it may be associated with irregular bowels, even diarrhea. Because the diarrhea is due to the cathartic action of blood, the stools will often be described as black, shiny and sticky, like tar (vide infra, p. 41).

Irritable Bowel Syndrome

Patients with the irritable bowel syndrome will sometimes have upper abdominal pain, but it will not have the characteristics described in the preceding paragraph. The diarrhea will be normal in color and not sticky. It tends to be loose and frequent, to contain mucus, and to be associated with a sense of incomplete evacuation. The abdominal pain may be relieved by the act of defecation, or even by passing gas. Recently, formal criteria for the irritable bowel syndrome have been proposed (Chaudhary & Truelove, 1962; Manning et al., 1978). However, many normal persons met the criteria although they had never sought medical help. Thus, it seems that part of the syndrome is help-seeking behavior. Until better criteria are available, the following types of questions should be asked of the patient suspected of having the irritable bowel syndrome:

1. Do you have more than three bowel movements a day? Or less than three bowel movements a week? (Empirically, these represent the normal ranges.)
2. Do your stools get loose when the pain begins?
3. Do you have more frequent bowel movements when the pain starts?
4. Is your pain often eased after you have had a bowel movement?
5. Do you have visible distention of your abdomen?
6. What seems to be going on in your life at times when you're having more pain or more frequent bowel movements?

Abdominal Pain Associated with Syncope

The painful abdominal conditions most likely to cause fainting are perforation of a peptic ulcer, acute pancreatitis, ruptured aortic aneurysm, and ruptured ectopic pregnancy ("Cope," Silen, 1979).

Pain Associated with Vomiting

When the leading symptoms are vomiting and pain, one should determine which came first. If the pain preceded the vomiting, one should think of diseases below the ligament of Treitz. An exception is a perforated gastric or duodenal ulcer, in which the pain and vomiting may occur close together; Cope points out that the vomiting in perforated ulcer is actually due to acid stimulation of the peritoneal surface. Viral gastroenteritis rarely causes this sequence of pain followed by vomiting, but may cause vomiting followed by pain.

Migratory Pains

The Durga Syndrome

Durga is the Hindu goddess sometimes depicted with six or eight arms. Some patients whose pain travels in anatomically unlikely pathways may remind the student of the goddess Durga, in that more than two arms seem to be required to point out the various routes of the pain.

There are actually two such syndromes. In the first, the pain actually moves along the path described. But in the second, the pain just appears first at one place (say, the right knee), and then in a second (possibly the left elbow), without actually being experienced along the pathway that the patient infers. (Since the pain is qualitatively the same in both locations, the patient tends to assume that it must be the same pain, traveling along the shortest distance between the two points. We use the same concept in referring to the migratory polyarthritis of rheumatic fever. The arthritis does not truly migrate across intervening tissues from one joint to another.)

One can distinguish between the two forms of the Durga syndrome by asking the patient to describe the migratory pain at a midpoint along its itinerary. Patients with the second type of Durga syndrome will become puzzled, and say that they do not actually feel the pain at this or that way station, possibly infuriating the interviewer who is not familiar with this phenomenon. In this situation, one does the differential diagnosis for pain in the right knee and left elbow, not pain moving from the right knee up the front of the right thigh, across the abdomen, ...

The Pseudo-Durga Syndrome: Radiating Pain

There are certain diseases in which the pain truly does move along a seemingly bizarre path, or may seem to jump from one point to another.

We have already alluded to the pain of ureteral colic, which can begin in the patient's "back" (the costovertebral angle), move around to the flank (which may be called anything from "my hip" to "my belly"), and then down into the testicles ("my privates"). Sometimes the pain ends in the groin ("in between my legs") or the medial part of the thigh (variously identified as the hip, or the "leg," which means the calf to some doctors). Without taking the time to be sure of the precise topologic path, a doctor trying to identify the pain syndrome from the words used above could easily become confused.

Gallbladder pain on occasion can begin in the right upper quadrant, but instead of radiating straight through to the back, it may migrate to the right side of the abdomen, then to the left upper quadrant, then back to the right upper quadrant. The patient might draw a circle on his ventral surface as he describes the pain. Because he looks calm, not having the pain at the moment that he is being examined, some physicians become quite frustrated by his story.

Upper quadrant pain can irritate the diaphragm and be referred to the neck or shoulder. This pattern of migration can also be a snare to the unwary.

Weight Loss

A statement about the appetite should always be included in the history of weight loss. In most cases, weight loss is accompanied by anorexia, as in depression and most cases of carcinoma, tuberculosis, and so forth.

However, if the weight loss is due to metabolic causes (such as hyperthyroidism, diabetes mellitus, or pheochromocytoma) or in some cases of collagen vascular disease, there may be no anorexia at all, and some patients with anorexia nervosa may actually have bulimia. (They eat voraciously, but then induce vomiting.) Patients with malabsorption may also exhibit considerable weight loss with no decrease in appetite, or even with an increase in caloric intake. Thus, weight loss without anorexia requires an additional statement about the presence or absence of diarrhea. Another cause of weight loss without anorexia (or even with voracious eating) can be Parkinson's disease, especially of the postencephalitic variety. This finding was first noted by Parkinson himself (Sacks, 1973).

A caveat.   Be careful to question the patient about appetite at the *beginning* of the illness. Many patients who originally had no anorexia will lose their taste for food in the course of becoming malnourished. This might be caused by a supervening zinc deficiency.

The Belt Sign

The belt sign is very useful in situations in which the patient's weight is thought to be changing. Examine the patient's belt. New holes punched, or a change in the hole that is used, may indicate decreasing or increasing girth. As a rule, the grooves near the most recently used holes tend to be sharper. The duration of use of any given hole can be estimated by the surface abrasion and width of its groove.

This principle can be extended in a number of ways. For instance, with goiter, collar size may change. In acromegaly, the glove, hat, and shoe size may change. The diagnosis of Cushing's syndrome, acromegaly, hypothyroidism, and a number of other entities may be easily made by inspecting photographs of patients taken over a period of years in their family albums.

These methods lie in the borderland between the history and the physical examination.

Vomiting

The time of onset of the vomiting and associated symptoms is very important in the differential diagnosis. Dr. Lee Hershenson of Pittsburgh used to visualize the entire gut as a tube with a craniocaudal gradient. Diseases that interrupted the gradient at the rear could cause some diarrhea, eventually constipation, and finally nausea and vomiting.

Diseases affecting the upper end of the gradient would cause nausea and vomiting early in the course of the disease. They would not cause early constipation (defined as the retention of feces), though a decreased amount of feces might eventually result from poor intake. Early diarrhea would not ordinarily be expected and so would suggest the cathartic action of blood or the large volume of acid secreted in the Zollinger Ellison syndrome.

The appearance of the vomitus should be carefully described. In order be considered "coffee-grounds emesis," the vomitus must meet three criteria: a dark brown color, a texture that resembles coffee grounds (due to blood poured into acid), and a shiny appearance (like the outside of a roasted coffee bean), due to the lipids in the red cell membrane. This permits the confident diagnosis of bleeding proximal to the ligament of Treitz.

•

One morning a resident announced at morning report that a patient had been admitted with a history of coffee-grounds bowel movements. This was an unprecedented occurrence. Outdated banked blood instilled through a nasogastric tube into the stomachs of healthy volunteers caused brown stools or black and tarry stools, or even (if the infusion rate was very fast) bright red blood in the stools, but no coffee-grounds stools. One suggestion was that a direct passage, a gastrocolic fistula, might permit coffee grounds to get from the stomach to the stool without the usual transformations along the way. But it was pointed out that the direction of flow in a gastrocolic fistula was from the colon to the stomach, not vice versa. Later, it developed that the patient's wife and the resident had both believed that "coffee grounds" simply meant brown. This illustrates the importance of a precise history.

•

Melena

The vomiting of blood of any kind is bad; its passage as excrement is not a good sign, nor is the passage of black stools.

Hippocrates, *Aphorisms* 4:25

Melena is derived from the Greek word meaning black. A black stool can result from blood originating below the ligament of Treitz (although more commonly the blood from such a location is maroon) if the blood has resided in the colon with fecal bacteria for a sufficient time. Thus, the expectation that melena means upper gastrointestinal blood loss is a statistical likelihood but not a completely reliable logical branch point. A black stool may also suggest the patient's use of charcoal, bismuth, black cherries, blueberries, or even licorice ice cream.

Two further descriptors signal that the blood did originate above the ligament of Treitz: the sticky consistency of *tar* and a glistening quality like tar or roofing pitch. These characteristics have not been reported in stools following a bleed into the colon.

Only 50 to 80 cc of blood are required to produce a tarry stool (Daniel & Egan, 1939). With larger amounts of blood (1,000 to 2,000 cc administered through a nasogastric tube), the tarry character may persist as long as 5 to 8 days (Schiff et al., 1942), especially if the patient receives an agent such as atropine or codeine that slows intestinal motility.

Other Characteristics of the Stool

Pencil Stools

It was formerly taught that stools the diameter of a pencil indicated the presence of rectal carcinoma. In fact, most patients who have an episode of such stools have proctitis or other irritation of the distal sigmoid and rectum. While the irritation might be due to a rectal carcinoma on some occasions, it most often is not.

Stool in Malabsorption

The stools in malabsorption are characteristically described as unusually greasy, floating, and malodorous. The patient might say, "Yes, around November it got oily looking and would stick to the sides of the bowl." Or he might have noticed that his stools have become more difficult to flush because of their tendency to float. Some patients with small-bowel disease but normal pancreatic function can hydrolyze much of the triglyceride into glycerol and fatty acid, and their stools may not appear extremely greasy.

Unfortunately, some patients do not observe their stools and so cannot state whether the appearance is greasy (due to undigested triglycerides) or floating (because of the high gas content). The first question you must ask is, "Do you usually look at your stools in the toilet bowl?" Do not ask, "Do you know what your stool looks like?" because many patients may examine the stool on the toilet paper, but do not look at it in the bowl, so that they cannot see whether or not it floats.

If the patient does not observe his stool, the question about its odor is particularly important. But if you simply ask, "Is your stool foul smelling?" he will usually reply in the affirmative. A better question is, "Have you noticed any change in the odor of your stools?" If the patient replies, "Yes, I now have to leave the bathroom window open even when it is snowing, just to get that smell out of the house," you can reliably infer that the stools are especially malodorous.

Impotence

Potency is the ability to develop and maintain an erection satisfactory for penetration and sufficient stimulation of the vagina. The impotent patient should be asked whether he wishes an evaluation. If he does not, he should be asked, "Why not?" If he does, he should be asked the questions suggested below.

First one must distinguish a decreased desire (decreased libido) from impotence (inability to perform, accompanied by adequate desire, at least in the early stages).

The differential diagnosis of decreased libido includes a wide variety of chronic debilitating diseases as well as psychologic conditions such as affective disorders (depressed type), adjustment reactions, and neuroses. Endocrine conditions and certain drugs can affect the libido. But peripheral neuropathy and vascular diseases should not do so initially. Some patients who repeatedly experience impotence develop a secondary decrease in attempted intercourse, not because of a primary decrease in libido per se, but rather because of the embarrassment and shame associated with the impotence. These emotional motivators can make even the thought of attempting intercourse seem noxious. These feelings can be dissected out with a few questions by a sensitive interviewer.

Impotence, on the other hand, basically involves the differential diagnosis shown in Table 3-1.

Associated symptoms are particularly important in assessing this problem. One should ask at least about temperature intolerance as a clue to a thyroid disorder, if one has not already done so in the review of systems. A neurologic condition will generally be associated with other neurologic symptoms as well. The sense of smell may be lost in Kallman's hypogonadotrophic hypogonadism as well as in zinc deficiency. Drugs frequently associated with impotence are listed in Table 3-2.

Patients with psychogenic impotence often have normal morning erections, and may perform satisfactorily with certain partners. If the patient has a sleeping partner, he can ask his partner about whether nocturnal erections occur. If the answer is in doubt, the patient should be instructed to place a roll of about four postage stamps *snugly* about the circumference of his penis upon retiring to sleep. The end stamp can be moistened to fasten the roll. If the circle of stamps splits at the perforation during the night, one knows that nocturnal tumescence has probably occurred, and that psychogenic impotence is the most likely diagnosis.

One study found 65% of cases of impotence to have a mixed

Table 3-1.   Causes of Impotence

Condition	% of Cases (after Morley, 1986)
Endocrine[a,b]	6–44
Hypogonadism	6–39
Hyperprolactinemia	2–8
Thyroid disorder	3–4
Diabetes mellitus	20
Neurologic[a]	2–7
Psychogenic	14–60
Vascular[c]	1–37

[a]*Includes drug-induced cases (see Table 3-2).*
[b]*Includes zinc deficiency.*
[c]*In addition to arterial insufficiency and "steal" syndromes, vascular causes include a corporeal venous shunt (Nelson, 1987), and the combined neural and vascular problem that may be induced by compression of the blood supply to the penis and the pudendal nerves due to bicycle seats (Solomon, 1987).*

etiology, neurologic plus vascular, or psychogenic plus a mild vascular disorder, for example (Collins et al., 1983).

For more details, consult Chapter 18 (p. 347), Chapter 21 (p. 392), and Chapter 26 (p. 504).

Frigidity

A sexist disclaimer. There is no large section on frigidity in this work to match the one on impotence in the male. This is because frigidity does not have the same broad semiophysiologic significance (in terms of the vascular, neurologic, and endocrine systems) as does impotence in the male. This is not to say that frigidity is always of cerebral origin (Levine, 1977). It can definitely

Table 3-2.   Drugs Frequently Associated with Impotence

Diuretics
　Thiazides
　Spironolactone
Other antihypertensive medications
　Methyldopa
　Reserpine
　Propranolol and other beta blockers
　Verapamil
Other noradrenergically active drugs
Other anorectics
Other psychoactive drugs (e.g., phenothiazines, cocaine, opiates, marijuana, alcohol)
Anticholinergic agents (including tricyclic antidepressants)
Proestrogens and antiandrogens (e.g., cimetidine, clofibrate)
Other commonly prescribed drugs
　Digoxin
　Phenytoin
　Indomethacin
　Metoclopramide
　Metronidazole
Tobacco smoking

Sources: *Morley (1986) and Nelson (1987).*
An extensive listing of drugs affecting libido and potency, with references, is available in The Medical Letter on Drugs and Therapeutics *(Anonymous, 1987).*

be conditioned from dyspareunia, which in turn could be due to local factors, some of which might have an endocrine (i.e., estrogen deficiency) basis. It is simply that the Leriche syndrome, for example (see p. 347), in the female is not accompanied by frigidity. An excellent protocol for investigating the complaint of frigidity is available (Levine, 1976).

Gynecologic Symptoms

Abnormal Menses

Abnormal menstrual periods are of several general types. Hypermenorrhea or menorrhagia means excessive or prolonged flow. The average amount of blood loss is from 25 to 70 cc over 3 or 4 days. The patient generally describes this in terms of number of pads or tampons, from which it is very difficult to estimate the actual amount of blood, but which may be useful for comparison with the patient's customary pattern. The cause of change may be systemic disease, such as leukemia, or gynecologic disease, such as a uterine leiomyoma or malignancy.

Irregular bleeding is called metrorrhagia. This often signifies anovulatory cycles. Menometrorrhagia means irregular and excessive bleeding.

Amenorrhea means the absence of menses, and oligomenorrhea means scant menses. Amenorrhea should be characterized as primary (if the patient has not experienced menarche) or secondary (if she has had menstrual periods that have now ceased).

Intermenstrual bleeding should raise suspicion of a cervical or endometrial polyp or malignancy, or an infection. Some staining may normally occur due to endometrial breakdown at the time of ovulation (Kistner, 1986).

Pain

Pain associated with menstrual flow is called dysmenorrhea. Severe dysmenorrhea may result from endometriosis, as the ectopic endometrial tissue bleeds into the peritoneum or into areas encapsulated by fibrous tissue. Generally, the history is of progressive increase in severity. The soreness in the abdomen and pelvis may be present throughout the month, but tends to increase premenstrually or during coitus. Endometriosis in the cul-de-sac or rectosigmoid region may cause pain on defecation or dyspareunia.

Pain associated with ovulation ("mittelschmerz") may be difficult to differentiate from appendicitis or other surgical emergency. The exact timing of the menstrual periods may be of great diagnostic help.

Infertility

The "male factor" is the single most common cause of infertility (Glass, 1976). Disorders of ovulation account for 10% to 15% of failures to conceive. Generally, the menstrual history will be abnormal (vide supra).

In an infertile woman with regular menses, inquire with particular care about past episodes of pelvic inflammation, induced abortions, and symptoms suggestive of endometriosis.

Other Symptoms

Inquire specifically about vaginal discharge or irritation and dyspareunia. Remember that the female organs are wedged between the bladder and the rectum, so that gynecologic diseases can present with genitourinary or bowel symptoms.

Urinary Incontinence

Urinary incontinence should be described as to volume and frequency. Simple bladder neck obstruction results in many passages of a relatively small amount, but a neurogenic bladder may result in the rare passage of a very large amount of urine. In the female, also ask about stress incontinence (i.e., involuntary passage of urine with cough or other mechanism that increases intraabdominal pressure), evidence of pelvic relaxation.

Tinnitus

Tinnitus simply means ringing in the ears. It is a sensation of noise, which tends to be temporally continuous, consistent in pitch, and constant in volume, most (but not necessarily all) of the time. Intrinsic tinnitus is most commonly associated with deafness, usually of the sensorineural variety. Tinnitus may be caused by irritation of the auditory portion of cranial nerve VIII or of the external auditory canal, eustachian tube obstruction, otitis media, or disturbances of the vascular supply to the auditory portion of the ear. Tinnitus accompanied by paroxysms of vertigo and deafness occurs in Meniere's disease.

Pseudotinnitus or extrinsic tinnitus is caused by something external to the ear (e.g., vascular tinnitus) (Ch. 18, p. 343).

Restless Legs

The restless legs syndrome is an example of a condition diagnosed exclusively on the basis of the history. The classic description is that of Thomas Willis in *The London Practice of Physick* (1685, p. 404):

> Wherefore to some, when being a Bed they betake themselves to sleep, presently in the Arms and Leggs, Leapings and Contractions of the Tendons, and so great a Restlessness and Tossings of their Members ensue, that the diseased are no more able to sleep, than if they were in a Place of the greatest Torture.

These patients have unpleasant creeping sensations, primarily affecting the legs, appearing only at rest, and accompanied by the irresistible urge to move the extremities. The condition may be familial and is often associated with a sleep-related disorder called nocturnal myoclonus. These patients have neither quinine-responsive night cramps nor hypochondriasis. They may respond to carbamazepine and perhaps clonazepam (see Ekbom, 1960; Montplasir et al., 1985; Telstad et al., 1984).

Self-Study. What other syndrome or disease would illustrate the principle, here exampled by the restless legs syndrome, of a diagnosis that can only be made by history?

A Philosophical Interlude on "Diseases" and "Syndromes"

"Disease" is defined by *Dorland's Illustrated Medical Dictionary*, 24th edition, as a definite morbid process having a characteristic train of symptoms. It may affect the whole body or any of its parts, and its *etiology*, pathology, and prognosis may be known or unknown (emphasis mine). It comes from the words meaning "without ease" or "uncomfortable."

"Syndrome" is defined as a set of symptoms that occur together; the sum of signs of any morbid state; a symptom complex. It comes from the words meaning "to run together."

To restate the above, a disease is a definite entity with a single etiology. A syndrome is a concurrence of events. A syndrome could occur in many different diseases; for example, malignant hypertension could be a syndrome occurring in the various diseases of pheochromocytoma, renoprival hypertension, polyarteritis nodosa, and so forth.

As the experienced reader may have guessed, many objections could be raised to this formulation. A substance abuser might be considered "nondiseased," and only become symptomatic and hence "diseased" when abstinent; yet we generally consider abstinence equivalent to health. Further, the idea that a disease has only one etiology works well for malaria, but not so well for ischemic heart disease, in which both mechanisms and etiologies may be diverse.

Do we demote myocardial infarction to a syndrome? And since there are different infarction syndromes, we could end up with a rather complicated outline (see the New York Heart Association Classification of Heart Disease). Notice, in the last sentence, we now have a single disease comprising several syndromes, and not a syndrome comprising several parts.

Worse, even when we know the specific etiology of a disease, such as the hepatitis B virus, there are many different clinical outcomes that are diverse and not at all "definite" or "characteristic," as Dr. Herbert Weiner of Los Angeles has pointed out. These range from an asymptomatic carrier state to aggressive forms of hepatitis, including those in which the body's own immune response produces disease in organs other than the liver (e.g., the kidneys). Thus, while the hepatitis virus is the etiology of one disease that causes the syndrome "hepatitis," the disease itself constitutes various syndromes.

In summary, with advances in knowledge, we should not be surprised if the defined use of "disease" and "syndrome" become less useful.

Use of Diagnostic Conclusions

You may include the previous diagnostic conclusions of other physicians in the history providing that you try to establish the basis of the diagnosis and indicate the level of certainty. For instance, duodenal ulcer removed at surgery would be of a higher level of certainty than a duodenal ulcer reportedly seen at endoscopy, which would be more certain than a "suspected" duodenal ulcer seen on a radiograph, although any of these might be acceptable. A diagnosis of duodenal ulcer made strictly on the basis of another doctor's history would not be at a comparable level of certainty, and might be placed in quotation marks in the write-up. However, if the patient says something like, "I have a gas pain," it is obviously a mistake to accept his diagnosis and record it in the chart, instead of asking something like, "What about it tells you that it is a gas pain?" While we are cautious in accepting the diagnoses of other physicians, we still ask about some of their findings, especially heart murmurs. Of course, this is secondhand information, but when we know that the patient has previously been under the care of competent physicians, we may wish to learn when a murmur (or other finding) was first noted. We again use the technique of bracketing (see p. 22), attempting to learn when the physician first heard the murmur as well as a previous time when the murmur was sought but not found.

To illustrate how this information might be useful, consider the usual time of onset of various types of murmur-producing heart disease. Murmurs appearing before the age of 5 tend to be due to congenital heart disease (although mitral valve prolapse and some other congenital lesions may not become evident until later in life, vide infra.) Murmurs appearing between the ages of 5 and 15 are usually caused by rheumatic heart disease; those

appearing between 15 and 30 are usually due to mitral valve prolapse; and those first heard after age 30 are most likely from idiopathic hypertrophic subaortic stenosis or bicuspid aortic valve stenosis (congenital lesions with tardy manifestation). While using these clues, do not slavishly surrender your good judgment to them. More than one cardiologist has inherited a patient diagnosed as mitral stenosis, who turned out to have an atrial septal defect. Of course, none of these rules apply if the patient has not been examined regularly and competently.

Past Medical History

Traditionally, this section contained a list of the patient's past medical and surgical hospitalizations. With changes in the use of hospitals resulting from government-encouraged rationing of medical care, it may be necessary to modify the past medical history to include important illnesses (not symptoms) that were evaluated in ambulatory care.

Students are frequently confused about what belongs in the past medical history, and what goes in the review of systems. As a rule, all hospitalizations and major medical events go in the past medical history. These will usually be listed by the date, name and location of the hospital, and diagnosis or operation, as outlined in Chapter 4. The review of systems, on the other hand, is a symptom review of all the symptoms pertinent to a particular system.

The past medical history should correlate with the physical examination. If the patient tells you of an operation, he should have a matching scar; conversely, if you find a surgical scar, you need to review the history. Sometimes patients forget about an operation until the scar reminds them. This may also be a clue to the presence of an organic brain syndrome (see p. 18).

The past medical history also includes immunizations. Always ask if the patient has been immunized against diphtheria, pertussis, tetanus, or poliomyelitis.

If the patient has not received tetanus toxoid in the past 10 years, now is a good time to update his immunity. If the patient has never had the primary series, that should be started now. It is surprising how many older patients are not immune to this frequently fatal disease. Women are more likely to be unprotected because they probably did not serve in the armed forces, and are less likely to have sustained an occupational injury. This part of the past medical history provides a good reminder to practice preventive medicine; unless the patient sustains an injury serious enough to require medical attention, this important matter will probably be neglected.

In the appropriate circumstances (which are constantly changing), one should also inquire about immunization against rabies, rubella, Pneumococci, hepatitis B virus, influenza, yellow fever, typhoid, and cholera. It is no longer necessary to inquire about smallpox vaccination. (See also the section on the immunization history in Ch. 4, p. 66.)

Social History

The information that should be included in the social history is given in Chapter 4, in the outlines for the case record. Some questions used to elicit the social history are these:

"What do you do on your day off?" or "What do you do on a typical Sunday?" (Dr. Lawrence Weed of Ohio liked to identify what the patient did on an average day, but that part of the Weed data base was the first part to be omitted.)

"When was the last time you took a vacation?"

"What happened to your hobby?" This is an open-ended question because at the time that it is asked, one does not know that the patient has discontinued an earlier hobby; or for that matter, that he has ever had a hobby.

"What do you do for fun?"

"Who cooks for you when you are sick?"

It is essential at the first interview that the physician determine what sort of ego defenses the patient uses and what sort of social support systems the patient has available. If this information is already at hand, it will help the physician convey catastrophic news in the least noxious and disruptive manner, should this become necessary.

In the absence of formal training in the assaying of ego defenses, the physician can simply ask, "What is the worst thing that ever happened to you?" and then listen attentively to the patient's description of how he dealt with it. To learn about social support systems, the physician should ask, "To whom would you go if you had a really terrible problem you could not deal with alone?" Many people with no apparent support systems have good answers, and many people with multigenerational families and intact marriages surprisingly can name no one. Assume nothing; be prepared.

If the patient has had a particularly traumatic experience (e.g., being held as a hostage, a prisoner of war, or a political prisoner), he should specifically be asked to recount that experience. You specifically need to know about torture, so that you do not unintentionally evoke associations to that experience.

Sexual History

Many would consider the sexual history to be a subsection of the social history, but the questions asked are like those that one asks about any other organ system. The customary dimensions are useful: quantity, quality, chronology, setting, aggravating factors, and alleviating factors. One needs to determine the patient's preferences and actions in terms of object, frequency, and mode, and whether the patient feels good or bad about his sexual activities, and in what specific ways.

•

In no other sphere is quantitation so important and adjectival labeling so potentially misleading, as illustrated by the following case:

A 68-year-old veteran was admitted 25 years after bilateral adrenalectomy, which was followed by the appearance of sellar enlargement and bitemporal hemianopsia. The patient shaved every other day, had a female escutcheon, and lacked axillary hair. The house staff was unwilling to accept the diagnosis of hypogonadism because the patient was "sexually active." On further inquiry, it was learned that his sexual activity consisted of cunnilingus with his wife about once a month. Testosterone and gonadotrophin levels later were found to be subnormal.

•

Sexual History in Women

Is the Patient Pregnant?

The possibility of pregnancy must *always* be kept in mind from the outset for women of childbearing years, because it affects all

diagnostic and treatment decisions. Therefore, young women should be asked the date of their last menstrual period at every office visit. The physician should also ascertain whether the flow occurred on time and was otherwise normal, and whether any recent menses have been abnormal or skipped.

Occasionally, menstrual flow still occurs during the early months of pregnancy. So the occurrence of periodic bleeding does not absolutely rule out pregnancy. Further, the most recent episode of bleeding might be the result of an obstetric complication, such as a tubal pregnancy, rather than a normal menstrual period. This is especially important in women presenting with abdominal pain.

Other symptoms of pregnancy include nausea, unusual fatigue, and breast soreness. Women who present with symptoms suggesting pregnancy should be asked whether they have been pregnant before, and whether they felt the same way then.

Of course, the sexual history (vide supra) should be obtained, including the type of contraception employed, if any. In a patient who might be pregnant, the past history of pelvic inflammatory disease is especially important, because it increases the likelihood of an ectopic pregnancy with its potential for catastrophe.

Drug History

The physician must know about all the patient's medicines: those that were prescribed by the physician, those which the patient obtained over the counter, and those that were taken for recreational purposes. Some women do not consider birth control pills to be medicines or drugs, and must be specifically asked about them.

Prescription Drugs

The important descriptors for drugs include the route, dose, and the frequency. One may wish to add the duration. And of course one always wants to comment on how the patient is actually taking the medication (as opposed to recounting the directions on the bottle). This aspect is often referred to by the misnomer "compliance." The word "compliance" may be stamped on the form one must submit to the motor vehicle division to certify that one's automobile meets the standards for emission controls. It is very frequently used in the context of adherence to the dictates of an authority. In medical contexts, it should be eschewed. The physician should remember that the patient is only purchasing advice, not an order or an instruction to which he must conform.

Over-the-Counter Medications

Sometimes the patient does not consider over-the-counter products worth mentioning, especially vitamins and "nutritional supplements," which he may be taking in toxic amounts, or his present illness could be due to the side effects of medications, particularly the anticholinergic effects of antihistamines, or the gastrointestinal irritation caused by aspirin. You should specifically ask about any such drugs that come to mind.

The issue of unorthodox remedies requires tactful handling, just as the problem of "compliance" does. Many patients have experienced anger or condescension from their physicians when they have admitted to taking nutritional supplements, "kidney pills," or other remedies from the health food store or the "natural healer." You need to examine your own attitude toward such remedies. Resorting to "quackery" is a normal human tendency, not a sign of personal rejection of the physician. Patients desperately need hope, and the therapeutic value of "doing something" should never be underestimated.

You need to communicate to the patient that the purpose of the inquiry is to obtain information so you can help him better, not to gather evidence for an indictment.

Illegal Drugs

The information we need about the patient's use of what our culture euphemistically calls "recreational drugs" is almost the same as is required for his prescription drugs. We need to know exactly what drugs are being taken, the route, and the dosage interval. We need a detailed history for the last week, in the event that the patient is taking a drug with a recognized withdrawal syndrome. Specifically, we need to know precisely when a narcotic analgesic or a sedative-hypnotic was stopped, since withdrawal may be akin to the abrupt stop at the pavement after a person has jumped off a building. The daily dose prior to the withdrawal is analogous to the height of the building.

If the patient dissolves oral medications and takes them parenterally, another frequently unappreciated question must be asked. The inert filler added for bulk during the manufacture of both legal and illegal drugs includes talc and starch. When these are injected, they form microemboli throughout the body, first in the lungs, where their cumulative effect is a disease known as angiothrombotic pulmonary hypertension, sometimes called "blue velvet lung." These microemboli can also reach the systemic circulation. They have been seen in vivo in the eyes and at autopsy in spinal cord, kidney, and other organs. Their presence in the brain is inferred from the neurologic findings.

So, if you determine the patient to be an intravenous drug user, you must ask, "When you shake the drugs up, or dissolve them in a spoon or cap, are they perfectly clear?" or, "When you look through the barrel of the syringe before you inject, is it perfectly clear like water, or is it cloudy?" or "Could you read a newspaper through it? Is it that clear?"

If the material is not perfectly transparent, then there is obviously something that is not solubilized. For a more complete discussion, see Sapira and Cherubin (1975).

There is too much detail in this chapter for you to have assimilated it all into your routine history. Accordingly, you should review the appropriate parts of this chapter, depending on which service you are on.

In your senior year, reread the section on the interviewing process, and use a tape recorder, even if you have already done so. Most physicians need the satisfaction of observing a significant improvement in their physical examination skills, before they can relax enough to utilize some of the lessons to be learned from auditing themselves with patients.

References

Anonymous: Drugs that cause sexual dysfunction. *Med Lett Drugs Ther* 29:65–70, 1987.

Beart RW, O'Connell MJ: Postoperative follow-up of patients with carcinoma of the colon. *Mayo Clin Proc* 58:361–363, 1983.

Bernhard JD: Itching as a manifestation of noncutaneous disease. *Hosp Pract* 22(1A):81–95, 1987.

Chaudhary NA, Truelove SC: The irritable colon syndrome: A study of the clinical features, predisposing causes, and prognosis in 130 cases. *Q J Med* 31:307–322, 1962.

Collins WE, McKendry JBR, Silverman M, Krul LE, Collins JP, Irvine AH: Multidisciplinary survey of erectile impotence. *Can Med Assoc J* 128:1393–1399, 1983.

Daniel WA Jr, Egan S: The quantity of blood required to produce a tarry stool. *JAMA* 113:2232, 1939.

Dennis C: Current procedure in management of obstruction of small intestine. *JAMA* 154:463–470, 1954.

Ekbom KA: Restless legs syndrome. *Neurology* 10:868–873, 1960.

Friedman M, Thoresen CE, Gill JJ, Powell LH, Ulmer D, Thompson L, Price VA, Rabin DD, Breall WS, Dixon T, Levy R, Bourg E: Alteration of type A behavior and reduction in cardiac recurrences in post-myocardial infarction patients. *Am Heart J* 108:237–248, 1984.

Glass RH: *Office Gynecology*. Williams & Wilkins, Baltimore, 1976.

Hampton JR, Harrison MJG, Mitchell JRA, Prichard JS, Seymour C: Relative contributions of history-taking, physical examination, and laboratory investigation to diagnosis and management of medical outpatients. *Br Med J* 2:486–489, 1975.

Kistner RW: *Gynecology: Principles and Practice*, ed 4. Year Book Medical Publishers, Chicago, 1986.

Levine SB: Marital sexual dysfunction: Introductory concepts. *Ann Intern Med* 84:448–453, 1976.

Levine SB: Marital sexual dysfunction: Female dysfunctions. *Ann Intern Med* 86:588–597, 1977.

Manning AP, Thompson WG, Heaton KW, Morris AF: Towards positive diagnosis of the irritable bowel. *Br Med J* 2:653–654, 1978.

Martin GJ, Adams SL, Martin HG: Evaluation of patients with syncope. *N Engl J Med* 309:1650, 1983.

Montplasir J, Godbout R, Boghen D, DeChamplain J, Young SN, Lapierre G: Familial restless legs with periodic movements in sleep: Electrophysiologic, biochemical, and pharmacologic study. *Neurology* 35:130–134, 1985.

Morgan WL Jr, Engel GL: *The Clinical Approach to the Patient*. WB Saunders, Philadelphia, 1969.

Morley JE: Impotence. *Am J Med* 80:897–905, 1986.

Nelson RP: Male sexual dysfunction: Evaluation and treatment. *South Med J* 80:69–74, 1987.

Nunes EV, Frank KA, Kornfeld DS: Psychologic treatment for the type A behavior pattern and for coronary heart disease: A meta-analysis of the literature. *Psychosom Med* 48:159–173, 1987.

Rosenman RH, Brand RJ, Jenkins D, Friedman M, Straus R, Wurm M: Coronary heart disease in the Western collaborative group study: Final follow-up experience of 8½ years. *JAMA* 233:872–877, 1975.

Sacks O: *Awakenings*. Vintage Books, New York, 1973.

Sapira JD: Medicine is a trust. *South Med J* 76:76–78, 1983.

Sapira JD, Cherubin CE: *Drug Abuse*. American Elsevier, New York, 1975.

Schiff L, Stevens RJ, Shapiro S, Goodman S: Observations on the oral administration of citrated blood in man: II. The effect on the stools. *Am J Med Sci* 203:409–412, 1942.

Silen W (ed): *Cope's Early Diagnosis of the Acute Abdomen*, ed 15. Oxford University Press, New York, 1979.

Solomon S: Impotence and bicycling: A seldom-reported connection. *Postgrad Med* 81:99–100, 1987.

Sternbach RA: *Pain Patients: Traits and Treatment*. Academic Press, New York, 1974.

Swartout R: Some pains I have known. *Lancet* 1:1133–1134, 1987.

Telstad W, Sorenson O, Larsen S, Lillevold PE, Stensrud P, Nyberg-Hansen R: Treatment of the restless legs syndrome with carbamazepine. *Br Med J* 288:444–446, 1984.

Williams RB: Hostility, anger, and heart disease. *Drug Ther* 16 (August):41–48, 1986.

Willis T: *The London Practice of Physick*, ed 1. Thomas Bassett and William Crooke, London, 1685.

4
The Case Record

Mephistopheles: I'll wait on you tonight, when you partake
Of college gaudy, where the doctors dine;
Only—since life, or let's say death's at stake—
I'll bring you back, please, a couple of lines to sign.
Faust: So, black and white you want? You've never heard
Good pedant, that a man may keep his word? . . .
A parchment, notwithstanding, signed and sealed,
Is bogey fit to make the bravest yield.

Faust: Part I: The Study (3)
Goethe, translated by Philip Wayne

Introduction

Pedagogy

When first seeing patients, it is hard to remember all the parts of the history and all the questions in the review of systems. Therefore, two outlines are given here (although the student may wish to substitute a different one supplied by his school). The first of the two is better for the student. After examining about 100 patients using this form, the student will know it by heart. At that time, a shorter form (such as the second one) may be substituted.

The educational principle is that initially one is well advised to be complete (even if it means being labeled "o-c," or obsessive-compulsive) and only later to use truncated approaches. This general principle of medicine applies to far more than just the case history. First of all, if one can perform, say, a complete neurologic examination according to the outline, then at any future date one can revert to this examination when confronted with a patient who has a neurologic problem and not be limited by the currently ubiquitous "grossly normal." Second, if one rigorously follows this outline, one incidentally gains a great deal of experience with the normal, enabling one to recognize variations of the normal and to pick up subtle abnormalities. Third, the use of this outline in conjunction with a differential diagnosis will quickly convince even the neophyte of the power of a thorough examination. Finally, as the repeated examination becomes faster and faster, the student gains a salubrious sense of mastery that must be experienced, literally, to be appreciated.

How Much Time Does the Examination Take?

When I was a junior medical student, it took 2 hours for me to obtain a complete history. A complete physical examination took another 2 hours. To record this information, to construct my dif-

ferential diagnosis, and then to add the laboratory tests that we were supposed to do ourselves (routine and microscopic urinalysis, hemoglobin and hematocrit, white count and differential, and electrocardiogram) took another 2 hours, for a total of 6 hours. I should add that most of these patients had but one major diagnostic problem; nevertheless, this problem was often a diagnostic challenge, and required the student to do considerable reading.

After three medicine rotations, we could perform and record a complete history and physical (without laboratory work) in the outpatient department in about 2 hours. At that time, I was once assigned a woman who was deaf and dumb. Because the entire history, questions and answers, had to be written longhand, it took me 4 hours. The 4 hours were well spent because, after visits to many doctors, the patient's diagnosis was finally made. She suffered from what would now be called neurocirculatory asthenia. Previously, she had received only incorrect diagnoses carrying an ominous prognosis. Her secondary neurosis was completely reversed after I saw her, one of my first solo transference cures.

By the time I was an intern, I could perform and record a good two-page history and physical in 1 hour, only occasionally missing nystagmus or failing to elicit muscular fasciculations. At the time of my oral examination in internal medicine, 7 years after graduation, I could do a complete history and physical on two patients in 1½ hours.

The student should not be discouraged by what at first seems an overwhelming task. Attention to detail at the beginning is time-consuming, but necessary and richly rewarding in the long run.

For faculty to say, "We can't teach this in our curriculum because there is not enough time" is analogous to a surgeon declining to insert an artificial heart valve because it would take more than 2 hours.

Model Outline of Gerry Rodnan, MD

The following is an abridgement and revision of the outline given to our class at the University of Pittsburgh in the fall of 1958 by our coursemaster, Dr. Gerry Rodnan. I used it with good results for 10 years, after which I became a consultant and was allowed to improvise.

A Biographical Note

Gerry P. Rodnan, MD, was a Professor of Medicine and rheumatologist at the University of Pittsburgh. He is known for Rodnan's Law (1959): "Corticosteroids will do anything if you give enough of them." Rodnan's Rule of Urine was stated in 1971: "In a contemporary teaching hospital, it takes 72 hours to collect a 24-hour urine specimen." Rodnan's Aphorism states: "All the great diagnosticians are not at the university center. And all the bad ones are not in the community hospitals."

Rodnan was also the inventor of the "professorial dozen." He noted that whenever a full professor was asked how many cases he had seen of some unusual entity, the professor would say, "Oh, about a dozen." Rodnan suggested that the dozen was generated in the following manner: the junior medical student saw a case at Grand Rounds. (Historically, patients were presented at Grand Rounds; today, the activity that goes by that name bears no resemblance to the patient-oriented sessions of bygone days.) He referred to that case in the senior year, thus making it two. By the time he was an intern, the case had multiplied to three. As a junior assistant resident, the very same case had become four; and so forth, as he rose through the ranks. By the time he was a professor, it was a professorial dozen.

A. *Identification*
Name, age, sex, marital status, color, occupation, religion, birthplace (state or country), referring physician and/or agency, date of examination (including year).
B. *Informant and Reliability*
C. *Chief Complaint*
D. *Present Illness*
The present illness is not simply a complete but disorganized catalog of statements and facts. The organization of the history is based on two principles:
  1. The major problem from which the patient is suffering must be dissected free of other unrelated information.
  2. The progression of the major disease from its inception must be made clear, culminating in an evaluation of the current effects of the illness upon the patient's life.
E. *Past History*
  1. *General health*: Give the patient's estimate of his health in general. Body weight: present, maximum, minimum, recent change. Any significant facts from previous physical examination (military, school, insurance, employment, etc.)
  2. *Serious illness*: Record any infectious disease or prolonged illness.
  3. *Injuries*: Broken bones, lacerations, or other injuries.
  4. *Operations*: Date, diagnosis, postoperative course, biopsy reports.
  5. *Admission to other hospitals*: Record chronologically, giving the name of the hospital and physician and the source of information. List admission and discharge dates, brief summary of presenting symptoms and significant physical or laboratory findings if known, diagnoses, and therapy.
  6. *Past admissions to this hospital and outpatient department*: If the patient has been seen frequently in the outpatient department, each visit does not need to be summarized but appropriate resumes of time intervals or change in symptoms must be recorded. Such hospital admissions and clinic visits should be summarized chronologically in the following form:
      Number of Admission (First, second, etc.):
      Service (Medical, ENT, Surgical, etc.):
      Date of Admission: Date of Discharge:
      Operations:
      Summary: This summary should be sufficiently detailed to contain all pertinent symptoms, physical findings, laboratory results, medications, and course in the hospital.
  7. *Current medications*
F. *Review of Systems*
The chief symptoms referable to each system are reviewed. Information that belongs with the present illness will frequently be obtained and should be recorded there. Repetitions are to be avoided by referring to preceding sections that contain the same information.
  1. *Skin*: Abnormal pigmentation, sweating pattern, bleeding, bruising, eruptions, or itching.
  2. *Lymph Nodes*: Enlargement, pain, sinuses, drainage.
  3. *Head*: Headache, injury, fainting, seizures.

4. *Eyes*: Vision, inflammation, pain, diplopia, scotomata, exophthalmos, glaucoma.
5. *Ears*: Hearing, pain, discharge, tinnitus, vertigo.
6. *Nose and Throat*: Abnormal odors, discharge, bleeding, obstruction, pain, sore throat, change in voice, hoarseness, goiter.
7. *Breasts*: Masses, pain, discharge.
8. *Cardiovascular, Respiratory*: General exercise tolerance, dyspnea, cough, sputum (amount, description), wheezing, hemoptysis, chest pain, fever, night sweats, orthopnea, edema, cyanosis, hypertension, palpitations, history of heart murmur, treatment with cardiovascular drugs (such as digoxin, diuretics, or nitroglycerin), intermittent claudication, leg ulcers.
9. *Gastrointestinal*: Appetite, condition of teeth and gums, sore tongue, dysphagia, nausea, vomiting, hematemesis, constipation, diarrhea, unusual stool color or consistency, abdominal pain, jaundice, results of gastrointestinal X rays, food intolerance, rectal bleeding.
10. *Endocrine*: Growth, body configuration, symptoms of increased or decreased metabolism. Polyphagia, polydipsia, polyuria, glycosuria. Sexual development, impotence, sterility, menstrual history (age at onset, cycle, duration, amount, amenorrhea, menorrhagia, metrorrhagia, dysmenorrhea, date of last period, premenstrual edema and tension, number of pregnancies, induced or spontaneous abortions, stillbirths, live births, obstetrical complications, age of menopause, hot flashes, postmenopausal bleeding).
11. *Allergic and immunologic*: Urticaria, angioneurotic edema, hay fever, asthma, eczema, sensitivity to drugs, foods, pollens, dander. Immunizations and skin tests.
12. *Musculoskeletal*: Pain, swelling, stiffness, limitation of motion of joints. Fractures, serious sprains.
13. *Neuropsychiatric*: Headache, convulsions, loss of consciousness, paralysis, weakness, atrophy, spasticity, tremor, involuntary movements, gait, incoordination, pain, change in sensation, paresthesias, incontinence, sweating pattern. Predominant mood; anxiety; phobias; sleep pattern; memory; judgment; thought content (delusions, hallucinations); history of psychiatric care, sexual adjustment, attitudes toward friends, associates, family, disease.

G. *Family History*
Record the age and health (or death and cause of death where appropriate) of parents, siblings, and children. Investigate the familial incidence of obesity, diabetes, cardiovascular and renal disease, cancer, neuropsychiatric disease, allergy, blood dyscrasias, arthritis, glaucoma, and infectious diseases such as tuberculosis. Many diseases are clearly heritable; many others have an important hereditary "tendency." A careful family history may suggest a good diagnostic possibility or may provide support for a tentative diagnosis.

H. *Social History*
Record the nativity, occupation, marital adjustment, and especially the patient's emotional relationship to the parents throughout his life. The patient's birthplace, residences, and education are important. The marital history includes age, health, occupation, education of the marital partner, number of children, and the marital adjustment. Describe the "extended family group." Also, who lives with the patient at home (not necessarily the same as the "extended family")? Learn exactly what the patient does in his occupation with particular reference to the degree of emotional tension or health hazard. What provisions are there for disability compensation and other marginal benefits? Are there debts or economic problems that will influence convalescence? How much does the patient participate in the civic, social, religious, and political activities of his particular economic and social group? How do his opinions or practices differ from those of the group (this presupposes previous knowledge or inquiry into the group opinion)? What are the medical opinions of the group? Find out in detail how the patient spends his day, what his hobbies are, how much he relaxes, how much he sleeps, how much physical activity there is. Learn the patient's dietary habits; this usually requires specific inquiries regarding each meal. Are tobacco, alcohol, narcotics, or other drugs used? If so, to what extent?

I. *Physical Examination*
1. *Vital signs*: Temperature, pulse, respiration, blood pressure (both arms and one leg, record position), height, weight.
2. *General appearance*: Development, nutrition, mental status, apparent age, race, sex, position in bed, comfort, attitude toward examination, degree of illness (acute or chronic), obvious abnormalities. A short statement embodying these features should always introduce the physical examination.

3. *Integument*: Skin: color (jaundice, pallor, cyanosis, pigmentation, erythema), temperature, texture, moisture, eruptions, petechia, telangiectasia, nodules, scars. Nails: color, shape, texture, subungal hemorrhages, paronychia. Hair: distribution, texture, quantity, color.
4. *Lymph nodes*: Size, consistency, tenderness, mobility, sinuses; describe for cervical, occipital, supraclavicular, axillary, epitrochlear, inguinal, and femoral nodes.
5. *Skull*: Size, contour, tenderness, bruit.
6. *Eyes*: Vision, protuberance; extraocular movements, nystagmus, strabismus; lids, sclerae, conjunctivae, cornea, ocular tension; pupillary size, equality, regularity, reactions to light and accommodation; ophthalmoscopic examination of lens, vitreous, discs, retina (scars, pigmentation, hemorrhages, exudates, macula), vessels.
7. *Ears*: Hearing, air and bone conduction; pinnae, external canal; drum, perforation, discharge.
8. *Nose*: Mucous membranes, obstruction, polyps, discharge, septum, sinus tenderness and transillumination.
9. *Mouth*: Color and lesions of lips; odor of breath; size, position, tremor, papillae, color, coating of tongue; number, condition, and alignment of teeth; pigmentation, ulceration, bleeding, infection of gums; eruptions or pigmentation of buccal mucosa.
10. *Throat*: Position of uvula; color, exudates, lymphoid tissue in posterior pharynx; tumors or ulceration; tonsils; voice, vocal cords.
11. *Neck*: Contour, mobility; tenderness, masses; thyroid size, consistency, bruit; tracheal position or tug; salivary glands.
12. *Breasts*: Size, contour, tenderness, masses, discharge, scars, nipples.
13. *Thorax and lungs*: inspection of thoracic contour and respiratory motion with special attention to the detection of diffuse obstructive or restrictive impairment of respiratory mechanics; palpation for tenderness, fremitus, rubs, wheezes; percussion, including descent of diaphragms; auscultation of breath sounds, spoken and whispered voice, adventitious sounds (râles, friction rubs).
14. *Cardiovascular*: Heart: inspect apical impulse, other pulsations. Palpate apical impulse, thrills, shocks. Percuss heart size, contour (describe in relationship to the midclavicular line). Auscult rhythm, quality, and intensity of heart sounds including 3rd and 4th sounds or gallops if present; murmurs (location, timing, intensity, character, transmission; relationship to position, respiration, or alterations in cardiac rhythm); friction rubs. Check for apical-pulse deficit (see Ch. 6, p. 000). Peripheral vascular system: thickening or tortuosity of peripheral arterial walls; abnormal or absent arterial pulses. Character and equality of carotid, brachial, radial, femoral, popliteal, dorsalis pedis, and posterior tibial pulses. Arterial bruits. Venous distention, pulsation, tenderness, or inflammation. Abnormal venous pattern over chest and abdomen.
15. *Abdomen*: Inspection: contour, abnormal venous structures, peristalsis, scars. Palpation: tenderness (local or rebound), spasm, masses, organs (liver, gallbladder, spleen, kidneys, uterus, bladder), heaviness of flanks, fluid wave, hernias. Percussion: organs, masses, shifting dullness. Auscultation: peristalsis, bruit, succussion splash.
16. *Genitalia*: Male: development, scars, discharge, tenderness or masses of epididymides and testes. Female: Perineum, labia, vagina, cervix, size and position of uterus and adnexae; examine for masses, tenderness, discharge, ulceration.
17. *Rectal*: Hemorrhoids, fissure, fistula, sphincter tone; prostate (size, contour, consistency), seminal vesicles; consistency and appearance of feces.
18. *Musculoskeletal*: Spine: contour, motion, tenderness. Muscles: tremor, atrophy, fasciculation. Joints; deformities, crepitation, range of motion, swelling, tenderness, heat, redness. Extremities: clubbing, edema.
19. *Mental status*: Behavior: appearance, facial expression, activity. Speech: rate, quality, quantity. Mood: depression, euphoria, resentment, fear, anxiety, lability. Content of thought: obsessions, delusions, ideas of persecution. Sensory deceptions: illusions, hallucinations. Sensorium: orientation (time, place, person), state of consciousness, memory (recent and remote). Intellectual endowment (not synonymous with education). Judgment and insight.
20. *Neurologic*: Every complete physical examination should include a brief survey of the cranial nerves, motor and sensory systems, and reflexes. If there is any indication from the history or physical examination that the patient has a neurologic defect or if the disease that he is suspected of having is frequently associated with neurologic complications, a detailed neurologic examination according to the following outline should be conducted and recorded:

Cranial nerves

I.	Recognition of odors
II.	Visual acuity and fields, optic discs
III, IV, VI.	Pupillary size and reactions, eyelid droop, extraocular movements, lid lag
V.	Sensations of face and tongue, corneal reflexes, chewing muscles
VII.	Facial muscles; taste of anterior two thirds of the tongue
VIII.	Hearing (bone and air conduction, Weber's test), nystagmus
IX.	Sensation of hard and soft palate, gag reflex; taste of posterior one third of tongue
X.	Weakness of soft palate, deviation of uvula, difficulty in phonation, vocal cord paralysis, rapid pulse (bilateral lesion)
XI.	Sternocleidomastoid and trapezius functions
XII.	Tongue muscles, protrusion and deviation

Skilled acts: Aphasia, apraxia, agnosia, asterognosis. Record if the patient is right- or left-handed.

Meningeal signs: stiff neck, Kernig, Brudzinski.

Posture, gait, and abnormal movements: Standing and reclining posture; circumduction, propulsion, ataxia; Tremors, tics, athetosis, chorea, localized muscle spasm

Coordination: Finger to nose, heel to knee, adiadochokinesia, rebound, past pointing, Romberg

Motor system: Muscle strength, tone, volume, contractures.

Reflexes: Biceps, triceps, radial, knee (clonus), ankle (clonus), abnormal, cremasteric, plantar response

Sensation: Pain (superficial and deep), temperature, touch, position, vibration

Autonomic: Sphincter tone, sweating, vasomotor changes, trophic disturbances

J.   Differential Diagnosis

Alternate Method: Model Outline of Ronald S. Banner, MD

This outline was developed by and is reproduced with the permission of Dr. Ronald S. Banner of Philadelphia. It has been slightly revised. It is presented, in part, to indicate that any practicing physician should wish to develop his own forms.

Accompanying Letter to Patient

Dear Patient:

If you are being asked to spend your time and effort completing this questionnaire, you deserve to know why I feel it is important. I believe in, and attempt to provide you with, personal and thorough health care. While this requires knowledge of medicine and compassion on my part, it also requires your participation and help. This questionnaire, which I devised, helps you give me needed information about your medical condition(s), your family, your medical habits, and you as a person. Although the questionnaire is long, the information is important—so please answer the questions as best you can. Some patients prefer to answer one or two questions in person rather than on paper; we can do that if you prefer.

During our appointment, we shall talk together, discussing your medical concerns and reviewing the questionnaire; together with a physical examination and laboratory tests, this information will help me provide you with the best possible, personal medical care.

The information in this questionnaire will be kept confidential.

Thank you for your cooperation.

A.   Identification Data

1.   Today's date _____

2.   Name_____

3.   Age _____   4.   Date of Birth _____

5. Home Address _____ Zip _____

6. Home Telephone _____

7. Occupation _____

8. Employer _____

9. Work Address _____ Zip _____

10. Work Telephone _____

11. Sex: ☐ male   ☐ female

12. Marital status: ☐ single ☐ married ☐ widowed ☐ separated ☐ divorced ☐ remarried for how many years? _____

13. Person to contact in case of emergency (include name, work and home addresses, and phone numbers _____

_____

B. Present Medical History

1. Explain in your own words your reasons for having this examination. Why now? Why with me?_____

_____

_____

_____

_____

_____

2. Please circle one:

    I wanted to come. My spouse/family insisted.

    My friends insisted. There is another reason.

    Please explain: _____

_____

3. I was referred by _____

4. If the problems above (in #1) are not new or have been treated before, please explain what was done (including when, where, and by whom). (Use other side if you need more room).

_____

_____

_____

5. When did you last see a doctor? _____

    For what reason? _____

6. When was your last thorough examination? _____

7. When was your last hospitalization? _____

8. When were you last sick in bed? _____

9. How is your present health? ☐ excellent ☐ good ☐ fair ☐ poor

C. Family History

Family background may be related to medical conditions. Please fill in all of the following chart:

	If Living Now				If Deceased			
	First name	Age	State of health (good, fair, or poor)	Where living	Age	Date: month, year	Cause of death	Your age then
Natural father:								
Natural Mother:								
Brothers and sisters, starting with the oldest (include yourself with a* by your name								
Spouse:								
Children:								

Please circle the names of all the people in the left-hand column with whom you are/were in close or frequent contact.

D. Illnesses in the Family

Check in the **Self** column if any one of the following has happened to you. Check the **Blood Relative** column if any of the following have happened to a blood relative, and state the relationship (mother, brother, aunt, etc.).

Self	Blood Relative		Self	Blood Relative	
____	_____	diabetes (sugar)	____	_____	bleeding problems
____	_____	high blood pressure	____	_____	epilepsy or seizures
____	_____	stroke	____	_____	glaucoma
____	_____	heart problem	____	_____	blindness before age 50
____	_____	cancer or tumor	____	_____	deafness before age 50
____	_____	emotional or nervous problems	____	_____	kidney problems
____	_____	arthritis	____	_____	bladder problems
____	_____	gout	____	_____	thyroid problems
____	_____	alcoholism	____	_____	migraine

Self Blood Relative

____	_____	asthma
____	_____	breathing problems
____	_____	tuberculosis
____	_____	cystic fibrosis
____	_____	allergies
____	_____	skin problems
____	_____	anemia
____	_____	sickle cell anemia

Self Blood Relative

____	_____	stomach problems
____	_____	bowel problems
____	_____	rectal polyp
____	_____	gallbladder problems
____	_____	liver problems
____	_____	genetic or inherited diseases
____	_____	other unusual diseases

E. Parents

	Father	**Mother**
Family (last name)	_____	_____
Birthplace	_____	_____
Country of grandparents or great grandparents (background)	_____	_____
Religion	_____	_____
Occupation (if deceased or retired, what did they do before?)	_____	_____
Favorite activities	_____	_____
What type of person is/was he/she?	_____	_____
	_____	_____
	_____	_____
Describe your relationship with each parent (even if deceased)	_____	_____
	_____	_____
	_____	_____

What were your parents' expectations of you? _____

_____

F. Past Medical History/Medical Habits

1. How would you describe your health as a child?

    ☐ excellent ☐ good ☐ fair ☐ poor

    If fair or poor, please explain: _____

    _____

2. When you were a child, did you have any life-threatening illnesses or accidents?

    ☐ no ☐ yes ☐ ?   If yes or ?, please

    explain _____

    _____

3. When you were ill, who provided most of the care?

    ☐ Mother ☐ Father ☐ Other _____

4. How did your parents, or the person who looked after you, react when you were sick?

    ☐ absent ☐ angry ☐ attentive ☐ indifferent ☐ panicked ☐ supportive ☐ other _____

5. Record of hospital stays (childhood and adulthood—surgery, observation, etc.): Please list chronologically, childhood events first and most recent events last:

Date in hospital or your age	Name of hospital and of doctor	Reason for hospital stay
_____	_____	_____
_____	_____	_____
_____	_____	_____

6. Record of separate tests (X rays, EKGs, scans, special)

Name of test and date	Place/person doing test	Reason for test and result
_____	_____	_____
_____	_____	_____

7. Please list all of the doctors that you see and reasons/conditions of yours that they treat.

_____   _____

_____   _____

_____   _____

8. People may see several doctors and may take medicine from some of them as well as over-the-counter medicine. Since there are interactions between some of the medicines, it is important to know all the medicines that you use (laxatives, vitamins, etc.) Please list names, strengths if known, and how often you take them.

_____

_____

_____

9. List all medicines or injections that you cannot take (because of allergy or reaction). What happened to you when you took them?

_____

_____

10. Please check any of the following if you think you may have received greater exposure to them than average:

   ☐ carbon monoxide   ☐ other gases   ☐ silica dust   ☐ lead   ☐ organic solvents

   ☐ coal dust   ☐ sulfur dioxide cyanides   ☐ hydrogen sulfide   ☐ asbestos   ☐ arsenic   ☐ mercury

   ☐ fluorine, fluorides, benzene   ☐ noise   ☐ radiation   ☐ other dusts, vapors, fumes, smoke

   (specify) _____   ☐ extreme temperatures or humidity   ☐ high or low pressures

   ☐ other hazards (specify) _____

11. When was the last time you had immunizations (shots) for tetanus _____ polio _____ German measles _____

12. Do you have dental problems? Explain _____

13. For Women Only: When did you last see your gynecologist for a Pap smear? _____
   Name of gynecologist _____

14. Check any of the following that have happened to you:

   ☐ chicken pox   ☐ German measles   ☐ scarlet fever   ☐ rheumatic fever   ☐ measles   ☐ polio

   ☐ mononucleosis   ☐ jaundice   ☐ herpes   ☐ pneumonia   ☐ venereal disease (VD)   ☐ phlebitis

   ☐ diverticulitis   ☐ hernia   ☐ hemorrhoids   ☐ tension/anxiety problems   ☐ depression

15. Do you follow a special diet? If yes, explain: _____

_____

16. Please describe your drinking of alcoholic beverages:

	Daily	Number of ounces Weekly	Monthly
Wine	_____	_____	_____
Beer	_____	_____	_____
Hard alcohol	_____	_____	_____

Do you think you have a drinking problem? _____

17. Coffee: Number of cups per day _____

Tea: Number of cups per day _____

How much chocolate do you eat: _____

18. Do you use anything to move your bowels? If yes, explain:

_____

19. Do you smoke? _____ How much? _____ If you smoked cigarettes and quit, date you quit _____,

number of packs per day _____, number of years _____.

20. When was your last chest X ray? _____ Where was it done? _____

21. What type and how much physical activity do you have? How frequently? _____

G. Personal History

Although this section may seem unnecessary to some, my experience has shown that this information can help me be a much more effective medical advisor for you.

1. Your birthplace _____

2. Where were you raised? _____

3. Last school attended and year _____

4. Armed forces? (if yes, explain) _____

5. Present job: Describe the work you do, your hours, and the effect it has on you: _____

_____

_____

6. If a housewife, or retired, describe how you spend your day. How does it affect you? Would you rather be doing something else? _____

_____

7. Earlier jobs _____

_____

8. List people living with you _____

9. What does your spouse do? _____

10. What words best describe your spouse? _____

11. Are there problems at home that disturb you? ☐ no   ☐ yes   ☐ maybe

If yes or maybe, please explain _____

_____

12. How do you spend your evenings and weekends?

    _____

    _____

13. Do you have any hobbies? If yes, what are they?

    _____

    _____

14. Do you belong to any organizations? _____ Your favorites _____

    What do you do for the organization(s), and what do(es) it (they) do for you? _____

    _____

15. Where and when have you traveled outside the USA? _____

    _____

16. Have you taken any vacations in the past year? ☐ no ☐ yes If yes, where did you go and for how long? If no, why not? _____

    _____

17. How is your sleep? ☐ good ☐ fair ☐ poor ☐ other _____

    _____

    When do you go to sleep? _____ When do you awaken? _____

    How often do you have a problem falling asleep? ____ (nights/week) Are you rested when you wake up? ____

    How many hours of sleep do you need? _____

18. List the major life events or changes that you have experienced (including but not limited to serious illnesses or injuries; separations from, or deaths of, persons close to you; losses of property or money; moves; unemployment; business/work crises; changes to different kind of work; family crises; marriage; births; violations of the law)

    _____

    _____

    How were you affected by these events? _____

    _____

    How did you adjust to these events? _____

    _____

19. What major events or changes have occurred in your life this past year? _____

20. Are there any major changes planned in the near future? _____

22. How are your coping abilities? ☐ excellent ☐ good ☐ fair ☐ poor

23. What do you do to relieve tension/anxiety/frustration? _____

24. Who are your heroes? After whom do you model yourself? What qualities in them do you try to imitate?

    _____

25. For the following items, check whether you feel each is beneficial, harmful, or without effect on you personally. *Star (*) those items that are a regular part of your life.*

	Beneficial	Harmful	No effect			Beneficial	Harmful	No effect
Daily family relationships	_____	_____	_____		Hobbies	_____	_____	_____
					Sex	_____	_____	_____

	Beneficial	Harmful	No effect		Beneficial	Harmful	No effect
Other family relationships	_____	_____	_____	Regular physical exertion	_____	_____	_____
Holiday functions	_____	_____	_____	Any physical exertion	_____	_____	_____
Religious activities	_____	_____	_____	Recreation	_____	_____	_____
				Vacations	_____	_____	_____
Social activities	_____	_____	_____	Vitamins	_____	_____	_____
Friends/ relationships	_____	_____	_____	Special diet	_____	_____	_____
				Prescribed medications	_____	_____	_____
Your work	_____	_____	_____				

26. What do you think will help you stay/become healthy? _____
_____

27. For the traits listed below, check the one word to the right of each trait that describes you best.

Competitive drive	☐ excess	☐ plenty	☐ minimal
Ambitious, like to achieve	☐ usually	☐ sometimes	☐ rarely
Need to display achievement	☐ usually	☐ sometimes	☐ rarely
Sense of urgency/impatience	☐ constant	☐ some	☐ rarely
Deadline oriented	☐ always	☐ sometimes	☐ rarely
Work results in worry or fear	☐ usually	☐ sometimes	☐ rarely
Drive yourself to accomplish	☐ usually	☐ sometimes	☐ rarely
Feel under pressure	☐ usually	☐ sometimes	☐ rarely
Tend to worry	☐ usually	☐ sometimes	☐ rarely
Can postpone thoughts about problems	☐ rarely	☐ sometimes	☐ usually
Recognize when you are tired	☐ rarely	☐ sometimes	☐ usually
Recognize fatigue and work harder	☐ rarely	☐ usually	☐ sometimes
Recognize fatigue and respond to it	☐ rarely	☐ sometimes	☐ usually
Able to relax	☐ rarely	☐ sometimes	☐ usually
Able to relax without guilt	☐ rarely	☐ sometimes	☐ usually
Interests outside of work	☐ many	☐ few	☐ rare
Family life	☐ chaotic	☐ varies	☐ stable
Get pleasure from daily activities	☐ usually	☐ sometimes	☐ rarely

H. Symptom Review

We all have occasional colds, fevers, belly pains, etc. This section is not for those things. Please read each question carefully and answer by placing a check in the appropriate column. If you are in doubt, check the "?" column.

Do you have now, or have you ever had?	**No**	**Yes**	**?**		**No**	**Yes**	**?**
Failing vision, not corrected by glasses	__	__	__	Other eye problems, such as eye pain	__	__	__
Double vision	__	__	__	Difficulty hearing	__	__	__

Do you have now, or have you ever had?   No Yes ?

	No	Yes	?
Ear infection or injury	—	—	—
Ringing or buzzing in your ears	—	—	—
Pain, swelling, or sores in your mouth	—	—	—
Recent change in taste	—	—	—
Severe sinus trouble	—	—	—
Frequent or severe nosebleeds	—	—	—
Other nose trouble	—	—	—
Frequent sore throats with fever	—	—	—
Hoarse voice without a cold	—	—	—
Lumps or swelling in your neck	—	—	—
Seasonal eye, nose, or throat problem	—	—	—
Coughing spells	—	—	—
Frequent chest colds	—	—	—
Coughing up phlegm (mucus)	—	—	—
Coughing up blood	—	—	—
Breathing problems	—	—	—
An abnormal chest X ray	—	—	—
Shortness of breath	—	—	—
Awakening at night with shortness of breath	—	—	—
More pillows needed to help you breathe at night	—	—	—
Palpitations (thumping or racing heart)	—	—	—
Discomfort, pressure, a tight feeling, or pain in the chest	—	—	—
Heart murmur	—	—	—
Cramps in your legs while walking	—	—	—
Swollen feet or ankles	—	—	—
Painful whitening of fingertips when cold	—	—	—
Difficulty swallowing	—	—	—
Frequent or severe heartburn	—	—	—
Frequent or severe indigestion	—	—	—
Frequent or severe belching	—	—	—
Bloating after meals	—	—	—
Gas	—	—	—
Nausea or vomiting (frequent or new)	—	—	—
Vomiting blood or black material	—	—	—

	No	Yes	?
Pain in your abdomen (belly)	—	—	—
Long-standing constipation	—	—	—
Recent onset of constipation	—	—	—
Frequent, loose, or watery bowel movements	—	—	—
Recent change in bowel movements (BMs)	—	—	—
Black or bloody BMs, except after taking spinach, beets, iron, or Pepto-Bismol	—	—	—
Gray or pale tan BMs	—	—	—
Bleeding from rectum	—	—	—
Rectal pain	—	—	—
Recurring severe headaches	—	—	—
Dizzy spells or lightheadedness	—	—	—
Fainting or blackout spells	—	—	—
Slurred speech, loss of speech	—	—	—
Trouble with memory	—	—	—
Coordination or balance problems	—	—	—
Repeated numbness or tingling in hands or feet	—	—	—
Hands shaking or trembling	—	—	—
Recent change in handwriting	—	—	—
Weakness in muscles	—	—	—
Aching muscles or joints	—	—	—
Swollen or stiff joints	—	—	—
Lasting or repeated back or shoulder pain	—	—	—
Painful feet	—	—	—
Any handicap or disability	—	—	—
A persistent skin problem	—	—	—
A mole that bleeds or has changed size or color	—	—	—
Any lumps, bumps, or swellings	—	—	—
X ray or radioactive medicine used for treatment (not for diagnosis)	—	—	—
A tendency to feel too hot	—	—	—
A tendency to feel too cold	—	—	—
Increased thirst or appetite	—	—	—
Loss of interest in eating	—	—	—
Weight loss over 10 pounds in past year	—	—	—

Do you have now, or have you ever had? No Yes ?

Weight gain over 10 pounds in last year   — — —

Tiredness without effort   — — —

Change in personality or behavior   — — —

A big change in sexual activity   — — —

Any sexual problem you want to discuss with the doctor   — — —

Inability to have children (that you see as a problem)   — — —

Many urinations, day or night   — — —

Burning when you urinate   — — —

Bloody, black, or brown urine   — — —

Difficulty holding your urine in   — — —

Constant feeling you have to urinate   — — —

Urinary infections or stones   — — —

For Men Only

A weak or slow urinary stream   — — —

Told of prostate problem by a doctor   — — —

Burning or discharge from penis   — — —

Swelling, lumps, or pain in your testicles   — — —

Feeling that you are losing your sex drive, potency, or nature   — — —

Any contraception used by you or your partner   — — —

For Women Only

Lump in breast   — — —

Discharge or bleeding from either nipple   — — —

No Yes ?

Persistent or severe vaginal discharge or itch   — — —

Recent trouble with menstrual periods   — — —

Apart from pregnancy, nursing, or menopause, have you ever gone more than 6 months without a period?   — — —

Bleeding between periods   — — —

Any bleeding after intercourse   — — —

Repeated pain during intercourse   — — —

Bloating or irritability before periods   — — —

If your periods have stopped, any bleeding since   — — —

Hot flashes   — — —

Are you pregnant or do you think you might be   — — —

Any ectopic (tubal) pregnancies   — — —

Any other serious or disabling female problems   — — —

If you are still menstruating, is any contraceptive being used by you or your partner?   — — —

If still menstruating, date of last menstrual period ____

Number of pregnancies _____ Miscarriages _____ Stillbirths _____

Induced abortions ____ Premature births ____

Number of children born alive ____

Number of Caesarian sections ____

Weight of your largest baby _____ Complications of pregnancy:
   (hemorrhage, toxemia, etc.) _____

I. Personal Reactions and Expectations

   1. Are there any additional experiences or reactions that you have had with illness, hospitals, doctors, etc. that you would like to describe. (Use other side if more space is required.) _____

_____

_____

   2. Looking to the next few years, what are the things that you are planning for and would like to see happen?

_____

_____

   3. What do you expect your health in the future will be? ☐ excellent ☐ good ☐ fair ☐ poor

4. What medical conditions do you think you'll get and at what age? _____

5. What illnesses are you most afraid of getting? _____

6. To what age do you expect to live? _____ years old.

7. I am interested in your thoughts and feelings about your present illness. What do you imagine is wrong with you? If you do not know, please guess. _____

8. Is there anything else you want to talk over with the doctor? _____

J. Problem List

Date list completed _____ updated _____

Current Problems

_____
_____
_____
_____
_____
_____
_____
_____

Past Problems

_____
_____
_____
_____
_____
_____
_____
_____

Potential Problems

_____
_____
_____
_____

K. Physical Examination

Name _____ Date _____ General description:

Weight _____ Height _____

BP right, supine _____ standing _____ left, standing _____

Pulse _____ Respirations _____ Temperature _____

Skin

    turgor/texture

    color/rash

    palms

    nails

    hair

HEENT

    eyes

    fundi

    ears

    nose

    pharynx

    teeth

    sinuses

Neck JVP   HJ
    bruit   carotid
           vertebral

    thyroid

Lymph Nodes

Breasts

Lungs

    inspection

    palpation

    percussion

    auscultation

Heart   0° 45° 90° LLD

    inspection

    palpation

    percussion

    S1 S2 gallop

    murmur

Abdomen

    bowel sounds

    liver

    spleen

    masses

    tenderness

    hernia

    rectal

    genitalia

    CVA tenderness

Extremities

    edema

    color

    temperature

    tenderness

    peripheral pulses

	Femoral	Popliteal	Posterior Tibial	Dorsalis Pedis
Right	/4	/4	/4	/4
Left	/4	/4	/4	/4

Neurologic

    cranial

    power

    DTRs   /4 return phase

    Babinski

    sensory
       position   touch
       pain   temperature

Rheumatologic

    hands

    elbows

    shoulders

    neck

back

hips

knees

ankles

feet

Explanatory Note: In the first line under heart examination, "0" refers to the patient lying recumbent, "45" to a 45-degree elevation of the top half of his body, and "LLD" to the left lateral decubitus position. Under the neck examination, "JVP" means jugular venous pressure and "HJ" means hepatojugular reflux.

L.   Summary

Date _____

_____ year old _____ of _____ stock,
age   race, sex   country, religion

_____ x _____ years, (ret) _____
marital status   job

referred by _____.

Initial Contacts _____

PT Requests   Q all/most/part
   extra info

                                         ROS + −
Central Core Complaints Issues
                                         DPI relationships

Sources of frustration,   Mental Status
breakdown, disenchantment
                                            Appearance, interview behavior

Ability to handle frustration   Mood
Ways of recovering, healing
and gaining satisfaction
                                         Thought, Stream of content

                                         Attention, orientation,
                                         memory, and comprehension

                                         Insights

                                         Heroes

                                         Goals

Explanatory Notes: This summary section is a brief encapsulation of the physician's understanding of the patient's illness. It may be placed on the front page of the patient's case record.

The categories after "Q" indicate to the physician how much of the questionnaire was filled out by the patient. This helps the physician determine what the patient wants from the encounter. The marks after "ROS" indicate whether that material was obtained. The physician uses that response to assure himself that the basic nuts and bolts of the total history have been obtained so he can refer to them later. Knowing that this material is already available may help him to proceed to the real issues that are of concern to the patient. "DPI relationships" refers to doctor-patient-illness relationships (Balint, 1957).

Under DPI, Dr. Banner might put a statement related to how the relationship between the doctor and the patient might affect the illness, or vice versa. For example, he might mention that the patient keeps showing up at prison sick call complaining of incapacitating headache, asking for narcotics. This behavior frustrates the doctor, who is attempting to relate to the patient as a physician but finds that he is being used as a flak catcher for the penal system.

Others might wish to use a different format, for example, making diagnoses at three levels, called medical, psychologic, and social. The medical might be the chart diagnosis (in a category that will satisfy the third party payer); the psychologic could be the patient's major ego defense or characterologic style; and the social might include anything from a list of measures available for social support to complicated analyses of interactions with the environment, which includes the doctor.

Comments

Reliability

Early in the case record, the examiner is asked to comment on the reliability of the informant. As discussed in Chapter 2, no patient should ever be described as a "poor historian."

If the interviewer has noticed that the patient has trouble remembering events, and if the physician has performed the cognitive portion of the mental status examination, as described in Chapter 2 (p. 18), and if, in fact, the patient is cognitively impaired, then it is fair to conclude that the patient either has retardation or an acute or chronic organic brain syndrome.

(Unfortunately, the cognitive portion of the mental status examination is performed by asking questions without touching or inspecting the patient's body. Therefore, some tyros omit this section of the neurologic examination from their physical examination, believing it to be part of the interview. Whatever the reason, this extremely important part of the physical examination is the part most frequently missing from the record.)

Examples:

"Reliability: the patient was a pleasant man who attempted to cooperate, but who was disoriented for time (missing the day and month, but not the year)."

"Reliability: the patient is disoriented to time but not to person or place. Most of the history of the present illness was obtained from his landlady. History of prior illness comes from our inpatient records, but the outpatient records were not available at the time of admission."

In the case of the comatose patient, the informant will be a person other than the patient. The informant's name and relationship to the patient, as well as the duration and frequency of contact with the patient, should be indicated in the upper right-hand corner of the first page of the case report.

Examples:

"The informant is the patient's consort, who has lived with her for 2 years."

"The informant is the patient's son, who had not seen the patient for 4 years up until the day of admission."

"The informant is a policeman who discovered the patient in the hallway."

At times, the old record may be the only source material for the history. In this instance, the informant statement might read: "Patient brought in by the police, who know nothing about him. The only historical material available is from our old inpatient records."

Abbreviations

Although some schoolmarms have attempted to drive abbreviations out of the medical record, human nature remains unchanged. Some institutions even have standing committees to designate certain abbreviations as acceptable, but their pronouncements are heeded about as well as those of the schoolmarms who preceded them.

Unless your preceptor has strong opinions, I would suggest the following: use abbreviations only when the context renders the abbreviation totally unambiguous.

Example of an acceptable abbreviation:

"The patient was treated with iv MS in 2-mg doses to a total of 12 mg in the first hour." Here, MS obviously means morphine sulfate.

Example of an unacceptable abbreviation:

"In 1986, he was told that he had a mild case of MS." In this context, the abbreviation is ambiguous, as it could mean either mitral stenosis or multiple sclerosis.

Chief Complaint

The chief complaint is discovered in the course of the interview (see p. 34), and is not necessarily the complaint that was written on the ER sheet by the nurse. Nor is it necessarily the first problem that the patient mentions. Some discussion may be required to elicit the problem that is really bothering the patient most.

The chief complaint is singular. On very rare occasions, one may wish to list two separate chief complaints. In such situations, one is also obligated to produce two separate histories of present illnesses, one to match each of the chief complaints. An exception to this rule is the presence of two symptoms that invariably accompany each other, such as polyuria and polydipsia, or nausea and vomiting.

Examples of two separate chief complaints:

1. "My arthritis has come back" (1 month duration).
2. "I have been drinking an awful lot of water and getting up five times a night to pee" (7 months duration).

In this example, the examiner had discovered, on review of systems, a second pair of problems that suggested one of the types of diabetes, with no apparent relationship to the patient's rheumatic complaints. Instead of making two chief complaints, the physician could have made the new, more exciting endocrine problem the chief complaint, and placed an asterisk beside the rheumatic problem in the past medical history section. (An asterisk beside an entry in the case record means that the problem will be dealt with in the "impressions" or the summary section, or in the case of the experienced physician, on the order sheet.)

Note that in the Weed "problem-oriented" system, it is usual to have multiple "problems" derived from patient complaints, each of which is supposed to have its own "SOAP" (subjective, objective, assessment, plan) in the record, though this requirement is usually honored by omission. Since those who are inept at preparing the traditional medical record are just as incompetent at operating the Weed system, we will not discuss it further.

The phrase "rule out" should never be used in a chief complaint, as in "the patient was admitted to rule out myocardial infarction." First, this type of statement does not give the patient's own description of his illness. Second, it puts the historian (the physician) in a logical dilemma. If he diagnoses a myocardial infarction, he has succeeded in making a diagnosis by failing at the appointed task of ruling it out. On the other hand, if he succeeds in that task, he has failed to make a diagnosis. Yet the patient still has chest pain or some other symptom. It is hardly desirable to send the patient home with nothing more than the negative statement, "You didn't have a heart attack."

Sometimes patients are referred into the hospital by their physician, and really do not know the reason. Sometimes they think they know and are mistaken; this can lead to interpersonal difficulties later in the hospitalization. It is a good idea to ask such patients, "Why do you think Dr. Jones sent you to the hospital?" A good follow-up question is, "Did he ever actually say that?"

Even patients who are in the hospital because of a doctor's request deserve to have a chief complaint, which should be stated in specific terms that indicate the level of certainty. For example: "The patient is admitted at the request of the cardiology service for elective coronary angiography." Such a statement of high certitude would be based either on a conversation with one of the cardiologists, or on a letter brought by the patient. An example of a still useful statement with a lesser degree of specificity and certitude is this: "Her local physician referred her to this institution to have her "gland problem" evaluated by Dr. Smith."

If you have not spoken to any of the referring physicians, do not assume that the "patient is here to get her digoxin and Lasix adjusted" on the basis of her flagrant signs of congestive heart failure. In reality, the patient might have high output heart failure due to masked thyrotoxicosis, and actually have been referred to the endocrinology service for definitive therapy (see Rodnan's Aphorism, p. 48).

The worst type of chief complaint is one that uses contemporary medical jargon without giving either the problem or the level of uncertainty. For instance, one medical resident's note said, "Patient admitted for tune-up." To say that this description would be more appropriate to the care of an automobile than of a human being would be unfair to automobile mechanics, who usually ask the customer what problem he has noticed.

History of the Present Illness (HPI)

Chronology

When composing the HPI, one wishes to tell the story in chronologic fashion. In order to avoid confusing the reader or listener, one of two available chronologic systems should be chosen, and used consistently. In the first system, all events are related to the time of admission.

For example:

"The history of the present illness began approximately 10 years prior to admission . . . (or PTA)."
    "However, 4 years prior to admission . . ."
    "Two months prior to admission . . ."
    "Three days prior to admission . . ."
    "A fever began 10 hours prior to admission, continuing up to 2 hours prior to admission, when . . ."
    "Forty-five minutes prior to admission . . ."
    ". . . 15 minutes prior to admission, when his wife decided to bring him to the emergency room."

The second system uses calendar dates. With this method, the history of present illness might proceed as follows:

". . . began in 1959."
    ". . . recurred in the fall of 1968 and continued into the next summer."
    In 1972, the patient first noticed . . ."
    "In February of 1980 . . ."
    "In March of 1981 . . ."
    "June 6, 1981, the patient first noticed . . ."
    "June 16th, the patient was admitted to the emergency room, kept for 6 hours, and discharged. At that time, . . ."
    "June 24, 1981, at 12 noon . . ."
    "Around 4:00, the patient noticed that . . ."
    "At 6:15 p.m., his wife insisted on bringing him to the emergency room. When he arrived at 6:45, he had no palpable pulses in his legs . . ."

The first system has the advantage for the listener or reader of being easier to follow. The calendar system has the advantage of placing the patient's history in its broader historical context, in terms of what diagnoses and treatment were available in that epoch, and may be more useful for longer histories. Also, the person who reviews the record several years later will not have to translate the times into a different reference system.

Pertinent Positives and Negatives

After the chronologic account of the present illness, there is sometimes an extra paragraph involving pertinent negative facts and/or positive facts that bear upon the history of the present illness. The emphasis on the word "pertinent" warns that this section is not to be an assortment of potentially interesting but possibly irrelevant facts that you could not build into the history of the present illness. (Such an assortment would only detract from the review of systems and confuse the auditor or reader who might just have been on the verge of arriving at a diagnosis.) In fact, most well-organized histories do not need a final statement of additional pertinent positives and negatives.

Some epidemiologic cardiologists enjoy the recitation of their favorite coronary risk factors. Some pulmonologists wish the presenter to produce at this point the date of the last chest film and a summary of its findings. Some infectious disease specialists want the presenter to give the results of the cultures drawn at the referring hospital (or the lack of same). If you have tried but really can't think of any pertinent positives, don't worry about it. They are probably unnecessary in that particular case.

Recently, the patient's drug regimen seems to have migrated

to the pertinent positives section, where it does not belong. See the section on past medical history, below.

Pertinent negatives are absent factors, which, had they been present, would have suggested another diagnosis. For example, a normal recent chest film might cause the presenter to doubt the diagnosis of tuberculosis. "The patient has never smoked" suggests the presenter's belief that the patient probably does not have bronchogenic carcinoma. "There has been no weight loss" is probably the most common pertinent negative. If the diagnosis of coronary artery disease is not completely clear, one might wish to include information suggesting that the cause of the chest pain was not something else, such as a hiatal hernia ("an upper gastrointestinal series was normal during the last admission"); pulmonary embolism ("no history of thrombophlebitis"); dissecting aneurysm ("no history of hypertension"); or costochondritis ("no tenderness to palpation of the costochondral junctions could be elicited during any of the last three admissions").

Pertinent positives and negatives of the type given above are global and almost matters of taste. However, more discrete pertinent positives and negatives are in common use. An example of a discrete pertinent positive is: "Four other persons attending the wedding were said to have been afflicted with a similar illness. Food served at the wedding dinner is currently being analyzed for Staphylotoxin A by the State Laboratories." (Of course, this information might just as well be incorporated into the narrative of the present illness, rather than be segregated as a pertinent positive.)

O   **Rule**: *Use pertinent positives and negatives only when they are relevant to items in your differential diagnosis.*

Information Obtained from Chart Review

In the better contemporary courses in clinical examination, the sophomore students are prohibited from reading the patient's chart until they have produced their own case record. While pedagogically valuable, this prohibition does impair the quality of the historical information available. In the usual clinical situation, one is obliged to read all of the old case records and to obtain copies of same from other hospitals as soon as it is humanly possible. In all instances, one must evaluate the information thus obtained in a critical manner, as explained in Chapter 3, and indicate its level of certainty.

Including Diagnoses in the Case Report

You may include the previous diagnostic conclusions of other physicians in the case report, with the caveats given in Chapter 3. However, you may not include your own diagnostic conclusions in the body of the history or physical report, no matter how high the level of certainty may be. The proper place to enter your conclusion is in the "impression" or on the list of differential diagnoses. To use it in the history would be circular reasoning. Thus, the tradition of the case record may be seen as an implied attempt to invoke the rules of logic at a clinical level.

Advice to the sophomore. Ordinarily, we attempt to perpetrate the fiction that the sophomore student saw the patient at the time and date of admission. This gives the student the opportunity to compare his case write-up with that of a more experienced person who saw the patient at the time of admission.

However, the patients selected for the student examination have generally been in the hospital for some time and in the course of a good interview will mention to the student potentially significant events that have happened during hospitalization. There are no hard-and-fast rules, but the general principle of intellectual honesty applies: any such postadmission information used in reaching your diagnostic conclusions or ordering your differential diagnoses should be mentioned, even if the patient volunteered it. For the neophyte, such unsolicited extra data could be entered into the history of present illness under a special section of unsolicited pertinent information (pertinent positives or negatives).

Expressions to Avoid

Two statements, rapidly becoming ubiquitous, that should never appear in a case write-up are "the patient stated" and "the patient denied." The former is a wasteful redundancy. Unless some other informant is being used, the entire history can usually be assumed to be stated by the patient. The second phrase is used in place of "there was no . . . ," but does not mean the same thing. In order for a patient to deny a statement, it must be true, and the patient must have some important unspoken reason for saying it is false. Of course the term "denial" also implies that the doctor knows what is true and what is not, in which case it is unclear why he is asking the patient questions to which the doctor already knows the answers. Worse, the term is better suited to an interrogation than to an interview, and hints at an adversarial relationship between doctor and patient (see Ch. 2, p. 13).

If the patient says he did not have a seizure, whereas in fact he had one but cannot remember it, his statement is not really a denial. If the doctor, whether at the bedside or in the case record (which is more and more frequently being read by patients), characterizes something told him in confidence as something that was "denied," imagine what the patient might think about that term were he to read the record. The implication is that the patient was lying.

Past Medical History

O   As a general guide to what goes in the past medical history, recall that this section is concerned with diseases and illnesses, whereas the review of systems is about symptoms.

Immunizations

The immunization record should be kept in a section of the chart where it is available for updating as the patient receives new immunizations. The date, dose, and source of the immunization should be listed for each (e.g., "Influenza: 1979, Cutter Labs split virus, triple vaccine, lot number _____, 0.5 cc, right deltoid"). For previous immunizations, one need only indicate their presence or absence, although a date is desirable, especially for tetanus toxoid. For children, precise dates are required, as the time of the vaccine may be important. For example, measles immunizations need to be repeated if the vaccine was given at an age less than 15 months, or before 1967 (when inactivated vaccine was used). For patients who engage in foreign travel, one should also indicate their status of immunization against yellow fever and cholera (e.g. "yellow fever +, cholera +, 1969 prior to Peace Corps trip"). For patients with special risk factors, particular attention should be paid to their immune status against rubella (women of childbearing age), pneumococcus (patients who have undergone splenectomy), hepatitis B (persons frequently exposed), and so on.

If you are having office forms printed up, be sure to leave sufficient space, as new vaccines are being introduced with some regularity.

Hospitalizations

In recording hospitalizations within the past medical history, it is important that one obtain the dates, location, and service. A wise physician has his office nurse prepare release forms that the patient should sign before leaving the office the first time. In the hospital, the same rule applies *mutatis mutandis*. For hospitals outside the city, it may be necessary to obtain addresses and postal (zip) codes. This "administrative" information about how to obtain the old records is valuable and often difficult to acquire. Therefore, it should be prominently placed in the medical record. Dr. John Bass of Alabama, stated that the most frequent and important service provided by his Pulmonary Division was not bronchoscopy but the retrieval and review of the patients' old records.

Drugs

The patient's medications should be listed in the past medical history, unless there was a good reason for mentioning a specific drug in the history of the present illness (e.g., digoxin in a patient with arrhythmia). (Include only the relevant drugs in the history of the present illness. If a patient is admitted for a cardiac complaint, the allopurinol for gout, the benzodiazepine for insomnia, and the estrogen for menopause all probably belong in the past medical history.)

Social History

The student should refer to Chapter 3 (p. 44) and the outlines for the information that should be included in a complete social history. Psychosocial data may be included here, or in the psychologic portion of the mental status examination, as you choose; however, you should be consistent, and the other persons in your practice should know where to find this information. (They may be obliged to give the patient bad news in your absence.) As a minimum, I consider it essential to have some notation about what the patient's most traumatic prior experience was, and how he reacted to it.

O   For sensitive information, you may wish to develop your own private coding system because the charts are increasingly available to persons outside the physician-patient dyad, and because physicians are increasingly hired by third parties. For example, I do not clearly enter material about sexual orientation in the case record, but rather write a heading word to the left for heterosexual, the right for homosexual, in the middle for bisexual, and in small letters for pedophilia.

Review of Systems

For recording the review of systems, it is particularly helpful to have a printed form that contains the questions that you usually ask, such as the one given in Banner's outline.

A diagnosis that can sometimes be made from taking the review of systems is a form of hysteria called De Briquet's syndrome (see the section on the mental status examination in Ch. 26). This diagnosis is based on finding 25 different symptoms in 9 of 10 symptoms, which had their onset before midlife and have no known medical explanation. This is a rather stable entity afflicting about 1% of the female population, so it is rather important that one be able to recognize it.

If a patient has many hospitalizations or illnesses, it is likely that much of the review of systems will have been "prerecorded." It is legitimate to refer to available portions of the old chart, including previous accounts of what was then the "present illness," but is now "past history." If one elects not to replicate the entire review, one should at least update it by doing an interim review of systems to see what formerly negative findings may have become positive. The rule is to save space and avoid redundancy, but to be sure that all the information is timely and present somewhere in the record.

Physical Examination

The student who is reading this work in sequence, without having performed any portion of the physical examination, would do well to skip through the pages of this chapter having to do with recording the physical examination.

However, don't forget to come back to this section as you begin to perform the physical examination. By the time you are handing in written case records to your preceptor, you should have read this chapter at least once. To get the most out of it, it will probably be necessary for you to work through it twice during your first year of doing case records: before and after studying the chapters on the various parts of the examination. Don't be discouraged if it seems a bit overwhelming at first.

This section presents "a method." If your preceptor or institution has strong feelings about some point, remember that, as in baseball, local ground rules are very important.

Vital Signs

Blood Pressure

The blood pressure notation should give the systolic pressure, the point at which the Korotkoff sounds become muffled, and the point at which they disappear, as follows: 140/92/85. Often the muffling cannot be detected, in which case one can record: 140/ /88.

One should state the extremity and the position in which the pressure was determined (e.g., LUE [left upper extremity], LA [left arm]); RL [right leg]). Lower extremity blood pressures will always be taken with the patient recumbent. However, for upper extremity blood pressures, one should say "recumbent," "sitting," or "standing," or draw stick figures. For recumbent as opposed to erect, two arrows would suffice: LA $\rightarrow$ 140/ /80, $\uparrow$ 90/ /50.

In some unstable patients, and others, it will not be possible to determine the blood pressure by auscultation. In that case, one should determine the systolic pressure by palpation. (There is a technique for determining diastolic pressure by palpation, but it usually doesn't work in unstable patients. See Ch. 6, p. 87.) Record such a pressure thus: BP LA recumbent inaudible, 90/? by palpation (*not* "90/palp" or "90 over palp").

It may be advisable to add the units mm Hg because there is an increasing tendency to express the pressure in kilopascals, millibars, newtons/m2, and other exotic units. Past workers have also published pressures expressed in cm Hg.

Pulsus Paradoxus

Pulsus paradoxus refers to a decrease in systolic blood pressure with inspiration. As is pointed out in Chapter 6, some inspiratory decrease is normal. The optimum way to record the observation in the case record is this: "pulsus paradoxus of _____ mm Hg." This shows that pulsus paradoxus of normal degree was actually sought, and gives the careful reader the opportunity to apply his own criteria (10 mm Hg or 10% of the expiratory systolic pressure) to the observation. The more common practice of noting pulsus paradoxus only if "present" and not if "absent" requires the reader to perform two separate acts of faith.

Respirations

Both the rate and character of the respirations should be described (e.g., 24 per minute and grunting; 13 per minute, regular and easy; 7 to 10 per minute and regularly irregular [Cheyne-Stokes]).

Skin

If there is a rash or an eruption, it must be described sufficiently to permit an expert dermatologist to make a diagnosis. The points to be included are these:

1. Is it macular, papular, herpetic, bullous? (A spot that is flat is called a macule. A lesion that is raised is called a papule. The differential diagnosis is completely different. If there are multiple lesions, some macular and some papular, the eruption would be described as maculopapular. There is no such thing as a single "maculopapular" lesion.)
2. Where is it located? If the distribution is uneven, where does it predominate? For example, is it palmar, or centripetal?
3. Describe an individual lesion. If it is a papule, does it have a white head, a black head, or no perceptible head? Is it surrounded by a halo? If there is a halo or any other type of border phenomenon, is the border sharp or gradual, smooth or serpiginous?
4. If possible, take a photograph or draw a diagram to include in the progress notes. At least provide a word picture indicating the most outstanding characteristics of the lesion even (or especially) if they are not listed here. For instance, some macules blanch on pressure, even though we would not describe other skin lesions in such a dimension. Nikolsy's sign and Koebner's phenomenon are other examples (see Ch. 7, p. 121).
5. The description must be sufficiently clear and detailed to provide a baseline for future progress notes. Sometimes one later observes a change in a dimension not initially described. It is permissible to add to your baseline description in another color ink, dating the addition.

An additional reason for describing skin lesions as precisely as possible is that a patient may develop a different eruption during his hospital stay. Consultants have sometimes been misled by assuming that the patient's rash was a recurrence of a previous one, rather than a new manifestation. This issue becomes increasingly important in teaching hospitals where members of the "team" change very frequently.

Lymph Nodes

A homunculus may be stamped in the record for showing the position and size of lymph nodes (Fig. 4-1).

Eyes

Describing Nystagmus

Some authors name nystagmus for the direction of gaze in which the nystagmus appears. Others name it for the quick return component. Since the former system will not work for fixation nystagmus and the latter will not work for pendular nystagmus, the method should be specified as part of the case report (e.g., "horizontal nystagmus on gaze to the right, quick component to the right" or "primary position vertical nystagmus, quick component down").

Diminution in optokinetic nystagmus is described in the record as being from that side of the patient in which the drum (or tape) was being rotated when the defective response was found. This is also the same side from which the slow initial phase of nystagmus moved, and the side towards which the rapid jerk recovery component was aimed. This is only an elementary description of optokinetic nystagmus. For a more advanced discussion, see Chapter 10 (p. 161) and Chapter 26 (p. 480).

Ears

A normal Rinne and Weber test would be described as follows: "AC > BC bilat. Weber midline." This "normal" finding can also be seen in bilateral partial sensorineural deafness. This il-

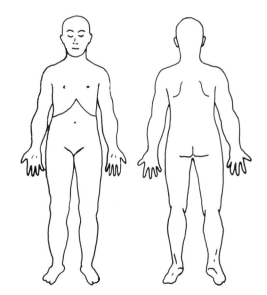

Figure 4-1. *Diagrams that may be stamped in the progress notes to record serial examinations of the lymph nodes. Courtesy of Dr. David Clarkson of Alabama.*

lustrates the point that one should never make an entry "normal" in the history and physical portion of the chart; "normal" is, after all, a conclusion from the data, not the actual data.

Auscultation of the Lungs

A diagram of the anterior and posterior aspects of the chest (see p. 275), is helpful for indicating the region in which findings are ausculted. For describing the breath sounds, an inverted "V" has traditionally been used. Inspiration is always shown on the left and expiration on the right. The relative duration of the phases may be demonstrated by altering the lengths of the two wings of the V (Fig. 4-2).

An Alternate Method

For adventitious sounds, Forgacs introduced the system of notation shown in Figure 4-3 (Forgacs, 1969). To understand his notation, you need to understand something about pathophysiology. After you have read the section on auscultation in the chest chapter, come back to this figure and identify the significance of each of these auscultatory patterns, before reading the correct answers, which appear in Appendix 4-1. Please note that there are at least two answers for the last pattern.

Auscultation of the Heart

Heart Sounds

In Chapter 17, you will learn how much information can be obtained from observing the intensity of the heart sounds and the

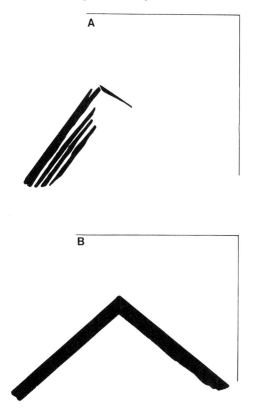

Figure 4-2. *One notation for breath sounds. The upslope of the inverted "V" represents inspiration, the downslope represents expiration. A, Soft (vesicular) breath sounds; B, loud tubular breath sounds.*

pattern of splitting of the second heart sound. It is important to record these observations. If the first heart sound (S1) is not louder than the second (S2) at the apex, or the first heart sound is not of a constant intensity, the finding is of great pathophysiologic significance. Most of the time these abnormalities are absent; the fact that they were sought and not observed should also be noted, by stating "S1 > S2 and constant."

The second heart sound splits into a pulmonic and an aortic component, P2 and A2, respectively (see pp. 293–297). Please note that P2 is not the total intensity of the second heart sound as heard in the pulmonic area, and A2 is not the total intensity of the second heart sound in the aortic area. (If one wished to record those, although such information is not at the optimal level of sophistication, they would be denoted "S2 at the pulmonic area" and "S2 at the aortic area," respectively.)

Most subjects have no abnormality in the splitting of the second heart sounds, and the pulmonic component will not be louder than the aortic component. The examiner should then record: "S2 splits normally; A2 > P2." This statement implies that S2 splitting was detectable with inspiration (sometimes it is not), and that its components have been compared at the pulmonic area (or wherever the distinct components are best heard). In some normal situations, the aortic and pulmonic components are equal, and the second part of the statement would be modified: "A2 = P2."

Murmurs

Dimensions. It is imperative that any cardiac murmur be described in all of the appropriate dimensions:

1. Timing: Is the murmur systolic, diastolic, continuous, or to-and-fro? (See also the Rule of Two Diastoles below.)
2. Shape: Is it decrescendo, decrescendo-crescendo, diamond shaped, or holosystolic?
3. Location: Where is the murmur loudest?
4. Radiation: Where else may it be heard? And where is it not heard (e.g., axilla, right midclavicle)?
5. Pitch: Is it high, low, rumbling, or other?
6. Timbre: Is it coarse, musical, or other?
7. Intensity: How loud is it, on a scale of 1 to 6 (see Ch. 17, p. 303)?
8. Special maneuvers: What was the effect of standing, rolling into the left lateral decubitus, leaning forward, squatting, releasing a Valsalva maneuver, and so forth?

Some murmurs are unremarkable in terms of pitch or timbre, and if this is your judgment, so state it. But do not omit the statement "unremarkable" in favor of no statement at all.

Rule of Two Diastoles

It is convenient to assume the fiction that there are two diastoles for every systole: an early diastole and a late diastole. In the section on cardiac examination, we will emphasize the importance of listening to them one at a time. Early diastole (protodiastole) is heard immediately after the second heart sound; late diastole is presystole and is heard just before the first heart sound. The timing is of great diagnostic significance, and all diastolic murmurs, gallops, snaps, plops, knocks, clicks, and rubs should be described as occurring in early or late diastole.

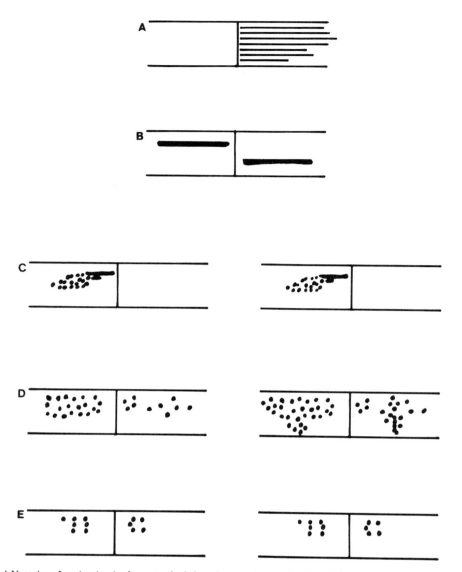

Figure 4-3.   *Forgacs' Notation. Inspiration is shown to the left and expiration to the right of the vertical bar. To indicate whether the events are recurring or random, show two sequential respirations, with either the same or different patterns. A, Expiratory polytonic wheeze; B, inspiratory and expiratory monotonic wheezes; C, end-inspiratory crackling and wheeze of recurrent pattern; D, inspiratory and expiratory crackling of random pattern; E, inspiratory and expiratory crackling of recurrent pattern.*

Vascular Examination

For grading the arterial pulses, there are several different systems. Some schools teach that the pulses should be graded so that 2 + is normal, 1 + is abnormal but palpable, and 0 is absent. Others teach that 3 + is normal, 4 + is bounding, 2 + is subnormal, and 1 + is palpable only after a careful search. Still other schools teach a system based on a scale of 0 to 6 + . Accordingly, it is important to note somewhere on the record which system is being used. Also, it is more important to find asymmetries than to obtain an exact gradation. Therefore, your recording system must have a place to indicate lateralization.

If your institution has no standard for gradation of pulses, I suggest the following:

0 = no palpable pulse found

+ / − = sometimes you don't feel it and sometimes you think you do. (Check your own pulse simultaneously and make sure it is not the pulse in your own fingers that you are feeling.)

1 + = you're sure that you can feel the pulse most of the time, but you would not be able to count it for a minute if the patient were in atrial fibrillation

2 + = you can feel the pulse all the time, but it seems weaker than your own

3 + = it feels like the pulse of a normal 25 year old

4 + = a bounding pulse that you expect to have a widened pulse pressure

Here is an example of a recorded examination of a male patient:

	R	L
Carotid	2/4	2 +
Subcl.	1 +	1 +
Brach.	3 +	3 +
Ulnar	1 +	1 +
Rad.	3 +	3 +

	R	L
Fem.	3 +	2 +
Pop.	1 +	0
DP	2 +	1 +
PT	2 +	1 +

The "2/4" notation for "carotid" indicates that the clinical grading scale ranges from 0 to 4. In this case it does not matter if the left posterior tibial (PT) is exactly as strong as the right ulnar or if the right dorsalis pedis (DP) is the same as the left carotid.

What we can see at a glance is that this patient needs some lower extremity blood pressure measurements, a DeWeese test (see Ch. 18, p. 351), careful auscultation of the left femoral, and detailed questioning about sexual potency and claudication of the buttock.

Joint Examination

A homunculus can be used to record serial examinations of the joints (Fig. 4-4).

Neurologic Examination

The cranial nerves are referred to by the appropriate Roman numerals. Deep tendon reflexes and the Babinski reflex may be recorded efficiently by means of a stick man (Fig. 4-5).

The phrase "decreased mental status" should never appear in the medical record. Persons who use this phrase to mean an impairment of cognitive function or an altered state of consciousness tend to forget that there are additional dimensions to the mental status examination. Once they omit proper recording of

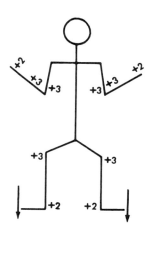

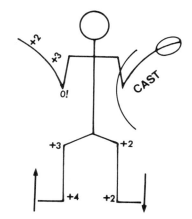

Figure 4-5. *A method of recording deep tendon reflexes and the Babinski reflexes.*

all dimensions, they soon omit the proper examination of these dimensions, and so fail to attend to the different types of disease that can be reflected in the examination. (This is a good example of an important and common semantic error, in Korzybski's true and correct sense of the term *semantic*: the study of meaning, connotative and denotative.)

Differential Diagnosis

The differential diagnosis is a list of alternate explanations for a given sign, symptom, or laboratory test, arranged in descending order of probability. Stated another way, it is a list of testable hypotheses. It is expected that one of the diagnoses on the list is the correct one, and that it can be established by specific laboratory tests or by excluding all the other items on the list.

It is possible to compose a differential diagnosis that explains not just one sign, symptom, or laboratory test, but multiple combinations of findings. However, the beginning student is advised to indicate formally which one finding is to be explained by each list. The use of differential diagnostic lists is explained more fully in the chapter on clinical reasoning (Ch. 27). For the present, let us simply point out some advantages of including the differential diagnosis in the case record.

The differential diagnosis structures the history of the present illness, and provides a guide for checking both the history and

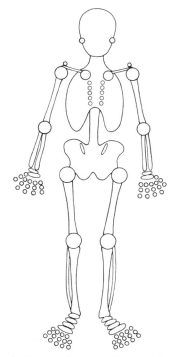

Figure 4-4. *A diagram for recording serial examinations of the joints. Reprinted from Polley and Hunder:* Rheumatologic Interviewing and Physical Examination of the Joints, *ed 2. With permission of WB Saunders.*

the physical examination for completeness. Much of the information pertinent to ranking the individual items in the differential diagnosis, or for excluding them, should be in the history of the present illness. The information may be in the chronologic section, or at the end in the pertinent positives and negatives. (In about 10% of the cases, the critical information will be derived from the physical examination rather than from the history of the present illness.)

Initially, the student will not know enough about diseases and medicine to utilize the differential diagnosis to its fullest capacity. However, it will serve him as a reading guide.

When I grade sophomore medical student papers, I begin by reading the chief complaint and history of present illness. As soon as I become confused, I skip all the way to the differential diagnosis, which should tell me what the student was thinking about when he composed his history.

The student is advised to spend a great deal of time developing the skill of composing an HPI that fits the differential diagnosis, with the aid of a preceptor. He should rewrite his histories of the present illness as many times as necessary, just as he rewrote essays in college composition classes. As with other skills, such as playing the piano, skiing, or fighting bulls (see epigram in Ch. 6), assiduous practice of the basic skills at the beginning will pay handsome dividends later.

For a skilled clinician, the interview itself contains a series of hypothesis tests concerning potential diagnoses.

In summary, the composed history of the present illness is a reflection of the implicit logic in the differential diagnosis. The ability to relate these topographically disparate portions of the case record is an acquired skill.

Acquired skills are learned through repetition.

Laboratory Data

At an earlier time, the only laboratory data that were initially entered into the case record were those that the medical student and house officer performed themselves. Thus, it was perfectly appropriate to give one's differential diagnosis and impressions right after the history and physical, and to use them as a guide to determine which diagnostic tests to perform. Times change.

More recently, I found an intern chastising a medical student for recording his impressions on the basis of "just" the history and physical. Only the laboratory tests were defined as "data" by this intern, even though they were either inappropriate or predictable from the clinical findings! This scene was a manifestation of the pecking order phenomenon, not of science.

Bedside Presentation

The student attending an institution without a tradition of bedside presentation can gather the essentials by reading the appropriate section in Morgan and Engel and using the form on page 34. Here we will point out a few basics.

First one should not read the case report at the bedside. The ability to present with at most a few notes is a sign that the student has taken sufficient time to organize his thoughts about the case in a coherent, logical manner. A poorly organized assortment of thoughts is difficult to remember.

Second, one wishes to avoid certain expressions at the bedside and substitute euphemisms. Syphilis is called lues or treponemes, cancer becomes mitotic activity, gonorrhea is referred to as Neisser's organism, and alcohol is called C_2H_5OH or two-carbon fragments. If one needs to intimate that there is pertinent information that cannot be discussed in front of the patient, one might say there is "concern about the number of eighth cranial nerve synapses at the present time." The thoughtful person is invited to invent his own euphemisms where necessary.

Also to be eschewed are "he pointed to" and "I asked him," which are redundant, and should be omitted. It is already assumed that the patient is the source of the information, unless another informant is named.

The general appearance section should be omitted during the bedside presentation unless it has changed since the original examination. Then one might say, for example, "He was as you see him now except that he was sitting straight up in bed, gasping for air."

Some are offended by the use of the terms "male" or "female." It is best to use "man" or "woman." Similarly, "black" is preferable to "Negro," although neither need be mentioned unless sickle cell disease or another race-related condition will be discussed. The correct adjective is "Jewish," not "Jew," although again the information is not pertinent unless Tay-Sachs or another disease occurring in Jews is to be a consideration. In that instance, one might need to proceed further and describe the patient as Ashkenazic or Sephardic.

Groups with wide phenotypic representation should not be grouped together, especially if they have experienced social repression. Swarthy Jews may not care to hear at the bedside that they are "Jewish appearing." An American who immigrated from Colombia may resent being called a Mexican. A nurse, who refers to herself as a Mexican (natal country), pointed out to me that older Mexicans often resent being called "chicanos," especially if female (the feminine form is *chicana*). Originally, the word was used as an insult by one group of Mexicans, who were in turn called *pochos* (faded, discolored) because they were losing their language and culture. The Spanish word *chicana* means "chicanery," and *chicanero* means "tricky" or "cunning" (Cuyás, 1940). The nurse was so offended to have the word "chicano" on her nursing license that she sent it back to the state capital to have it changed. Younger persons may not find the term objectionable. When you feel it is necessary to describe the patient's race or ethnic group, and are in doubt about the proper term, it is best to inquire of the patient. Common sense, courtesy, and *willingness to listen to the patient* are the main requirements for successfully handling sensitive issues.

Rules for the Attending
Conversing with a Resident About a Patient

1. Statements beginning with any of the following phrases are least likely to contain information useful in diagnosis and treatment:
    "They say that . . ."
    "I heard that you should . . ."
    "Omphalology (or the name of any other specialty) said . . ."
    "Dr. Smith said . . ."

"We were told . . ."

"It's taught that . . ."

"Because they say that you're always supposed to . . ."

And my all-time favorite: "My roommate is dating a cardiology fellow at St. Noodnik, and she said that he said . . ."

2. Statements beginning with any of the following phrases are highly likely to contain information useful to diagnosis and treatment:

"Because . . ."

"If you are willing to assume . . ."

"I saw . . ."

"I heard . . ."

"I found a . . ."

"The nurse noticed . . ."

"I thought so too, but when we measured it . . ."

Appendix 4-1. Forgacs Notation: Pathophysiologic Explanations

The sounds diagrammed in Figure 4-3 can be explained as follows:

1. Expiratory polytonic (polyphonic) wheezing is due to expiratory collapse of the lobar bronchi in diffuse airway obstruction.

2. The inspiratory and expiratory monotonic pair of wheezes is due to a single rigid airway narrowed to the point of closure.

3. Recurrent end inspiratory crackling and/or a terminal inspiratory wheeze, alone or together, are due to the delayed opening of small airways in deflated territories of the lung.

4. Inspiratory and expiratory crackling of random pattern is due to the inspiratory and expiratory gurgling of liquid in airways.

5. Inspiratory crackling of recurrent pattern is due to the delayed inspiratory opening of small airways. The expiratory crackling of recurrent pattern is due to expiratory air trapping in deflating territories of the lung. Taken together they are either a combination of the above, or, according to Forgacs, they may be a sign of pleural friction.

References

Balint M: *The Doctor, His Patient and the Illness*. International Universities Press, New York, 1957.

Cuyás A: *Appleton's New English-Spanish, Spanish-English Dictionary*. Appleton-Century-Crofts, New York, 1940.

Forgacs P: Lung sounds. *Br J Dis Chest* 63:1–12, 1969.

Appendix 4-2. A Spanish-English Case Record

The patient may be asked to fill out the form prior to the visit. The English terms are technical for brevity, the Spanish idiomatic.

Historia Médica

Información sobre su salud previa es muy importante para el doctor. Por favor conteste las siguientes preguntas antes de ver al doctor. Indique (√) bajo sí o no.

Fecha _____ (Date)

Nombre _____ (Name) Edad _____ (Age)

¿Qué clase de trabajo hace? _____ (Occupation)

Estado civil: casado, soltero, divorciado, viudo (M, S, D, W)

¿Cuántos hijos tiene? _____ (No. children)

¿Cuánto fuma? _____ (Amt. smoked)

¿Cuánto alcohol toma? _____ (Amt. alcohol)

Enfermedades en su familia: (Illnesses in your family)

    Padre: _____ (Father)

    Madre: _____ (Mother)

    Hermanos: _____ (Siblings)

    Hijos: _____ (Children)

    Otros: _____ (Others)

Alérgias: sí   no

penicilina   —   —   (penicillin)

otras drogas   —   —   ¿Cuáles? _____ (other drugs)

comidas   — —   ¿Cuáles? _____ (foods)

¿Qué medicinas toma ahora? (Current medications) _____

_____

Indique (√) si ha tomado algunas de estas medicinas:
(Have you ever taken . . . ?)

___ píldoras anticonceptiva   ___ anticoagulantes ___ diuréticos
    (oral contraceptives)   (anticoagulant) ___ (diuretics)

___ medicinas para el corazón   ___ medicinas para tuberculosis
    (heart medicine)   (drugs for tuberculosis)

___ medicinas para glaucoma   ___ calmante ___ cortisoma
    (glaucoma medicine)   (tranquilizers) ___ (cortisone)

Operaciónes: ¿Qué operaciónes ha tenido? _____

_____

_____

Accidentes o heridas: _____ (injuries)

Otras hospitalizaciónes (no incluyan embarazos normales)
(Approx. date and reason for hospitalization, excluding normal deliveries)

Fecha (approximativa)   Causa

_____   _____

_____   _____

_____   _____

_____   _____

Inmunizaciónes: Fecha

tétanos   _____

polio   _____

sarampión (rubeola)   _____

sarampión de tres días (rubella) _____

papera (mumps)   _____

otras   _____

¿Cuáles son sus problemas ahora? (What are your problems now?)

_____

_____

_____

_____

_____

Salud General	Sí	No	General Health	Comments
Aumento o pérdida de peso recientemente	—	—	Weight change recently	
Fiebre, escalofríos, o sudor de la noche	—	—	Fever, chills, night sweats	
Pérdida de apetito	—	—	Anorexia	

Sistema Endocrina			Endocrine System	
Intolerancia al calor o al frío	—	—	Heat or cold intolerance	
Enfermedad de tiroides	—	—	Thyroid disease	
¿Ha tenido tratamientos de radiación en el cuello?	—	—	Neck irradiation	
¿Ha tenido diabetes, o azúcar en la orina?	—	—	Diabetes, glucosuria	
Historia de diabetes en la familia	—	—	Family history of diabetes	

Piel			Skin	
Rascazón	—	—	Itching	
Sarpullido	—	—	Rash	
¿Tiene lunares negros o marrónes que han cambiado?	—	—	Change in mole	

Musculoesqueletal			Musculoskeletal	
Dolor en las articuladiónes, o artritis	—	—	Joint pain	
Hinchazón en las articuladiónes	—	—	Joint swelling	
Tiesura por la mañana	—	—	Morning stiffness	

Ojos			Eyes	
Cambio de su visión	—	—	Change in vision	
Halo alrededor de luces	—	—	Halos around lights	
Otros síntomas	—	—	Other symptoms	

Otorrhinolaringológia			ENT	
Pérdida de oído	—	—	Loss of hearing	
Zumbidos del oído	—	—	Tinnitus	
Hemorragia nasal	—	—	Nosebleed	
Ronquera, cambio de voz	—	—	Hoarseness	
Vértigo, o sensación de dar vueltas; mareo	—	—	Vertigo	

	Sí	No		Comments
Sistema Respiratorio			*Respiratory System*	
Resuello, asma, jadeo	—	—	Wheezing, asthma	
Tos	—	—	Cough	
¿Al toser, escupe?	—	—	Sputum	
¿Ha sido expuesto a tuber-culosis	—	—	Tuberculosis exposure	
¿Ha tenido prueba de la piel para tuberculosis?	—	—	PPD done?	
¿Fué positiva la prueba de la piel?	—	—	PPD positive?	
¿Ha escupido sangre?	—	—	Hemoptysis	
Radiografía del pecho anormal	—	—	Abnormal chest film	
Corazón y Circulatión			*Cardiovascular*	
¿Respira con dificuldad?	—	—	Dyspnea	
¿Tiene que sentarse por la noche para poder respirar?	—	—	Paroxysmal noctural dyspnea	
Palpitación de corazón	—	—	Palpitations	
¿Se desmaya?	—	—	Syncope	
Hinchazón de las piernas o los tobillos	—	—	Pedal edema	
Dolor en las piernas al andar	—	—	Claudication	
Fiebre reumática	—	—	Rheumatic fever	
Coágulo de la sangre	—	—	Blood clots	
Murmullo del corazón	—	—	Heart murmur	
Enfermedad previa del corazón	—	—	History of heart disease	
Enfermedad del corazón en su familia	—	—	Family history of heart disease	
Alta presión de la sangre	—	—	Hypertension	
Gastrointestinal			*GI*	
Náusea	—	—	Nausea	
¿Ha vomitado?	—	—	Vomiting	
¿Ha vomitado sangre?	—	—	Vomiting blood	
Ulcera péptica	—	—	Peptic ulcers	
Acedías, agruras de estómago	—	—	Heartburn	
Problemas al tragar	—	—	Dysphagia	
Dolor del vientre	—	—	Abdominal pain	
Hinchazón del vientre	—	—	Abdominal swelling	
Piel amarilla, ojos amarillos, orina marrón	—	—	Jaundice, brown urine	

	Sí	No		Comments
Cambio al obrar	—	—	Change in bowels	
Estreñimento	—	—	Constipation	
Diarrea	—	—	Diarrhea	
Excremento negro o al-quitranado	—	—	Melena	
Enfermedad de vesícula	—	—	Gallbladder disease	
Pancreatitis	—	—	Pancreatitis	
Hepatitis	—	—	Hepatitis	

Hematológico   *Hematologic*

	Sí	No		
Bolitas en los sobacos, el cuello, o la aldilla	—	—	Lumps in axilla, neck, or groin	
Anemia	—	—	Anemia	
Tendencia al sangramiento	—	—	Bleeding tendency	

Genitourinario   *Genitourinary*

	Sí	No		
¿Se despierta en la noche para orinar?	—	—	Nocturia	
Molestia al orinar	—	—	Dysuria	
Pérdida del control de la orina	—	—	Incontinence	
Sangre en la orina	—	—	Hematuria	
Infección en la orina o los riñónes	—	—	Urinary infections	
Cálculos o piedras en los riñónes	—	—	Stones	
Enfermedad venérea	—	—	Venereal disease	
Historia en su familia de enfer-medad de los riñónes	—	—	Family history renal disease	

Para Hombres Solamente   *For Men Only*

	Sí	No		
Disminución del chorro de la orina	—	—	Diminished stream	
Hinchazón o molestia en el es-croto o testículos	—	—	Swelling, discomfort in scrotum, testes	
Problemas sexuales	—	—	Sexual difficulties	
¿Le supura el pene?	—	—	Penile discharge	

Neurológico   *Neurologic-Psychiatric*

	Sí	No		
Dolor de cabeza	—	—	Headache	
Visión doble	—	—	Double vision	
Ataques (convulsiónes)	—	—	Seizures	
Cambio en sensación	—	—	Changed sensation	

	Sí	No		Comments
Debilidad de alguna parte del cuerpo	—	—	Weakness in any body part	
Desmaña	—	—	Clumsiness	
Cambio de personalidad	—	—	Change in personality	
Pérdida del equilibrio	—	—	Loss of equilibrium	
¿Se despierta muy temprano en la mañana?	—	—	Early awakening	
¿Pérdida de interés en actividades divertidos?	—	—	Anhedonia	
¿Considera el suicidio?	—	—	Suicidal thoughts	

Para Mujeres Solamente   *For Women Only*

	Sí	No	
Secreción o descargo de la vagína	—	—	Vaginal discharge
Irritación de la vagína	—	—	Vaginal irritation
Regla anormal	—	—	Abnormal menses
Manchas de sangre entre reglas	—	—	Spotting between periods
¿Si las reglas han terminado, ha ocurrido más sangramiento desde entonces?	—	—	Postmenopausal bleeding
Bolitas en los senos	—	—	Lumps in breasts
Dolor durante las relaciónes sexuales	—	—	Dyspareunia
¿Usa algún método para evitar embarazo?	—	—	Use of any birth control method
Aborto provocado	—	—	Induced abortion
Alguna complicación del embarazo	—	—	Complications of pregnancy

---

Fecha de la última regla _____ Date of last menses

¿Cuántos embarazos? _____ Number of pregnancies

¿Cuántos abortos naturales? _____ No. of spontaneous abortions

¿Cuántos niños han nacido vivos? _____ No. of live births

¿Cuántos niños han nacido muertos? _____ No. of stillbirths

¿Cuántas operaciónes cesáreas? _____ No. of Caesarian sections

5
General Appearance

"You can observe a lot by watching," said Yogi Berra.
taught by Dr. Ben Friedman of Alabama

Before beginning the sequential physical examination, it is important to take a moment just to look at the patient. Unless one's brain has been designed by nature to be like that of Arthur Conan Doyle's medical school teacher, Dr. Bell (see Ch. 26, p. 459), one must systematically seek and record specific observations about the patient's general appearance. I still suggest to medical students that they read the stories about Sherlock Holmes (who was modeled on Dr. Bell) to learn the excitement of drawing inferences from precise observations; but the student will continue the practice only if reinforced by success. Unfortunately, he will not achieve that success unless he knows what to look for. As Goethe said, "Was man weiss, man sieht" (what one knows, one sees).

On a piece of scratch paper, write down what season of the year is referred to in the phrase in Figure 5-1.

If you wrote down the word "spring," you are correct. No doubt, you read the sign as saying "Paris in the spring." However, that is not what it says. Go back and read it again, and if you still see the same thing, read it aloud, word by word, pointing at each word on the sign with your finger.

Most students feel that this sign is but a trick. They see their patients every day and cannot believe that something repeatedly exposed to their careful gaze would escape them. Accordingly, I suggest that you perform the following experiment on yourself, carefully following the steps in sequence.

1. Get a large piece of paper and a pen or pencil.
2. Take off your wristwatch and put it in your pocket or purse.

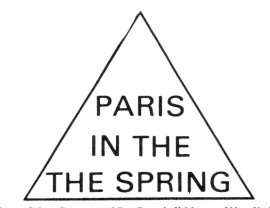

Figure 5-1. *Courtesy of Dr. Campbell Moses of New York.*

3. Draw the face of your wristwatch on the piece of paper. (If you have a digital watch, think of a clock face that you often see, such as your night table or kitchen clock.)
4. Now draw the hands, specifically indicating their shape and any markings upon them.
5. Indicate the color of the hands and the color of the background.
6. Show the markings for the hours. What color are they? Are they Roman numerals, or Arabic numerals? Are any numerals omitted, and what kind of mark is used at their position, if any?
7. Mark exactly on your drawing any words printed on the face of your watch, and any other outstanding marks.
8. Finally, take your watch out and compare its face to your drawing. How many false-positive memories did you have (i.e., markings on your sketch that do not actually exist on the face of the watch)? How many false-negative memories (markings on the face of the watch that you did not draw on your sketch)? How many thousands of times do you think you have glanced at this watch?

This exercise is intended to demonstrate that mere unstructured examination will not yield the most obvious of data, no matter how many times it is repeated, unless one is specifically looking for something. Although the outstanding diagnostician differs from the mediocre more in the way that he handles data than in the data that he collects, the importance of observation cannot be overemphasized: the superior clinician cannot gather too much information.

A Method

The principle of having a methodical search in mind before you begin the examination will be an underlying implicit emphasis of the remainder of this text. One sees what one looks for. Ironically, the general appearance section per se lends itself least to a methodical scheme.

Take care to observe the following aspects of the general appearance when first meeting the patient (see Rodnan's outline in Ch. 4): development, nutrition, apparent state of consciousness, apparent age, race, sex, posture or position in bed, comfort, attitude toward examination, degree of illness (acute or chronic), movements, habitus, and body proportions.

Morgan and Engel taught that the general appearance section of the write-up should contain sufficient succinct material to permit a stranger, should he walk upon the wards, to immediately identify the patient you are describing. It may include features of the patient that might also be included in a specific part of the physical examination (especially the skin, facial appearance, or the neurologic examination), but that are apparent to the methodical observer who is meeting the patient for the first time. Some syndromes, especially congenital ones, make the patient unusual (i.e., "funny looking"). It is the observer's job to describe just what is unusual about the patient's looks.

This text will focus on just three aspects of the general appearance for illustrative purposes: position and posture; movements; habitus and body proportions. Additional illustrations are given in Chapter 9.

This text will not follow the pattern of most other clinical diagnosis textbooks, that is, reciting a list of descriptions for the "cousin diseases" (so called because all the patients with the disease seem to have family resemblance): hyperthyroidism, hypothyroidism, Addison disease, Cushing disease, acromegaly, gargoylism, and so forth. First, the pictures of very advanced cases that appear in textbooks are obsolete in that we now usually make the diagnoses much earlier. Second, if you are experienced enough to be able to recognize these patients from their textbook photographs, you don't need a verbal description repeated here.

For the attending. Look at the devices attached to and the medications flowing into the patient. Professor Ask-Upmark would inspect the patient's bedside table for diagnostic clues and information about the patient's personality. Look at the orderliness with which things are arranged. What type of reading material is present? Inspect the clothing. Dr. Bill Domm of Virginia inspected the shoes of patients he suspected of malingering to see if the soles were worn in the pattern predicted from the abnormal gait that they displayed.

There is no specific place in the record for such observations. They might be placed in the history or the physical examination, under the general appearance, according to the taste of the individual.

Position and Posture

Patients with Abdominal Pain

In patients with abdominal pain, the position may be of particular value in the differential diagnosis. Patients with a perinephric abscess tend to bend toward the side of the lesion (see p. 389 and Fig. 20-7). Patients drawn up in the fetal position often have pancreatitis. Patients who are restless in their agony probably have some form of obstruction, whereas patients with peritonitis tend to hold themselves quite still ("Cope," Silen, 1979).

A patient who is lying on his back with his knee flexed and his hip externally rotated is said to have the "psoas sign" (Fig. 5-2). Formerly considered a sign of peritoneal irritation (resulting, for example, from appendicitis, or an abscess associated with regional ileitis or diverticulitis), in modern medicine it is more frequently seen with disease inside the psoas muscle itself, such as an abscess or iatrogenic hemorrhage due to anticoagulation. (See also the reverse psoas maneuver in Ch. 20, p. 379).

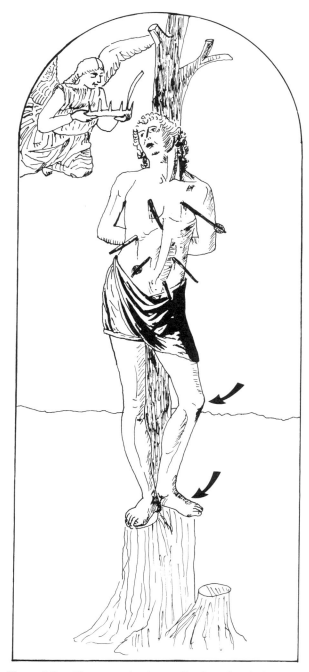

Figure 5-2. *The psoas sign is usually elicited with the patient supine, not erect. After Andrea del Castagno's* Saint Sebastian.

Patients with Breathing Difficulty

Posture may also be a helpful clue for diagnosing conditions that cause breathing difficulty. Several positions, each with pathophysiologic significance, have been described.

Orthopnea

Cardiac orthopnea. Orthopnea (literally, "straight up breathing") signifies left-sided congestive heart failure more than 95% of the time. The pathophysiology of orthopnea is rooted in the anatomic fact that in the erect posture, only the left heart remains centered in its (pulmonic) venous system, whereas the right heart becomes higher than most of the (systemic) venous system that supplies it. (In the supine posture, both the right and left heart are centered in their respective venous systems.) In other words, when the patient is erect (standing or sitting), the right ventricle experiences a lowering in its filling pressure relative to the left ventricle. This may selectively decrease right ventricular output to the point that the fluid filled lungs can now be cleared by the (weakened) left ventricle. This mechanism also explains why patients with pure right-sided heart failure do not experience orthopnea, and why patients with left heart failure experience some relief of their breathlessness when right heart failure supervenes.

Patients with pulmonic stenosis may say that they can breathe better with the head propped up on several pillows than when lying flat. There are also situations in which an increase of abdominal contents will make it easier for the patient to breathe when sitting up. While technically these are examples of orthopnea, they do not signify left ventricular failure and do not result from the pathophysiologic mechanism described above.

Pulmonary orthopnea.   If there is severe bilateral apical disease with relative sparing of the bases of the lungs, the patient may have orthopnea, since assuming the recumbent position will increase perfusion to the unventilated part of the lung and decrease oxygenation. Upon sitting up, such patients will again preferentially perfuse the better ventilated bases of their lungs, increase oxygenation, and decrease the sensation of breathlessness, thus mimicking the orthopnea of congestive heart failure.

Patients with severe obstructive pulmonary disease may also sit up in order to brace themselves (see Fig. 7-1A) to immobilize the thorax proper and improve the efficiency of the accessory muscles of inspiration. Leaning forward also helps by compressing the abdomen. The increase in the intraabdominal pressure pushes the flattened diaphragm of the emphysematous patient back up into a more rounded dome, increasing its efficiency as the piston of respiration (Sharp, 1986). Over a long period, this posture may lead to pigmented patches where the patient has braced his elbows on the thighs (see Fig. 7-1B).

Orthopnea can also occur in asthma. In fact, asthmatic patients who are sweating and sitting up have worse pulmonary functions than those who are not (Brenner et al., 1983).

Paroxysmal Nocturnal Dyspnea

To obtain relief of cardiac paroxysmal nocturnal dyspnea, patients may report going to the window for "better air." In reality, leaning upon the window only helps to support the fatigued body in an erect position; it is the standing that is important, the rest being cerebral elaboration.

Patients with pulmonary disease brace themselves against the window sill.

Patients with either cardiac or pulmonary dyspnea may also get up and go to the window just to have some cold air blow on their faces, since this reduces breathlessness even in normal subjects studied under conditions of hypercapnea and loaded breathing (Schwartzstein et al., 1987).

Platypnea

Platypnea (literally, "flat breathing") refers to the sensation of breathlessness when erect, with relief in the recumbent position. It is usually accompanied by orthodeoxia, which is a decrease in oxygen saturation in the erect posture when compared with the recumbent (vide infra). Platypnea was first described by Eugene D. Robin and co-workers, who found it in a coal miner with severe pulmonary emphysema (Altman & Robin, 1969).

In any pulmonary disease that afflicts primarily the basal segments of the lungs, assumption of the erect or sitting position increases the ventilation/perfusion mismatch, and causes the arterial oxygen saturation to decrease. Platypnea has been described in patients with multiple recurrent pulmonary emboli (Seward et al., 1984), necrotizing pneumonia with pneumatocele formation (Khan & Parekh, 1979), bilateral staphylococcal pneumonia, pleural effusion, tuberculosis (Limthongkul et al., 1983), and other conditions.

Obviously, any arteriovenous communication in the bases of the lungs could also be considered a ventilation/perfusion mismatch, which could be aggravated in the erect position (Robin et al., 1976). Thus, platypnea with orthodeoxia has even been seen in the absence of any apparent pulmonary disease, but in the presence of cirrhosis (Santiago & Dalton, 1977), in which case the existence of acquired arteriovenous malformations has been inferred.

Platypnea from any cause can disappear following the onset of the superior vena caval syndrome (see p. 366).

Very advanced.   In patients with an atrial septal defect, platypnea may occur if the right to left shunting is increased during the assumption of the erect posture. (This may be because the right atrium is higher than the left.) However, a sufficient increase in shunting seems to occur only when something else has happened to the lungs, for example, after a pneumonectomy (especially on the right), or a pleural effusion (which can also cause platypnea of itself), or a lesion in the lungs (Begin, 1975; Franco et al., 1984; LaBresh et al., 1981). The lesion need not even be in the lower lobe to produce platypnea, because in the case of the atrial septal defect, the lung lesion itself is not causing the ventilation/perfusion mismatch, but simply embarrassing the system that already has a shunt present at the atrial level.

Trepopnea

Trepopnea (literally, "twisted breathing") was coined by Dr. Richard A. Kern to indicate the preference of certain patients for the lateral recumbent position. This may result either from a pulmonary or a cardiac cause.

As a rule, with unilateral lung disease, pulmonary gas exchange is maximized by placing the normal lung in the dependent position. There are exceptions (vide infra).

Although recently popularized as a sign of pulmonary disease, trepopnea had earlier been observed in a large series of patients with congestive failure (Wood & Wolferth, 1937). In these patients, right trepopnea (right side down) was usual. It was suggested that the predominance of right-sided pleural effusions in congestive heart failure might be a result of the patient's preferred position.

One exception to the "good side down" rule is pleural disease accompanied by pleuritis, in which the patient uses the bed as a way of splinting the painful side of the chest. A second exception in which the abnormal lung may be placed in the inferior position was reported in a patient with a recurrent bronchial carcinoma, postresection, in the left upper lobe stump. The mass occluded the remaining left lobar lobe when the patient was in the right lateral decubitus position, so the patient had left lateral decubitus trepopnea, with the normal lung up (Mahler et al., 1983). Infants are a third exception (Davies et al., 1985). Another potential exception would be patients with chronic obstructive pulmonary disease, in

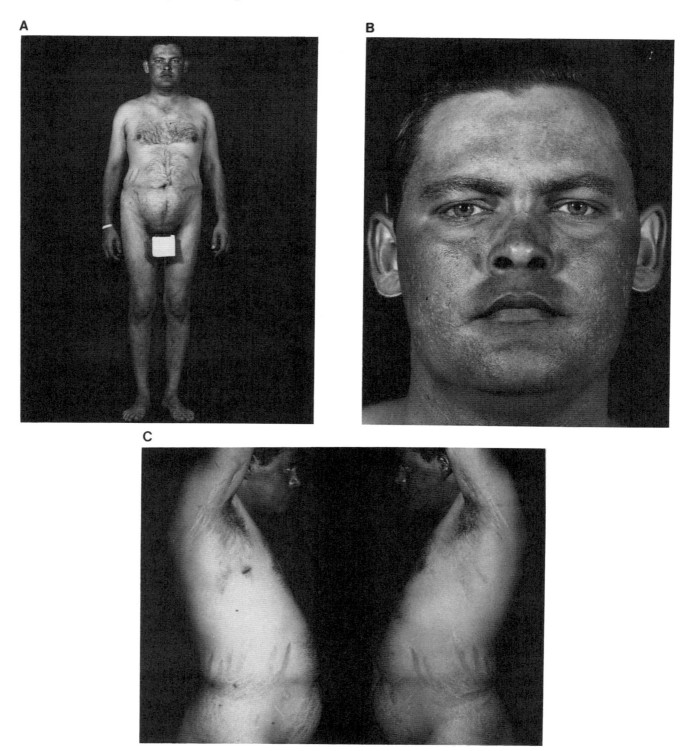

A

B

C

Figure 5-3.   A patient thought to have Cushing's syndrome.

whom ventilation to the superior lung increases, as ventilation to the dependent, supposedly better perfused lung, decreases. If this study, based upon only four patients and two controls, can be confirmed, it would suggest that patients with mild to moderate chronic obstructive pulmonary disease should never assume a lateral decubitus position (Shim et al., 1986).

Rare causes of trepopnea include atrial myxomas, and hepatocellular and renal carcinomas if they grow into the right atrium (Yasuhiro et al., 1983). The latter cause left trepopnea.

Movements

Although gait is discussed later under the neurologic examination, Dr. Albert I. Mendeloff of Maryland points out that it is very useful to observe the patient's gait for nonneurologic as well as for neurologic conditions. Dr. Mendeloff suggests weighing the patient yourself. Observe the patient's gait as you walk to the scale together, and pay attention to the manner in which the patient climbs onto the scale and off again. It is also useful to observe the patient's attempt to climb onto the examining table unassisted. These observations are in the tradition of the great French neurologist Charcot, who placed his examining room at the end of a long hall, and arranged his desk so that when he opened the door he could see the patient walking down the hall. In many cases, he had made the diagnosis before the patient had even entered the room.

Habitus and Body Proportions

Symphysis Pubis-to-Floor Measurements

Since the days of Herodotus, it has been known that a man's fingertip-to-fingertip span is approximately the same as his height ("crown to heel"). The length from the pubic symphysis to floor is about the same as from the pubic symphysis to the crown (i.e., about half the total height). More precisely, the ratio pubic symphysis to crown/pubic symphysis to floor is normally 0.92 (SD = 0.04) in whites and 0.85 (SD = 0.03) in blacks (McKusick, 1970).

Abnormalities in this ratio are characteristic of certain conditions. Achondroplastic dwarfs, but not persons who are constitutionally short statured, have a ratio greater than 1.0 (the symphysis pubis-to-floor span is much less than half the total height). Patients with Marfan's syndrome or "marfanoid habitus" (common in normal black persons) have a lower than normal ratio (the symphysis pubis-to-floor measurement is greater than half the height), while equally tall acromegalics do not. In Marfan's syndrome, the arm span is also greater than the height (McKusick, 1970). For other findings characteristic of this syndrome, see Chapter 25, page 441.

In achondroplastic dwarfs, the humeri and femora are relatively shorter than the forearms and lower legs.

Since these diagnostic distinctions can easily be made on other grounds, I personally do not use these measures very often.

In children, the skeletal changes may be the first sign of Marfan's syndrome to be expressed. Tables of normal values are available, but for sitting and standing heights, rather than the ratios we have mentioned. In childhood Marfan's, the sitting height remains normal, while the standing height is in the highest percentiles for age. Body measurements in children are extremely important, but a full discussion is beyond the scope of this book.

Weight: Distribution and Changes

The patient's weight and its distribution are important aspects of the body habitus. The examiner should look for evidence of changes in weight. New holes in the belt, or a change in the hole that is used (the "belt sign"), may show that the patient has lost weight, or that, conversely, he has had an increased abdominal girth due to ascites.

As a rule, the sharpest buckle groove indicates the most recent hole. The most worn buckle groove indicates the customary hole.

1. Individuals with abdominally located ("apple") obesity are likely to be at risk for type II diabetes and also for atherosclerotic vascular disease. Equally overweight persons with thigh ("pear") obesity are less likely to have type II diabetes. A formula for expedient differentiation of the two types is:

$$\text{Diameter of waist/diameter of hips} = 0.7$$
(in normals)

A result of less than 0.7 indicates "pear" obesity, and one of more than 0.85 indicates "apple" obesity (Malcolm et al., 1988)

2. A patient with "centripetal" obesity is pictured in Figure 5-3. This gentleman was correctly diagnosed as having Cushing's syndrome at the Cleveland Clinic in the late 1950s. In Figure 5-3A you may be able to see the abdominal scar (slanting above the umbilicus) from his one and seven-eighths adrenalectomy, which was then the treatment of choice. At first he did well, but a few years later all his symptoms returned. Oddly enough, he no longer had the facial appearance of a typical patient with Cushing's syndrome; his buccal fat pads had shrunk to the point that they no longer obscured his ears (Fig. 5-3B). But otherwise he had the signs, symptoms, and laboratory findings of that condition. Also note the obvious striae in Figure 5-3C. The diffuse hyperpigmentation, most notable in the striae and the face, is inexplicable. It is not simply suntanning, plethora, or a photographic trick. At this point, what diagnosis would you care to make? Write it down before reading on.

The patient had the remaining one-eighth adrenal gland removed, and later his pituitary gland as well, all to no avail. (The diagnosis until then had been hypersecretion of ACTH, which was supposedly driving his remaining adrenal cortical tissue and causing the hyperpigmentation.) At autopsy, no adrenal cortical tissue was found! There was also no residual pituitary tissue or tumorous or other apparent source of "ectopic" ACTH production. To this day, it is not known what other disease this patient had. What does this patient teach us? Reflect on this question, and write down your answer.

One thing it teaches is that one cannot diagnose diseases that have not yet been described.

Self-Study: Speculation

Without reading the legend, speculate on Figure 5-4.

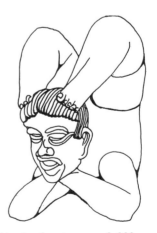

Figure 5-4. *This clay figurine, over 2,000 years old, may represent the first reported case of tetanus in meso-America. It shows severe opisthotonos and what seems to be a highly stylized risus sardonicus (sardonic grin) in an awake patient. Unfortunately, the arms are in the wrong position, as a patient suffering from tetanus would never be able to flex the upper extremities to the point of bringing the hands under the chin. Other observers have suggested that this piece of funeral statuary is an acrobat. This teaches us that what you see depends upon what you are looking for. Drawn from a figurine in the National Anthropological Museum in Mexico City.*

References

Altman M, Robin ED: Platypnea (diffuse zone I phenomenon?) *N Engl J Med* 281:1347–1348, 1969.

Begin R: Platypnea after pneumonectomy. *N Engl J Med* 293:342–343, 1975.

Brenner BE, Abraham E, Simon RR: Position and diaphoresis in acute asthma. *Am J Med* 74:1005–1009, 1983.

Davies H, Kitchman R, Gordon I, Helms P: Regional ventilation in infancy: Reversal of adult pattern. *N Engl J Med* 313:1626–1628, 1985.

Franco DP, Kinasewitz GT, Markham RV, Tucker WY, George RB: Postural hypoxemia in the postpneumonectomy patient. *Am Rev Respir Dis* 129:1021–1022, 1984.

Khan F, Parekh A: Reversible platypnea and orthodeoxia following recovery from adult respiratory distress syndrome. *Chest* 75:526–528, 1979.

LaBresh KA, Pietro DA, Coates EO, Khuri SF, Folland ED, Parisi AF: Platypnea syndrome after left pneumonectomy. *Chest* 79:605–607, 1981.

Limthongkul S, Charoenlap P, Nuchprayoon C., Songkhla YN, Hanvanich M: Platypnea and orthodeoxia: A Report of three cases and hypothesis of pathogenesis. *J Med Assoc Thai* 66:417–424, 1983.

Mahler DA, Snyder PE, Virgulto JA, Loke J: Positional dyspnea and oxygen desaturation related to carcinoma of the lung. *Chest* 83:826–828, 1983.

Malcolm R, Von JM, O'Neil PM, Currey HS, Sexauer JD, Riddle E: Update on the management of obesity. *South Med J* 81:632–638, 1988.

McKusick VA: The Marfan syndrome. In Wintrobe MM, Thorn GW, Adams RD, Bennett IL Jr, Braunwald E, Isselbacher KJ, Petersdorf RG (eds): *Harrison's Principles of Internal Medicine*, ed 6. McGraw-Hill, New York, 1970.

Robin ED, Laman D, Horn BR, Theodore J: Platypnea related to orthodeoxia caused by true vascular lung shunts. *N Engl J Med* 294:941–943, 1976.

Santiago SM Jr, Dalton JW Jr: Platypnea and hypoxemia in Laennec's cirrhosis of the liver. *South Med J* 70:510–512, 1977.

Schwartzstein RM, Lahive K, Pope A, Weinberger SE, Weiss JW: Cold facial stimulation reduces breathlessness induced in normal subjects. *Am Rev Respir Dis* 136:58–61, 1987.

Seward JB, Hayes DL, Smith HC, Williams DE, Rosenow EC III, Reeder GS, Piehler JM, Tajik AJ: Platypnea-orthodeoxia: Clinical profile, diagnostic workup, management, and report of seven cases. *Mayo Clin Proc* 59:221–231, 1984.

Sharp JT: The respiratory muscles in chronic obstructive pulmonary disease. *Am Rev Respir Dis* 134:1089–1091, 1986.

Shim C, Chun KJ, Williams MH, Blaufox MD: Positional effects on distribution of ventilation in chronic obstructive pulmonary disease. *Ann Intern Med* 105:346–350, 1986.

Silen W (ed): *Cope's Early Diagnosis of the Acute Abdomen*, ed 15. Oxford University Press, New York, 1979.

Wood FC, Wolferth CC: The tolerance of certain cardiac patients for various recumbent positions (trepopnea). *Am J Med Sci* 191:354–378, 1937.

Yasuhiro K, Nobuyoshi T, Kobayashi K, Ikeda T, Hattori N, Nonomura A: Growth of hepatocellular carcinoma in the right atrium. *Ann Intern Med* 99:472–474, 1983.

6
The Vital Signs

"At this point it is necessary that you see a bullfight. If I were to describe one it would not be the one that you would see, since the bullfighters and the bulls are all different, and if I were to explain the possible variations as I went along the chapter would be interminable. There are two sorts of guidebooks, those that are read before and those that are to be read after, and the ones that are to be read after the fact are bound to be incomprehensible to a certain extent before, if the fact is of enough importance in itself. So with any book on mountain skiing, sexual intercourse, wing shooting, or any other thing which it is impossible to make come true on paper, or at least impossible to attempt to make more than one version of at a time on paper, it being always an individual experience, there comes a place in the guidebook where you must say do not come back until you have skied, had sexual intercourse, shot quail or grouse, or been to the bullfight so that you will know what we are talking about. So from now on it is inferred that you have been to the bullfight."

Ernest Hemingway, *Death in the Afternoon*

Blood Pressure

History of Indirect Blood Pressure Measurement

The introduction of the sphygmomanometer is attributed to Potain, who is probably best remembered by cardiologists as the discoverer of cardiac gallops, and best remembered by the literate as the great Parisian diagnostician in Marcel Proust's *Remembrance of Things Past*. Potain's pupil, Riva Rocci, invented the mercury manometer, which led to the dissemination of indirect sphygmomanometry for the systolic pressure, and, once Korotkoff had discovered the sounds known by his name, for the diastolic as well. The latter story is a fable of medicine, well worth telling.

●

Korotkoff was a surgeon in the Czar's army, not an internist. He was doing experimental work on posttraumatic arteriovenous fistulas in the surgical dog laboratory. Pirogoff, his teacher (referred to in Dostoevsky's *The Idiot*), had taught him always to auscult over any area before performing an incision. On one occasion, while ausculting over an artery just as he was releasing a tourniquet, he heard thumping sounds! Abandoning his original scientific problem, he attempted to quantitate the amount of pressure required to make these auscultated sounds appear and disappear. He noticed that the sounds correlated with systole and diastole as determined by direct inspection of the flow of blood from the distally severed artery of the dog.

It is worth noting that when Korotkoff first found these sounds in humans and reported his research, some thought him to be quite mad. At the very least, his auditors found his suggestion that the sounds originated from pressure changes in the artery to be unacceptable because they "knew" that all such sounds had to emanate from the heart. Korotkoff's response that the sounds could not come from the heart since they disappeared when the artery was completely occluded (Geddes et al., 1966) convinced no one, although apparently none of his critical professors had bothered to understand, let alone to replicate, his experiment. Returning to the panel of experts a second time, Korotkoff produced more evidence supporting the concept that the sounds came from the artery, not the heart, but they remained unconvinced (Segall, 1980). This story, a part of the oral tradition in which I was intellectually raised, was later confirmed by the written record (Multanovsky, 1970).

The final chapter of the story is unknown. Just as Lavoisier was guillotined during the French Revolution,* Korotkoff was said to have been arrested after the Russian Revolution. One version holds that he finally died during a Stalinist purge; another that he perished in 1920. Since Stalin didn't seize power until the late 1920s, this teaches us that history repeats itself, and historians repeat each other.

●

Blood Pressure Cuffs

Shortly after the dissemination of the blood pressure cuff, workers realized that some cuffs were of insufficient length or width to efficiently transmit the bladder pressure through the intervening tissues to the brachial artery (Geddes et al., 1966). Pioneer after pioneer increased either the length or the width of the bladder in his cuff. (The length is the dimension of the bladder that is wrapped around the arm.) Then suddenly the march of progress stopped short: short of a length or width sufficient to guarantee that arm circumferences greater than 27 cm would not generate spuriously hypertensive readings on occasion.

---

*The decapitation device named for Dr. Joseph-Ignace Guillotin was neither invented nor christened by him. It was perfected by the Perpetual Secretary of the Academy of Surgery, Antoine Louis (Weiner, 1972).

The above is the historical basis for the belief that one should use as long or wide a blood pressure cuff bladder as possible. I use a thigh cuff. The scientific basis for this preference is reviewed on page 88.

I disagree with the recommendations of the American Heart Association's committee (AHA, 1980), which would have the medical student purchase no fewer than seven different blood pressure cuffs. Why, the neophyte might ask, should I believe the sole author of this book when there is a distinguished committee that has made recommendations to the contrary? My answer is that my own opinions are based upon data to be presented, while a camel has been defined as a horse built by a committee. In this regard, the neophyte should be aware that the first committee of the American Heart Association recommended that the fourth phase (muffling) of the Korotkoff sounds be adopted as the correct locus for diastolic pressure. In 1959, a second committee recommended that it be the fifth phase (disappearance). In 1967, a third committee switched back to recommending the muffling (fourth phase), but the published recommendation included an appendix stating why disappearance (fifth phase) was superior! In fact, one of the members of that committee used disappearance for determining the diastolic blood pressure in the famous Veterans Administration Cooperative Study. The next committee recommended using disappearance in adults and muffling in children. My own position is presented on page 88, but it should be clear to the casual observer that at least some of these expert committees must be incorrect.

A Warning to the Neophyte

$$ Many authors, when discussing the proper size of the bladder, refer to the blood pressure "cuff," when they really mean the bladder, which is inside the cuff. While the bladder, as a rule, has exactly the same width as the cloth covering (the cuff), the bladder is usually much shorter than the total cuff. Thus, *before purchasing* or making assumptions about a blood pressure cuff, one should inflate the bladder to see what its true dimensions are. (Recommended dimensions are given on p. 88 at the $$ sign.)

Calibrating the Manometer

$$ For your black bag, you will probably purchase a sphygmomanometer with an aneroid pressure gauge. Be sure that it is a kind that does *not* have a pin stop, that is, a device that keeps the gauge from reading below zero when the cuff is deflated. The pin stop keeps you from being able to see that the gauge is out of calibration.

The aneroid gauge should periodically be checked for accuracy, preferably against a mercury sphygmomanometer. You will need a Y-connector and tubing so that the bladder in your cuff can be simultaneously connected to both the mercury manometer and the aneroid gauge. Alternately, you can roll up two blood pressure cuffs together, inflate them partially, and squeeze them, checking their gauges against each other (whether one is a mercury manometer, or both are aneroids).

Ten to thirty-five percent of aneroid manometers are defective, yielding significant variances in accuracy when compared to the mercury manometer (Thulin et al., 1975).

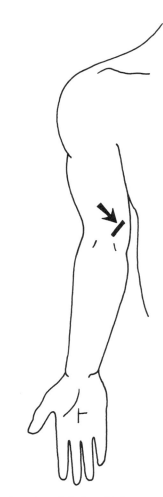

Figure 6-1. *Location of the brachial artery.*

Making an Indirect Blood Pressure Measurement: A Method

There are two steps here: first, measuring the palpable systolic blood pressure, and second, the more customary auscultatory determination, also called the indirect determination of the systolic and diastolic pressures.

1. A blood pressure cuff of the appropriate size is wrapped snugly around the biceps. Be sure it is high enough so that your stethoscope bell can be applied right over the brachial artery (Fig. 6-1). (There is no evidence that putting the stethoscope under the cuff, as is done in many automatic devices, gives a spurious reading.) To ensure this, you might wish to locate the brachial artery by palpation and mark it with chalk or a washable ink. (Be sure to ask the patient's permission to mark the arm.) Doing this the first dozen times is a good beginner's practice, as it may prevent your placing the cuff too low on the biceps. In that case, you would have to remove and reapply it between the determinations of the palpable and auscultatory systolic pressure.

2. Now look at the mark. Is it level with the patient's heart? If the patient is lying down, it probably is, unless you have allowed the arm to hang over the edge of the bed. In that instance, you would get a falsely elevated value, because the height of the blood column between the heart and the brachial artery would be added to the actual pressure inside the vasculature.

$$1.3 \times \text{cm} \, \Delta \, \text{height} = \text{mm Hg artifact}$$

If the patient is sitting with his arm resting on your desk, the marked brachial artery will probably not be beneath the level of the heart, but it might well be above that level. This could produce a falsely *decreased* blood pressure measurement, since the pressure generated during systole is partly expended in climbing the vertical distance up the arterial tree to the brachial artery where you are making your measurements (Mitchell et al., 1964).

Please remember these simple plumbing rules, as they are the basis for understanding several artifacts and caveats to be presented later.

3. Be sure that the blood pressure cuff is not applied over clothing. The addition of a layer of anything increases the diameter of the arm and also increases the chance for "slippage," that is, lateral displacement of the pressure generated by the cuff. In fact, the presence of clothing is similar to the model used for studying "cuff hypertension," another form of spuriously elevated blood pressure which is discussed on page 88. As with the arm position, the addition of a layer of thin clothing *usually* has a *small* effect on the blood pressure, but why introduce *any* indeterminate variable into your measurements if it is so easily avoided?

4. Notice that the pressure bulb has a screw valve that can be manipulated by the thumb and fingers with the bulb resting in the palm of your hand. Try screwing the valve into each of its two extreme positions. In one of these extreme positions, the air you squeeze from the bulb will go into the cuff and not come out. In the other extreme position, any air pumped into the cuff will immediately come out when you stop pumping. If neither position allows all the air to be retained, there must be a loose connection or a leak somewhere in the system.

To inflate the cuff, turn the screw valve to the position that allows all the air to be retained. To deflate the cuff, turn the screw valve *very slightly* so that the pressure drops at the rate of 1 mm per second. (Most of the time you will actually allow it to go faster than that, but there are situations in which it is necessary to go this *slowly*, for example, the determination of pulsus paradoxus.)

5. Put your right hand on the sphygmomanometer bulb and your left hand where you can feel either the brachial artery distal to the cuff, or the radial artery. This is for the purpose of determining the systolic pressure by palpation. Pump the pressure in the cuff as high as you need to in order to make the pulse disappear. Then slowly lower the pressure to see at what point the pulse returns. That point (expressed in mm Hg read from the manometer dial) is the systolic blood pressure "by palpation." Usually, this is not recorded unless it is not possible to obtain the systolic pressure by auscultation. In such a circumstance, both the positive and negative findings may be noted (e.g., "BP not auscultable; systolic 90 by palpation").

6. Lower the pressure all the way to zero, and pick up your stethoscope. The use of the stethoscope is discussed in more detail in Chapters 16 and 17. At this point you need know only the following: 1) The earpieces are to be placed in your ears so that they point slightly forward. Otherwise, depending on the anatomy of your ear canals, you may not be able to hear anything at all. 2) The earpieces should not hurt your ears. If they do, you must replace them with a style that fits comfortably as soon as possible. 3) The bell should be used for taking the blood pres-

sure. Tap or breathe alternately on the bell and the diaphragm to see which one is "on line." You switch from one to the other either by pressing a lever or rotating the head, depending on the model of your stethoscope. Although the diaphragm is usually satisfactory for taking the blood pressure, the bell is preferable for hearing the low-pitched Korotkoff sounds, especially when they are faint. Of course, if you press heavily with the bell (as evidenced by the circular indentation left in the skin), it is converted into a diaphragm.

7. Place the bell of the stethoscope lightly over the brachial artery, but in contact with the skin over its entire circumference.

8. With your other hand, pump up the cuff as before, quickly going about 10 mm above the systolic pressure, as determined by palpation. Gradually lower the pressure at a rate of about 2 mm Hg per heart beat or 1 mm Hg per second. The point at which you hear the Korotkoff sounds appear is the systolic pressure by auscultation.

9. Continue deflating the pressure until the sounds disappear. That is the diastolic pressure. If you were lowering the pressure too fast to determine the exact point of the diastolic, deflate the cuff, allow the veins to drain (so as to avoid producing an auscultatory gap, see p. 92) and again pump the cuff up to just above the "guesstimated" diastolic to obtain an exact measurement.

10. If you happened to notice a point at which the sounds became muffled, record that also (see p. 88). But if you did not notice the muffling, it is probably not worthwhile to go back and find it. As we shall see, it is probably not a useful number under ordinary circumstances. In addition, many normal people do not have a point of muffling.

It is possible to measure both systolic and diastolic pressure by palpation. The procedure was independently discovered by Ehret in 1909 and by Segall in 1940 (Enselberg, 1961). In Segall's original study (Segall, 1940), using *light* palpation over the vessel to sense the Korotkoff vibrations, it was possible to get values within 10 mm of the auscultatory measurements of both systolic and diastolic pressures in all 100 subjects. In over half the cases, there was no difference between the pressures as determined by palpation versus auscultation.

Variability of Blood Pressure

There is really no such thing as "*the*" blood pressure. A person's blood pressure varies throughout the day. Try the following as a self-study:

1. Go to the library and consult one of the better texts on hypertension, such as Kaplan's *Clinical Hypertension*. Read the portions indexed under "variation," "variability," or "diurnal variation," and the summarized literature. Has anyone ever made multiple measurements of the blood pressure, and found *the* blood pressure, or has everyone who has made multiple measurements found variability to be the rule?

2. Take your partner's blood pressure, then have him take yours. Repeat several times. Do the pressures change, or stay the same?

3. Put your partner at complete rest and take his pressure several times, until sequential readings are within 5 mm Hg of the last reading (systolic and/or diastolic). Now simply leave the room and return immediately to make another measurement. Or by prearranged signal have someone else enter the room while you are making a measurement. What happens to the blood pressure? Alternately, do not tell your partner one of the readings, but look at him with astonishment, and quickly begin to measure the pressure again. What happens to the pressure?

4. Go onto the wards and pick up a chart containing blood pressure determinations (by the nurses) more than once a day. Are they ever the same? How often?

5. Go to the intensive care unit where a patient is at complete rest and has a continuously reading intraarterial blood pressure monitor. Pick a patient whose medication is not being changed. Write down the displayed blood pressure every 10 seconds. How many are the same? How many are different? How many of the patients are like this?

6. Which of the above maneuvers showed the greatest variability? The least? Did you calculate the standard deviations?

What are the standard errors of the means? Which should be used for comparisons, standard deviation or standard error? Which varies inversely with the size of the sample?

(*Answer*: The standard error of the mean varies inversely with the size of the sample, so it should not be used alone for comparisons if the two groups are of different sizes.)

Determining Diastolic Pressure

There has long been a controversy as to whether the muffling or the disappearance of the Korotkoff sounds should be used as the diastolic pressure. A thorough review of the literature clearly indicates to me that in most persons, the disappearance of the sounds should be used for the diastolic (vide infra). The various drug studies proving the value of antihypertensive therapy have all used diastolic pressures determined by disappearance.

Admittedly, there are situations of high stroke volume in which the disappearance gives an artifactually low pressure, sometimes even an impossible 0 mm Hg. (Apparently, in such cases, the artery continues to return toward baseline throughout diastole.) Examples include severe aortic insufficiency; patent ductus arteriosus; and high output cardiac failure, as in pregnancy, fever, anemia, thyrotoxic heart disease, and beriberi. If you suspect one of these entities, you should follow the American Heart Association's current recommendation of recording all three pressures (i.e., systolic, muffling, and disappearance, e.g., 140/80/0). But which one should be "used"?

In aortic insufficiency, at least, we know that muffling best approximates the directly measured intraarterial pressure when the indirect diastolic blood pressure is "zero" (Goldstein & Killip, 1962). Since muffling was only 2 mm different from the directly measured pressure, we may assume that in other situations with an impossible "zero" diastolic, muffling should also be used as the diastolic pressure.

The muffle point may also be used for the diastolic in severe bradycardia, in which the disappearance point may be nearly zero, although the high stroke volume is not accompanied by a high cardiac output (Goldstein & Killip, 1962).

I had originally intended to write an entire chapter on the confusion about the indirectly determined diastolic blood pressure, not only to clarify and convince, but because the history of the subject is an example of how fuzzy thinking and sloppy scholar-

ship can confound such a common activity. However, intraarterial lines are now so ubiquitous that the student is advised to measure indirect blood pressures on such monitored patients and convince himself of the truth. Accordingly, I will simply cite a few examples of well-done experiments that demonstrate disappearance to be closer to the true diastolic pressure than muffling, except in situations of high stroke volume (Karvonen et al., 1964; London & London, 1967; Raftery & Ward, 1968).

The Fat Arm

The standard adult blood pressure cuff has a bladder of the correct size for arms whose brachial circumference is up to 27 cm. If the circumference is greater than 27 cm, the larger the arm, the greater the overestimation of both systolic and diastolic pressures if the indirect blood pressure is performed with a standard cuff (King, 1967). The pharmacologic treatment of normotensive patients who have "cuff hypertension" may actually increase their mortality (Kaplan, 1983).

Some authors have attempted to apply epidemiologic formulas to correct the systolic and diastolic pressures in patients with large arms (Pickering et al., 1954). The epidemiologic corrections were derived from experimental data (Ragan & Bordley, 1941), which were faulted in several ways, according to the original report. In any event, the correction factors are invalid in individual patients because of variability in pulse wave contour, radius of the brachial artery, brachial artery to biceps ratio, and so forth, all of which affect the exact degree of blood pressure overestimation from an undersized cuff.

Some workers (Devetski, 1963) have suggested wrapping the arm cuff around the forearm and taking the blood pressure at the radial artery, with the arm in a supinated position. (The mean arterial blood pressure at the radial is from 3 to 5 mm less than at the brachial.) My own preference is to obtain a very large cuff. **$$** One can use either a very wide (20 cm) cuff such as a thigh cuff, or a very long (42 cm) bladdered cuff (King, 1967). Despite statements to the contrary, I know of no good evidence that the use of a large cuff in an adult can produce a spuriously low blood pressure. In fact, there is evidence to the contrary (Karvonen et al., 1964; King, 1967; Linfors et al., 1984; Montfrans et al., 1987; Nielsen & Janniche, 1974).

For the attending.   As a teaching exercise, pick a medical student with large biceps and take his blood pressure. Then take some foam rubber padding, about 1 inch thick, and wrap it around the upper extremity to imitate the mechanical effect of fat. (Alternately, use a few turkish towels, a lab coat, or any pliable material that resembles normal fat in being compressible.) Note that you have not actually altered the subject's cardiovascular system. Place your blood pressure cuff around the foam rubber "fat" and take the blood pressure again. Remove the "fat" and take the blood pressure yet again. What is the effect of increasing the upper arm circumference on the indirectly determined blood pressure?

Admittedly, obesity tends to increase the blood pressure even beyond the effect on circumference. But here we are concerned only with the effect of arm circumference on the accuracy of the indirectly determined blood pressure.

Many clinicians have very sharp cutoff points above which they treat the blood pressure and below which they do not. You can estimate from this experiment that a large number of people with fat arms are being treated for a disease, essential hypertension, which they in fact do not have.

I regretfully use the word "essential" to modify the noun "hypertension" for convenience in communicating. With Sir George Pickering, I do not believe that hypertension is a disease *sui generis*. But if it is, I do not see how it can be "essential."

Back at the turn of the century, arterial occlusive disease could be diagnosed at autopsy. As some of these patients were found to have elevated blood pressures, as determined by the newly popular sphygmomanometer, some prestigious authorities hypothesized that the hypertension was secondary to the diffuse arterial occlusive disease, and that it was an adaptive response, "essential" in that it provided a high head of pressure for driving the blood through the stenotic vessels. The ghost of this disproven hypothesis lingers among those who fear that lowering the blood pressure in malignant hypertension will deprive vital organs of blood flow.

As various specific etiologies of hypertensive states were discovered, the adjective "essential" came to refer to those forms of hypertension of unknown etiology. It should be distinguished from hypertension of unexamined etiology.

Oddly, the new adjectival meaning of "essential" has metastasized to a variety of other conditions. For instance, one reads of an entity called "essential migraine," although one is hard pressed to explain to the migrainous patient exactly what is essential about his suffering. (Migraine itself is a useful word only if you know that it is derived from "hemicrania." It then becomes a diagnosis that suggests itself when evaluating a patient with unilateral cephalalgia.)

A Note to the Sophomore

Have you noticed how the text is changing? Words and concepts that you have not previously encountered are starting to spring up. The material is no longer oriented to the layperson. If you are a sophomore reading this in sequence, you are confronted with a problem that will continue for the next few years: what to do when you are no longer sure that you understand all the words.

My advice is to stop and look up the strange words in a medical dictionary or textbook. Remember this is not a textbook of medicine. This is like a book on how to sail your boat; you still have to buy some maps to see exactly where you are sailing to.

On the wards, you will also hear residents and staff using words and phrases that you do not know. You can raise your apparent IQ by 10 points simply by carrying with you at all times a small notebook for recording all the strange words of the workday. Each night look up all the words you collected during the day.

Where to Measure Blood Pressure

Upper Extremities

Begin by taking the blood pressure in both upper extremities. This is usually done at the right and left brachial arteries. The difference in the systolic blood pressure between the two arms is due to any intrinsic abnormality present in at least one arm, *plus* the amount of neurovasomotor change (either excitement or relaxation) that has occurred as you move from one extremity to the other. Such change will affect both systolic and diastolic pressures. Any significant intrinsic vascular obstruction will cause a difference of at least 10 or 15 mm in the systolic pressures. To be sure that a significant difference is present requires two observers who measure at the same time, then switch sides to remeasure. Dr. Alvin Shapiro of Pennsylvania reports, "I have 'ruled out' coarctation and subclavian steals 'detected' by

house officers and students by using this maneuver at the bedside, on many occasions."

Once you have determined that both arms have the same blood pressure, you usually need to take the pressure in only one arm. If the pressures are unequal, the arm with the *lower* pressure is the abnormal one, most often because of an obstruction due to atherosclerosis (see, for example, subclavian steal syndrome, Ch. 18, p. 342), or more rarely from a dissecting aneurysm.

Lower Extremities

With the patient recumbent, take a lower extremity *systolic* blood pressure, by palpation or auscultation, over the popliteal artery (using a thigh cuff) or the dorsalis pedis (placing a cuff around the calf). The difference between the arm and leg systolic pressures is due to any change in neurovasomotor tone occurring between the two measurements plus any intrinsic abnormality. Note that *paired leg and arm pressures must both be taken with the patient recumbent*. Never take a lower extremity blood pressure with the patient sitting or standing because the height of the blood column between the artery and the heart would add to the blood pressure and confound your data.

Brachial-Popliteal or Brachial-Dorsalis Pedis Systolic Pressure Gradients

Normally the *indirect* systolic blood pressure can be *up to* 10 mm Hg *higher* in the lower than in the upper extremity in the absence of any structural abnormality. The difference may even be as great as 20 mm Hg (Frank et al., 1965; Sapira, 1981). However, *direct* intra-arterial measurements reveal that the systolic and diastolic pressures, as well as the mean pressures, are normally the same in upper and lower extremities (Pascarelli & Bertrand, 1964).

The systolic blood pressure in the lower extremity is found to be *significantly less* (*at least* 6 mm Hg) than in the upper extremity in cases of obstruction in the vascular tree. The most common cause of obstruction in the elderly Westerner is atherosclerosis (see also Ch. 18, p. 350). The most common cause in the young hypertensive is coarctation of the aorta (see pp. 345 and 347).

The systolic blood pressure in the lower extremity is significantly *higher* than in the upper extremities in patients with occlusion of the upper extremity vasculature as in Takayasu's disease, Buerger's disease, or other selective disease of the upper extremity; in some cases of dissecting aneurysm; and in conditions of high stroke volume (Hill's sign). In Hill's sign, especially due to aortic insufficiency, the indirect lower extremity systolic pressure may be 20 to 60 mm Hg higher than that in the upper extremity. (The mechanism for Hill's sign is given in Ch. 17, p. 311).

Once you have the recumbent blood pressures recorded in all four limbs, you have a perfect baseline for the later detection of dissecting aortic aneurysm. Depending on the location of the dissection, any one or more of the extremities might have a damped arterial pulse wave. In fact, suspicion of this life-threatening disease is the one situation in which you *must recheck* all four extremity blood pressures in the recumbent position.

Postural Hypotension

Postural hypotension refers to hypotension in the erect position relative to the recumbent position. The two main causes are volume depletion (due to anything from gastrointestinal hemorrhage to adrenal cortical insufficiency to diuretics) and neurogenic (e.g., due to certain antihypertensive medications; the various forms of autonomic vasomotor dysfunction; or even pro-longed bedrest or weightlessness, as with the original astronauts). Less common causes include heart failure (the heart being unable to increase output when the patient stands) and pheochromocytoma (a rare disease in which hypovolemia compounds the problem caused by down regulation of the noradrenergic receptors).

A Method

Take the systolic and diastolic blood pressure in an upper extremity with the patient recumbent. Have the patient stand, and immediately repeat the measurement, with his arm by his side. Normally, the diastolic pressure remains the same or rises slightly, and the systolic pressure stays the same or drops slightly. The calculated *mean arterial blood pressure*

$$BP_{mean} = BP_{dias} + 0.4 (BP_{sys} - BP_{dias})$$

does not normally drop more than a few mm Hg during standing. Note that the normal diastolic pressure almost never drops, and when it does, the drop is slight and the systolic will rise. Conversely, many normal persons drop their systolic pressure on standing, but their diastolic rises so that the mean arterial pressure is maintained.

As a teaching exercise, take your partner's blood pressure and pulse recumbent, then erect. Calculate the mean arterial blood pressure changes (if any) with orthostasis. Have your partner repeat the exercise on you.

Some authorities recommend multiplying the pulse pressure ($BP_{sys} - BP_{dias}$) by one third or one half. I use 0.4 as my correction factor because that yields values that most closely correlate with simultaneous *direct* mean arterial blood pressure measurements. In actual practice for assessing postural hypotension, any of the formulas may be used.

○   If the patient has postural hypotension, don't forget to check the pulse simultaneously. Failure of the pulse rate to rise in response to an orthostatic drop in pressure is a valuable clue that the problem is neurogenic, and not due to volume depletion. However, beta blockers can prevent the orthostatic pulse increase despite the presence of volume depletion. The presence of an *increase* in pulse tells you nothing; some neurologic lesions impair the pressor response without preventing a rise in the pulse rate. And some patients (e.g., some diabetics, patients with Wernicke's encephalopathy, and recipients of cardiac transplants) have a predominant vagal insufficiency so that the pulse is always high.

Sometimes, you will attempt to find postural hypotension in a patient who is too ill to stand by himself. In that case, the blood pressure may be taken in the sitting position, and compared with that in the recumbent position. (Here try, if possible, to get the legs in a dependent position to promote blood pooling in the lower extremities.)

If it is difficult to obtain the standing blood pressure because you are moving too slowly due to inexperience, try pumping up the blood pressure cuff to a point just above the recumbent systolic immediately before having the patient stand. The same maneuver can be used for the diastolic. However, you must still move quickly because pain, including that produced by an inflated blood pressure cuff, can act as a pressor stimulus.

Tilt Tables

If you have access to a tilt table, you can use it to obtain orthostatic pressures in a patient who is very ill. Simply *strap the patient* in with his feet against the footboard, measure the blood pressure with the patient in the horizontal position, and tilt him to the erect position for the second blood pressure measurement. Remember that normal persons may have an initial orthostasis if passively tilted in such a way that they *cannot* use their leg muscles for standing, or that weak persons may have orthostasis if they do *not* contract their leg muscles (since muscle contraction increases venous return). That is why the patient should be observed to be sure that his feet are positioned properly against the footboard, and that he is using his legs.

Sensitivity and Specificity

In phlebotomy, an orthostatic rise in pulse rate of 30 per minute *or* lightheadedness sufficiently severe to cause the patient to lie down or experience syncope was associated with the loss of 1,000 ml. The sensitivity was 98% and the specificity was 98%. However, the test did not work for 500 ml blood loss, or if the subject only sat up instead of standing (Knopp et al., 1980). Using a tilt table, the cutoff was 25 per minute regardless of symptoms, with 100% sensitivity and specificity (Green & Metheny, 1948).

A Caveat

If you already know that the patient is volume depleted or in shock, you might *not* want to perform the testing for postural hypotension. There are two reasons for this.

The first reason is derived from one of the first rules of medicine: *primum non nocere* (variously translated as "first, do no harm" or "whatever you do, don't make things worse, even if it means doing nothing very much"). If the patient is hypotensive to the point of having marginal perfusion to some of his tissues, standing him up might do temporary or permanent harm by decreasing perfusion further. It is rare for a patient in shock to have a stroke because he was tilted up, but it is impossible to predict which patient that might be.

The second reason is that any risk of harm must be justified by an expected benefit. If one already knows the patient to be in shock, adducing more evidence in favor of the diagnosis is wasteful at best. Initially, treatment can be titrated against blood pressure, pulse rate, urine output, and so forth, until these are normalized. At that point, one can more safely switch to more sensitive measures of homeostasis, such as orthostatic hypotension.

Delayed Orthostatic Readings

In order to improve the specificity of the postural hypotension test for *extreme* conditions of volume depletion or neurogenic orthostatic hypotension, some speakers have recommended keeping the patient in an erect position for 5, 10, or 15 minutes, and continuing to measure the blood pressure. It has been stated, in the absence of any data of which I am aware, and contrary to my experience, that those individuals who are able to compensate by the end of 10 or 15 minutes are experiencing neurogenic orthostatic hypotension, and specifically do not have volume depletion.

The absence of normal values is one source of confusion. An additional problem is a modification that certain young clinicians have made: omitting the initial measurement on standing, when the patient's symptoms are at a maximum. I have seen *both false positives and false negatives* with this latter technique, and therefore strongly warn against it. Because there is no such thing as "the" blood pressure, the mean arterial pressure changing gradually over the course of the day, there is a 50% chance that the 15-

minutes-later blood pressure will be lower than the baseline pressure, even if there was no initial orthostatic drop (a false positive). The false negatives occur in individuals with milder degrees of volume depletion, who increase cardiac output by increasing venous return through "walking in place." Also, the noxious subjective experience of the initial (but unmeasured) orthostatic hypotension stimulates the autonomic nervous system. For these reasons, many persons are able to compensate, and even overcompensate, for orthostasis, after 10 to 15 minutes of standing.

The rollover test for predicting hypertension during pregnancy is discussed in Appendix 6-2.

Blood Pressure in Atrial Fibrillation

The blood pressure depends on cardiac output and peripheral resistance, and the cardiac output, in turn, depends upon stroke volume and heart rate. Since indirect blood pressure determinations are made on a beat-by-beat basis, anything that changes the stroke volume from beat to beat will alter the blood pressure measurement. Although we willingly take advantage of this phenomenon when measuring pulsus paradoxus (vide infra), we tend blithely to ignore it in the case of atrial fibrillation.

An isolated indirect blood pressure reading is completely unreliable in a patient who has atrial fibrillation with irregular ventricular responses and highly variable R-R intervals. Since a short R-R interval permits a minimal amount of ventricular filling, the stroke volume will be quite low at the time of the next ventricular contraction, and hence the indirectly measured blood pressure (systolic and diastolic) will be low. Conversely, when the R-R interval is extremely prolonged, the ventricular filling will be great and the apparent systolic (and diastolic) pressures will be quite high. Thus, while rough estimations of the general range of blood pressure can be made during atrial fibrillation, the more exact measurements needed for diagnosis and therapy of high or low blood pressure must await more regular R-R intervals. Of course, the same is true for all other arrhythmias in which there are wide variations in R-R intervals.

What should the practitioner do? I suggest averaging three blood pressures obtained in the following manner:

1. Drop the cuff pressure *very slowly* until you can hear three beats in a row (i.e., three beats with a *relatively* constant R-R interval). The pressure at the first beat is the systolic.
2. After having previously "guesstimated" what the diastolic might be, quickly drop down to about 10 mm Hg above that value, then lower the pressure very slowly. Whenever you last find three audible beats in a row, the diastolic is obtained from the last beat you heard.

This method is not scientifically validated, and would no doubt produce different results than a "two-in-a-row" method. Different observers will get different pressures, not only because of sampling differences but because they will decompress the cuff at different rates. Thus, while this is a fairly good adaptation of the indirect blood pressure method for measuring changes in a given individual, it is not so good for measuring the exact, absolute diastolic pressure, an important issue for those who believe that a diastolic of 90 mm Hg requires lifelong treatment, while one of 89 mm Hg does not.

Arthur Mirsky used to tell me that there were no brittle diabetics, only brittle physicians. Maybe atrial fibrillation is God's way of making some hypertensionologists less brittle and more humble.

Blood Pressure in Ventricular Tachycardia

In ventricular tachycardia with AV dissociation, there is irregular ventricular filling and hence irregular stroke volume, depending upon the chance position of the atrial contraction in relationship to the ventricular contraction. Thus, the first Korotkoff sound may be irregularly heard at a higher pressure than that at which the sound is heard with every beat. This finding may help to distinguish the rhythm from a supraventricular tachycardia (Wilson et al., 1964).

Pulsus Paradoxus

When the sphygmomanometer was disseminated, observers began quantitating the degree of drop in systolic blood pressure that normally occurs during inspiration. Many pathologic conditions were found to cause an exaggeration of this normal phenomenon, even though the pulse was still palpable (i.e., contemporary pulsus paradoxus).

•

Historical Note

You are probably wondering why this phenomenon is called "pulsus" when it generally refers to a drop in blood pressure during inspiration. In fact, it was discovered by Richard Lower (1631–1691), a Cornish physiologist, before the sphygmomanometer was even invented. He noticed the weakening of a patient's pulse with inspiration. He reasoned that the phenomenon was caused by adhesions, since the necropsy showed a thickened pericardium, which was adherent to the diaphragm. Lower's observation remained unappreciated, and the phenomenon awaited rediscovery by Kussmaul, who gave it its name (Kussmaul, 1873). (The title of his work, "Concerning Callous Mediastinopericarditis and the Paradoxical Pulse," possibly contributed to the erroneous belief that constrictive pericarditis produces pulsus paradoxus. The patient who was described in the paper actually had an exudative component to his pericardial disease discovered at autopsy, and today this would be stressed in titling the report.) In the patient that Kussmaul examined, the pressure change was so dramatic that the palpable pulse itself disappeared during inspiration. The paradox was that the pulse went away, whereas the central heartbeat continued.

•

Pathophysiology

The normal systolic pressure drop during inspiration is due to a number of factors (Guntheroth et al., 1967). First, the high negative intrapleural pressure sucks blood into the venae cavae and increases filling of the right atrium, and hence of the right ventricle. Some workers have suggested that with increased right ventricular volume, the interventricular septum may bulge into the left ventricular outflow tract, decreasing the stroke volume. Other workers have pointed out that during inspiration the highly negative intrapleural pressure increases the pulmonary blood volume and therefore momentarily decreases left atrial and left ventricular filling, decreasing the stroke volume in that way. Most authorities feel that an abnormal pulsus paradoxus is usually produced by accentuations in these basic mechanisms. Distortion of the abnormal pericardial sac by descent of the diaphragm (Dock, 1961) and various other subsidiary mechanisms (Spodick, 1964) may sometimes be operant in pericardial disease.

Criteria

Since pulsus paradoxus is, to some degree, a normal phenomenon, at what point does it have clinical significance? At the present time, almost all authorities define an inspiratory fall in the systolic pressure of greater than 10 mm Hg as abnormal. A dissenting minority has presented data suggesting that it should actually be a fall greater than 10% of the (expiratory) systolic blood pressure (Reddy et al., 1978).

A Method

To determine the pulsus paradoxus, repeat the blood pressure measurement, lowering the mercury ever so slowly while approaching the previous systolic blood pressure. At first, you will hear the Korotkoff sounds only during expiration; this is the first number to record. Continue to lower the cuff pressure (1 mm per heartbeat) to the highest value at which the Korotkoff sound is heard with each beat, including those that occur during inspiration. This is the second figure. The difference between the two is the value of the pulsus paradoxus in mm Hg.

A Self-Study

While you measure his systolic blood pressure, have your partner breathe in and out against resistance, for example, through the center cardboard from a toilet paper roll, with the distal end squeezed together. If he generates significant inspiratory and expiratory intrapleural pressures, an abnormal pulsus paradoxus will be produced (Sapira & Kirkpatrick, 1983). One might prefer, for aesthetic reasons, to use one's fist to generate the resistance. When done properly, this exercise also slows up the phases of respiration, giving the novice more time to make the measurements.

In many normal people, it is even possible to appreciate a drop in the systolic blood pressure by palpation at the radial artery as the subject takes a very deep breath. Try it on yourself: While palpating your radial pulse, suddenly take a deep breath. Pay attention to the pulse during the next two beats. What happens to the wave amplitude?

Many people can detect a difference. If you are not sure you can feel the change, repeat the experiment by breathing in and out against a strong airway resistance as described above.

For the attending. This is probably one of the most important parts of the teaching of pulsus paradoxus both because it uses a physiologic approach and because the discussion of pulsus paradoxus can be wrong even in a standard textbook (Chamberlain & Ogilvie, 1974).

Causes of Abnormal Pulsus Paradoxus

➧ Between 70% and 100% of patients with pericardial tamponade exhibit this finding (Kuhn, 1976; Reddy et al., 1978). The lower figure probably includes cases of chronic pericardial tamponade in which the pericardium has had an opportunity to distend; acute cases, in which the pericardium has not been stretched, probably all have the finding.

Abnormal pulsus paradoxus has been described in 80% of cases of asthma (Vaisrub, 1974); it appears when the FEV1 is reduced to about 0.5 to 0.7 liters (Rebuck & Pengelly, 1973). It also occurs in 50% of cases of shock, especially those with an increased peripheral resistance and a decreased blood volume (Cohn et al., 1967); 30% to 45% of cases of effusive, "constrictive" pericarditis (Braunwald, 1980; Wise & Conti, 1976) but not in true dry constrictive pericarditis (Spodick, 1984); about 30 percent of cases of pulmonary embolism (Cohen et al., 1973); and occasionally in right ventricular failure (McGregor, 1979), severe congestive failure (Salel et al., 1973), right ventricular infarction (Greenberg & Gitler, 1983), obesity (Kuhn, 1976), and possibly patent ductus arteriosus (Gauchat & Katz, 1924). Some of the above etiologies are actually classes of etiology that may subsume specific mention of myocarditis, tumors of the mediastinum (Major, 1975), pulmonary emphysema, paramediastinal effusion, endocardial fibrosis, fibro-

elastosis, myocardial amyloidosis, scleroderma, mitral stenosis with right sided cardiac failure, and tricuspid stenosis (DeGowin, 1965).

False Negatives

There are certain situations in which one would expect pulsus paradoxus, but an intervening problem interferes with the requisite mechanism; either both ventricles do not fill against a common pericardial stiffness or else the respiratory changes alternately favoring the right and left heart do not occur. Examples of these intervening confounders that produce false negatives are: far advanced left ventricular hypertrophy, severe left heart failure, atrial septal defect, severe aortic insufficiency, severe tamponade with *extreme* hypotension, "right heart tamponade" (from a low compliance left ventricle), loculated pericardial fluid (which prevents equalization of ventricular diastolic pressures), and low-pressure tamponade (Spodick, 1983).

Reversed Pulsus Paradoxus

An inspiratory *rise* of the systolic blood pressure is seen in idiopathic hypertrophic subaortic stenosis, isorhythmic ventricular rhythms, and with intermittent inspiratory positive-pressure breathing in the presence of left ventricular failure (Massumi et al., 1973).

Unusual Pulse Pressures

An extremely *widened pulse pressure* (i.e., $[BP_{sys} - BP_{dias}] > 50\%\ BP_{sys}$) may be seen in conditions associated with a high stroke volume (see Ch. 17). While aortic insufficiency is the best known example, others are hyperthyroidism, beriberi, pregnancy, fever, anemia, patent ductus arteriosus, severe Paget's disease with extensive arteriovenous shunting through the diseased bone, and severe exfoliative dermatitis with shunting through the diseased skin. If an extremely wide pulse pressure is found in only one limb, one should search for an arteriovenous fistula in that limb. Branham's sign (see p. 94) will be confirmatory even without angiography.

It should be noted that patients with high stroke volume will not always have a widened pulse pressure. Patients with hepatic cirrhosis, for instance, so rarely have sufficient arteriovenous shunting to cause a widened pulse pressure that cirrhosis never appears in the differential diagnosis of the finding.

Many of the signs associated with aortic insufficiency are really signs of high stroke volume, and so may also be associated with other diseases in the latter's differential diagnosis.

A *narrowed* pulse pressure may be defined as one that is less than 25% of the systolic pressure. It suggests decreased stroke volume and may be seen in pericardial tamponade, constrictive pericarditis, tachycardia, or aortic stenosis (see Ch. 17, p. 313). (Artifactually narrowed pulse pressure may sometimes be produced in conditions of severely heightened vasomotor tone with increased peripheral vascular resistance, e.g., cardiogenic shock. Like other blood pressure artifacts, it can be unmasked with a direct measurement of the intraarterial pressure.)

A Chrestomathy of Artifacts

Auscultatory Gap

The auscultatory gap is fortunately a rare phenomenon of indirect blood pressure determination. At some pressure below the systolic pressure, the Korotkoff sounds fade out, to fade in again

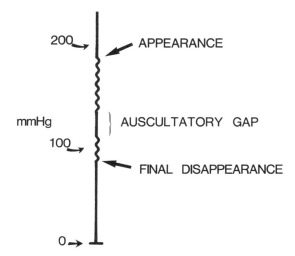

200 → ← APPEARANCE

mmHg   } AUSCULTATORY GAP

100 →

← FINAL DISAPPEARANCE

0 →

Figure 6-2.   The auscultatory gap.

at a lower pressure, persisting then down to the true diastolic, where they disappear for the last time. Figure 6-2 shows a blood pressure determination that has an auscultatory gap. The points of first disappearance and of second reappearance mark the borders of the auscultatory gap.

The danger of the auscultatory gap lies in not realizing that it is there. In that instance, one might conclude that the diastolic pressure is much higher than is really the case. Alternately, if one did not detect the true systolic by palpation first, one might begin searching for the systolic pressure inside the auscultatory gap, taking the point of reappearance of the Korotkoff sounds to be the systolic pressure. Either way, inappropriate and dangerous therapy might be instituted.

The auscultatory gap is most likely to appear in the obese arm, especially if the physician pumps up the blood pressure cuff slowly and traps a great deal of blood in the arm's venous compartment (Ragan & Bordley, 1941). Another way to trap blood is to pump the blood pressure cuff up a second time immediately following the first determination, without allowing a minute or two for the trapped blood to escape. The mechanism suggests the remedy. Having the patient with an obese arm hold the arm straight up in the air when you pump up the cuff the first time, and quickly inflating the cuff above the palpable systolic, would help to prevent the initial venous pooling.

Effects of Vessel Wall Stiffness

The stiffness or laxity of the vessel wall affects the propagation of the pressure waves, and may cause either an artifactual increase or decrease in the indirectly determined pressure, depending on the circumstances. In Hill's sign (discussed in Ch. 17, p. 310), the apparent systolic pressure is higher than the actual pressure because of the extra pressure waves that may be propagated or reverberated along a very lax vessel wall. As you might expect, a stiff wall could have the opposite effect (Cohn, 1967, vide infra). Further, just as a lax wall can produce an artificially low diastolic blood pressure in conditions of high stroke volume such as aortic insufficiency, a stiff wall might produce an artifactually high value (Messerli et al., 1985).

Pseudohypotension.   When simultaneous direct and indirect blood pressure measurements were made upon patients in shock (Cohn, 1967), it was found that subjects with a high peripheral vascular resistance had damping of their arterial wall sound-

boards, and the Korotkoff sounds were produced so poorly that both the systolic and diastolic pressures were significantly underestimated by the indirect technique (i.e., pseudohypotension). The low cuff pressures were not simply due to a low cardiac output, because in the patients with shock and a *low* peripheral vascular resistance, the direct and indirect methods gave equivalent results. Furthermore, Cohn could reproduce the pseudohypotension by infusing vasopressors into the arm circulation of normal volunteers.

Pseudohypertension.   This stiff wall artifact, unlike the above, is not related to sound generation, but results from the fact that the arterial wall is difficult to compress. The cuff pressure will be the sum of the pressure required to collapse the artery plus the pressure of the column of blood. Both the systolic and diastolic pressure measurements will be artifactually high (Messerli et al., 1985). The phenomenon is analogous to cuff hypertension.

You can judge the stiffness of the arteries by feeling the pulse, then occluding the artery proximal to the pulse with a blood pressure cuff or your finger, a maneuver described by Osler (Mishriki, 1987). If the distal artery can still be felt unchanged, even after the pulse is obliterated, the patient has sufficient arteriosclerosis to produce some degree of pseudohypertension.

The remedy for both pseudohypotension and pseudohypertension is the touchstone of science: an independent covariable—in this case, the direct intraarterial blood pressure determination.

Other Vagaries of Blood Pressure Measurement

Nurses often obtain lower blood pressures than physicians (Moutsos et al., 1967). Some psychosomatic studies reveal that pleasant conversation will lower the blood pressure, but that the pressure will rise if an unpleasant or tension-filled subject is introduced, as in the so-called "stress interview." These phenomena are further examples of the point made earlier: there is no such thing as "the" blood pressure.

Finally, there is the unconscious bias of the physician, manifest in the fact that physicians tend to record the terminal digits "8" and "0" more often than could be accounted for by chance. Further, this tendency can be eliminated by giving the same physicians a random-zero blood pressure machine (Pemberton, 1963).

Other Tests That Use a Blood Pressure Cuff

Any of the tests involving the assessment of an arterial pulse may be made quantitative by employing the blood pressure cuff. Most of these will be found in the chapter concerned with the arterial circulation (e.g., Adson's sign), although a few (e.g., pulsus alternans) will be found in the next section.

The Trousseau test is done with a blood pressure cuff, but does not involve measuring the blood pressure. Accordingly, it is described under the neurologic exam, Chapter 26, page 488. Sternbach's pain thermometer (see Ch. 3, p. 38) also employs a blood pressure cuff, as does a test for thrombophlebitis (Ch. 19, p. 367).

The Pulse

Doctor Pinch: Give me your hand and let me feel your pulse. (William Shakespeare, *Comedy of Errors*, Act 4, Scene 4)

This section discusses the frequency and regularity of the heartbeat as detected peripherally. It does not consider the arterial pulse wave contour which is best detected at the carotid artery and is recorded under the "arterial" part of the peripheral vascular examination (see pp. 331–333). Similarly, the palpable consistency of the arterial wall itself (which contributes to the estimation of the biologic, as opposed to the chronologic age) is also recorded under the "arterial" part of the peripheral vascular examination (see Ch. 18).

Frequency

The pulse is universally expressed in beats per minute.

A Method

At the radial artery (or the carotid, if both radials are impalpable), count the number of impulses in a 1-minute period. Later one can shorten this time to 30 seconds and double the counted beats if they are between 30 and 50. However, whenever one decreases the sampling time, one decreases the opportunity to find abnormalities.

Normals

A rate faster than 100/minute is considered a tachycardia. A rate below 50/minute is a bradycardia by the usual definition. However, since the physical examination is a screening method, we want to accept many false positives, but not have any false negatives. Therefore, we will consider a pulse rate below 60/minute to be abnormal; that is, worthy of further consideration with the understanding that it may turn out to be a normal variant.

An epistemologic note. If, after further searching, nothing else can be connected with a finding, it is considered of peripheral significance, rather than of critical significance. When assembling all the findings at the end of the examination, one would use the critical findings to compose the differential diagnosis. One does not know in advance whether a finding will be critical or peripheral, so initially all must be taken seriously (and not assumed to be peripheral). Examples would be a bradycardia in a healthy young sprinter applying for insurance (peripheral) versus bradycardia in an untreated cretin (critical).

Regularity

The pulse may be described as regular when every beat comes at the expected time. An irregular pulse may be *regularly* irregular (when the irregularities can be predicted) or *irregularly* irregular (when they cannot).

Although the study of arrhythmias in the modern era correctly requires an electrocardiograph machine, much can still be learned from an examination of the pulse, including which patients need an electrocardiographic recording. Additional information about arrhythmias can be obtained from auscultation of the first heart sound (Ch. 17, p. 292), carotid sinus massage (Ch. 18, p. 337), and observation of the jugular venous pulses (Ch. 19, p. 363).

Regular Tachycardias

The rate and regularity are clues to the most probable type of arrhythmia. If there is a regular tachycardia, it is most likely sinus tachycardia if the rate is between 100 and 125; atrial flutter with 2:1 block if the rate is from 125 to 165; paroxysmal atrial tachycardia if the rate is from 175 to 200.

Above 200/minute, the prognosis becomes ominous either because of the etiology or because of the physiologic effects of the rapid rate itself. Ventricular tachycardia may have a rate of about 250, at which there is often no measurable blood pressure.

A Note on Sinus Tachycardia

Sinus tachycardia may be seen in a wide variety of abnormal conditions: any type of congestive heart failure or any high-output state, such as fever, anemia, or thyrotoxicosis. As a sign, sinus tachycardia is sensitive for pathology, so it is important not to disregard it. (For example, a pulse rate of 90 or greater has a sensitivity of 84% for hyperthyroidism in patients aged 10 to 29, 79% in patients aged 30 to 39, and 75% in patients aged 60 to 83 (Nordyke et al., 1988).) However, there are many false positives.

The sinus tachycardia of excitement disappears during sleep. Most other sinus tachycardias lessen during sleep, but that from thyrotoxicosis sometimes continues unabated.

•

As an example of the potential importance of this finding, sinus tachycardia was once noticed in a research subject. Her "innocent" systolic murmur was rediscovered, as well as her wide fixed split second heart sound. This led to the erroneous but testable hypothesis that she had an atrial septal defect. Instead, at cardiac catheterization she was found to have a partial anomalous pulmonary venous return, a condition that was of great significance in the study because it might have affected the metabolism of the experimental drugs. In this case, the tachycardia was a central finding.

•

One feature that may help distinguish sinus tachycardia from paroxysmal atrial tachycardia (PAT) is that the former begins with gradual acceleration and ends by gradual deceleration (Fig. 6-3A), whereas PAT classically has an abrupt onset and termination (Fig. 6-3B). (However, the excitement caused by the arrhythmia might increase circulating catecholamines. The PAT could then convert to a sinus tachycardia, which would slowly decelerate as the catecholamines waned.)

There are two types of sinus tachycardia that have eponyms. In patients with chronic lung disease or other causes of right-sided hypertension, stretching of the right atrial receptors initiates a reflex resulting in chronic sinus tachycardia. This is known as the *Bainbridge reflex.*

Branham's sign is a sinus tachycardia due to an arteriovenous fistula in which the heart rate can be slowed to normal upon occlusion of arterial flow (by means of a blood pressure cuff) to the limb containing the fistula. When the blood pressure cuff is deflated and blood flow to that limb resumes, the heart rate immediately rises.

Regularly Irregular Pulses

Second-degree heart block. If some, but not all, of the atrial impulses are blocked and do not reach the ventricles (the definition of second-degree heart block), a regularly irregular pulse may result. One way of naming the second-degree heart blocks is by ratio (e.g., 5:4, 4:3, 3:2, and 2:1). The first number in the ratio is the number of atrial impulses in a recurring sequence, and the second number is the number of times (in each series) that the atrial impulse activates the ventricle. Since there is almost never time for a ventricular escape beat (unlike third-degree heart block, in which the ventricles are never excited by the atrial impulses), there is simply a skipped beat. The ratio of the block is usually very regular.

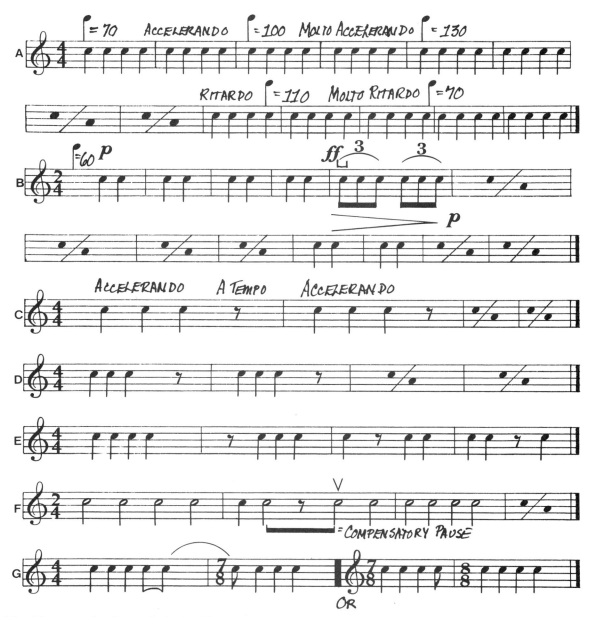

Figure 6-3. *The meter of various arrhythmias. The notation ./. means to repeat the previous measure. A, sinus tachycardia; B, paroxysmal atrial tachycardia (PAT); C, Mobitz type I second-degree heart block (4:3 Wenckebach); as the PR intervals lengthen before the dropped beat, the RR intervals decrease; D. Mobitz type II second-degree heart block (4:3); E, Mobitz II second-degree heart block (5:4); F, premature ventricular contraction with compensatory pause; G, premature atrial contractions. (In real life the time value of the first eighth note is not always exactly half a quarter note.)*

What one feels is a series of regular pulses, then a missing beat. Then again the same number of regular pulses, and—right on cue—the missing one. With 5:4 block, there are four pulses, then a skipped one; with 4:3 block, three beats then a miss (see Fig. 6-3C).

Whenever one feels such a series, with the missed beat coming right on time, one should think of second-degree heart block, examine the neck veins immediately (see Ch. 19), and do an electrocardiogram as soon as possible.

With 2:1 block, there is no way to know that a beat is missing, unless one looks at the neck veins; thus, this particular rhythm is actually a regular one.

In addition to naming the second-degree heart blocks by their ratios of atrial to ventricular activities, they may also be named in terms of what the electrocardiographic PR interval is doing. If it is being gradually prolonged until the atrial impulse fails to be transmitted to the ventricles, it is called a Wenckebach phenomenon, after the doctor who first described it (Wenckebach, 1906), or Mobitz type I block (Fig. 6-4). If, on the other hand, there is no lengthening of successive PR intervals prior to the skipped beat, it is called a Mobitz type II block (Fig. 6-3, D and E).

In Mobitz type I, there is a slight acceleration not seen in Mobitz type II. See the legend to Figure 6-4 for the explanation.

Sinus arrhythmia. The subtlest, and least important, of the regular irregularities is sinus arrhythmia. It is simply the clini-

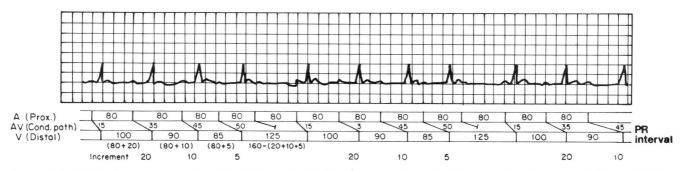

A (Prox.)		80		80		80		80		80		80		80		80		80		80		80		80			
AV (Cond. path)	15		35		45		50		15		3		45		50		15		35		45	**PR**
V (Distal)		100		90		85		125		100		90		85		125		100		90			**interval**

(80+20) (80+10) (80+5) 160−(20+10+5) 100 90 85 125 100 90

Increment 20   10   5   20   10   5   20   10

Figure 6-4. *Mobitz I second-degree heart block (Wenckebach). This shows why Figure 6-3C is marked accelerando and Figure 6-3D is not. In Mobitz type I (but not type II), the amount of PR prolongation decreases on successive beats ("increments"). This makes successive RR intervals shorter.*

cally noticeable exaggeration of a normal phenomenon: the speeding of the heart rate with inspiration and the deceleration of the heart rate during expiration.

•

A self-experiment: Take a deep breath while feeling your pulse. What happened? Now exhale, and note what happens to the rate. If you do a Valsalva maneuver during expiration, the pulse will slow even more.

Sinus arrhythmia is most frequently observed in healthy young persons, especially well-conditioned athletes.

•

Ectopic beats. *Bigeminy,* which comes from the Latin word for twin, means that every other beat is an ectopic beat—either atrial or ventricular—so that the beats seem to come in pairs. Usually, bigeminy is caused by ventricular premature contractions, and may be a sign of digitalis intoxication (though it is neither very sensitive nor specific for that diagnosis). *Trigeminy* means that every third beat is ectopic, so that the pulse seems to be divided into triads. *Quadrigeminy* means that every fourth beat is ectopic.

Pulsus alternans. Pulsus alternans is a regular irregularity in amplitude, a weak beat alternating with a strong beat. If it occurs during a tachycardia, pulsus alternans may be quite benign, depending upon the underlying disease. But when it occurs with sinus rhythm, as in left ventricular failure due either to ischemic heart disease or hypertensive cardiovascular disease, it is of ominous significance, because the heart apparently is unable to pump out an adequate stroke volume on alternate beats.

The meter of pulsus alternans *may* also be regularly irregular because the weak beat can be slightly early or late, playing off the rhythm in the manner of Errol Garner. But usually the pulse feels regular because the premature occurrence of the weak beat (Friedman, 1956) is compensated for by its prolonged transit time to the periphery (Friedberg, 1956).

A better method for detecting pulsus alternans than simple palpation of the pulse is to pump the blood pressure cuff up above the systolic. Deflating it slowly, search for a point at which only alternate beats are felt (and heard). This will be above the point at which all beats are felt (heard). (This method is analogous to that used for determining pulsus paradoxus [p. 92], except that the alternation is not related to the respiratory cycle.)

Pulsus alternans may or may not be associated with electrical alternans, the electrocardiographic alternation in the height of the QRS in any given lead. In cases of tachycardia, such an associa-

tion is neither surprising nor ominous. However, in cases of congestive heart failure, the occurrence of electrical alternans with pulsus alternans has a serious prognosis.

Irregularly Irregular Pulses

There are basically four irregularly irregular pulses that are of concern at the bedside: premature atrial contractions (PACs), premature ventricular contractions (PVCs), atrial fibrillation, and multifocal atrial tachycardia.

The two types of premature contractions are easy to identify when episodic (vide infra). However, when combined or frequent, the pulse can be so confusing that a confident determination cannot be made without the ECG.

Atrial fibrillation is highly chaotic in its usual form. It has been called delirium cordis because the only thing predictable about the beat was its unpredictability.

These irregular irregularities are best learned at the bedside. If you will prepare yourself by reading, you will be able to take advantage of learning opportunities that present themselves, and can return to these pages later for a leisurely review.

For the attending. There is also a fifth type of irregularly irregular pulse, sinus arrest, and a sixth, sinus exit block. In these situations, a sinus impulse never reaches the atria. If the pause between beats is exactly two RR intervals, there is no way to distinguish the two, even with an ECG strip (since this does not show sinus node events, only atrial and ventricular activity). If the interval is less than exactly two RR intervals, the pulse taker could make a diagnosis of sinus arrest. However, the arrest might be for longer than two RR intervals, albeit not an exact multiple. To make things more confusing, the longer a sinus pause, the greater the likelihood of an escape beat from a lower pacemaker. Thus, some very confusing pulses can be generated. Because of the episodic nature of these pulses, their rarity, and the ubiquity of Holter monitoring, I have abandoned the teaching of these pulses.

There is also no way to distinguish 2:1 sinus exit block from 2:1 atrioventricular block, a distinction that can be significant both in terms of underlying diagnosis, and in the case of the latter, the use of drugs that could further slow the atrioventricular conduction. If carotid sinus pressure (see Ch. 18, p. 337) should geometrically increase the block (slow the pulse), the diagnosis of atrioventricular block would seem secure. Conversely, if there were no effect, it would be suggestive of exit block, although the test would not be definitive.

Premature ventricular contractions. This type of ectopic beat is followed by a *fully compensatory pause.* The pause permits the beat *after* the ectopic to occur just on time, that is, at two normal RR intervals after the last *normal* beat. In other

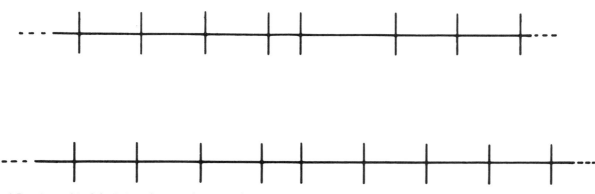

Figure 6-5. *A graphical depiction of ectopic beats, each vertical stroke representing one pulse beat. Can you identify the ectopic beat in each tracing? Is the ectopic beat atrial or ventricular? (See text.)*

words, the shortened RR interval before the ectopic plus the lengthened RR interval after the ectopic are exactly equal to twice the normal interval. Demonstrate this fact to yourself on Figure 6-5.

One effect of the compensatory pause is to allow a longer filling period and hence greater stroke volume. Thus, the postextrasystolic pulse amplitude should normally be greater. In fact, it is usually this postextrasystolic contraction that attracts the patient's attention, rather than the extrasystole itself. It is often described by saying "my heart flipped over."

There are two situations in which the postextrasystolic pulse amplitude is less than expected. The first is a state of impaired contractility, as in congestive heart failure. The second is idiopathic hypertrophic subaortic stenosis. If the Starling-Frank curve is still normal, the greater filling increases the strength of contraction of all the cardiac muscle, including the obstructing ring. The net effect is to blunt the expected rise in stroke volume.

Unfortunately, in both cases we are attempting to compare the actual beat with "what should have been." The absence of an increase over normal may be difficult to detect, since the natural comparison is with the preceding (extrasystolic) beat, which is of diminished amplitude. However, in the rare cases in which the postextrasystolic beat is definitely less than the following beat, the differential diagnosis is reduced to two possibilities. Though perhaps not worth searching for, this phenomenon may be, to those capable of appreciating it, the free gift of circumstance.

Very advanced. Sometimes one may wish to induce a premature ventricular contraction, especially when one wants to auscult for the effect of the postextrasystolic beat upon a murmur (see Ch. 17, p. 315), or to let the patient identify such a beat as the cause of his palpitations. Some physicians have actually struck the patient sharply on the precordium. I have not had success with that technique, but have had some luck with the noxious stressor of mental arithmetic, when vigorously applied to susceptible patients (Lown et al., 1978).

Note that the fully compensatory pause is longer than the pause after the skipped beat in Mobitz type I block. In the latter instance, the exact length of the interval containing the skipped beat is twice the PP interval minus the sum of the increments in PR intervals before the dropped beat (Cabeen et al., 1978), or twice the PP minus the difference between the first PR interval after the missed beat and the last PR interval before it (Fig. 6-4).

Premature atrial contractions. With PACs, there is no compensatory pause. The RR interval after the ectopic beat is equal to the normal RR interval. As shown in Figure 6-6, the PAC's ventricular contraction is preceded by a normal activation

sequence, including a His bundle spike, and followed by a "resetting" of the sinus node.

For musicians, the difference between PVCs and PACs is illustrated in Figure 6-3F. The PVC is simply a syncopated beat; the fourth note in measure two comes in exactly "on the down beat." You can make this diagnosis by tapping your foot in time at the bedside. On the other hand, the PAC initiates a new time signature, although the conductor's tempo does not change. If you attempt to tap this out at the bedside, you will find yourself out of synch following the premature contraction; the heart will now be beating on the "up beat" (Fig. 6-3G).

In point of fact, electrocardiographic PACs with fully compensatory pauses do occur, rarely and inexplicably.

Atrial fibrillation. One bedside trick that helps to identify atrial fibrillation is the *apical-radial pulse deficit*. If one simultaneously measures the apical ventricular rate and the radial pulse, one will find the radial rate to be the lesser in all cases of atrial fibrillation except those at very slow rates (under 50/ minute). This is due to the fact that some of the ventricular contractions are preceded by short diastoles with such poor ventricular filling that there is insufficient stroke volume to transmit the pressure wave out to the radial pulse. Occasionally, patients with frequent multifocal premature atrial contractions and multifocal premature ventricular contractions can also generate small apical-radial pulse deficits.

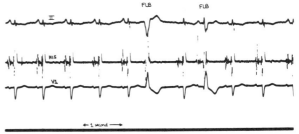

Figure 6-6. *Simultaneous electrocardiographic (leads II and V1) and His bundle tracings. The first FLB (funny-looking beat) is a premature ventricular contraction; the second FLB is a premature atrial contraction. Considering the second FLB, note that 1) the QRS is preceded by a P wave, 2) the His bundle recording (middle) shows the same activation sequence as the normal beats, and 3) there is no compensatory pause. With the first FLB, none of the above are true. Tracing courtesy of Drs. M. Fisher and R. Peters of Maryland.*

1. If a digitalized patient with a prior diagnosis of chronic atrial fibrillation presents with a perfectly regular pulse, one should suspect digitalis intoxication with a regular nodal rhythm and atrioventricular dissociation. (Note that in this form of "regularized" atrial fibrillation, the apical-radial pulse deficit also disappears.)
2. When the ventricular rate is speeded by drugs or exercise, atrial fibrillation usually becomes more irregular and ectopy tends to become more regular. However, this test has fallen into disrepute because there are many false negatives unless one gets the heart rate up to 140/minute. Also, ectopy due to an "anoxic focus" may worsen with exercise, producing a false positive.
3. The following aphorisms apply to atrial fibrillation:
   a. Atrial fibrillation plus stroke suggests cerebral embolism.
   b. Atrial fibrillation plus acute abdominal pain suggests a superior mesenteric artery embolism.
   c. Atrial fibrillation by itself suggests ischemic heart disease, long-standing mitral valve disease (especially mitral stenosis), long-standing hypertensive heart disease, or recent onset of masked hyperthyroidism. If these etiologies are excluded, one might consider hypoxia, Wolff-Parkinson-White syndrome, or chronic myocardiopathy.

An exercise in clinical reasoning.   Although clinical reasoning is discussed in Chapter 27, it is important to introduce some ideas now, so that you will be circumspect about the aphorisms that are offered, and so that you will remember that you are learning to collect data for a logical process.

Given that 85% of patients with new-onset atrial fibrillation can be shown to have ischemic heart disease, long-standing hypertensive heart disease, thyrotoxicosis, or rheumatic or mitral heart disease, could documented absence of the last three in a patient with recent-onset atrial fibrillation be used as evidence for ischemic heart disease? Write down your answer before reading Appendix 6-1.

Multifocal atrial tachycardia.   An important difference between this rhythm and atrial fibrillation is that this rhythm is "regular enough" to permit valid blood pressure measurements because the filling is equal for most beats. Similarly, there may be no apical radial pulse deficit with multifocal atrial tachycardia.

A Note on the History of Arrhythmias

When the patient has had an arrhythmia, you can often diagnose the type by beating out rhythms on the top of your desk and asking the patient to identify the one he experienced. Often, it is possible at least to exclude some arrhythmias. However, patients who had a very strong chronotropic stimulus, say from endogenous catecholamines, tend in retrospect to overestimate their heart rate.

Valsalva Maneuver

The Valsalva maneuver was invented in the 18th century by Valsalva for the laudable purpose of clearing the eustachian tubes (Nishimura & Tajik, 1986). It is still used for that purpose by divers. However, in medicine it consists of expiration against a closed glottis (not against the occluded nares), sustained for about 10 to 25 seconds, depending upon the specific protocol.

In research protocols, the subject blows into a mouthpiece connected to a mercury manometer, and generates the desired pressure (about 40 mm Hg). At the bedside, the patient is instructed to take a deep breath and strain as if to have a bowel movement or to lift something very heavy. Alternately, he can be asked to push against the examiner's hand, which is placed on the abdomen.

In the 20th century, physiologists discovered that this maneuver produced a variety of cardiovascular effects. The response has four phases (Fig. 6-7 and Table 6-1).

Abnormalities in the autonomic nervous system cause aberrations in this response. However, as you will notice, some of the blood pressure changes last but a few beats, so they cannot be detected at the bedside with an indirect blood pressure measurement. Accordingly, the Valsalva maneuver never gained in clinical popularity until phonocardiologists discovered that the change in murmurs during certain phases of the Valsalva response could help identify their etiology (see Ch. 17).

I have abandoned the teaching of the pulse and blood pressure responses, despite the fact that many books allude to them, because they cannot be measured using the contents of a black bag. However, some of the pulse changes can be picked up at the bedside by an astute clinician or even a sophomore equipped with a portable electrocardiograph machine.

For the attending.   These three methods should each detect the same autonomic dysfunction, produced by the same diseases.

1. *Method of Dr. Gerhard Muehlheims of Missouri*   Look for the post-Valsalva overshoot reflex bradycardia (phase IV). It is lost in altered sympathetic states, such as congestive heart failure and the faithful ingestion of noradrenolytic drugs.
2. *Method of Ewing*   The post-Valsalva bradycardia is also lost in the autonomic neuropathy of diabetes and in end-stage renal disease (Blake et al., 1989). One way of quantitating this requires an ECG machine. The subject performs the Valsalva maneuver for only 15 seconds, and the shortest RR interval during this time (phase II) is taken as the "tachycardia," or the denominator of the ratio to be calculated. The longest RR interval in the post-Valsalva overshoot period (phase IV "bradycardia") is the numerator. A ratio of 1.21 or more is the arbitrarily stated normal, 1.11 to 1.20 is borderline, and 1.10 or less is abnormal. The ratios are determined for three trials and averaged (Ewing et al., 1973).
3. *Method of Thomas*   The Mayo Clinic uses this method (Thomas et al., 1981) in the evaluation of orthostatic hypotension, which often has an autonomic etiology. Patients with orthostatic hypotension due to volume depletion should have a normal Valsalva response by this method.

   The RR interval is converted into a pulse rate. The maximum instantaneous heart rate observed during phase II is divided by the minimum heart rate obtained during phase IV, the post-Valsalva overshoot period. A ratio of 1.25 or above is taken to be normal, while ratios of less than unity are abnormal.

A Caveat

The tests are said to be invalid (Schatz, 1984) in congestive heart failure or obstructive lung disease. I suspect that this is because of

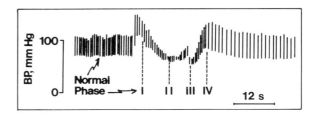

Figure 6-7.   The Valsalva response.

Table 6-1. Phases of the Valsalva Response

Phase	Action	BP	Pulse	Mechanism
I	Onset of strain	Increase	Stable	Compression of aorta
II	Continued strain	Decrease	Increase	Decreased venous return; increase in sympathetic tone
III	Release	Decrease	Stable	Blood pools in pulmonary vasculature
IV	Recovery	Increase	Decrease	Increased cardiac output due to increased venous return with continued vasoconstriction due to sympathetic activity; reflex bradycardia

Sources: Schatz (1984) and Thomas et al. (1981).

the sympathetic abnormalities that may occur in the former, and the Bainbridge reflex (p. 94) in the latter.

Respiration

His breathing was irregular; it would entirely cease for a quarter of a minute, and then it would become perceptible though very low, then by degrees it became heaving and quick, and then it would gradually cease again. This revolution in the state of his breathing occupied about a minute, during which there were about 30 acts of respiration. (Cheyne, 1818)

A Method

After taking the pulse rate, continue holding the patient's wrist. While looking toward your watch, observe the patient's chest for another minute, without speaking, counting the respiratory rate. If one counts for a full minute, one will not miss an irregularity such as Cheyne-Stokes or Biot's respirations (vide infra).

Respiratory Rate

The normal mean resting respiratory rate for recumbent healthy young men is 13/minute in the morning and 15/minute after lunch. No normal subjects had rates over 19/minute.

Bradypnea may be defined as a respiratory rate less than 10/minute. It can be seen in severe hypothyroidism and in central nervous system disease, especially that due to pharmacologic agents (e.g., narcotic analgesics and hypnotics). Bradypnea does not always mean alveolar hypoventilation, which is now operationally defined as an elevated arterial partial pressure of carbon dioxide.

Apneustic breathing is a bradypneic form of preterminal respiration seen in comatose patients. The patient will hold the breath at end inspiration before the Hering-Breuer reflex initiates the next cycle with expiration. Apneustic breathing is most often a sign of pontine disease (e.g., hemorrhage or basilar artery occlusion, but it occasionally accompanies hypoglycemia, anoxia, or severe meningitis) (Plum & Posner, 1972).

Tachypnea may be defined as a respiratory rate of 20/minute (or greater.) It is abnormal except in chronic care patients over the age of 67 years, in whom the normal range of respirations is 16–25/minute (McFadden et al., 1982). Tachypnea is seen in a wide variety of cardiac, pulmonary, metabolic, central nervous system, and infectious diseases.

1. The above definition of tachypnea may permit too many false negatives. A stricter definition would be more sensitive for pulmonary embolus: only 8% of patients with pulmonary embo-

lism breathe at a rate less than 16/minute (Fulkerson et al., 1986).
2. Cope (Silen, 1979) pointed out that a respiratory rate twice normal in a patient with suspected acute abdomen is evidence of primary thoracic disease with secondary referral of symptoms to the abdomen.
3. Tachypnea may be of value in the differential diagnosis of hypovolemic shock versus the hypotension of sepsis. If the respiratory rate is elevated, some clinicians favor the diagnosis of sepsis.
4. Tachypneic patients who are in congestive heart failure have waterlogged lungs and pant like a dog from respiratory midposition. Tachypneic patients who have obstructive lung disease "breathe off the top" from a position of chest expansion, and additionally sometimes have "door stopping" when air trapping occurs during expiration. The best way to learn to make these observations is in the company of an older clinician.
5. The hyperventilation syndrome may be diagnosed by reproducing the symptoms (such as lightheadedness and paresthesias), then showing that they can be relieved by breathing into a paper bag. Have the patient follow your respiratory rate and exaggerated respiratory excursion. When you start to become lightheaded, continue to move your shoulders and arms as if still taking deep breaths, but breathe only on about one third of the excursions.

This diagnostic maneuver is actually therapeutic in that the patient learns that you truly understand what is happening to him and that you are calm about it. That mastery spreads to him, especially when he learns that the paper bag works.

Effort

In addition to rate, one should observe the ease of respiration. Patients with severe emphysema attempt to prevent terminal respiratory airway closure by pursing their lips. Other types of pulmonary and cardiac tachypnea can be accompanied by a variety of audible sounds ranging from intentional vocalizations to grunting, stridor, wheezing, and audible breathing. Some patients may grunt because of sputum, blood, or tumor occluding an airway; others from pleuritis, whenever they take a deep breath. Some patients who grunt with respiration have an acute abdomen and no intrathoracic pathology. Grunting, like pursed lip breathing, may help to prevent terminal airway closure. Grunting is also a useful clue to the presence of pneumonia or pulmonary fluid in infants. Patients are said to have labored breathing when they are concentrating their efforts on breathing, even if they make no noise.

The most common abnormalities seen on the medical ward are labored breathing and Kussmaul respirations (vide infra).

Patients may assume a particular position in order to breathe better. (Orthopnea, platypnea, and trepopnea are discussed in Ch. 5.)

Respiratory Pattern

Cheyne-Stokes Respiration

Cheyne-Stokes respiration (periodic breathing) is a regularly irregular pattern in respiratory volume, which ranges from apnea to hyperpnea and back again (Fig. 6-8A.) The classic description (Cheyne, 1818) is quoted at the beginning of this section.

Cheyne's original patient had both a diseased heart and enlarged cerebral ventricles, and the debate over whether Cheyne-Stokes has primarily a cardiovascular or a neurologic etiology continues to the present time.

Brown and Plum studied 28 patients with Cheyne-Stokes respiration, plus control subjects from the following groups: normal, patients with congestive heart failure, and patients with unilateral and bilateral cerebral vascular disease. Every subject with Cheyne-Stokes respiration had an increased respiratory sensitivity to CO_2 resulting from bilateral supramedullary brain dysfunction. Peak ventilation coincided with maximal $PaCO_2$ and apnea with low $PaCO_2$. The authors concluded (Brown & Plum, 1961) that periodic breathing is apparently neurogenic posthyperventilation apnea and that extracerebral abnormalities are not the primary cause. However, they also referred to an experiment in which it was possible to induce Cheyne-Stokes respiration in animals by artificially increasing the length of their carotid arteries, without otherwise altering brain function. Such an experiment could support either etiology, neurogenic or cardiovascular.

Karp confirmed and extended the blood gas determinations of the previous workers, and also noted that the circulation time across the brain was relatively prolonged during periods of apnea (Karp et al., 1961). The alteration in cerebral circulation was felt to be the most important factor, but the converse possibility, that the changes in circulation were secondary events, could not be excluded.

Neurologists supporting the primacy of the central nervous system etiology of Cheyne-Stokes respirations have also reported similar fluctuations in other neurologic events. A most interesting example is the series of three patients with periodic breathing who demonstrated pupillary dilatation during hyperpnea and constriction during the apneic phase (Sullivan et al., 1968).

When apparently contradictory evidence supports each of two opposing theories on pathophysiology, time usually proves both of them to be right in some way.

It was formerly believed that Cheyne-Stokes respirations could only occur with an intact brain stem, but the classic pattern has been seen in partial pontine hematomas (Kase et al., 1980).

With this background, we can better understand the clinical differential diagnosis of Cheyne-Stokes respiration.

The causes of Cheyne-Stokes respiration are: congestive heart failure, meningitis, pneumonia, hypoxia (DeGowin, 1965), brain tumor, chronic nephritis, some poisonings, high-altitude mountain sickness, bilateral or unilateral cerebral infarction, damage to the central pontine tegmentum, bilateral disease of the descending motor pathways, pseudobulbar palsy, mild congestive heart failure accompanying some motor pathway disease, posthyperventilation in patients without neurologic or cardiovascular disease (Brown & Plum, 1961), and the obesity cardiorespiratory syndrome (Karp et al., 1961).

Seemingly normal persons may have Cheyne-Stokes respiration during sleep. Although today we would suspect that such persons might have the sleep-apnea syndrome, the abruptness with which a full inspiratory effort appears in the sleep-apnea syndrome is not seen in Cheyne-Stokes syndrome, but rather in Biot's breathing, another form of irregular breathing.

Biot's Breathing

Biot's breathing (Fig. 6-8B) is an irregularly irregular breathing, characterized by more abrupt starts and stops than Cheyne-Stokes respiration and by an absence of periodicity. Biot's breathing is much less common and has been less well studied. I consider them to be equally ominous, directing attention to the central nervous system, the meninges, and their blood supply.

In point of fact I have seen tracings supposed to represent Cheyne-Stokes respiration that were sufficiently irregular to resemble those published by Biot (Karp et al., 1961, Figs. 4 and 5). Conversely, some of the tracings from Biot's patients closely resemble those of Cheyne-Stokes respiration, and Biot's paper was actually entitled "A Contribution to the Study of the Cheyne-Stokes Respiratory Phenomenon" (Biot, 1876).

Cheyne-Stokes breathing rarely leads to sudden apnea and cardiorespiratory arrest, whereas Biot's breathing commonly does (J. Bass, personal communication, 1986).

Kussmaul Respirations

Kussmaul respirations are regular, deep, and usually fast. Unlike the other eponymous forms of breathing, the pattern is basically an exaggeration of the normal. It results from central hyperventilation, and is a response to any type of acute metabolic acidosis.

In metabolic acidosis, the loss of bicarbonate and resulting rise in the pH could be compensated for by removing proportional amounts of carbon dioxide, as the Henderson-Hasselbach equation shows. The only feasible way to achieve this is hyperventilation.

Patients with cardiac or pulmonary disease may also hyperventilate, not to eliminate carbon dioxide, but to increase the oxygenation of their blood. They will also appear to have "air hunger" or Kussmaul respirations.

In patients with Kussmaul respirations but a normal respiratory rate, the increase in tidal volume can be detected by noting that the patient has trouble with conversation. The respirations cannot be inhibited for speech, so that the patient must pause in mid-phrase to breathe.

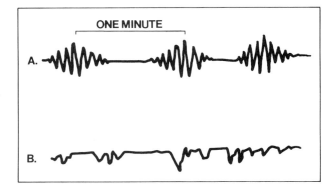

ONE MINUTE

A.

B.

Figure 6-8. *A, The classic spirogram of Cheyne-Stokes respiration, a regularly irregular pattern. The flat lines represent periods of apnea. Notice that when the patient is breathing, the amplitude changes, but not the frequency. B, An example of Biot's breathing in a patient with tuberculosis meningitis, traced from Figure 4 in Biot's paper. The respiratory activity is irregularly irregular in that frequency, respiratory depth, and periodicity vary in an irregular manner.*

Parkinson's Disease

Peculiar respiratory patterns may occur in patients with postencephalitic Parkinson's disease (Sacks, 1973). Without warning, one such patient experienced a sudden inspiratory gasp, followed by forced breath holding for 10 to 15 seconds, then a violent expiration, and finally an apneic pause for 10 to 15 seconds.

Temperature

"He is so shaken of a burning quotidian tertian that it is most lamentable to behold."

William Shakespeare, *King Henry the Fifth*, II, i

Temperature Measurement

The temperature may be measured rectally or orally. The latter should be performed by placing the thermometer bulb under the tongue with the lips kept closed. With a mercury thermometer that has been well shaken down, equilibration requires about 3 minutes. With newer instruments using a thermistor, less than 60 seconds may be required. (*A self-study*: Try sticking the probes from several of these under your tongue at the same time. With your mouth closed, do the instruments record the same temperature?)

The rectal temperature is usually about 1°F (0.55°C) higher than the oral temperature. In patients who are tachypneic (breathing more than 20 times per minute), the difference averages 1.67°F (0.93°C.), increasing with the respiratory rate, and becoming independent of whether the patient is mouth breathing (Tandberg & Sklar, 1983).

Other causes for falsely low oral temperatures include recent ingestion of cold substances or failure to keep the lips closed. Falsely high oral temperatures may result from failure to shake down the thermometer, ingestion of hot substances, or smoking.

Axillary temperatures are extremely inaccurate.

Although the scientific literature has adopted the convention of expressing temperatures in degrees Centigrade, many clinical thermometers are still calibrated in degrees Fahrenheit. The conversion formula is: $T°F = 9/5 (T°C) + 32$; Or, $T°C = 5/9 [(T°F) - 32]$.

Factitious fever may be produced by the patient surreptitiously applying heat to the thermometer. If factitious fever is suspected, the patient should be observed throughout the process of taking the temperature. Patients have been known to switch glass thermometers, substituting a preheated one, so the serial number on the original thermometer should be noted (Murray, 1979). The technique of holding hot liquids in the mouth before the temperature taking could be foiled by measuring the rectal temperature. Another method is to use an electronic thermometer to measure the temperature of the urine as it is voided. Data and nomograms are available (Murray et al., 1977). If the oral temperature is 38°C, the expected urine temperature is 37.3°C (lower 99% confidence limit = 36.15°C). For an oral temperature of 39°C, the comparable figures are 38.15°C and 36.95°C. Thus, if the patient's measured oral temperature is 40°C, and the urine temperature is only 37.7°C, one should suspect factitious fever.

Factitious fever is to be distinguished from factitious infection, in which fever is a secondary but genuine phenomenon.

Normal Temperature

Although most thermometers give 98.6°F (37°C) as the upper limit of normal, many normal persons have a higher temperature, especially in the afternoon or after strenuous activity or a very warm bath. An *oral* temperature greater than 100.2°F (37.9°C) is definitely considered a fever (Hoeprich, 1972).

The normal temperature has a diurnal variation of from 0.5°F to 2°F (0.28°F to 1.11°C). There is also a cyclical variation in ovulating women, with the early morning temperature (taken with the patient still in bed, just after awakening) dropping slightly just before the onset of menstruation. There may be a further drop just prior to ovulation, followed by a rise coincident with ovulation. Thereafter, the temperature remains at that level until just prior to the next menstruation.

Fever

An elevation in temperature is usually a sign of an infectious or inflammatory condition, although it may also result from thyrotoxicosis, heat stroke, neoplasia, drugs, and many other entities. Several fever patterns have been described.

Relapsing fevers have afebrile days alternating with days of fever. Diseases characterized by relapsing fevers include familial Mediterranean fever; brucellosis, in which the fever is associated with physical activity and disappears on days of bed rest; Hodgkin's disease; Borrelia infections; tuberculosis, especially extrapulmonary; and malaria.

The Pel-Ebstein relapsing fever of Hodgkin's disease occurs in about 16% of cases, and is quite variable. It may last for hours to days, followed by days or weeks without fever.

The fever pattern in malaria may indicate the organism involved. Tertian fevers return on the 3rd day and so have a periodicity of 48 hours. They signify infection with *Plasmodium vivax* or *P. ovale*. Quartan fever is one that returns on the 4th day, so that it has a 72-hour periodicity. It is seen with *P. malariae*. A double quartan fever returns every other day, but the recurrences are alternately severe and mild. But triple quartan fever results from infection with three different strains of *P. malariae*, resulting in daily (quotidian) fever. (Of course, not all such fevers are due to malaria.)

A double quotidian fever occurs twice a day, and is seen in about half the cases of gonococcal endocarditis.

A double-humped ("saddle-backed") fever curve (with two peaks during 1 week, and a low grade fever in the valley) is seen in some viral diseases such as West Nile fever, dengue, and Bornholm's disease.

A remittent fever is one that falls each day, but not quite to normal, remaining at 99.2°F (37.3°C) or above. An intermittent fever falls to normal or below each day. In remittent or intermittent fever, the excursion in temperature is more than 0.3°C (0.5°F) and less than 1.4°C (2.5°F). A hectic fever is a remittent or intermittent fever with a difference of 1.4°C (2.5°F) or more between peak and trough. A sustained fever has less than 0.3°C (0.5°F) fluctuation during a 24-hour period.

The latter four fever patterns are of minimal diagnostic value, as shown in a study of 200 patients with single episodes of fever (Musher et al., 1979). A sustained fever occurred frequently enough in cases of Gram-negative pneumonia and of central nervous system damage (and infrequently enough in other conditions) to suggest but not establish one of these two diagnoses. The absence of the usual diurnal effect (maximum temperature between 4 p.m. and midnight) supported but did not prove a noninfectious etiology, especially central nervous system damage. Impairment of hypothalamic control of temperature was thought to be the mechanism of the fever associated with central nervous system damage.

The most common hypothalamic fever is part of the hypnotic-sedative withdrawal syndrome. It appears only during acute abstinence, and abates with treatment.

Paroxysmal hypothalamic fevers occur in syndromes with other centrally mediated events such as insomnia, hypersomnia, hyperphagia, restlessness, and electroencephalographic abnormalities. When the fever abates, so do the associated findings. The condition is fortunately extremely rare, since it is generally either over-diagnosed or underdiagnosed.

Extremely high fevers (in excess of 106°F or 41.2°C) are rarely due to infection, with the exception of central nervous system infections such as bacterial meningitis or viral encephalitis. They suggest central lesions such as heat stroke. In my own experience, stroke has been the most common cause. The temperature obtained with a regular thermometer may be a dangerous underestimate. Such patients should be monitored immediately with a thermistor placed high in the rectum.

Fever is usually accompanied by an increase in the pulse rate approximately 10 beats per minute per degree Fahrenheit. With some infections, the pulse is characteristically slower than expected: salmonelloses (including typhoid fever), tularemia, brucellosis, bacterial meningitis complicated by increased intracranial pressure, mycoplasmal pneumonia, rickettsialpox, Legionella pneumonia, mumps, infectious hepatitis, Colorado tick fever, and dengue. A disproportionately low pulse may also be seen in factitious fever, or in patients taking digitalis glycosides or beta blockers.

Assessing Change in Fever: A Cusum Plot

For any rapidly changing variable, which moves widely about a mean (such as platelet count or temperature), a cusum (cumulative sums) plot will help you determine when a real change has taken place. To make such a plot, arbitrarily define a standard value, such as 100° for the temperature. Make a list of the temperatures and of their deviations from the standard value, and calculate the cusum, which is the cumulative sum of the deviations (Table 6-2). Plot the cusums on a graph (Fig. 6-9). The change point is the point at which there is a change in the slope. This may help you determine which antibiotic made a difference in the fever.

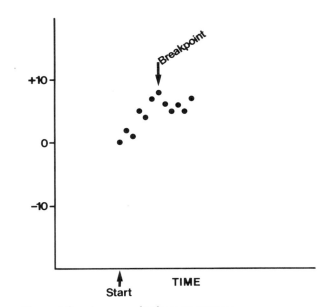

Figure 6-9. *A cusum plot for temperatures.*

Another technique is to record the maximum temperature for each 24-hour period.

Hypothermia

Hypothermia is defined as an oral temperature less than 95°F (35°C). Because routine thermometers do not read temperatures this low, it may be missed unless the examiner suspects it, and checks the temperature with a thermistor.

There are six specific causes of severe hypothermia that are reversible and may require emergency treatment: hypoglycemia, hypothyroidism, hypoadrenocorticism, overwhelming infection (Bryant et al., 1971), intoxications, and exposure.

With severe depression of body temperature, metabolic processes slow and the patient may resemble a person with myxedema, or may even appear to be dead.

Appendix 6-1. Answer to the Question on Atrial Fibrillation on Page 98

From the information given, the answer is "probably not." To answer yes, you would need evidence that the entities comprising the residual 15% were collectively less frequent than ischemic heart disease alone. (Otherwise ischemic heart disease might not be at the top of the list.)

Appendix 6-2. The Rollover Test for Predicting Pregnancy-Induced Hypertension

After the patient has rested 15 minutes in the left lateral decubitus position, a baseline blood pressure is obtained from the right arm. The patient then rolls into the supine position and after 5 minutes another pressure is taken. An increase in the diastolic blood pressure when the patient is supine is a positive test. See Table 6-3.

Table 6-2. Temperatures and Cusums

Hourly temperature (°F)	Deviation	Cusum
100	0	0
102	+2	+2
99	−1	+1
104	+4	+5
99	−1	+4
103	+3	+7
101	+1	+8
98	−2	+6
99	−1	+5
101	+1	+6
99	−1	+5
101	+1	+6
102	+2	+7

Table 6.3. The Rollover Test

Reference	Weeks of Pregnancy	mm Hg Rise Used as Criterion	Results
Gant et al., 1974	28–32	20	Predictive value of a positive test = 93% Predictive value of a negative test = 91%
Phelan et al., 1977	28–32	20	Sensitivity = 78% Specificity = 96%
Schiff et al., 1989	28–29	15	Predictive value of a positive test = 35% Predictive value of a negative test = 91%

References

American Heart Association, Report of the Subcommittee of the Postgraduate Education Committee: Recommendation for human blood pressure determination by sphygmomanometers, 1980.

Biot MC: Contribution a l'etude du phenomene respiratoire de Cheyne-Stokes (A contribution to the study of Cheyne-Stokes respiration). *Lyon Medicine* 23:517–528, 561–567, 1876.

Blake JW, Solangi KB, Herman MV, Goodman AA, Meggs LG: Left ventricular response to exercise and autonomic control mechanisms in end-stage renal disease. *Arch Intern Med* 149:433–436, 1989.

Braunwald E: *Heart Disease*. WB Saunders, Philadelphia, 1980, p. 1543.

Brown HW, Plum F: The neurologic basis of Cheyne-Stokes respiration. *Am J Med* 30:849–860, 1961.

Bryant RE, Hood AF, Hood CE, Koenig MG: Factors affecting mortality of Gram negative rod bacteremia. *Arch Intern Med* 127:120–128, 1971.

Cabeen WR Jr, Roberts NK, Child JS: Recognition of the Wenckebach phenomenon. *West J Med* 129:521–526, 1978.

Chamberlain EN, Ogilvie C: *Symptoms and Signs in Clinical Medicine*, ed 7. John Wright & Sons. Distributed in the USA by Year Book Medical Publishers, Chicago, 1974. [See p. 243. Apparently, no student has challenged the authors.]

Cheyne J: A case of apoplexy in which the fleshy part of the heart was converted into fat. *Dublin Hospital Reports* 2:216, 1818.

Cohen SI, Kupersmith J, Aroesty J, Rowe JW: Pulsus paradoxus and Kussmaul's sign in acute pulmonary embolism. *Am J Cardiol* 32:271–275, 1973.

Cohn JN: Blood pressure measurement in shock: Mechanism of inaccuracy in auscultatory and palpatory methods. *JAMA* 199:972–976, 1967. [This citation is sometimes given as pp 118–122. The confusion results from the dual pagination used by some journals, especially those published by the American Medical Association. This article is on pp 972–976 of the bound volume, and on pp 118–122 of one of the twelve issues in that volume. There is no easy way to find out which issue this is, a particularly frustrating problem in progressive libraries which have replaced the bound journal with microfiche.]

Cohn JN, Pinkerson AL, Tristani FE: Mechanism of pulsus paradoxus in clinical shock. *J Clin Invest* 46:1744–1755, 1967.

Davidson E, Weinberger I, Rotenberg Z, Fuchs J, Agmon J: Atrial fibrillation: Cause and time of onset. *Arch Intern Med* 149:457–459, 1989.

DeGowin EL: *Bedside Diagnostic Examination*. Macmillan, New York, 1965.

Delp MH, Manning RT: *Major's Physical Diagnosis*. WB Saunders, Philadelphia, 1975.

Devetski RL: A modified technic for the determination of systemic arterial pressure in patients with extremely obese arms. *N Engl J Med* 269:1137–1138, 1963.

Dock W: Inspiratory traction on the pericardium: The cause of pulsus paradoxus in pericardial disease. *Arch Intern Med* 108:837–840, 1961.

Enselberg CD: Measurement of diastolic blood pressure by palpation. *N Engl J Med* 265:272–274, 1961.

Ewing DJ, Campbell IW, Burt AA, Clarke BF: Vascular reflexes in diabetic autonomic neuropathy. *Lancet* 2:1354–1356, 1973.

Frank MJ, Casanegra P, Migliori AJ, et al: The clinical evaluation of aortic regurgitation: With special reference to a neglected sign: The popliteal-brachial pressure gradient. *Arch Intern Med* 116:357–365, 1965.

Friedberg CK: *Diseases of the Heart*, ed 2. WB Saunders, Philadelphia, 1956.

Friedman B: Alteration of cycle length in pulsus alternans. *Am Heart J* 51:701–712, 1956.

Fulkerson WJ, Coleman RE, Ravin CE, Saltzman HA: Diagnosis of pulmonary embolism. *Arch Intern Med* 146:961–967, 1986.

Gant NF, Chand S, Worley RJ, Whalley, PJ, Crosby UD, MacDonald PC: A clinical test useful for predicting the development of acute hypertension in pregnancy. *Am J Obstet Gynecol* 120:1–7, 1974.

Gauchat HW, Katz LN: Observations on pulsus paradoxus (with special reference to pericardial effusions): I. Clinical. *Arch Intern Med* 33:350–370, 1924.

Geddes LA, Hoff HE, Badger AS: Introduction of the auscultatory method of measuring blood pressure—including a translation of Korotkoff's original paper. *Cardiovasc Res Cent Bull* 5:57–74, 1966.

Goldstein S, Killip T: Comparison of direct and indirect arterial pressures in aortic regurgitation. *N Engl J Med* 267:1121–1124, 1962.

Green DM, Metheny D: Estimation of acute blood loss by the tilt test. *Surg Gynecol Obstet* 8:145–150, 1948.

Greenberg MA, Gitler B: Left ventricular rupture in a patient with coexisting right ventricular infarction. *N Engl J Med* 309:539–542, 1983.

Guntheroth WG, Morgan BC, Mullins GL: Effect of respiration on venous return and stroke volume in cardiac tamponade. *Circ Res* 20:381–390, 1967.

Hoeprich PD, ed: *Infectious Diseases*. Harper & Row, New York, 1972.

Kaplan NM: Hypertension: Prevalence, risks and effective therapy. *Ann Intern Med* 98 Part II:705–709, 1983.

Karp HR, Seiker HO, Heyman, A: Cerebral circulation in Cheyne-Stokes respiration. *Am J Med* 30:861–870, 1961.

Karvonen MJ, Telivuo LJ, Jarvinen JK: Sphygmomanometer cuff size and the accuracy of indirect measurement of blood pressure. *Am J Cardiol* 13:688–693, 1964.

Kase CS, Maulsby GO, Mohr JP: Partial pontine hematomas. *Neurology* 30:652–655, 1980.

King GE: Errors in clinical measurement of blood pressure in obesity. *Clin Sci* 32:223–237, 1967.

Knopp R, Claypool R, Leonardi D: Use of the tilt table in measuring acute blood loss. *Ann Emerg Med* 9:29–32, 1980.

Kuhn LA: Acute and chronic cardiac tamponade. In DH Spodick (ed): *Pericardial Diseases*. FA Davis, Philadelphia, 1976, pp 177–195.

Kussmaul A: Ueber schwielige Mediastino-Pericarditis und den paradoxen Puls (Concerning callous mediastinopericarditis and the paradoxical pulse.) *Berl Klin Wochenschr* 10:433–435, 1873. [Other cases followed in other issues of this journal.]

Linfors EW, Feussner JR, Blessing CL, Starmer CF, Neelson FA, McKee PA: Spurious hypertension in the obese patient. *Arch Intern Med* 144:1482–1486, 1984.

London SB, London RE: Critique of indirect diastolic end point. *Arch Intern Med* 119:39–49, 1967.

Lown B, DeSilva RA, Lenson R: Roles of psychologic stress and autonomic nervous system changes in provocation of ventricular premature complexes. *Am J Cardiol* 41:979–85, 1973.

Massumi RA, Mason DT, Vera Z, Zelis R, Otero J, Amsterdam EA: Reversed pulsus paradoxus. *N Engl J Med* 289:1272–1275, 1973.

McFadden JP, Price RC, Eastwood HD, Briggs RS: Raised respiratory rate in elderly patients: A valuable physical sign. *Br Med J* 284:626–627, 1982.

McGregor M: Pulsus paradoxus. *N Engl J Med* 301:480–482, 1979.

Messerli FH, Ventura HO, Amodeo C: Osler's maneuver and pseudo-hypertension. *N Engl J Med* 312:1548–1551, 1985.

Mishriki YY: Back to the future. *Arch Intern Med* 147:2089–2090, 1987.

Mitchell PL, Parlin RW, Blackburn H: Effect of vertical displacement of the arm on indirect blood pressure measurement. *N Engl J Med* 271:72–74, 1964.

Montfrans GA, van der Hoeven GMA, Karemaker JM, Wieling W, Dunning, AJ: Accuracy of auscultatory blood pressure measurements with a long cuff. *Br Med J* 295:354–357, 1987.

Moutsos SE, Sapira JD, Scheib ET, Shapiro, AP: An analysis of the placebo effect in hospitalized hypertensive patients. *Clin Pharmacol Ther* 8:676–683, 1967.

Multanovsky MP: The Korotkov's method: History of its discovery and clinical and experimental interpretation, and contemporary appraisal of its merits. *Cor Vasa* 12:1–7, 1970.

Murray HW: Factitious fever updated. *Arch Intern Med* 139:739–740, 1979.

Murray HW, Tuazon CU, Guerrero IC, Claudio MS, Alling DW, Sheagren, JN: Urinary temperature: A clue to early diagnosis of factitious fever. *N Engl J Med* 296:23–25, 1977.

Musher DM, Fainstein V, Young EJ, Pruett, TL: Fever patterns: Their lack of clinical significance. *Arch Intern Med* 139:1225–1228, 1979.

Nielsen PE, Janniche H: The accuracy of auscultatory measurement of arm blood pressure in very obese subjects. *Acta Med Scand* 195:403–409, 1974.

Nishimura RA, Tajik AJ: The Valsalva maneuver and response revisited. *Mayo Clin Proc* 61:211–217, 1986.

Nordyke RA, Gilbert FI, Jr, Harada ASM: Graves' disease: influence of age on clinical findings. *Arch Intern Med* 148:626–631, 1988.

Pascarelli EF, Bertrand CA: Comparison of blood pressure in the arms and legs. *N Engl J Med* 270:693–698, 1964.

Pemberton J: *Epidemiology*. Oxford University Press, Oxford, 1963, pp 271–281.

Phelan JP, Everidge GJ, Wilder TL, Newman C: Is the supine pressor test an adequate means of predicting acute hypertension in pregnancy? *Am J Obstet Gynecol* 128:173–176, 1977.

Pickering GW, Roberts JAF, Sowry GSC: Aetiology of essential hypertension: Effect of correcting for arm circumference on growth rate of arterial pressure with age. *Clin Sci* 13:267–271, 1954.

Plum F, Posner JB: *The Diagnosis of Stupor and Coma*, ed 2. FA Davis, Philadelphia, 1972.

Raftery EB, Ward AP: The indirect method of recording blood pressure. *Cardiovasc Res* 2:210–218, 1968.

Ragan C, Bordley J: The accuracy of clinical measurements of arterial blood pressure. With a note on the auscultatory gap. *Bull Johns Hopkins Hosp* 69:504–528, 1941.

Rebuck AS, Pengelly, LD: Development of pulsus paradoxus in the presence of airways obstruction. *N Engl J Med* 288:66–69, 1973.

Reddy PS, Curtiss EI, O'Toole JD, Shaver JA: Cardiac tamponade: Hemodynamic observations in man. *Circulation* 58:265–271, 1978.

Sacks O: *Awakenings*. Vintage Books, New York, 1973.

Salel A, Amsterdam EA, Zelis, R: Pseudopulsus paradoxus. *Chest* 64:671–672, 1973.

Sapira JD: Quincke, de Musset, Duroziez, and Hill: Some aortic regurgitations. *South Med J* 74: 459–467, 1981.

Sapira JD, Kirkpatrick MB: On pulsus paradoxus. *South Med J* 76:1163–1164, 1983.

Schatz IJ: Orthostatic hypotension: II. Clinical diagnosis, testing, and treatment. *Arch Intern Med* 114:1037–1041, 1984.

Schiff E, Peleg E, Goldenberg M, Rosenthal T, Ruppin E, Tamarkin M, Barkai G, Ben-Baruch G, Yahal I, Blankstein J, Goldman B, Mashiach S. The use of aspirin to prevent pregnancy-induced hypertension and lower the ratio of thromboxane A_2 to prostacyclin in relatively high risk pregnancies. *N Engl J Med* 321:351–356, 1989.

Segall HN: A note on the measurement of diastolic and systolic blood pressure by the palpation of arterial vibrations (sounds) over the brachial artery. *Can Med Assoc J* 42:311–313, 1940.

Segall HN: *Experiments for Determining the Efficiency of Arterial Collaterals by N. S. Korotkoff*. Preface, biographical notes and editing of translation from Russian. Privately printed: IBSN 0-9690339-0-7 Montreal, 1980.

Silen W (ed): *Cope's Early Diagnosis of the Acute Abdomen*, ed 15. Oxford University Press, New York, 1979.

Spodick D: *Chronic and Constrictive Pericarditis*. Grune & Stratton, New York, 1964, pp 63–64.

Spodick DH: The normal and diseased pericardium: Current concepts of pericardial physiology, diagnosis and treatment. *J Am Coll Cardiol* 1:240–251, 1983.

Spodick DH: Pulsus paradoxus. *South Med J* 77:804, 1984.

Sullivan KN, Manfredi F, Behnke RH: Hippus in Cheyne-Stokes respiration: observations in three patients with rhythmic respiratory pupillary changes. *Arch Intern Med* 122:116–121, 1968.

Tandberg D, Sklar D: Effect of tachypnea on the estimation of body temperature by an oral thermometer. *N Engl J Med* 308:945–946, 1983.

Thomas JE, Schirger A, Fealey RD, Sheps, SG: Orthostatic hypotension. *Mayo Clin Proc* 56:117–125, 1981.

Thulin T, Andersson G, Schersten B: Measurement of blood pressure — a routine test in need of standardization. *Postgrad Med J* 51:390–395, 1975.

Vaisrub S: Pulsus paradoxus pulmonale. *JAMA* 228:1030–1031, 1974.

Weiner DB: The real Doctor Guillotin. *JAMA* 220:85–89, 1972.

Wenckebach KF: Beitrge zur Kenntnis der menschlichen Herzttigkeit. *Archives für Anatomie und Physiologie*. Physiologische Abteilung 297–354, 1906.

Wilson WS, Judge RD, Siegel JH: A simple diagnostic sign in ventricular tachycardia. *N Engl J Med* 270:446–448, 1964.

Wise DE, Conti CR: Constrictive pericarditis. In DH Spodick (ed): *Pericardial Diseases*. FA Davis, Philadelphia, 1976, pp 197–209.

7
Integument

"We reflect far too little on the fact that a sign really cannot mean more than it is."

Wittgenstein, *Philosophical Remarks*

Skin

The skin is the most accessible organ in the body, and can provide many diagnostic clues for the examiner who knows what he seeks. The skin should be inspected methodically, with adequate exposure, preferably in direct sunlight. The texture should be felt, and any lesions should be palpated, making careful observations of the details listed in Chapter 4 (p. 50).

It is not possible to give an exhaustive description of all the lesions that might be observed in the skin. *We are not concerned with a compendium of dermatology but rather with a method and some illustrations* of skin manifestations of medical diseases. The sampling is chosen partly to illustrate epistemologic principles. The student who has learned to observe and describe precisely will then be able to make effective use of textbooks of medicine and dermatology. Even if you haven't a clue about the etiology of a skin lesion, if you can describe it accurately, a dermatologist, with his highly developed pattern recognition skills, may be able to diagnose it over the telephone.

Dermatologic findings fairly specific to one region of the body are found in the "inspection" portion of appropriate chapters (e.g., pretibial myxedema, erythema nodosum, and some other skin lesions usually associated with the pretibial region are in Ch. 25 (p. 442).

(A MS 24 first became aware of how much time he had spent looking at the patient's skin when he got bifocals and could no longer see it at the usual focal length. He found he had to do the examination close up, peering all around the body like a dog sniffing for a scent.)

Color

Pigmentation

A method. In Caucasians, pay particular attention to the abdomen, which has been protected from the sun. The excess pigment will be more obvious there, although it may *not* be as pronounced as in the sun-exposed areas. Pressure points, such as the belt line, will often show an exaggeration of pigmentation due to a chronic process. Be sure to check the mucous membranes.

Diffuse. The most common cause of diffuse endogenous pigmentation is jaundice. (Also see Ch. 10, p. 162).

Diffuse hyperpigmentation can occur in chronic adrenocortical insufficiency or other states characterized by chronically high levels of ACTH, such as the so-called ectopic ACTH syndrome, a paraneoplastic syndrome in which the tumor makes huge amounts of pro-ACTH along with the carboxypeptidase to cleave it (Fig. 5-3). A diffuse brown hyperpigmentation may occur in some patients with melanoma.

A pale yellow color not simply due to anemia is seen in pernicious anemia (due to indirect bilirubin from intramedullary hemolysis), in some cases of myxedema (due to carotene), and in some cases of the nephrotic syndrome (due to urochrome and carotene). This color is not so striking in simple chronic uremia, which also has the pallor of anemia. In nephrotic syndrome, the hypoalbuminemia is accompanied by a compensatory hyperglobulinemia, including an increase in the carotene-binding globulin. (However, hypercarotenemia does not occur in cirrhosis, presumably because of a concurrent problem with hepatic metabolism.)

Progressive systemic sclerosis is also stated to cause diffuse pigmentation, but this occurs only when the skin lesions are truly diffuse, by which time there is little diagnostic challenge.

In hemochromatosis, the skin is greyish or bronze or appears dirty.

Other diffuse hyperpigmented states due to naturally occurring pigments are chronic jaundice with bile salt retention, and some cases of malabsorption syndrome.

I once saw a family in which the children suffered a green coloration of the skin occurring maximally about 30 minutes after exercise. I assumed that the exercise produced hemolysis and deduced that there must have been a congenital defect in biliverdin reductase, since biliverdin would be the only green substance that could be endogenously produced in sufficient quantity to color the skin. I was not able to persuade the doctors in charge to perform the proper studies to test this hypothesis. Still, such cases are a useful reminder that the book is not closed on unusual skin pigmentations.

Various types of drugs or poisons can induce a diffuse hyperpigmentation. Examples include atabrine (which causes a yellowish color), phenol, busulfan, and heavy metal poisoning. In contrast to adrenal cortical insufficiency, most heavy metals (mercury, lead, arsenic, and bismuth) do not cause pigmentation of the mucous membranes. The silvery blue-gray pigmentation of argyria is so striking that once seen it is never forgotten.

A striking yellow or orange pigment, most noticeable in the palms or soles, can occur with ingestion of excessive amounts of carotene-containing foods or with isoretinoin or rifampin overdose. Food faddists who eat massive amounts of tomatoes develop the red-tinted lycopenemia. In both, the skin is tinted more than the scleral conjunctivae.

An excessive melanin deposition can occur after many years of high-dose chlorpromazine therapy due to the photosensitizing and melanin-binding effect of phenothiazines. About 2% to 5% of patients taking amiodarone develop hyperpigmentation. In both cases, the pigment is more dirty gray than brown.

Focal.   In chronic adrenocortical insufficiency, pigmented spots may appear in the buccal mucosa in addition to the diffuse hyperpigmentation (see Ch. 13, p. 225). Scars also become hyperpigmented in chronic adrenocortical insufficiency.

Acanthosis nigricans is discussed on page 118. The skin signs of pregnancy are included in Table 22-2.

Hyperpigmented, sometimes callused, patches above the knees (Dahl's sign, Fig. 7-1A) may be seen in chronic obstructive lung disease (Dahl, 1970). They are produced by the patient's posture (Fig. 7-1B), a common one in patients with chronic obstructive lung disease because such bracing of the musculoskeletal bellows

improves the efficiency of the muscles of respiration (see Ch. 5, p. 81).

Ochronosis primarily affects cartilage, especially that of the ears. It is more brownish or yellowish than other pigmented states, hence the name, which derives from ochre.

"Porphyria" is stated to cause pigmentation; however, the types that do so are also associated with hypersensitivity to light. The skin abrades and blisters easily, and may also show healed depigmented scars over the exposed areas, such as the hands (see Fig. 25-2). However, the most common type of porphyria seen in medical practice in the United States, acute intermittent porphyria, is not associated with hyperpigmentation.

Uremic Frost

Uremic frost is a white crystalline deposit seen especially on the faces of undialyzed patients with uremia, particularly those who are comatose. It exactly resembles frost, or the salt film seen in some of those who exercise in the sun, and then allow their sweat to dry. It is not seen in patients who wash their faces or in those institutions in which the nurses regularly bathe the comatose patients.

Erythema

Erythema means "redness" and can occur as a generalized phenomenon in vasodilatory states (such as scarlet fever), or it may be localized (also see exanthems, p. 111). The erythema may

A

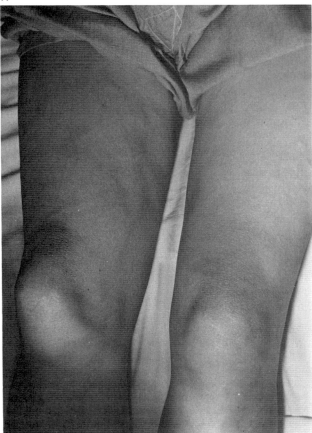

B

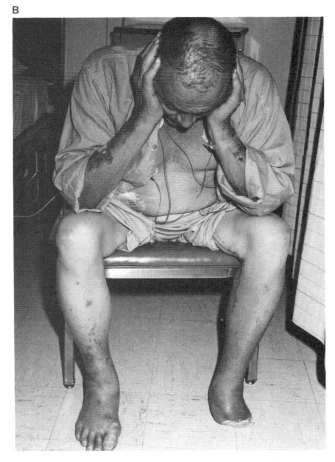

Figure 7-1.   A, *Hyperpigmented patches above the knees in a patient with chronic obstructive lung disease (Dahl's sign). This patient reported that his father, who also suffered from chronic obstructive lung disease, had similar patches. B, Typical posture of such patients. Photographs courtesy of Dr. Gretchen Meyer of California.*

be followed by exfoliation, as in staphylococcal scalded skin syndrome.

If localized to sun-exposed areas of the body, the erythema may be part of a photosensitivity syndrome. (The part of the neck shaded by the chin is often spared.) On the other hand, exposed areas (e.g., the face and hands) can also be involved by contact dermatitis. Systemic lupus erythematosus and discoid lupus erythematosus have probably displaced pellagra as the most common etiologies of photosensitivity. Xeroderma pigmentosa and porphyria (other than acute intermittent porphyria) may also cause this phenomenon. In a fixed drug eruption, either local or systemic medication sensitizes skin to subsequent light exposure. Drugs that can cause photosensitivity include amiodarone, demeclocycline, nalidixic acid, thiazides, and sulfonylureas, to name just a few. Polymorphous photosensitivity is a diagnosis of exclusion of the above.

Erythema confined to the extensor surfaces is a sign of dermatomyositis (called Gottron's sign—see also Gottron's knuckle patches in Ch. 25, p. 441).

An erythema resembling sunburn is the first skin sign of pellagra. The skin lesions tend to be symmetric and localized over exposed areas. In addition, the scrotum, vulva, and perianal area may be involved, especially as the dementia and diarrhea supervene. The skin later develops vesicles or peeling, a dirty-brown color, and a rough scaly texture.

The "red neck syndrome," also called the "red man syndrome" may result from too rapid infusion of vancomycin, among other causes (e.g., the Sezary syndrome, see p. 113, or histamine release as from intravenous codeine administration).

Cyanosis

Cyanosis means "blue-colored." Generalized cyanosis is due to deoxyhemoglobin, methemoglobin, or sulfhemoglobin. Methemoglobinemia and sulfhemoglobinemia are very rare causes of cyanosis and are usually due to drug exposure and/or certain congenital metabolic abnormalities. Most cases of deoxyhemoglobin are due to insufficient oxygenation, either because of shunting, hypoventilation, diffusion defect, or ventilation/perfusion mismatch. Except where noted, the remainder of the discussion refers to cyanosis due to such deoxyhemoglobinemia, the most common cause of cyanosis.

In order to get cyanosis due to deoxyhemoglobinemia, there must be at least 5 g/dl of unsaturated hemoglobin (deoxyhemoglobin). Thus an anemic patient with only 5 g/dl of hemoglobin cannot become cyanotic. With 7.5 g/dl of hemoglobin, a patient would have to be 67% unsaturated to show the same bluish color as a patient with a normal hemoglobin (15 g/dl) and 33% unsaturation. (This does not hold for methemoglobinemia and sulfhemoglobinemia, which cause cyanosis at 1.5 g/dl and 0.5 g/dl, respectively. And, of course, it does not hold for carboxyhemoglobinemia due to carbon monoxide poisoning, which never causes cyanosis even as the patient succumbs to cellular anoxia.)

The presence of cyanosis is often recorded under "general appearance" in the physical examination, rather than under "integument." If restricted to the extremities, it might also be in that section. (See nail beds for acrocyanosis, p. 127.)

Differential cyanosis refers to the appearance of cyanosis in both lower extremities (and sometimes the left upper extremity—"harlequin" cyanosis) with a normally pink right upper extremity. This is seen in patent ductus arteriosus, when secondary pulmonary hypertension has supervened. The cyanotic blood in the pulmonary artery then goes through the patent ductus arteriosus, empties into the aorta, and flows to the lower half of the body. The upper half of the body continues to get oxygenated blood from the left ventricle. If the patent ductus enters the aorta below the left subclavian artery, the left arm is pink; if it enters above the left subclavian artery, the left arm is blue.

This lesion initially has the cardinal sign of a continuous, "machinery" murmur in the second left intercostal space (Gibson murmur, Ch. 17, p. 305), which is so characteristic that few books also mention the differential cyanosis. However, if the diagnosis is initially missed, the unoperated patient develops pulmonary hypertension, and the shunt reverses direction. The murmur is now altered, and the sign of differential cyanosis appears. In practical terms, the appearance of the latter finding means that it is now too late to operate on the patient.

In reverse differential cyanosis, the arms are more cyanotic than the legs. This is caused by transposition of the great vessels with ventricular septal defect and patent ductus arteriosus. (In this disease, both the pulmonary artery and the aorta arise from the right ventricle, causing the cyanosis.) Oxygenated blood from the left ventricle can cross the ventricular septal defect into the right ventricle and the pulmonary artery, which sits just above the septal defect. When pulmonary hypertension supervenes, this oxygenated blood flows back through the patent ductus arteriosus into the descending aorta, "pinking up" the feet (Perloff, 1982).

Differential cyanosis due to other vascular lesions, including dissecting aortic aneurysm, is discussed in Chapter 18.

Livedo reticularis. Latin for "skin discoloration in the form of a small net," this pattern is usually found on the extremities, but possibly on the trunk. It is characterized by connected bluish-purple streaks without discrete borders.

True livedo reticularis might be a sign of a collagen vascular disease such as polyarteritis nodosa, dermatomyositis, rheumatoid arthritis, systemic lupus erythematosus (and, by extension, Raynaud's "disease," if this entity exists—see Ch. 18, p. 345 for an epistemologic discussion), as well as in association with a variety of states such as pancreatitis shock or bacterial endocarditis (Bishop et al., 1981). It may also be seen in association with leg ulcers, or as part of congenital phlebectasia (Fitzpatrick et al., 1979) or Sneddon's syndrome (Levine et al., 1988).

Livedo reticularis may be confused with *cutis marmorata* (literally, "marbled skin"), which might or might not have bright pink splotches between the blue-purple lines. Unlike livedo reticularis, cutis marmorata characteristically appears in response to cold and disappears with warming, and has no strong associations with serious disease.

Livedo reticularis may also be confused with *erythema ab igne*, which literally means "redness from the fire." Again, there is a netlike appearance, but *erythema ab igne* is not blue-purple but red, or, when chronic, simply pigmented. It results from chronic exposure of the limb to heat, for example, from a fireplace (especially when seen over the legs) or from a heating pad (Bean, 1976).

Vitiligo

Vitiligo is a condition manifested by white spots on the skin. It begins before age 18 in half the patients. Usually, the hands, feet, or face are affected first. Like a forest fire, the process of death of the pigment cells spreads, and then burns out.

An associated autoimmune endocrine disorder, such as thyroiditis, diabetes mellitus (Dawber, 1968), or chronic adrenocortical insufficiency is found in about 20% to 30% of patients with vitiligo. Perhaps another 25% have elevated serum levels of one of the autoantibodies associated with such a disease, although not the disease itself.

Vitiligo is also seen in association with multiple myeloma, Hodgkin's disease, mycosis fungoides, autoimmune hemolytic anemia, dysgammaglobulinemia, mucocutaneous candidiasis, and in some melanoma patients who have metastases (Nordlund & Lerner, 1982).

Vitiligo is to be distinguished from hypomelanosis (Table 7-1). The difference in degree is most evident when the skin is $\$\$$ examined under ultraviolet light filtered through a Wood's glass (Wood's light); vitiligo has an ivory-white appearance.

The occurrence of vitiligo with anterior uveitis (iritis), poliosis (premature greying of some or all of the hair), alopecia, and/or dysacusia (the experience of pain caused by certain sounds) is the Vogt-Koyanagi-Harada syndrome (Nordlund & Lerner, 1982). Such patients may also have posterior uveitis (chorioretinitis).

Fluorescence

Examination under Wood's light reveals fluorescence in some lesions (e.g., a golden color due to tinea versicolor, orange-red due to erythrasma, or green due to a *Pseudomonas* infection, especially in burns).

Telangiectasia

"Telangiectasia" is Greek for "dilatation of the ends of the vessels." Like a foolish parrot, I repeated for years the error that I had been taught: that the "tel" came from the Latin meaning "woven, like a web." In fact, there is nothing at all weblike in the telangiectasia seen in the CREST variant of scleroderma or the red spots of hereditary hemorrhagic telangiectasia (Osler-Weber-Rendu disease). The latter are located on the fingers, tongue, and mouth. They resemble senile hemangiomas, (see p. 117), except for the distribution and the fact that the latter are raised.

Table 7-1.   Types of Hypomelanosis and Amelanosis

	Amelanotic	Hypomelanotic
Scattered, discrete, various sizes	Vitiligo	
	Hyperthyroidism	
	Addison's disease	
	Pernicious anemia	
	Hypoparathyroidism & Addison's disease	
	Vogt-Koyanagi-Harada	
	Tuberous sclerosis	
	Tinea versicolor	
	Leprosy (tuberculoid)	
	Postinflammation depigmentation	
	Psoriasis	
	Atopic dermatitis	
	Pityriasis alba	
Segmental, in quasi-dermatomal pattern	Vitiligo	Nevus depigmentosus
		Tuberous sclerosis

Source: Fitzpatrick et al. (1979).

Turn to Chapter 24 (p. 416) and look at Figure 24-2A, without reading the legend. What is the lesion indicated by the arrow? After you have written down your answer, read on.

Spider telangiectasia (Bean, 1958) are arterial telangiectasia appearing in the region drained by the superior vena cava (the chest and upper arms). They appear to have legs radiating spider-like out from a body. The body is actually the central arterial supply of the lesion, as can be shown by a simple bedside diagnostic test. If a glass slide is placed on top of the spider, the pressure can be gradually increased to a point at which the spider will blanch only during diastole, and will be seen to pulsate in time with the heartbeat. If the lesion is blanched completely, and the pressure is gradually reduced, the central spot will fill with blood first. Conversely, the entire spider can be blanched by exerting pressure on the central arterial supply either with a pencil point or the edge of the glass slide. (A little immersion oil sometimes makes it easier to see the pressure phenomena.)

Spider telangiectasia are usually considered a sign of hyperestrogenism, either physiologic as in a pregnant female, or pathologic as in a cirrhotic male (Bean, 1958).

Telangiectasis involving the ears, neck, and flexor creases at the elbows and knees (as well as the bulbar conjunctiva) is a sign of ataxia telangiectasia, one of the neurocutaneous syndromes or phakomatoses (see Table 10-24, p. 195).

Corona radiata is the name given to a corona or halo of easily observed superficial vessels that radiate longitudinally along the lower chest in the general vicinity of the diaphragmatic insertions. The entire halo may also be called the zona corona or the costal fringe. The finding is believed to be of no diagnostic significance (Bean, 1958).

The individual lesions comprising the corona radiata are called venous stars. They range from blood red to venous purple and can range from less than 1 mm to over 2 mm in their individual long axes. They are bilateral and may cover most of the anterior chest, or just a few inches of the circumference on each side. Venous stars may occur all over the body, and are also of no significance, except when they suddenly appear over the thorax, in which case they should suggest significant obstruction of the veins of the superior mediastinum (Fred et al., 1962).

The inspection of venous patterns may be aided by the use of red-tinted glasses (see Ch. 19, p. 366).

Lesions Due to Bleeding Problems

Petechiae

A petechia is a pinpoint (less than 1 mm) red hemorrhage (Fig. 7-2), which does not blanch with pressure. Petechiae signify a capillary or platelet disorder, although the involvement of the capillary may be only secondary, for example, due to endocarditis or fat embolism.

In the preantibiotic era, petechiae were found in 29% to 88% of patients with *bacterial endocarditis*. In the postantibiotic era, the prevalence is said to be 19% to 40% (Bishop et al., 1981).

Skin petechiae are actually found in only about half of the patients with *fat embolism*, and in some series less than a quarter, depending upon the criteria used for diagnosis (i.e., clinical or autopsy). This holds even for series reported from the same institution (Dines et al., 1975; Thomas & Ayyar, 1972). But the same sort of prevalences also occur for conjunctival petechiae, retinal findings, and lipiduria. Far from diminishing the importance of petechiae, this emphasizes their diagnostic utility as part of a systematic search for findings.

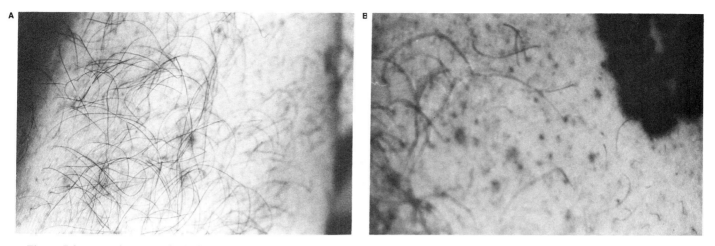

Figure 7-2. Petechiae. A, The little speckles beneath the hairs are slightly out of focus to remind you that in real life you must actively search for them. B, These petechiae are easier to see because there is less hair in the way. The large dark spot is a coincidental tatoo. This patient had prostatic carcinoma invading his marrow, causing thrombocytopenia. The petechiae were important in drawing attention to his platelets since he had other explanations for his presenting epistaxis and hematuria.

Capillaritis, a member of the set of petechial disorders, is an inflammation of the capillaries as in necrotizing vasculitis (after Zeek) or as secondary capillaritis as in the various collagen vascular disorders. On the rare occasion when the capillaritis is seen acutely, tiny red flecks (capillary hemorrhages) are apparent all over the surface of the involved skin. It is as if someone had thrown rough ground cayenne pepper at the patient's skin. In a few days, the red pepper turns brown, the color of cinnamon or allspice, and the fine speckled appearance remains. (This latter appearance may also be seen in chronic venous disease. Apparently, the high venous pressure can sometimes cause blood to leak through the capillaries.)

The perifollicular hemorrhages of *scurvy*, which occur in up to 84% of cases, are often mistaken for petechiae (Vilter et al., 1946).

A method. The Rumpel-Leede test is a provocative bedside test for capillary disease or platelet dysfunction.

1. In the middle of the flexor surface of the forearm, about 4 cm distal to the antecubital fossa, outline in ballpoint pen a United States quarter (2.5 cm diameter).

2. Place the sphygmomanometer cuff around the biceps of the same arm, and pump the cuff up to halfway between the systolic and diastolic blood pressures. Keep it inflated for 5 minutes.

3. Count the number of petechiae that appear within the circle. Normal is five or fewer for men, 10 or fewer for women and children.

To improve the results of the Rumpel-Leede test in cases of scurvy, delay the reading of the petechiae for 30 minutes (Vitamin C Subcommittee, 1953).

(For other bedside studies of platelets and platelet function, see "blood clot tests" [Ch. 28, p. 543] and "platelets" [Ch. 28, p. 545].)

Ecchymoses

An ecchymosis is also a bloody extravasation, distinguished from a petechia by size greater than 1 mm. Ecchymoses generally signify large-vessel bleeding from trauma or clotting factor deficiency, although they may also result from a confluence of petechiae, which then turn purple. There are several types of ecchymosis that are considered pathognomonic: 1) and 2) See

Figures 7-3, 7-4, and 7-5; 3) an iatrogenic ecchymosis is caused by subcutaneous heparin or insulin administration in the anterior abdominal wall; 4) the paramalleolar ecchymosis due to a ruptured popliteal cyst is shown in Figure 25-11; 5) Battle's sign and raccoon eyes are shown in Figure 9-1; 6) Grey Turner's sign and Cullen's sign are discussed in Chapter 20 (p. 372). Bryant's sign is discussed in Chapter 24. Corticosteroid therapy may cause "steroid bruising," especially over the forearms. If the patient has not been forewarned, this can be a source of anxiety.

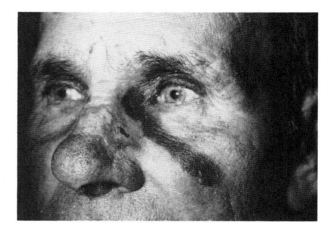

Figure 7-3. This suborbital ecchymosis is the first of the several types of ecchymosis that permit a specific diagnosis. Dr. David Dobmeyer of Missouri reported that this patient was placed in the knee-chest position for a sigmoidoscopy, and the examining table was tilted, so that the patient's head remained dependent for a considerable period of time. The medical student was the first to notice the ecchymosis, and since he had prepared himself by reading about the patient's underlying disease, he was able to explain the finding. The cause of this pathognomonic ecchymosis was the increased capillary fragility of the periorbital tissues, which enabled the increased venous pressure from the head-down position to produce the lesion. Can you make the diagnosis? (Answer is in Appendix 7-1.) This ecchymosis must be distinguished from "raccoon eyes" (see Fig. 9-1B).

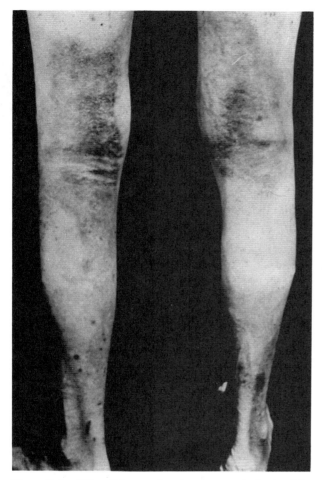

Figure 7-4.   *This solid mass of ecchymoses on the backs of the legs extended up to the buttocks and perineum. This is called the "saddle" distribution, since this portion of the body of a horseback rider would touch the saddle. The disease is scurvy, due to vitamin C deficiency. It is the second type of ecchymosis that permits an etiologic diagnosis. It is an empiric, but not a scientific fact (see p. 4) since there is as yet no scientific explanation for the peculiar distribution.*

Purpura and ecchymoses are seen in up to 90% of scorbutic patients. They may occur elsewhere in addition to the saddle distribution (Vilter et al., 1946). Photograph courtesy of Cliggot Publishing Company.

In scurvy, the ecchymoses begin with follicular hyperkeratoses, which develop petechiae that enlarge and become confluent to form purpura. In one study of experimental scurvy in a surgical resident (Crandon et al., 1940), the petechiae and ecchymoses began on the lower legs, but in another study of full-time volunteers (Vitamin C Subcommittee, 1948), they began on the trunk and upper arms.

Thus, the old idea that purpura always signify a clotting problem must be wrong because in at least this disease, petechiae evolve into purpura. I have seen the same evolution in vasculitis and cryoglobulinemia.

Although scurvy is thought to be rare, it is not. It is simply unrecognized. I saw two cases and was shown two more in a 10-month period while this chapter was in preparation. Unfortunately, this potentially lethal and completely reversible disease must be diagnosed clinically and not by the laboratory. Serum ascorbate levels may be zero, weeks before the disease appears (Crandon et al.,

1940), while some patients with the disease have had measurable serum and leukocyte ascorbate levels (Thomas et al., 1984). Further, leukocyte ascorbate levels equivalent to those found in patients with scurvy may be found in 3% of healthy elderly persons and in 20% to 50% of hospitalized and institutionalized patients (Cheraskin, 1985). Urine levels are only helpful if performed as part of the ascorbic acid loading test, but you have to make the diagnosis clinically before ordering that test.

Can you think of some other diseases that can only be diagnosed by clinical acumen?

Purpura

Purpura simply means purple. Any type of large hemorrhage undergoes characteristic changes in color. As the red blood gives up its oxygen, it becomes deoxyhemoglobin, which is purple. In a few days, it is degraded to biliverdin (green) and bilirubin (orange).

Some diseases in which purpura are the most obvious physical finding include: idiopathic thrombocytopenic purpura, thrombotic thrombocytopenic purpura, Henoch Schoenlein purpura, and purpura fulminans.

Purpura should be palpated. If they can be differentiated from normal adjacent skin by the fingertip with your eyes closed, they are called palpable purpura. Such lesions imply an antigen-antibody complex. Palpable purpura are *never normal* (Fig. 7-6).

In a febrile patient with purpuric macules, papules, or vesicles, consider bacteremia (meningococcemia, gonococcemia, staphylococcemia, *Pseudomonas*), enterovirus infections (ECHO and Coxsackie), and rickettsial diseases (Fitzpatrick et al., 1979).

An entity called autoerythrocyte sensitization purpura has been described, but every case that has been referred to me turned out to be factitious purpura. My assertion that the disease does not exist is tolerated with courteous bemusement by Dr. David Agle of Ohio, who along with Ratnoff has done some of the best investigation of this disorder. (They believe the condition to be psychosomatic in the true sense of the word.) Dr. Agle knows that it would be logically fallacious for me to offer a negative proposition as a provable conclusion. But to encourage the reader always to consider the possibility of factitious purpura, let me explain why I doubt that autoerythrocyte sensitization purpura is any more than a collection of self-administered love-bites or pinches.

1.   Skin tests in which the lesion develops in response to injections of the patient's own erythrocytes, but not to saline, have been considered highly significant. But this finding is quite variable (Hersle & Mobacken, 1969; Levin et al., 1969). (Since the patients are supposed to be sensitive to DNA, which is not present in erythrocytes, I propose that the function of the erythrocytes is to color the solution so that the patient will know which one is saline. As a rule, positive skin tests occurred with erythrocyte concentrations greater than 20%, i.e., sufficient to be visible to the patient [Hersle & Mobacken, 1969].)

2.   The personality characteristics of the patients tend to be the same as are seen in factitious purpura and in surreptitious warfarin ingestion (Agle et al., 1967).

3.   Purpuric lesions that were purportedly induced by hypnosis required the passage of hours before the lesions would appear (Agle et al., 1967).

4.   When patients were carefully observed, some were found to be inducing the lesions, although they would deny this both before and after the fact (Levin et al., 1969, Stefanini & Baumgart, 1972). (Of course, no patient can be truly observed for 24 hours, especially under conditions in which both hands are visible at all times.)

A

B

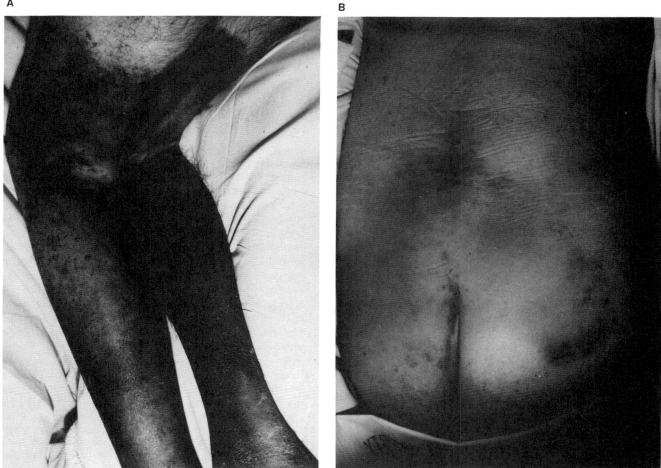

Figure 7-5. *Another patient with scurvy. In this patient, the "saddle" is relatively free of ecchymoses when compared with the lower extremities, which show huge confluent hemorrhages. See also Figure 7-24.*

5. Skin that is out of reach of the patient's mouth or fingers, such as that in the interscapular area, is never afflicted. Furthermore, that skin can become involved when it is transplanted to an accessible area (Schwartz et al., 1962), and previously involved skin becomes "disease resistant" when transplanted to the interscapular area. Bandaging or casting an area (Levin et al., 1969; Stefanini & Baumgart, 1972) is another effective and less draconian method of conferring "resistance."

Exanthems

Dimensions

An exanthem* is a temporary skin eruption or rash occurring as a symptom of a general disease, resulting either from direct invasion of the skin by an infectious agent, or from a toxin or an immune response. A careful description of the rash in all its dimensions (including time course and distribution) can lead directly to diagnosis and timely initiation of therapy (Cherry, 1982).

○ Repeated examination may be necessary to see rashes that are delayed or transient. The rash of Still's disease is best seen dur-

---

*According to Gibbon, during the Dark Ages exanthemata were the "outflowerings" of raised embroidery upon silk, in the form of flowers done in silver or gold thread.

ing a fever, or may be brought out by a hot bath. The same is said to be true for the rash of other febrile illnesses, such as rheumatic fever and Lyme disease. The macular erythematous rash of toxic shock syndrome may be confined to a small area, and may change with blood pressure or blood flow to the skin (Smith & Jacobson, 1986).

The characteristic rash of *erythema chronicum migrans* was one of the clues to the infectious etiology of Lyme arthritis. The skin lesion begins as a red macule or papule that expands to form a large ring with central clearing (Mast & Burrows, 1976; Steere et al., 1977). A similar lesion may occur in the necrolytic migratory erythema of glucagonoma syndrome (Fitzpatrick et al., 1979).

Vesicular, Bullous, and Pustular Eruptions

Vesicles are blisters containing clear fluid. Bullae are blisters larger than 0.5 cm in diameter. Pustules are blisters that contain purulent fluid.

Grouped vesicles on an erythematous base are characteristic of herpetic infections, both *Herpes zoster* and *Herpes simplex*. The former mostly involves skin in a dermatomal distribution, usually but not always unilaterally (see Fig. 9-1). For the latter, see Chapter 13 (p. 226) and Chapter 21 (p. 391).

Large tense clear bullae surrounded by erythema with histologic evidence of sweat gland necrosis (Fig. 7-7) were originally described in association with barbiturate-induced coma. These

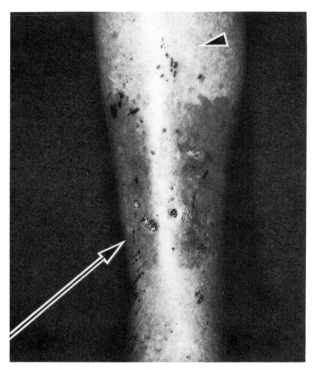

Figure 7-6. *The arrow head points to a collection of purpura high on the shin. The examiner could detect them with his eyes closed, hence they were palpable purpura. More distally, in a band of stasis pigmentation, the arrow points to some punched-out ulcers, due to vasculitis. This patient had vasculitis due to cryoglobulinemia, the etiology of which I could never determine. Others called it "agnogenic," "essential," "crypto-genic," "idiopathic," or "mixed" cryoglobulinemia. Which of these modifiers is falsifiable? (Answer is in Appendix 7-2.)*

bullae are found over pressure points and areas likely to be trau-matized. The lesions occur in approximately 6.5% of barbi-turate-intoxicated patients. They have been noted in glutethi-mide coma, carbon monoxide poisoning, narcotic "overdose," methamphetamine abuse, 4% of cases of pure tricyclic overdose (Noble & Matthew, 1969), and cerebral vascular accidents with hemiplegia. Coma itself is apparently not a prerequisite, but neural damage of one sort or another appears to be the common factor (Sapira & Cherubin, 1975).

Vesiculobullous lesions scattered on an erythematous base with significant golden crusting are due to impetigo, a bacterial (staphylococcal or streptococcal) infection of the skin.

Other mucocutaneous conditions with vesicular or bullous le-sions comprise in part the Stevens-Johnson syndrome (a severe form of erythema multiforme, often resulting from a drug re-action), pemphigus (see p. 122 and Ch. 13, p. 226), bullous pemphigoid, dermatitis herpetiformis, contact dermatitides such as that due to poison ivy and other *Rhus* plants, and occa-sionally lupus erythematosus. Isolated pustules on the ex-tremities, surrounded by purpuric macules, represent septic em-boli and are cutaneous signs of bacteremia (e.g., disseminated gonorrhea). Red papular pustules with white centers tend to be staphylococcal.

There is no illustration of *the* skin lesion of disseminated gonococcal infection because there is no such thing. Skin lesions

seen in gonococcemia and in the dermatitis-arthritis syndrome may be petechial, erythematous macular, vesicular, or bullous. The larger lesions may show a necrotic center, and the bullae may be hemorrhagic. Unfortunately, all or some of these may also be due to *Neissenia meningitidis*, *Haemophilus influenzae*, and *Streptobacillus moniliformis* infections.

Skin Cancers

Malignant Melanoma

Malignant melanomas are said to be differentiable from other lesions by examining them for red color (a sign of immunologic reactivity against a "foreign" substance?), white color (amela-notic sites indicating depigmentation due to tumor atavism), or blue color (said to be peculiar to some melanomas, but also oc-curring in the benign blue nevus). Whatever the correct patho-physiologic explanations for these colors, the clinical signifi-cance is correct; they are flags for a possible malignancy. (The mnemonic might be the colors of the flags of the United States, the United Kingdom, New Zealand, or Australia.) Malignant pigmented tumors also tend to have a notch and to be asym-metrical.

Stretching a suspicious nevus between two fingers may make erythema and irregular pigmentation more obvious. It is also important to use adequate lighting, such as direct sunlight or a strong incandescent or quartz halogen light.

Try guessing the malignancy of the various lesions shown in Figure 7-8. Do not read the legend until you have written down your answers.

In a study of patients with dysplastic melanocytic nevi, which may develop in-situ melanoma (Kelly et al., 1986), the red, white, and blue flag—with a notch—was also found. Erythema was present in 68%, irregular pigmentation (also blue or amelanotic areas) in 84%, and a notch or irregular border in 47%.

The rare but completely benign dermatofibroma may be distin-guished from malignant melanoma by means of the dimple sign. The dermatofibroma will indent (dimple) if you squeeze it from the sides; the melanoma will not. Alas, this sign cannot be used to distinguish the other lesions from melanoma, and so we are left with the red-white-blue-notch asymmetry system.

Squamous Cell and Basal Cell Carcinomas

Squamous cell carcinomas are also dangerous. Location in an area caudad to lines running from the angles of the mouth to the earlobes suggest this diagnosis.

Above that line, nonpigmented skin cancers are more likely to be basal cell carcinomas, which are less malignant. These can-cers tend to have a "pearly" border, that is, a light-colored area somewhere on the edge of the tumor with the color and reflec-tance of pearl. These findings, coupled with any vessel or tel-angiectasia apparent anywhere on the lesion, almost guarantee that it is a basal cell carcinoma.

Kaposi's Sarcoma

This lesion usually consists of purple masses, which are some-times scaly. Formerly a rare, slow-growing malignancy confined mostly to the lower extremities of older men, usually of Mediter-ranean stock, the disease is now commonly seen in association with the acquired immune deficiency syndrome (AIDS). The new form of the disease tends to affect younger persons, to be faster growing, and to become more widely disseminated (Fig. 7-9, A and B).

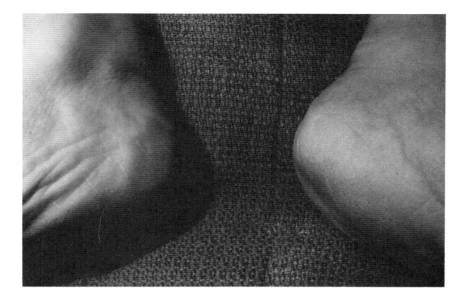

Figure 7-7. *The "barb blister," a lesion first described with barbiturate-induced coma. See text for other causes.*

Metastatic Tumors

Tumors may metastasize to the skin. The most common are colon, ovary (in women), oat cell (in men), melanoma, and breast, supposedly in that order, forming the acronym COMB. The word "comb" reminds us of the scalp, where the differential diagnosis does not hold, the most common metastasis to the scalp being renal cell carcinoma.

About one fifth of B-cell lymphocyte tumors will migrate to the skin at some time in the course of the disease, although T-cell tumors are better known for this behavior. Of the latter, mycosis fungoides is the best known, and most pleiomorphic. The Sezary syndrome has a characteristic cell, the Sezary cell, which is identifiable in the peripheral blood as well as the skin. Inflammation from the Sezary syndrome may produce the "red man," a Caucasian who looks as if he had just received a large dose of histamine (see p. 107 for other causes of the red man syndrome).

Lesions Resembling Carcinoma

The annular lesion of blastomycosis may mimic carcinoma when it appears on the face. It is never caused by direct inoculation, but rather by dissemination of a pulmonary focus. The skin lesion may be the only evidence that dissemination has occurred, and may be of great importance in deciding to initiate therapy. Other organisms, including histoplasmosis, coccidioidomycosis, and *Mycobacterium marinum* (*Balnei*), may also produce indolent, epithelialized lesions.

Excrescences

Keratoses

A keratosis is a hyperkeratotic papule, varying from yellow or flesh colored to quite dark, even black in the case of the seborrheic keratosis. Seborrheic or senile keratoses are a common but benign occurrence in old age. The lesions are of variable color and have a greasy, stuck-on appearance. In fact, they may be easily removed with a sharp curette, as they involve only the superficial layer of the skin.

Palmar keratoses are discussed in Chapter 25 (p. 437).

Solar keratosis is a waxy buildup of keratinous skin, which preserves some of the major skin creases, often found on the

back of the neck of sailors, outdoor stoop laborers, and others with chronic sun exposure (before long hair styles), and has been stated (incorrectly) to be the origin of the term *redneck*.* However, if this type of "chicken skin" is seen in the front of the neck or in the axillae, especially without a history of sun exposure, one is entitled to diagnose pseudoxanthoma elasticum (also see Ch. 10, p. 182).

•

I once had a patient who had lost weight due to lung cancer, giving the skin in the axillae a chicken-skin-like appearance. This myopic former lumberman also had solar keratoses on the back of his neck, and pseudoangioid ("lacquer crack") streaks in his fundi (see Ch. 10, p. 183). This then was a case of pseudopseudoxanthoma elasticum.

•

Lesions resembling senile keratoses or freckles, that suddenly appear and/or expand, often with pruritus, comprise the sign of Leser and Trelat (Fig. 7-10), which is of serious significance. Originally described by two European surgeons in the 19th century, the world's literature long consisted of only 10 cases. However, for some reason, the sign has been increasingly recognized in the past decade as one of the dermatologic signals of internal malignancy. Most common are abdominal carcinomas, usually gastric adenocarcinoma, but any type of neoplasm can occur, including leukemia or lymphoma (Greer et al., 1978; Kaplan & Jegasothy, 1984; Lynch et al., 1982; Safai et al., 1978; Schwartz, 1981). This association with occult malignancy is reminiscent of acanthosis nigricans, with which the sign of Leser and Trelat has coexisted.

Neurofibromas

These fleshy, pedunculated tumors (see Fig. 10-29) permit the diagnosis of neurofibromatosis (von Recklinghausen's disease).

---

*Redneck first appeared in Mississippi during the rise of a populist politician whose supporters, most of whom were poor rural whites, wore red bandanas around their necks (Rogers, 1986).

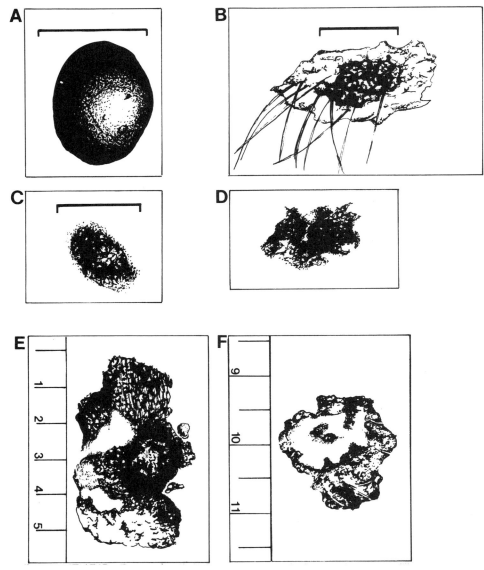

Figure 7-8.   *A, Seborrheic keratosis, also called the senile wart. It has no red spots, white spots, or notching, and occurs after middle age. It is symmetrical. The bar in this and the other photographs indicates 10 mm. B, Intradermal nevus, the common adult mole. This same type can be very large, as in a bathing trunk nevus. Note the hairs in the lesion, a statistical sign of benignity. C, Compound nevus. Its only resemblance to malignant melanoma is the elevated center; it lacks amelanotic white spots, red spots, or a notch. Rarely, it may develop into a melanoma. D, Hutchinson's melanotic freckle (lentigo maligna). This premalignant lesion usually begins as a brown macule on the face of middle aged persons. It usually grows very slowly and remains flat. However, when it demonstrates changes such as the development of a plaque, papule, or nodule, it may be undergoing malignant transformation. Notice the irregular notched edge. E and F, Two malignant melanomas. Both E and F have amelanotic segments within them; none of the other four do. Note the many notches in the edges of the asymmetrical lesions in E and F. Drawings courtesy of Jane Clanton.*

   Management: *Using the rule of "red, white, blue, or notch," the rule of "when in doubt, cut it out," and the rule of the hairs, you would ignore A and B, but would have to excise C, D, E, and F.*

Before the actual appearance of the tumors, the diagnosis is suggested by the finding of at least six café-au-lait ("coffee with milk") spots at least 1.5 cm in diameter. In a group of 6,856 normal adults, only 10% had café-au-lait spots, and never more than five; while 75% of 223 individuals with proven neurofibromatosis had six or more spots greater than 1.5 cm in diameter (Crowe, 1964).

Some say that axillary freckles also are diagnostic. They were found to be present in 22% of neurofibromatosis patients, all of

whom had other evidence of hyperpigmentation such as café-au-lait spots or diffuse duskiness (Crowe, 1964). However, I have seen such freckles in the absence of any other sign of neurofibromatosis. One might say "all that proves is that the patient does not have the rest of the syndrome . . . yet." The epistemologic problem is that "yet" can be stretched, if not to infinity, at least past the lifetime of the physician, or patient. (This relates to the general problem of statements that are not falsifiable. See the discussion regarding Raynaud's phenomenon versus Raynaud's disease, Ch. 18, p. 346.)

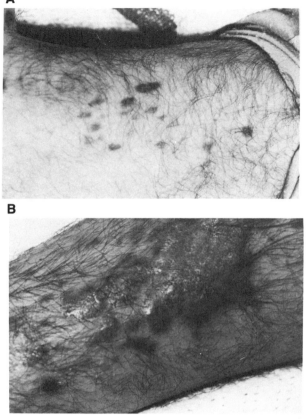

Figure 7-9. *A, Kaposi's sarcoma on the arm of a young AIDS patient. B, An older lesion on the thigh of the same patient. At first, this lesion was similar to the one shown in A.*

Tuberous Sclerosis

Small groups of fleshy tumors, seeming at first glance to be acne, may be found in the nasal creases of patients with tuberous sclerosis, also known as epiloia, or Bourneville's disease. The paranasal tumors are called adenoma sebaceum and are actually hamartomas. Hamartomas also afflict the heart, kidney, and brain, the last being responsible for the seizures with which these patients often present.

Other skin signs of tuberous sclerosis include a depigmented area in the shape of an ash leaf (best seen under a Wood's light), periungual fibromas like those seen in the Sipple syndrome, shagreen (shark skin) patches, and café-au-lait spots with borders said to resemble the smooth coast of California (in contrast to the café-au-lait spots in Albright's polyostotic fibrous dysplasia, which are likened to the rugged coast of Maine). Of these, the ash leaf is the earliest sign to appear (O'Brien 1973), if it appears.

Skin Tags (Acrochordons)

Acrochordons (Fig. 7-11) are simple papillomatous lesions at least 2 mm in height, often pedunculated, most easily found on the upper trunk, in or near the axilla or neck, but also seen on the head near the skin folds of the eyes and on the lower half of the body. In patients referred (for other reasons) for colonoscopy, these skin tags are about 75% sensitive and about 75% specific in predicting the demonstration of colonic polyps (Chobanian et al., 1985; Leavitt et al., 1983). Can colonic polyps—a precursor of colonic carcinoma—be predicted simply from the presence of acrochordons?

To evaluate the usefulness of this sign, we also need to know that the prevalence of colonic polyps in asymptomatic persons over the age of 50 is 5%. Using these numbers in a 2 × 2 table (see Ch. 1, p. 6), the predictive value of a positive test is only 14%. Thus, the presence of skin tags alone is not an indication for colonoscopy (Flegel et al., 1984). Even in kindreds with familial colonic polyposis, skin tags do not predict the existence of colonic polyps (Luk et al., 1986). However, the predictive value of a *negative* test (i.e., the probability that a patient without skin tags will not have polyps) is 98% (assuming that the patient is from the general population, not from the population that has been specifically selected for colonoscopy by some other criterion). The student should verify these numbers for himself, using his own 2 × 2 table (see Appendix 7-3).

Keratoderma Blenorrhagica

This lesion (Fig. 7-12) is considered to be pathognomonic of Reiter's syndrome. The example shown is the fully developed form, which resembles the top of a carrot with the greens cut off. Notice especially the one on the patient's left knee and the two near the calcaneus. If an astute observer had not remembered to examine the soles of the feet, this patient's urethritis and arthritis might have gone undiagnosed. The lesion is often associated with circinate balanitis (see Ch. 21, p. 392).

Atypical cases may be misdiagnosed as pustular psoriasis, even by experts.

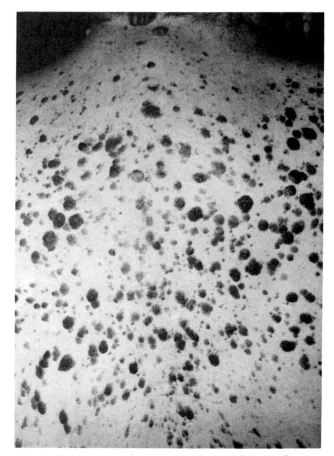

Figure 7-10. *The sign of Leser and Trelat. Photograph courtesy of Dr. Cliff Dasco of California.*

A

B

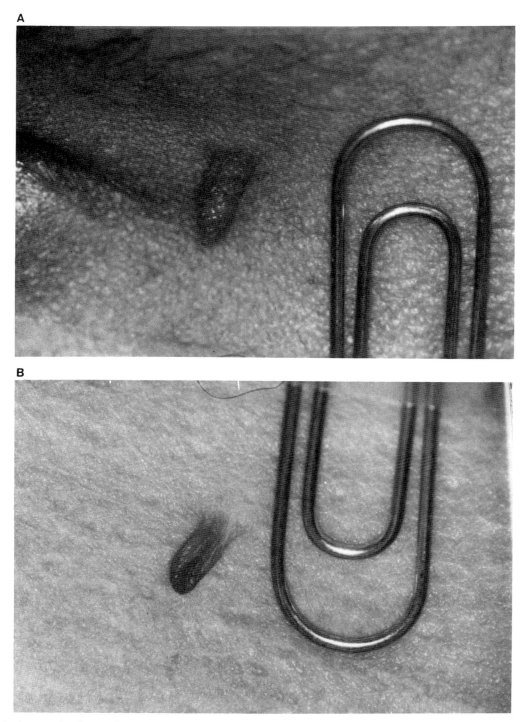

Figure 7-11.   *A, An acrochordon or skin tag next to the lateral canthus. B, An acrocordon on the neck. This patient has been followed for over 10 years without any colonoscopic evidence of cancer or polyps. The paper clip is shown for size comparison.*

Xanthomas

Xanthomas are collections of cholesterol and other fats. They have a shiny surface and a consistency like rheumatoid nodules and syphilitic gummas—firm but not hard. Some are located on the extensor surfaces and others over pressure points such as the elbow, knee, heel, and ischial tuberosities (Fleischmajer & Schragger, 1971; Polano et al., 1969).

With the possible exception of xanthelasma (vide infra), xanthomas are never normal, although some types are not diagnostic of a particular type of hyperlipidemia.

Even if the lipids are normal, the patient might have either: 1) local tissue abnormalities; 2) an associated systemic disorder, especially a lymphoproliferative disease; or 3) altered lipoprotein structure or function (Parker, 1986).

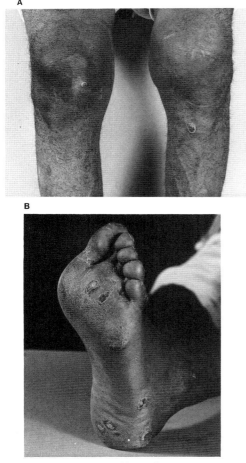

Figure 7-12. *Keratoderma blenorrhagica.*

Table 7-2. Types of Xanthomas

Lesion	Type of Hyperlipoproteinemia
Xanthelasma	II, III, IV, and supposed normals
Xanthomas	
Tuberous	Any type
Eruptive	Any type
Finger-fold	II or III
Palmar	III, rarely IV, or paraproteinemia
Tendon	II or III

Sources: *Fleischmajer and Schragger (1971), Parker (1986), and Polano et al. (1969).*

There are several types of xanthomas (Table 7-2). *Xanthelasma* are fatty, yellowish deposits beginning in the periocular skin folds. They occur in 25% of patients with type III hyperlipoproteinemia but are also common in types II and IV. Since the latter are so much more prevalent than type III hyperlipoproteinemia, most of the time xanthelasma signify the presence of type II or IV. Some apparently normal individuals may also have xanthelasma; but these persons may actually have apoprotein abnormalities (Douste-Blazy et al., 1982).

Tuberous xanthomas are shaped like tubers or potatoes (Fig. 7-13A). The individual tubers tend to be grouped together, and may appear and disappear over periods of weeks, depending on the state of the patient's blood lipids. These lesions always signify a hyperlipoproteinemia. A look at the serum may help to distinguish the type. If the serum is clear, the patient has hypercholesterolemia rather than high triglycerides, and thus probably has hyperlipoproteinemia type II (Parker, 1986). See also Chapter 28.

Eruptive xanthomas look like an eruption; that is, they are characterized by their inflammatory component, and are too small to resemble tubers. Those eruptive xanthomas secondary to the hyperlipemia of diabetes are given a special name, *xanthoma diabeticorum*. Patients with eruptive xanthomas will have turbid serum from the excess triglycerides.

If the xanthomas have the shape of tubers, but also occur in crops like an inflammatory eruption, they may be called *tubero-eruptive* (Fig. 7-13B).

Xanthomas can also be flat (therefore nontuberous) and bland (therefore noneruptive), in which case they are named by their location: finger-fold, palmar, tendon, and so forth. Finger-fold xanthomas are seen in type III hyperlipoproteinemias, and very rarely in type II. Palmar xanthomas are little fatty beads that appear in the palmar creases. These are seen in only half the patients with type III, but rarely in type IV or in the paraprotein hyperlipoproteinemias (Parker, 1986). They have also been seen in a child with hyperlipidemia due to biliary cirrhosis. *Tendon xanthomas* are the hallmark of type II hyperlipoproteinemia. Rarely, they may also be seen in type III. Christian's dictum applies: common manifestations of common diseases are more common than uncommon manifestations of uncommon diseases. If you see tendon xanthomas, diagnose type II over type III.

One can go no farther with the physical examination in these conditions. The xanthomatous patient deserves a laboratory examination (see Ch. 28, p. 547).

For the attending. What Christian actually said was this: "Uncommon manifestations of common diseases are more common than common manifestations of uncommon diseases." However, I find that reciting the perverted form first is pedagogically useful, since it is more obvious and helps make the transition to the correct form of Christian's dictum.

The perverted form is a truism, but, paradoxically, Christian's original dictum is not necessarily true. For instance, if a common disease had a prevalence of 30/100, and a rare disease had a prevalence of only 5/100, and the word "common"—used as a modifier of "manifestation"—means 95% of the cases, and "uncommon" means 5% of the cases, then the dictum would not hold.

Rigorously stated, the original dictum would be as follows:

Where

a = the prevalence of the common disease A,
b = the prevalence of the uncommon disease B,
c = the frequency of the uncommon manifestation of A,
d = the frequency of the common manifestation of B,

Then

$$(a \times c) > (b \times d)$$

This is obviously not true for all possible values of a, b, c, and d, as the above example shows.

Senile Hemangiomas

These small (about 1 mm) raised red lesions, also called cherry hemangiomas or de Morgan spots, differ from papules in having

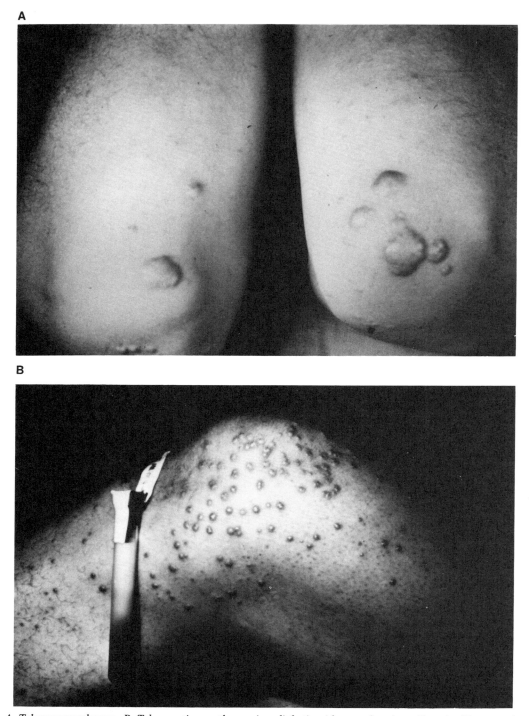

Figure 7-13.   *A, Tuberous xanthomas. B, Tuboeruptive xanthomas in a diabetic with secondary hyperlipemia. Photographs reproduced by permission of* Consultant Magazine, *Cliggott Publishing Company, Greenwich, Connecticut.*

a perfectly discrete border with surrounding normal skin. They are usually found on the chest and upper abdomen, and are perfectly benign. Unlike a red melanoma, they have a perfectly symmetrical and smooth dome.

At one time it was thought that senile hemangiomas were a sign of visceral carcinomatosis. This was due to a statistical artifact: the senile hemangiomas appeared in middle-aged subjects at the time they were entering the high risk decades for visceral carcinomas.

Acanthosis Nigricans

Acanthosis nigricans is a black hyperkeratotic but velvety lesion, appearing in the axillae and other intertriginous areas. It is seen as a harbinger of occult malignancy or in association with metabolic abnormalities, especially resistance to exogenous insulin in diabetes mellitus. Rarely, it is familial.

The history of this abnormality gives an interesting perspective on the progress of knowledge about clinical examination. In 1959, an evening with the *Quarterly Index* revealed only a few papers on acanthosis nigricans as a sign of internal malignancy, most by a New York private dermatologist named Curth. After several decades of searching among my own patients, I still had not used the information. Then there was an explosion of interest in this sign in metabolic abnormalities. A 5-minute computer search of the literature from 1984 to 1986 produced several feet of citations. In addition to the association with at least three different types of insulin resistance (both alone and together with hypothyroidism, obesity, systemic lupus erythematosus, polycystic kidneys, or acral hypertrophy), acanthosis nigricans had been described in the Lawrence-Seip syndrome (generalized lipodystrophy), cutaneous insulin reaction, nonneoplastic masculinization of females, and Crouzon's disease (both alone and in further association with periapical cemental dysplasia.) The original association with malignancy had now become so unusual that there were only isolated case reports of acanthosis nigricans with mycosis fungoides and adenocarcinoma of the stomach or gallbladder.

Supernumerary Nipples

Supernumerary nipples are sometimes confused with other skin lesions, such as nevi (see Ch. 15, p. 239).

Umbilicated Papules

The most common conditions causing umbilicated papules are molluscum contagiosum and prurigo nodularis. The former is caused by a virus, which may be sexually transmitted or spread by autoinoculation. The lesions generally occur on the face, the trunk, or the anogenital region. Prurigo nodularis is an eczematoid lesion.

Reactive perforating collagenosis. This condition is characterized by umbilicated papules, which microscopically are bundles of collagen fibers being extruded through the epidermis. Such papules, 0.2 to 1.0 cm in diameter, may be found, usually on the extensor surfaces, in association with diabetes mellitus and renal failure (Poliak et al., 1982). Koebner's phenomenon is present (see p. 121).

Kohlmeier-Dagos's disease (malignant atrophic papulosis). This progressive arterial occlusive disorder afflicts almost any organ of relatively young males, but especially the intestine. The skin lesion, which is conveniently displayed on the abdomen, usually in crops, is an umbilicated papule. Each central umbilicus is porcelain white and surrounded by an erythematous halo (Strole et al., 1967).

Scars

Signs of Drug Abuse

Scars are extremely useful signs of drug abuse, as shown in Figures 7-14 to 7-21. A more encyclopedic treatment is found in *Drug Abuse: A Guide for the Clinician* (Sapira & Cherubin, 1975).

Other Scars

In Caucasians, postsurgical scars show inflammation for up to 2 years. They then blend with the normal skin for about 8 years. Only after 10 years do they begin to develop pigmentation. Black skin has a tendency to heal any lesion with either hyper- or hypopigmentation.

Exuberant collagenosis in a scar, more commonly seen in blacks, is called keloid formation.

Sarcoid may appear in scars as localized irregularities, like microkeloids.

Tissue-paper scars are seen in porphyria, Ehlers-Danlos syndrome, and homocystinuria (Carey et al., 1968).

Excoriations

Signs of excoriation can be correlated with a history of itching (see Ch. 3, p. 39). Excoriations should prompt a careful search for other signs of skin disease. In the absence of visible skin disease, one should consider internal diseases. The most common etiologies are the secondary hyperparathyroidism of uremia, polycythemia rubra vera, lymphoma (especially Hodgkin's disease), and obstructive liver disease. In the last, itching due to the retention of bile salts may precede the appearance of jaundice.

If the itching is chronic and has produced scars and scratches, Dr. Frank Iber suggests searching inside the scratches for white fat infiltrates, which would favor chronic obstructive liver disease as the cause of the pruritus.

Ulcers and Open Sores

Ulcers arise from external trauma (e.g., scratching), the unroofing of vesicular or bullous lesions, or from necrosis due to ischemia (see Ch. 25, p. 447 for rheumatoid vasculitis).

The early lesions of *pyoderma gangrenosum*, which may appear following minor trauma, consist of pustules, vesicles, boils, or inflammatory nodules, which rapidly break down to form burrowing ulcers. The advancing, irregular border is raised, purple-red, and undermined. Large areas of the abdomen, trunk, and extremities may become involved.

Over a third of cases of pyoderma gangrenosum occur in association with inflammatory bowel disease (ulcerative colitis or regional enteritis) and about another third in association with immune arthritis, although there is some overlap between these two groups. In about 30% of cases there is no underlying disease. The few remaining are accounted for by a wide variety of seemingly unrelated disorders including multiple myeloma, biliary cirrhosis, malignancy, thyroid disease, pulmonary disease, systemic sarcoidosis, diabetes mellitus, spider bite, and iodine ingestion (Walling & Sweet, 1987).

The lesion must be differentiated from fungal lesions (histoplasmosis, blastomycosis, cryptococcosis, sporotrichosis, mucormycosis, candida, and cryptococcus), vascular lesions, neoplasms, and acute neutrophilic dermatosis (Sweet's disease).

Lupus profundus is the panniculitis that supervenes in 2% to 3% of cases of systemic lupus erythematosus (Diaz-Johnson et al., 1975; Tuffanelli, 1971). Beginning as nodules, these break down and leave full-thickness ulcers, as if a punch biopsy had been performed with an odd-shaped punch (Fig. 7-22, p. 127). Healing is, as usual, from the edges, often leaving pigment behind.

Findings on Palpation

Texture

The skin of primary hypothyroidism is coarse and dry. In contrast, hypothyroidism secondary to panhypopituitarism may be associated with fine skin, which may appear wrinkled like cigarette paper. Patients under 50 with hyperthyroidism have warm, moist, fine skin, likened to that of a baby. Patients with acro-

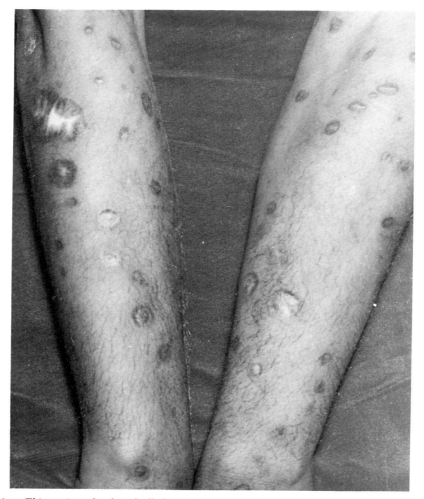

Figure 7-14. *Skin popping. This patient developed all these sharply demarcated, punched-out, hypopigmented scars from the subcutaneous injection of a single batch of contaminated heroin. They were not due to an allergic reaction, as shown by subsequent challenge with subcutaneous injections of pure morphine, without sequelae. Courtesy of the* American Journal of Medicine.

megaly have excessive sebaceous activity, resulting in a greasy or waxy feel to the skin. (Patients who have coincidental facial resemblance to acromegaly, but no greasy skin, tend to have normal growth hormone studies.) Parkinsonian patients also have greasy skin. The skin texture in scleroderma is described under "Sclerodactyly" on page 441.

Scleredema adultorum of Buschke is a hard, nonpitting skin that cannot be picked up by the examiner's fingers. It begins as an induration on the posterior neck and then spreads to other areas in the distribution of the superior vena cava. Those cases that follow infection usually remit, but those that occur in the diabetic may persist (Cohn et al., 1970).

Turgor

Skin turgor is traditionally tested for by plucking up a fold of skin and observing whether or not it tents ("poor turgor") or returns to normal ("good turgor"). Poor turgor is now equated with dehydration. There is an important caveat: Although this sign works well in young people with normal elastic fibers, in old people it may only work on forehead skin, which for some reason retains its elasticity for a long time. Try comparing the forehead turgor with the buccolabial fold moisture (see p. 226).

Temperature

Throughout this work, the student is instructed to palpate the skin overlying various portions of the body. When comparisons can be made between the sides, it is assumed that some pathologic process is occurring on one side but not the other. However, if the patient has been lying in a decubitus position, or if one portion of his body has been covered and not the other, the retained heat can produce a false positive. Accordingly, you should not check for skin temperature until the patient has been under your observation for some time.

Special Maneuvers

Flaying

I have heard of a technique in which the skin is examined for nodules by "flaying" the skin with the back of the hand. That is, the back of the hand is rapidly passed over the torso, arms, legs, and so forth, pressing as firmly as is compatible with rapid motion. Nodules, lipoatrophy, and other findings which are otherwise not readily apparent, are easily picked up, it is said. Several professors of medicine at Johns Hopkins, who were born before 1925, use this method, but I have no reference.

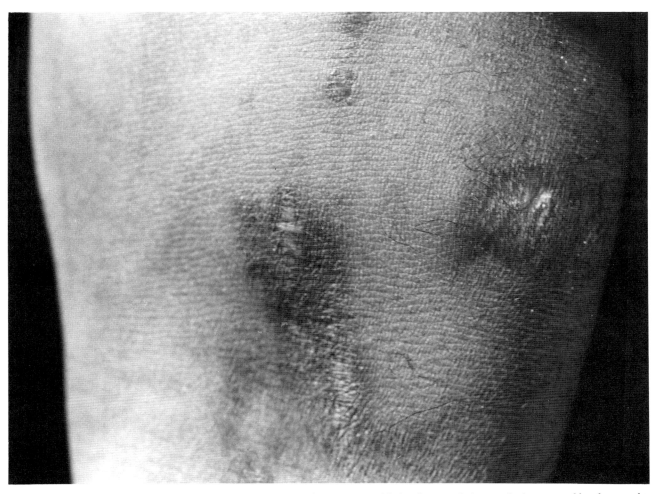

Figure 7-15. *This drug user's antecubital fossa shows two post abscess scars with the characteristic, poorly demarcated borders, and two short segments of "railroad tracks" (not "tracts"). Courtesy of the* American Journal of Medicine.

The Triceps Skin Fold

A variety of tables and formulas using height and weight are available for estimating obesity, and these are beyond the scope of this work. However, the triceps skin-fold test may be performed by pinching the skin overlying the triceps, and measuring the thickness of the doubled skin fold. Formerly, drug companies selling anorectics provided calipers (see Ch. 8, p. 139; Ch. 15, p. 240; and Ch. 21, p. 396 for other uses) with cutoff lines to dichotomize this continuously distributed unimodal variable (see Ch. 16, p. 277). **$$** Calipers for measuring skin-fold thickness are now available from Cambridge Scientific Industries, P.O. Box 265, Cambridge, MD 21613, Ross Laboratories, 625 Cleveland Ave., Dept. 441, Columbus, OH 43216, and Adria Laboratories, Columbus, OH 43215. "You can't pinch an inch" is an advertising slogan that is part of the USA's current craze for thinness, but an inch (2.54 cm) is actually a generous cutoff. The severe constructionists of yesterday's advertising calipers gave the value of 1.5 cm. Nowadays we can use the diameter of a dime, 1.7 cm, as a convenient metric standard in a nonmetric country.

Dermatographism

Dermatographism is an exaggeration of the normal response (wheal and erythema) to cutaneous trauma. Writing on the skin with a dull point gives rise to raised, red letters. It may be associated with atopic disease, or it may simply be a curiosity.

Koebner's Phenomenon

If an old established skin lesion appears to "jump" to a new *noncontiguous* location following trauma to that previously normal-appearing skin, the lesion is said to exhibit Koebner's phenomenon. This has been traditionally associated with psoriasis, scabies, lichen planus (see Ch. 13, p. 226), warts, and a number of rarer dermatoses. However, it is not highly diagnostic, and has even been reported in the eruptive xanthomas of hyperlipidemia (Barker & Gould, 1979).

A schoolboy once drew the name of his beloved on the extensor surface of his arm with a compass during a boring geometry class. At the time of the infatuation, the name remained private. However, he later developed vitiligo, which made the girl's name visible, in a dramatic manifestation of the Koebner phenomenon (Sweet, 1978).

Darier's Sign

Rubbing the reddish-brown macular lesions of urticaria pigmentosa results in urticaria with a pinkish halo in the otherwise normal skin surrounding the lesions.

Nikolsky's Sign

In patients with Nikolsky's sign, a firm lateral pressure will produce a sliding of superficial layers of the epidermis over the deeper

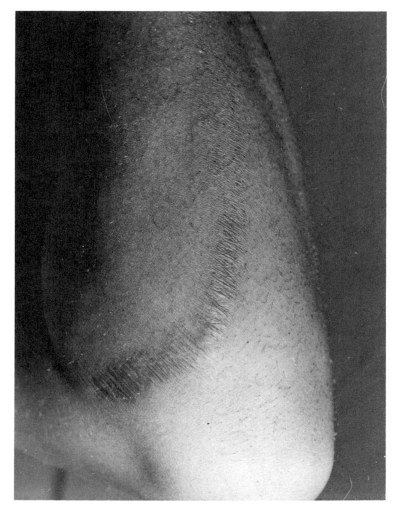

Figure 7-16. *Here is an extremely broad venous "railroad track" seen on the extensor surface of the upper extremity. The antecubital fossae were clear in this case, as the patient had no veins there. All accessible veins were, or had been, under this scar.* Courtesy of the American Journal of Medicine.

layers. In normal persons, this sign cannot be elicited. (Try it on yourself.)

The test is positive in pemphigus vulgaris, pemphigus erythematosus, epidermolysis bullosa dystrophica, the staphylococcal scalded skin syndrome, and other epidermolytic diseases. Thus, it is not a highly specific test. (In fact, a method of screening for epidermal toxins is by injecting substances into the newborn mouse and attempting to produce a Nikolsky sign by lightly stroking the skin [Todd et al., 1978].)

The test reflects disease activity since clinical and serologic remission is often accompanied by reversion of the sign to normal.

The test is painful if positive. Nevertheless, it has been done in the same way, using the thumb, since 1895. Recently, two Israeli dermatologists accidentally discovered a modification while attempting to test for dermatographism by stroking with the round end of a paper clip (Hacham-Zadeh & Even-Paz, 1980). The paper clip is held at a 45-degree angle to the firmly stroked skin. A smaller, less painful Nikolsky sign can be produced in this way.

Very advanced. The history of Nikolsky's sign is useful for teaching how correct Hippocrates was when he wrote that the art of medicine was "long." In fact, it seems that Hippocrates himself first described the sign!

In the late 19th century, there was great confusion about the dif-

ferent pemphigoid disorders. (Pemphigus comes from the Greek word for "blister." Note that herpes, another blistering disease, comes from the Greek word for "wander.") To help sort out the confusion, Nikolsky described the sign that bears his name (although he had learned it from his professor Stoukowenkow). The sign was offered as a way to distinguish pemphigus foliaceus (which is Nikolsky positive) from pemphigus vulgaris (which did not meet the criteria for a positive test in Nikolsky's doctoral thesis, the original publication!). Later, Nikolsky changed the criteria when he published the second edition of his dermatology textbook in 1927. Using various criteria, a wide variety of pemphigoid diseases, other bullous diseases, and even a nonbullous disease (gas gangrene) have been reported to have a positive Nikolsky sign (Polifka & Krusinski, 1980).

Worse, even some of the widely accepted etiologies for a positive Nikolsky sign, such as bullous pemphigoid, do not give a true Nikolsky sign. Biopsies reveal not the sliding of one layer of the epidermis on another, but rather a sliding of the entire epidermis upon the dermis (Grunwald et al., 1984). Not unexpectedly, this has been christened the pseudo-Nikolsky sign.

Given the confusion among the experts, one is tempted to quote Thomas "Fats" Waller's reply to the society lady who asked him to explain syncopation. "Lady," he said, "if you don't know what it is, you ain't got no business messing with it."

A **B**

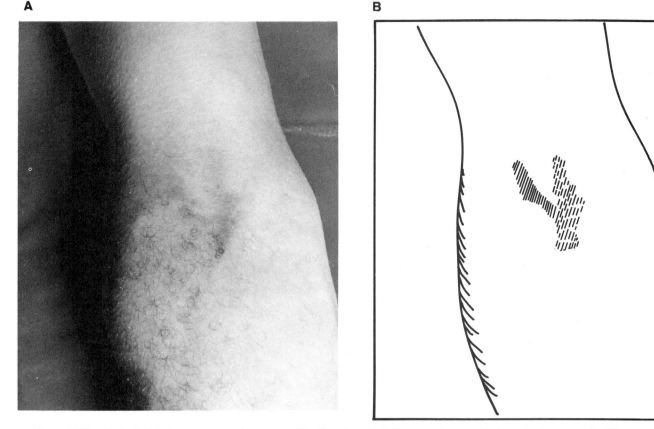

Figure 7-17. *A, A slightly hyperpigmented segment of "railroad tracks." If you can't see it, look at the diagram in B. Pigmentation over the veins has also been reported in severe malnutrition, pellagrous dermatitis, stasis dermatitis, and injury to the vein following the injection of nitrogen mustard (Bean, 1976).* **Photograph courtesy of the** American Journal of Medicine.

Transillumination

If a penlight is placed against one side of a lump, and the light can be seen from the other side, we say that the lump is translucent, or, vulgarly, that it transilluminates. (Actually, the penlight transilluminates.) Cysts, lipomas, chondromas, and xanthomas may transilluminate, in this sense.

Odor

Certain skin conditions are associated with an unpleasant smell, such as infected eczema, hidradenitis suppurativa, pemphigus, herpes labialis and *Herpes zoster*, and Darier's disease. Leg ulcers that have become infected may emit an unpleasant odor. A *Pseudomonas* skin infection produces a musty odor; so do some cancers, possibly from the sweat.

The sweat in scurvy is said to have a putrid odor, and patients with scrofula are said to have a smell like that of stale beer. The sweat of some schizophrenic subjects, but not that of normals, contains trans-3-methyl-2-hexenoic acid, adding weight to the theory that some schizophrenia is an inborn error of metabolism (Liddell, 1976). In maple syrup urine disease, the sweat smells like maple syrup, and in hypermethioninemia, like fish, rancid butter, or boiled cabbage (Hayden, 1980).

Other odors are discussed in Ch. 13 (p. 228).

Hair

The examiner should note the hair distribution, texture, and appearance.

(I do not examine individual hairs unless I am considering the diagnosis of scurvy [see p. 110].)

Distribution

Sexual Hair

Three sites of body hair should be examined for clues to the patient's endocrine status: the face, the axilla, and the pubic region.

Face. Sexual hair formation is stimulated by androgens, so facial hair may occur in some women with a constitutional predisposition (e.g., androgen receptor sensitivity), or as a sign of elevated androgen levels. Conversely, in men, damage to the testes or the development of hypogonadotropic insufficiency for any reason will cause the facial hair to become sparse and slow growing.

Because of the normal constitutional variability, a good history is necessary for interpreting the physical findings. *Change* is more important than the actual amount of hair. In some women of Mediterranean background, a significant amount of facial hirsutism may be quite normal, and among Amerindians and some Asians, very sparse facial hair is the norm in men.

Axilla. In both men and women who are hypogonadotropic, the axillary hair will slow its growth and become sparse compared with baseline.

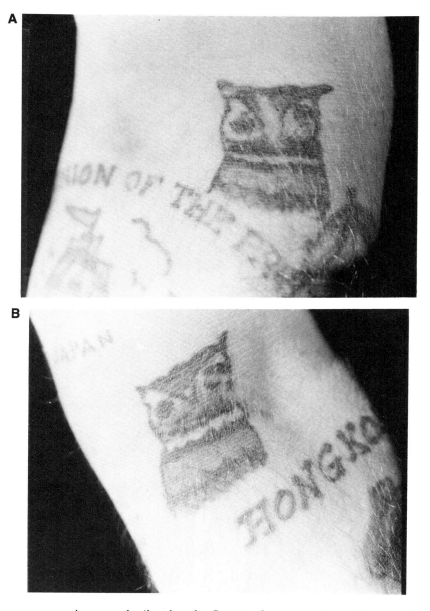

Figure 7-18. *Sometimes tattos are used to conceal railroad tracks. Compare the noses and eyes of the two owls, from the two antecubital fossae (A and B) of the same patient, who injected bilaterally. Courtesy of* Excerpta Medica.

Before the development of good assays for gonadotrophic hormones, research subjects participated in the bioassay of experimental preparations by weekly measurements of the weight of their shaved, acetone-defatted axillary hair (and in the case of men, facial hair also).

Pubis.   The shape of the pubic hair distribution is called "female" if it forms a triangle with the apex pointed toward the perineum, and "male" if it is in the shape of a diamond, with the superior tip of the diamond pointing to the umbilicus. It responds to the excess or lack of androgens effect on hair in the same way as the other sexual hair described above. (Also see p. 401).

Eyebrows

Thinning of the lateral third of the eyebrows is a form of local acquired alopecia that is suggestive of the diagnosis of hypothy-

roidism. Eyebrows that are sparse laterally, and normal medially, are called Queen Anne's eyebrows (see Fig. 9-2).

In addition to hypothyroidism, causes of lateral thinning of the eyebrows include trichorhinophalangeal syndrome, trichodental syndrome (Fitzpatrick et al., 1979), leprosy ("Bailey," Clain, 1973), normal aging (De Groot et al., 1984), and subacute thallium intoxication (Grunfeld & Hinostroza, 1964).

Systemic lupus erythematosus may cause total loss of the eyebrows, not just of the lateral third, as may syphilis (Fitzgerald, 1982).

Eyebrow pencil may obscure these findings, unless one looks closely.

It is not certain that Anne of Denmark (Fig. 7-23) had goitrous hypothyroidism, although she seems to have had a goiter, the dull facies of hypothyroidism, and in some reproductions of her por-

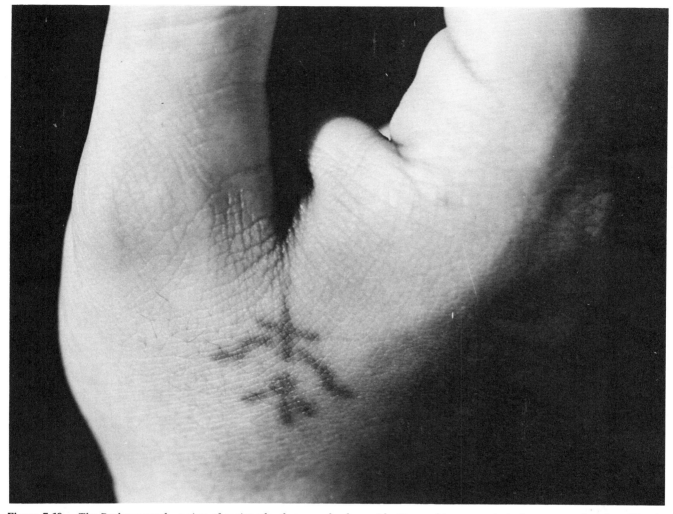

Figure 7-19.   *The Pachuco mark, a sign of sociopathy that can also be an identity card in some criminal segments of society. That is, someone from the drug-using demi-monde can help establish his credentials as a member of the subculture by displaying his tattoo on entering a strange community . For someone seeking to buy illegal drugs, the tattoo serves the same purpose as a credit card or curriculum vitae does for a traveling professor. Courtesy of the* American Journal of Medicine.

traits, lateral thinning of the eyebrows. She had three miscarriages and seven sickly children, ceasing sexual activity at age 32. Her arthritic complaints could have been the musculoskeletal complications of myxedema although they were diagnosed as gout. Hyperuricemia can occur secondary to myxedema (as can pseudogout), or in her case it might have been saturnine gout from Spanish sherry. Queen Anne also had the "dropsy," which possibly was congestive heart failure due to myxedema heart. Her "leg ulcers" were probably secondary to pedal edema. She responded to only two attempts at therapy: a visit to the waters of Bath, and a potion made for her by Sir Walter Raleigh, either of which might have relieved an iodide deficiency state. In later life, she became torpid, withdrawn, and depressed. Her death was compatible with myxedema (Williams, 1970).

Once I was shown a patient with a low-serum thyroxine, in whom Queen Anne's eyebrows were the only evidence of hypothyroidism that could be found on the physical examination. Alas, they were constitutional, not acquired, and the low-serum thyroxine was eventually ascribed to the euthyroid sick syndrome. This illustrates an important principle, especially in regard to general appearance, facies, skin, habitus, and in this case, hair. If at all possi-

ble, have the patient or a member of the family bring in an old snapshot, or even better, the family photograph album.

Very advanced. Blepharospasm may be differentiated from apraxia of lid opening by the fact that chronic contraction of the orbicularis oculi causes the eyebrow to be below the superior orbital rim in blepharospasm, whereas the eyebrow is positioned normally in apraxia of lid opening (Jones et al., 1985).

Hair on the Feet

Loss of hair on the toes, feet, and ankles has been presented as evidence of arteriolar sclerosis or diabetes mellitus. However, when 40 patients with diagnosed arterial occlusive disease were compared with 40 controls, no difference was found in any measure regarding hair on the toes and anterior shins (Parfrey et al., 1979).

Alopecia

The causes of hair loss are legion. To shorten one's library time, I suggest describing alopecia as diffuse or patchy. In the case of

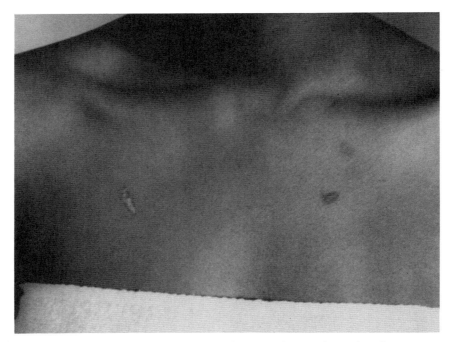

Figure 7-20. *The "necklace" of heroin use is composed of individual cigarette burns. The smoking heroin user nods off during the drug effect, and the head, cigarette in the mouth, falls forward. The burn is not perceived because of the analgesic effect of the heroin, as demonstrated by the length of some of the scars. This is a very early, yet common form of the necklace; a full-blown form would be composed of 15 or 20 individual burns.*

patchy hair loss, one should also describe it as occurring with normal-appearing scalp or secondary to scarring or lesions of the scalp.

Many patients with diffuse alopecia will wear a wig, which must be noticed and removed by the examiner. Unfortunately for the diagnostician, the most common causes for wearing a wig are vanity and senescent hair loss, the latter having no significance beyond itself.

Another reason for always removing turbans and wigs is to examine the scalp. I once missed an obvious case of herpes zoster (in a patient I allowed to be presented while she was receiving a shampoo) because I believed the house officer's incorrect description of a bilateral pustular lesion, when there was actually a unilateral herpetic one.

Diffuse hair loss may be seen in hypothyroidism, panhypopituitarism, hyperthyroidism, some cases of hypoparathyroidism, lupus erythematosus, heavy metal toxicity (e.g., thallium), and as a sequel to treatment with retinoids (Ellis, 1987) or cer-

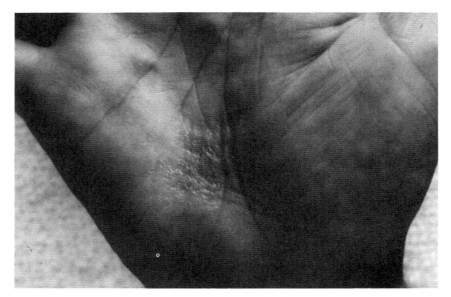

Figure 7-21. *The scars in the palm of this heroin user have the same basic pathophysiology as the necklace. This unusually neat heroin user did not like to spill his cigarette ashes on the floor and so used his hand as an ashtray. The good analgesic effect of the heroin is shown by the degree of scarring.*

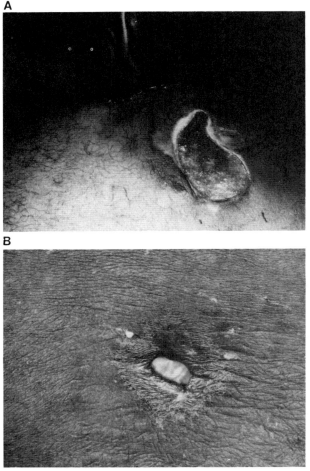

A

B

Figure 7-22. *Lupus profundus.*

tain drugs used to treat hyperthyroidism or cancer. The scalp will appear normal. Currently, the most common cause of complete alopecia (total baldness) is cancer chemotherapy.

The most common cause of patchy hair loss with normal-appearing scalp is alopecia areata, a disease that has kept many pre-minoxidil hair restorers in business by providing dramatic visual "proof" through before-and-after pictures (although the alopecia is irreversible in some cases). Female patients with alopecia areata may cover their hair, but tend not to buy wigs. Alopecia areata does not suggest presence of another disease. However, patchy hair loss with normal-appearing scale can also occur in misdiagnosed and untreated syphilis.

Patchy hair loss with scalp lesions is seen in tuberculosis, systemic lupus erythematosus, and sarcoidosis, *inter alia.*

Color

Canites (greying of the hair) occurs in pernicious anemia, with chloroquine treatment, and in some of the etiologies of vitiligo (see p. 107). Poliosis (premature canites) occurs in patients with thyroid disease and their kindreds.

Brown hair in orientals is not always a sign of protein calorie deficiency, or of phenylketonuria. It may also be a result of chemical exposure from swimming pool chlorine or cosmetics.

Scalp hairs in tinea capitis caused by *Microsporum canis* and *M. audouini* display a green fluorescence under Wood's light.

Texture

The hair is very fine in hypermetabolic conditions such as hyperthyroidism, and in some patients with chronic obstructive pulmonary disease. Coarse hair is found in hypothyroidism.

Brittle hair occurs in Menke's kinky-hair syndrome, a disease of copper transport, and in the Sabinas syndrome, which is so far confined to one town in Mexico.

Appearance

Corkscrew hairs (Fig. 7-24) are pathognomonic for scurvy provided that they occur in persons who do not normally have corkscrew hairs (i.e., straight-haired people) and in parts of the body where the hairs are not normally curled (i.e., on the arms and legs but not in the pubic areas of those with naturally curly pubic hair). The etiology and semiophysiology of this type of hair can be deduced from Figure 7-25.

False positives have been seen in situations (e.g., thrombocytopenia) in which the follicles have become plugged with blood, but this phenomenon is restricted to areas of hemorrhage.

Nails

From the fingernails, the astute clinician can make meaningful estimates of the results of laboratory tests such as the hematocrit, serum albumin, and blood urea nitrogen. In addition, the nails give clues to various congenital anomalies as well as to numerous systemic diseases.

Color of the Nail Bed

Acrocyanosis

Cyanosis may be due to deoxyhemoglobin, methemoglobin, or sulfhemoglobin, as previously noted (see p. 107). Acrocyanosis may be due to slowing of the peripheral circulation as in erythrocytosis, but the rest of the body remains pink. Local venous disease can produce focal acrocyanosis.

Pallor

With practice, one can estimate the hematocrit to within a few points by simply examining the nail beds.

Self-Study. The best way to learn to recognize and quantify pallor is to go to the medical ward and look at a patient's fingernails. Estimate the hematocrit, committing yourself in writing, and then look up the measured hematocrit. Repeat at the next bed. By the time you have been once around the ward, you should be pretty accurate. (Note that the electronic counter does not measure the hematocrit, but rather calculates it from the red cell count and the mean corpuscular volume, and this reported hematocrit may be inaccurate by three to five points.)

Even if you miss the hematocrit by a few points most of the time, it does not matter. What you want to know is whether the patient has anemia or not. Whether the hematocrit is actually 20, 24, or 28, you will proceed to evaluate the anemia.

False positives. In patients with leukonychia or if the fingernails congenitally compress the distal nail bed vasculature, the

A

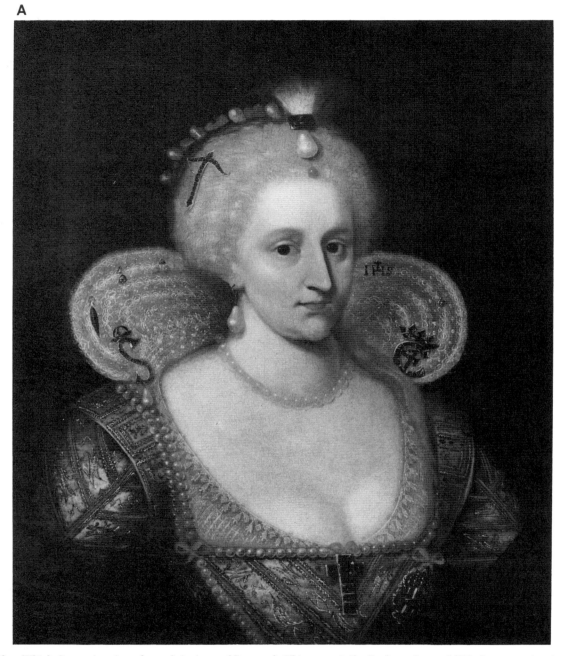

Figure 7-23. *Which Queen Anne's eyebrows? A, Anne of Denmark. This portrait (by Paul van Somer, 1617) shows a goiter, but does not show Queen Anne's eyebrows. Normal eyebrows are also seen in the portraits of Anne of France, Anne of Brittany, Anne of Great Britain, Anne of Austria, Anne of Cleve, and Anne Boleyn. B, Anne of England, the daughter of James II, does not have Queen Anne's eyebrows in this painting, even though she looks a little puffy. Some have seen a portrait in which the lateral thirds of the eyebrows are missing, but the issue is not resolvable because during the period when she reigned (1707–1714) it became fashionable to shave the lateral eyebrows. Photographs courtesy of the National Portrait Gallery, London.*

nails look pale despite a normal hematocrit. The latter phenomenon can be detected by lifting the nail from the nail bed and observing the filling phenomenon (see Ch. 18, p. 331). Nail bed pallor is also seen in the vascular insufficiency of shock and of arterial obstruction.

One can also routinely estimate the hematocrit from the conjunctivae, oral mucosa, and tongue (Jacobs et al., 1979) to obviate such interfering circumstances of the nail beds. A study that compared the pallor of the conjunctivae, nail beds, and palmar creases with a photograph of a tint scale, using a color tint selector, showed a significant correlation (Strobach et al., 1988).

A patient was presented with a stated hematocrit of 39. He looked quite pale, and his nail beds were pale. All agreed that he was paler than on admission. I announced that the stated hematocrit must be wrong, and was confronted with an identical repeat value. I took the patient to the sunlight and examined his conjunctivae, which were also quite pale, so I bet a lunch. The next morning I was presented with another electronic hematocrit of 39 and also a spun hematocrit of 39. Puzzled, I went back to look at

B

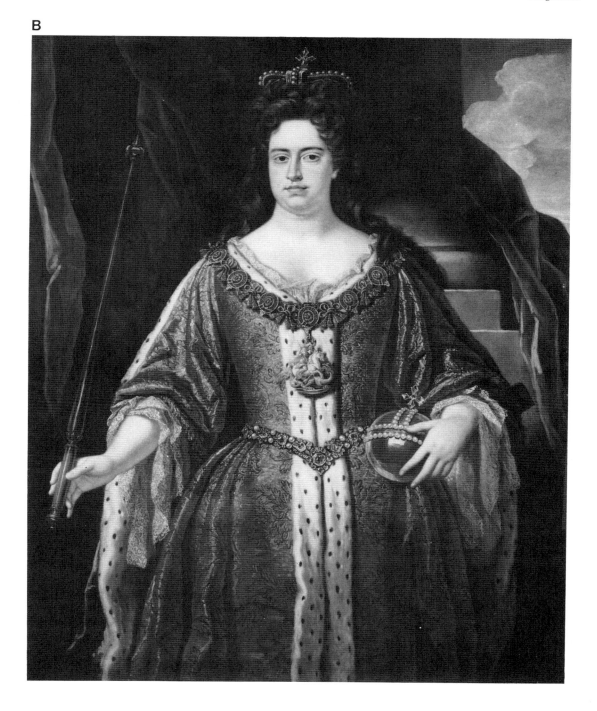

the patient, who was now quite pink, as were his nail beds and conjunctivae. When I told him what puzzled me, he stated that he often became pale under circumstances of excitement or fright.

"You mean," I asked, "that when we all came in here the other morning to examine you, you became upset."

"Yes," he said.

"Oh," I said. "That's what caused the pallor."

The patient looked up at me and smiled. "You didn't know you were that ugly, did you?" he laughed.

Moral: **When all else fails, go back and ask the patient.**

False negatives. Many non-Caucasians have sufficient pigmentation in their nail beds to prevent the appearance of pallor even in the presence of a low hematocrit. (This was first pointed

out to me by Dr. Bruce Singh of Australia, and emphasized by Dr. Liz Torres of Texas.) This error can be avoided by inspecting the degree of redness and ignoring the total amount of pigmentation.

Lighting. Another common cause of difficulty is the use of indoor lighting. The most accurate predictions of hematocrit values are made in direct sunlight (see similar comments on scleral icterus, Ch. 10, p. 162). To convince yourself of the truth of this statement, on a bright, sunny day examine several patients under incandescent lights in an inner hallway, and then immediately walk them to a window where their hands can be examined in direct sunlight.

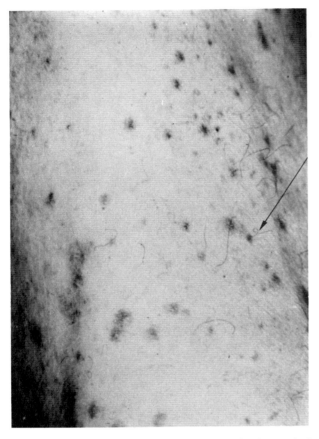

Figure 7-24. *Corkscrew or pigtail hair on a background of perifollicular hemorrhages is pathognomic for scurvy. What other characteristic hemorrhage is seen in this disease? (See p. 110.) Photograph courtesy of Cliggott Publishing Company.*

Abnormalities of the Nail

Leukonychia Totalis

Leukonychia totalis (a completely white nail) may result from a variety of causes (Zaias, 1980), listed in Table 7-3.

Some of the familial cases of leukonychia totalis may also have knuckle pads and deafness in a dominant pattern (Bart & Pumphrey, 1967). Others have multiple sebaceous cysts and renal calculi (Zaias, 1980).

Incomplete Leukonychia

Incomplete leukonychia, in the form of bands or spots, may be acquired or inherited. The etiologies include trauma, heavy metal poisoning, typhoid fever, ulcerative colitis, and for unknown reasons, myocardial infarction in some patients.

Transverse white bands. Mees' lines, seen in arsenical polyneuropathy, consist of a single transverse white band (Mees, 1919). The same transverse single bands, when they occur in infectious fevers, are called Reil's lines. Without an eponym, these same bands have been seen in acute and chronic renal failure, thallium toxicity (Grunfeld & Hinostroza, 1964), leprosy, malaria, fluorosis, psoriasis, cardiac insufficiency, pellagra, Hodgkin's disease, pneumonia, myocardial infarction,

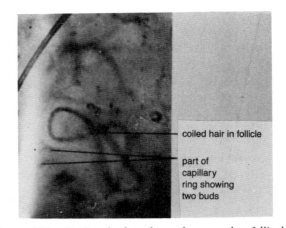

coiled hair in follicle

part of capillary ring showing two buds

Figure 7-25. *During the first phase of scurvy when follicular hyperkeratosis supervenes, the mouth of the hair follicle becomes plugged. But the hair continues to grow within it, becoming curled up. This is shown as "coiled hair in follicle" in microphotos of the hair follicle of a World War II conscientious objector who volunteered for the world's only double-blind experimental scurvy study. (Half the volunteers were given vitamin C and half placebo tablets as a supplement to their scorbutic diet.) When the follicle's plug is eventually knocked loose, the coiled hair springs out fully formed, like Zeus's wife from his head. There is nothing intrinsically wrong with the hair itself; its odd form is due to growing in a plugged follicle (Vitamin C Subcommittee, 1953). Photograph reproduced with permission of the Controller of Her Britannic Majesty's Stationery Office.*

and sickle cell disease (Hudson & Dennis, 1966). (Given the excess of causes over eponyms for what is essentially the same sign, the ambitious student may wish to attach his own name to some eponymously vacant etiology.)

Hypoalbuminemia, especially if intermittent, may also cause white transverse opaque bands. A pair of transverse lines (see Fig. 7-26) were described in hypoalbuminemic patients suffering from the nephrotic syndrome (Muehrcke, 1956). These lines are pathognomonic for hypoalbuminemia (Conn & Smith, 1965).

Other Transverse Bands in the Nail

Periods of (intermittent) catabolism due to fever, cachexia, malnutrition, and so forth, will produce Beau's lines: nonpigmented indented transverse bands best seen in oblique light. These were first described by Hillier (Wilks, 1869).

No false positives were seen if Beau's lines were defined as transverse grooves running across the greater part of each nail and occurring simultaneously in all (Robertson & Braune, 1974).

Yellowish bands can be seen after parenteral gold therapy (Fam & Paton, 1984).

Nail Bands as Calendars

Most of these bands (but not Muehrcke's lines) can be used to time an illness by noting their distance from the proximal nail bed. The nails of the upper extremities grow out in about 120 days (Bean, 1968). However, the rate of growth slows with age and with local afflictions of the nail bed as well as with systemic diseases. Toenail growth is much slower than fingernail growth.

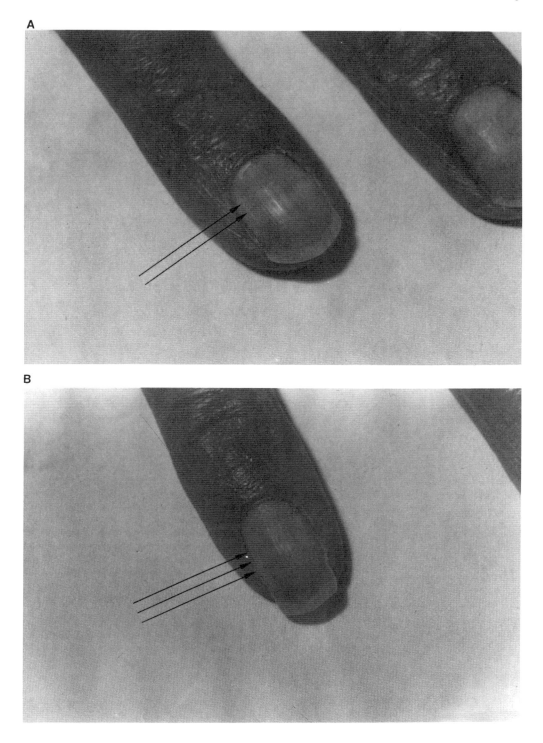

Figure 7-26. *While there is no reason that someone could not be twice poisoned with arsenic, Mees' lines are usually single. Double bands (A) are generally Muehrcke's lines, and diagnostic for hypoalbuminemia, in that they may be reversed with albumin infusions without waiting for the nail to grow out. Thus, they are not in the nail itself as the other lines are, but in the nail bed. Accordingly, they do not grow out with the nail like the other bands do and so may* not *be used for timing illness. A triple Muehrcke line (B) was found in a patient with an albumin of 3.1 g/dl, below normal but above the ceiling of 2.2 g/dl given in the original paper (Muehrcke, 1956). What other sign of disease do you see here? Where are the lunulae? (See Terry's nails in text.) One trick useful in seeing the lines is to concentrate on the dark bands separating the light Muehrcke lines.*

Table 7-3.   Differential Diagnosis of Leukonychia Totalis

Familial
    Autosomal dominant
Local dystrophic disease
    Leprosy
    Herpes zoster
    Fungal infection
    Trophic diseases of the upper extremity
Systemic diseases
    Adrenocortical insufficiency
    Cancer chemotherapy
    "Cardiac insufficiency"
    Exfoliative dermatitis
    Hodgkin's disease
    Pneumonia
    Tuberculosis
    Trichinosis
    Chronic arsenic poisoning
    Hepatic cirrhosis
Nutritional deficiencies
    Zinc deficiency
    Pellagra
    Hypoalbuminemia, chronic

4–7% of normal persons (Harrington, 1964)

Sources: *Terry (1954a) and Zaias (1980).*

Half-and-Half Nail

The half-and-half nail (Lindsay, 1967) consists of a nail whose proximal portion is white to pink and whose distal portion, always well demarcated, is a dirty red or brown. Originally believed to be a sign of chronic renal disease, in some populations it is much more commonly seen with chronic hepatic failure. The finding is not necessarily abnormal on toenails.

Pigmentary Changes

Darkening of the nails has been reported with many chemotherapeutic drugs (Furth & Kazakis, 1987), including azidothymidine, bleomycin, doxorubicin, fluorouracil, melphalan, nitrogen mustard, nitrosoureas, methotrexate, cyclophosphamide, and mitoxantrone (Speechly-Dick & Owen, 1988). Black nails have been seen after radiation and exposure to photographic developer and hair dye, and in Peutz-Jeghers' disease, vitamin B_{12} deficiency, malignant melanoma, and pinta.

Green nails have been seen with *Pseudomonas* infection (Fitzpatrick et al., 1979).

Also see "Yellow nail syndrome" on page 133.

The Lunula

The lunula should be sought on the thumbnail, where normally it is easily observed. (On small nails with abundant cuticles, the lunula may not be so apparent.) The lunula disappears or undergoes "reversal" in catabolic and hypoalbuminemic states. Reversal refers to a red lunula with a white distal nail. (The latter is the second type of Terry nail.)

The Terry nail has caused an unrecognized confusion because Terry published two articles on two different abnormal fingernails in the same journal and year (Terry, 1954a, 1954b). In the first, he described the white nails of hepatic cirrhosis. Although the distal few millimeters were usually pink, the lunula was usually obscured. This Terry nail was observed in 82% of patients with he-

patic cirrhosis. Additional causes were chronic congestive heart failure, diabetes mellitus (especially in the young), pulmonary tuberculosis, rheumatoid arthritis, viral hepatitis in convalescence, multiple sclerosis, and some forms of carcinoma. A few apparently healthy children and adolescents also had these nails.

In the second type of Terry nail, the lunula was suffused a deep red. Over half the patients with this finding suffered from congestive heart failure. The rest had pulmonary disease, cirrhosis, polycythemia vera, malnutrition, Hodgkin's disease, or other lymphoma. These nails were specifically sought and not found in 150 healthy young women nor in patients with nonsystemic diseases such as hernia or peptic ulcer.

Very advanced.   A bluish discoloration of the proximal portion of the nails is termed the azure lunule. It has been seen in Pseudomonas infections of the nails, Wilson's disease (Bearn & McKusick, 1958), and argyria, as well as following the local application of mercury, or therapy with quinacrine, chloroquine, or phenolphthalein (Whelton & Pope, 1968).

Longitudinal Lines

Splinter hemorrhages in the fingernail *beds* have their long axes parallel to the long axis of the finger. Their color should be described. Broad (greater than 1 mm width), red splinter hemorrhages are seen in trichinosis, Darier's disease, psoriasis, or infective endocarditis (in which they result from embolic material or large antigen-antibody complexes). Thin (less than 1 mm width), black or brown splinter "hemorrhages"—often in the nail, not the nail bed—are most commonly due to incidental trauma and are seen in manual laborers.

Splinter hemorrhages (color unmentioned) have been reported in 10% to 66% of all hospital admissions (Bishop et al., 1981; Kilpatrick et al., 1965), and in from 0% (Platts & Greaves, 1958) to as many as 56% of normals (Robertson & Braune, 1974). Thus, "splinter hemorrhages" of unspecified color are not pathognomonic for endocarditis (see Table 7-4), although many think so. (In over 25 years of carefully examining the fingernails of all comers, I have never seen anything like the figures in Table 7-4, which must be referring to the incidental thin brown and black splinters that are of little use in the diagnosis of endocarditis or anything else. In the literature, as far as I have been able to find, the critical distinction is not made between these "splinters" and the rare, highly diagnostic broad red type.)

Brown or black streaks, too wide to be splinter hemorrhages (1 mm or more), have been reported in chronic primary adrenocortical insufficiency (Bondy & Harwick, 1969), but may also be seen normally in highly pigmented persons. Black streaks could also be from a junctional nevus or malignant melanoma (Fitzpatrick et al., 1979).

Dots

The fingernail beds should be examined for round red spots the size of a pinhead. When single, such a spot should suggest the extremely rare diagnosis of a glomus tumor (Phalen & Mouroulis, 1966). (Such tumors tend to be very painful, which will help to make the diagnosis.) When multiple, they suggest the possibility of hereditary hemorrhagic telangiectasia.

Pits

Small "pits" in the nail, 1 mm or less in size, are seen in psoriasis, and the conditions listed in Table 7-5. Deep wide pits (about 5 mm in size) are diagnostic of *psoriasis.*

Table 7-4. Prevalence of "Splinter Hemorrhages" Reported in Various Conditions

Mitral stenosis	67–86%
Rheumatic fever	27–44%
Purpura	25% (1 of 4)
Nonrheumatoid arthritis	20% (1 of 5)
Renal disease	20%
Hemodialysis	20% (1 of 4)
Heart disease	15%
Pulmonary disease	12%
Cancer	17%
Hypertension	18%
Hematologic disease	20%
Scurvy (Vilter et al., 1946)	26%
Bacterial endocarditis (Bishop et al., 1981)	13%

Sources: *Platts and Greaves (1958) and Zaias (1980).*

A Pedagogic Note for Sophomores

Table 7-5 is *only for reference, not for memorization.* It certainly is an impressive list of diseases. But if the truth be known, I have only seen pitting of the nails in psoriasis and in the last entry on the list. In fact, I have never seen (recognized?) most of the diseases listed. A few I had never even heard of before.

This note is for sophomores only, because they have not yet acquired the perspective that comes with experience. More advanced students have already come to appreciate the lamentation of Hippocrates: "The art* is long, life is short."

The reader may well ask whether other authors and other compilers of lists sometimes describe that which they have not seen. Yes. That is called scholarship. Are some lists comprised of secondhand information? Yes. Does that mean that some of the entries on the list may be wrong? Yes. And are the lists incomplete? Yes, it must be so. Why, then, should one read the literature?

Hippocrates also wrote that "experience is deceiving." It can only be corrected by further experience. The person who reads critically and assiduously will vicariously increase his experience exponentially, and so increase his ability to correct his own errors.

Dysplastic Nails

Onycholysis. Onycholysis is a frayed appearance to the distal nail accompanied by an irregular separation of the distal nail from the nail bed, averaging at least a millimeter or more in length. Excluding local dermatoses and fungal infections of the finger, it is seen in hypermetabolic conditions, of which hyperthyroidism is the best known.

I have also seen onycholysis as a sequela of chronic amphetamine use, and, very rarely, as a manifestation of chronic obstructive lung disease. In the last, it could be due to a hypermetabolic state produced by the increased work cost of breathing or by the phenylethylamines that such patients received. (In former years, the most popular phenylethylamine was ephedrine, which is hydroxylated methamphetamine.)

Onycholysis is also seen in some porphyrias and photosensitivities (Zaias, 1980), in psoriasis (with and without arthropathy), in Reiter's syndrome, and after treatment with mitoxantrone, doxorubicin (Speechly-Dick & Owen, 1988), or captopril (Borders, 1986).

---

*Hippocrates used the word *techne*, which means art, profession, and craft, all at once.

Table 7-5. Causes of Shallow Pitting of the Nails Other Than Psoriasis

Reiter's syndrome
Pityriasis rubra pilaris
Acrodermatitis continua of Hallopeau
Psoriasiform acral dermatitis
Parakeratosis dermatitis
Hyponychial dermatitis
Alopecia areata
Some normal individuals

Source: *Zaias (1980).*

Onycholysis in association with a brownish discoloration of the distal third of the fingernails has been seen following erythematous photosensitivity induced by tetracycline (Segal, 1963). Onycholysis with greenish discoloration suggests *Pseudomonas*, which may coexist with a candidal infection (Zaias, 1980).

Koilonychia. Koilonychia is Greek for "hollow nails"; we now call them spoon nails. The distal and lateral edges of the nail are lifted up so as to leave a valley or hollow in the center of the nail. This characteristic contour gives a neat operational definition: a spoon nail is sufficiently concave so that a drop of water placed on the nail will not roll off.

Koilonychia is best known as a sign of hypochromic anemia, being found in 4% of adult patients with iron deficiency anemia (Kalra et al., 1986).

The figures are somewhat different for infants: In a well-baby clinic, 22 out of 400 infants were found to have koilonychia (Hogan & Jones, 1970). Of these 22, 19 had iron deficiency (true positives) and three did not (false positives). Of 15 age-matched controls from the group of 378 patients without koilonychia, three had iron deficiency (false negatives) and 12 did not (true negatives.) If we assume that the prevalence of iron deficiency among all the infants without koilonychia was the same as in the infants who were studied (i.e., 3/15 or 20%), what is the prevalence of iron deficiency in the entire population of 400? The sensitivity of koilonychia for the diagnosis of iron deficiency? The specificity? The predictive value of a positive test? The predictive value of a negative test? The diagnostic accuracy? Make a 2 × 2 contingency table, as shown in Chapter 1 (p. 6). See Appendix 7-4 for the answer.

It is most interesting that the hypochromic anemias associated with koilonychia may also be associated with esophageal webs. This is called Plummer-Vinson syndrome in the United States and the Paterson-Kelly syndrome in England (Schetman, 1972). But this precancerous esophageal condition has almost disappeared with improved nutrition (Larsson et al., 1975). In fact, in one 1975 study there were no cases of Plummer-Vinson syndrome; patients in the United States with esophageal webs had no higher incidence of iron deficiency anemia than the controls (Nosher et al., 1975).

Koilonychia may also be familial (Bumpers & Bishop, 1980). It may be a marker of various congenital disorders, such as Turner's syndrome or the leukonychia-renal calculi-multiple sebaceous cysts syndrome. It may be associated with other ectodermal findings, such as palmar keratoses, monolithrix, and steatocystoma multiplex (Leung, 1985). Finally, it may be acquired, due to carpal tunnel syndrome, fungal infection, intestinal diseases, or thyroid dysfunction (Leung, 1985).

Yellow nail syndrome. Yellow or yellow-green nails, which are also thickened, smooth, slow growing, excessively curved from side to side, and possibly onycholytic or ridged transversely, form part of a triad. The second part is lymphedema due to lymphatic insufficiency (see Ch. 25, p. 446), and the third is pleural effusion with a high pleural fluid protein concentration (i.e., above 1.5 g/dl).

Only two of the three findings need be present in any given case, so it is possible for a patient to have the yellow nail syndrome without the yellow nails (Eastwood & Williams, 1973; Hiller et al., 1972).

Other.   Dysplastic fingernails can be seen in an autosomally inherited disorder in association with rudimentary patellae, dysplastic elbows and anterior iliac horns, and a renal disease affecting some but not all of the glomeruli (Perkoff, 1967).

Clubbing

The fingernails become curved and the fingers become warm, especially at their tips. Hippocrates, *Prognosis* 17

A Method

1.   To detect clubbing, observe the angle between the nail bed and the base of the finger, the unguophalangeal angle (Lovibond's angle). This should be less than 180 degrees. (Some clinicians have the patient place the right and left fingers against each other, knuckle to knuckle and fingernail tip to fingernail tip. If there is no abnormality of the angle, a definite rhombus will be seen between the distal phalanges. But if the unguophalangeal angle is greater than 180 degrees, no such rhombus will be seen (Schamroth, 1976). (Try it on yourself.)

2.   As a double check, one should see whether the nail "floats." The technique is a simple form of ballottement: press the distal nail with a finger of one hand, while holding a finger of the other hand over the proximal nail. If the proximal nail rises easily through the spongy soft intervening tissue, the nails are said to "float."

It is essential to note the presence or absence of clubbing on the initial workup since many patients, especially black patients, have clubbing on a congenital basis. It is my distinct impression that such congenital clubbing (which obfuscates the use of this sign in signaling the presence of new disease) is not accompanied by a floating nail. However, I have not prospectively collected data on this point, nor have I seen the additional criterion of a floating nail sufficiently documented in the literature to give certainty to the similar claims of others on this point.

Clubbing may also be known by the misnomers of pulmonary osteodystrophy or osteoarthropathy—a misnomer because chronic pulmonary disease is not the only cause. Congenital heart disease is another cause that may involve chronic hemoglobin unsaturation. However, some of the diseases associated with clubbing are not accompanied by significant cyanosis (e.g., endocarditis, chronic renal disease, and severe ulcerative colitis). Finally, patients with the Marie-Bamberger syndrome have clubbing of all extremities; thick, redundant skin (so-called pachydermatosis or elephant skin); and possibly the radiologic bone signs without any of the disease entities associated with clubbing.

Can clubbing be identified reproducibly? Pyke had 12 physicians and four medical students examine 12 patients and state whether clubbing was present or not (Pyke, 1954). One finger was selected from each patient for examination, and unlabeled photographs of the same finger (front view and profile) were offered to the same panel. Only one physician was consistent in identifying the actual fingers and their photographs in exactly the same way. In only two of the 12 fingers was there any reliable consistency between examiners. Most of the finger-photograph pairings were described in a discordant manner by some examiners. That is, only

the photograph was called clubbing, or only the finger was called clubbing. But there was no clear trend toward misreading one more often than the other.

How should one interpret these results? I suggest that it is always possible to find someone who cannot do a particular task. Also, the clinically inept operate with no predefined criteria, whereas the clinically skilled arrive at the bedside with certain expectations. In Pyke's experiment, the examiners were required to produce at exit a written definition of the term "clubbing," although none knew beforehand that this would be asked of them. The 16 observers offered 14 different definitions!

Pyke's results should be contrasted with those of a later experiment, in which almost 100% agreement was achieved by nine observers of 20 patients, who were evaluated for 20 stable physical signs (Smyllie et al., 1965). In fact, their agreement on clubbing was superior to the interobserver rating of tachypnea (which, as an externally counted event, would presumably be as objective as one could get).

Plaster casts of the fingers have been used to quantitate the ratio of the distal phalangeal depth (DPD) to the interphalangeal depth (IPD). The normal DPD/IPD averages 0.895 for the index finger, independent of age, sex, and race. A ratio of 1.0 exceeds the normal average by about 2.5 standard deviations. The DPD/IPD is greater than 1.0 in 85% of children with cystic fibrosis, and less than 5% of children with chronic asthma (Hansen-Flaschen & Nordberg, 1987).

Very advanced.   Unilateral clubbing is most commonly caused by aneurysm of the aorta, or the innominate or subclavian artery. It has been seen in recurrent subluxation of the shoulder, axillary tumor, Pancoast syndrome, unilateral erythromelalgia, and lymphangitis. Unilateral accentuation of clubbing has been seen in apical tuberculosis, empyema, ulnar neuritis, and brachial plexus neuroma (Mendlowitz, 1942).

Unidigital clubbing has been seen after trauma to the finger or the median nerve, in palmar arteriovenous fistulas, in sarcoid, with felons, and with tophaceous gout (Mendlowitz, 1942). Symmetric but homolaterally unequal clubbing of the fingers is something I have observed in many black patients, as has Dr. H.J. Roberts of Florida.

Shape of the Nail: Handedness

Methods for determining handedness in patients who have suffered a stroke are discussed in Chapter 26 (p. 468).

Nail-Fold Capillaries

If one puts immersion oil on the nail-fold, the nail-fold capillary loop may be visualized with the ophthalmoscope. However, to get meaningful information from the examination, I strongly advise using a dissecting microscope.

Two different types of abnormalities (see Table 7-6) have been described (Kenik et al., 1981). The first, seen in scleroderma and dermatomyositis, consists of dilated segments, which have a "bushy" appearance. The second type has a convoluted, tortuous, "meandering" loop, which in its most extreme form reminds me of a cylindrical bunch of grapes. These abnormal nail-folds may help make a specific diagnosis instead of "undifferentiated rheumatic disease" or "Raynaud's phenomenon, unknown etiology."

Simply being able to distinguish abnormal from normal is also helpful, particularly when a history of Raynaud's phenomenon (see Ch. 18, p. 345) is remote and ambiguous. (Challenge with a bucket of ice water may also serve as a useful diagnostic maneuver.)

Table 7-6. Abnormal Nail-Fold Capillaries

	Dilated and "Bushy"	Tortuous and Meandering
PSS	82–94%	0(!)
Dermatomyositis	>87%	0(!)
SLE	3%	42–75%
MCTD	54%	12%
Raynaud's disease	9%	36%
Normal	0%	0%

Source: *Kenik et al. (1981).*

PSS, scleroderma (progressive systemic sclerosis); SLE, systemic lupus erythematosus; MCTD, mixed connective tissue disease.

Appendix 7-1. Answers to the Question in Figure 7-3

In Figure 7-3, the name of the disease is derived from the name of the material that infiltrated the capillaries of the periorbital tissue: amyloidosis and amyloid, respectively.

Appendix 7-2. Answer to the Question in Figure 7-6 and a Note on Terminology (Expressions of Ignorance)

In Figure 7-6, only the word "mixed" is falsifiable. It refers to observable physical and immunologic characteristics of the cryoglobulin. You should train yourself to be constantly self-conscious about what you are thinking. Asking whether a hypothesis is "falsifiable" (see Ch. 1, p. 4) is a helpful device.

All the other words in the diagnosis given to that patient are cloaks for ignorance. "Cryptogenic," which means that the cause is hidden (as in a secret message or cryptogram) is a good word to use when one means to imply that a bright physician can decipher the clinical signs and symptoms and eventually discover the correct diagnosis. But when one means to say lost or permanently buried (like a body that is sealed in a crypt), a better word would be "agnogenic,"which says that the cause is unknown (cf. "agnostic"). "Agnogenic" is a good, honest word if it comes at the end of a thoughtful, thorough evaluation, but not if it comes before or in place of such an evaluation.

The term "essential" has been discussed in the section on blood pressure measurement (pp. 89–89).

"Idiopathic" is related to "idiot," which comes from the Greek word *idios*, meaning self. It originated among the Greeks as a term of opprobrium for any person interested in himself to the total exclusion of his involvement in the common good. The word "idiot" thus carries no inherent connotation of imbecility or stupidity. An idioventricular rhythm is a rhythm generated by the ventricle itself (actually, a "smart" rhythm in cases of complete heart block, in which the alternative is no rhythm at all). The term "idiopathic" is really an oxymoron, since it means literally that the thing causes itself. The student should avoid this mind-warping adjective, and substitute the phrase "of unknown cause." (Remember, half of medicine is knowing what you know, and the other half is knowing what you don't know.)

These prefatory words should be sufficient to satisfy obscurantists, who can use them as pedantic preludes to any number of medical terms, thus disguising ignorance with vacuous euphony. However, there has recently been a new entry to the list, "spontaneous" bacterial peritonitis, which is apparently a bastard of spontaneous pneumothorax. With the latter, we know at least the exact instant of the onset of illness, and the hyperbole is justified to indicate that no etiology was known to its original describers, who thought the book of etiologies closed. However, considering the length to which Spallanzani went to prove to Bishop Needham that bacteria were not spontaneous (thus helping to prepare the way for the age of microbiology), it is especially ironic to apply this adjective to an infectious disease.

Appendix 7-3. Predictive Value of Skin Tags for the Presence of Colonic Polyps

Given that the prevalence of colonic polyps in an asymptomatic population over the age of 50 is 5% and that the sensitivity $[TP/(TP + FN)]$ and specificity $[TN/(TN + FP)]$ of skin tags as a test for polyps are both 0.75, a 2×2 table is constructed as follows for a population of 100:

		Polyps	
		Yes	No
Skin Tags	Yes	TP = 3.75	FP = 23.75
	No	FN = 1.25	TN = 71.25

Thus, the predictive value of a positive test = $[TP/(TP + FP)]$ = 13.6%. The predictive value of a negative test = $[TN/(FN + TN)]$ = 98.3%.

A study in a primary care setting found the predictive value of a positive test to be 10.2% (Gould et al., 1988). In this study, the prevalence of colonic polyps was 8.7%. Please note that the predicted and observed predictive values of a positive test in unselected populations are so low as to make this a useless test in practice.

Although the predictive values of a negative test initially look appealing, this is not relevant to the issue of which patients should be further investigated. Stated another way, if the prevalence of polyps is 5%, then the prevalence of "no polyps" is 95%. A diagnosis of "no polyps" on every single patient would be right 95% of the time, and the absence of skin tags increases that percentage very slightly.

These facts would not have been apparent from the initial papers unless one made prevalence-dependent calculations, which showed the limits of the sign and turned out to be extremely close to what was finally found in practice.

Appendix 7-4. Koilonychia in a Well-Baby Clinic

The prevalence of disease is 94.6/400 or 23.65/100. The sensitivity is 19/94.6 or 20%, the specificity $[TN/(TN + FP)]$ is 302.4/305.4 or 99%, and the predictive value of a positive test is 19/22 or 86%. The predictive value of a negative test is 302.4/(302.4 + 75.6) or 80%. The diagnostic accuracy = (302.4 + 19)/400 or 80.3%.

References

Agle DP, Ratnoff OD, Wasman M: Studies in autoerythrocyte sensitization purpura: The induction of purpuric lesions by hypnotic suggestion. *Psychosom Med* 29:491–503, 1967.

Barker DJ, Gould DJ: The Koebner phenomenon in eruptive xanthoma. *Arch Dermatol* 115:112, 1979.

Bart RS, Pumphrey RE: Knuckle pads, leukonychia and deafness: A dominantly inherited syndrome. *N Engl J Med* 276:202–207, 1967.

Bean WB: *Vascular Spiders and Related Lesions of the Skin.* Charles C Thomas, Springfield, IL, 1958.

Bean WB: Nail growth: Twenty-five years' observation. *Arch Intern Med* 122:359–361, 1968.

Bean WB: *Rare Diseases and Lesions: Their Contribution to Clinical Medicine.* Charles C Thomas, Springfield, IL, 1976.

Bearn AG, McKusick VA: Azure lunulae: An unusual change in the fingernails in two patients with hepatolenticular degeneration (Wilson's disease). *JAMA* 166:903–906, 1958.

Bishop H, Nelson SC, Ravreby WD: Case report: Livedo reticularis in endocarditis. *Am J Med Sci* 282:131–135, 1981.

Bondy PK, Harwick JH: Longitudinal banded pigmentation of nails following adrenalectomy for Cushing's syndrome. *N Engl J Med* 281: 1056–1057, 1969.

Borders JV: Captopril and onycholysis. *Ann Intern Med* 105:305–306, 1986.

Bumpers RD, Bishop ME: Familial koilonychia: A current case history. *Arch Dermatol* 116:845, 1980.

Carey MC, Donovan DE, Fitzgerald O, McCauley FD: Homocystinuria: I. A clinical and pathologic study of nine subjects in six families. *Am J Med* 45:7–25, 1968.

Cheraskin E: The prevalence of hypovitaminosis C. *JAMA* 254:2894, 1985.

Cherry JD: Viral exanthems. *DM* 28(May), 1982.

Chobanian SJ, Van Ness MM, Winters C, Cattau EL: Skin tags as a marker for adenomatous polyps of the colon. *Ann Intern Med* 103: 892–893, 1985.

Clain A (ed): *Hamilton Bailey's Demonstrations of Physical Signs in Clinical Surgery,* ed 15. Williams & Wilkins, Baltimore, 1973.

Cohn BA, Wheeler CE, Jr., Briggaman RA: Scleredema adultorum of Buschke and diabetes mellitus. *Arch Dermatol* 101:27–35, 1970.

Conn RD, Smith RF: Malnutrition, myoedema and Muehrcke's lines. *Arch Intern Med* 116:875–878, 1965.

Crandon JH, Lund CC, Dill DB: Experimental human scurvy. *N Engl J Med* 223:353–369, 1940.

Crowe FW: Axillary freckling as a diagnostic aid in neurofibromatosis. *Ann Intern Med* 61:1142–1143, 1964.

Dahl MV: Emphysema. *Arch Dermatol* 101:117, 1970.

Dawber RPR: Vitiligo in mature-onset diabetes mellitus. *Br J Dermatol* 80:275–278, 1968.

De Groot LJ, Larsen PR, Refetoff S, Stanbury JB: *The Thyroid and Its Diseases,* ed 5. John Wiley, New York, 1984.

Diaz-Johnson E, DeHoratius RJ, Alarcon-Segovia D, Messner RP: Systemic lupus erythematosus presenting as panniculitis (lupus profundus) *Ann Intern Med* 82:376–379, 1975.

Dines DE, Burgher LW, Okazaki H: The clinical and pathologic correlation of fat embolism syndrome. *Mayo Clin Proc* 50:407–411, 1975.

Douste-Blazy P, Marcel YL, Cohen L, Giroux J-M, Davignon J: Increased frequency of apo E-ND phenotype and hyperapobetalipoproteinemia in normolipidemic subjects with xanthelasmas of the eyelids. *Ann Intern Med* 96:164–169, 1982.

Eastwood HD, Williams MB: Pleural effusions and yellow nails of late onset. *Postgrad Med J* 49:364–365, 1973.

Ellis CN: Retinoids in dermatology. *Mayo Clin Proc* 62:1161–1164, 1987.

Fam AG, Paton TW: Nail pigmentation after parenteral gold therapy for rheumatoid arthritis: "Gold nails". *Arthritis Rheum* 27:119–120, 1984.

Fitzgerald F: The bedside Sherlock Holmes. *West J Med* 137:169–175, 1982.

Fitzpatrick TB, Eisen AZ, Wolff K, Freedberg IM, Auston KF (eds.): *Dermatology in General Medicine,* ed 2. McGraw-Hill, New York, 1979.

Flegel KJ, Dunn PM, Bentley RW, Miller MN: Skin tags and colonic polyps. *Ann Intern Med* 100:159–160, 1984.

Fleischmajer R, Schragger AM: Familial hyperlipoproteinemias. *Modern Medicine,* April 15: 97–104, 1971.

Fred HL, Castle CH, Cancilla PA: Venous stars in mediastinal disease. *Arch Intern Med* 109:290–296, 1962.

Furth PA, Kazakis AM: Nail pigmentation changes associated with azidothymidine (zidovudine). *Ann Intern Med* 107:350, 1987.

Gould BE, Ellison C, Greene HL, Bernhard JD: Lack of association between skin tags and colon polyps in a primary care setting. *Arch Intern Med* 148:1799–1800, 1988.

Greer KE, Hawkins H, Hess C: Leser-Trelat associated with acute leukemia. *Arch Dermatol* 114:1552, 1978.

Grunfeld O, Hinostroza G: Thallium poisoning. *Arch Intern Med* 114:132–138, 1964.

Grunwald MH, Ginzburg A, David M, Feuerman E: Nikolsky's or pseudo-Nikolsky's sign in bullous pemphigoid. *Int J Dermatol* 23: 629, 1984.

Hacham-Zadeh S, Even-Paz Z: A modified technique for eliciting Nikolsky's sign. *Arch Dermatol* 116:160, 1980.

Hansen-Flaschen J, Nordberg J: Clubbing and hypertrophic osteoarthropathy. *Clin Chest Med* 8:287–298, 1987.

Harrington JF: White fingernails. *Arch Intern Med* 114:301–306, 1964.

Hayden GF: Olfactory diagnosis in medicine. *Postgrad Med* 67(4):110–118, 1980.

Hersle K, Mobacken H: Autoerythrocyte sensitization syndrome (painful bruising syndrome). *Br J Dermatol* 81:574–587, 1969.

Hiller E, Rosenow EC, Olsen AM: Pulmonary manifestations of the yellow nail syndrome. *Chest* 61:452–458, 1972.

Hogan GR, Jones B: The relationship of koilonychia and iron deficiency in infants. *J Pediatr* 77:1054–1057, 1970.

Hudson JB, Dennis AJ: Transverse white lines in the fingernails after acute and chronic renal failure. *Arch Intern Med* 117:276–279, 1966.

Jacobs HD, Farndell PR, Grobbelaar PS, Smith DJ, Bromfield ME: Observer bias and error in the integumentary clinical diagnosis of chronic anaemia. *S Afr Med J.* 55:1031–1034, 1979.

Jones TW Jr, Waller RW, Samples JR: Myectomy for essential blepharospasm. *Mayo Clin Proc* 60:663–666, 1985.

Kalra L, Hamlyn AN, Jones BJM: Blue sclerae: A common sign of iron deficiency. *Lancet* 2:1267–1268, 1986.

Kaplan DL, Jegasothy B: The sign of Leser-Trelat associated with primary lymphoma of the brain. *Cutis* 34:164–165, 1984.

Kelly JW, Crutcher WA, Sagebiel RW: Clinical diagnosis of dysplastic melanocytic nevi. *J Am Acad Dermatol* 14:1044–1052, 1986.

Kenik JG, Maricq HR, Bole GG: Blind evaluation of the diagnostic specificity of nailfold capillary microscopy in the connective tissue diseases. *Arthritis Rheum* 24:885–891, 1981.

Kilpatrick ZM, Greenberg PA, Sanford JP: Splinter hemorrhages—their clinical significance. *Arch Intern Med* 115:730–735, 1965.

Larsson L-G, Sandstrom A, Westling P: Relationship of Plummer-Vinson disease to cancer of the upper alimentary tract in Sweden. *Cancer Res* 35:3308–3316, 1975.

Leavitt J, Klein I, Kendricks F, Van Thiel DH: Skin tags: A cutaneous marker for colonic polyps. *Ann Intern Med* 98:928–930, 1983.

Leung AKC: The many causes of koilonychia. *Hosp Pract* 20:29, 1985.

Levin RM, Chodosh R, Sherman JD: Factitious purpura simulating autoerythrocyte sensitization. *Ann Intern Med* 70:1201–1206, 1969.

Liddell K: Smell as a diagnostic marker. *Postgrad Med J* 52(March): 136–138, 1976.

Lindsay PG: The half-and-half nail. *Arch Intern Med* 119:583–587, 1967.

Luk GD, the Colon Neoplasia Work Group: Colonic polyps and acrochordons do not correlate in familial colonic polyposis kindreds. *Ann Intern Med* 104:209–210, 1986.

Lynch HT, Fusar RM, Pester JA, Lynch, JF: Leser-Trelat sign in mother and daughter with breast cancer. *J Med Genet* 19:218–221, 1982.

Mast WE, Burrows WM, Jr: Erythema chronicum migrans in the United States. *JAMA* 236:859–860, 1976.

Mees RA: Een verschijnsel bij polyneuritis arsenicosa. *Ned Tijdschr Geneeskd* 63:391–396, 1919.

Mendlowitz M: Clubbing and hypertrophic osteoarthropathy. *Medicine* 21:269–306, 1942.

Muehrcke RC: The finger-nails in chronic hypoalbuminaemia: A new physical sign. *Br Med J* 1:1327–1328, 1956.

Noble J, Matthew H: Acute poisoning by tricyclic antidepressants: Clinical features and management of 100 patients. *Clin Toxicol* 403–421, 1969.

Nordlund JJ, Lerner AB: Vitiligo: It is important. *Arch Dermatol* 118:5–8, 1982.

Nosher JL, Campbell WL, Seaman WB: The clinical significance of cervical, esophageal, and hypopharyngeal webs. *Radiology* 117:45–47, 1975.

O'Brien M: The use of ultraviolet fluoroscopy (Wood's light) in the diagnosis of tuberous sclerosis. *Irish Coll Physicians Surgeons* 3:19–20, 1973.

Parfrey N, Ryan JF, Shanahan L, Brady MF: Hairless lower limbs and occlusive arterial disease. *Lancet* 1:276, 1979.

Parker F: Normocholesterolemic xanthomatosis. *Arch Dermatol* 122:1253–1257, 1986.

Perkoff GT: Hereditary renal diseases. *N Engl J Med* 277:129–138, 1967.

Perloff JK: *Physical Examination of the Heart and Circulation.* WB Saunders, Philadelphia, 1982.

Phalen GS, Mouroulis DI: The diagnosis and treatment of glomus tumor. *Cleve Clin Q* 33:73–79, 1966.

Platts MM, Greaves MS: Splinter haemorrhages. *Br Med J* 2:143–144, 1958.

Polano MK, Baes H, Hulsman AM, Querido A, Pries C, Van Gent M: Xanthomata in primary hyperlipoproteinemia. *Arch Dermatol* 100:387–400, 1969.

Poliak SC, Lebwohl MG, Parria A, Prioleau PG: Reactive perforating collagenosis with diabetes mellitus. *N Engl J Med* 306:81–84, 1982.

Polifka M, Krusinski PA: The Nikolsky sign. *Cutis* 26:521–525, 1980.

Pyke DA: Finger clubbing: validity as a physical sign. *Lancet* 2:352–354, 1954.

Robertson JC, Braune ML: Splinter haemorrhages, pitting, and other findings in fingernails of healthy adults. *Br Med J* 4:279–281, 1974.

Rogers DE: Red in the face. *Reason* 18(Nov):8, 1986.

Safai B, Grant JM, Good RA: Cutaneous manifestations of internal malignancies II: the sign of Leser-Trelat. *Int J Dermatol* 17:494–495, 1978.

Sapira, JD, Cherubin CE: *Drug Abuse.* American Elsevier, New York, 1975.

Schamroth L: Personal experience. *S Afr Med J* 50:297–300, 1976.

Schetman D: The Plummer-Vinson syndrome: A cutaneous manifestation of internal disease. *Arch Dermatol* 105:720–721, 1972.

Schwartz RA: Acanthosis nigricans, florid cutaneous papillomatosis and the sign of Leser-Trelat. *Cutis* 28:319–322, 326–327, 330–331, 1981.

Schwartz RS, Lewis FB, Dameshek W: Hemorrhagic cutaneous anaphylaxis due to autosensitization to deoxyribonucleic acid. *N Engl J Med* 267:1105–1111, 1962.

Segal BM: Photosensitivity, nail discoloration and onycholysis. *Arch Intern Med* 112:165–167, 1963.

Smith CB, Jacobson JA: Toxic shock syndrome. *DM* 32 (2):1118, 1986.

Smyllie HC, Blendis LM, Armitage P: Observer disagreement in physical signs of the respiratory system. *Lancet* 2:412–413, 1965.

Speechly-Dick ME, Owen ERTC: Mitozantrone-induced onycholysis. *Lancet* 1:113, 1988.

Steere AC, Malawista SE, Hardin JA, Ruddy S, Askenase PW, Andiman WA: Erythema chronicum migrans and Lyme arthritis: The enlarging clinical spectrum. *Ann Intern Med* 86:685–698, 1977.

Stefanini M, Baumgart ET: Purpura factitia: An analysis of criteria for its differentiation from auto-erythrocyte sensitization purpura. *Arch Dermatol* 106:238–241, 1972.

Strobach RS, Anderson SK, Doll DC, Ringenberg S: The value of the physical examination in the diagnosis of anemia. *Arch Intern Med* 148:831–832, 1988.

Strole WE Jr, Clark WH Jr, Isselbacher KJ: Progressive arterial occlusive disease (Kohlmeier-Degos): A frequently fatal cutaneosystemic disorder. *N Engl J Med* 276:195–201, 1967.

Sweet RD: Vitiligo as a Koebner phenomenon. *Brit J Dermatol* 99:223–224, 1978.

Terry R: White nails in hepatic cirrhosis. *Lancet* 1:757–759, 1954a.

Terry R: Red half-moons in cardiac failure. *Lancet* 2:842–844, 1954b.

Thomas AJ, Briggs R, Monro P: Is leucocyte ascorbic acid an unreliable estimate of vitamin C? *Age Ageing* 13:243–247, 1984.

Thomas JE, Ayyar DR: Systemic fat embolism: A diagnostic profile in 24 patients. *Arch Neurol* 26:517–523, 1972.

Todd J, Fishaut M, Kapral F, Welch T: Toxic shock syndrome associated with phage group I staphylococci. *Lancet* 2:1116–1118, 1978.

Tuffanelli DL: Lupus erythematosus panniculitis (profundus): Clinical and immunologic studies. *Arch Dermatol* 103:231–241, 1971.

Vilter RW, Woolford RM, Spies TD: Severe scurvy: A clinical and hematologic study. *J Lab Clin Med* 31:609–630, 1946.

Vitamin C Subcommittee of the Accessory Food Factors Committee of the Medical Research Council: Vitamin-C requirement of human adults: Experimental study of vitamin-C deprivation in man. *Lancet* 1:853–858, 1948.

Vitamin C Subcommittee of the Accessory Food Factors Committee: *Vitamin C Requirement of Human Adults.* Medical Research Council Special Report Series No. 280. Her Majesty's Stationery Office, London, 1953.

Walling AD, Sweet D: Pyoderma gangrenosum, *Am Fam Practitioner* 35(1):159–164, 1987.

Whelton MJ, Pope FM: Azure lunules in argyria. *Arch Intern Med* 121:267–269, 1968.

Wilks S: Markings or furrows on the nails as a result of illness. *Lancet* 1:5–6, 1869.

Williams EC: *Anne of Denmark.* Longman, London, 1970.

Zaias N: *The Nail in Health and Disease.* Spectrum Publications, New York, 1980.

8
Lymph Nodes

"It showed its first signs in men and women alike by means of swellings in the groin or under the armpits, some of which grew to the size of an apple or an egg, and these were called buboes."

G. Boccaccio, *The Decameron*, Introduction

The lymph nodes were discovered not by a physician, but by a Swedish zoologist and botanist named Olof Rudbeck (1630–1702). They were confirmed by the Danish physician Bartholin, whose son discovered the glands of that name (see Ch. 22, p. 401).

The search for lymph nodes is easily one of the most important parts of the physical examination, especially in patients with a fever of unknown origin, weight loss, or known or suspected carcinomas. For example, on reviewing the oncology records in his practice, Dr. David Clarkson of Alabama found that 21% had measurable nodes.

Dimensions

Although this chapter emphasizes the locations of lymph nodes and some techniques for finding them, there are four dimensions that must be described for any lymph node that is detected: 1) size, 2) tenderness, 3) consistency, and 4) matting. This is especially important for persons using this text, who will tend to find more lymph nodes than others do.

1. As a general rule, lymph nodes bigger than the terminal phalanx of your little finger are significant. However, the benign chronic lymphadenopathy of intravenous drug users can occasionally cause larger nodes (Sapira, 1968), and a small node may be highly significant if it occurs in an unusual location (e.g., in the preauricular area). In cancer patients, the precise measurement of lymph nodes is an important index of response to treatment.

\$\$ Plastic calipers for measuring nodes (or skin-fold thickness) may be purchased from the sources referenced in Ch. 7 (p. 121).

2. Tenderness usually indicates inflammation. Tender nodes are usually of clinical importance.

3. Nodes that are stony hard are felt in metastatic neoplasia. Nodes that are not stony hard but very firm like the rubber on a pencil tip eraser are often due to Hodgkin's disease or other lymphomas.

The adjective "shotty" (not "shoddy") refers to small nodes that feel like buckshot under the skin. The size of the shot may be large, but the nodes all feel firm, disconnected (not matted), and generally of the same size.

4. Matted nodes feel as if they are connected, and when one is moved, the others seem to move with it. Such nodes are found in metastatic neoplasms and sometimes in primary lymphatic malignancy. However, matting also occurs in nonneoplastic conditions such as chronic inflammation and occasionally sarcoidosis.

Lymph Node Groups

Axillary Nodes

Normally, lymph nodes cannot be palpated in the axilla. However, with the following method it is occasionally possible to find very small nodes, whose normality is indicated by small size, lack of tenderness, and lack of matting (if multiple).

A Method

To examine the patient's left axilla, place your right hand with your fingers in the roof of the axilla and your palm turned naturally toward the patient. With your other hand, passively abduct the patient's arm, advancing your examining fingers superiorly. Then, to relax the skin folds and give you the best opportunity to palpate the roof of the axilla, bring the patient's arm back down toward his side. Continue by pressing your fingers superiorly and medially. Next, work your fingertips down the medial wall of the axilla, trying to catch any lymph nodes in the fat pad and, lastly, those beneath the fat pad and against the chest wall. Examine the other side in a mirror image fashion.

Epitrochlear Nodes

A Method

To feel the epitrochlear nodes at the patient's right epitrochlear area, grasp the patient's right hand with your right hand, and place the palm of your left hand around the distal insertion of the triceps, as if you were a politician shaking hands (Fig. 8-1). The fingers of your left hand will now curl medially, pointing anteriorly (back at you). With your little finger on the medial epicon-

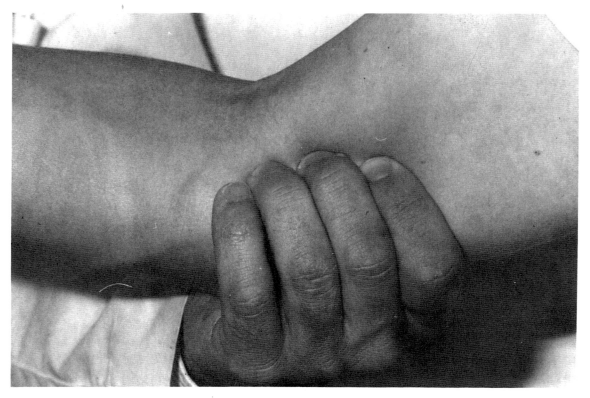

Figure 8-1. *Palpating for epitrochlear nodes. The examiner's right hand is shaking hands with the patient's right hand, while the examiner's left hand (shown) palpates correctly.*

dyle of the humerus, the remainder of your fingers should fall in or near a groove at the brachialis muscle. This is where the epitrochlear nodes will be if they are enlarged (or, *rarely*, normally palpable, as in a very thin person). Another reason for calling this a politician's handshake is that it is sometimes necessary to use your hand-grasping hand to pump the arm (extend and flex the elbow joint) 10 or 15 degrees so as to maximize the exposure of the subcutaneous anatomy to the palpating fingers. An incorrect method is shown in Figure 8-2.

Reverse the procedure for examining the epitrochlear nodes on the other side.

In the absence of dermatitis or other inflammation of the hands or forearms, the presence of epitrochlear nodes is an extremely valuable clue to systemic diseases, such as sarcoid.

Teaching Hint

The best persons in whom to search for epitrochlear nodes are intravenous drug abusers. (Drug abuse is, of course, a systemic disease.)

•

I was told that the type of handshake described above was invented by Sir William Osler when he was Regius Professor of Medicine at Oxford. Supposedly, he would shake hands in this way with young men who came to call on his daughter, in order to search for epitrochlear nodes sometimes found in the systemic lymphadenopathy of syphilis. Additionally, from this position the palpating fingers can slip a short distance to feel for the bounding Corrigan pulse of luetic aortic insufficiency at the brachial artery.

Question: *What is wrong with this story? (See Appendix 8-1 for the answer.)*

•

Cervical Nodes

A Method for Posterior Cervical Nodes

1.   Standing in front of the patient, put your fingers over the posterior cervical area and move quickly from top to bottom, searching for easily palpable nodes (Fig. 8-3). If you cannot see the nodes, this doesn't usually work.

2.   Then, start again at the skull, putting your fingers in the groove behind the sternocleidomastoid and in front of the trapezius. Work your way down the groove, palpating deeply with almost a scratching motion. Once you have felt such lymph nodes in a patient, you will unconsciously adopt this type of motion from then on.

As Stern has pointed out, posterior cervical lymphadenopathy, in the 20th century United States, is very often due to dandruff.

Anterior cervical nodes are found in front of the sternocleidomastoid. Search for them just after checking for submandibular nodes.

Other Nodes in the Head and Neck

1.   I do not routinely palpate for the preauricular, postauricular, or occipital nodes. These can usually be seen if significant. When I

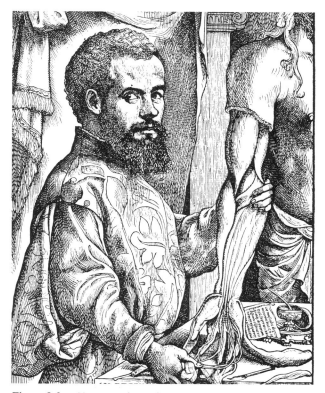

Figure 8-2. *No matter how often Dr. Vesalius dissects the arm, he will continue to miss the epitrochlear nodes unless he moves his hand higher and more posteriorly. See text and legend to Figure 8-1 for the correct method for palpating for epitrochlear nodes. Reproduced from* Medicine and the Artist (Ars Medica) *by permission of the Philadelphia Museum of Art.*

am on a zebra hunt (p. 530), I may palpate for the trapezial nodes, anterior to the trapezius near its inferolateral insertion, but I do not remember ever having found critical nodes in that location. (That is, either there were no nodes, or I had already found nodes elsewhere.)

2. The preauricular node may be enlarged in lymphoma or ipsilateral to conjunctivitis in Parinaud's oculoglandular syndrome. This condition has been variously associated with Leptothrix infection, cat-scratch fever, viral epidemic conjunctivitis (Ch. 10, p. 166), and American trypanosomiasis following its inoculation at the outer canthus by the kissing bug. (In the latter situation, the syndrome may be called Romaña syndrome. To heighten the confusion, Parinaud's syndrome (see Ch. 26, p. 455) is also the name given to paralysis of conjugate vertical gaze, especially upward gaze, which results from damage in the region of the posterior commissures, a hallmark of pinealoma.)

3. There are nodes in the hypothyroid membrane that are normally not palpable. These nodes may become enlarged and palpable in tracheal carcinoma, in carcinoma of the thyroid, in de Quervain's thyroiditis or in Hashimoto's thyroiditis. In association with carcinoma, they are called delphian nodes, in honor of the Greek oracle that would foretell disaster to those clever enough to correctly interpret its usually cryptic messages.

4. The submandibular nodes are arranged along the underside of the mandibles in a zone extending a few centimeters medially. The best way to learn to feel the submandibular nodes is to find a patient with infected teeth. The submandibular nodes under the chin have their own adjective, submental. Bimanual palpation may be useful for detecting submaxillary and submental nodes, according to Adams (1958).

○ Intraabdominal malignancies do not metastasize to submental nodes. If present and there is no dental pathology, one would do better to diagnose an independent lymphoma, even in the presence of known intraabdominal neoplasia.

Supraclavicular Nodes

A Method

1. When searching for lymph nodes in the supraclavicular fossa, have the patient sit up.

○ 2. It is a good idea to have the patient perform the Valsalva maneuver (Kuiper & Papp, 1969), which occasionally brings out an otherwise inapparent node.

3. Wiener and Nathanson (1976–77) point out that one should always palpate for supraclavicular nodes with the patient's head straight forward and the arms down so as to keep from "finding" cervical vertebrae or the omohyoid muscle, either of which might be incorrectly identified as a node.

In addition to the usual systemic diseases that cause lymphadenopathy, cancer of the breast and bronchus may metastasize to the ipsilateral supraclavicular nodes. But the left supraclavicular nodes may additionally be involved by metastases from the abdominal organs. In that case, even a single lymph node may herald an intraabdominal carcinoma, and so is called a sentinel node. (This is the same thing as Troisier's node or Virchow's node.) While gastric carcinoma is the usual cause, the primary may be as far away as the testis.

Sentinel nodes may rarely appear in the retrosternal notch.

Inguinal and Femoral Nodes

The locations of these two groups of lymph nodes (Table 8-1) are shown in Figure 8-4. When enlarged, they can be seen in a thin patient. Even in an obese patient, they are easily palpable when enlarged; no specific method is required.

This text makes the distinction between the femoral and inguinal nodes because an old chestnut taught that the former, but not the latter, would become enlarged in cases of pedal dermatophytoses and other nonspecific inflammations involving the nodes secondarily. While this hypothesis, elegant in its simplicity, has never to my knowledge been tested, it seems to work. The converse would state that inguinal nodes are highly predictive of genital or pelvic disease, or depending on the other findings of the case, a systemic disease. In fact, it is my distinct impression that inguinal nodes meeting the criteria for significance implicit in the four dimensions tend to produce biopsy material helpful in the evaluation of the patient. But femoral nodes, especially if they do not meet the criteria, tend to be interpreted histologically as "reactive hyperplasia."

While the "hedge" has been called the national flower of pathologists, the problem with "reactive hyperplasia" may result from the tendency of the surgeon to choose the node that is most easily accessible, rather than the one that is most deviant according to the four dimensions.

Very advanced. In massive inguinal lymphadenopathy, there may be a groove running between the nodes. This occurs because the fold of the groin is not obliterated between the superior and inferior inguinal nodes. According to Bailey (Clain, 1973), this groove is pathognomonic for lymphogranuloma venereum.

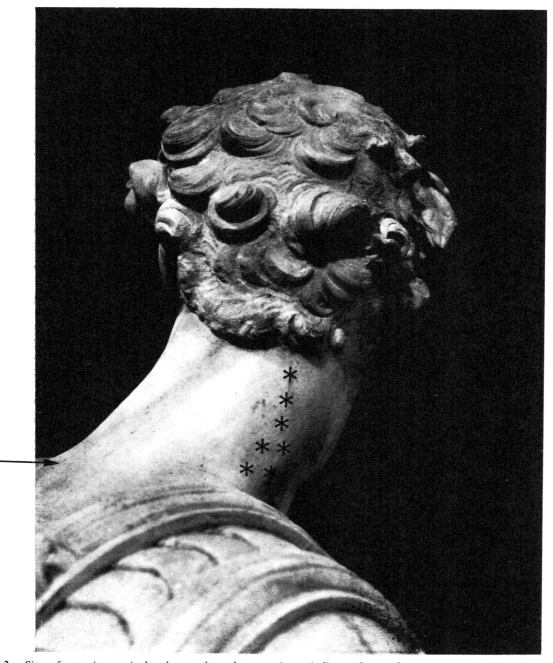

Figure 8-3.   *Sites of posterior cervical nodes are shown by stars. Arrow indicates the vertebra prominens (See Ch. 16, p. 267). Detail of Guilliano de Medici by Michelangelo.*

I have also seen this groove in a case of squamous carcinoma of the skin with metastases to the two sets of lymph nodes. This teaches us that most of the findings in medicine that are well known for being diagnostic of a disease are in fact not so diagnostic. (Conversely, most of the signs that are diagnostic are not well known.)

For the attending.   It has been suggested (Desprez-Curley, 1979) that biopsy of the inguinal and femoral nodes may now be delayed until attempts to reach a diagnosis by other means (such as lymphangiography or cytologic examination of aspirates) fail.

Further improvements in diagnostic techniques as well as the increasing influence of the legal and economic professions will probably further change the workup of a palpable lymph node. The point to be made to students is that if you cannot find the nodes, you cannot do any type of workup.

A word on nomenclature is in order. I have divided the lymph nodes into two groups according to the way in which I was taught. Please note the absence of uniformity among systems of nomenclature (see Table 8-1). Gray's system has no nodes called "femoral," and one contemporary system has none called "inguinal." Neither system recognizes nodes above the inguinal ligament, without which Bailey's groove (vide supra) could not exist.

Table 8-1. A Concordance of Nomenclature for Lymph Nodes in the Groin

Location	Gray (1954)	Wapnick et al. (1973)	This Text
Above the inguinal ligament	(None!)	(None!)	Inguinal nodes, superior
Just below the inguinal ligament and horizontal	Superficial inguinal	Horizontal femoral	Inguinal nodes, inferior
Superficial vertically grouped nodes	Superficial subinguinal nodes	Vertical femoral nodes (?)	Femoral nodes
Deep vertically grouped nodes including node of Cloquet	Deep subinguinal nodes	Vertical femoral nodes	Femoral nodes

Popliteal Nodes

I do not routinely check for popliteal nodes. The current teaching is that lesions on the heel drain to the popliteal nodes before they drain to those in the groin (vide infra). Presumably, this information would somehow let one distinguish an anterior foot problem from a

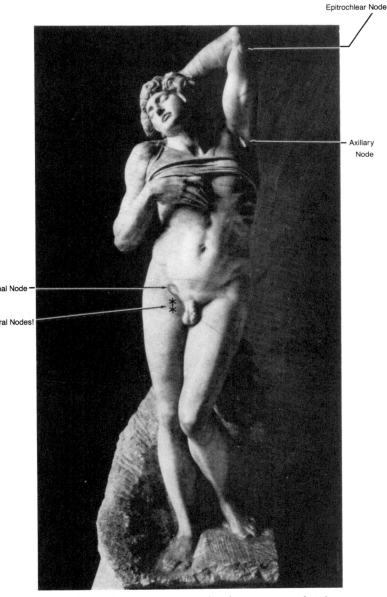

Figure 8-4. *Axillary and inguinal nodes are present, but there are no femoral nodes visible. Monument of Pope Julius II by Michelangelo: The dying slave.*

posterior foot problem (a distinction presumably feasible on other grounds), or it might help in staging lesions of the heel. However, a lymphangiographic study (Riveros & Cabanas, 1972) of normals and persons with lesions of the heel supports my disinterest. Popliteal lymph nodes may be impalpable because the examiner is inept, because they are so deep, because they are not involved, or because they do not exist in a given patient. Furthermore, the invasion of popliteal nodes may either precede or follow the involvement of other groups. The various possibilities cannot be resolved without lymphangiography.

The lesson is that the physical examination must not be stretched beyond its limits.

Paraumbilical Nodes (Sister Joseph's Node)

Patients with intraabdominal or pelvic neoplasms may have metastases to a paraumbilical node that is easily palpable through the navel. This node is named after Sister Joseph, who, according to the legend, became proficient at predicting the results of the celiotomy based upon the presence of this node. She felt it while hand-prepping the abdomen! This node is often called, incorrectly, "Sister Mary Joseph's nodule," perhaps because Sister Joseph was the superintendent at St. Mary's Hospital, a unit of the early Mayo Clinic (Schwartz, 1987) or because Catholic nuns have traditionally taken the name of Mary in addition to another name.

Hilar Adenopathy

Posterior hilar adenopathy may be detected on the physical examination of the chest (see d'Espine's sign, p. 267).

Evaluating the Clinical Significance of Lymph Nodes

In observing master clinicians, I have noticed that they do three things that the jejune do not. First, they describe the nodes according to the four dimensions. In the case of obvious deviations from normal, they immediately promote the lymphadenopathy to the top of the list of findings that must be explained. Second, they evaluate the lymph nodes within the context of the total set of clinical findings. Junior students tend to forget this principle in the rush of clinical duties. (They might want to read about diagnostic strategies (Ch. 27) before doing the assessment of a patient with lymphadenopathy.) Third, they distinguish between local and generalized lymphadenopathy (involving more than two separate anatomic regions), which have a separate differential diagnosis. Some of the causes of local adenopathy have been mentioned above or are discussed in the chapters pertaining to the specific region. Some causes of generalized lymphadenopathy are listed in Table 8-2.

Table 8-2. Some Causes of Generalized Lymphadenopathy

Infectious
  Scarlet fever
  Rheumatic fever
  Brucellosis
  Secondary syphilis
  Rubella
  Tularemia
  Bubonic plague
  Infectious mononucleosis
  Tuberculosis
  Cat-scratch fever
  Measles
  Toxoplasmosis
  Sporotrichosis
  African sleeping sickness
  Chagas' disease
  Kala-azar
  Acquired immune deficiency syndrome (AIDS) and AIDS-
    related complex (ARC)
Metabolic
  Gaucher's disease
  Niemann-Pick disease
  Hyperthyroidism
Neoplastic
  Lymphatic leukemia
  Hodgkin's disease
  Other lymphoreticular malignancies
Collagen-vascular disease
  Still's disease
  Rheumatoid arthritis
  Systemic lupus erythematosus
  Dermatomyositis
Miscellaneous
  Phenytoin ingestion
  Amyloidosis
  Serum sickness
  Sarcoidosis
  Scabies infestation
  Intravenous drug abuse

Appendix 8-1. What Is Wrong with the Story About Osler?

First, epitrochlear nodes are not completely sensitive nor pathognomonic for secondary syphilis. Second, Corrigan's pulse is not completely sensitive or pathognomonic for aortic insufficiency, whether of luetic or other etiology. Third, this method cannot detect the primary luetic chancre, which would be the most likely way to transmit syphilis in the course of an evening. Secondary lues *might* not be genitally infectious, and tertiary cardiovascular lues might well be noninfectious. Fourth, would Osler have palpated through a jacket? Finally, Osler and his wife never had a daughter.

References

Adams FD: *Physical Diagnosis*, ed 14. Williams & Wilkins, Baltimore, 1958.

Clain A (ed): *Hamilton Bailey's Demonstrations of Physical Signs in Clinical Surgery*, ed 15. Williams & Wilkins, Baltimore, 1973.

Desprez-Curley JP: Ne biopsiez plus d'emblée les ganglions inguinaux. *Nouvelle Presse Med* 8:1391, 1979.

Gray H: *Anatomy of the Human Body*, 26th ed Goss CM (ed), Lea & Febiger, Philadelphia, 1954, pp 778–780.

Kuiper DH, Papp JP: Supraclavicular adenopathy demonstrated by the Valsalva maneuver. *N Engl J Med* 280:1007–1008, 1969.

Riveros M, Cabanas R: A lymphangiographic study of the popliteal lymph nodes. *Surg Gynecol Obstet* 134:227–230, 1972.

Sapira JD: The narcotic addict as a medical patient. *Am J Med* 45: 555–588, 1968.

Schwartz IS: Sister (Mary?) Joseph's nodule. *N Engl J Med* 316:1348, 1987.

Wapnick S, MacKintosh M, Mauchaza R: Shoelessness, enlarged femoral lymph nodes, and femoral hernia: A possible association. *Am J Surg* 126:108–110, 1973.

Wiener SL, Nathanson M: *Med Times*, 1976–1977. [See reference in Chapter 29.]

9
The Head

"At the place where this battle was fought I saw a very odd thing, which the natives had told me about. The bones still lay there, those of the Persian dead separate from those of the Egyptian, just as they were originally divided, and I noticed that the skulls of the Persians are so thin that the merest touch with a pebble will pierce them, but those of the Egyptians, on the other hand, are so tough that it is hardly possible to break them with a blow from a stone. I was told very credibly, that the reason was that the Egyptians shave their heads from childhood, so that the bone of the skull is indurated by the action of the sun—this is also why they hardly ever go bald, baldness being rather less common in Egypt than anywhere else. This, then, explains the thickness of their skulls; and the thinness of the Persians' skulls rests upon a similar principle: namely that they have always worn felt skull-caps, to guard their heads from the sun."

Herodotus, *The Histories*, Book Three

Inspection

Self-Study

Before reading this chapter, inspect the first six illustrations without reading the legends. For each, commit to writing: 1) what you see and 2) a diagnosis (if you can).

Trauma

In cases of trauma or coma of unknown cause, examination of the skull is especially important. Look for bruises, swellings, and cerebrospinal fluid otorrhea or rhinorrhea (see Ch. 12, p. 218).

A bruise over the mastoid signifies a middle fossa hemorrhage (Fig. 9-1A) from a basal skull fracture. In Great Britain, this is called *Battle's sign*, although it was first noted by Sir Prescott Hewett. (In the United States, the same eponym and significance have been attached both to blood behind the eardrum and a bruise posterior to the mastoid.) Battle's sign may be on the same side as the fracture, or on the opposite side, or, in the case of some fractures close to the midline, can actually be bilateral. It does not appear until 3 to 12 days after the trauma. The sensitivity of the sign is only 2% to 8%, but the predictive value of a positive test is essentially 100% (Alter et al., 1974).

False negatives were noted by Battle, who stated that "it is necessary for the production of this sign that there should be a complete fracture, one penetrating both tables" (Battle, 1890).

He also discussed false positives due to external trauma to the mastoid. These were invariably accompanied by ecchymosis over the parietal area and the external ear. Furthermore, the false-positive ecchymosis appeared almost immediately, without the previously described delay in true Battle's sign, in which the blood migrates from a distant point. Experiments supporting this idea are also recounted in his original paper.

Battle's paper was actually a compendium of signs of basal skull fracture, including anterior basal skull fracture (presenting with conjunctival and eyelid hemorrhage, epistaxis from one nostril, unilateral proptosis (p. 158), unilateral conjunctival chemosis (p. 164), or cranial nerve dysfunction) and what Battle called "optic neuritis," but would today probably be called papilledema (see p. 179).

Raccoon eyes (Fig. 9-1B) could come from either external trauma with no skull fracture, or from a skull fracture, or from intracranial bleeding. Thus, the raccoon eyes are of less diagnostic value than Battle's sign.

Raccoon eyes should be distinguished from amyloid eyes (Ch. 7, p. 109).

Since head injury is frequently associated with cervical spine injury, the presence of any of these signs reinforces the importance of protecting the cervical spine until injury to that region can be ruled out.

A Comment on Contemporary Terminology

The head is presently described, when it is described at all, as normocephalic. (Actually, the head is "normal." It is the patient who is normocephalic!) However, if everyone is "normocephalic," it seems superfluous to say so.

"Normocephalic" was previously used as a descriptor that meant that the patient was not brachycephalic or dolichocephalic, anthropologic terms defined by specific measurements of the cranial dimensions. These were erroneously thought to have diagnostic import, but have now been abandoned.

Later, "normocephalic" was used to mean that the skull did not have burr holes or frontal bossing. (Burr holes were formerly

A

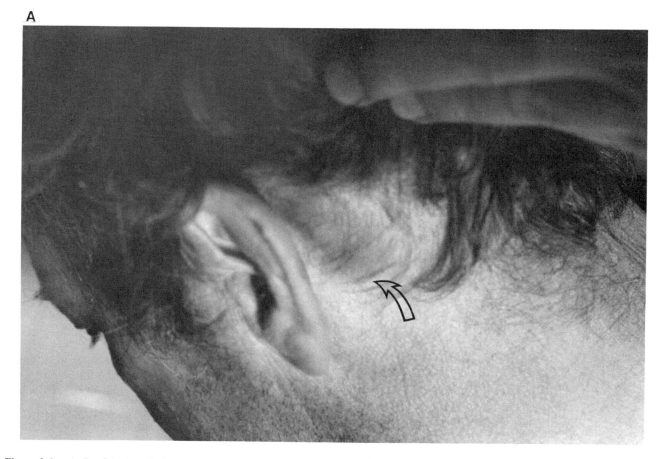

Figure 9-1. *A, Battle's sign. B, Raccoon eyes. This gentleman returned home late one night after a symposium, awakening the next morning amnestic for the events of the evening and unable to recognize his wife. The further discovery that his wallet was missing suggested that he had been set upon by villians, a suspicion that was heightened with the appearance of these skin signs. The herpetic outbreak (which is bilateral) was posttraumatic. Additionally, there was blood behind the left tympanic membrane (ipsilateral to Battle's sign), and left papilledema, presumably due to hemorrhage down the optic nerve sheath. The initial CAT scan revealed bifrontal intracerebral hemorrhages and a right temporal hemorrhage, but missed his basal skull fracture, which was later seen on a repeat skull film taken after the Battle's sign was recognized.*

B

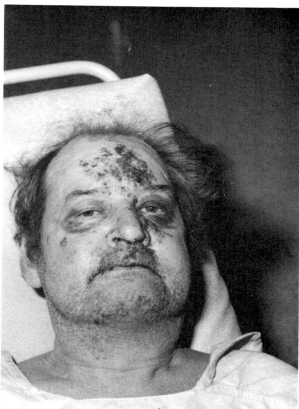

placed as a diagnostic for subdural hematomas, a procedure made obsolete by the CAT scan.)

Frontal bossing is a sign of *congenital heart disease, syphilis,* or, in the elderly, *Paget's disease.* Unfortunately, such diagnostically useful bumps have been thrown out with the bath water of phrenology.

Note that normocephaly, as a diagnostic sign, is 100% sensitive for almost all diseases. However, it is of approximately zero predictive value, either in the positive or the negative sense.

Movements of the Head

The bobbing of the head fore and aft during systole is called de Musset's sign (see Ch. 17, p. 311). It may be seen in aortic insufficiency or any other high stroke volume condition. Lateral systolic head bobbing is a sign of severe tricuspid regurgitation.

Dyskinetic movements or dystonic posturing of the head are seen in primary neurologic diseases and in both the dystonias and the tardive dyskinesia associated with dopaminergic blockers such as the phenothiazines (see Ch. 26, p. 476).

Torticollis is discussed in Chapter 24 (p. 415).

Facies

A Pedagogic Note

The appearance of the face is quite characteristic in a number of congenital disorders and systemic illnesses. Only a few examples can be presented here.

Scleroderma

Patients with scleroderma (progressive systemic sclerosis, or PSS) have a pinched nose, a mouth that will not open far (see Ch. 13, p. 222), and a shiny, tight skin. The usual wrinkles of time can become obliterated, but because of the pinched nose women so affected still do not look younger than their age.

Morphea or localized scleroderma (to be distinguished from PSS) may present with a vertical patch of scar over the skull. This "duelling scar" looks like a healed saber blow or *coup de sabre.*

Endocrine Disorders

Myxedema. The patient shown in Figure 9-2 has myxedema (primary hypothyroidism). In addition to the coarse hair and dry rough skin (see Ch. 7, pp. 127 and 119), there is a puffy appearance and a yellow hue (from increased carotene). (The nephrotic syndrome has a similar appearance, in which the puffiness is due to hypoproteinemic edema, and the yellow hue is due to urochromes.)

Sipple's syndrome. The typical facies of a patient with Sipple's syndrome, one of the multiple endocrine adenomatosis syndromes, is shown in Figure 9-3. Notice the thickened tarsal plates, the triangular shaped face, and the thick lips. (This patient's mucosal neuromas may be seen in Fig. 13-1.) Such patients also tend to have a Marfanoid habitus. They are at risk for bilateral medullary carcinoma of the thyroid and bilateral pheochromocytomas.

Cushing's syndrome. Obese persons with diabetes and hypertension are frequently suspected of having Cushing's syndrome, although the vast majority of them do not. Buccal fat pads and moon facies are considered to be reliable signs of Cushing's syndrome. To check for buccal fat pads, stand directly in front of the patient and try to see his ears. Facial fat sufficient

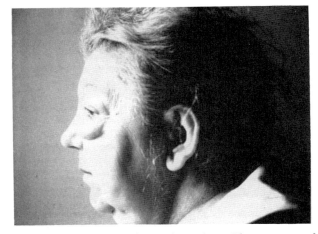

Figure 9-2. *The classic facies of myxedema. Photo courtesy of Dr. Chris Casten of Illinois and Cliggott Publishing Company.*

to obscure normal ears is a positive sign (although the patient still may not have Cushing's). Protuberant ears can be the cause of a false negative. The patient pictured in Figure 5-3 has the diagnosis of Cushing's, but does not have buccal fat pads obscuring his ears (hence he has a false negative). The specificity of this test is still high because most of the patients who do not have this sign will also not have the disease. This reemphasizes the importance of the prevalence of disease and shows why specificity is a less useful concept than predictive value.

For the attending. One is probably safe in "ruling out" Cushing's syndrome based on any physical finding that you wish to offer, because it is so rare. (When betting, always bet that the patient does not have Cushing's. It is such a rare disease that you will usually be correct.) But in all fairness to the students, you should point out that you are playing the prevalence game.

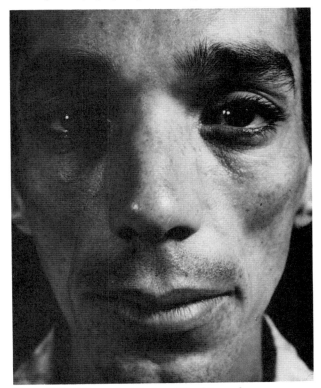

Figure 9-3. *The typical facies of Sipple's syndrome.*

Polycythemia Rubra Vera

The facies of the patient with polycythemia rubra vera have been described as "man in the moon" or "nutcracker" (Fig. 9-4). The patient tends to be thin-faced, almost dolichocephalic ("fish-headed"; narrow, deep skull), with a prominent nose looking down over the mouth toward a prominent, thin chin, which points upwards. The last two patients presented to me as "proven" polycythemia rubra vera, in whom I "predicted" these facies before seeing the patient, were actually brachycephalic ("short headed"; the skull has a broad face, relative to the A-P dimension). Their pseudonutcracker facies were caused by their being without their dental plates. Interestingly, both patients were later shown to have secondary forms of erythrocytosis.

Congenital Syphilis

The facies of congenital syphilis, including Hutchinson's teeth, is described in this case report (Hutchinson, 1859):

> Henry C., aged 14, admitted on account of the remains of chronic keratitis in both eyes. All congestion had long since disappeared and only dim white interstitial clouds of opacity remained. The bridge of his nose was broad and rather flat; teeth most characteristic, being notched and tuberculated. There were wide spaces between the incisors, and all the four canines showed a central tubercle. [The teeth are better described in Ch. 13, p. 224; the nose in Ch. 12, p. 215.]

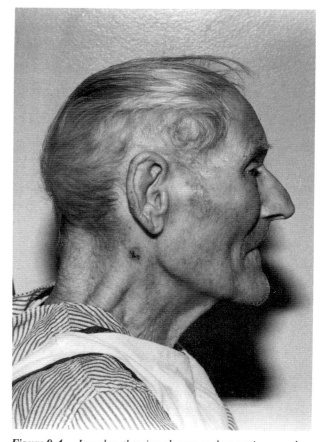

Figure 9-4.   *In polycythemia rubra vera, but not in secondary polycythemia, there is a "nutcracker" face. That is, when viewed in profile, the nose and the chin seem to be pointing at each other. Some prefer to call this a "man in the moon" face (a quarter moon). However, this particular patient is quite pale. Why? Write down your reason. (Answer is in Appendix 9-1.) Photograph courtesy of Dr. A.K. Sharma of Missouri.*

Bruegel's Syndrome

The dyskinetic facial movements of Bruegel's syndrome are illustrated in Figure 9-5.

Smoker's Face

About half the people who have smoked cigarettes for 10 years will have a characteristic facial appearance. The features appear gaunt, and the skin is wrinkled, atrophic, and gray. The complexion may be plethoric, with a slightly orange, red, or purple cast. Age, exposure to sun, and recent weight change failed to account for the differences between the smoking and the control groups (Soffer, 1986).

Hippocratic Facies

Hippocrates described the facies of a patient dying after an exhausting illness thusly: "the nose sharp, the eyes sunken, the temples fallen in, the ears cold and drawn in and their lobes distorted, the skin of the face hard, stretched, and dry, and the color of the face pale or dusky" (Lloyd, 1978).

Facial Expression

Observe the face while checking for pain during the physical examination, especially when evaluating a patient with abdominal pain. Gentle pressure over an inflamed appendix is both painful and nauseating, so that in some cases of acute appendicitis, the patient not only grimaces or winces but also curls the upper lip (see Fig. 20-8) (Odom, 1982).

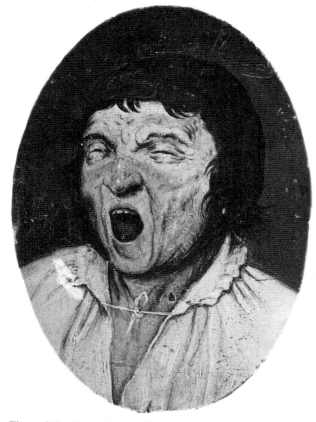

Figure 9-5.   *Brueghel's syndrome, an apparently isolated dyskinesia presenting in middle life, may actually be a focal manifestation of the syndrome of adult-onset torsion dystonia (Marsden, 1976). Photograph of "The Gaper" by Brueghel, the Elder, courtesy of the Musées Royaux des Beaux-Arts, Brussels.*

Of course, the facial expression can also give important clues to emotional states (see Ch. 26, p. 522).

An expressionless or masklike face is characteristic of Parkinson's disease.

Rash

Rashes that involve the face are generally described under the examination of the skin. There is one rash that may occur only on the face that is of particular diagnostic importance, the malar rash of systemic lupus erythematosus (SLE).

The malar rash is one of the 11 criteria of the American Rheumatism Association for the diagnosis of SLE (Tan et al., 1982).* Four of the 11 are required to make the diagnosis. However, the diagnosis may be made with a probability greater than 96% in the presence of only three criteria, if malar rash (or discoid rash, photosensitivity, renal disorder, neurologic disorder, or immunologic disorder) is one of them (Manu, 1983).

The malar rash of SLE can, on occasion, spare the bridge of the nose. The presence of a malar rash in a patient with a clinical picture compatible with either SLE or thrombotic thrombocytopenic purpura makes the diagnosis of the former disease.

The malar rash needs to be distinguished from the malar flush, which may be seen in mitral stenosis or pulmonic stenosis (Fig. 9-6A and Ch. 17, p. 321).

Tuberculosis involving the malar area is called lupus vulgaris (Fig. 9-6B).

Patients with the chronic metastatic ileal (classic) carcinoid syndrome may have a vascular, violaceous malar rash. However, patients with the gastric variant of carcinoid do not seem to get that lesion, but rather a bright-red geographic erythema, not confined to the malar area, with serpentine borders. Patients with the third (bronchial) form of the carcinoid syndrome get yet another facial lesion, including chemosis (see p. 164), facial swelling, parotid swelling, periorbital edema, and lacrimation. These are here presented as empiric findings; you may wish to read about their biochemical bases in a specialty text.

A Note on the Case Record

When one of the above diagnostic facies is recognized, it is often moved into the "general appearance" section of the case record. Similarly, if the face suggests a certain affective disorder, then the information is usually moved from the "head" section and inserted into the "mental status" section. (Other examples of "highlighting" the findings by moving them out of their customary portion of the case record are discussed in Ch. 4.) The important teaching point is that when the examiner fails to present negative findings in their proper topologic place, they are soon dropped from his routine, and are later missed even when positive.

---

*The others are: 2) discoid rash, 3) photosensitivity, 4) oral or nasal ulcerations, 5) nonerosive arthritis of at least two joints, 6) serositis (pleuritis or pericarditis), 7) renal disorder (persistent proteinuria of more than 500 mg/day or the presence of cellular casts), 8) neurologic disorder (seizures or psychosis), 9) hematologic disorder (hemolysis or WBC < 4,000/mm³ on two measurements, or lymphocytes < 1,500/mm³ on two measurements, or platelets less than 100,000/mm³, 10) immunologic disorder (LE cells, anti-native DNA antibodies, anti-Smith antibodies, or a biologic false-positive test for syphilis for more than 6 months), and 11) antinuclear antibodies.

Palpation

Palpation of the skull is most important in the examination of the infant, which is beyond the scope of this text. In the adult, the fontanelles have closed, and the major purpose of skull palpation is to find unexplained lumps in the scalp. Having never found one (not previously reported by the patient) that was not either a wen or lipoma, I have dropped this procedure from my *routine* examination. (Some may object to dropping parts of the routine, on the basis that "if two generations stop it, it becomes lost.")

Palpable crepitus is found in association with skull rarefaction diseases, such as syphilis, infantile rickets, and hydrocephalus ("French," Hart, 1985).

Formerly, we palpated all skulls for burr holes to see if the patient had ever been investigated for subdural hematomas, especially if the patient was comatose or suspected of having Munchausen's syndrome (see Ch. 2, p. 24).

The areas over the maxillary and frontal sinuses may be tender if the sinuses are infected. The mastoid may be tender to palpation in postauricular lymphadenitis, otitis media, and acute (but not chronic) mastoiditis. (The lymphadenitis may be diagnosed simply by finding the involved node, leaving only the other two to be differentiated, as follows.)

Just above the auditory meatus, the temporal bone contains a recess shaped like a quarter moon (dark side down). This is called the suprameatal triangle of McEwen. Try feeling this on your own temporal bones right above the insertion of the external ear. The recess is a little posterior to the uppermost part of the external ear insertion, at 1 o'clock on the left and 11 o'clock on the right. This area is tender in mastoiditis, but not in otitis media, assuming that you have not disturbed the external ear while performing the test.

The posterior aspect of the junction of the external ear and the mastoid forms an angle that is obliterated in some cases of mastoiditis, but never in external otitis, even if complicated.

Very advanced. Mastoiditis in the presence of a sixth cranial nerve palsy is called Gradenigo's syndrome. There may also be pain in the distribution of the ophthalmic branch of the fifth cranial nerve. Rarely, mastoiditis may be associated with an ipsilateral seventh nerve palsy with sparing of the lateral rectus. These are not seen in adequately treated cases of petrositis, mastoiditis, or meningitis, and their occurrence during treatment should be a warning that the advantages of the antibiotic era are being lost, usually through injudicious trust in a son of ceph du jour.

Percussion

1. In children, tapping a hydrocephalic skull produces a sound like that from a "cracked pot."

2. Some old-time clinicians believed that the skull overlying a mass lesion was decidedly more tender to percussion than the normal side. Thus, they would percuss the skull to see if one (and only one) side was tender enough to make the patient wince. The clinician who did this was trying to lateralize the lesion, but not based upon the percussion note. On the other hand, auscultatory percussion may be able to lateralize such lesions regardless of whether or not the patient winces to percussion.

3. Percussion of the head can also be used to detect disease of the vertebral column:

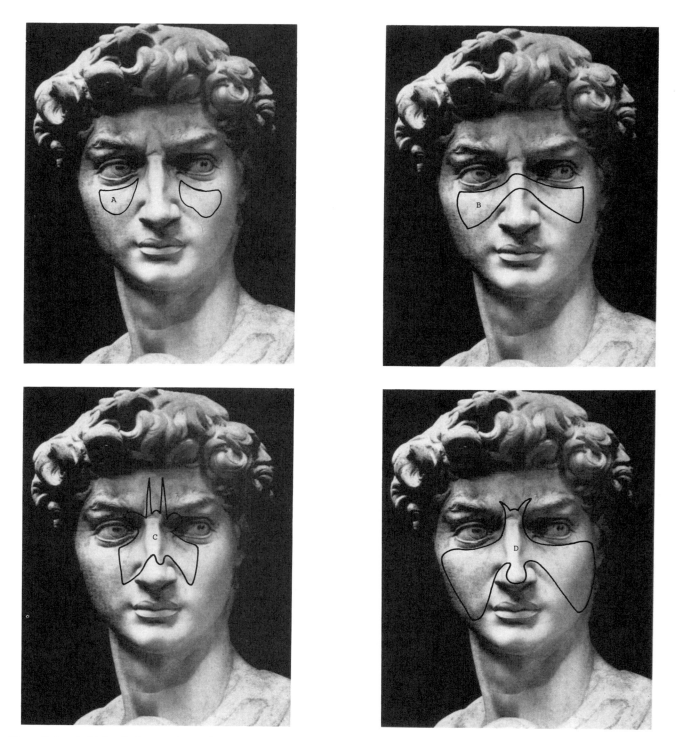

Figure 9-6.   *A, Malar flush. Note the erythema (not a scaling rash) that does not cross the bridge of the nose. B, The malar or "wolf" rash. (This is a scaling rash, not just an erythema. "Wolf" is English for "lupus." In some parts of the world, the most common cause of the lupus rash is lupus vulgaris, which is due to tuberculosis. But in the United States, systemic lupus erythematosus is more "vulgaris" (common) than facial tuberculosis. Note that the rash crosses the bridge of the nose (in this case) but does not extend above the eyebrows. (Dr. René Wegria of Missouri had considerable experience with lupus vulgaris. It was the custom to make the diagnosis by placing a glass slide against the lesion and exerting downward pressure on the lesion. When viewed through a slide thus held, lupus vulgaris had the appearance of cooked kernels of corn.) C, A true butterfly rash of systemic lupus erythematosus, sketched from a patient of Dr. Joe Hardin of Alabama. The rash extends above the eyebrows. Although quite rare, this true butterfly rash is probably pathognomonic for systemic lupus erythematosus. D, Another butterfly rash from a patient with acute systemic lupus erythematosus. Photo: David, by Michelangelo, with superimposed lesions.*

A Method

Have the patient sit or stand erect. Place one of your hands on top of his head and strike it with your other hand. (Interposing one hand minimizes the patient's direct discomfort from the blow.) If the patient is properly positioned, the impulse wave from the blow will travel down his vertebral column. If the patient has vertebral column disease, this maneuver may cause remote pain at the site of the affected vertebra. (False negatives occurred in patients with small vertebral metastases, in whom the cortex of the bone was radiographically intact.)

Auscultation

A Method

In a quiet room, listen over the frontal regions of the skull, the temples, the mastoid processes, and the atlantooccipital regions (Fisher, 1957). Also listen over the eyeballs (see Ch. 10, p. 202).

Significance of Bruits

Skull bruits in apparently normal children were first described in 1834. They were found by Still in 4% of children from age 4 to 16 years, by Bell in 6% of "young children," by Osler in 13% of children under 3 years after the fontanelles had closed, and by Henoch in 73% of rachitic children with delayed closure of the fontanelles. They have also been described over the unclosed fontanelles of 5% to 19% of children between 1 and 1.5 years old, but none over 2.5 years (Dalsgaard-Nielsen, 1939); in 42% of those under 4 years; and in 84% of children with "delayed dentition." The authors who reviewed these studies confirmed that spontaneous bruits were frequent in children, but decreased after age 10.

In adults, spontaneous bruits were found in 0% (Mackby 1942); 1% (Wadia & Monckton, 1957); and 6% (of 16), only some of whom had angiograms (Allen & Mustian, 1962). Such spontaneous bruits should suggest an intracranial angioma, the prevalence of the sign being reported, in various series of angiomas, as 5.5%, 19%, 38%, 50%, 82%, and, by Cushing, 89% (Wadia & Monckton, 1957). True positives have also been observed in medulloblastoma (1), craniopharyngioma (1), astrocytoma (1), glioma (1), subdural hematoma (1), and hemangioblastic (arteriovenous) malformation (Mackby, 1942).

Some have demonstrated evoked bruits in children by alternately compressing each carotid artery in turn, a technique not used by others (Wadia & Monckton, 1957). Such evoked bruits are also quite common in adults.

The causes of systolic murmurs over the skull are summarized in Table 9-1. Causes related to carotid vascular disease are discussed in Chapter 18. But the sensitivity of a skull bruit for carotid occlusion was 0% in one series (Silverstein et al., 1960).

Continuous murmurs, with systolic accentuation, are heard in carotid artery-cavernous sinus fistula and in 50% to 82% of intracranial angiomas (Allen, 1965). In both cases, the diastolic component can be made to disappear and the systolic component to decrease remarkably by bilateral jugular venous compression. With the former, compression of the ipsilateral carotid artery will decrease the murmur but will not abolish it completely. In older persons, the increased blood flow through the hypervascular frontal bone of Paget's disease may produce a continuous murmur over the affected area.

The sensitivity of a loud harsh machinery murmur was found to be 18% to 29% for arteriovenous malformation, 8% for angioma, 17% for tumors involving the fourth ventricle and producing hydrocephalus, and 0% for glioma, meningioma, Lindau-Hippel disease, pituitary tumor, or acoustic neurinoma. The total prevalence

Table 9-1. Differential Diagnosis of a High-Pitched Systolic Bruit Over the Skull

Common
Occlusion of the contralateral internal carotid artery
Arteriovenous fistula
Cerebral angioma
Glomus jugulare tumor
Radiating aortic murmur
Scalp angioma
Rare
Saccular aneurysms
Vascular meningioma
Arteriosclerotic plaques
Brain tumor compressing an artery
Paget's disease
A vascular thyroid gland
Coarctation of the aorta
Increased intracranial pressure in children
Subdural hematoma (one case) (Allen, 1965)
Intracerebral hematoma (one case) (Allen, 1965)
Migraine during the attack (one case) (Allen, 1965)
Normal persons

Source: *Fisher (1957).*

in a large neurologic experience was only 0.5% (Dalsgaard-Nielsen, 1939).

Significance of Breath Sounds and Voice Sounds

Breath sounds may be louder over an area of Paget's disease than over normal skull. Voice sounds ausculted over the skull are louder and of greater clarity when the stethoscope is over an osteolytic metastasis than when it is over the normal skull (Green & Joynt, 1961).

Special Maneuvers

Thermal Palpation

It is sometimes possible to detect a palpable generalized warmth emanating from the scalps of patients with hypermetabolic states, such as hyperthyroidism.

A Method (modified from that taught to me by Dr. Ted Danowski of Pennsylvania)

Place one hand lightly on top of the patient's hair, not touching the skin, and your other hand (the "control" hand) on top of your own hair, each hand equidistant from the scalp. (This method is based on the same principle used by grandmothers for detecting fever.)

In Paget's disease, there may be a local warmth. To detect this, the fingers must actually touch the skin.

Transillumination

A Method

To transilluminate the *frontal* sinuses, sequentially place a *very bright* penlight in the patient's supraorbital notches and compare the sides. (The light from the otoscope or the penlights supplied by drug detail men is not bright enough).

To transilluminate the *maxillary* sinuses, have the patient hold a very bright penlight midline in his mouth while the examiner observes the relative intensity of the glows at the lower eyelids.

If the light is not strong enough, the bulb may be sequentially placed at the gum line medially to the last upper molar on each side, directed toward the sinus. Alternatively, the penlight may be placed externally at the inferior portion of each orbit, and the glow observed through the palate.

It should be obvious that the test must be performed in a completely darkened room, but I have seen its supposed uselessness demonstrated by performing it in daylight!

Interpretation

A unilaterally opaque maxillary sinus is always abnormal (Evans et al., 1975).

Another Method

Transillumination is another example of the need for a special textbook of physical diagnosis for black persons. It can be very difficult to see the skin transillumination in a highly pigmented patient. If both sides fail to transilluminate well, is this due to bilateral disease, or bilateral normality beneath a dark skin?

1. Have the patient close his eyes.

2. Transilluminate from the mouth (as above).

3. Ask the patient to give a hand signal if he has a perception of light, and if so, in which eye (or eyes).

4. Have the patient open his eyes and fix at a far point. If both eyes show a pupillary red reflex (with the light shining in the mouth), the sinuses transilluminate bilaterally. *Caveat:* again a *very strong* lamp is needed to make this test work.

The method given above for shining the light from the inferior orbital position and observing at the palate also works well for black patients.

Diagnostic Accuracy

While still getting good correlation between transillumination of the frontal sinuses and subsequent roentgen examination, others have noted less success with transillumination of the maxillary sinuses (Spector et al., 1981).

From the earlier literature, the diagnostic accuracy of transillumination of the maxillary sinuses was 68% in one large series (McNeill, 1963). But false positives and false negatives have both emerged, the exact numbers varying with whether radiologic examination or puncture fluid analysis was used as the gold standard. The latter is an important issue, as radiologic examination has a diagnostic accuracy (when compared with fluid analysis) of only 76%, 86%, and 89% in three series (Ballantyne & Rowe, 1949; Burtoff, 1947; McNeill, 1963). Further, there is an inter-rater variability between examiners of the roentgenograms, so these figures are subject to further variability in attempted replication.

At the present time, transillumination is a convenient, accessible, noninvasive diagnostic method, although it is not intended as a substitute for sinus films. If positive, it should be followed by roentgen examination. Either imaging procedure should be repeated if the clinical picture becomes disparate with an initially negative result.

Auscultatory Percussion

Guarino has adapted the technique of auscultatory percussion (see Ch. 16, p. 271; Ch. 20, p. 381; and Ch. 24, p. 430) to examination of the head and brain (Guarino, 1982a,b).

A Method

1. Imagine a horizontal plane across the upper border of the helices of the ears, extending bilaterally from the forehead to the occiput (Fig. 9-7). The anterior starting place is the palpable vertical ridge on the side of the forehead.

2. Apply the diaphragm of the stethoscope (Guarino, personal communication, 1984) to the patient's head, methodically alternating, from one side to the other, at corresponding anatomical points along the plane. If the hair is exceptionally thick or is matted by hair spray, place the rubber edged bell beneath the hair (Guarino, 1982b).

3. Apply direct percussion lightly and with equal intensity, using the pulp of a finger (not the fingertip), at a point marked in the midline of the upper forehead, well above the frontal sinuses. (The frontal sinuses extend about 3 cm above the supraorbital ridge and have a breadth of about 2.5 cm. They normally produce dullness and can confound the examination).

4. Listen for differences in sound between the two sides of the head as you continue tapping.

5. With the same technique, progress toward the vertex in additional planes, less than the diameter of the stethoscope diaphragm apart.

Interpretation

An intracranial mass lying in the path of the generated sound will produce a distinct dullness over time compared with the other side. Some listeners do not hear a dullness so much as they hear a difference in sound intensity (Guarino, 1982b). A decrease in dullness over time suggests resolution and a favorable prognosis. The technique is particularly useful in following patients with a subdural hematoma (Guarino, personal communication, 1988).

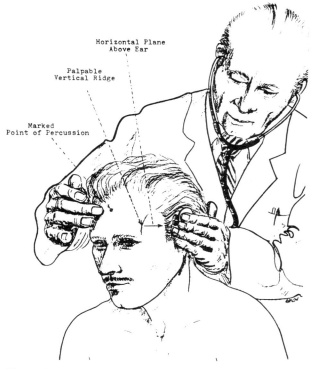

Figure 9-7. *Auscultatory percussion of the head. (The diaphragm piece with a double-lumen stethoscope is preferable to the single-lumen stethoscope shown here.) Figure courtesy of Dr. John Guarino of Idaho.*

Results

False negatives occurred in 14% of 51 patients with abnormal computerized axial tomography (CAT) scans. These seven instances were due to four cases of diffuse cerebral atrophy, one case of a small left parietal infarct, one case of a 1 cm pontine tumor, and one case of a 2-cm thalamic mass near the midline. (Auscultatory percussion became positive when that lesion reached 4 cm [Guarino, 1982a].)

However, fewer false negatives occurred with this method than with the CAT scan. There were 11 patients with hemiparesis from a stroke, who still had a normal CAT scan at the time that auscultatory percussion was positive for a lesion on the side opposite the hemiparesis.

False Positives

Of the 27 patients with normal CAT scans and no hemiparesis or other evidence of stroke, two had abnormal findings on auscultatory percussion, giving a 7% false positive rate. (These 27 patients were referred to as "healthy," but it is not clear why they underwent a CAT scan.)

Comments

1. Other workers have been able to confirm the utility of auscultatory percussion (Campbell & Wren, 1982; Weinhold, 1983).
2. Of the patients suspected of having subdural hematoma, there were no false negatives by auscultatory percussion.
3. The best place to search is in the fronto-parietaltemporal areas within 6 cm above the helices of the ears.
4. Continued refinement of this technique has involved the visual recording of the sound waves. Unilateral dullness can now be seen as well as heard in meningitis, encephalitis, multiple sclerosis, coma of metabolic origin(!), and contusions with localized edema. That this is not due to inherent asymmetry of the cranium is shown by the fact that the percussion note changes may be altered with time, as in brain tumors undergoing treatment with radiation or steroids (Guarino, personal communication, 1984).
5. As with auscultatory percussion of other parts of the body, musicians who play percussion instruments such as the drums, guitar, piano, and so forth, may tend to miss differences by changing the intensity of percussion. They must learn to swing the percussing finger a given distance each time, and not adjust the blow to the sound as they would if they were playing a musical instrument.

Very advanced. A patient discovered that scratching an area of skull over an osteolytic metastasis produced a "hollow feeling" (Wei, 1984).

Appendix 9-1. Answer to Question in Figure 9-4.

The patient is anemic due to the marrow failure of agnogenic myeloid metaplasia, his polycythemia rubra vera having burned out.

References

Allen N: The significance of vascular murmurs in the head and neck. *Geriatrics* 20:515–538, 1965.

Allen N, Mustian V: Origin and significance of vascular murmurs of the head and neck. *Medicine* 41:227–247, 1962.

Alter M, Steigler P, Harshe: Mastoid ecchymosis: Battle's sign of basal skull fracture. *Minn Med* 57:263–265, 1974.

Ballantyne JC, Rowe AR: Some points in the pathology, diagnosis and treatment of chronic maxillary sinusitis. *J Laryngol Otol* 63:337–341, 1949.

Battle WH: Three lectures on some points relating to injuries of the head. *Br Med J* 2:75–81, 1890.

Burtoff S: Evaluation of diagnostic methods used in cases of maxillary sinusitis, with a comparative study of recent therapeutic agents employed locally. *Arch Otolaryngol* 45:516–542, 1947.

Campbell, WD, Wren DR: Auscultatory percussion of the head. *Br Med J* 284:1556, 1982.

Dalsgaard-Nielsen T: Studies on intracranial vascular sounds. *Acta Psychiatri Neurolog* 14:69–87, 1939.

Evans FO, Sydnor JB, Moore WEC, Moore GR, Manwaring JL, Brill AH, Jackson RT, Hanna S, Skaar JS, Holderman LV, Fitz-Hugh GS, Sande MA, Gwaltney JM Jr.: Sinusitis of the maxillary antrum. *N Engl J Med* 293:735–739, 1975.

Fisher CM: Cranial bruit associated with occlusion of the internal carotid artery. *Neurology* 7:298–306, 1957.

Green D, Joynt RJ: Auscultation of the skull in the detection of osteolytic lesions. *N Engl J Med* 264:1203–1204, 1961.

Guarino JR: Auscultatory percussion of the head. *Br Med J* 284:1075–1077, 1982a.

Guarino JR: Auscultatory percussion of the head. *Br Med J* 285:295, 1982b.

Hart FD (ed): *French's Index of Differential Diagnosis,* ed 12. John Wright & Sons, Bristol, 1985.

Hutchinson J: On the different forms of inflammation of the eye consequent on inherited syphilis. *Ophthalmol Hosp Rep* 2:54–105, 1859.

Levine SR, Langer SL, Albers JW, Welch KMA: Sneddon's syndrome: An antiphospholipid antibody syndrome? *Neurology* 38:798–800, 1988.

Lloyd GER (ed): *Hippocratic Writings.* Penguin Books, Middlesex, England, 1978.

Mackby MJ: Cephalic bruit: A review of the literature and a report of six cases. *Am J Surg* 55:527–533, 1942.

Manu P: Serial probability analysis of the 1982 revised criteria for classification of systemic lupus erythematosus. *N Engl J Med* 309:1460, 1983.

Marsden CD: Blepharospasm-oromandibular dystonia syndrome (Brueghel's syndrome): A variant of adult-onset torsion dystonia. *J Neurol Neurosurg Psychiatry* 39:1204–1209, 1976.

McNeill RA: Comparison of the findings on transillumination, x-ray and lavage of the maxillary sinus. *J Laryngol Otol* 77:1009–1013, 1963.

Odom NJ: Facial expression in acute appendicitis. *Ann R Coll Surg Engl* 64:260–261, 1982.

Silverstein A, Lehrer GM, Mones R: Relation of certain diagnostic features of carotid occlusion to collateral circulation. *Neurology* 10:409–417, 1960.

Soffer A: Smoker's faces: Who are the smokers? *Arch Intern Med* 146:1496, 1986.

Spector SL, Lotan A, English G, Philpot I. Comparison between transillumination and the roentgenogram in diagnosing paranasal sinus disease. *J Allergy Clin Immunol* 67:22–26, 1981. [This paper contains a good review of all the other authors who have been dissatisfied with this technique.]

Tan EM, Cohen AS, Fries JF, Masi AT, McShane DJ, Rothfield NF, Schaller JG, Talal N, Winchester RJ: The 1982 revised criteria for the classification of systemic lupus erythematosus. *Arthritis Rheum* 25:1271–1277, 1982.

Wadia NH, Monckton G: Intracranial bruits in health and disease. *Brain* 80:492–509, 1957.

Wei N: The "hollow scratch," sign. *Arthritis Rheum* 27:116, 1984.

Weinhold S: Auscultatory percussion of the head after trauma. *Med Tribune* 29:2, 1983.

10
The Eye

"The eye is the window on the soul."

Talmud

Order of the Examination

Although the examination of the eyes is recorded after the examination of the head, one might want to proceed directly to examination of the pupils, after checking the vital signs, particularly in a patient who has an altered mental status or is severely ill.

For medicolegal reasons, visual acuity should be checked before proceeding with the rest of the eye examination, especially if any instruments are to be used or any medication is to be instilled into the eye, so that impaired acuity cannot be attributed to your manipulation. In addition, medications used to dilate the pupils tend to impair accommodation of the lens, blurring the vision.

Once you have examined the pupils (see p. 169), measured the acuity, and ascertained that the patient does not have a contraindication to dilating the pupils (see pp. 167 and 175 [pupils and anterior chamber]), instill one drop of a mydriatic into each conjunctival sac, as described on page 175. Proceed with the rest of the physical examination. By the time you finish, the pupils should be dilated, ready for the funduscopic examination.

Visual Acuity

Snellen Chart

Visual acuity is generally tested by having the patient read a Snellen chart from a distance of 20 feet, alternately covering one eye, then the other. If the patient has read a line correctly with one eye, he may be asked to read it backward when testing the other eye. Where there is no such wall chart, you may substitute a pocket-size card (obtainable at a medical supply store) for the Snellen chart. Such cards are designed to be held 14 inches from the patient's eyes. If the patient misses one or two letters on a line, record the results as "20/20 − 1," "20/30 − 2," and so on.

You should test the patient while he is wearing his own corrective lenses. If these are unavailable, or if the vision is still poor, see whether the patient does better looking through a pinhole, which corrects refractive errors by focusing the light on the retina regardless of the focal length of the eyeball. (Just poke a hole in an index card, and have the patient hold it very close to his eye. Note that the illumination has to be strong.) If the patient cannot read the largest letter on the eye chart, determine whether he can count fingers, detect hand motion, or perceive light.

For the resident. Look through the patient's glasses at your finger, a pencil, or any object of fairly constant size that can project beyond the glasses. If the object appears smaller through the glasses, then they belong to a myope (a person whose eyeball is "too long" for its lens to focus perfectly on the retina). If it appears larger, the glasses belong to a hypermetrope, whose eyeball is "too short." If the glasses are bifocals, always look through the top lenses; the bottom lenses are simply magnifying glasses, for presbyopes (persons whose lens has lost its ability to accommodate well due to age).

Ocular Malingering and Ocular Hysteria

Is this the world's first description of blindness as a conversion symptom?

> During the action a very strange thing happened: Epizelus, the son of Cuphagoras, an Athenian soldier, was fighting bravely when he suddenly lost the sight of both eyes, though nothing had touched him anywhere—neither sword, spear, nor missile. From that moment he continued blind as long as he lived. I am told that in speaking about what happened to him he used to say that he fancied he was opposed by a man of great stature in heavy armour, whose beard overshadowed his shield; but the phantom passed him by, and killed the man at his side. (Herodotus, *The Histories*)

In persons claiming to have markedly decreased vision, check several times, and look for variable results from reading the Snellen chart. If the patient claims total blindness, check for pupillary responses (see p. 171) and optokinetic nystagmus (p. 162). Some malingerers will be unwilling or apparently unable to perform the test of touching their fingertips together, although a truly blind person can perform this maneuver with ease, using proprioception.

Many other tests have been used (Kramer et al., 1979). The first two described below can be used in patients claiming blindness in both eyes, or with the good eye patched in patients claiming poor vision in only one eye. The remaining tests are specifically for patients claiming poor vision in one eye.

The Mirror Test

1. A mirror, of dimensions greater than 1×2 feet, is held close to the patient's face, so that the examiner can look over the top of the mirror at the patient's eyes.
2. The mirror is either rocked from side to side or up and down.
3. If the patient has the ability to fixate (and thus can see formed objects), the eyes will move in a direction corresponding to the motion of the mirror.

The Briefcase Test

1. Walk 40 feet down the hall and tell the patient to look at your nose. (Do not ask him if he can see it.)
2. Lift up a briefcase, a large book, a typewriter, or a large piece of colored cardboard. Ask the patient if he can see anything.

If the patient says no, his vision is so restricted that he should be unable to walk without bumping into things.

The Tropicamide Test

1. While instilling the drops for the intraocular pressure check (vide infra), also place some tropicamide in the putative good eye. (Of course this must be done after the patient has read with both eyes open, near and far.)
2. After at least 30 minutes, the patient is again asked to read at a distance and close up. If he is able to perform the near-vision test the second time (a "positive test"), he must be using the eye alleged to be poor. Of course, the test is only useful when positive, because a malingerer might detect the change in accommodative ability.

A caveat. Tropicamide is a relatively weak cycloplegic, even though it is a relatively good mydriatic. It is conceivable that the drop might not be effective and, therefore, the test might be "positive" simply because the drug is not working as an effective cycloplegic.

Psychologic Techniques

Of course, one way to support the diagnosis of conversion reaction or malingering is to have the impairment disappear, simply with the physician's encouragement. Methods developed in a military practice could be adapted. One method is to tell the patient that he will see much better if he scans the letters on the Snellen chart from the upper left to the lower right-hand corner, instead of staring directly at them. The patient is encouraged to describe anything he can about the letter in question, even whether it is square or round. Some patients will have to be asked to guess the shape. The subject is then led to see the component parts (square or round) of each letter (even by guessing) until he is able to "see" the entire letter. He is constantly reminded to keep scanning the letter and not to stare at it.

Another such technique (Kramer et al., 1979) is "retinal rest," in which the patient is placed at bed rest in a private room, patched bilaterally, without sedatives, television, radio, company, or interaction with the ward personnel. Daily checks of the patient's vision are said to produce dramatic results within 3 days.

Visual Fields

Just imagine; there are those nerves in the head, I mean in the brain . . . and those nerves have some kind of little tails which vibrate . . . And whenever I look at something with my eyes, those little tails vibrate and the image appears; it doesn't appear at once, though. It takes a while, a second maybe, and then there comes a moment, no I don't mean a moment. . . . I mean an image, that is, the object or the event or whatever it is. That's how I perceive things and how I think. . . . So I think because of those little tails and not at all because I have a soul or because I've been made in God's image, which is all nonsense. . . . I understand all that very well. But I am unhappy about God—I miss Him! (Dostoevsky, *The Brothers Karamazov,* Part 4, Book 11, Ch. 4)

Checking visual fields by confrontation is a very crude screening test that is in no way as sensitive as the formal testing of visual fields by tangent screen or Goldmann perimetry, but it is inexpensive, quick, and convenient. The method assumes that the examiner's own visual fields are normal.

A Method

1. Instruct the patient to look at your nose.

2. Stretch your arms out, placing your hands in a plane equidistant from the patient and yourself.

3. With your fingers held in the V-for-Victory sign, move your hands to the periphery of your own vision as you watch the patient's eyes.

4. Wiggle one set of fingers and ask the patient whether he sees anything move. If he says yes, ask which side.

5. Change the position of your hands, keeping them always at the periphery of your own visual fields and in the plane equidistant between yourself and the patient, checking superiorly and inferiorly. On successive trials, it is a good idea to vary the pattern, wiggling the right only, the left only, or both.

Interpretation

This crude test might detect the bitemporal defects of sellar and chiasmal disease, the homonymous hemianopsia of optic tract disease, the monocular anopsia of retinal or optic nerve disease, and the field cuts of late glaucoma. (Of course, glaucoma should be diagnosed by other means before the onset of blindness, see pp. 167 and 181).

False negatives will occur, for example, in patients with small defects due to retinal degeneration. The method will also miss nasal scotomata, such as that caused by early glaucoma. The latter could be detected by checking each eye individually, temporally and nasally, but remember to take into account the fact that your nose does not have the same shape as the patient's. Both defects can be detected by Goldmann perimetry or tangent screen testing. When in doubt, always proceed to such formal testing. The time to do it is the time that you first think of it.

Wiener and Nathanson (1976–77) noted that visual field testing was limited by failure to include tests for "impairment of color, identification of common objects and form," leading to failure to pick up significant visual field defects. Identification of common objects is more a test of cortical function than of the visual fields. On the other hand, the failure to use colored objects may be an important criticism because changes in color field ("color desaturation") precede gross field changes. However, at the present time color field testing is thought to be an issue only for the formal perimetrist. Even DeJong (1979) suggests that the field for all colors might well be the same if one could control for color intensity. In other words, a field defect can be picked up with a red marker before it is evident with a white marker, not because of the color but because the red object is less intense than the white object. If true, female medical students with red nail polish should be superior examiners.

We must emphasize that the physical examination is composed of individual screening maneuvers. The fact of the matter is that formal perimetry is superior to visual fields by confrontation for the purpose of detecting all field cuts. The advantage of visual fields by confrontation, with its lesser sensitivity, is that it is quick, cheap, and convenient in the sense that is immediately accessible to the information processor—the physician. Were the components of the physical examination to be divided among different physicians without each having immediate access to the findings of the other, there would be no point in performing physical examinations, since some technologic substitute could be found for each specific maneuver. This is an important principle, a corollary of which is that in such a world certain diagnoses could never be made.

An Alternate Method
(De Juan, personal communication, 1987)

Rather than wiggling the fingers, hold up a different number of fingers in each hand. Ask the patient to total the number of fingers being held up.

For example, if you hold up one finger on the left eye hand (your right) in the superotemporal quadrant, and two fingers in the right eye hand in the inferotemporal, each of the possible answers "zero," "one," "two," or "three" has immediate diagnostic significance.

Additionally, this method prevents the patient from orienting to one finger or the other, and it is a more sensitive test for retinal function. For example, a patient with a retinal detachment may be able to see hand motions, but will not be able to count fingers in the quadrants corresponding to the detached retina. Finally, this is an objective measure, not relying upon the patient guessing the hand motion. However, it does require a cognitively intact patient.

○ *A caveat.* Do not use methods that fail to present peripheral targets or that present large targets in the center of the field (such as the palm of the hands) as these will consistently *fail* to pick up *large* defects that are detectable, equally consistently, by the methods above.

Central Scotomata

At the bedside, it is possible to have the patient draw out his own central scotoma on a piece of graph paper. (The patient is instructed to delimit the area in which he can see nothing.) Dr. Simon Horenstein of Missouri uses a piece of newspaper for the same purpose.

●

A Case Report

I once was presented a patient who was said to have bitemporal hemianopsia. Indeed, he could see no fingers wiggling in any temporal quadrant. After a negative pituitary workup, formal visual fields were reported back: the patient had nearly total blindness from long-standing glaucoma!

The house staff had omitted the Snellen card test because "he didn't wear glasses, and he didn't look like he was blind." I, in turn, had failed to proceed to monocular and nasal field testing because formal visual fields were to be done. That was a reason of sorts, but less excusable was my failure to feel the patient's eyeballs or to examine the fundus for glaucomatous cupping (see p. 181). In turn, my "excuse" was that the house staff had already "examined" the patient, and they didn't look like *they* were . . .

●

The Lacrimal Apparatus

Inspect the lacrimal puncta (located medially) and the lacrimal sac (inferiorly). Infection of the lacrimal sac may cause uni-lateral swelling. The lacrimal glands, located superiorly and laterally, may be enlarged unilaterally from a mixed tumor, or bilaterally from sarcoidosis or the Mickulicz syndrome (a variant or precursor of Sjögren's syndrome).

The function of the lacrimal apparatus is checked in patients complaining of dry eyes by means of the Schirmer test. (This may also serve as a test of facial nerve function, see p. 460). Bend a strip of filter paper so that the proximal portion can be inserted between the palpebral and scleral conjunctivae. Take care not to touch the cornea. After 5 minutes, remove the filter paper and measure the distance that the tears have migrated. Normal is 15 mm in persons under age 40, and 10 mm in persons over 40. Less than 10 mm is suspicious, and less than 5 mm is clearly abnormal. A standardized kit is available from SMP Division, Cooper Laboratories (PR) Inc., San German, Puerto Rico 00753. If you wish to use your own filter paper, you will have to standardize it, since different types have different absorbencies.

The Eyelids and Other Periorbital Tissue

Inspection of the eyelids might reveal clues to the patient's personality (the use of dramatic eye makeup) or to the presence of various systemic diseases, as well as local diseases of interest to the ophthalmologist but beyond the scope of this discussion. Look for xanthelasma in patients who might have hyperlipidemia (see Ch. 7, p. 116). A heliotrope rash on the eyelids is seen in dermatomyositis. Can you diagnose the patient shown in Figure 10-29?

Periorbital Edema

Periorbital edema is considered a useful sign for distinguishing the edema of the nephrotic syndrome from the edema of congestive heart failure, which generally spares the eyelids. The theory is that the high-protein ultrafiltrate of cardiac edema sinks, whereas the low-protein edema of the nephrotic syndrome does not. Of course, if this were the sole explanation, one would expect to see periorbital edema in severe cirrhosis, and one does not.

Other causes for periorbital edema are given in Table 10-1.

Palpebral Fissure

Unilateral ptosis, or drooping of the eyelid, may be a component of Horner's syndrome (see p. 170), and unilateral or bilateral ptosis in a young person should always suggest myasthenia gravis.

Wiener and Nathanson (1976–77) noted that many patients who were squinting were erroneously thought to have ptosis. This misadventure can be avoided by examining the patient without having him face into the light and by carefully observing the lids when performing the "up" movement of the cardinal directions of gaze. Squint is voluntary, and ptosis is not. Further, ptosis is unchanging, except in the Marcus Gunn jaw-wink and its variants, which are discussed in the following paragraphs.

Robert Marcus Gunn was a British ophthalmologist who described a benign phenomenon probably due to a congenital aberrancy of innervation. It consists of unilateral lid ptosis, which lid can be hyperelevated upon opening the jaw and moving the jaw to the opposite side. This is also known as the jaw-winking reflex. Gunn also first described the Gunn pupil (see p. 171).

Table 10-1.   Differential Diagnosis of Periorbital Edema

Systemic edema (e.g., nephrotic syndrome)
Infectious (including sinusitis)
    Bacterial: maxillary osteomyelitis, diphtheria, scarlet fever,
      syphilitic gumma, cavernous sinus thrombosis,
      mycobacterial
    Viral: infectious mononucleosis
    Fungal: aspergillosis, sporotrichosis, mucormycosis,
      actinomycosis
    Parasitic: trichinosis, ascariasis, onchocerciasis, malaria,
      syphilitic gumma
Endocrinologic
    Graves' disease (may be euthyroid at presentation)
    Hypothroidism (no indentation with pressure)
Traumatic
    Fracture of sinuses (crepitance on palpation)
    Foreign body
Allergic (e.g., Angioneurotic edema)
Neoplastic
    Acute myelocytic leukemia
    Rhabdomyosarcoma
    Retinoblastoma
    Sarcoma
    Lymphoma
    Melanoma
    Metastatic tumor (e.g., breast, lung)
    Superior caval syndrome

Source: *Phillips and Frank (1987).*

The inverse Gunn phenomenon is the abnormal movement of facial musculature on intention to close the eyes. Alternately, the subject may find that his eye closes when he attempts to open his mouth (Marin Amat's phenomenon). This is due to aberrant facial nerve regeneration or in some cases follows therapeutic transplantation of the facial nerve.

Other peculiar eponymic synkinesias have been catalogued (Duke-Elder & Leigh, 1965).

A widening of the palpebral fissure may be due to proptosis (vide infra), hypertonus of the eyelid, or a combination of the two, as in Graves' disease. These factors may also cause Graefe's lid lag, in which the eyelids of the hyperthyroid patient seem to lag behind the globe as the patient quickly changes his direction of gaze from the ceiling to the floor. (This sign may be easier to discern with the patient lying down, looking up toward the top of his head, and then toward his toes. If he is seated, be sure that your eye level is no higher than the patient's. Try this maneuver with a control subject available the first few times.)

The eye signs of Graves' disease are summarized in Table 10-2.

Table 10-2.   Eye Signs of Graves' Disease

Graefe's lid lag (p. 158)
Rosenbach's tremor (p. 158)
Griffith's sign (p. 158)
Boston's sign (p. 158)
Means' sign (p. 158)
Exophthalmos (proptosis) (p. 158)
Chemosis (p. 164)
Stellwag's sign (p. 158)
Joffroy's sign (p. 158)
Möbius' sign (p. 160)
Periorbital edema (see Table 10-1)
Bruit over the globe (see p. 202)

Some authors limit Graefe's sign to a lag of the upper lid during downward gaze, calling the lag of the lower lid during upward gaze Griffith's sign, lagging of the globe during upward glance Means' sign, and any jerking of the laggard lid Boston's sign.

Patients with Graves' disease may also have chemosis (see p. 164), which may be partly responsible for the infrequency of blinking in some such patients. The combination of infrequent blinking and proptosis is called Stellwag's sign, or Stellwag's stare. A hyperthyroid patient with exophthalmos is said to be able to look up at the ceiling, with the head held straight, without wrinkling the forehead (Joffroy's sign). There may be an element of frontalis myopathy, or this may simply be another version of the test for proptosis (Naffziger's method) in which the physician looks down upon the patient's face from a vantage point above his head to see whether the eyeballs can be observed from such a position. Another sign of hyperthyroidism is Rosenbach's tremor of the lightly closed eyelids.

○   *As a general rule in medicine, a plethora of signs or tests or therapies suggests that no one of them is perfect, and that possibly none of them are very excellent. Usually, one should choose a few, try them on one's own patient population, and see what seems to work best.*

Exophthalmos (Proptosis)

The degree of exophthalmos may be measured by using the Luedde exophthalmometer (Fig. 10-1); the 99th percentiles are 19 mm for white females, 21 mm for white males, 23 mm for black females, and 24 mm for black males. An evaluation for unilateral exophthalmos is indicated if there is a measured discrepancy of at least 2 mm in white subjects or 3 mm in black subjects (De Juan et al., 1980).

The most common medical causes of unilateral exophthalmos are, in approximate order of decreasing prevalence (Grove, 1975): Graves' disease; metastatic carcinoma, including paranasal sinus carcinoma in extension; hemangioma; lymphangioma; idiopathic orbital inflammation; lymphoma; neural tumors (including neurofibromas); meningioma; rhabdomyosarcoma, lacrimal gland epithelial tumor; malignant melanoma; dermoids; and epidermoid tumors. Of these, rhabdomyosarcoma leads the list of children's tumors. Unilateral exophthalmos can also be a sign of basal skull fracture (see Ch. 9, p. 145). Pulsating unilateral exophthalmos is a sign of carotid-cavernous sinus fistula.

Bilateral orbital involvement is most commonly caused by Graves' disease. Other etiologies in adults include lymphoma, and less frequently acute orbital pseudotumor, Wegener's granulomatosis, and mycotic infections. In children, bilateral disease is most frequently the result of metastatic neuroblastoma or leukemia.

Acute orbital pseudotumor is the sudden onset of ocular pain, proptosis, chemosis, impaired ocular mobility, and optic neuropathy, usually unilateral. It is a medical emergency (Phillips & Frank, 1987).

Some individuals have the ability to produce voluntarily an extreme form of proptosis, called propulsion of the eyeballs (Fig. 10-2) or the "double whammy" syndrome (Berman, 1966). An abnormality of the extraocular muscles was found at autopsy of one such person.

Extraocular Movements

Cardinal Directions of Gaze

By testing only six directions of gaze, one can test six different ocular muscles, and the three cranial nerves that control them.

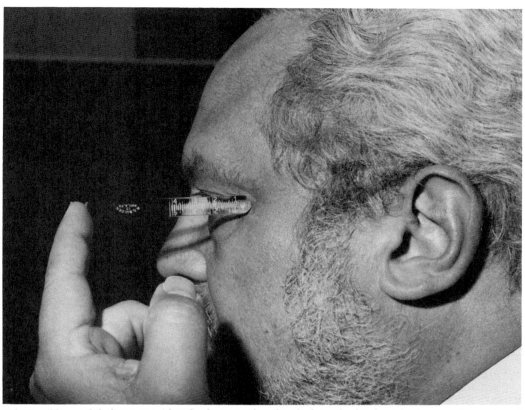

Figure 10-1. *The Luedde exophthalmometer. After the device is placed in the lateral orbital notch (the posteriormost portion of the lateral orbit), the anterior cornea is sighted through the graded plastic rod, which has markings on both sides to avoid parallax. The device need not be held with just the forefinger.*

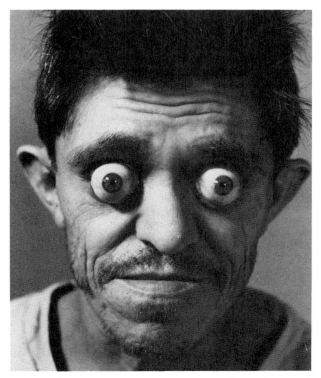

Figure 10-2. *Voluntary propulsion of the eyeball. Photograph courtesy of Dr. Barnett Berman of Maryland.*

These directions are northeast, east, southeast, southwest, west, and northwest, but *not* directly north or south (up and down). These directions are shown on the right eye in Figure 10-3, at which you may now glance *briefly*, only for the purpose of seeing the six directions.

There are times when we test the subject's ability to look directly up or down, but these are not cardinal directions of gaze. For additional information, see the neurologic examination (p. 454).

The six muscles are arranged to move around three axes, so oriented as to allow medical students to read large volumes of print without having to move their heads continuously in the fashion of a cobra following a mongoose.

The lateral rectus moves the globe laterally, and the medial rectus moves it medially, corresponding to the east and west directions. This much is not in dispute.

The superior oblique, despite its name and its reputation among morbid anatomists, actually moves the eyeball down and in. This has been a mystery to some (mysteries often have a spiral staircase, which goes *down and in*), but nonetheless is clearly true (Sapira, 1979; Younge and Sutula, 1977).

The inferior oblique moves the globe up and in (superiorly and medially). The superior rectus moves the globe up and out (superiorly and temporally). The inferior rectus moves the globe down and out (inferiorly and temporally). This much is true. The following statements are *generally* true, but incomplete. They will generally lead to the correct answer, or one that is not entirely wrong: the "upward" movement of the globe is by the superior rectus, and the "downward" movement by the inferior rectus. (To understand why these statements are not false, but not exactly true, you need to review the anatomy and physiology of the eye.)

The testing of the cranial nerves is done by inference from a knowledge of the anatomy of the muscles. All are supplied by cranial nerve III, except for the superior oblique (SO), which is supplied by cranial nerve IV, and the lateral rectus (LR), which is supplied by cranial nerve VI. The mnemonic is "LR sulfate," spelled LR_6SO_4.

Superior Oblique Palsy

A patient with a right superior oblique palsy, due to an isolated lesion of the trochlear nerve, is shown in Figure 26-3A, which illustrates the spontaneous Bielschowsky head tilt sign (Younge & Sutla, 1977). The head is tilted down towards the side away from the lesion. This spontaneous sign has a 50% sensitivity. However, if you remember to tilt the head back the other way (down towards the side of the lesion), and look for the iris on the bad side to move superiorly, the test is positive in 94% of the cases (Fig. 26-3B).

False positives. A *spontaneous* head tilt could also be idiopathic, or due to torticollis (see Ch. 24, p. 415).

Apparent Inferior Oblique Palsy

Very advanced. Brown's syndrome (Figs. 10-4 and 10-5) is an unusual manifestation of rheumatoid arthritis, which is probably due to a stenosing tenosynovitis* of the superior oblique tendon and sheath. The patient intermittently has vertical diplopia, a clicking sensation, and an apparent inferior oblique palsy. The eye is able to look down and medially but sometimes becomes trapped in that position. When the patient then attempts to look up and medially, the trapped eye acts as if it has an inferior oblique palsy. With continued effort, the eye sometimes is able to pop loose, snapping all or part of the way up. The patient feels a click, and the physician might be able to palpate it at the orbit's upper medial corner (Killian et al., 1977).

Because there is no true inferior oblique palsy, and because both the intermittency and the clicking sensation sound unusual, the unaware skeptic might be tempted to dismiss the patient or administer an unneeded psychotropic medication.

Weakness of Convergence

Möbius' sign of hyperthyroidism is weakness of ocular convergence during near accommodation (about 5 inches away). This occurs because of a myopathy involving the medial recti.

---

*The word "synovium" comes from the Greek "syn" (with) and the Latin "ova" (egg). The synovial fluid, originally called the synovium, looked like the white of an egg, that is, the stuff that came *with the egg.* Later, the word was transferred to the lining of the joint, which was thought to make the synovium, and the lining came to be called the synovium (instead of synovial lining, i.e., the lining that makes the synovium), and that which was previously called the synovium became the synovial fluid. (This is very similar to what happened to "ventricle," which means sack, and is used by cardiologists, alternately to mean the sack itself or the space (cavity) contained by the sack.)

Brown's syndrome could also be called a tenovaginitis. The word "vagina" underwent a similar evolution. The vagina was the sheath or scabbard that the Roman carried around his waist to hold his sword. As defined in the older anatomy books, there were many vaginas, only one of which is now called by that word. To have said "gonorrhea is a common disease of *the* vagina" would have been incorrect, because there was in those past days no single vagina to justify use of the singular definite article.

Self-Study

Complete Figure 10-3.

Strabismus

Strabismus is a disorder of gaze in which one eye deviates from parallelism with the other. It may be paralytic or nonparalytic, the former being caused by specific oculomotor palsies. In nonparalytic strabismus, the relative abnormality of the two globes appears to remain constant over a fairly wide angle of vision, and each eye can move in all four quadrants.

A Method

An easy way to check for strabismus is to have the subject look at a penlight about 3 feet away. The reflection of the light should come from approximately the same part of each pupil. A more sensitive test is the "cover test" (see p. 161).

Nonparalytic convergent strabismus (cross eyes) is called esotropia. Divergent strabismus (wall eyes) is exotropia. In the vertical dimension, the aberrant eye may point up to the ceiling (hy-

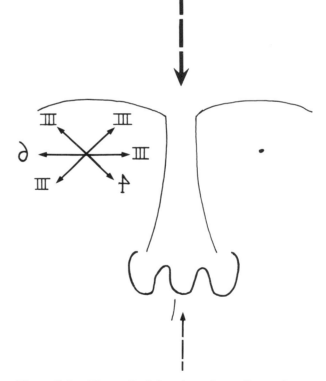

Figure 10-3. *The cardinal directions of gaze. Instructions:*
1. *Place a hand mirror on the arrows down the middle of the nose, the reflecting surface to your left (the face's right eye). Keep that side hidden, while you work on the face's left eye.*
2. *Draw in the cardinal directions of gaze, on the face's left eye.*
3. *For those directions that are* unique *to a cranial nerve, write the number of the cranial nerve in Arabic numerals.*
4. *Designate the remainder of the cranial nerves in Roman numerals.*
5. *Now, you may look at the right eye. The correct answers for the left eye will be given in the mirror.*

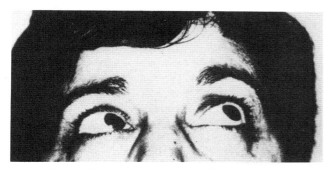

Figure 10-4. *Right pseudo-inferior oblique palsy due to Brown's syndrome, in a patient of Dr. Bruce McClain of Washington, D.C.*

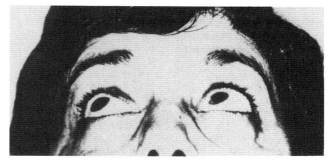

Figure 10-5. *Same patient as in Figure 10-4. The left eye is normal.*

pertropia, not to be confused with hypermetropia [hyperopia] p. 155), or down at the floor, hypotropia.

The various tropias may result in amblyopia, which is reduced vision due to suppression of the image from the deviating eye so as to avoid the discomfort attendant upon diplopia (double vision). It is extremely important to discover tropias very early in childhood in order to prevent permanent loss of vision.

Latent Strabismus

Latent strabismus is given the suffix "phoria" instead of "tropia." It is usually not detected by routine physical examination, and is often of no clinical significance. However, in some cases (e.g., superior oblique palsy, Brown's syndrome, etc.), there are some fields of gaze in which there is single vision. But in other fields of gaze, the phoria becomes manifest or tropic. Therefore, in any patient who complains of double vision, a cover test may give the first clue to an underlying cranial nerve lesion or other etiology of the diplopia.

The Cover Test

A method:

1. Sit directly in front of the subject and ask him to look at a light 2 to 3 feet away, with one eye covered.

2. Now move the cover across to the other eye and watch for motion of the eye that is uncovered. (Actually, this test might better be called the "uncover test.")

3. Re-cover the first eye, and watch for motion of the eye that is now being uncovered.

Interpretation. Motion of either eye *as it is uncovered* is a sign of strabismus. With *esophoria,* the eye moves outward as it is uncovered. With *exophoria,* the eye moves inward as it is uncovered.

Nystagmus

Nystagmus refers to slight, rapid, rhythmic, "spontaneous" movements of the eyes. The movements often have a slow (vestibular) deviation component and a quick (cerebral) return component. Some authors name nystagmus for the direction of gaze in which the nystagmus appears; others name it for the quick return component (see Ch. 4, p. 68). For this reason, it is probably best simply to describe the nystagmus.

Nystagmus is basically a neurologic sign, but is included here because it is discovered in the routine examination of the extra-ocular movements. It indicates disease somewhere in the vestibular-cerebellar-oculomotor system, either structural or toxic. Other brain stem signs involving the central control of ocular position, such as doll's eyes, and caloric stimulation are discussed in Chapter 26.

A Method

Nystagmus may occur (ominously) in the primary position (at rest), but it is usually evoked by holding the patient's head and having him visually follow a *rapid* finger movement, first horizontally, then vertically. When testing for nystagmus on lateral gaze, you do not have to go very far laterally. Significant nystagmus will occur within 30 degrees of the primary position.

Some Definitions

In *horizontal nystagmus,* the oscillation is from side to side (as in patients given hypnotic-sedatives). In vertical nystagmus, the oscillation is up and down (usually due to a midline lesion or Wernicke's encephalopathy), and in *rotatory nystagmus,* the motion is circular. *Fixation nystagmus* is present only when looking at an object. *Pendular nystagmus* is a side-to-side motion lacking a quick or slow component (i.e., both movements are equal in rate and speed.)

Downbeat nystagmus, a vertical jerk occurring in primary position and usually exacerbated by lateral or downward gaze, is presumptive evidence of dysfunction at the lower end of the brain stem or cerebellum. Structural causes include platybasia and the Arnold-Chiari malformation. Metabolic causes include magnesium depletion, lithium intoxication, alcoholic cerebellar degeneration, Wernicke's encephalopathy, anoxia, and anticonvulsant toxicity (phenytoin or carbamazepine.) Inflammatory causes include encephalitis, syphilis, and multiple sclerosis. Other causes include hereditary and paraneoplastic cerebellar degeneration, encephalitis, brain stem infarction or vertebrobasilar insufficiency, and bilateral internuclear ophthalmoplegia (Alpert, 1978; Chrousos et al., 1987; Cogan, 1968).

Monocular nystagmus is almost always due to pontomedullary disease.

Nystagmoid movement is a false nystagmus of up to three beats, never more, which can occur in normal individuals on initially looking to an extreme position.

Blind-eye nystagmus refers to the irregular oscillations sometimes seen in a blind eye. These go away if the blind eye is asked to "look" at a fixed point, and is thus a false nystagmus.

Paretic nystagmus is also a false nystagmus, due to weakness of the oculomotor muscles. It resembles the post-disuse weakness of larger striated muscles. It is best elicited by having the patient look in a direction that requires the use of the paralyzed muscle.

In *gaze paretic nystagmus,* both eyes show more nystagmus to one end position than to the other. This accompanies lesions that produce paralysis of conjugate gaze, and has no significance beyond that of the paralysis.

Physiologic nystagmus occurs when persons in a moving vehicle stare past a fixed portion such as the edge of the windshield at a repetitive, quickly moving background, such as poles, tunnel arches, trees, and so forth.

Optokinetic nystagmus is a physiologic response elicited by having the patient gaze at a rotating vertically striped drum. The unilateral absence of this nystagmus is a clue to abnormality of the ipsilateral oculomotor nucleus and nerve. Cerebral lesions have loss of nystagmus only when the drum is moving towards the affected side. It is also useful in a patient who claims total loss of vision, who therefore should not have any optokinetic nystagmus, but in fact does.

An optokinetic drum can be constructed out of a roll of chart labeling tape if the labels have a colored stripe (a method shown to me by Dr. Cheolsu Shin of North Carolina). The tape is placed around a pencil, held erect on its axis, and the tape is unwound at a constant rate.

Saccadic Eye Movements

Saccadic eye movements, which may be confused with nystagmus, are 10 to 15 per second square wave jerks. In fact, the word "saccadic" comes from a French term meaning to stop a horse by giving its reins (and head) a quick jerk. Saccadic eye movements are most frequently encountered during the ophthalmoscopic examination as one cause of the "uncooperative" patient syndrome, but saccadic movements are not volitional. Some saccadic eye movements have special names, such as ocular flutter, opsoclonus, and saccadomania (Leigh & Zee, 1983).

In a general medical practice, saccadic movements may be encountered most frequently in the very old and in a small number of schizophrenics, many of whom also have abnormal eye pursuit in research studies (Anonymous, 1983). Saccadic movements may also be seen in infants less than 6 months of age. Saccadic movements seem normal in AIDS patients, but are actually slowed (Nguyen et al., 1989).

If the saccadic oscillations do not have an intersaccadic interval (that is, a pause between the jerks), they may be caused by viral encephalitis, hydrocephalus, cranial trauma, intracranial tumor, thalamic hemorrhage, chemicals such as lithium or thallium, and as part of the "dancing eyes and dancing feet" syndrome of infantile myoclonic encephalopathy (Leigh & Zee, 1983).

The Sclera

Scleral Icterus

Scleral icterus is a misnomer because one actually is observing icterus of the bulbar conjunctiva, against the white background provided by the sclera. A whole school of one-upmanship has evolved around the question, "Where is the best place to look for jaundice?" Some say the palms of the hand, others say the roof of the palate, and still others champion the tympanic membranes. I usually answer "in the parking lot." By this I mean that the most important issue is not which portion of the body is being examined (although I still favor the scleral conjunctiva), but the quality of the light that is used. As a student, I missed icterus in patients with a measured serum bilirubin as high as 8 mg/dl if I examined them at night in a room dimly lit by incandescent bulbs in the ceiling. Fluorescent light bulbs at night are not much better. In natural daylight, one can perceive levels of 4 mg/dl (on a cloudy day or in a poorly lit room). In the Midwest, in direct sunshine filtered through haze, one can get into the range of 2.3 to 2.1 mg/dl of bilirubin. In sunny Southern climes on the side of the building struck by the sun, one can detect as little as 1.5 to 1.7 mg/dl.

Self-Teaching Exercise

On a sunny day, find a patient with a total serum bilirubin around 2 to 3 mg/dl. First, examine the scleral conjunctivae in artificial light in a poorly lit room. Then walk the patient to a window on the sunny side of the building and reexamine his eyes in *direct* sunlight.

Black patients may normally have a brown or muddy pigmentation, which appears to be scleral but is actually conjunctival. Ignore this. Instead, have the patient gaze superiorly or inferiorly and examine the portion of the bulbar conjunctiva that is not usually exposed to sunlight. Those portions will not have the brown muddy pigmentation, but will clearly show the yellow pigment of icterus, if present.

For the attending. The pigment that is observed is not the serum bilirubin, but the bilirubin deposited in tissues. When the serum bilirubin is rapidly changing, the scleral icterus will tend to lag behind. This will improve your roundsmanship when the patient's bilirubin is dropping, because you may be able to see scleral icterus at a time when the serum bilirubin has dropped almost to the upper limit of normal. On the other hand, you will be less impressive when the serum bilirubin is rising.

Spots on the Sclerae

Pingueculae and pterygia (see p. 163) actually arise from the conjunctiva; they are frequently misperceived to be scleral in origin.

Pigmented spots medial and lateral to the limbus may be seen in ochronosis or in Gaucher's disease. The spots shown in Figure 10-6 are senile hyaline plaques, which are a simple degenerative phenomenon occurring after the age of 50. They have no systemic or ocular significance. They are characteristically found at the insertions of the medial and lateral rectus muscles, and so are more discrete and rectangular than the pigment spots of the two diseases mentioned first in this paragraph.

White spots like Brie cheese, usually located only on the temporal side, are called Bitot's spots. They are seen in vitamin A deficiency and are thus exceedingly rare in developed countries.

Blue Sclerae

Blue sclerae have been called pathognomonic for osteogenesis imperfecta, but this is not true. In 1908, Osler described the association between blue sclerae and iron-deficiency anemia. A study of 169 hospitalized patients showed blue sclerae in 87% of patients with iron-deficiency anemia, 7% of patients with other anemias, and 5.3% of patients without anemia (Kalra et al., 1986). Blue sclerae are also seen in 3% of patients with Marfan's syndrome (Cross & Jensen, 1973; Hanno & Weiss, 1961), 15% of cases of pseudo-pseudohypoparathyroidism (Scheie & Albert, 1977), 5% of cases of homocystinuria (Cross & Jensen, 1973), occasionally in Ehlers-Danlos syndrome (Paton, 1972; Thomas et al., 1954), and very rarely in pseudoxanthoma elasticum (Paton, 1972; Roy, 1972; Scheie & Albert, 1977). They may be seen with mitoxantrone therapy (Anonymous, 1988), corticosteroid therapy, myasthenia gravis, and various collagen vascular disorders (Kalra et al., 1986). Other very rare causes of blue sclerae that are of potential interest to the nonophthalmologist include oxycephaly (Walsh & Hoyt, 1969), incontinentia pigmenti, Turner's syndrome, hypophosphatasia, Crouzon's disease, Hallerman-Streiff syndrome, pyncnodysostosis, and the ocular staphylomas (Roy, 1972).

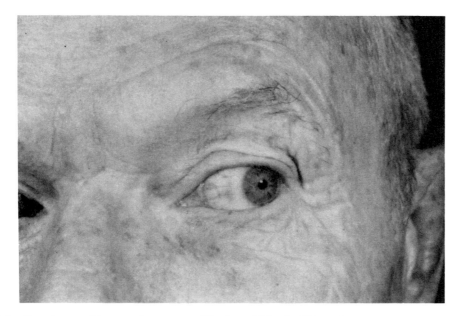

Figure 10-6. *Senile hyaline plaques. Photograph courtesy of Dr. Franck Mocek of Kentucky.*

Possibly blue sclerae are also seen in pseudohypoparathyroidism, but ophthalmologists have unsuccessfully sought such an association (Hanno & Weiss, 1961). It may have gained entry to the differential diagnosis when a well-meaning medical secretary decided that the proper diagnosis, pseudo-pseudohypoparathyroidism, was a *lapsus linguae* of the dictator and so amputated one of the "pseudos."

Finally, this discussion is concerned with truly, abnormally blue sclerae. Many persons have a light-blue tinge to their sclerae, and with a good light an attending physician can probably find a bluish scleromalacia in patients with rheumatoid arthritis, or (with a little imagination) even in red-haired persons with hypertension. (By the 16th century, portrait painters knew to add blue to the white of the eyes of normal subjects (Burckhardt, 1929).) Don't push the physical examination beyond its capacity.

The Conjunctiva

Examining the Conjunctivae

The conjunctiva covers the entire anterior eyeball, with the exception of the cornea. For convenience, one may speak of the bulbar conjunctiva, which covers the sclera, and the palpebral conjunctiva.

A Method

Inspect the fornices and the lower palpebral conjunctiva by simply pulling down the lower eyelid. This is done, *not* by touching the lower eyelid but by pressing the skin overlying the inferior orbital maxilla against its underlying bone and then tugging this skin inferiorly. The eyelid will evert.

If there is inflammation of the eye, or any other reason to suspect a foreign body, the conjunctiva of the upper lid must also be inspected, by everting the eyelid. Ask the patient to look down, and grasp the upper eyelashes gently with the thumb and forefinger of one hand. Using a cotton swab placed at the upper border of the tarsal plate as a fulcrum, pull up on the lashes and push down on the tarsal plate. Later, when the patient looks up, the eyelid will flip back to its normal position.

Findings

Examining the palpebral conjunctiva in bright direct sunlight will enable you to estimate the hematocrit, and is especially helpful in patients in whom fingernail abnormalities complicate the examination of the nail bed.

A pterygium (from the Greek word for "wing") is a fan-shaped or wing-shaped proliferation of opaque fibrovasacular conjunctival tissue almost always medial to the iris and in some cases growing over the cornea, where it may interfere with vision.

A pinguecula (from one of the Latin words for "fat") is a collection of fat medial or lateral to the iris. It is not ophthalmologically ominous or systemically significant.

Hemorrhages on the palpebral conjunctiva may be a sign of systemic infection, such as bacterial endocarditis.

Nothing is so dramatic as a large bright-red bulbar conjunctival hemorrhage that suddenly blossoms where none was seen before, but where it cannot be ignored.

The most common cause is local trauma, although it may be a sign of remote trauma, as in subarachnoid hemorrhage. If it appears more than 1 day after the trauma, it is pathognomonic for basal skull fracture. (The sensitivity for basal skull fracture is 10% (Duke-Elder & Leigh, 1965).) It may also appear after acute venous hypertension (severe coughing) or sustained venous hypertension (e.g., superior vena caval syndrome); or as a local manifestation of a systemic vasculitis, thrombocytopenia, or clotting disorder. In the latter conditions, conjunctival hemorrhage never occurs in isolation but always in the presence of other signs.

There is evidence (Duke-Elder & Leigh, 1965) that the vessels of the conjunctiva become more fragile with diabetes mellitus, hypertension, or simply aging. Thus it is not surprising that one of the most common conclusions in investigating isolated conjunctival hemorrhage is "no known explanation and no known pathology."

The ophthalmoscope may be used to inspect that bulbar conjunctiva usually covered by the lower lid for the corkscrew vessels of the sickle hemoglobinopathies. The test is 91% sensitive for hemoglobin S disease, less sensitive for heterozygotes, and has no false positives (Comer & Fred, 1964).

Chemosis

Chemosis is a Greek word meaning conjunctival edema, derived from the classic Greek word meaning to yawn, gape, or stare, which became a slang word meaning mollusc or bivalve (whose shell might gape apart). This was considered a fine analogy to conjunctival edema, with the two shells corresponding to the eyelids.

Sometimes the chemosis is unaccompanied by lacrimation, so that the conjunctiva looks wet, but no tearing can be seen. Hence, the wetness is within the conjunctival tissue per se.

A Method

To demonstrate chemosis, rub the palpebral conjunctiva of the lower lid upwards against the bulbar conjunctiva, keeping your finger on the skin of the lower lid. This will cause the boggy, water-logged bulbar conjunctiva to heap up on itself. The corrugated appearance may be easily seen when obliquely illuminated with a good light.

Etiologies of chemosis include increased vascular permeability, increased venous pressure, decreased plasma albumin, and metabolic afflictions of the periorbital tissue.

Increased vascular permeability may either be systemic or local (from inflammation of the eye or neighboring tissues, possibly including the meninges). The systemic causes include infections, hypersensitivity reactions, and Quincke's angioneurotic edema. It is said that chemosis may be a valuable early sign of meningitis (Duke-Elder & Leigh, 1965).

Venous congestion may result from a cause within the orbit, or it may be a very valuable sign of the superior vena caval syndrome (see p. 366). In pure right-sided heart failure (due to tricuspid stenosis, constrictive pericarditis, cardiac tamponade, etc.), rarely, very mild chemosis may be seen. It may occur in nephrotic syndrome, but is not seen in pure left-sided ("backward") congestive heart failure, which produces edema of a high protein concentration. In chronic cases, the conjunctiva takes on a yellow hue.

The two metabolic afflictions of the orbit that cause chemosis are Graves' ophthalmopathy and myxedema.

Unilateral chemosis can be a sign of anterior basal skull fracture (see Ch. 9, p. 145).

The Iris

Findings in the iris are often associated with pupillary findings (see p. 169), since the function of the iris is to regulate pupillary size.

Spots on the Iris

Check the iris for nevi, which if elevated may actually be melanomas. Also check for Koeppe's nodules (which are most easily seen as projections into the pupil). These may be a clue to sarcoidosis, although they are also seen in tuberculosis and other uveitides.

Brushfield spots are white spots in the iris, which at one time were thought to be diagnostic of Down's syndrome. Although they are indeed present in 85% to 90% of those so afflicted, they have also been found in 10% to 24% of normal subjects (Donaldson, 1961).

The Brushfield spots in Down's syndrome are more numerous than in normal individuals. (Normals have about 11, patients with Down's syndrome have about twice as many.) The normal subject's spots tend to be in the periphery, whereas at least some of the spots tend to be located in the middle third of the iris in Down's syndrome. The spots are more distinct in patients with Down's syndrome. Finally, the spots are associated with hypoplasia of the iris in 50% to 95% of patients with Down's syndrome, while only 9% of normals have this hypoplasia. The hypoplasia may be detected by searching the periphery of the iris for a tangential missing piece (Donaldson, 1961.)

A note on nomenclature. The term *mongolism* was offensive alike to Caucasians with the disease and Asians without it. The eponym is preferred to "trisomy 21," since a small percentage of cases have translocations rather than an extra chromosome.

The Cornea

Band Keratopathy

Band keratopathy is a white cloudiness of the afflicted area of the cornea, resembling the fine precipitate of calcium phosphate (in a test tube) or the haze of a London sunrise. It can be seen with the naked eye if one examines the cornea in a good light. The horizontal band of the cornea that is exposed to sunlight is afflicted, while the protected portion usually remains as sparkling clear as aspic. Sometimes the keratopathy extends to the conjunctiva, but only in severe cases.

Band keratopathy is seen in many hypercalcemic states, including primary hyperparathyroidism, sarcoidosis, vitamin D intoxication, and milk-alkali syndrome (Cogan et al., 1948); berylliosis, multiple myeloma, Hodgkin's disease (Walsh & Hoyt, 1969); and most quickly (within 4 months) in infantile hypercalcemia (Duke-Elder & Leigh, 1965). Band keratopathy remains even after the serum calcium has returned to normal.

Other causes of the dystrophic calcification type of band keratopathy include secondary hyperparathyroidism (Cogan et al., 1948), Paget's disease, hypophosphatasia (Duke-Elder & Leigh, 1965), "acute osteoporosis" (Roy, 1972), and renal failure with nephrocalcinosis or nephrolithiasis, due to the milk-alkali syndrome, secondary hyperparathyroidism, or perhaps cystinosis (Roy, 1972).

Band keratopathy has also been seen in juvenile rheumatoid arthritis (Scheie & Albert, 1977; Walsh & Hoyt, 1969), but in fewer than 1% of cases of adult rheumatoid arthritis (Roy, 1972; Smith, 1957). It has occurred in discoid lupus erythematosus (Roy, 1972), and, on one occasion, in gout (Fishman & Sunderman, 1966). Very rarely, it has been reported in tuberous sclerosis (Duke-Elder & Leigh, 1965), ichthyosis (Roy, 1972), Rothmund's syndrome, Parry-Romberg syndrome (Roy, 1972), and pulmonary tuberculosis (Duke-Elder & Leigh, 1965), although the last is now known to produce hypercalcemia on occasion (Shai et al., 1972).

Ocular disorders that can cause band keratopathy include 3% to 5% of cases of peripheral uveitis (pars planitis) (Brockhurst et al., 1960; Schlaegel, 1978), interstitial keratitis, phthisis bulbi, chronic iridocyclitis (Roy, 1972), sympathetic ophthalmia (Pau, 1978), absolute glaucoma* (Pau, 1978), and toxoplasmosis (Schlaegel, 1977). Band keratopathy can be associated with any type of corneal injury, whether toxic, thermal, traumatic, or so on (De Juan, personal communication, 1987). Among the posttraumatic ocular causes are postburn and postperforation (Pau, 1978), toxic fumes (mercury, calomel, calcium bichromate), and particle irritation, for example in hatters who cut rabbit fur with scissors (Duke-Elder & Leigh, 1965). Finally, there are recognized families with band keratopathy (Duke-Elder & Leigh, 1965), as well as instances of "idiopathic" band keratopathy (Roy, 1972).

The Limbus Sign

While band keratopathy is the best-known sign of hypercalcemia, I am personally more impressed with the utility of the limbus sign (Fig. 10-7), a ring of dystrophic calcification best seen as a milky precipitate at the limbus (Pau, 1978; Roberts, 1958; Schumacher & Scheler, 1969). The limbus sign has almost been forgotten among modern professors of medicine, and even when stumbled upon by the thorough is usually misinterpreted as arcus senilis, which it closely resembles. This sign may be present in situations like chronic renal insufficiency wherein the absolute value of the serum calcium is within the normal range, yet still inappropriately high for the clinical situation, as demonstrated by the elevated calcium-phosphate product (Schumacher & Scheler, 1969). The limbus sign is permanent and persists even after the calcium-phosphate product is returned to normal.

Arcus Senilis

Arcus senilis is a white ring at the limbus, which begins as an arc, hence its name. The modifier indicates the belief that the finding is a degenerative sign, although, more accurately, it correlates with aging. It was found to be absent in hospitalized black men under age 15, in white men under 50, in black women under 30, and in white women under 40. In a steel mill, arcus senilis was absent in black men under 20 and white men under 30 (Macaraeg et al., 1968). Thus, the term is inaccurate for

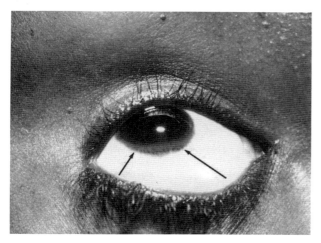

Figure 10-7. *This 24-year-old woman had an elevated calcium-phosphate product due to renal disease, but no lipid abnormalities. A milky arc (the limbus sign) can be seen obscuring the underlying dark iris, sweeping inferiorly between the two arrows. Photograph courtesy of Dr. David Johnson of Tennessee.*

*Absolute glaucoma means a totally blind eye, which is very often painful.

blacks, who develop the sign earlier than whites and also for women, for whom the Latin term for aging is *anilis*.

It was thought that arcus senilis signified vascular disease, which also covaries with age, through what I refer to as the Bayesian fallacy, a belief that all findings are independent of each other. Thus, young people have little vascular disease and rarely have arcus senilis, and older people frequently have both, hence the arcus is taken to be a sign of disease. However, if this were true often enough to be clinically useful, it should be easy to show the claimed correlation, and it is not, although there is some evidence for it. At the present time, the best correlation seems to be with ECG abnormalities (Macaraeg et al., 1968; Rodstein & Zelman, 1963), which are still one step removed from specific diseases with specific names.

Kayser-Fleischer Ring

The occurrence of a brownish-*green* ring, at or near the limbus, represents copper deposition in Descemet's membrane. This ring, described by Kayser and Fleischer, has high positive and negative predictive value for the diagnosis of untreated Wilson's disease. It is visible to the naked eye without special arrangements, time, equipment (i.e., a slit-lamp), or cost, although slit-lamp examination is more sensitive.

False Positives

The emphasis here is first on the color green. Bilirubin and carotene have produced false-positive Kayser-Fleischer rings, by "staining" a white arcus senilis background (Weinberg et al., 1981). We can thus predict the subsequent report of a similar false positive due to lycopenemia in a tomato juice addict with arcus senilis. Yet none of these pigments is truly green. Bilirubin is yellow-orangish, carotenes are orange, but lycopenes are reddish. Finally, all three pigments stain the skin, and bilirubin tends to produce more "scleral" (conjunctival) pigmentation. The copper of Wilson's disease does not pigment the sclera or the skin.

So far, no one has managed to confuse the green Kayser-Fleischer ring with the brown limbal ring of Addison's disease (Straub & Russman, 1966). This latter ring is more obvious at the superior and inferior arcs than it is medially and laterally.

Another key descriptor for the Kayser-Fleischer ring is "visible to the naked eye without the use of a slit-lamp." It is true that patients with a wide variety of hepatic diseases, other than Wilson's disease, apparently have a secondary abnormality of copper metabolism, which although different from that of Wilson's disease, eventually results in the deposition of enough copper in Descemet's membrane to be visualized by slit lamp examination (Rimola et al., 1978; Weinberg et al., 1981). Among these liver diseases are posthepatitic cirrhosis, primary biliary cirrhosis, cryptogenic cirrhosis, neonatal liver disease, active chronic hepatitis, and progressive intrahepatic cholestasis. But in these cases, the green rings were reported only on slit-lamp examination.

Alas, nothing is perfect. A truly green ring, visible to the naked eye, has been reported in one case of multiple myeloma associated with hypercupremia due to an unusual circulating copper-binding protein (Gordon et al., 1967). And I have seen a tiny, thin, brownish-green ring, visible to the unaided eye, in a patient with Laennec's cirrhosis.

We now know that up to 16% of the patients with Wilson's disease in some series (Nazer et al., 1986) may have normal amounts of ceruloplasmin, although the material is functionally inept. Such patients should have hepatic copper determinations or measurement of radiocopper absorption. Since these steps were not taken in the patient described in the last paragraph, he can no longer be considered a proven case of non-Wilson's disease. Heraclitus, the pre-Socratic philosopher who believed that the first principle of the universe is unceasing change, would be a good mentor for medical authors.

False Negatives

The recent claim that the Kayser-Fleischer ring is only 74% sensitive for the diagnosis is based upon family populations with a mean age of 15 years and a range of 6 to 33 (Nazer et al., 1986). In the older population, the Kayser-Fleischer is more confounded by false positives (vide supra) than false negatives, although one 58-year-old patient with neurologic impairment due to Wilson's disease, yet no Kayser-Fleischer ring, has been reported (Ross et al., 1985). Of course, the sign disappears with treatment of the disease.

Special Maneuvers

The dendritic-appearing corneal lesion of herpes simplex is best seen if the tears are stained by touching the palpebral conjunctiva with a moistened fluorescein strip. (Fluorescein staining is also helpful for seeing corneal abrasions due to trauma.)

The corneal reflex is discussed in Chapter 26 (p. 457). Ophthalmoscopic examination of the cornea is given on page 177.

The Red Eye

The differential diagnosis of the red eye is given in Table 10-3. Although this is the accepted differential, I have yet to see my first case of *acute* angle closure glaucoma, despite dilating the pupils of nearly all comers. Accordingly, the remainder of the discussion will refer just to acute conjunctivitis and acute iritis.

The major historical clue is that true pain, as opposed to a scratchy discomfort, signifies iritis, not conjunctivitis.

The most discriminating physical finding is the distribution of the injected vessels. To see whether the involved vessels are the superficial conjunctival ones, check whether they move when you place your finger below the lower lid and press upwards, as you did when testing for chemosis by displacing the conjunctiva.

Although posterior keratoprecipitates make the diagnosis of iritis (see the ophthalmoscopic examination, p. 177), most patients with acute iritis do not yet have these at the time they initially present.

While pus makes the diagnosis of acute conjunctivitis, many cases of acute conjunctivitis have such watery secretions that you will not be able to tell whether or not pus is present. Gram and Wright stains of conjunctival scrapings are extremely useful in the diagnosis of the red eye.

Viral (epidemic) conjunctivitis will frequently be associated with palpable preauricular lymph nodes (see Ch. 8, p. 141).

When in doubt about the distinction between iritis and conjunctivitis, proceed to the Au-Henkind test (Au & Henkind, 1981). The patient closes the eye to be tested, leaving the other eye open. Shine a penlight into the open eye and ask the patient whether or not he has experienced a sensation in the closed eye. Pain in the closed eye is a positive test for iritis. This test presumes that a normal consensual pupillary response to light is present. The test is 100% sensitive and highly specific.

Patients with iritis will also experience pain during testing for accommodation, and the pain will occur at a reproducible distance. Thus, the examiner begins with the patient focusing on a distant (3 feet) finger as it moves closer to the eyes (Talbot, 1987). The sensitivity was 74%, the specificity 97%, and the positive predictive value 50% in an outpatient ophthalmology clinic, where the prevalence of the disease was 4.5% as judged from biomicroscopy.

A problem seen more often in real life than in books is the patient with *both* iritis and conjunctivitis. Thus, it is important to use more than one discriminator so as not to miss a diagnosis. When both are present, one should begin with the differential diagnosis of acute iritis because it includes more medically important and treatable entities than conjunctivitis, which itself can be secondary to iritis. (Iritis is almost never secondary to conjunctivitis, except in the case of infectious etiologies.)

Medical conditions associated with iritis include systemic lupus erythematosus, ankylosing spondylitis, Still's syndrome, inflammatory bowel disease, HLA B27 positivity in and of itself, Behçet's syndrome, polyarteritis, granulomatosis, and sarcoidosis.

The differential diagnosis of conjunctivitis includes gram-positive cocci, gram-negative cocci, gram-negative rods, some chlamydia, viruses, and allergies. Only Reiter's syndrome, among the seronegative spondylarthropathies, is associated with conjunctivitis.

Table 10-3. Differential Diagnosis of the Red Eye

Descriptor	Acute Iritis	Acute Conjunctivitis	Acute Narrow-Angle Glaucoma
Onset	Gradual	Gradual	Abrupt
Pain	Moderate and noxious; may be likened to a headache	No true pain; burning or itching	Severe
Injection	More intense near limbus; individual vessels often not distinguished; less pink	Most intense in fornices; topical epinephrine (1:1000) lightens eye; superficial vessels move with conjunctiva; pinker	As for iritis
Pupil	May be miotic with sluggish or absent reflexes	Always normal	Somewhat dilated; does not respond to light
Cornea	May have posterior surface keratoprecipitates or may be clear	Always clear	Foggy; iris out of focus
Secretions	Watery	May have pus	Watery
Vision	May be reduced	Never reduced	Markedly reduced

Source: *Newell (1982).*

The Anterior Chamber

Introduction to Glaucoma

Glaucoma is a disease of intraocular (*not* arterial) hypertension, which insidiously produces irreversible blindness. Just as war is too important to be left to the generals, glaucoma is too important to be left to the ophthalmologists.

Glaucoma will not be diagnosed early by checking the visual acuity, or by checking the visual fields by confrontation (see p. 156). It does not affect the ability to focus, and the early visual field cuts are usually nasal, where they are least likely to be detected by confrontation. (Later the field cuts become nasal arcuate, then they spread temporally; central vision is the last to be lost.) Over 50% of the nerve tissue may be lost before visual field changes can be detected. It is partly for these reasons that glaucoma is so pernicious and insidious.

Glaucomatous changes in the optic disc are discussed on page 181. There are basically three forms of glaucoma (all of which eventually cause the same type of changes in the visual fields and optic discs): 1) wide angle or open angle (the most common), in which the depth of the anterior chamber is normal; 2) narrow angle (rare), also called acute angle (pupillary block) or angle closure glaucoma, in which the anterior chamber is shallow; and 3) a miscellany including "normal pressure" glaucoma.

"Normal pressure glaucoma" is metaphysical. Just as there is no such thing as "the" blood pressure, there is no such thing as "the" intraocular pressure. If an individual has high intraocular pressure at one point in time, but his pressures when actually measured at another time happen to be normal, then he might be said to have "normal pressure" glaucoma, which may be likened to "labile hypertension."

Checking the Anterior Chamber Depth

Because dilating the pupil can acutely precipitate an attack of narrow-angle glaucoma, it is essential to check the depth of the anterior chamber before instilling a mydriatic, if one is concerned about narrow-angle glaucoma (Fig. 10-8).

A Method

1. Have the patient look forward at the examiner's eyes.

2. Aim the beam of a flashlight or a penlight from the temporal side at the patient's lateral limbus, in a plane perpendicular to the patient's axis of vision. The light should shine across the iris in a plane that just barely illuminates the entire iris. Anterior displacement of the lens and central iris forms a nipple-like protrusion that casts a medial (nasal) shadow (Fig. 10-9).

Another method of estimating anterior chamber depth uses the slit aperture on the ophthalmoscope (see p. 174.)

Positive Tests

Note that the check for shallow anterior chamber tells you nothing about whether or not the patient might have glaucoma without a narrow-angle. In fact, it does not really detect narrow-angle glaucoma, but only the shallow anterior chamber that co-exists with nearly all cases of narrow-angle glaucoma. Thus, about 90% of all positives will be false positives for the disease since the test picks up all cases of central shallowing of the ante-

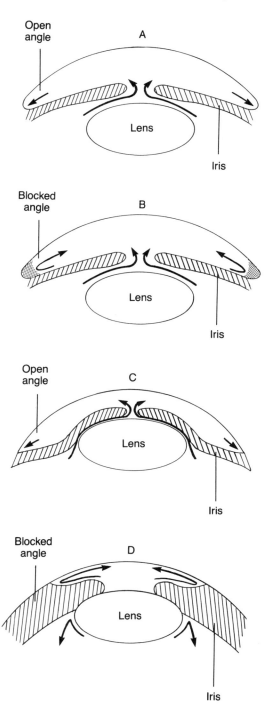

Figure 10-8. *A, A normal eye, showing the flow of the aqueous into the anterior chamber and thence egressing through the Canal of Schlemm in the angle. B, The common wide-angle or open-angle glaucoma showing the block at the egress from the anterior chamber. There is no anterior displacement of the lens and so the anterior chamber depth will be normal with this kind of glaucoma. C, Anterior displacement of the lens in senescence or in someone with a propensity to acute-angle glaucoma. D, Anterior displacement of the lens in someone developing an attack of acute-angle glaucoma following pupillary dilation. As the iris dilates, it occludes both the entrance of the fluid to the anterior chamber and its egress thence. Since the fluid continues to form, the pressure can only rise. Compare to C.*

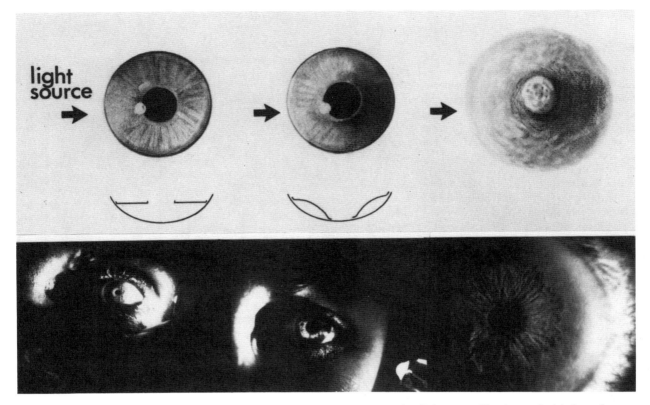

Figure 10-9.   *Method of checking the depth of the anterior chamber. In the top panel, a light source illuminates the iris from the temporal side. There is no shadow on the normal eye. The eye in the center demonstrates a positive test because of the anterior buckling of the lens and central iris (see the coronal section in the center of the top panel). On the right is a photograph of a nipple, for comparison. The bottom panel shows the following: left, a positive test on the left eye of a patient with untreated narrow angle glaucoma; center, a negative test on normal eye with a nevus on the nasal iris (not a shadow); right, a closeup of a positive test, provided by Dr. Eugene De Juan, Jr. of North Carolina. Courtesy of Year Book Medical Publishers.*

rior chamber, which is common in older persons with enlarged lenses. So, if the test is positive for a shallow anterior chamber, you *must* arrange for the intraocular pressure to be measured. If the pressure is normal, you may dilate the pupil. But if the pressure is high and the patient actually has narrow-angle glaucoma, he can be treated appropriately, with laser or surgical iridectomy, after which the pupil can be dilated with impunity.

Negative Tests

If the test is negative, I proceed to dilate the pupils. However, there are very rare false negatives for narrow-angle glaucoma. Therefore, because an attack of angle glaucoma could come hours later, all patients should be cautioned to be alert to the development of pain or blurred vision, and to call immediately should one of these supervene.

Screening for Glaucoma

Because the increase in intraocular pressure occurs long before the patient experiences any symptoms, and because the disease is so eminently treatable, screening for glaucoma is extremely important for preventive medicine. A 2-year study in which patients on a general medical service were screened by Schiotz tonometry (Fig. 10-10) revealed a 3.3% prevalence of glaucoma (Robertson, 1977). Unfortunately, tonometry is no longer ubiq-

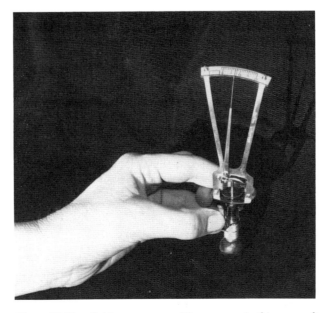

Figure 10-10.   *Schiotz tonometer. The pressure in this very soft grape is 10.2 mm Hg, corresponding to the scale reading of 8, according to the chart that comes with the instrument. Courtesy of Susan Edmiston of Arizona.*

uitous in the training and practice of all primary care physicians. A method for estimation and a comment on measurement follow.

Estimating the Intraocular Pressure

A Method

1. Have the patient close his eyes lightly.

2. Rest your hand on the patient's forehead and lightly press on the eyeball through the relaxed lid with one or two fingers. How does it compare with your own? Is it soft, like a ripe grape, or hard, like an unstuffed green olive with the seed still in place? The latter is abnormal and suggests one of the three forms of glaucoma. The former is usually normal, although extreme softness can also be a sign of advanced volume depletion.

3. As with all paired organs, you must check both sides, and compare them with each other. Some of the secondary forms of glaucoma may afflict only one eye.

Eyeball palpation is making a comeback in nursing homes, whose inhabitants may be unable to cooperate for tonometry. However, it is more often used to check for the soft eyeballs of dehydration than for the hard eyeballs of glaucoma.

This estimate cannot be performed with 100% confidence until one has accrued substantial experience, with feedback from actual tonometry readings.

Measuring the Intraocular Pressure

\$\$ Instructions for the use of the Schiotz tonometer will not be given here. They come with the instrument, which can be obtained at medical supply stores, or through a mail-order catalog. Formerly, medical students performed the test on each other, demonstrating that it was simple to perform, and painless.

In older patients, the Schiotz tonometer may give a falsely high reading due to scleral rigidity.

Today, most ophthalmologists prefer the use of applanation tonometry; however, that equipment is far more expensive and not available to the general physician.

•

A Pedagogic Note

Dr. Andy Lonigro of Missouri was visiting his sister, when his brother-in-law complained of blind spots.

"Then you better go directly to the doctor. This needs to be checked into immediately," advised Dr. Lonigro.

"Oh, I did. The doctor told me it was my contact lenses and that I should stop wearing them for awhile."

"I'd go see another doctor if I were you."

"Well, I did. And the second one told me the same thing."

"Look, you better go see an ophthalmologist."

"I did. They were both ophthalmologists."

"You mean optometrists?"

"No. They were both ophthalmologists, not optometrists."

Dr. Lonigro arranged for his brother to be examined, and an intraocular pressure of 60 mm Hg was found (the upper limit of normal being 20 mm).

This story illustrates two principles: 1) Good medicine does not require a giant intellect, but it does require thoroughness. 2) Certificates on the wall don't make diagnoses, physicians do.

•

Pupils

In the middle of the eye there is a hole which constricts with strong light and dilates with darkness. (Rhazes, 850–932)

Measuring Pupil Size

Pupil size should either be measured accurately, or not at all. If measurements are not made, one is restricted to describing the pupils as widely dilated, mid-position, or pinpoint. These descriptions are far too vague to be used as baseline points when attempting to assess changes over time or differences between the two pupils. (The descriptor "pinpoint" pupils tends to be used inaccurately for anything less than 2.5 mm. True pinpoint pupils are very rare, even in an overdose of a narcotic analgesic).

A Method

1. Photocopy Figure 10-11 and tape it to a piece of cardboard. Since some photocopy machines will change the scale a little bit, you might measure the size of the dots. (However, since you are usually interested only in differences, repeated use of the same inaccurate card will give precise* measurements.)

2. Hold the card next to the patient's iris, and move it up and down until the patient's pupil matches a black spot of the same

---

*As in physics, precision is defined by reproducibility, and accuracy by reference to an external standard.

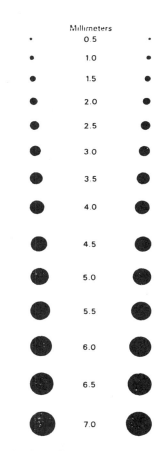

Millimeters
0.5
1.0
1.5
2.0
2.5
3.0
3.5
4.0
4.5
5.0
5.5
6.0
6.5
7.0

Figure 10-11. *Card pupillometer. See text for instructions for use. Courtesy of Excerpta Medica.*

size. With practice, you will easily be able to appreciate 0.5-mm gradations.

For comparisons to be meaningful, measurements must be made in the same amount of ambient light and with the same accommodation distance.

Pupillary dilatation of as little as 0.5 mm in response to injection of a narcotic antagonist, such as naloxone, is a legal definition of addiction in some states (Sapira & Cherubin, 1975). Pupil dilation from baseline can similarly be sought, for medical purposes, as evidence for precipitated abstinence when a patient is given naloxone in the emergency room.

Anisocoria

"Anisocoria" simply means inequality of the pupils. In addition to the "benign" and factitious causes given in Table 10-4, up to 20% of normal persons will have anisocoria (pupillary inequality ≥ 0.4 mm in *dim* light) at any given point in time (Lam et al., 1987).

If one requires that the pupillary inequality be 0.5 mm or more in bright light and that it be present more than once, there will be few cases of benign causes and relatively more bona fide cases detected.

In long practice, one will even see cases of bona fide anisocoria that last for days to weeks and then disappear. These benign cases do not have associated neurologic signs although they may produce anxiety when they occur among the neuroanatomically sophisticated. The best treatment is to be sent to a very old clinician.

Horner's Syndrome

Horner's syndrome consists of anisocoria (the smaller pupil homolateral to the lesion) plus unilateral (homolateral) enophthalmos, ptosis, anhidrosis, and decreased pilomotor response (see Table 10-5). (Also see Ch. 26, p. 451.)

A tumor in the superior sulcus (Pancoast's syndrome) can produce Horner's syndrome (most frequently on the left), in association with neurologic manifestations in the homolateral arm. The latter consist of sensory changes (paresthesia, hypesthesia, hyperesthesia, thermoanesthesia); autonomic changes (anhidrosis, decreased piloerection, warmth, digital dystrophy, and dependent cyanosis); and motor changes, including fibrillations, fasciculation, pseudo-ulnar signs (inability to oppose the thumb and little finger, with interosseus atrophy); and other muscle atrophy and weakness.

Pancoast was not the man who discovered the syndrome that bears his name, but the one who popularized it (Pancoast, 1932). The first case (Freeman, 1921) was described 3 years before Pancoast wrote his first paper (Pancoast, 1924). Most ironically, Pancoast was the radiologic consultant to that first case, and missed the diagnosis both prospectively and retrospectively! Table 10-4 is a modified differential diagnosis of the type described in Chapter 27, page 534. The entities are grouped under the processes that one might have originally encountered in pathology. Tables 10-4 and 10-5 illustrate another principle discussed in that chapter, the concept of levels. Once one has decided that the etiology of anisocoria is the Horner's syndrome, one is then forced to perform in turn the differential diagnosis of the latter. If one then diagnoses the Pancoast syndrome as the cause of Horner's, one might proceed even further to determine what type of superior sulcus tumor was involved.

Table 10-4.   Differential Diagnosis of Anisocoria on the Medical Service

| | The abnormal pupil is the one that is relatively | |
	Dilated	Constricted
Factitious and benign	Mydriatic in one eye Unilateral blindness Prosthetic eye Unequal lighting Ipsilateral unilateral cataract	Miotic in one eye Prosthetic eye Unequal lighting
Mechanical	Iris diseases, trauma, or aniridia Unilateral narrow-angle glaucoma	Posterior synechiae
Inflammatory	Uveitis	Uveitis Keratitis Tabes dorsalis
Vascular	Internal carotid insufficiency (or other anterior ocular segment ischemia) Aneurysm Carotid sinus thrombosis Subdural hematoma Epidural hematoma	
Neurologic	Pupillary sphincter paralysis Cerebral Encephalitis Neoplasms Other Infections Botulism Diphtheria Herpes zoster Syphilis Toxic Alcohol Lead Arsenic Others Diabetes	Midbrain lesion Horner's syndrome (see Table 10-5)

Sources: *Newell (1982) and Roy (1984).*

Pupillary Shape

The acronym PERRLA, found in the records of a bygone day, meant that the pupils had been examined for *equality* of size, *regularity* (or *roundness* of shape), *reactivity* to *light*, and *accommodation*. Abnormalities of shape are listed in Table 10-6; the important ones are set in boldface type.

Pupillary Responses

Pupillary Response to Light (Reaction)

The response to light is generally easy to test; it just involves shining a penlight into the patient's eyes. Check both the direct and the consensual response. (The consensual response is the constriction induced by shining the light in the opposite pupil.) On the routine examination, if both pupils react directly, a consensual response to light need only be observed in one pupil.

In patients with dark-brown eyes, it may be difficult, in the

Table 10-5. Differential Diagnosis of Horner's Syndrome

Congenital
Inflammatory
   Multiple sclerosis
   Other demyelinating diseases
Mechanical
   Syringomyelia
   Trauma
   Thyroid adenoma
   Mediastinal tumors
Vascular
   Posterior inferior cerebellar artery syndrome
   Internal carotid artery aneurysm
Neoplastic
   Brain-stem tumor
   Cervical cord tumor
   Neurofibromatosis
   Part of the Pancoast syndrome

Sources: *Newell (1982) and Roy (1984).*

dimly lit room, to discern the difference between the pupil and the iris.

A method. To get around this problem, illuminate the pupils stroboscopically at the rate of twice per second.

1. Stare at where the pupil will be and quickly sweep the penlight beam over the patient's eye while attending to the briefly illuminated pupil size.

2. On the first sweep, you will actually see the pupil *before* a response to the light, and on the second sweep, the normally reacting pupil will be smaller. (It is easier to see this way, because if the light is maintained on the pupil, the examiner must try to remember the original size of the pupil while watching it constrict.)

Sometimes, it is easier to see the pupil dilate after the light is removed than it was to see it constrict.

The consensual reflex can be tested in a similar manner:

1. Sweep past the test eye quickly for a baseline observation.

2. Shine the beam into the opposite eye for half a second (though not looking at *its* pupil, but rather keeping the baseline pupil in eye and in mind).

Table 10-6. Abnormalities of Pupillary Shape Seen on the Medical Service

Shape	Etiologies
Oval	**Neurosyphilis** **Glaucoma** (dilated) Congenital corectopia (eccentric) **Adie's Pupil** (dilated)
Pear-shaped	Postsurgery Old anterior synechiae Congenital coloboma **Neurologic Disease**
Scalloped	Rupture of the sphincter muscle **Amyloidosis**
Polygonal	**Neurosyphilis**
Other irregularity	**Argyll Robertson Pupil** **Posterior Synechiae,** especially after prior uveitis

Source: *Roy (1972).*

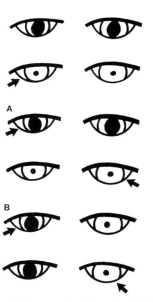

Figure 10-12. *In all the panels, the patient is looking at you. The top pair of eyes illustrates the baseline. The second pair of eyes shows the normal response. In all panels, the arrow indicates from which side the light is being shined. Write down your diagnoses for the conditions illustrated in situations A and B (answers in Appendix 10-1).*

3. Sweep the light back to the test eye to see if constriction has taken place.

Self-Test. To be sure you understand this section, do the self-test shown in Figure 10-12.

Marcus Gunn pupil. If the pupil of the test eye dilates when the penlight shines on it in step 3, then the consensual light reflex is more pronounced than the direct reflex. The patient is said to have a Marcus Gunn pupil or a positive "swinging flashlight test."

This apparently paradoxical reaction to light is really due to the fact that the affected side has an intact motor system but a defective sensory system (i.e., there is an afferent pupillary defect in the eye that dilates with direct illumination [Miller, 1985]). The affected eye's normal efferent response is seen with the light shining on the contralateral eye. (The sign can also be elicited by covering the normal side.)

The Marcus Gunn pupil is seen in any unilateral disease of the retina or optic nerve (e.g., retrobulbar optic neuritis or ipsilateral monocular blindness).

Pupillary Accommodation

To test for accommodation, have the patient look at something a long distance away, then focus on something just in front of his eyes, such as your finger or a pencil. Constriction is the normal response to the near object.

Importance of Pupillary Responses

We check the pupillary responses because the loss of accommodation, reaction to light, or consensual reaction is indicative of ocular or nervous system disease (Table 10-7).

The converse can also be helpful. If a patient has total loss of vision in both eyes, the pupillary reactions to light should be appro-

Table 10-7.   Abnormal Pupils

Name	Size/Shape	Accommodation	Reaction	Laterality	Comments
Argyll Robertson	Usually miotic Possibly irregular	Normal	Absent (late) Sluggish (early)	95% bilateral	Formally usually CNS lues (Also see Table 10-8) Incomplete dilation with atropine
Adie's tonic pupil	Not always miotic	Absent or sluggish	Absent or sluggish	80% unilateral	Never CNS lues Tendon jerks may be absent Methacholine constricts; normal response to mydriatics
Fixed		Absent	Absent	Unilateral or bilateral	Meningovascular syphilis or blindness
Paradoxical			Dilates		Seen in CNS syphilis, tumors, and "normals"
Paradoxical		Dilates	Normal		Same as above
Horner's	Miotic			Unilateral	Seen in Pancoast's syndrome, inter alia
Parinaud	Never miotic	Variable (see p. 455)	Sluggish	99% bilateral	Never benign; seen with Parinaud's syndrome

Sources: *Duke-Elder and Scott (1971) and Maciewicz (1983).*

priately missing. See the section on ocular malingering or hysteria, page 155.

However, one should not be too quick to diagnose ocular malingering. I was once presented a patient who claimed adult-onset total blindness, but in whom the pupillary direct and consensual responses to light were both well preserved. The house officer had failed to examine the fundi. The patient had bilateral macular degeneration and was for all intents and purposes legally blind. But the surrounding retinal tissues were normal, accounting for the normal light reflexes.

Fixed dilated pupils are a well-known sign of brain stem disease. Less well known are the fixed pupils that fail to dilate in the dark. These are also an ominous indicator of brain stem disease.

In increased intracranial pressure, there is a loss of hippus (the one-per-second pupillary dilation–constriction sequence), even before the gross light response is lost.

Argyll Robertson Pupil

The Argyll Robertson pupil is likened to a woman of easy virtue: it accommodates, but doesn't react. The Argyll Robertson pupil is never benign. It is seen in central nervous system syphilis, and in other conditions (Table 10-8).

For purposes of winning coffee money from those who believe there was a Dr. Argyll, the full name of the one physician who is commemorated in the Argyll Robertson pupil is Douglas Moray Cooper Lamb Argyll Robertson. A more complete description than the one in the table above was given in his case reports (Robertson, 1869a, 1869b). An even better explication of the Argyll Robertson pupil was made by Adie (who has a different pupil named for him).

1. The retina is quite sensitive; that is, the vision is intact. This is important because the pupil of the blind eye in many unilaterally blind patients accommodates but does not react to light; that alone does not make it an Argyll Robertson pupil. The pupil of a blind eye may react consensually, whereas the true Argyll Robertson pupil never does (Adie, 1931b). Similarly, if the vision is defective from some other cause than retinal disease, some reaction to light will persist as long as any vision remains. Such pupils react sluggishly to light, but well to convergence (accommodation). However, this should *not* be called "incomplete" Argyll Robertson pupil, for the

blindness and pupillary changes in this situation have nothing to do with central nervous system syphilis.

2. The Argyll Robertson pupil contracts briskly during accommodation and dilates again briskly if the subject again looks far away.

3. Alteration in the amount of light admitted to the eye does not influence the size of the pupil. Therefore, the Argyll Robertson pupil is fixed, not in the sense that it exhibits pupil atonia, but in that it can remain the same size for days, weeks, or months.

4. Slow and only partial dilation occurs with the application of mydriatics.

Table 10-8.   Other Causes of Argyll Robertson Pupils

Tumors
  Mesencephalic location
  Craniopharyngioma

Infections and inflammation
  Encephalitis lethargica
  Polio encephalitis
  Cerebral malaria
  Herpes zoster
  Lyme disease

Metabolic causes
  Diabetes mellitus
  Alcoholism
  Carbon disulfide poisoning

Other
  Syringomyelia
  Pressure on cranial nerve III trunk by cerebral aneurysm!
  Trauma
  Multiple sclerosis
  Hypertropic interstitial neuritis
  Charcot-Marie-Tooth disease
  Sarcoid
  Hemorrhage in the periacqueductal gray rostral to the Edinger-Westphal nucleus

Sources: *Duke-Elder and Scott (1971) and Dacso and Bortz (1989).*

Adie's Pupil

The tonic pupil, or Adie's pupil, may be described as a bored housewife: it may neither react nor accommodate, or it may react only after a great deal of preparation in a dark room; in any case, it will be sluggish. The Adie's pupil is always benign, unless the physician can't make the diagnosis, and erroneously diagnoses syphilis. To continue the mnemonic, one would expect to find more syphilis in women of easy virtue than in housewives.

Adie's pupil was originally described by a number of other people, but we credit Adie for bringing these descriptions together (Adie, 1931a). In the initial six cases, the pupils were said to "react on accommodation but not to light." As ankle jerks and knee jerks were missing in most of the original cases, it was thought that these patients might be syphilitic, a fear that was disproved by testing. A few months later, Adie had correctly refined his pupil description as follows (Adie, 1931b):

1. The myotonic pupil is most often unilateral; it is then almost always larger than its mate.

2. It may be oval, with the long axis either horizontal or vertical.

3. It is often large, occasionally small, but never miotic.

4. When ordinary bedside methods are used, the reaction to light, direct and consensual, appears to be completely or almost completely abolished. However, after a sojourn in a dark room, the pupil dilates, and on reexposure to strong daylight again contracts very slowly. The emphasis is on a long exposure to diffuse strong daylight after proper preparation in a dark room.

5. During the act of accommodation for a near object (convergence), the pupil after a short delay would began to contract very slowly but through a range in excess of normal. This originally larger (abnormal) pupil could thus end as smaller than the normal pupil on the opposite side! With convergence, the abnormal pupil might remain small for seconds to minutes after convergence has ceased.

6. However, prompt and full dilatation occurs with those mydriatics, cocaine and atropine, which are so stunted in their effect on the Argyll Robertson pupil.

An odd additional finding has been rediscovered regarding the Adie's pupil. In every Adie's pupil that has any remaining light reaction, a segmental palsy of the iris sphincter will be found. This is characteristic of Adie's pupil, though not pathognomonic, since it can also be seen in traumatic iridoplegia, postganglionic denervation, preganglionic third-nerve diseases, aberrant regeneration of the third nerve, midbrain ocular motor involvement, and Parinaud's syndrome if that occurs posttrauma (Thompson, 1978).

Other Abnormal Pupils

Sluggish responses to light and accommodation are sometimes seen in myotonic dystrophy (Duke-Elder & Scott, 1971).

Among the British who were caught in the fall of Singapore and interned during World War II, Wernicke's encephalopathy was said to produce the loss of accommodation, with a normal light response. This would be the reverse of an Argyll Robertson pupil.

The Ophthalmoscopic Examination (Sapira, 1984)

History

In 1847, Babbage, an eccentric British millionaire, had one of his engineers construct a device consisting of a silvered surface (a mirror) that reflected light into the eye. A scratch in the silvered surface permitted one to peek for the first time into the illuminated interior of the living eye. Babbage gave the device to his personal physician, who never realized its utility, apparently because Babbage was a known practical joker and because the physician, who was myopic, found that Babbage's device, lacking a lens system, did not work for him. Three years later, apparently independently, Helmholtz used the same principles, added a lens system, and published his invention.

The ophthalmoscope used today is basically the same as that of Helmholtz, except that the light source is battery operated and the lens system is mounted on a wheel, which permits rapid focusing.

Method

Parts of the Ophthalmoscope

$$ Before attempting to look through the ophthalmoscope, it is a good idea to learn its component parts. First, switch on the light. If your ophthalmoscope has a rheostat, push in the button that unlocks the rheostat and rotate it to maximum brightness. Smaller ophthalmoscopes simply have an on-off switch.

If you are holding the instrument properly (with the diopter numbers pointing toward you, the light shining *away* from you), you will be able to shine the light on your palm. If you move the aperture selector dial, which usually lies between the lens wheel and the on-off rheostat, you can observe various shapes and colors of light. Under normal circumstances, you will use the round circle of white light. Some ophthalmoscopes have a second smaller circle, which decreases the amount of light. This may be used to decrease the amount of reflex pupillary constriction in the unusual circumstance that the pupils have not been pharmacologically dilated. Sometimes it is also useful to decrease reflected glare from the cornea and anterior lens. Some older ophthalmoscopes had an aperture that produced a half-moon of light that could be used for the same purpose. But the best device to reduce glare is a little window of polarizing glass, mounted on the part of the ophthalmoscope head facing the patient, which can be slid into place with a flick of the finger. (Some students do not even realize that their ophthalmoscopes are so equipped.)

The grids are intended for localization, but are rarely used because of the common custom of describing lesions in terms of distance from the disc along radial coordinates (e.g., "1½ disc diameters out at 8 o'clock, "3 disc diameters at 12 o'clock," etc.). Lesions may also be located in terms of their relationship to specific retinal vessels and their branchings, and in some cases a drawing in the chart is used.

Most ophthalmoscopes also have a bluish-green filter that provides "red-free" light. (This is *not* the lens used in fluorescein angiography, a special procedure performed only by those trained in its use. Specifically, one should *never* try to improvise any fluorescein examination of the eye that involves shining an ultraviolet light into the eye, since this could cause blindness.) Some experts can make judgments about retinal arteriolar medial and adventitial thickening by using the "red-free" light (see p. 187). It has also been stated that "red-free" light is helpful in finding hemorrhages, which will appear black on a green field. However, hemorrhages generally appear dark red on a light orange field and are easy to see in any case. Missed hemorrhages result from a failure to look systematically, not from the color of the light.

Red-free light is also said to be useful for identifying early neovascularization (fine vessels) in patients with diabetes mellitus, since it changes the red-on-orange contrast to black-on-green. Some skilled workers are also able to make estimates about damage to the outer nerve fiber layer based upon inspection with the red-free light. Other uses of red-free light are discussed on page 187.

Finally, there is an aperture that casts the light as a slit. This aperture provides a means for determining fundal contour, and for estimating the depth of the anterior chamber (see p. 167). This is not the light used in a slit-lamp examination. That is a special instrument used by ophthalmologists for studying the lens, Descemet's membrane, and other anterior structures.

It is often very difficult to use the slit aperture for determining the contour of the optic disc, because if one looks at the stripe directly *en face,* monocular vision may not permit the appreciation of any contour. Sometimes, one can move one's eye laterally, still peering through the viewing area, and so create an angle between the axis of inspection and the axis of illumination. The most frequent reason for wanting a measure of elevation is in the question of a "choked disc," or papilledema. But for this purpose the slit is inferior to measuring the elevation of the disc in diopters, which is a useful way to follow the progress of papilledema (or its resolution with treatment) on a day-to-day basis. This requires focusing on the disc with the ophthalmoscope, rather than with your eye (vide infra).

The other dial on the ophthalmoscope is used for changing the lenses, from high positive (magnifying), usually numbered in black, to high negative, usually numbered in red.

For the attending.   Some persons can do much of the focusing with the lens in their own eye, but use of the focusing wheel should be encouraged. The autofocusing ability is one more thing for the student to have to master initially, and it will eventually be lost with age.

Finally, when you have finished using your ophthalmoscope, don't forget to switch it off. In the case of an ophthalmoscope with a rheostat, you must rotate the dial to the point at which you hear or feel a click. Otherwise your batteries will often be drained, producing a light that is too dim. Although the rheostat, like the smaller peephole, is advertised as a method of decreasing the light in sensitive patients, it is just one more thing that can break, and it increases the cost of the instrument. I don't remember when I last tried to use mine; probably before I finally learned that one sees best with a bright light and that most compromises in clinical examination are to be eschewed.

Practicing with the Ophthalmoscope

Instruct your partner to remove his spectacles and to stare at a fixed distant point. Remove your own spectacles, and select the round circle of white light. (You may wish to examine the patient through his spectacles if he wears a highly "minus" set of lenses. Likewise, if either member of the doctor-patient dyad has a distorting abnormality of the lens, such as a severe astigmatism, leave the spectacles on for the examination that involves the abnormal eye.)

○ *Very advanced.*   Bifocals are an especially difficult problem for physicians with severe astigmatism. The near lenses cannot be used because of the angle, but taking the glasses off leaves the astigmatism uncorrected. If you anticipate this problem, save your last pair of glasses before getting the bifocals, and try using them only during ophthalmoscopy.

To examine your partner's right eye, place the ophthalmoscope as close as possible to your own right eye, peer through the hole, and shine the light into your partner's right pupil until you see the red reflex. Repeat, using your left eye to observe the red reflex in your partner's left eye. It is very important to learn to use the correct eye (i.e., both of your eyes), even if you have a strong monocular dominance. Otherwise, you will have to hang over the top of the patient's head to examine one of his eyes, a contortion not always permitted by the clinical situation or hospital architecture.

For the next step, it is best to use a teaching device such as an artificial eye or mannequin. If your school does not have such a device, volunteers should be solicited from the Curriculum Committee. In either case, begin examining the dummy by finding the red reflex as before. Next, move as close to the eye as you can, all the while keeping the red reflex in view through the ophthalmoscope. Turn the lens wheel until detail begins to appear. If you go too far, back up by reversing the lens wheel, just as you would with a microscope.

Looking into the eye with an ophthalmoscope is, in fact, looking through an in vivo microscope. (The optic disc in reality is only 1.5 mm in diameter, although it appears larger through the ophthalmoscope. The relative sizes of other structures and lesions are given in Table 10-9.) The main difference is that the traditional microscope focuses continuously, and the ophthalmoscope lens wheel discontinuously. Similarly, when you first looked through a microscope, you learned, perhaps unconsciously, to relax your eye so as to look *through* the lens toward a point beyond it, rather than accommodating so as to look *at* the lens as if it were a small television set. Now, in using the ophthalmoscope, also allow your eye to adjust grossly to the different focal length needed to approach the fundus. Don't look *at* the lens; look *through* it. Then, perform the fine-focus adjustment with the focusing wheel on the instrument. (Some persons like to shift their own viewpoint slightly during the procedure. If they then see something red flash by, they know it is a blood vessel, and this gives them a target to focus on.)

Once you are able to focus on structures of the fundus, return to your partner. (Later you should go back to the mannequin to practice examining the four vascular axes, as described below).

When you are first practicing, but only then, you may omit the examination of the cornea and the lens (see pp. 176–177). Your partner is presumably a healthy young person with no opacities there. Just find the red reflex, and focus in.

Some hints include the following:

1. You should be cheek to jowl with your partner. As in looking through a keyhole or a window, you must be as close as possible.
2. You may want to hold the partner's head from behind with your left hand.

Table 10-9.   Size of Various Structures and Lesions in the Fundus Oculi

Optic disc	1.5 mm
Width of the arterial blood column exiting the disc	0.1 mm (100 μm)
Average microaneurysm	0.05 mm (50 μm)
Average Drüsen[a]	0.01 mm (10 μm)

[a]*Drüsen can go to 100 μm and beyond.*

3. Are you in a comfortable position? If your partner is sitting, and you are standing crouched over him, you are learning a habit that will give you low back strain in later years. Worse, it is hard to concentrate on the examination, if you are also concentrating on keeping your balance.

4. The subject needs a fixed object to look at with his unobstructed eye.

For the attending. In yesteryear, one of the better institutions had little penciled "x's" marked on the ceilings of rooms where generations of house staff had examined the fundi. Once, in a new institution, the department chairman instructed the house staff not to so mark the ceilings, because the cost of painting them was allegedly causing the hospital to run a deficit. Later, I cared for a patient whose proliferative diabetic retinopathy had become irreversible under that chairman's "tight," nonophthalmoscopic control.

I always attempted to examine the fundi at least once when I was a visiting professor. I would ask someone to hold up a finger for the patient to look at. If, after a few seconds, the patient's eye began to wander, I checked to see if the host's finger was still in place. When it was not, I knew that the fundi were examined so infrequently that the average participant in rounds did not even understand the need for a fixed point of gaze. This occurred much more often than accrediting agencies lead one to believe.

Once you have focused on a vessel, follow the natural arrows formed by the branchings of the blood vessels to find the disc (Fig. 10-13). Then follow the vessels away from the disc in this sequence, returning to the disc each time: superior temporal vessels, superior nasal vessels, inferior nasal vessels, and inferior temporal vessels. (If you are unable to do this with your partner, you need more practice on the mannequin.) Then, without leaving the view, see if you can change the aperture, finding the control wheel with your finger without looking at it. (Most people have to practice this on the mannequin also.) Repeat the procedure with your left eye, examining your partner's left eye.

O It is very important to establish, from the beginning, a methodical sequence of examination, which you adhere to as rigidly and

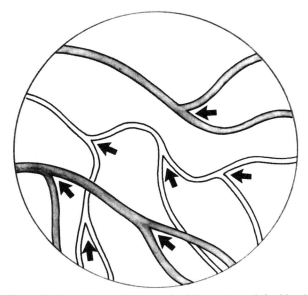

Figure 10-13. *A law of nature: the bifurcations of the blood vessels always form arrows that point to the optic disc. Courtesy of Year Book Medical Publishers.*

thoroughly as possible. Once you have practiced finding the disc and following the blood vessels, you can begin using the entire routine, given on page 176.

Dilating the Pupil

An illustration of how I made myself look stupid by not dilating the pupils is given on page 195. (Also see Appendix 10-4.)

Contraindications. There are few contraindications to dilating the pupils. 1) The most important one is presence or suspicion of a cerebrovascular or other neurologic disease, in which evolving pupillary signs might be of diagnostic value. (Remember that the effects of the medication may persist for a variable length of time, and that asymmetry of the pupils may result, even if you are careful to put the same number of drops in each eye.) 2) Certain lens implants are an absolute contraindication to pupillary dilatation. 3) Anterior uveitis is a *relative* contraindication. 4) As mentioned above (p. 167), if the patient has *narrow-angle* glaucoma, dilating the pupil could precipitate an acute attack. If that results in an earlier diagnosis of the problem, the patient might ultimately benefit, provided that the physician is capable of recognizing and treating it.

A method (Practice first on yourself and your partner):

$$ 1. Be sure that your black bag is supplied with a mydriatic agent. I have used 10% phenylephrine (Neosynephrine ophthalmic) for 30 years without difficulty. However, if I were starting over today, I might choose tropicamide 0.5% or 1% (Mydriacil ophthalmic) instead.

There is no doubt that these medications are absorbed systemically. Because much of the absorption seems to be via the nasal mucosa (as a result of tearing, with passage of the drug through the nasolacrimal duct), the problem can be minimized by having the patient press on the inner canthi to block the ducts for a few minutes after instillation.

Phenylephrine, an alpha-1 adrenergic agonist, has been associated with hypertension, presumably causing an intracerebral hemorrhage in one adult case (Adler et al., 1982). The ocular effects can be reversed with thymoxamine (if you live where it is available) or any other ophthalmic alpha blocker. You could use phentolamine or prazosin as specifics to reverse systemic effects, but in most cases one would simply let the drug wear off.

Tropicamide, a very short-acting antimuscarinic agent, might be preferable in a patient in whom you are worried about cardiovascular reactions. However, it occasionally fails to produce a brisk pupillary dilation. In one instance, it caused a systemic reaction of opisthotonos, pallor, and cyanosis in a child, presumably due to anaphylaxis (Wahl, 1969). The ocular effects can be reversed with pilocarpine ophthalmic solution.

2. With the patient seated, have him maximally extend his head on the neck, and instruct him to stare at the ceiling. If the patient is recumbent, have him stare at the head of the bed.

3. Hold the dropper of mydriatic solution about 1 inch above the conjunctival sac, so that it does not touch the globe, the skin, or even (especially) the eyelashes.

4. Pull down on the subpalpebral skin, and drop one drop into the conjunctival sac, not onto the globe. (Once the skin under your finger has been rolled down over the general area of the maxillary zygomatic bony suture, firm pressure will hold the eye open in such a way as to maintain painless exposure of the conjunctival sac against the patient's best efforts. Try it on yourself.)

5. Rarely, if the patient is uncooperative and has long upper lashes, one may rarely have to resort to dropping the fluid on the globe, which may be further exposed by pulling the upper lid superiorly away from the globe. Simply press on the skin above the supraorbital bone, and roll the skin superiorly until the eyeball is exposed. Then press your finger more firmly so that the eye cannot be closed.

6. *Make a note in the record*, especially if you dilate unilaterally. This may save the patient an investigation for neurologic causes of a "blown pupil" when someone else makes rounds at night.

7. If sufficient dilatation has not occurred after 10 minutes, instill a second drop.

Methods for Improving Patient Cooperation

During the ophthalmoscopic examination, some patients will close their eyes or abruptly turn their heads away just when you think you have found something of interest. They may say, "The light is too bright." How should you respond in a situation like that? (Write your answer down.)

Obviously, you should not say, "It's not bright," since it isn't shining into *your* eye. Nor should you lecture the patient about the difficulty he is causing you. Also, you should not give up, since that is unfair to both the present and future patients.

You can smile at the patient and say, "I know it's bright. I'll turn it down a little." Turn it to a smaller aperture or try the red-free light. You may wish to add, "But it still may be bright for you, so try to stare at the spot as long as you can. You are doing a good job."

Neophytes tend to blame problems on themselves, often correctly. Sometimes they wantonly sweep the light back and forth over the macula before they even have a chance to orient themselves topographically, and the patient is naturally troubled by the repeated macular stimulation. To avoid hitting the macula early, while you are "going in," approach the patient's pupil from the temporal side, rather than directly from the front.

Synopsis of Routine Ophthalmoscopic Examination

This section gives an overview of the order of the examination, and the general observations to be made. The remainder of the chapter is concerned with the ophthalmoscopic findings and their significance, and with specific techniques as they relate to specific findings.

1. *Checking for anterior (corneal and lenticular) opacities.* This part of the examination is done first because it informs us about those central opacities that interfere with subsequent examination of the fundus oculi. When the retinal structures are in focus, the obstructing opacity cannot be in focus and therefore is not seen. The examiner who is not aware of this will become confused and frustrated by the seemingly inexplicable difficulty experienced in visualizing a relatively large area of the fundus.

A method: After the red reflex is obtained, with the examining eye and ophthalmoscope held at 2 or 3 feet from the patient's eye, focus on the iris to ascertain that you are in the approximate focal plane of the cornea and lens. Returning your attention to the red reflex, move your head slightly, looking for sharp black opacities to appear in front of the red reflex. You may also focus up and down a few lens settings.

The better mannequins have plastic devices that mimic anterior opacities. These can be inserted, and you can practice looking for them.

2. One can next examine the vitreous for opacities and abnormal structures, as an ophthalmologist does. However, this is rarely useful in an asymptomatic patient and almost never produces useful information about the medical condition of the nonophthalmologic patient, except in the case of vitreous hemorrhages (p. 198), which are almost impossible to miss, even if one is not looking for them. Therefore, most diagnosticians proceed from the anterior structures directly to the fundus.

3. *Focusing on the fundus.* Once you have located the optic disc, there are several features for which you must consciously look. Note the color, the size of the optic cup, the presence or absence of papilledema, and the presence or absence of retinal vein pulsations (p. 178). While following the blood vessels in the sequence previously given (superior temporal, superior nasal, inferior nasal, inferior temporal), observe the arteriovenous crossings (p. 186), the retinal background (p. 183), and the size and appearance of the vessels themselves. Then swing from the disc temporally about 2 disc diameters to find the macula, which is examined last because it is the most uncomfortable for the patient. The macula is the best place to look for microaneurysms and hard exudates. Do not forget to examine the macula itself (p. 198). It is somewhat darker than the surrounding retina. At its center is the fovea centralis, which may appear as a small circle with a reddish center, a spot of light, a shifting crescent, a shining line, or a moiré pattern. Small vessels appear to converge toward the macula, but not to actually enter it.

If the patient does not have cataracts, and one still can't clearly see the fundus, have the patient put on his spectacles and repeat the examination; the problem may be a severe astigmatism.

Finally, repeat this sequence for the other eye.

A philosophical note. For some reason, the most dramatic findings in the fundus, such as choroidal sclerosis (p. 191) and large black areas due to burned-out chorioretinitis (p. 192) are never really urgent or acute, while the most ominous findings, for example, splinter hemorrhages appearing around the disc (p. 197), loss of spontaneous retinal venous pulsations (p. 178), posterior pole Drüsen in beginning senile macular degeneration (p. 194), and microaneurysms and exudates in preproliferative diabetic retinopathy (p. 201), tend to be quite subtle in appearance. (See Appendix 10-4).

Ophthalmoscopic Findings

Findings in the Anterior Part of the Eyeball

Opacities of the Cornea

Interstitial keratitis. While looking for the lens, one can sometimes see a haze in the cornea, obscuring the view of the iris. This sign of interstitial keratitis can often be detected by a clinician (although that diagnosis usually requires the special techniques of an ophthalmologist.) Sometimes new vessel formation occurs in the healing process, resulting in salmon colored patches.

Interstitial keratitis was formerly seen along with two other signs—labyrinthine deafness and Hutchinson's notched incisors—in congenital syphilis (Hutchinson, 1859). However, the other two signs, in the absence of the characteristic teeth, may be acquired in the adult as part of Cogan's syndrome (Vollerstein et al., 1986). The above instances of keratitis are bilateral. However, unilateral, isolated keratitis may rarely occur due either to acquired (not congenital) syphilis or tuberculosis.

Posterior keratoprecipitates. These round gray spots on the posterior cornea are also called mutton fat bodies. Contrary to popular wisdom, posterior keratoprecipitates, though seen in some cases of ocular sarcoidosis, are not pathognomonic. They may also be seen in the retinopathies of candidiasis (Chumbley, 1981), toxoplasmosis (Havener, 1973; Schlaegel, 1978), cyto-megalovirus (Chumbley, 1981), tuberculosis, brucellosis (Scheie & Albert, 1977), Entamoeba histolytica brain abscess (Walsh & Hoyt, 1969), and Boutonneuse fever (Rickettsia conori) (Lebas & Bernaerts-Lebas, 1962). In fact, if searched for, they would probably be found in many other retinopathies and uveitides.

Opacities in the Lens

Cataracts are the most common finding on ophthalmoscopic examination of the anterior eyeball. They may actually be more of a problem for the physician than for the patient. If the cataract is impairing the patient's vision, he should be referred.

Anterior capsular cataracts (indicated by A in Fig. 10-14A) and corneal opacities can be distinguished from posterior capsular opacities (indicated by P in Fig. 10-14A). Look through the ophthalmoscope and through a theoretical point in the center of the lens. Then, instruct the patient to look upward as you continue to maintain a line of sight through the center of the lens (not the globe). This will require you to tilt your line of sight somewhat upward (not shown). Anterior opacities will tend to move up, and posterior opacities down (Fig. 10-14B).

Ectopic Lens

A simple check for ectopic lens is to examine the red reflex with a penlight. In ectopic lens, there will be an incomplete appearance in the form of an ellipsoid below where one expected the full circle of light, somewhat as if a light shade of concave inferior surface had been pulled down halfway across the pupil (Chan et al., 1987).

Ectopic lens occurs in patients with Marfan's syndrome inter alia (see Ch. 25, p. 441).

Anterior Chamber Depth

Another method of estimating anterior chamber depth (see also p. 167) uses the slit aperture on the ophthalmoscope. Shine the light so that you can see the slit reflected from both the cornea and the lens, and observe the distance between the two reflections. In order to be able to judge that a chamber is abnormally narrow, you will have to have examined a number of normal eyes. Myopic patients tend to have deep anterior chambers.

The Vitreous

The major vitreous finding is vitreous hemorrhage (see p. 198). Another, unexpected finding that may interfere with the examiner's view is asteroides hyalosis ("planet-like structures that are glassy"), which are white or yellowish-white spheres made of calcium containing compounds. These are primarily seen in men of middle age. Oddly enough, they do not impair the patient's vision as much as they impair the physician's inspection, so a complaint of visual impairment should prompt a search for another entity.

Asteroides hyalosis may be mimicked by other diseases which produce a "snowstorm in the vitreous" and which are of significance. These include the ophthalmologic diseases pars planitis (a peripheral uveitis) and retinoblastoma; "medical" diseases such as Behçet's syndrome and sarcoid; or any severe form of uveitis (Roy, 1984).

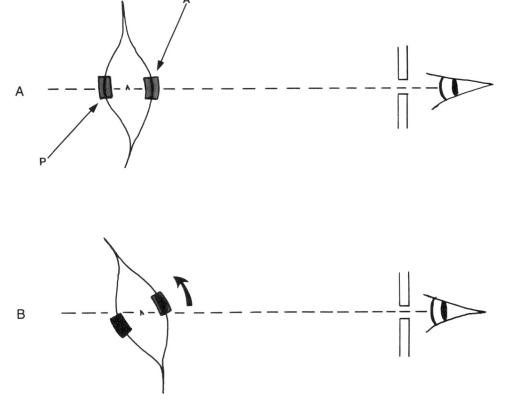

Figure 10-14. *Distinguishing anterior and posterior lenticular opacities. See text.*

The Disc

Spontaneous Retinal Venous Pulsations

A method.   Look at the largest retinal veins as they course up from the cup of the disc. A momentary tapering or flickering may be seen in the portion of the vein that is almost parallel to the axis of inspection. Retinal venous pulsations are probably never seen in the peripheral venous tree beyond the disc.

Digital compression of the eyeball may elicit retinal venous pulsations in some normal persons who do not initially have them. This may be done for teaching and learning purposes, but it should never be part of a patient examination, for it may produce a false sense of security, as explained below.

Physiology.   As shown schematically in Figure 10-15A, there is normally a pressure differential between the intraocular pressure and the retinal venous pressure, the latter obviously being higher (or the veins would empty and not be seen). During systole, the pulse pressure is briefly transmitted to the intraocular pressure through the expansion of the retinal artery, and this may permit the intraocular pressure briefly to exceed the retinal venous pressure. At that moment, the retinal veins begin to *collapse.* As the retinal artery pressure peaks and then drops, the intraocular pressure also drops to normal, allowing *reexpansion* of the retinal vein to its customary diameter. This is seen as retinal vein "pulsation."

If the retinal artery is sclerosed and does not transmit pressure well by expansion, retinal venous pulsations may be absent (even with normal retinal venous pressures). This may explain the fact that the incidence of spontaneous retinal venous pulsations decreases with age (Lo Zito, 1977).

An increase in retinal venous pressure will cause the loss of spontaneous retinal venous pulsations, all other things being equal (see Fig. 10-16). In cases of increased intracranial pressure, the retinal venous pressure is elevated because the retinal veins traverse the subarachnoid space surrounding the optic nerve. "Nonspontaneous" retinal venous pulsations (Fig. 10-16C), elicited by pressing on the patient's eyeball, could give a false sense of

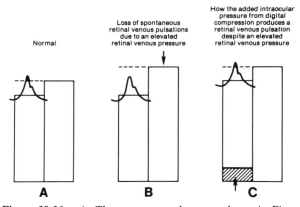

Figure 10-16.   *A, The same normal eye as shown in Figure 10-15. B, Loss of spontaneous retinal venous pulsations due to the pathologic increase in the retinal venous pressure. C, "Nonspontaneous" retinal venous pulsations inappropriately elicited by means of finger pressure on the eyeball. This should not be done in clinical practice. Courtesy of Year Book Medical Publishers.*

security prior to performing a lumbar puncture. Therefore, this maneuver is contraindicated.

Experimental evidence.   The relationships diagrammed in Figures 10-15 and 10-16 have been experimentally studied in humans. In all of 50 patients with spontaneous retinal venous pulsations, the intracranial pressure was less than 195 mm water (Kahn & Cherry, 1950). In all 18 patients with intracranial pressures greater than 195 mm water, spontaneous retinal venous pulsations were absent. In another experiment, 10 subjects with spontaneous retinal venous pulsations underwent lumbar puncture. The highest opening pressure was 170 mm water. The cerebrospinal fluid pressure was acutely raised with a digital Queckenstedt maneuver, and the cerebrospinal fluid pressures at which the spontaneous retinal venous pulsations disappeared, and then returned, were observed. The respective means were 204 and 202 mm water, and the highest individual value was 236 mm (Walsh et al., 1968). A study of 400 consecutive neurology consultations in which 65 lumbar punctures were performed revealed no spontaneous retinal venous pulsations in any of the 19 patients with opening pressures greater than 200 mm water. In the 22 patients who had spontaneous retinal venous pulsations, the highest cerebrospinal fluid opening pressure was exactly 200 mm water (Lo Zito, 1977). In still another study, 180 mm water was the highest opening cerebrospinal fluid pressure in 29 patients with spontaneous retinal venous pulsations, and in nine patients with increased cerebrospinal fluid pressures, the spontaneous retinal venous pulsations disappeared at 190 mm water (Levin, 1978).

The evidence cited above would suggest that 180 to 205 mm water is the general level of cerebrospinal fluid pressure above which one would not expect to see spontaneous retinal venous pulsations. A single letter to the editor (Van Uitert & Eisenstadt, 1978) reported four patients with opening cerebrospinal fluid pressures of 210 to 280 mm water despite the presence of spontaneous retinal venous pulsations. Unfortunately, the letter does not state how many total patients were seen in order to collect these four. These lumbar punctures were uncomplicated as were two others of the same nature (unreported) of which I have heard.

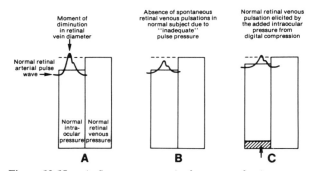

Figure 10-15.   *A, Spontaneous retinal venous pulsations occur in this normal eye during the brief moment that the intraocular pressure plus the transmitted arterial pressure exceed the normal retinal venous pressure. B, Spontaneous retinal venous pulsations do not occur in this normal eye because the normal retinal venous pressure is always greater than the sum of the normal intraocular pressure plus the transmitted arterial pressure. C, "Nonspontaneous" retinal venous pulsations can be brought out, for pedagogic purposes only, in the normal eye by finger pressure on the eyeball. This maneuver artificially increases the intraocular pressure to a point at which the addition of the transmitted arterial pressure is now sufficient to briefly exceed the normal retinal venous pressure. Courtesy of Year Book Medical Publishers.*

○ *Significance.*   In summary, the presence of spontaneous (without digital compression) retinal venous pulsations suggests that the cerebrospinal fluid pressure is unlikely to be elevated. The absence of spontaneous retinal venous pulsations is of no diagnostic utility.

For the attending. Because spontaneous retinal venous pulsations are synchronous with the heartbeat and dependent upon the stroke volume, they may be lost or irregular in conditions in which the stroke volume is not constant, for example, atrial fibrillation or atrioventricular dissociation. Although cardiac monitors have removed much of the suspense from the bedside examination of patients, they also give one the opportunity to confound the unsuspecting ignorant by describing to them the events on the monitor as you look into the patient's eye, with the monitor outside your range of vision. This maneuver is commended to you as a way to obtain wager money to help pay for this text.

Spontaneous retinal venous pulsations are also helpful in distinguishing *diabetic papillopathy*, in which they are present (Barr et al., 1980; Pavan et al., 1980), from papilledema due to increased intracranial pressure, in which they are absent. This is an important issue since many diabetic patients also have hypertension, and the diabetic hemorrhages and exudates, in the presence of swelling of the disc (vide infra), could suggest malignant hypertension, unless spontaneous venous pulsations are observed.

However, while the presence of spontaneous venous pulsations tells you that the cerebrospinal fluid pressure is currently low enough to permit lumbar puncture, theoretically it does not guarantee the absence of brain edema. The sine wave of intracranial pressure might just happen to be at a normal trough value at the moment of your examination.

Can arterial hypertension produce false normal spontaneous retinal venous pulsations in the presence of elevated intracranial pressure, according to the mechanism in the figures? Although theoretically possible, this has not been reported. Even the more likely occurrence, false normal spontaneous venous pulsations (in the presence of elevated intracranial pressure) due to a wide pulse pressure, has not occurred. In cases of very wide pulse pressures (such as those seen in aortic insufficiency and severe hyper-thyroidism) what one sees is retinal *arterial* pulsations (Roy, 1984). When this happens in aortic insufficiency (see Ch. 17, p. 312), it is called Becker's sign.

Papilledema

When papilledema is experimentally produced in animals by creating an increased intracranial pressure, the first observable static changes are loss of the disc margin and swelling of the nerve head (Walsh & Hoyt, 1969), as shown in Figure 10-17.

Splinter hemorrhages around the disc are also a sign of papilledema. Although they do not develop as early as the other signs, they have the advantage of persisting at the nadir of the intracranial pressure, unlike the loss of spontaneous retinal venous pulsations (discussed above). Probably no single sign should ever be relied upon for making the diagnosis of papilledema. Etiologies of papilledema are listed in Table 10-10.

You may have noticed that the light reflex of the retina's nerve fiber layer, which gives the retina its appearance of having texture, is more easily visualized with red-free than with white light. In papilledema, the nerve fiber layer around the disc loses its usual sharpness, and the examiner, using red-free light, gets the impression that his scope is out of focus because he cannot perfectly sharpen the image of the individual nerve bundle's central light reflexes.

Optic neurities or papillitis is often accompanied by papilledema. The distinction is made because papillitis also causes a blind spot, not seen in simple papilledema. (Retrobulbar neuritis, which afflicts the optic nerve behind the globe, produces a blind spot without papilledema.)

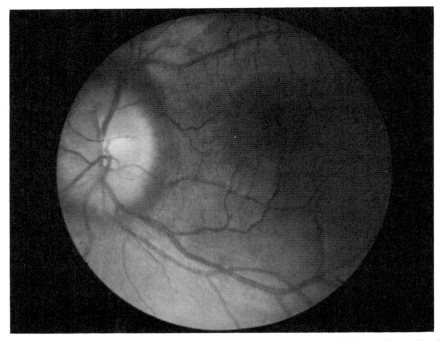

Figure 10-17. *Blurring and loss of a distinct disc margin are two of the very first signs of papilledema. Normally, there can be slightly less distinction to the temporal margin of a disc without papilledema as compared with its nasal margin. But no normal disc would have this much blurring, especially at the superior and inferior margins. What else do you see?*

No, the dark spot is simply the way the macula photographs. How about the vessels? Although this is a two-dimensional representation, can you see how the vessels are coming off a protruding disc, rather than up from a deep disc?

This is the only picture of papilledema in the book. Compare the disc margins in this picture with the disc margins in any other. After a few trials, you should be able to see the difference clearly. Now try the same thing with the vessels exiting the disc.

Table 10-10. Causes of Papilledema

With visual impairment
  Papillitis of any cause

Without visual impairment
  Idiopathic intracranial hypertension
  Intracranial tumor of any type
  Intracranial infection of any type
  Vascular disease
    Subarachnoid hemorrhage
    Subdural hematoma
    Hypertensive encephalopathy
  Retinal vascular disease
    Central retinal vein thrombosis
    Cavernous sinus thrombosis
    Retinal vasculitis of any type
  Metabolic
    Hypervitaminosis A
    Ethylene glycol poisoning
    Lead poisoning
    Arsenic poisoning
    Carbon dioxide retention
    Hyperthyroidism (?)
  Guillain-Barré syndrome
  Decreased intraocular pressure of any cause
  Congenital malformations
  Hematologic disease
    Severe anemia
    Polycythemia
    Leukemia
    Thrombotic thrombocytopenic purpura

Sources: *Duke-Elder and Scott (1971), Havener (1984), Newell (1982), and Roy (1984).*

Pseudopapilledema

Many conditions can imitate papilledema, for example, hypermetropia, in which the disc border may appear indistinct, especially temporally. There is no true protrusion of the disc, as can be shown by using the light stripe or by simply focusing up and down on the nerve head. The discs of some patients with astigmatism may have a similar appearance.

The following listing is doubtless incomplete, especially for conditions that would be seen on the ophthalmology service (see Roy, 1984).

Myelinated (also called medullated) nerve fibers, a congenital defect, also mimics papilledema. The myelinated nerve fibers arising from the disc are opaque, the color of white eggshell, rather than transparent. They are usually unilateral, while papilledema is usually bilateral. ("Usually" here means 80% of the time.) The disc margins in myelinated nerve fibers will *always* have a feathery edge, as if someone had taken a paintbrush and swept white paint out from the disc. The feather is composed of a bundle of myelinated nerve fibers, each individual fiber making a barb. (The only other ocular finding that has a feathery edge is the red flame hemorrhage [see p. 197].) Although myelinated nerve fibers may rarely be seen with neurofibromatosis or with cranial dysostosis, they otherwise have no association with any medical disease.

A variety of tumors can obscure the disc, fooling the unwary or inexperienced. These include tumors of the eye tissue itself (gliomas, meningiomas, and neurofibromas, or the hamartomas of tuberous sclerosis), or metastatic tumors.

Pseudopapilledema may also be caused by Bergmeister's papilla, a glial sheath that surrounds the first one third of the hyaloid artery. It is a normal embryonic sheath that occasionally persists in the adult as a small tuft of tissue replacing the physiologic optic cup of the disc.

Colloid bodies of the disc (also called hyaloid bodies) may cause cuneate visual field defects and obscure the disc borders. The appearance is like that of small (50 to 100 μm) and later large blobs (500 to 600 μm in diameter) of pineapple gelatin on the disc.

Although they may simply be inherited as an autosomal dominant with no systemic significance, colloid bodies are also seen variously in association with retinitis pigmentosa, Friedrich's ataxia, Wilson's disease, glaucoma, syphilis, pseudoxanthoma elasticum, and hypermetropia with disc elevation. Tuberous sclerosis is often listed in the differential diagnosis, but there the apparent hyaloid bodies turn out to be little hamartomas on histologic examination.

•

Colloid body: A case report. A 48-year-old Professor of Medicine presented himself to the eye clinic with a chief complaint of, "I've got a quadrant field cut on the right," of less than 1½ years duration. The professor had just been teaching visual fields by confrontation to his sophomore physical diagnosis students, as had been his habit for several decades. After his standard lecture, which included the facts that temporal brain tumors caused an upper quadrantanopsia, while parietal brain tumors caused a lower quadrantanopsia, he proceeded to the practicum. To his amazement, he could no longer see his own fingers when they were in the right lower quadrant.

The onset of this change could be dated within the prior 1½ years, when he had moved to an Eastern medical school where physical examinations were no longer performed with any care or skill, and so he had not been presented a single case of a visual field cut to be checked by confrontation.

Physical examination revealed a sweating, apprehensive, middle-aged white man who had a cuneate monocular right lower quadrant field cut with central sparing. On funduscopic examination, the right disc had a colloid body. Extensive studies, including computerized axial tomography of the brain, revealed nothing. Repeated Goldmann perimetry revealed stability of the lesion over a 6-month period, an important issue, because due to his peculiar occupation the professor was able to date the appearance of the quadrantanopsia, and so was suspected of being hysterical by one of his consultants, who had not grasped the significance of the colloid body.

•

For the attending. Colloid bodies (also misnamed "disc Drüsen") are acellular concretions of PAS-negative material, which has a whorled appearance on electron microscopy. On chemical analysis, it yields a positive test for sphingomyelin. True Drüsen (see p. 193), much smaller structures not found on the disc, are PAS-positive accretions on Bruch's membrane, and show no whorling or sphingomyelin. Other differences will no doubt be discovered. Without knowing that these two completely dissimilar structures have been called by the same names, it becomes impossible to understand the ophthalmologist's literature or consultation notes.

Retinal Neovascularization

Neovascularization is a proliferation of very small new vessels into an area where they formerly did not exist and are not normally seen. This usually occurs around the disc. When it involves the macula, it may cause blindness.

Normally, the retinal vasculature does not send new sprouts into territory that it does not usually supply. Furthermore, the normal vitreous and retina contain a substance that inhibits new growth of vessels. Thus, neovascularization implies both an abnormality of the microvasculature and a disease of the retina. The most common causes are diabetes mellitus, the various hemoglobinopathies, sarcoid, and Eales' syndrome (see p. 201).

Glaucoma

The word *glaucoma* is thought to come from the Greek word meaning "shining" or "sparkling." It is believed that this was intended to distinguish those who were blind from cataracts (whose eyes were no longer shining) from those who were blind from glaucoma. The importance of this etymology is to remind you of the insidiousness of glaucoma: to an untrained observer, the eyes seem to be normal, while the blindness progresses. As the painless increase in intraocular pressure jeopardizes the blood flow to the eye, the peripheral fields constrict. Because central vision is preserved to the end, the patient may not notice the problem until all other vision is lost (Johnson & Brubaker, 1986).

Despite the effective surgical and pharmacologic remedies available these days, glaucoma is the leading cause of blindness in the United States. If someone does not make the diagnosis, the patient might as well be living in ancient Greece as far as the preservation of his sight is concerned.

Glaucomatous changes in the disc are listed below. After studying this portion of the text, you should be able to screen all your patients for glaucoma and selectively refer suspected glaucoma victims for consultation. Your batting average will improve with practice and good consultants. The funduscopic findings should heighten your index of suspicion for glaucoma, but you should proceed to a pressure measurement at the drop of a hat.

1. Deepening of the Optic Cup. As the glaucomatous globe sustains its chronic hypertension, the optic cup begins to excavate, and the blood vessels exiting the disc come to be concealed beneath the lip of the disc (see Figs. 10-18, A and B, and 10-19). This sign, like many of the others, has a good specificity, but a lesser sensitivity. The only potential false positive is the cilioretinal vessel, which is easy to identify once one knows of it (see legend to Fig. 10-18C).

2. Cup/Disc Ratio. With increasing pressure over time, the cup/disc ratio may increase, and this can be clinically estimated with sufficient intraobserver reliability to be useful (see Fig. 10-19).

The disc is the entire creamy yellow structure. The cup is the part of the disc from which the vessels emerge. Its focal plane is farther away from the examiner. Determining exactly where the cup begins is somewhat arbitrary; your job is to be arbitrary in the same way each time.

The average cup occupies only 30% of the disc surface. However, some normal persons can have very large cups. Accordingly, this sign, like the others, is not pathognomonic for glaucoma. A few facts (Armaly, 1967) will provide perspective. Of normal subjects, 99% have optic cups that occupy less than 70% of the disc. If your patient has a cup bigger than 70% of the disc, he probably has glaucoma. An inter-eye discrepancy between the two cups of greater than 20% of the respective disc area also suggests glaucoma. Many patients with glaucoma do not have increased cup/disc ratios, so the sign is not highly sensitive, although it is the one that best predicts future damage.

3. Nasalization of the Vessels. A peculiar phenomenon of glaucoma is that most of the vessels seem to be coming from

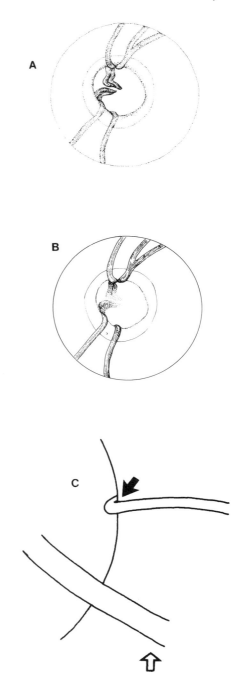

Figure 10-18. *A and B show a disc whose cup is quite deep. In A, one can focus on the vessel emerging from the deep cup but not as clearly see the vessels as they exit the disc. In B, one sees the vessel going under the lip of the disc and the distal vessel emerging, but one cannot see the proximal vessel clearly. In C, we see a normal vessel exiting the disc at the bottom (hollow arrow). We also see a "false-positive" cilioretinal artery exiting the disc in a manner faintly suggestive of a true glaucomatous vessel (solid arrow). This cilioretinal artery is always smaller than the normal artery. Furthermore, although it exits the disc by coming over the edge like a glaucomatous vessel, the more proximal portion of the cilioretinal artery cannot be identified, as would be the case with a true glaucomatous vessel (compare with B, above).*

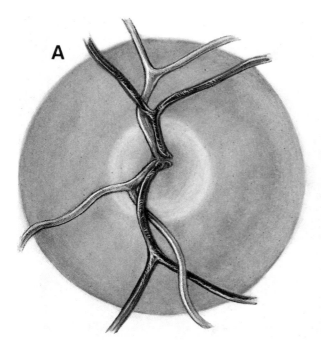

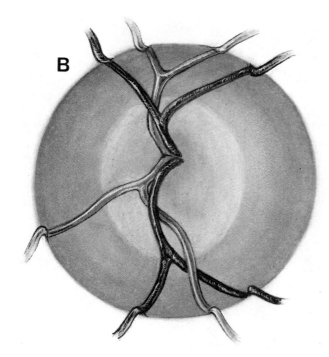

Figure 10-19. *A, The disc at the top is normal. The vessels exit the disc normally. B, The disc at the bottom shows glaucomatous changes in the vessels exiting the disc, similar to those in Figure 10-18B. However, this figure also shows the change in cup/disc ratio. A cup/disc ratio like this one makes one consider the diagnosis of glaucoma. In these drawings, the focal plane relationships have been doctored so that everything appears to be simultaneously in focus. Actually, the ophthalmoscope could not simultaneously focus on the lip of the disc and the depths of the cup. Now try Figure 10-20.*

the nasal side of the disc, whereas usually they radiate from both the nasal and temporal sides (Fig. 10-20A).

4. Pallor. Pallor of the disc is a relatively late sign.

5. Vertical Ovality of the Optic Cup. Ordinarily, the optic cup, if oval in shape, has a horizontal long axis. In glaucoma, the oval tends to have its long axis vertical (see Fig. 10-20A).

Other "soft" signs include: 6) notching of the disc (either inferior temporal or superior temporal), 7) flame or splinter hemorrhages on the disc (see Table 10-28), and 8) the appearance of laminar dots (due to the exposure of the lamina cribosa, which is stippled).

The list is incomplete, and none of the signs is perfect (Heilmann & Richardson, 1978). However, it is arguable that any two items in the above list should be considered reasonable evidence of glaucoma, and the higher the finding on the list, the more certain it is that the tentative diagnosis is correct.

The diagnostic accuracy of inspection of the disc alone was evaluated for 372 normal eyes and 132 glaucomatous eyes in a blinded study that used stereophotographic slides, measurement of intraocular pressure, and Goldmann perimetry to detect peripheral visual field loss. The sensitivity of the test (inspection of the disc) was 89%, and the specificity was 93% (Hitchings & Spaeth, 1977). Another study of 22 patients found direct ophthalmoscopy to have a sensitivity of only 48%, and a specificity of 73% (Wood & Bosanquet, 1987).

Special equipment:

1. Stereoscopic viewing is probably the earliest and best method for detecting optic nerve damage from glaucoma before 50% loss of nerve tissue has occurred. But the special equipment is usually not available to the nonspecialist.

2. Blind spots on perimetry might be placed just after changes in the cup/disc ratio on the list above. Visual field testing by confrontation (see p. 156) is simply not sensitive enough to pick up the early blind spots, which occur in the mid-periphery, and later become arcs, surrounded by good visual fields on all sides.

Formerly, one would have recommended a tangent screen examination, done with a black velvet backdrop into which pins with white or red heads could be inserted. These screens have disappeared, to be replaced by Goldmann perimetry, done by specialized technicians, which in turn has been supplanted by computerized perimetry. The middle has been vacated, so there is no longer a reasonably good technique available to the frontline undifferentiated physician for picking up small nasal defects.

Optic Atrophy

The disc is usually a creamy yellow, like Hollandaise sauce. In optic nerve atrophy, it becomes bone white, like Bechamel sauce. Causes are listed in Table 10-11.

Hyperemia of the Disc

The normal color of the disc varies considerably. It is described as being somewhat redder than usual in a variety of conditions (Table 10-12).

In the bourbon country of Kentucky, the special bourbon barrels are cleaned with methanol so that they can be reused. The material that comes out of the cleaned barrels (smoky, bourbon-colored methanol) is called "heads" and is a cheap but dangerous form of beverage alcohol, since it can be lethal. Oddly, some patients who have survived a bout of methanol poisoning from the ingestion of "heads" have been known to reappear in the hospital after a second ingestion.

Some of the patients do not die from the methanol, but instead have retinal poisoning. At first, the disc is hyperemic, but later with death of the retinal cells there is edema and finally pallor of the disc. The patient is left blind. (It has been suggested that this is the origin of the term "blind staggers.")

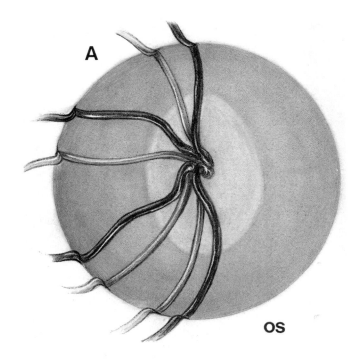

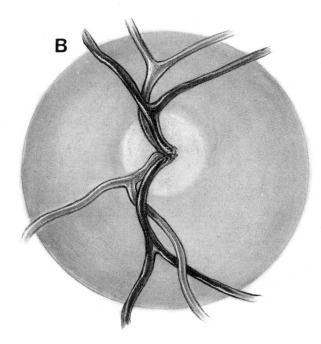

Figure 10-20. *Which of the two discs is more likely to be glaucomatous? (Answer is in Appendix 10-2.)*

Retinal Streaks and Stripes

Angioid Streaks

These fault lines in Bruch's membrane are usually lighter than the retinal background. Because they radiate out from the disc and are of relatively constant diameter, they may look like ves-

Table 10-11. Causes of Optic Atrophy

Consequent to optic neuritis, including:
  Multiple sclerosis
  Other diffuse sclerotic diseases (Schilder's and the leukodystrophies)

Hereditary/congenital

Secondary to papilledema

Vascular
  Temporal arteritis
  Post ischemia (as in thrombosis of either the central artery or vein of the retina)
  Syphilis

Traumatic
  Surgery
  Blows on the head
  Avulsion of optic nerve

Compressive
  Glaucoma
  Neoplasm
  Craniometaphyseal dysplasia
  Aneurysm

Toxic and Metabolic (temporal pallor more prominent)
  Vitamin deficiencies
  Carbon monoxide poisoning
  Tobacco-alcohol amblyopia
  Ethylene glycol intoxication (Ahmed, 1971)
  Post-methanol poisoning

Ophthalmologic
  Optic nerve colloid bodies

Source: *Roy (1984).*

sels (hence the term *angioid*). They may be much shorter than vessels. They will *always* appear to be under the real retinal vessels (Fig. 10-21).

Conditions associated with angioid streaks are given in Table 10-13.

Pseudoangioid Streaks

Pseudoangioid streaks (Fig. 10-22) do not appear to radiate from the disc.

The most common cause of pseudoangioid streaks is a misinterpretation of the light spaces in between the dark spaces in patients with a tigroid fundus, a background appearance common in highly pigmented individuals, which has no clinical significance.

Table 10-12. Causes of Hyperemia of the Disc

Papilledema

Polycythemia

Hypermetropia

Optic neuritis

Neovascularization

Central retinal vein thrombosis

Hemangioma

Ischemic optic neuropathy

von Hippel-Lindau disease

Methanol ingestion

Sources: *Duke-Elder and Scott (1971) and Roy (1984).*

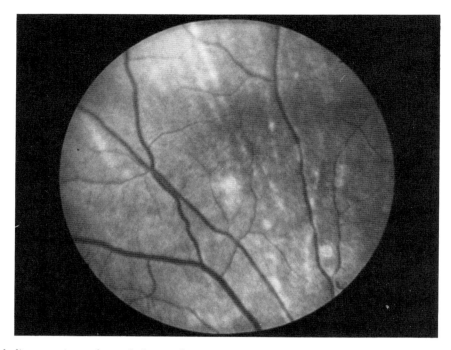

Figure 10-21.   *The light lines running underneath the vessels are angioid streaks.*

Lacquer cracking has been reported in myopia. The cracks radiate about the disc as well as from it, and they all run together just like lacquer cracks (Sapira, 1984). For an idea of what lacquer cracks look like, see the old man's forehead in Figure 12-1.

In "choroidal sclerosis" (see p. 191), which has as its outstanding feature the atrophy of the retinal pigment epithelium, the choriocapillaris may become visible, and this can resemble angioid streaks (Fig. 10-22).

Retinal Detachments

🖘 Occasionally you will see an unusual streak, which is not due to a change in color or background, but to a change in contour, as if

Table 10-13.   Angioid Streaks

Diagnostic Entity	% cases (of this entity) that have streaks	% all cases of angioid streaks caused by this entity
Pseudoxanthoma elasticum	85%–87%	59%
Paget's disease	8%–15%	14%
Sickle hemoglobino-pathies	0%–27%	7%
Pituitary tumors	Rare	Very rare
Familial hyper-phosphatemia with metastatic calcification	All	So rare it's reportable

Associations of uncertain significance: calcinosis, optic atrophy, systemic lupus erythematosus, ipsilateral facial angiomatosis, posthemorrhagic retinal hemorrhages.

Highly questionable associations: carotid aneurysm, hemolytic anemia, posttraumatic, retinitis albuminuria, lead poisoning, diffuse lipomatosis, dwarfism, epilepsy, senile actinic elastosis.
Source: Sapira (1984).

the retina were folded up, somewhat like a bath mat whose edges had been pushed slightly towards the center. This is a retinal detachment, which requires immediate ophthalmologic consultation to prevent irreversible loss of vision.

Retinal Pigment Epithelium Detachments

Some retinal pigment epithelium detachments have discrete borders. The color is often a variant shade of the normal background color of that patient. (It looks as if someone had painted on the fundus a spot that had not yet weathered, so that the spot appears to be an off-brand shade of the correct normal background color.) They have no systemic significance.

Arteriosclerosis of the Retinal Arteries and Arterioles

Caveat Lector

The statements made in the next section have aroused the ire of many a medical schoolmarm, and the politic reader may wish to skip this entire section. However, the student is warned that the instruction of the "experts" will leave him just as confused as I was at his age, and he might be better off to swallow the following passages whole.

One of the beauties of physical diagnosis is that the tools are available to all, not just those skilled in fine tuning separatory devices and radioligands. Thus, any reader, as a good scientist, can decide the truth or falsity of these passages. The material is fully referenced elsewhere (Sapira, 1984) so that any reader with scholarly skills and tenacity can make his way back through the labyrinth of scientific discovery and penetrate the curtains of our regularly recurring professional amnesia.

Introductory Summary

"Arteriosclerosis" refers to any one of the forms of hardening of the arteries (Table 10-14). One of these, atherosclerosis, rarely shows up in the fundus, and when it does, it affects only the

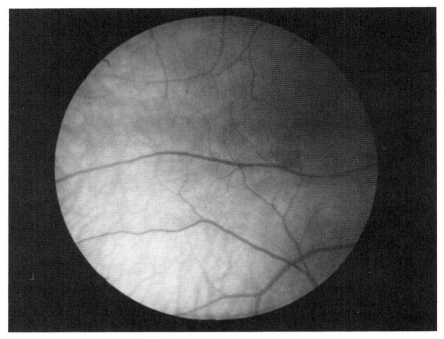

Figure 10-22. *These are the pseudoangioid streaks seen in choroidal thinning (called "choroidal sclerosis"). But note that these do not radiate from the disc, but appear to cross under the retinal vessels at right angles. Courtesy of Year Book Medical Publishers.*

vessels near the disc since only these are still true arteries (i.e., they have a muscularis layer.)

Another one, arteriolar sclerosis, refers to the name of both a process and certain ophthalmoscopic findings. This normal aging process is so accelerated by untreated chronic moderate hypertension that its ophthalmoscopic appearance can be clinically useful.

From the 1950s to the 1980s, there was pathetically little research with the pink hyaline of arteriolar sclerosis, whereas every medical school or hospital with more than 10 residents had at least one local authority on atherosclerosis. Accordingly, atherosclerosis was the predominant type of arteriosclerosis mentioned in the clinical literature, and those two words became synonymous in the minds of many. As these minds aged and began to write chapters in textbooks, the error became institutionalized. Naive readers, their sophomore pathology concept of arteriolar sclerosis unreinforced, slowly abandoned arteriolar sclerosis, as perhaps only the memory of a dream. Yet the pictures in the ophthalmologic literature (Scheie, 1953) and in Robbin's textbook of pathology are not hallucinations.

Atherosclerosis is a fat-mediated disease. *Au contraire*, arteriolar sclerosis is a "wear-and-tear" disease. Fig. 10-23 shows how the two different diseases have two different histologic bases producing two different ophthalmoscopic appearances.

Table 10-14.   The Pathologic Subdivisions of Arteriosclerosis[a]

1. Arteriolosclerosis (literally, hardening of the arterioles) of hypertension
   a. Arteriolar sclerosis (see text)
   b. Hyperplastic arteriosclerosis (The famous "onion skinning" seen in renal biopsies. It cannot be seen ophthalmoscopically and so is not discussed in the text.)
   c. Fibrinoid necrosis of the arterioles (A sign of acute accelerated hypertension, it cannot be seen ophthalmoscopically, although it undoubtedly covaries with the hemorrhages and exudates of neuroretinitis.)
2. Atherosclerosis (literally, porridge-hardening, because the fatty plaques look like porridge). Although accelerated by hypertension, it may occur independently of hypertension. (See text.)
3. Mönckeberg's medial calcific sclerosis (It has no relationship to hypertension and it cannot be diagnosed ophthalmoscopically, so it is not discussed in the text.)

Sources: *Sapira (1984).*

[a]*Literally, hardening of the arteries.*

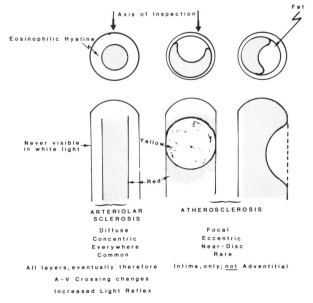

Figure 10-23. *Arteriolar sclerosis compared with atherosclerosis. Courtesy of Year Book Medical Publishers.*

The major retinal findings of arteriolar sclerosis are: 1) arteriovenous crossing changes, 2) changes in the arteriolar light reflex, 3) tortuosity of the arterioles, 4) focal narrowing of the arteriolar blood column, and 5) diffuse arteriolar narrowing.

1. Arteriovenous Crossing Changes in Arteriolar Sclerosis

Thesis.   As a rule of thumb, complete arteriovenous crossing changes more than 2 disc diameters away from the disc are due to chronic, moderate hypertension.

Method and criteria.   Each of the four major vascular systems is examined in the sequence given above. Once the examiner is *more than 2 disc diameters* away from the disc, the arteriovenous crossings are specifically examined for *complete* nicking (Fig. 10-24). This requires a perfectly clear space on each side of the arteriole (not due to arteriolar sheathing (see p. 191).

If one does not require precise criteria for arteriovenous crossing changes, one will do no better in terms of replication than the experts did in the four World Health Organization (WHO) studies, summarized in Table 10-15. Because arteriolar sclerosis is a normal accompaniment of aging, albeit accelerated by hypertension, it is important for us to require the extreme case in order to accurately relate the finding to chronic moderate hypertension per se.

Of course, the strictness of the criteria will decrease the sensitivity of the crossing changes for detecting chronic hypertension. However, it will increase the specificity and positive predictive value of the observations, by decreasing the number of false positives. Another way of looking at this is that changing the criteria substitutes one type of error for another, as shown in Fig. 10-25. In this case, the use of stricter criteria accepts a beta (type II) error so as to be free of alpha (type I) errors, as defined in Table 10-16.

Etiology.   The revealed wisdom (on and off since 1905) is that the artery has occluded the vein. In fact, this could not be so, or

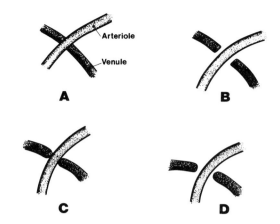

Figure 10-24.   *Arteriovenous crossings. A and C do not show "arteriovenous nicking" or "arteriovenous changes" by our strict criteria, even though the ends of the vein are tapered in C. B and D do show the crossing change that is evidence of chronic moderate hypertension if more than 2 disc diameters out. Courtesy of Year Book Medical Publishers.*

there would be signs of segmental venous occlusion. Histopathologic study of crossing changes previously examined in vivo has shown repeatedly that the "compression" is more apparent than real.

The disappearance of the vein in the vicinity of a retinal artery or arteriole is, like the disappearance of the magician's assistant in the stage cabinet, merely an optical illusion. And just as the magician uses mirrors to produce the illusion, so an altered refractile property of the retinal tissues at the AV crossing produces the illusion that the vein has disappeared (Sapira, 1984).

This material of altered refractile property may be of several origins. First, it may be due to scarring of the common arteriovenous adventitia at the arteriovenous crossing (the only place in the body where there is a shared adventitia). This is produced by arteriolar sclerosis (a process that is accelerated by chronic hypertension). Second, it may consist of very dense glial elements; this is the etiology of the normal arteriovenous crossing changes near

Table 10-15.   Four WHO Studies of Clinical Ophthalmoscopy and Arterial Hypertension

	Study			
	1	2	3	4
Technique	Ophthalmoscopy	Black & white photos	Color photos	Color photos
No. of experts	6	7	37	7
No. of fundi examined	48 (twice)	33 (twice)	50 (twice)	156 (55 twice)
	Mean Interobserver Disagreement (%)			
	(Mean Intraobserver Disagreement) (%)			
Diffuse arteriolar narrowing	29 (21)	33 (15)	34 (22)	42 (33)
Localized arteriolar narrowing	31 (25)	24 (14)	37 (27)	20 (19)
Increased light reflex	24 (14)	21 (10)	31 (21)	Not done
AV crossing changes	33 (26)	43 (23)	24 (21)	23 (22)

Source: *Kagan et al. (1966).*

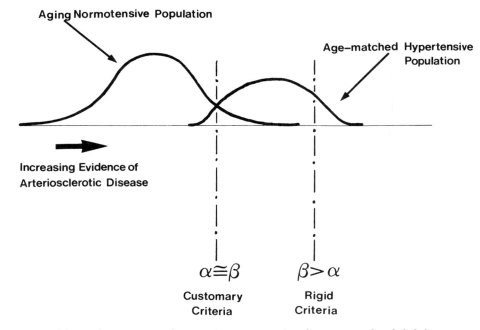

Figure 10-25.   *A comparison of the rigid criteria (complete arteriovenous crossing changes more than 2 disk diameters away from the disk) with the customary criteria (which are not well defined) for arteriovenous crossing changes. The alpha error is given by the area under the Gaussian curve for the aging normotensive population that lies to the right of the cutoff point (for either set of criteria). The beta area is the area under the curve for hypertensives that lies to the left of a cutoff point.*

the disc (Seitz, 1964; Shelburne, 1965). Third and rarely, tumors in the fundus oculi may produce arteriovenous crossing changes in nearby vessels, by the glial mechanism, or by retinal edema. ("Rarely" here means about once in an examiner's decade.) Fourth, and also rarely, retinal edema as in very severe cases of anasarca from undialyzed Kimmelstiel-Wilson disease or acute tsutsugamushi disease have caused the alteration in the normal refractile properties of the retina.

Additionally, what is called "arteriolar sheathing" (see Table 10-20 and p. 191) may produce pseudo-arteriovenous crossing changes, but these are easy to detect because the arteriolar sheathing consists of white stripes at the edge of the red arteriolar stripe; the other types of arteriovenous crossing changes do not have such an easily observed change. Myelinated nerve fibers can have the same effect, but again the correct diagnosis is obvious on other grounds.

Red-free light.   To learn to use the red-free light to make judgments about adventitial thickening (and medial thickening also), find a hypertensive patient with complete arteriovenous crossing changes more than 2 disc diameters away from the disc. After locating such a crossing change with the usual white light, slip your finger down to the aperture selector and flick the red-free light into position, as you continue to observe the crossing. Concentrate on the area of the arteriole near the crossing, especially just outside the arteriolar blood column. You will notice a refractile or ghostly appearance parallel to the blood column. It may be necessary to flick the white light back on and off a few times to convince yourself that the refractile quality is only observable under the red-free light.

To convince yourself that this appearance is specific for vessel-wall thickening, examine two other types of vessels, which will not show this phenomenon: the arteriovenous crossing changes of normal persons, near the disc; and the distal arterioles of a normotensive person's fundus.

Significance of arteriovenous crossing changes.   About 96% of those hypertensive patients who have arteriovenous crossing changes by the strict criteria will also have cardiomegaly (including left ventricular hypertrophy) caused by chronic moderate hypertension (Shelburne, 1949). This finding can be helpful in assessing the duration of uncontrolled hypertension in a patient seen for the first time, when no records are available. It can also be helpful in definitely assigning a hyper-

Table 10-16.   Definitions: Alpha and Beta Errors

Null hypothesis	The hypothesis that there is *no* difference between the experimental group and the control group, or in terms of sampling theory, that both sets of observations could have been randomly drawn from the same sampling universe.
Alpha or type I error	The rejection of the null hypothesis when the null hypothesis is actually true. (This corresponds to the erroneous belief that there is a significant difference between experimental and control groups when there actually is no such difference.) Clinically, the situation in which the examiner believes the sign signifies abnormality, when the patient is actually normal.
Beta or type II error	The acceptance of the null hypothesis when the null hypothesis is actually false; that is, a significant difference between the experimental and the control groups is missed. Clinically, the situation in which the examiner believes the patient to be normal, when in fact the patient is not.

tensive etiology to a patient who has cardiomegaly (although hypertensive cardiomegaly *can* occur before the arteriovenous crossing changes).

Similarly, the arteriovenous crossing changes can be useful in a patient suffering both hypertension and renal failure. The azotemia of hypertensive arteriolar sclerosis does not supervene until there has been enough chronic moderate hypertension to produce the arteriovenous crossing changes (Shelburne, 1949). Thus, in a hypertensive patient with renal failure but no arteriovenous crossing changes, one should think either of primary renal disease with secondary hypertension, or an episode (current or remote) of malignant hypertension inducing renal failure; the latter is easily diagnosed on other grounds.

The arteriovenous crossing changes are permanent (Sapira, 1984; Shelburne, 1965), and thus constitute permanent records of what has happened to the patient's vascular system.

Because the hypertension merely accelerates the arteriolar sclerosis that accompanies aging, even the strict criteria should eventually break down in a nonagenarian with a high normal diastolic pressure. For instance, if these changes appear with only 10 years of 40 mm Hg excess pressure (say a diastolic of 120 minus a "normal" of 80 mm Hg), there is no reason why it should not appear with 50 years of 8 mm Hg excess pressure (a diastolic of 88 mm Hg)—both patients have 400 "mm Hg years." Of course, it is not possible to prove a negative proposition (e.g., "complete arteriovenous crossing changes are not found in normals"). Yet a critical review of the literature (Sapira, 1984) found little if any evidence that the rigid criteria do break down in practice (Table 10-17).

Our knowledge of the evolution of arteriovenous crossing changes is largely derived from the observations of Shelburne between 1929 and 1969. For most of his career, there were no efficacious treatments for hypertension, and Shelburne was willing to do that which most clinical scientists avoid today: make careful long-term clinical observations on patients with a (currently) untreatable disease. Today, it would not be ethical to so study the natural history of arteriovenous crossing changes (i.e., to withhold treatment for 10 to 15 years).

A buccolingual* pedagogic note: the miracle of the right eye. After discussing arteriovenous crossing changes, I must recount one of those rare medical experiences that truly deserve to be described as miraculous.

●

I saw a patient who had, some 20 years earlier, undergone enucleation of the right eye following trauma. Initially, he had a glass prosthesis placed, but some short time after this, the right eye apparently grew back in. The evidence for this last statement comprises the many subsequent notations in the chart that stated the eyes to be normal. One careful observer found that the pupils had become equal and reactive to light *and* accommodation, so even the nerves must have grown back into the new eye. Furthermore, the new eye developed the same retina as the old eye; the patient's old arteriovenous crossing changes recurred within 1 year, according to the notes of two observers, although it usually takes from 7 to 10 years of chronic moderate hypertension to produce such changes. This miracle was documented for some 20 years, but shortly before I saw the patient in the fall of 1985, the second eye apparently evaporated, and it became necessary for him to again begin wearing a prosthesis. It was truly providential that the records of these many interesting eye examinations had not been lost, because by this time the patient had become demented and could not tell us what had happened to him.

---

*From the Latin "tongue 'n cheek."

Table 10-17.   Do Normal Persons Ever Have Complete AV Crossing Changes More Than 2 Disc Diameters Out from the Disc?

Study	Population	Findings	Were Changes Complete?	Location?
Van Buchem et al. (1964)	908 men, age 40–60	"Changes" in 26% of normotensives (13%–43%, varying with age)	Not stated	Not stated
Aurell & Tibblin (1965); Svarrdsdudd et al. (1978)	855 men, age 50; Same cohort, age 55	80 (9%) had "changes," but only 5 of these persons normotensive	Not stated	Not stated
Bechgaard et al. (1950)	Several hundred hypertensive patients	9% had "changes"	Yes	Not stated
Vogelius & Bechgaard (1950)	124 normotensive patients >age 60	2 had "changes"	Yes	Not stated
Wendland (1966)	217 diabetics	2 (1%) had "changes"; 1 "normotensive" (diastolic <100 mm Hg)	Yes	Not stated
Hofman et al. (1973)	974 nondiabetic patients (some hypertensive); 1,080 normotensive patients; 540 hypertensive patients	11% had "changes" (all hypertensive; addition of focal narrowing to criteria confounded the data	Yes	Not stated
Ralph (1974)	57 eye clinic patients who had electrocardiograms in their charts	Appears to confirm Shelburne, but data are confounded	Yes	At least 1 disc diameter out

Source: *Sapira (1984).*

For the attending.   Other clinicians in teaching hospitals have also seen examples of this phenomenon. I had previously seen two others, but none so well documented.

2. Changes in Arteriolar Light Reflex

Changes in the light reflex have been described as "copper" or "silver wiring." Figure 10-26 offers a schematic explanation of how such changes come about. For the changes to be attributed to arteriolar sclerosis, they must be diffuse, since many segmental arterioles that have once experienced an occlusion will also show silver wiring.

While these descriptions, which refer to an external standard, are acceptable, the light reflex should not simply be called "increased" without criteria. Using such a vague description, one cannot expect to do much better than the experts in the World Health Organization studies (see Table 10-15).

3. Tortuosity of the Arterioles

If the retinal arterioles are subjected to chronic moderate hypertension, they will no doubt become tortuous, like a garden hose, occluded at the nozzle, which twists and becomes ectatic when the luminal water pressure is up. This has been demonstrated in Japanese studies using a fundus camera and measures of the curvature of the vessels, a technique that does not lend itself to bedside clinical examination at the present time.

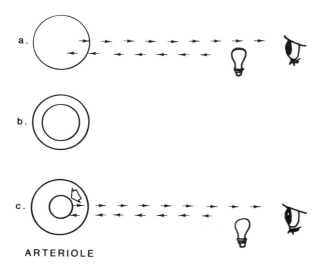

ARTERIOLE

Figure 10-26.   *Cross-sectional diagrams of retinal arterioles. A normal arteriole is shown in a. Light rays penetrate the thin vessel wall, illuminate the blood column within, and return to the observer's eye. In c, the arteriolar wall is so much thickened that the light rays cannot reach the column of blood within. Instead, the thick, scarred arteriolar sclerotic vessel acts as a mirror, reflecting pure white light back to the observer, who sees a silver vessel. The reflecting surface is probably that between the vessel lumen and the interior vessel wall (see the hollow-headed arrow), explaining the relative "narrowing" of the silver wire. The copper wire vessel in b has an intermediate degree of wall thickening. The reflected red light is made up partly of reflected silver light and partly of light from the blood column, which combine to produce a shiny orange or copper color. Courtesy of Year Book Medical Publishers.*

Such "soft curves" of the arterioles, which looked as if they were too long for the veins and tended to cross the veins at right angles, were described in 14% of 500 hypertensive subjects (Bechgaard et al., 1950). The same workers found this sign present in only two of 124 normotensive subjects (Vogelius & Bechgaard, 1950). (This is probably the same as the Salus S sign, which Salus thought was diagnostic for hypertension; the arteriole is "banked" as it crosses over the vein, and so describes the letter "S."

This sign of chronic moderate hypertension is the only one not dependent upon the pathologic process of arteriolar sclerosis, and so it is potentially most useful for distinguishing the hypertensive fundus from the normotensive but aged one.

4. Focal Narrowing of Arteriolar Blood Column

Focal or localized narrowing of the arteriolar blood column is another of those findings that stumped the experts (Table 10-15). Furthermore, despite the trouble taken above to distinguish atherosclerosis and arteriolar sclerosis, this is one finding that can be due to atherosclerosis (Scheie, 1953), especially if the narrowing is eccentric. This has been proven by histopathologic examination of the previously photographed fundus, an opportunity that arises when a hypertensive patient must undergo enucleation for some other reason.

5. Diffuse Arteriolar Narrowing

Diffuse arteriolar narrowing is another source of difficulty. Fundus photographs have shown that after the infusion of vasoactive substances, the retinal arteriolar blood column can undergo a reversible narrowing (Dollery et al., 1963). Thus, arteriolar narrowing could be seen in the fundus of the acutely hypertensive patient who has not yet developed arteriolar sclerosis (see also the discussion of the two retinopathies of hypertension, p. 200). Furthermore, most of us do not obtain fundus photographs with measuring grids, for comparison with baseline. Without such an objective measure, we cannot expect to do any better than the World Health Organization experts (Table 10-15).

The attempt to estimate this diffuse narrowing from the ratio of the diameters of arteriole and venule (the AV ratio) is also fraught with problems. A review of the literature revealed that a wide variety of AV ratios had been preferred ex cathedra. Unfortunately, they were so different (varying from 2:1, 3:2, 4:3, and 5:4) that all of them could not possibly have been correct, even if one had been experimentally determined (which was not done). In fact, there is considerable normal variation in the anatomy of the retinal vasculature. Additionally, even given a situation in which the AV ratio was clearly abnormal in the judgment of all observers, how could one know that the arteriolar diameter was the abnormal one? There are many circumstances in which the retinal veins become engorged (Table 10-18). Furthermore, a Scandinavian study reported a 6% prevalence of venous engorgement in hypertensive men and a 2% prevalence in hypertensive women (Bechgaard et al., 1950). These findings were separate from the higher than normal prevalences of arteriolar narrowing reported in the same paper. Since no fundus camera was used in this study, it is not clear to me how the ophthalmologist could, in the case of an increased AV ratio, know whether the arterial blood column was small or the venous blood column enlarged. Furthermore, even if such judgments were made with a camera, what would the criteria for normality be? One should remember that a 5% prevalence of a finding such as arteriolar narrowing could be expected if the common definition of normality (plus or minus two standard deviations from the mean) is used.

Ophthalmoscopic Changes in Patients with Coronary Artery Disease

Unfortunately, nothing seems to be perfect in biology. An interesting paper appeared in 1979, whose results cannot easily be under-

Table 10-18.   A Partial List of Reported Etiologies of Retinal Venous Engorgement

Hematologic diseases
    Sickle hemoglobinopathies (10%–96%), other severe anemias, Waldenström's macroglobulinemia, cryoglobulinemia, multiple myeloma, thrombotic thrombocytopenic purpura, polycythemia, leukemia (33%), lymphoma, hereditary hemorrhagic telangiectasia

Metabolic diseases
    Fabry's disease, diabetes mellitus

Infectious diseases
    Scrub typhus (67%), Rocky Mountain spotted fever, murine typhus, lymphogranuloma venereum

Congenital heart disease

Internal carotid-cavernous sinus aneurysm

?Coarctation of the aorta

Dermatomyositis

Cystic fibrosis

Behçet's syndrome

von Hippel-Lindau disease

Wyburn-Mason disease

Stasis retinopathies
    Arterial
        Internal carotid occlusion
        Takayasu's disease
    Venous
        Retinal vein occlusion
        Increased intracranial pressure
        Superior vena caval syndrome
        Congestive heart failure
        Cardiac tamponade
        Tricuspid stenosis

Hypertension (see text)

Source: *Sapira (1984).*

stood within the present framework. Seventy patients undergoing coronary arteriography were independently evaluated for retinal arteriolar changes. The results, which are statistically significant, are shown in Table 10-19. Study the table, and write down your explanation of the results.

Answer 1.   If you said that the correlations occurred because hypertension accelerates both atherosclerosis and arteriosclerosis, it must be pointed out that all of these patients were normotensive. Try again.

Answer 2.   If you said that age accelerates both atherosclerosis and arteriolar sclerosis, it must be noted that the authors checked this point, and claimed that they could not show an age effect. Try again.

Answer 3.   If you said that a power function test was not done, and there might not have been sufficient patients to demonstrate the age correlation, you gave a good answer. However, one is still left with the puzzle that there were sufficient patients to demonstrate a correlation between (coronary) atherosclerosis and some signs of (retinal) arteriolar sclerosis. Try again.

Answer 4.   If you said there is a third factor, neither age nor blood pressure, which predisposes to or covaries with vascular damage of both types, you gave a good answer since it suggests a line of experimentation and points out the weakness in present concepts. However, it is not presently falsifiable (see definitions, p. 187). Try again.

Table 10-19.   Signs of Arteriolar Sclerosis in 70 Patients Undergoing Coronary Arteriography

Sign	Sensitivity[a]	Specificity[a]
Light reflex	98%	61%
Vessel tortuosity	19%	98%
Vessel caliber	53%	87%
AV crossing changes (criteria unspecified)	68%	70%

Source: *Michelson et al. (1979).*

[a]For coronary artery disease (i.e., atherosclerosis).

Answer 5.   If you said the conversion of continuously distributed variables (vascular findings and retinal findings) into dichotomized and therefore discontinuously distributed variables (plus/minus ratings of vascular disease) may have confounded some correlations so that they were no longer apparent, while leaving other correlations apparent, you gave an educated answer. While this is my favorite explanation, it is not necessarily the correct one. Based on the data presented, it is not possible to test it effectively.

The point of this lengthy discussion is to show you the excitement of experiment that can be attained by anyone who is adept at clinical examination, and to indicate some of the epistemologic questions that can be generated by the results of such an experiment, particularly if they do not seem to "fit" into the current revealed wisdom.

It is also important for your education for you to be exposed to differing viewpoints, especially in a single-author textbook.

Plaque of Hollenhorst

Up to this point, we have been concentrating on the funduscopic signs of arteriolar sclerosis, noting that these may be clearly distinguished from atherosclerosis with the occasional exception of focal and eccentric narrowing of the blood column. There is, however, one true sign of atherosclerosis that cannot possibly be confused with arteriolar sclerosis: the plaque of Hollenhorst. This is a glistening, golden-yellow fixed spot in the arterial blood column, which, as its name implies, was once thought to be an atheroma. Actually, all or most of them are not plaques arising in situ, but cholesterol emboli from an ulcerating atheromatous plaque in the ipsilateral carotid (Brownstein et al., 1973; Pfaffenback & Hollenhorst, 1973).

The plaque of Hollenhorst is associated with generalized vascular disease. Patients with this finding succumb to either myocardial infarction or stroke at a much higher rate than the age-matched population; their 10-year survival rate is only half that expected (Pfaffenback & Hollenhorst, 1973).

The Hollenhorst plaque is 11% sensitive for the detection of occlusive disease of the carotid system. It is 4% sensitive for the detection of vertebrobasilar disease, not because the vertebrobasilar system serves the fundus (it does not) but rather through common atherosclerotic involvement. The Hollenhorst plaques may also appear during 14% of carotid endarterectomies (Hollenhorst, 1961).

A perfect distinction between cholesterol emboli and plaques arising in situ is sometimes, but not always, possible. Since an atheroma can only arise in an artery, we need to ask ourselves where the retinal arteries are. Remembering that the retinal artery must by definition have a recognizable muscularis layer, we learn that only the retinal arterial vasculature very near the disc is truly arterial; the remainder is arteriolar. Thus plaques of Hollenhorst at the periphery and not near the disc must be embolic. This is easy to visualize because many of these are lodged at bifurcations or are wedged into the arteriolar lumen of ever-decreasing diameter. Similarly, an eccentric plaque in a true retinal artery near the disc, which is too small to be wedged in place, and is clearly growing on the side of the vessel wall, is probably a true atheromatous plaque (see Fig. 10-23, right-hand panel). A back-lit plaque (Fig. 10-23, middle panel) might be an atheroma. However, if it appeared to be wedged into the retinal artery at a bifurcation or if seen moving through the arterioles, it is undoubtedly a plaque of Hollenhorst.

Other Emboli

White plaques moving through the retinal vasculature may be platelet emboli or valvular emboli from rheumatic, marantic, endocarditic, or myxomatous disease (Sapira, 1984). One might also see tissue emboli from cardiac neoplasms, foreign microdispersoids (Lee & Sapira, 1973), or fat emboli from long bone fractures, which have found their way to a retinal arteriole.

"Choroidal Sclerosis"

"Choroidal sclerosis" (Fig. 10-22), sometimes confused with atherosclerosis because of paronymy, does not involve blood vessels at all, although it may expose to view the normally inapparent choroidal vessels as the retinal pigment epithelium thins over large areas of the fundus. Sometimes these are the vessels of the choriocapillaris, which look like multiple angioid streaks except that they bear no relation to the disc. But sometimes one sees the large choroidal arteries, which look like a tangle of snakes (Paton et al., 1976) or a jumble of macaroncelli (Waldo, 1964). The neophyte might think that the large choroidal vessels are actually the retinal vessels, though the latter can still be seen in front of the choroidal vessels, providing that one does not panic, and looks for them. Choroidal sclerosis does not have any significance in terms of vascular or other systemic disease.

Other Changes in the Renal Vasculature

"Box-carring" and "Sausaging" (Fig. 10-27)

"Box-carring" refers to the segmentation of the blood column within the vessel. It obviously requires that there be no motion within the vascular tree, and is therefore a valid sign of death (i.e., the cessation of cardiac function).

"Sausaging" of the veins is a hallmark of macroglobulinemia, although also seen in other hyperviscosity syndromes. The vein swells in diameter between arteriovenous crossing points, and thus resembles a string of sausages (more like bratwurst, knockwurst, or boudin, than andouille).

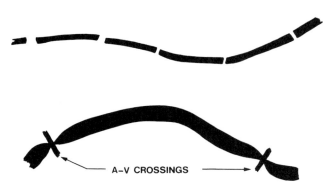

Figure 10-27. *Above, box-carring. Below, sausaging of the veins.*

Sheathing

Sheathing may be arteriolar or venous, and refers to the appearance of a pair of white stripes on either side of the blood column, as if it were a red or purple highway (seen from above) with sidewalks alongside. Causes of sheathing are given in Table 10-20. Arteriolar sheathing is the most common retinal vessel abnormality in sickle hemoglobinopathy, occurring in 51% of children with hemoglobin SS and 30% of children with hemoglobin SC (Talbot et al., 1982).

Light Spots on the Retina

Cotton Wool Exudates

The name for these fluffy, nonglistening, pale white (to gray) spots derives from their generally fuzzy appearance and nondiscrete borders (which distinguish them from the "hard exudates," described below). Cotton wool exudates (also called soft exudates) are actually not white blood cell exudates, but rather microinfarctions of the retina. Histologically, they are called "cytoid bodies." Their size varies up to 1 mm in diameter (Table 10-9). There are many causes of cotton wool exudates, some of which are listed in Table 10-21.

Cotton wool exudates are important for two reasons: 1) They are never normal, so their presence encourages a search for the underlying diagnosis. (However, as should be apparent from Table 10-21, and contrary to what is suggested in many texts, cotton wool exudates are not diagnostic for any one, or even two diseases.) 2) In patients whose diagnosis has already been made, cotton wool exudates are special in their ability to reveal the vasculopathic severity of the disease in that individual patient.

Hard Exudates

Hard exudates are proteinaceous (or sometimes lipoproteinaceous) deposits, due to transudation (as in "albuminuric retinitis"). This results from a breakdown of the blood retinal barrier so that serum leaks within the retina. Rarely, hard exudates

Table 10-20. Causes of Sheathing

Arteriolar
Hypertension
Kimmelstiel-Wilson disease
Leukemia
Mycosis fungoides
Syphilis
Onchocerciasis
Polyarteritis nodosa
Eales' syndrome
Posttraumatic
Sickle hemoglobinopathy
Venous
Hypertension
Diabetes mellitus
Myelocytic leukemia
Syphilis
Tuberculosis
Candidiasis
Coccidioidomycosis
Sarcoidosis
Multiple sclerosis
Normal variant

Source: *Sapira (1984)*.

Table 10-21.   Some Causes of Cotton Wool Exudates

All types of acute severe hypertension
   Renal disease, vasculopathic
   Toxemia of pregnancy

Collagen vascular diseases (even without hypertension)
   Systemic lupus erythematosus (3%–28% of cases)
   Polyarteritis nodosa
   Progressive systemic sclerosis (even without renal disease)
   Dermatomyositis (especially in children, rarely in adults)
   Wegener's granulomatosis

Infections
   Septic retinitis (including bacterial endocarditis)
   AIDS[a] (Newsome et al., 1984)
   See chorioretinitis, Table 10-23

Diabetes mellitus (especially accompanied by hypoglycemia, hypertension and/or nephropathy)

Conditions that cause papilledema (see p. 180, Table 10-10)

Increased intracranial pressure, even before papilledema appears

Stasis retinopathies (see p. 199 and Table 10-29)

Microembolization
   Intravenous drug abuse
   Postcardiac surgery
   Fat embolism or Purtscher's retinopathy (see p. 199–200)

Adult anemia, when the hemoglobin is < 6.6 to 8.0 g/dl (up to 33% of cases from some historical epochs)

Neoplasia
   Leukemia
   Carcinomatosis
   Hodgkin's disease

Eales' syndrome

Pseudoxanthoma elasticum

Posthemorrhagic retinopathy (see p. 200)

Source: *Sapira (1984).*

[a]*AIDS causes a microvascular disease apparent in the fundus and not related to ocular candidiasis, cytomegalovirus, or toxoplasmosis.*

Table 10-22.   Some Common Etiologies of Hard Exudates

Severe hypertension, especially with renal disease

Renal disease

Severe diabetes mellitus, especially with renal disease

Infections
   Measles, influenza, meningitis, erysipelas, psittacosis, parasitic infections, coccidioidomycosis, candidiasis, chronic syphilis, tuberculosis

Collagen vascular diseases
   Normotensive dermatomyositis, Behçet's syndrome, polyarteritis nodosa, systemic lupus erythematosus (<13%), progressive systemic sclerosis, "rheumatic polyarthritis"

Hematologic diseases
   Pernicious anemia, other severe adult anemias (hemoglobin less than 8 g/dl), multiple myeloma, leukemia

Eye diseases
   Disciform macular degeneration, Coats' syndrome, Eales' syndrome

Cerebral trauma

After strangulation

Fat embolism

Lead poisoning

Old central vein thrombosis

Papilledematous states

Sarcoidosis

Hypercholesterolemia, especially with nephrotic syndrome[a]

Residual of prior hemorrhage (see Tables 10-25 to 10-27)

Source: *Sapira (1984).*

[a]*It is not clear from the literature that hypercholesterolemia ever causes hard waxy exudates in the absence of renal disease.*

are revealed after the resorption of (previously identified) hemorrhages.

Hard exudates have discrete borders. They vary in color from yellow all the way to pure white. They often resemble candle drippings, in that they are shiny like wax or soap. Sometimes they are arranged about the macula like the spokes or the rim of a wagon wheel (or a portion of such a wheel); in that case one can be certain that they are indeed hard exudates.

Hard exudates should suggest the presence of severe albuminuria, until proven otherwise. They are seen in severe hypertension and in renal disease with or without hypertension (and sometimes without proteinuria). They are also seen in 10% of severe cases of diabetes mellitus. A partial list of etiologies is given in Table 10-22.

Like soft exudates, hard exudates are never normal. They are most useful for evaluating the progress and severity of a previously diagnosed disease in the *individual* patient.

Pseudoexudates

Pseudoexudates are fundus lesions that are neither hard nor soft exudates but that visually could be confused with either. Causes are given in Table 10-23. The most important of the pseudoexudates is chorioretinitis.

Chorioretinitis.   This lesion can be easily confused with exudates, especially at the most important time—when the chorioretinitis is still in the acute stage and has not yet acquired the distinctive black pigmentation of the chronic stage (see p. 194). (Cotton wool exudates and hard exudates do not have black pigmentation.)

The selection of the causes listed as major is somewhat arbitrary. For example, *onchocerca* infections blind 3% to 5% of the 20 to 40 million persons infected, but are not a problem in the United States. Conversely, *ocular histoplasmosis* is most common in those portions of the United States where the systemic disease is endemic but is rarely the cause of a similar retinal picture in the experiences of European workers. Its ophthalmoscopic features are: 1) white to yellowish lesions, 2) a grouping of the lesions right around the disc, 3) peripapillary atrophy, 4) macular hemorrhage that can evolve into macular degeneration, and 5) equatorial streaks in about 5% of cases. The last are perfectly even bands or stripes thought to result from the coalescence of multiple lesions. But there is still no explanation for their perfect geometry. Despite their rarity, they are important because they may be pathognomonic for histoplasmosis.

Choroidal tubercles can be single and unilateral or multiple and of varying size. Although not clustered around the disc as tightly as the lesions in histoplasmosis, they still are often found within only 5 mm of the disc (a little more than 3 disc diameters). And although found in less than one third of cases of pulmonary tuberculosis, choroidal tubercles are stated to be present in over half the cases of miliary tuberculosis. They are often of great diagnostic utility since they appear quite early in the miliary disease.

Acquired *toxoplasmosis*, when acute, produces a white lesion

Table 10-23. Some Etiologies of Pseudoexudates

Chorioretinitis
Major
Histoplasmosis
Tuberculosis
Toxoplasmosis
Syphilis
Onchocerca volvulus
Sarcoidosis
Laser therapy for diabetic retinopathy
Minor
Other parasites
e.g., *toxocara*, leptospirosis, *E. histolytica*
Other fungi
e.g., *Sporotrichosis, Candida, Coccidioides,
Cryptococcus*
Other bacteria
e.g., *Brucella*, leprosy
Rickettsial diseases
e.g., typhus, Q fever, boutonneuse fever
Other viruses
e.g., Herpesvirus, cytomegalovirus, chickenpox,
measles, influenza, Rift Valley fever
Other Pseudoexudates
Major
Drüsen
Myelinated nerve fibers
Minor
Leukemic infiltrates
The phakomatoses (Table 10-24, Figs. 10-29 and 10-30)
Choroidal tumors
Metastatic tumors
Rare
Secondary oxalosis
Fundus xerophthalmicus (vitamin A deficiency)
Thrombosed microaneurysm

Source: *Sapira (1984).*

that is not located near the disc. When congenital, the lesions are usually bilateral, pigmented, and large (>1 mm), with small satellite lesions surrounding the larger ones.

Syphilis often but not always has a salt-and-pepper appearance, especially in the congenital form.

Sarcoidosis is shown in Figure 10-28. The retinal findings are the most classic of all the eye signs of sarcoidosis. The patient whose fundi are shown had granulomas on liver biopsy, which might have been due to any one of 14 causes. The fundal findings clinched the diagnosis. Such sarcoid tubercles, which are clearly neither hard nor soft exudates, may eventually progress to black scars. See Appendix 10-5 for a syllabus of sarcoidosis.

Drüsen. Drüsen are little clusters of discrete white, yellow, or gray spots, which are actually excrescences on Bruch's membrane. (Drüsen, the German word for "glands," was apparently chosen because these little dots resemble apocrine glands.) They are very small, beginning at about 10 μm. In most cases, they do not indicate any underlying ocular or systemic disease, and do not have the more serious significance of true exudates.

Table 10-24. The Phakomatoses

Eponym	Descriptive
von Recklinghausen	Neurofibromatosis (see Figs. 10-29 and 10-30)
Bourneville	Tuberous sclerosis (epiloia)
Sturge-Weber	Encephalotrigeminal angiomatosis (port wine stain)
von Hippel-Lindau	Cerebelloretinal angiomatosis
Louis-Bar	Ataxia telangiectasia (with immunodeficiency)
Wyburn-Mason	Encephaloocular arteriovenous fistulae or angiomas

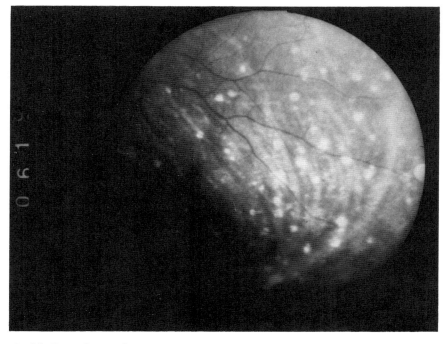

Figure 10-28. *Classic retinal findings of sarcoidosis. Recognition of these findings might have saved this patient a liver biopsy (see text).*

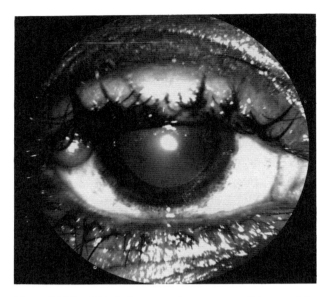

Figure 10-29. *This is the external appearance of the eye of the patient whose fundi are shown in the next figure. Without this additional clue, it would be almost impossible to make the correct diagnosis from looking at the fundus photographs in a two-dimensional manner. Note the pedunculated fleshy protuberance on the upper lid. There were many of these all over the patient's body. Can you make the diagnosis? (See Ch. 7, p. 113.)*

Drüsen, especially when grouped around the posterior pole, can be an adumbration of senile macular degeneration in the elderly. And they may rarely signify serious ocular disease in children. Finally, they may be seen as a degenerative phenomenon (after Duke-Elder) occurring secondary to a number of diseases such as pseudoxanthoma elasticum, Bloom's syndrome, Osler-Weber-Rendu disease, scleroderma, recurrent polyserositis, chronic leukemia, lipoid proteinosis, dysproteinemia, and phthisis of all causes. Still, in most clinical situations, Drüsen are of no diagnostic importance.

Myelinated nerve fibers.   Also known as medullated nerve fibers, these have already been discussed in connection with pseudopapilledema (p. 180). They resemble cotton wool exudates (see p. 191) only in that they are white and may obscure an underlying retinal vessel. However, myelinated nerve fibers are the *only* white structures that have a feathery edge.

Minor and rare causes of pseudoexudates.   Leukemic infiltrates are yellow, white, and/or gray, and are heaped up in masses. Like the phakomatoses, they may obscure the retinal vessels, whereas the large choroidal tumors and metastatic tumors do not. All of the minor group of pseudoexudates are relatively large lesions, compared with those lesions described as rare in Table 10-23. The latter are scattered about as tiny yellow crystals in the case of secondary oxalosis and as white spots in the other two cases. The fundus xerophthalmicus occurs in 20% to 46% of patients with vitamin A deficiency; the white spots are beneath the vessels and spare the macula.

Black Spots

Healed Chorioretinitis

The acute lesions of chorioretinitis, which are white or yellow, have been described above. However, with the passage of time, the chorioretinitis from any of the causes listed above will begin to heal. Then previously unseen cells from the retinal pigment epithelium migrate into the lesion. It is these cells, normally pigmented, but not usually visible, that produce the startling black appearance of old chorioretinitis. Despite their ominous appearance, the lesions do not interfere with vision, unless they happen to involve the macula.

The round, regular, isometric pigmented scars of laser photocoagulation are so characteristic that its recognition should not be a problem, providing that one remembers to look through dilated pupils. The patient's history confirms the diagnosis.

I was once fooled in a case of laser photocoagulation (Fig. 10-31) by breaking my own rules: 1) Never accept the findings of another

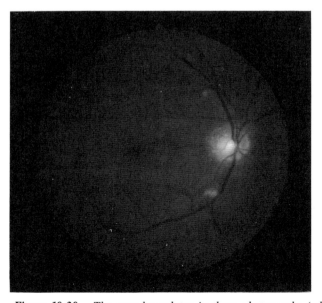

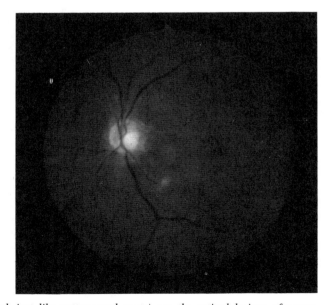

Figure 10-30.   *The pseudoexudates in these photographs (which look just like cotton wool spots) are the retinal lesions of neurofibromatosis. In addition to the pseudoexudates, one can see pseudoangioid streaks. Both angioid streaks and pseudoangioid streaks are always beneath the real blood vessels.*

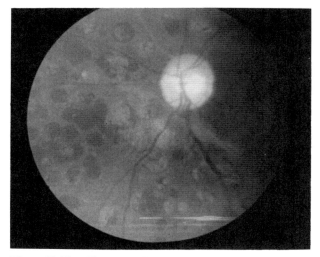

Figure 10-31.   *The scars of laser photocoagulation (see text).*

examiner, and 2) never examine through undilated pupils (if at all possible). I was told that the patient had a single white exudate, and I foolishly agreed to look through undilated pupils. I then saw a single white lesion near the disc, which I thought was the "single lesion" the house staff had seen, so I discussed the diagnosis of histoplasmosis (compare with the description on p. 192). But when the pupils were correctly dilated, the picture shown in Figure 10-31 was revealed. (Because some of the lesions were fresh, they were still white.) The erroneous diagnosis of histoplasmosis thus suggested in this patient from the endemic zone of riparian Missouri could have been avoided if only the pupils had been dilated! (Oddly enough, the patient had no recollection of the laser therapy.)

Retinitis Pigmentosa

Many peripheral black spots, arranged in the shape and aggregation of bone spicules, are characteristic of retinitis pigmentosa (Heckenlively & Ellis, 1984). The term is a misnomer, because the syndrome is not an infection or an inflammation, but rather a degenerative process. Furthermore, about 10% of the cases lack pigmentation.

In some cases, the most prominent finding is the choroidal degeneration that permits the choriocapillaris and/or the choroidal blood vessels to appear in the fundus view just as with choroidal "sclerosis" (discussed on p. 191).

There are at least five or six forms of retinitis pigmentosa that are considered "primary," that is, without known etiology, although about half are familial and of an autosomal inheritance. In addition, retinitis pigmentosa is said to be secondary to about 20 known diseases.

Unless the patient has one of the few medical diseases for which effective therapy is available (e.g., vitamin A deficiency), the retinal condition is untreatable. Thus, ironically, the only treatable cases of retinitis pigmentosa are those that must be discovered by the primary physician. Usually, by the time the patient comes to the attention of the ophthalmologist, most peripheral vision, and in some cases, central vision, is already gone.

Retinal Pigment Epithelium Hypertrophy

Retinal pigment epithelium hypertrophy results in discrete black-to-brown, round, oval, or kidney-shaped spots, ranging in size from 0.15 to 1.5 mm or more, usually bilateral. Small (less than 0.15 mm) bilateral or unilateral lesions may be seen in normal controls, but no control ever had more than four lesions total.

These spots are a useful sign of Gardner's syndrome. Using bilaterality and multiplicity (more than four) as criteria, the spots were 78% sensitive and 95% specific (Traboulsi et al., 1987). Colorectal carcinoma develops in 100% of patients with Gardner's syndrome, which also includes colonic polyposis, benign soft-tissue and bone tumors, dental abnormalities, extracolonic cancer, and desmoid tumors. The syndrome is inherited as an autosomal dominant.

The fundal lesions are *not* seen in Peutz-Jeghers' disease, which does not lead to carcinoma.

Choroidal Hemorrhages

Choroidal hemorrhages occur behind the pigment layer. Therefore, instead of being red, they appear to be purple, black, or gray. Some have imitated a malignant melanoma so well that the eye was enucleated. A valuable clue, in addition to its color, is that the retinal vessels will *always* cross over the top of this type of hemorrhage. The reason for this can best be understood by reviewing the sagittal section of the fundus shown in Figure 10-32.

These hemorrhages come from the choroidal vessels, not from the retinal vessels, and so do not necessarily result from the same etiologies (vide infra) as the hemorrhages that are discussed later (pp. 196–198).

Etiologies include but are not limited to subarachnoid hemorrhage, chorioretinitis, polyarteritis of the choroidal (not retinal) vessels, thrombotic thrombocytopenic purpura, leukemia, entamoeba histolytica brain abscess, pernicious anemia, diabetes mellitus, Paget's disease, and eye diseases including senile macular degeneration (Sapira, 1984).

Melanomas

Melanomas may appear to be less black and more grayish if they are choroidal (behind the pigment layer) and not retinal. Amelanotic (white) melanomas are as unusual in the fundus as they are elsewhere.

Benign Choroidal Nevi

These must be distinguished from melanomas. Benign choroidal nevi are sometimes gray.

The Benign Melanocytoma

This lesion is seen in blacks and is characteristically located on the nerve head.

"Bear Tracks"

This term refers to a benign collection of pigment epithelium rests with perfectly discrete borders. A large lesion is accompanied by a few smaller ones of the same general (oval) shape, falling more or less along a line, as if a bear had stepped in some black paint and started to walk across the fundus.

All of the above (except for the last two benign lesions) may sometimes create difficulties in diagnosis, requiring referral to an experienced ophthalmoscopist.

Red Spots

Microaneurysms

Capillary microaneurysms (Fig. 10-33) are small, perfectly round, red dots, with distinct edges, 20 to 60 μm in diameter. They are most common near the macula. Capillary microaneurysms should be considered due to diabetes mellitus until proven otherwise (Sapira, 1984).

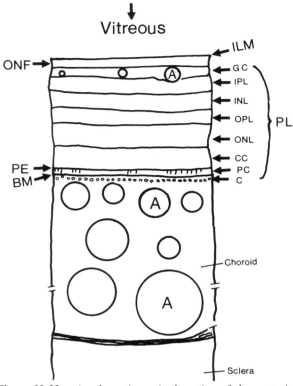

↓
Vitreous

Figure 10-32. *A schematic sagittal section of the posterior pole: the arrow at the top indicates the axis of inspection. Starting from the bottom of the diagram, we move anteriorly or inwardly. First comes the sclera; then the choroid with artery* A. C *represents the small choriocapillaris, which is the smaller choroidal vasculature that best imitates angioid streaking in choroidal thinning (see Fig. 10-22).* BM *is Bruch's membrane, also known as the lamina vitrea,the anterior delimitation of the choroid. This is where angioid streaks and Drüsen occur.* PE *is the pigment epithelium. Only hemorrhages anterior to this layer will appear red.* PC *denotes the pigment cells. The next six layers are the connecting cilium* (CC), *the outer nuclear layer* (ONL), *the outer plexiform layer* (OPL), *the inner nuclear layer* (INL), *the inner plexiform layer* (IPL), *and the ganglion cell layer* (GC). *These are collectively labeled* PL, *or parallel layers. This is to emphasize that hemorrhages in these layers will tend to align themselves along the nerve fiber layers in an axis parallel to the axis of inspection, producing blot hemorrhages. The round structures lying among the ganglion cells, one of which is labeled* A, *are retinal arterioles in cross section.*

Since the peripheral arterioles and venules tend to lie in the ganglion cell layer, it becomes obvious that hemorrhages posterior to this layer will not obscure these larger vessels, and hemorrhages in layers anterior to these vessels must always obscure them. ONF *is the optic nerve fiber layer (also called the inner nerve fiber layer) or stratum opticum. Here the nerve fibers run perpendicular to the axis of inspection so that hemorrhages between nerve fiber bundles will appear splinter- or flame-shaped.* ILM *is the internal limiting membrane that holds back preretinal or subhyaloid hemorrhages. Hemorrhages that burst through the internal limiting membrane anteriorly would become subhyaloid (preretinal). If they could next penetrate the hyaloid membrane (not shown but immediately anterior to the internal limiting membrane), they would become vitreous hemorrhages. Courtesy of Year Book Medical Publishers.*

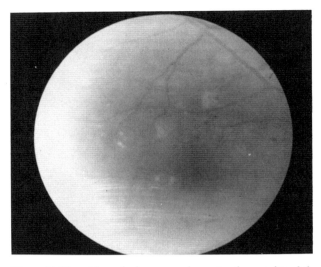

Figure 10-33. *Above the large vessel crossing from right to left are two microaneurysms fortuitously backlit by an exudate. Below the vessel are more dark spots that were bright red in vivo. These were also due to diabetes mellitus. The light spots in the photograph are exudates; some look like discrete drops of wax, and others are softer in appearance. Courtesy of Year Book Medical Publishers.*

Microaneurysms have also been reported in up to 40% of cases of sickle cell disease and other sickle hemoglobinopathies and, rarely, in other anemias, when severe. They may also be seen in AIDS (Newsome et al., 1984) Very rarely, microaneurysms may be seen in bacterial endocarditis, in the other arterial or venous forms of stasis retinopathy (see p. 199), and in Coats' syndrome. I have never seen them in uncomplicated hypertension. Actually, the ones that occur in hypertension and polyarteritis (pictured in Fig. V, Shelburne, 1965) are aneurysms of the arterioles. They look different from diabetic microaneurysms, which occur away from vessels, mostly in the perimacular area. I have seen microaneurysms in normoglycemic recovering addicts who could have been prediabetic (Sapira & Cherubin, 1975). In Scandinavia, they have been reported in unaffected relatives of diabetics, and in one study were considered to be "idiopathic" (Sapira, 1984). Other very rare associations include posterior uveitis and loa loa infection (Sapira, 1984).

Blot Hemorrhages

Blot hemorrhages are the result of bleeding somewhere deep among the parallel layers (see Fig. 10-32). Blot hemorrhages are usually cylindrical but appear round when viewed "down the barrel." They vary in size from 100 μm to 10 times that large. If you initially have trouble distinguishing them from microaneurysms, remember that the latter are smaller, more perfectly round, and have a perfectly distinct border. Blot hemorrhages actually look like a blot. With practice, these differences become obvious, although even the "experts" did not clearly distinguish microaneurysms and blot hemorrhages until this century.

Some causes of blot hemorrhages are listed in Table 10-25.

There is also a subretinal hemorrhage that is just in front of the pigment epithelium and therefore red. It is called subretinal because it is under the parallel layers, and so instead of forming a blot hemorrhage, it may actually spread out and form a wide hemorrhage. The retinal vessels are, of course, always on top of this hemorrhage. It has the same significance as the blot hemorrhage.

Table 10-25.   Some Common Causes of Blot Hemorrhages

Severe hypertension

Diabetes mellitus

Collagen vascular disease
  Systemic lupus erythematosus
  Progressive systemic sclerosis (even without hypertension)
  Dermatomyositis (even without hypertension)

Intracranial hemorrhage (10%–40%)

Stasis retinopathies, both arterial and venous forms (see p. 199)

Hematologic disorders
  Anemias (severe: hemoglobin < 8g/dl if no associated
  thrombocytopenia)
    Aplastic (about 30%)
    Pernicious, untreated (about 25%)
    Iron deficiency (about 10%)
    Hemolytic, specifically excluding thalassemia (about 10%)
  Leukemia (about 33%)
  Waldenström's macroglobulinemia
  Multiple myeloma (about 33%)
  Amyloidosis
  Myelofibrosis (<33%)
  Polycythemia rubra vera
  Thrombotic thrombocytopenic purpura
  Other thrombocytopenia if associated with anemia
    (Hgb < 12 g/dl)

Infections
  Bacterial endocarditis
  Scrub typhus and other rickettsial diseases (5%–33%)
  AIDS (Newsome et al., 1984)

Sarcoidosis

Traumatic
  Strangulation
  Decompressive barotrauma (caisson disease)
  Posthemorrhagic retinopathy
  Fat embolism
  Other embolizations, as from talc in intravenous drug abuse

Eales' syndrome

Purtscher's retinopathy (see p. 199)

Source: *Sapira (1984).*

Flame and Splinter Hemorrhages

Within the area seen by direct ophthalmoscopy, hemorrhages in the outer nerve layer may look like splinters or flames (see ONF in Fig. 10-32). The individual splinter is a line of blood pooling between nerve fibers oriented with their long axes perpendicular to your axis of inspection. A larger collection of blood will have a flame-shaped or feathery edge; thus, the flameshaped hemorrhage is just a coalescence of splinter hemorrhages.

■ The causes of flame and splinter hemorrhages are listed in Table 10-26. *Splinter hemorrhages found only on or near the disc are always important.*

White-Centered Hemorrhages

There are three common but erroneous beliefs (Sapira, 1984) concerning the white-centered hemorrhage (see Fig. 10-34). The first is that its correct eponym is the "Roth spot."

Roth, in 1872, did describe retinal red spots (previously described by Bowman), as well as retinal white spots, in septic retinitis (Roth, 1872). But he did not describe red spots with white centers in bacterial endocarditis or any other illness. The

Table 10-26.   Some Common Causes of Flame or Splinter Hemorrhages

Dangerous Hemorrhages
  Splinter hemorrhages found only on or near the disc
    Glaucoma
    Papilledematous states
    Increased intracranial pressure
    Retinal vein obstruction
    Subdural hematoma
    Subarachnoid hemorrhage
  Other emergencies
    Intracranial hemorrhage (10%–40%)
    Accelerated (malignant) hypertension
    Posthemorrhagic retinopathy

Additional Causes
  Any of the causes of blot hemorrhages (see Table 10-25) can
    also cause flame or splinter hemorrhages
  Polyarteritis nodosa
  Behçet's syndrome
  Takayasu's disease
  Paget's disease
  Atrial myxoma
  Uncomplicated thrombocytopenia
    (platelet count less than 50,000/mm³)
  Malnutrition

Source: *Sapira (1984).*

white-centered hemorrhage was first described in endocarditis by Litten in 1878, 6 years later.

Here, in the same sequence in which they published, are the two authors:

Roth, in 1872, discussing retinitis septica: " . . . *Kleine weisse Flecke in verscheidener Zahl, meist auf beiden Seiten, oder auch rothe Flecke* . . . " (Roth, 1872). (" . . . Small white spots in varying number, mostly on both sides or also red spots. . . . ")

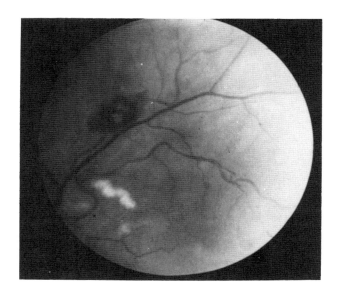

Figure 10-34. *A flame hemorrhage with two white centers, from a patient who did not have infectious endocarditis. If you share the misconceptions that these lesions should be called Roth spots, have a center composed of white cells and microorganisms, and are diagnostic of endocarditis, please see the text. Courtesy of Year Book Medical Publishers.*

Litten, in 1878, discussing the bilateral retinal hemorrhages seen in Charlotte Lewald, 1 day before she died of endocarditis: *"Viele von ihnen lassen in ihren Centrum eine helle weisse Stelle erkennen."* (Litten, 1878). ("Many of these showed in the center a light white place.")

The second common erroneous belief is that the white-centered hemorrhage, by whatever name, is specific for endocarditis. This is not true, as shown by Table 10-27.

The third erroneous belief is that the white centers are the result of the presence of white cells. However, except for the leukemias and some cases of bacterial endocarditis, the white centers are not white cells but fibrin (Duane et al., 1980; Mahneke & Videbaek, 1964, Van Uitert & Solomon, 1979). Accordingly, any flame-shaped hemorrhage could come from a vascular leak, which presumably could also leak protein and so permit the hemorrhage to become a white-centered hemorrhage (Litten spot). Thus, Table 10-27 is undoubtedly too short.

A red-centered white spot has been reported in neurodermatitis diffusa and bronchial asthma. I have also seen one in diabetes

Table 10-27.   Causes of White-Centered Hemorrhages

Infections
    Endocarditis (may be embolic)
    Other bacterial septicemias (may be embolic)
    Rocky Mountain spotted fever
    Kala-azar
    Candidiasis
    Psittacosis
    Typhoid fever
    Viral infections
    AIDS (Newsome et al., 1984)

Hematologic diseases
    Severe anemia
    Multiple myeloma
    Leukemia

Cardiovascular diseases
    Postcardiac surgery
    Syphilitic aortitis
    Rheumatic valvulitis
    Hypertension

Vasculitis, specifically including that due to systemic lupus
    erythematosus

Neurologic disorders
    Intraventricular hemorrhage
    Ruptured arteriovenous malformation
    Ruptured mycotic aneurysm
    Ruptured nonmycotic aneurysm
    Subdural hematoma

Other
    Metabolic
        Diabetes mellitus
        Scurvy
        Hypoxia of mountain climbing
        Carbon monoxide poisoning
    Lung cancer with cyanosis retinae
    Posthemorrhagic retinopathy
    Neonatal birth trauma
    Battered children
    Difficult or prolonged anesthetic intubation
    Oral contraceptives
    Central hemorrhagic retinopathy

Source: *Sapira (1984).*

mellitus. Any blot hemorrhage surrounded by retinal edema could produce that same appearance, as could an exudate with a hemorrhage in the middle.

Preretinal (Subhyaloid) Hemorrhage

These hemorrhages have one of two very characteristic appearances, depending on the patient's position (see Fig. 10-35). When the patient is erect, the preretinal hemorrhage serves as nature's own carpentry level.

These hemorrhages can arise by anterior extension of any retinal hemorrhage, or from the etiologies listed in Table 10-28.

There is now evidence that these hemorrhages can actually be in two anatomically different spaces. But the preretinal and subhyaloid hemorrhages are of identical etiology and appearance, so the difference can be considered moot for our purposes.

Vitreous Hemorrhage

The most anterior of the hemorrhages, the vitreous hemorrhage, can arise by extension from any preretinal or subhyaloid hemorrhage and so, by extension, from any flame or blot hemorrhage. (See Fig. 10-32 for a review of the anatomy.) The appearance can vary from a small amount of ill-defined blood to a mass of blood so large as to obscure even the red reflex. A vitreous hemorrhage is an indication to call the ophthalmologist, immediately after putting the patient at rest, since an underlying retinal detachment may be present. As for determining the etiology, the most important information is the premorbid appearance of the fundus (i.e., before the vitreous hemorrhage obscured the view). This is another reason why all primary care physicians should perform and record baseline ophthalmoscopy regardless of the reason for the patient's initial physical examination.

The Macula

Cherry-Red Macula

The medical causes of a cherry-red macula are listed in Table 10-31. The cherry-red macula may occur with vascular syndromes because the macula receives a separate blood supply, permitting it to glow red against the pale ischemic background of the remainder of the fundus. Alternately, the remainder of the fundus may become pale, not from ischemia, but from neuronal infiltration by the substances of the various storage diseases.

Macular Degeneration and Destruction

Macular degeneration is protean in appearance. It may simply appear, in white light, as an absence of the macula. The situation is more obvious in those degenerations in which the macula is replaced by Drüsen, colloid bodies, pigment, or even plaques.

A patient was presented as having a past history of blindness due to glaucoma, which supposedly had not been treated because he was thought to be cortically blind from an old stroke. Inexplicably, he claimed to have some vision remaining on the right. No one could place a lesion that would account for such a constellation of chart diagnoses, and after a fruitless quarter hour of drawing visual pathways, someone decided to examine the patient.

The patient explained that he could still see objects on the periphery of the visual field of his right eye, a fact that had been misunderstood to mean hemianopsia. Examination revealed that the patient had a direct pupillary response to light on the right (but not on the left), peripheral but no central vision on the right, and no

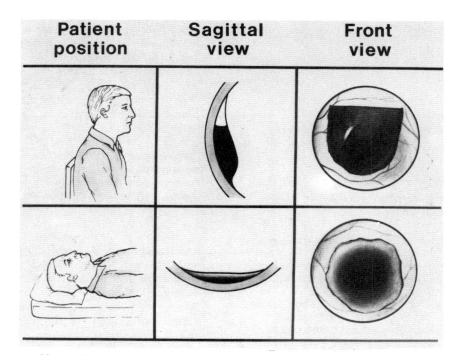

Patient position	Sagittal view	Front view

Figure 10-35. *Are preretinal hemorrhages round, or do they have straight tops? It depends on whether the patient is sitting or recumbent. Patients who are well enough to walk into the ophthalmologist's office will have their hemorrhage layer out as shown in the top sagittal view. Thus, in the frontal view, they will have a straight edge superiorly, like a cup of borscht (a Russian beet soup served in a glass cup). This is the way that the hemorrhages are usually illustrated in ophthalmology textbooks.*

However, if the patient has had a major vascular accident and is taken to the emergency room, his posterior pole hemorrhage will layer out as shown in the bottom panels, and will appear as a saucer of wine. Thus, neurosurgeons and neurologists describe these hemorrhages as round, illustrating the rule of: "What you see depends on where you stand" —or in this case, on whether the patient is able to stand. (Note that regardless of whether the preretinal hemorrhage has the cup-of-borscht or the saucer-of-wine appearance, the retinal vessels are always obscured by the hemorrhage.) Courtesy of Year Book Medical Publishers.

For the attending: *The erect position is preferable for roundsmanship since with time the components of the blood begin to sediment, providing that the patient is not disturbed. Thus, the observant attending can not only make an estimation of the erythrocyte sedimentation rate, the size of the buffy coat, and the icterus index, but he can also occasionally estimate the degree of lipemia.*

vision on the left. The anterior chambers were not shallow, and the eyeballs were soft. So far, one could diagnose nonglaucoma, and noncortical blindness, but there was no explanation for the peculiar findings, until the fifth physician to examine the patient on this one admission used the ophthalmoscope to find obvious old chorioretinitis, diffuse on the left and involving the maculae bilaterally.

Very advanced. In patients whose macular degeneration is secondary to macular edema or cystoid macular degeneration, white light may reveal flecks, holes, honeycombing, or nothing, as noted above. However, in the last case, red-free light may reveal a rough, cobblestone type of reflection in the area of the macula, which can be the first sign of macular degeneration of the honeycomb type.

Table 10-28.   Some Etiologies of Subhyaloid and Preretinal Hemorrhages

Any of the causes listed in Table 10-25 or 10-26

Infectious diseases
  Histoplasmosis
  Pertussis

Ruptured diabetic neovascularization
  Sickle hemoglobinopathies

  Source: *Sapira (1984).*

Synthesis: Retinopathies

Stasis Retinopathy

Stasis retinopathy results from any condition that impairs venous drainage from the eye, or that impedes arterial flow. The various etiologies are listed in Table 10-29.

The retinopathy seen ipsilateral to occlusive disease of the carotid artery includes: 1) cotton wool exudates, 2) yellow plaques of Hollenhorst (see p. 190), and 3) dilation of the arterioles. Additional features recognized in 1963 (Kearns & Hollenhorst, 1963) were called venous stasis retinopathy, although they could also be seen in association with carotid artery occlusion. These consisted of: 1) microaneurysms in close proximity to the retinal veins, 2) small blossom-shaped (blot) hemorrhages always less than 1/8 disc diameter in size, and 3) dilation of the retinal veins. In the subset of these patients who had an elevation in the erythrocyte sedimentation rate, spontaneous sludging of the blood in the retinal veins was sometimes observed. Except for the absence of waxy (hard) exudates, this retinopathy was felt to mimic diabetic retinopathy exactly.

Purtscher's Retinopathy

Patients suffering severe trauma may experience a sudden loss of vision hours after the accident. The fundus shows the picture of Purtscher's retinopathy: arterial spasm, retinal edema, cotton wool exudates, and hemorrhages confined to an area limited by the optic discs and macula. The changes may progress over several

Table 10-29.   Some Causes of Stasis Retinopathy

Hyperviscosity syndromes
    Multiple myeloma (6% of cases, especially with hypertension)
    Cryoglobulinemia
    Macroglobulinemia
    Polycythemia
    Sickle cell disease
Venous stasis (e.g., retinal vein occlusion)
Arterial occlusions (e.g., carotid occlusion [atherosclerosis];
    Takayasu's disease)
Embolization (e.g., fat emboli, specifically including pancreatitis;
    atheromatous emboli)

Source: *Sapira (1984).*

days, and resolve slowly. Sometimes vision improves to a varying degree.

Purtscher's retinopathy was originally described in patients who had sustained head trauma. The mechanism was thought to be a rapid rise in intravascular pressure caused by the force of deceleration. However, this retinopathy can also result from other types of trauma. Embolism due to air, fat, or aggregates of granulocytes are the postulated mechanisms (Kincaid et al., 1982).

Purtscher's retinopathy has also been reported in patients with acute pancreatitis. Here, complement-induced leukoembolization (Jacob et al., 1981) and/or fat emboli (Inkeles & Walsh, 1975) are thought to play a role. In fact, it is not certain that Purtscher's retinopathy is anything more than the ophthalmoscopic part of systemic "fat embolism."

Hypertensive Retinopathies

There are actually two different types of retinopathy associated with hypertension (see Table 10-30), the individual component parts of each having already been presented.

The first type, called "neuroretinitis," is that of accelerated hypertension, including acute malignant hypertension or hypertensive crisis of any etiology. It occurs without regard to the presence or absence of the other type of hypertensive retinopathy, and may develop in a matter of hours or days. It can resolve in days or weeks, with resolution of the hypertension. The retinal findings reflect an acute generalized vasospasm. The find-

Table 10-30.   The Two Retinopathies of Hypertension

Finding	Neuroretinitis	Arteriolar Sclerosis
Type of hypertension	Acute, accelerated	Chronic, moderate
Hemorrhages	Usually	No
Exudates	Usually	No
Papilledema	Possible	No
Diffuse narrowing	?Vasospasm	Yes
Focal narrowing	?Vasospasm	?Yes
Complete AV crossing changes more than 2 disc diameters away from the disc	No	Possible
Copper or silver wiring	No	Possible

Source: *Sapira (1984).*

ings that distinguish this type are the hemorrhages, exudates, and papilledema. However, only the hemorrhages are required to make the diagnosis, and the papilledema appears only after the hemorrhages and exudates, if at all. Of course, the findings (Fig. 10-36), individually and collectively, could also be due to some other process, and must be interpreted in the light of the clinical picture, especially including the measurement of the blood pressure.

Normotensive patients who have experienced severe hemorrhage may acutely develop an ischemic retinopathy, complete with hemorrhages and exudates, which exactly resembles the neuroretinitis of accelerated hypertension (Pears & Pickering, 1960). This is called "posthemorrhagic retinopathy."

The second hypertensive retinopathy, due to chronic moderate hypertension, has been called arteriolar sclerosis (see p. 186), an unfortunate term because it is also the name of the pathologic process that underlies most of the various ophthalmoscopic components. It takes years for the signs of arteriolar sclerosis to develop, and once they develop, they never resolve. At this point, the sophomore should review the material on pages 184 to 189. To summarize, the hallmarks of arteriolar sclerosis are AV

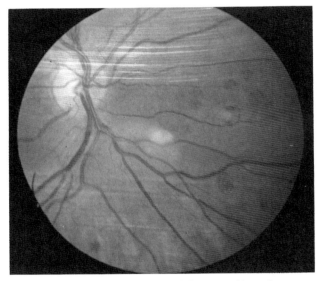

Figure 10-36.   Many persons will diagnose this as hypertensive retinopathy, and some will bet on that (in case you are short of coffee money). For the record, this photograph is from an otherwise healthy 23-year-old drug abuser I cared for, who specifically had had no episodes of hypertension or any of the arteriosclerotic diseases. Furthermore, repeated follow-up photographs (not shown) documented the complete resolution of all the hemorrhages and exudates. Note that these changes are not specific. (The white-centered hemorrhages, which the observant reader may have spotted, are likewise nonspecific, see p. 197) What disease caused these events, if not an acute hypertensive episode? (See Appendix 10-3.)

To those who claim that there are arteriovenous crossing changes, we note that the distal changes are incomplete and the ones near the disc are perfectly normal, being found in about half of the normal population (see criteria, p. 186). Some think that there is arteriolar narrowing; we refer them to page 189. Photograph courtesy of Charles B. Slack, Inc.

crossing changes, copper or silver wiring ("increased light reflex"), tortuosity of the arterioles, and diffuse arteriolar narrowing. (The last may also occur due to the vasospasm in the first type of hypertensive retinopathies. Focal narrowing can occur in both types as well.)

Note that the findings of arteriolar sclerosis may be seen in a fundus that also shows neuroretinitis, if the patient has the acute process of accelerated hypertension superimposed on chronic moderate hypertension. Conversely, a patient with newly occurring mild hypertension might have *neither* type of retinopathy.

When Scheie distinguished the two retinopathies in 1953, he chose the unfortunate terms "hypertension" for one and "arteriolar sclerosis" for the other. He published diagrams of two different gradings at the same time. These were, for a time, reprinted in physical diagnosis textbooks without the long accompanying discussion or the histopathology. In this way, the wrong idea arose that the "hypertensive" changes were from hypertension, but that the "arteriolar sclerosis" was *not* due to hypertension, but rather came from *athero*sclerosis.

It will be noticed that no grading system from Roman numerals I to IV (although a tradition in texts of physical diagnosis) has been preferred. There are a variety of such systems, some of which combine the acute and chronic changes, and some of which do not. Scheie's 1953 system, which separates the two, could be recommended, but it requires two gradings for each patient, and no one seems to do that any longer. The Wagener system of the 1930s was used to predict prognosis, but would have to be adjusted each decade to allow for changes in prognosis due to improvements in therapy.

For the attending. The two empiric patterns of neuroretinitis and arteriolar sclerosis are useful in the individual patient. Gradings, on the other hand, are statistical associations useful only for group prognostication. And there are also other statistical associations. For example, hypertension is associated with senile macular degeneration in some studies (Sperduto & Hiller, 1986).

Diagnosticity of hypertensive retinopathy. How good are the experts at diagnosing hypertension from the examination of the fundus? Only two studies have attempted to answer this question in a blind fashion. In a European study performed before World War II, Salus had a sensitivity of 70%, with no false positives (Salus, 1958). This stands as a world record. In a WHO study published in 1966, the sensitivity of a group of seven experts was only 12% (SD 6.5%), and the false positive rate was 7.4% (SD 5.2%) (Kagan et al., 1966). Clearly, the diagnosis of hypertension is made with a stethoscope and a blood pressure cuff. But for understanding the vasculopathic effects of the blood pressure in the individual patient, an intelligent observation of the fundus has no superior.

Diabetic Retinopathy

To summarize, diabetic retinopathy is characterized by microaneurysms, hemorrhages, exudates, and eventually neovascularization. By the time hemorrhages and exudates occur, microaneurysms are generally present; their absence would make one reconsider the etiology of the former signs.

There is an interesting statistical correlation between diabetic retinopathy and Kimmelstiel-Wilson disease. While not all patients with retinopathy will have Kimmelstiel-Wilson disease, the reverse correlation is so good that if one finds no retinopathy in a diabetic with the nephrotic syndrome, one should search for another etiology for the renal disease.

Table 10-31. Some Causes of a Cherry-Red Macula[a]

The sphingolipidoses (including the gangliosidoses GM_1-type 2 and GM^2-type 2)
Retinal artery occlusion (or very severe arterial stasis retinopathy)
Mucopolysaccharidoses type VIII and I-H
Temporal arteritis
Cryoglobulinemia
Traumatic retinal edema
Sandhoff's disease
Hemorrhage at the macula, which has been misidentified
Severe hypertension
Quinine toxicity
Hallevorden-Spatz disease
Disseminated lipogranulomatosis
Cherry-red spot-myoclonus syndrome (Rapin et al., 1978)

[a]Full list in Roy (1984).

Diabetic papillopathy is discussed on page 179.

Patients with diabetes should have a thorough ophthalmoscopic examination annually. Patients with hemorrhages, exudates, and (possibly) microaneurysms are candidates for fluororetinography (Diabetic Retinopathy Study Research Group, 1978, 1981).

In patients with diabetes, a single cotton wool spot is associated with an increased chance of developing proliferative diabetic retinopathy over the next year, and thus is a strong indication for ophthalmologic referral (Diabetic Retinopathy Study Research Group, 1981).

There are data supporting the concept that tight regulation of diabetes mellitus is actually accompanied by increased retinopathy, especially cotton wool exudates (Brinchmann-Hansen et al., 1985; Lauritzen et al., 1983).

Eyes with neovascularization plus preretinal or vitreous hemorrhage must be treated. Neovascularization alone is an indication for treatment if it occurs on or within 1 disc diameter of the optic disc and exceeds one quarter of the disc in area. Laser photocoagulation can help prevent devastating loss of vision due to diabetic retinopathy.

Sickle Cell Retinopathy

Peripheral retinal capillary occlusion by sickled red cells initiates a proliferative retinopathy, which commonly leads to vitreous hemorrhage and retinal detachments (Talbot et al., 1982). Unfortunately, the results of laser photocoagulation have not been good (Condon & Serjeant, 1980).

Eales' Syndrome

Very advanced. In 1880, Henry Eales published an article entitled "Retinal hemorrhage associated with epistaxis and constipation" (Eales, 1880). By 1882, other workers had reported what was apparently the same syndrome, and Eales himself published another paper (Eales, 1882), in which he decided that a better name for the disease would be "primary recurrent retinal hemorrhage." He also added to the syndrome the presence of bradycardia, and noted that the disease primarily and initially affected the left eye of young (14- to 20-year-old) men. "Probably females are saved from retinal hemorrhage by their menstruation" (Eales, 1880). He noted that the disease was rare; he himself had a total experience of only seven cases, and saw no new ones among 12,000 admissions to the Birmingham and Midland Hospital in the year prior to publication.

During the subsequent century, the epistaxis evaporated and the constipation dropped out, the diagnosis being made in those cases of intraocular hemorrhage and periphlebitis for which no cause was apparent. Yet, various etiologies were invoked, including tuberculosis (many patients were treated with the first antitubercular drugs) and rickettsia (in the French and Belgian literature, based on serologic data). At the present time, the diagnosis should not be made unless no other known cause of blot, flame, or vitreous hemorrhage can be found (see Tables 10-25 and 10-26).

Retinal Artery Occlusion

■ If the *central* retinal artery is occluded, the patient will experience a sudden loss of vision, and on examination the entire retina will appear edematous and pale, except for the cherry-red macula (see p. 198) plus any part of the retina that is supplied by the cilioretinal artery that is present in 15% to 20% of people (see Fig. 10-18C). Sometimes a hemorrhage may be superimposed. The etiologies are the same as for any arterial occlusion.

Peripheral arteriolar and arterial occlusions are often caused by the plaques of Hollenhorst and the white emboli already described above (see p. 190). The findings will be similar to those described in the last paragraph, except they will be segmental and possibly associated with the characteristic intraarteriolar findings.

After the acute occlusion and during healing, all or part of the arteriole or artery that was occluded may show arterial sheathing or even silver wiring.

Some teach that massage of the eyeball may salvage vision in cases of acute retinal artery occlusion. Movement of the embolus, as observed through the ophthalmoscope, has been reported after this maneuver (De Schweinitz, 1915).

Retinal Venous Occlusion

In contrast to the usual rather bland appearance of the fundus in a central retinal artery occlusion, a retinal venous occlusion will regularly cause a horrendous appearance of the fundus (see stasis retinopathy, p. 199), although the prognosis for recovery of vision is actually fairly good. Initially, one sees preretinal hemorrhages, splinter hemorrhages, and/or blot hemorrhages, especially around the nerve head. The veins may be engorged, the disc edematous, and exudates may appear.

Segmental retinal vein occlusion has the same horrible appearance, confined to one quadrant (usually the superior temporal one) or even a smaller segment.

Retinal vein occlusions can be caused by anything that will externally compress the vein, internally inflame it, or simply promote thrombosis within the vascular system in general.

Auscultation Over the Globe

A Method

Listen over the eyeballs by applying the bell of the stethoscope lightly so as to make an airtight seal. In alert patients, vigorous reflex blinking may cause so much adventitious noise that faint vascular sounds are obscured. To overcome this problem, the patient is asked to open his eyes after the stethoscope is in place. Blinking then becomes greatly reduced, while the stethoscope holds one eyelid shut. At the same time, ask the patient to fix his gaze on some object to prevent random extraocular movements, and to hold his breath lest respiratory sounds interfere with auscultation (Fisher, 1957).

Significance

Murmurs over the eyeball may be found in hyperthyroidism or in diseases that produce murmurs in the internal carotids (see Ch. 18, p. 343), including but not limited to (contralateral) internal carotid stenosis, carotid-cavernous fistula, and severe anemia (Wadia & Monckton, 1957). Other causes include cerebral infarction, glioma, migraine (during attack), and increased intracranial pressure (Allen & Mustian, 1962).

False Negatives

The sensitivity of auscultation over the globes for the diagnosis of carotid occlusion was 0% in one series (Silverstein et al., 1960)!

False Positives

Globe murmurs may also be found in normal persons (Berry, 1965; Wadia & Monckton, 1957). The false positive rate (i.e., the percent of murmurs in which no etiology or vascular symptoms were found) is about 11% (Allen & Mustian, 1962).

Appendix 10-1.
Answers to Questions on Pupillary Light Reflex

In Figure 10-12, situation A shows a pure right afferent lesion. Since both pupils respond when the light is shined into the left eye, both efferents must be intact, as well as the left afferent. Therefore, the absence of any response when the light is shone into the right eye must be due to an isolated right afferent defect. In situation B, the left efferent must be intact because that pupil constricts. Furthermore, since it constricts no matter which eye the light is shining in, both afferents must be intact. Thus, this must be, by logical process of elimination, a pure right efferent lesion.

Appendix 10-2. Ophthalmoscopic Signs of Glaucoma

In Figure 10-20, diagram A shows nasalization of the vessels and verticalization of the cup, two of the "soft" signs of glaucoma.

Appendix 10-3. Answer to Question in Figure 10-36

The patient had prepared an oral medication for intravenous injection, causing talc embolization (Lee & Sapira, 1973).

Appendix 10-4. Six Pearls of Clinical Ophthalmoscopy for the Primary Care Physician and Medical Consultant

1. Attempting to inspect the fundi through constricted pupils is like eating spaghetti with your fingers.
2. Exudates and hemorrhages are *never* normal.
3. No exudate or hemorrhage is specific (in the diagnostic sense) for any disease. But these findings tell you the vasculopathic and neural effects of the disease in that patient at that particular time better than anything else.
4. Microaneurysms = diabetes mellitus, until proven otherwise.

5. Arteriovenous crossing changes that are complete and more than 2 disc diameters out = chronic moderate hypertension, until proven otherwise.

6. The fact that you don't know its significance doesn't mean that it doesn't have significance.

Appendix 10-5. Sarcoidosis

Eye findings in sarcoidosis may include Koeppe's iris nodules; conjunctivitis; corneal scarring; band keratopathy (due to the hypercalcemia); keratoconjunctivis sicca (from lacrimal gland involvement); ocular palsies; anterior uveitis (sometimes nodular); vitreous opacity in the dependent vitreous, sometimes seen as a string-of-pearls shadow on the lower retina; retinal hemorrhages; posterior uveitis, including the retinal granulomas shown in Figure 10-28; periphlebitis with venous sheathing; and disease of the optic nerve, from simple optic neuritis to papilledema or optic nerve atrophy (Chumbley, 1981).

References

Adie WJ: Pseudo-Argyll Robertson pupils with absent tendon reflexes. *Br Med J* 1:928–930, 1931a.

Adie WJ: Argyll Robertson pupils true and false. *Br Med J* 2:136–138, 1931b.

Adler AG, McElwain GE, Merli GJ, Martin JH: Systemic effects of eye drops. *Arch Intern Med* 142:2293–2294, 1982.

Ahmed MM: Ocular effects of antifreeze poisoning. *Br J Ophthalmol* 55:845–855, 1971.

Allen N, Mustian V: Origin and significance of vascular murmurs of the head and neck. *Medicine* 41:227–247, 1962.

Alpert JN: Downbeat nystagmus due to anticonvulsant toxicity. *Ann Neurol* 4:471–473, 1978.

Anonymous: Smooth pursuit impairment in schizophrenia—what does it mean? *Schizophr Bull* 9:37–43, 1983.

Anonymous: Mitoxantrone. *Med Lett Drugs Ther* 30:67–68, 1988.

Armaly MF: Genetic determination of cup/disc ratio of the optic nerve. *Arch Ophthalmol* 78:35–43, 1967.

Au YK, Henkind, P: Pain elicited by consensual pupillary reflex: A diagnostic test for acute iritis. *Lancet* 2:1254–1255, 1981.

Aurell E, Tibblin G: Hypertensive eye-ground changes in a Swedish population of middle-aged men. *Acta Ophthalmol* 43:355–361, 1965.

Barr CC, Glaser JS, Blankenship G: Acute disc swelling in juvenile diabetes: Clinical profile and natural history of 12 cases. *Arch Ophthalmol* 98:2185–2192, 1980.

Bechgaard P, Porsaa K, Voeglius H: Ophthalmological investigation of 500 persons with hypertension of long duration. *Br J Ophthalmol* 34:409–424, 1950.

Berman B: Voluntary propulsion of the eyeballs: The double whammy syndrome. *Arch Intern Med* 117:648–651, 1966.

Berry JN: Benign intracranial and neck bruits in an adult. *Ann Intern Med* 63:661–663, 1965.

Brinchmann-Hansen O, Dahl-Jørgensen K, Hanssen KF, Sandvik L, the Oslo Study Group. Effects of intensified insulin treatment on various lesions of diabetic retinopathy. *Am J Ophthalmol* 100:644–653, 1985.

Brockhurst RJ, Schepens CL, Okamura ID: Uveitis: II. peripheral uveitis: Clinical description, complications, and differential diagnosis. *Am J Ophthalmol* 49:1257–1266, 1960.

Brownstein S, Font RL, Alper MG: Atheromatous plaques of the retinal blood vessel: Histologic confirmation of ophthalmoscopically visible lesions. *Arch Ophthalmol* 90:49–52, 1973.

Burckhardt J: *The Civilization of the Renaissance in Italy.* Harper & Row, New York, 1929.

Chan K-L, Callahan JA, Seward JB, Tajik AJ, Gordon H: Marfan syndrome diagnosed in patients 32 years of age or older. *Mayo Clin Proc* 62:589–594, 1987.

Chrousos GA, Cowdry R, Schuelein M, Abdul-Rahim AS, Matsuo V, Currie JN: Two cases of downbeat nystagmus and oscillopsia associated with carbamazepine. *Am J Ophthalmol* 103:221–224, 1987.

Chumbley LC: *Ophthalmology in Internal Medicine.* WB Saunders, Philadelphia, 1981.

Cogan DG: Down-beat nystagmus. *Arch Ophthalmol* 80:757–768, 1968.

Cogan DG, Albright F, Bartter FC: Hypercalcemia and band keratopathy: Report of nineteen cases. *Arch Ophthalmol* 40:624–638, 1948.

Comer PB, Fred HL: Diagnosis of sickle-cell disease by ophthalmoscopic inspection of the conjunctiva. *N Engl J Med* 271:544–546, 1964.

Condon PI, Serjeant GR: Photocoagulation in proliferative sickle retinopathy: Results of a 5-year study. *Br J Ophthalmol* 64:832–840, 1980.

Cross HE, Jensen AD: Ocular manifestations in the Marfan syndrome and homocystinuria. *Am J Ophthalmol* 75:405–420, 1973.

Dasco CC, Bortz DL: Significance of the Argyll Robertson pupil in clinical medicine. *Am J Med* 86:199–202, 1989.

De Juan E Jr, Hurley DP, Sapira JD: Racial differences in normal values of proptosis. *Arch Intern Med* 140:1230–1231, 1980.

De Schweinitz GE: *Diseases of the Eye: A Handbook of Ophthalmic Practice for Students and Practitioners.* WB Saunders, Philadelphia, 1915.

DeJong RN: *The Neurologic Examination*, ed. 4. Harper & Row, New York, 1979.

Diabetic Retinopathy Study Research Group: Photocoagulation treatment of proliferative diabetic retinopathy: The second report of diabetic retinopathy findings. *Ophthalmology* 85:82–105, 1978.

Diabetic Retinopathy Study Research Group: Photocoagulation treatment of proliferative diabetic retinopathy: Clinical application of diabetic retinopathy study findings, DRS Report Number 8. *Ophthalmology* 88:583–600, 1981.

Dollery CT, Hill DW, Hodge JV: The response of normal retinal blood vessels to angiotensin and noradrenaline. *J Physiol* 165:500–507, 1963.

Donaldson D: The significance of spotting of the iris in mongoloids. *Arch Ophthalmol* 4:50–55, 1961.

Duane TD, Osher RH, Reden R: White centered hemorrhages: Their significance. *Ophthalmology* 87:66–69, 1980.

Duke-Elder S, Leigh AG: *Diseases of the Outer Eye:* VIII. In: Duke-Elder S (ed), *System of Ophthalmology.* CV Mosby, St. Louis, 1965. ["Duke-Elder" is the definitive review of the entire ophthalmology literature published between 1958 and 1976 by Mosby and in London by Henry Kimpton, with helpful illustrations. The nonophthalmologist should consult vol 15, which is an index to the other 14 volumes, arranged by medical disease. Highly recommended.]

Duke-Elder S, Scott GI: *Neuroophthalmology*: XII. In: Duke-Elder S (ed), *System of Ophthalmology.* CV Mosby, St. Louis, 1971.

Eales H: Cases of retinal hemorrhage associated with epistaxis and constipation. *Birmingham Med Rev* 9:262–273, 1880.

Eales H: Primary retinal hemorrhage in young men. *Ophthalmol Rev* 1:41–46, 1882.

Fisher CM: Cranial bruit associated with occlusion of the internal carotid artery. *Neurology* 7:298–306, 1957.

Fishman RS, Sunderman FW: Band keratopathy in gout. *Arch Ophthalmol* 75:367–369, 1966.

Freeman W: Endothelioma of pleura simulating spinal cord tumor. *Int Clin Ser 31.* 4:159–166, 1921.

Gordon SI, Rodgerson DO, Kauffman J: Hypercupremia in a patient with multiple myeloma. *J Lab Clin Med* 70:57–62, 1967.

Grove AS Jr: Evaluation of exophalthmos. *N Engl J Med* 292:1005–1013, 1975.

Hanno HA, Weiss DI: Hypoparathyroidism, pseudohypoparathyroidism, and pseudopseudohypoparathyroidism. *Arch Ophthalmol* 65:238–242, 1961.

Havener WH: *Synopsis of Ophthalmology: The Ophthalmoscopy Book*, ed 6. CV Mosby, St. Louis, 1984.

Heckenlively Jr, Ellis DS: Retinitis pigmentosa: Distinguishing its many forms from other retinopathies. *Consultant* 24(5):51–73, 1984. [Excellent photographs.]

Heilmann C, Richardson KD (eds): *Glaucoma: Conceptions of a Disease.* WB Saunders, Philadelphia, 1978.

Hitchings RA, Spaeth GL: The optic disc in glaucoma: II. Correlation of the appearance of the disc with the visual field. *Br J Ophthalmol* 61:107–113, 1977.

Hofman O, Kamancova E, Kolar M, Reisenauer R, Metousek V: Significance of the difference in the prevalence of certain ophthalmoscopic findings between normotensive and hypertensive subjects. *Acta Univ Carol Med* 19:635–650, 1973.

Hollenhorst RW: Significance of bright plaques in the retinal arterioles. *Trans Am Ophthalmol Soc* 59:252–273, 1961. [One of the few papers containing a published discussion worth reading: Dr. V. (concluding a lengthy discussion based upon philosophy): "I have discussed this matter without knowing a damned thing about it." (Laughter.) Dr. Hollenhorst: "Dr. V., I think you have settled it, at least to my satisfaction." (Laughter.)]

Hutchinson J: On the different forms of inflammation of the eye consequent on inherited syphilis. *Ophthalmol Hosp Rep* 2:54–105, 1859. (Actually, only 8 of the 64 cases had deafness, but all 64 had both keratitis and notched incisors.)

Inkeles DM, Walsh JB: Retinal fat emboli as a sequela to acute pancreatitis. *Am J Ophthalmol* 80:935–938, 1975.

Jacob HS, Goldstein IM, Shapiro I, Craddock PR, Hammerschmidt DE, Weissman G: Sudden blindness in acute pancreatitis: Possible role of complement-induced retinal leukoembolization. *Arch Intern Med* 141:134–136, 1981.

Johnson DH, Brubaker RF: Glaucoma: An overview. *Mayo Clin Proc* 61:59–67, 1986.

Kagan A, Aurell E, Dobree J, Hara K, McKendrick C, Michaelson I, Shaper G, Sundaresan T, Tibblin G: A note on signs in the fundus oculi and arterial hypertension: Conventional assessment and significance. *Bull WHO* 34:955–960, 1966.

Kahn EA, Cherry GR: The clinical importance of spontaneous retinal venous pulsation. *Univ Mich Med Bull* 16:305–308, 1950.

Kalra L, Hamlyn AN, Jones BJM: Blue sclerae: A common sign of iron deficiency. *Lancet* 2:1267–1269, 1986.

Kearns TP, Hollenhorst RW: Venous-stasis retinopathy of occlusive disease of the carotid artery. *Staff Meet Mayo Clin* 38:304–312, 1963.

Killian PJ, McClain B, Lawless OJ: Brown's syndrome: An unusual manifestation of rheumatoid arthritis. *Arthritis Rheum* 20:1080–1084, 1977.

Kincaid MC, Green WR, Knox DL, Mohler C: A clinicopathological case report of retinopathy of pancreatitis. *Br J Ophthalmol* 66:219–226, 1982.

Kramer KK, LaPiana FG, Appleton B: Ocular malingering and hysteria: Diagnosis and management. *Surv Ophthalmol* 24:89–96, 1979.

Lam BL, Thompson HS, Corbett JJ: The prevalence of simple anisocoria. *Am J Ophthalmol* 104:69–73, 1987.

Lauritzen T, Frost-Larsen K, Larsen H-W, Deckert T, the Steno Study Group. *Lancet* 1:200–203, 1983,

Lebas MP, Bernaerts-Lebas MA: Rickettsioses et affections oculaires. *Bull Soc Belge Ophtalmol* 131:437–464, 1962.

Lee J, Sapira JD: Retinal and cerebral microembolization of talc in a drug abuser. *Am J Med Sci* 265:75–77, 1973.

Leigh RJ, Zee DS: *The Neurology of Eye Movements.* FA Davis, Philadelphia, 1983.

Levin BE: The clinical significance of spontaneous pulsation of the retinal vein. *Arch Neurol* 35:37–40, 1978.

Litten M: Über akute maligne Endocarditis und die dabaei vorkommenden retinal Vernderungen. *Charite Ann* 3:137–190, 1878.

Lo Zito JC: Retinal spontaneous venous pulsations in neurologically ill patients: Incidence and significance. *J Fla Med Assoc* 64:355–357, 1977.

Macaraeg PVJ, Lasagna L, Snyder B: Arcus not so senilis. *Ann Intern Med* 68:345–354, 1968.

Maciewicz RJ: Case records of the Massachusetts General Hospital. *N Engl J Med* 309:542–549, 1983.

Mahneke A, Videbaek A: On changes in the optic fundus in leukemia. *Acta Ophthalmol* 42:201–209, 1964.

Michelson EL, Morganroth J, Nichols CW, MacVaugh H III: Retinal arteriolar changes as an indicator of coronary artery disease. *Arch Intern Med* 139:1139–1141, 1979.

Miller NR: *Walsh and Hoyt's Clinical Neuro-Ophthalmology*, ed 4. Williams & Wilkins, Baltimore, 1985.

Nazer H, Ede RJ, Mowat AP, Williams, R: Wilson's disease: Clinical presentation and use of prognostic index. *Gut* 27:1377–1381, 1986.

Newell F: *Ophthalmology: Principles and Concepts*, ed 8. CV Mosby, St. Louis, 1982, p 559.

Newsome DA, Green WR, Miller ED, Kiessling LA, Morgan B, Jabs DA, Polk BF: Microvascular aspects of acquired immune deficiency syndrome retinopathy. *Am J Ophthalmol* 98:590–691, 1984.

Nguyen N, Rimmer S, Katz B: Slowed saccades in the acquired immunodeficiency syndrome. *Am J Ophthalmol* 107:356–360, 1989.

Pancoast HK: Importance of careful roentgen-ray investigations of apical chest tumors. *JAMA* 83:1407–1411, 1924.

Pancoast HK: Superior pulmonary sulcus tumor. *JAMA* 99:1391–1396, 1932.

Paton JD: *The Relation of Angiod Streaks to Systemic Disease.* Charles C Thomas, Springfield, IL, 1972, p 82.

Paton JD, Hyman BN, Justice J Jr.: *Introduction to Ophthalmology.* Upjohn Co, Kalamazoo, MI, 1976. [This excellent monograph has superb color illustrations of various fundi. Although I sometimes disagree with the text, (e.g., in its discussion of the hypertensive fundus), this is still a useful overview of ophthalmoscopy. An additional virtue of this work is its gratis distribution to sophomore medical students by the pharmaceutical company that published it.]

Pau H: *Differential Diagnosis of Eye Diseases.* Translated by G Cibis. WB Saunders, Philadelphia, 1978.

Pavan PR, Aiello LM, Wafai MZ, Briones JC, Sebestyen JG, Bradbury MJ: Optic disc edema in juvenile-onset diabetes. *Arch Ophthalmol* 98:2193–2195, 1980.

Pears MA, Pickering GW: Changes in the fundus oculi after hemorrhage. *Q J Med* 29:153–178, 1960.

Pfaffenback DD, Hollenhorst RW: Morbidity and survivorship of patients with embolic cholesterol crystals in the ocular fundus. *Am J Ophthalmol* 75:372–375, 1973.

Phillips SL, Frank E: Acute orbital pseudotumor: Ocular emergency on a general medical service. *South Med J* 80:792–793, 1987.

Ralph RA: Prediction of cardiovascular status from arteriovenous crossing phenomena. *Ann Ophthalmol* 7:323–326, 1974.

Rapin I, Goldfischer S, Katzman R, Engel J Jr., and O'Brien JS: The cherry-red-spot-myoclonus syndrome. *Ann Neurol* 3:234–424, 1978.

Rimola A, Brunguera M, Rodes J: Kayser-Fleischer-like ring in cryptogenic cirrhosis. *Arch Intern Med* 138:1857–1858, 1978.

Roberts HJ: *Difficult Diagnosis. Atlas.* WB Saunders, Philadelphia, 1958.

Robertson A: On an interesting series of eye-symptoms in a case of spinal disease, with remarks on the action of belladonna on the iris. *Edinburgh Med J* 14:696–708, 1869a.

Robertson A: Four cases of spinal miosis, with remarks on the action of light on the pupil. *Edinburgh Med J* 15:487–493, 1869b.

Robertson D: Tonometry screening on the medical service. *Arch Intern Med* 137:443–445, 1977.

Rodstein M, Zelman FD: Arcus senilis and arteriosclerosis in the aged. *Am J Med Sci* 245:70–78, 1963.

Ross ME, Jacobson IM, Dienstag L, Martin JB: Late-onset Wilson's disease with neurological involvement in the absence of Kayser-Fleischer rings. *Ann Neurol* 17:411–413, 1985.

Roth M: Über Netzhautaffectionen bei Wundfiebern. *Dtsche Z Chir* 1:417–484, 1872.

Roy FH: *Ocular Differential Diagnosis.* Lea & Febiger, Philadelphia, 1972.

Roy FH: *Ocular Differential Diagnosis*, ed 3. Lea & Febiger, Philadelphia, 1984. [A comprehensive unillustrated listing of differential diagnoses of the eye, with no discussion of the lesions or estimation of their relative frequency.]

Salus R: A contribution to the diagnosis of arteriosclerosis and hypertension. *Am J Ophthalmol* 45:81–92, 1958.

Sapira JD: Why is medical school difficult? Or, if it isn't difficult, why it should be. *South Med J* 72:1453–1455, 1979.

Sapira JD: An internist looks at the fundus oculi. *DM* 30(14):1–64, 1984.

Sapira JD, Cherubin CE: Nalorphine and naloxone testing. In: *Drug Abuse*. American Elsevier, New York, 1975.

Scheie HG: Evaluation of ophthalmoscopic changes of hypertension and arteriolar sclerosis. *Arch Ophthalmol* 49:117–138, 1953.

Scheie HG, Albert DM: *Textbook of Ophthalmology*, ed 9. WB Saunders, Philadelphia, 1977.

Schlaegel TF Jr: *Ocular Histoplasmosis*. Grune & Stratton, New York, 1977.

Schlaegel TF Jr: *Ocular Toxoplasmosis and Pars Planitis*. Grune & Stratton, New York, 1978.

Schumacher J, Scheler F: [Metastatic calcification of the cornea and conjunctiva in chronic renal insufficiency]. *Klin Monatsbl Augenheilkd* 154:815–819, 1969.

Seitz R: *The Retinal Vessels*, translated by FC Blodi. CV Mosby, St. Louis, 1964.

Shai F, Baker RK, Addrizzo JR, Wallach S: Hypercalcemia in mycobacterial infection. *J Clin Endocrinol* 34:251–256, 1972.

Shelburne SA: Retinal arteriovenous nicking: A long term study of the development of arteriovenous nicking in hypertensive patients. *Arch Intern Med* 83:377–381, 1949.

Shelburne SA: *Hypertensive Retinal Disease*. Grune & Stratton, New York, 1965.

Silverstein A, Lehrer GM, Mones R: Relation of certain diagnostic features of carotid occlusion to collateral circulation. *Neurology* 10:409–417, 1960.

Smith LH: Ocular complications of rheumatic fever and rheumatoid arthritis. *Am J Ophthalmol* 43:535–582, 1957.

Sperduto RD, Hiller R: Systemic hypertension and age related maculopathy in the Framingham study. *Arch Ophthalmol* 104:216–219, 1986.

Straub W, Russman H: *Atlas of Diseases of the Anterior Segment of the Eye*. McGraw-Hill, New York, 1966.

Svarrdsdudd K, Wedel H, Aurell E, Tibblin G: Hypertensive eye ground changes. *Acta Med Scand* 204:159–167, 1978.

Talbot EM: A simple test to diagnose iritis. *Br Med J* 295:812–813, 1987.

Talbot JF, Bird AC, Serjeant GR, Hayes RJ: Sickle cell retinopathy in young children in Jamaica. *Br J Ophthalmol* 66:149–154, 1982.

Thomas C, Cordier J, Algan B: (Ocular changes in Ehlers-Danlos syndrome). *Arch Ophthalmol* (Paris) 14:690–697, 1954.

Thompson HS: Segmental palsy of the iris sphincter in Adie's syndrome. *Arch Ophthalmol* 96:1615–1620, 1978.

Traboulsi EI, Krush AJ, Gardner EJ, Booker SV, Offerhaus GJA, Yardley JH, Hamilton SR, Luk GD, Giardiello FM, Welsh SB, Hughes JP, Maumenee IH: Prevalence and importance of pigmented ocular fundus lesions in Gardner's syndrome. *N Engl J Med* 316:661–667, 1987.

Van Buchem FSP, Heuvel-Aghina JWM, Heuval JEA: Hypertension and changes of the fundus oculi. *Acta Med Scand* 176:539–548, 1964.

Van Uitert RL, Eisenstadt ML: Venous pulsations not always indicative of normal intracranial pressure. *Arch Neurol* 35:550, 1978.

Van Uitert RL, Solomon GE: White centered retinal hemorrhages: A sign of intracranial hemorrhage. *Neurology* 29:236–239, 1979.

Vogelius H, Bechgaard P: The ophthalmoscopical appearance of the fundus oculi in elderly persons with arteriosclerosis and normal blood pressures. *Br J Ophthalmol* 34:404–408, 1950.

Vollerstein RS, McDonald TJ, Younge BR, Banks PM, Standon AW, Halstrup DM: Cogan's syndrome: 18 cases and a review of the literature. *Mayo Clin Proc* 61:344–361, 1986.

Wadia NH, Monckton G: Intracranial bruits in health and disease. *Brain* 80:492–509, 1957. [Good historical review with emphasis on children.]

Wahl JW: Systemic reaction to tropicamide. *Arch Ophthalmol* 82:320–321, 1969.

Waldo M: *The Art of Spaghetti Cookery*. Doubleday, Garden City, NY, 1964.

Walsh FB, Hoyt WF: *Clinical Neuroophthalmology*, vol 1, ed 3. Williams & Wilkins, Baltimore, 1969.

Walsh TJ, Garden J, Gallagher B: Relationship of retinal venous pulse to intracranial pressure. In: Smith JL (ed), *Neuro-ophthalmology*, ed 4. CV Mosby, St. Louis, 1968.

Weinberg LM, Brasitus TA, Lefkowitch JH: Fluctuating Kayser-Fleischer-like rings in a jaundiced patient. *Arch Intern Med* 141:246–247, 1981.

Wendland JP: Retinal arteriosclerosis in age, essential hypertension, and diabetes mellitus. *Trans Am Ophthalmol Soc* 64:735–761, 1966.

Wiener SL, Nathanson M: *Med Times*, 1976–1977. [See reference in Chapter 29.]

Wood CM, Bosanquet RC: Limitations of direct ophthalmoscopy in screening for glaucoma. *Br Med J* 294:1587–1588, 1987.

Younge BR, Sutula, F: Analysis of trochlear nerve palsies: Diagnosis etiology and treatment. *Mayo Clin Proc* 52:11–18, 1977.

11
The Ear

"Nature, I am persuaded, did not without a purpose frame our ears open, putting thereto no gate at all, nor shutting them up with any manner of inclosures, as she hath done upon the tongue, the eyes, and other such out-jetting parts of the body. The cause as I imagine, is, to the end that every day and every night, and that continually, we may be ready to hear, and by a perpetual hearing apt to learn. For, of all the senses, it is the fittest for the reception of the knowledge of arts, sciences, and disciplines."

Rabelais, *Gargantua and Pantagruel*, III, 16

External Inspection

It is best to examine the patient sitting up, if possible, so that his ears are approximately at your eye level.

Deformities of the External Ear

Look for low-set ears, a sign of Down's syndrome. Ears are considered to be low set when they are completely beneath a coronal plane passing through the pupils and palpebral fissures. (Do not use this for neonates, as it will produce false positives.)

Benign isolated abnormalities of the ears, such as bat-wing ears, Aztec ears, and Darwinian tubercles, will not be considered here because they are not presently known to be associated with disease.

Deformities of the ear, including those of just the earlobe, are said to correlate with renal abnormalities, predicting the side(s) of the lesion. In order to demonstrate this, one needs a patient in whom an intravenous pyelogram has been obtained. Since this is not a routine screening test, this clinical correlation is at least partly based upon a biased sample, leading to an artifactually increased predictive value of a positive test. (In other words, no intravenous pyelogram would have been performed unless there had been some reason to suspect a renal problem.) Still, the correlation seems to be a useful one, although many of the anomalies are benign and asymptomatic ones such as reduplication of the ureter on the side of the ear malformation.

Earlobe Creases

Earlobe creases (also called Frank creases for their discoverer) are a risk factor* for coronary artery disease (Elliott, 1983; Frank, 1973) (Fig. 11-1). Since they may occur on only one side, be sure to look at both earlobes.

A study of 340 consecutive patients undergoing coronary arteriography has shown that the Frank sign, if present in either ear

---

*Remember, a risk factor is a statistical phenomenon. A risk factor is not necessarily an etiologic factor.

and extending for a distance greater than half the diagonal length of the earlobe, correlated with coronary artery disease, age, and arcus senilis (Pasternac & Sami, 1982). The sensitivity of the sign was 60%. (Review Ch. 1, p. 6, and write down definitions for sensitivity, specificity, and positive predictive value on a piece of paper). The specificity of the test was 82%. (Recall that specificity refers to the chance that a person who does not have the disease will not have the sign.) The positive predictive value of the sign was 91%. This suggests that the test is fairly good.

Dr. A.I. Mendeloff of Maryland points out that 75% of the subjects (in this study) had coronary artery disease. That is, the study population had a very high prevalence of the disease in question, much higher than the prevalence that would be seen in a supposedly random population presenting at a physician's office. Since the prevalence of the disease would actually be much less in a nonselected population, would you expect a study of the Frank earlobe crease, using the same criteria but a randomly selected population, to produce a different result for sensitivity, specificity, or positive predictive value? Write down your answers at this point. (*Hint*: Ask yourself which items in the equations would be increased by diluting out the numbers in the present study with persons who have no coronary artery disease.)

In a review of the world literature (Elliott, 1983), involving 6,414 cases with varying criteria for the diagnosis of coronary artery disease, 1,721 cases had a true positive earlobe crease, 1,034 had a false positive, 1,112 had a false negative, and 2,547 had a true negative. In 1,000 consecutive personal cases, including 843 general medical admissions and 157 patients from a cardiac catheterization lab, there were 275 true positives, 98 false positives, 101 false negatives, and 526 false negatives (Elliott, 1983).

Exercise for the student: Construct 2 x 2 contingency tables, and calculate the sensitivities, specificities, and positive predictive values for the literature review and for Elliott's series. What are the predictive values of a negative test? (The answer is in Appendix 11-1.)

Age is a confounding variable. The degeneration of elastic substance around arterioles, which is thought to be the cause of the crease, is an accompaniment of arteriolar sclerosis and also occurs with aging. But the association with coronary artery disease exists in all age groups (Elliott, 1983).

A smaller subsequent study failed to find a significant association between earlobe creases and coronary artery disease (Brady et al., 1987). In analyzing such papers, students should ask the following questions: 1) What is the power of the study? Were suffi-

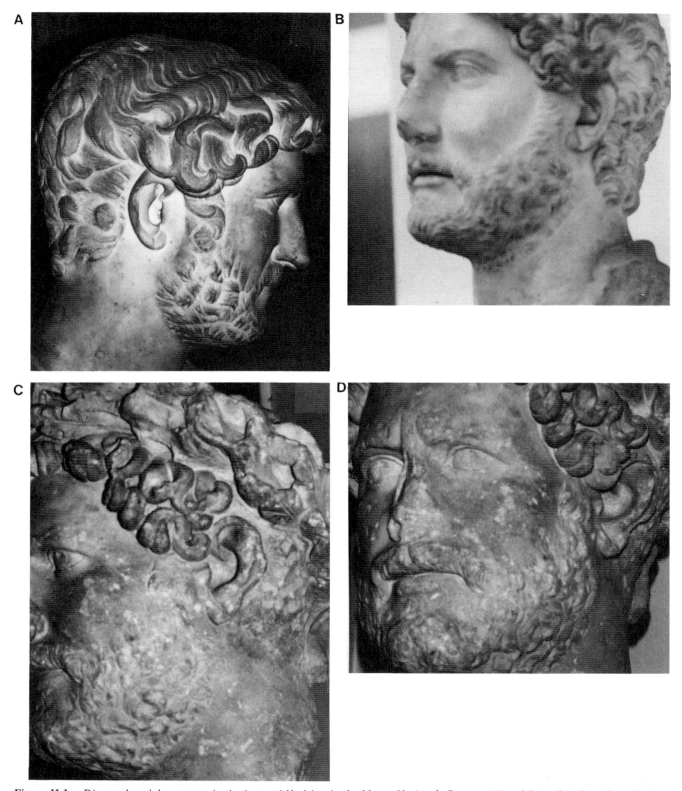

Figure 11-1.   *Diagonal earlobe creases in the busts of Hadrian in the Museo Nazionale Romano (A and B) and in the Athens National Museum #3729 (C and D). Photographs reproduced, with permission, from the masterful essay on the diagonal earlobe crease, type A behavior, and the death of Emperor Hadrian (Petrakis, 1980).*

cient patients included to have a reasonable chance of finding an association, if it exists? 2) Were confounding variables, such as hypertension, age, and smoking, handled appropriately (as by a multivariate analysis)? 3) Was there a selection bias? If the risk factor is associated with disease at a young age, a noncohort study of an elderly population may be negative because of premature "die-out" of affected individuals. (This may also account for negative results in some of the later studies of type A personality). 4) Is there publication bias? (That is, doctors who believe in modifying risk factors might not want to suggest operating on asymptomatic earlobes.)

Skin Lesions

The external ear may be affected by skin lesions, including solar keratoses and carcinomas, both basal cell and squamous cell.

The skin of the pinna and external canal is frequently involved in seborrheic dermatitis and other dermatoses, which cause scaling, edema, and inflammation.

A vesicular rash on the pinna occurs in Ramsay Hunt syndrome, caused by a *Herpes zoster* infection of the facial nerve; it should be specifically sought in patients presenting with a facial paralysis (see Ch. 26, p. 458).

Other Findings

Collections of urate in the form of tophi may be seen in the external ear, but these are quite rare these days due to the combination of automated uric acid analyses and effective hypouricemic drugs. Nevertheless, if found in an arthritic patient, they could be a valuable clue to a gouty etiology.

See Chapter 17 (p. 323) for the winking earlobe signs.

Palpation

Feel the external ear and tug on it. Is it painful? Many patients with otitis cannot stand to have the external ear touched even though it looks normal. Check the mastoid process for tenderness (see Ch. 9, p. 149, "Mastoiditis").

Floppy ears may be felt in relapsing polychondritis. However, not all patients with this disease actually have floppy ears; sometimes the ears simply show inflammation of the pinna. In one series collected in a single institution, 85% of 112 patients with relapsing polychondritis had some evidence of such auricular chondritis at some point during their illness (Michet et al., 1986).

A note to sophomores. You have probably not heard of the disease, relapsing polychondritis. Thus, it is a "border phrase": a phrase on the border of this work and another, a textbook of medicine. This is a good time to apply the technique for increasing your apparent IQ suggested in Chapter 6 (p. 89). Jot down this unfamiliar term and look it up before you go to sleep tonight.

Dr. A. I. Mendeloff of Maryland, who has seen many patients with Addison's disease, notes that stiffening of the earlobe is a useful sign favoring that diagnosis. This phenomenon is distinct from the Addisonian calcification of cartilage, which is nondiagnostic, having also been reported in other endocrine disorders such as hyperthyroidism, pseudo-pseudohypoparathyroidism, diabetes mellitus, acromegaly, and hypopituitarism, and in metabolic disturbances including ochronosis and hypercalcemia. In the

two cases of acromegaly that had such calcification, pituitary and adrenal insufficiency were not excluded. It has also been seen in sarcoid, presumably due to hypercalcemia. Furthermore, it may occur in conditions that produce localized injury to tissue, such as frostbite, trauma, and inflammation (bacterial chondritis, nonbacterial chondritis, and perichondritis). Miscellaneous etiologies are senile keratosis and idiopathic calcification in the aged (Randall & Spong, 1963).

Internal Inspection

A Method

1. From your collection of specula, select one that is the correct size for the patient. Use the largest one possible for the best view and the least chance of hurting the patient. Place a plastic or paper disposable cover over the speculum, if you have one. Otherwise check that the speculum was cleaned (by washing in hot soapy water and rinsing with alcohol) since its last use.

2. Turn the light on. For examining the patient's right ear, place the otoscope in your right hand, so that your left hand is free to lift the patient's external ear superiorly, posteriorly, and away from the head, in order to straighten the canal of adults and older children. (In infants, you will need to pull inferiorly on the auricle.)

For the left ear, hold the otoscope in your left hand, so that you can manipulate the ear with your right hand, without having to cross hands.

3. Hold the otoscope so that you are comfortable. Most people grasp it like a hammer. Others cradle the battery compartment in the "V" between the thumb and forefinger, with the handle pointing up. The latter has the advantage that in an uncooperative patient or excitable child, you can rest the ulnar edge of your hand against the patient's head, so that you will automatically move the otoscope if the patient moves his head, and so avoid injuring the ear canal. Examining such a patient in the lateral decubitus position will also reduce the potential movement of the head.

4. Look through the otoscope. Insert the speculum in the canal, as you tug on the ear with your other hand (see step 2). (If you are performing this examination correctly, it should be nearly painless, unless the patient has a furuncle or foreign body in his ear canal.)

5. If there is cerumen in the canal, clean it out with warm mineral oil or warm olive oil and a cotton-tipped swab. Do not use a swab to remove hardened wax as you may impact it against the eardrum. You may be able to lavage wax from the canal with water and an ear syringe (after softening it with over-the-counter drops such as Debrox). Do not lavage the canal if a perforated eardrum is suspected. In any case, be sure to use water of approximately body temperature; cold or hot fluids will set up thermal currents in the endolymph, induce nystagmus, and induce vomiting in some patients. (See caloric testing, Ch. 26, p. 480). If you use a blunt cerumen spoon to remove wax, do it only under direct vision, preferably using a head mirror (a skill accrued only by considerable practice, usually from working in the ENT clinic).

In truth, many physicians simply do not clean out the canal if it is occluded with cerumen. Sometimes one can get a partial look. If the Weber and Rinne (see below) are normal, and the patient has no complaints referable to the ear, examination of the eardrum is less critical. But otherwise, you must visualize the eardrum.

Note: Don't forget to clean the speculum on your otoscope before putting it away.

Ear Canal

Inspect the external canal for foreign bodies, such as errant insects, pieces of food (in the toddler set), or pieces of stored hashish among adolescents of all ages. Blood in the external canal can be a useful sign of fracture of the middle fossa.

An exquisitely tender red spot is a furuncle, even if it does not have a white center.

In external otitis, the canal may be edematous, inflamed, and coated with an exudate. It may be difficult to distinguish infectious from noninfectious etiologies. "Swimmer's ear" due to a variety of bacteria, but especially *Pseudomonas*, is a common external otitis. It is often accompanied by tenderness over the tragus and tender regional adenopathy. In fungal infections, tiny fungus particles may be seen in the canal. These may be white, grey, black, tan, yellow, or blue-green in color. External otitis in an elderly diabetic is of very serious concern, as it may progress to malignant external otitis and osteomyelitis of the temporal bone.

A bony exostosis in the canal is a rounded nodule of hypertrophic bone. It is to be distinguished from an osteoma, a benign tumor that is attached to the inner third of the canal wall by a bony pedicle.

Tympanic Membrane

Look for the landmarks on the tympanic membrane. Figure 11-2 is a highly schematic diagram. The shadows are seldom seen; it is quite rare to see all three of them in the same patient. Similarly, the flaccid part is usually not as well visualized as the diagram suggests.

Manubrium is the Latin word for handle. The *umbo* was the protuberance in the middle of a Roman shield; the umbo of the *malleus* (hammer) is a similar protuberance. *Annulus* means rim or ring.

If the tympanic membrane is retracted, as with blockage of the eustachian tube, the umbo will stand out greatly.

If the membrane is bulging outward and the landmarks are obscured, the diagnosis of acute suppurative otitis media can be made.

If bubbles are seen *behind* the eardrum, one may diagnose acute serous otitis media. There may also be a fluid level behind the drum. If the fluid is high enough to reach the manubrium of the malleus, this line, which is actually a meniscus, may break in two and appear as two slightly curved lines (menisci) bowed out from the manubrium. Sometimes, both the meniscus and the bubbles may be seen.

Blisters, looking like bubbles on the near surface of the drum, are bullae or vesicles. Bullous otitis media is not diagnostic of mycoplasma infection, also being seen with bacterial infections or even viral infections as in the Ramsay Hunt syndrome.

Blood behind the tympanic membrane is seen in fractures of the skull. The sign was discovered by the British surgeon W.H. Battle (1855–1936), who also described several other signs of similar significance (see Ch. 9, p. 145).

The annulus must be carefully inspected over its entire circumference, because very small perforations sometimes begin there. (Perforations are usually evidence of trauma or a prior episode of otitis media.) Also, a cholesteatoma may perforate there. A cholesteatoma is an accretion of squamous cells that seems to take on a life of its own, penetrating through the tympanic membrane and sometimes even eroding bone in the middle ear. It may appear as a little pearly or fatty fleck, as if a bit of Brie had stuck to the annulus. The cholesteatoma can be a clue to the presence of a brain abscess.

At times, you may want to check the mobility of the tympanic membrane. An immobile eardrum results from a perforation, old middle-ear adhesions, a blocked eustachian tube, a middle-ear

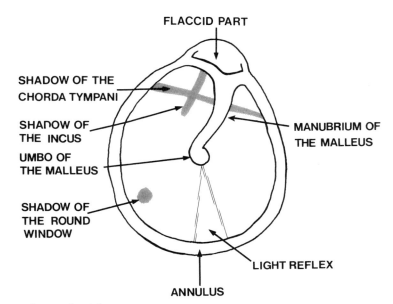

Figure 11-2. *The tympanic membrane of a right ear.*

effusion, or acute otitis media (presumably due to a combination of edema, inflammation, and fluid).

One should especially perform pneumatoscopy in children because decreased eardrum mobility can result in impairment of hearing and language acquisition. Some otoscopes are equipped with a little nipple that accepts a rubber tube attached to a squeeze bulb (Politzer bag). With the lens and ear speculum in place, an airtight system can be obtained. Observe the patient's eardrum through the otoscope as you squeeze the bulb to vary the air pressure. (Also see "The Politzer Maneuver" on p. 214.)

Alternately, you can ask the patient to hold his nose and swallow. Sometimes you can see eardrum motion in this way (without the fancy equipment).

Auscultation

If the patient complains of a whooshing sound, he may be hearing the noise of an arteriovenous fistula anywhere from the carotid up into the temporal lobe. Alternately, he may be describing the vascular tinnitus that afflicts the elderly and that is not pathophysiologically based upon arteriovenous fistula but rather upon a vascular stenosis with a high-grade obstruction maintained throughout systole and sometimes part or all of diastole.

In the case of the arteriovenous fistula, one can sometimes auscult the very same sound that the patient is hearing, while with vascular tinnitus, one usually cannot hear the sound. But one can still make the diagnosis by temporarily occluding the carotid artery ipsilateral to the ear in which the patient reports the sound. That will stop the blood flow and therefore stop the tinnitus.

A continuous sound, like water running, that the patient can hear but the doctor cannot, may be due to a ventriculoperitoneal shunt. To make the diagnosis, clamp the shunt for a time. The sound should immediately disappear, to recur when the occlusion is released (Ordia et al., 1987).

A consultant was once asked to examine a patient in whom the sound of a ticking watch could be heard emanating from the left ear, so as to determine whether a ticking watch was present in the ear. It was not. On auscultation of the left preauricular area, a clicking sound was heard, which differed from the sound of a watch in that it was variable in rhythm and would begin and stop abruptly. (The sound could actually be heard without a stethoscope.) If respiration was suspended, the clicking would cease after a slight slowing of rate, and would never resume during held inspiration.

The consultant diagnosed cyclic obstruction of the left eustachian tube, because he could think of nothing else. This unproved diagnosis was accepted, without any effort to refute it, when radiographs confirmed the absence of a ticking watch.

Study question: *What might have been done to refute the diagnosis? (See Appendix 11-2.)*

Special Maneuvers

Checking for Hearing Loss

Those who believe they can detect hearing defects by simply observing a patient's behavior are usually wrong. For example, who would have thought that a totally deaf person could compose the score illustrated in Figure 11-3?

Walk *behind* the patient and whisper an instruction such as, "raise your right arm." If the patient responds appropriately, he has passed a very crude screening test for total or severe *bilateral* hearing loss.

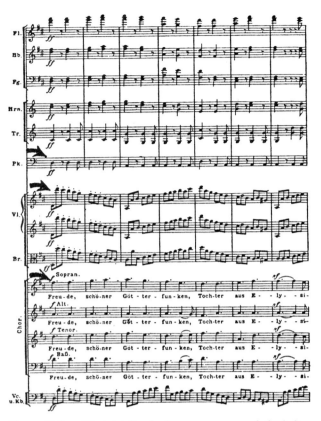

Figure 11-3. *What totally deaf person composed this? See Appendix 11-3.*

Alternately, ask him in a natural voice to repeat "the following numbers," then whisper a random set of numbers, such as your unlisted telephone number. To test the ears *separately,* you *must* have him occlude first one ear, then the other.

To distinguish a conduction from a sensorineural hearing loss, you *must* perform the Rinne and Weber or Schwabach tests (vide infra).

Often, persons who will not take a few seconds to do a Weber and a Rinne cannot think of anything more original to whisper than "1, 2, 3," and thus the patient can transfer the "sound" information from the good ear to a good guess on the bad side. Or if the numbers are whispered in front of the patient, he may be able to read the examiner's lips. If you stand in front of the patient and hold your wristwatch near his ear, he may respond affirmatively to your query about ticking—even if he is deaf, and even if you have a digital watch.

I personally perform the Weber and Rinne tests on all comers as my screening tests.

The Weber Test

If one ear is occluded and one ear is open, the tone will be stronger in the occluded ear than in the open ear. (Translated from E.H. Weber, *De Pulsu Resorptione, Auditu et Tactu*, 1834) (During a discussion of the tuning fork, which, while vibrating, had been applied to the teeth.)

Self-Study

Normally, vibrations are transmitted through solid matter quite well. Strike your tuning fork (preferably 1024 Hz or 512 Hz) and hold the base against your skull in the midline. You may hold the fork against the top of your skull or your forehead or the front incisors; the important factor is that the fork be equidistant from your two ears. Notice that the sound is heard in both ears. Obviously, if you had sufficient neural damage on one side, you would not hear the hum on that side. The Weber would then be said to have lateralized to the good side.

What makes the Weber test so valuable is that in cases of conduction deafness (e.g., middle-ear disease), which spare the neural tissue, the Weber lateralizes to the bad side! To demonstrate this, give yourself a temporary left conduction loss (sparing neural tissue) by occluding your left external canal with a finger. Now place the vibrating fork against your skull in the midline, and note that the sound is louder on the left side, where the canal is occluded. If you cannot appreciate this, rapidly occlude and unocclude the external canal on that side (about once per second), as the midline tuning fork vibrates.

A Method

1. Place the vibrating tuning fork on the patient's skull, in the midline.

2. Ask, "What do you feel?" The patient may say, "buzzing," "tingling," or some phrase that refers to vibration. Note that the feeling of vibration has nothing to do with the Weber test per se, but gives the patient a reference point for later testing of vibratory sensation. Without such a reference point, patients may feel the pressure of the tuning fork and say, "Yes, I feel it" (with reference to the tactile sensation), even though they cannot perceive the vibrations. (Although vibratory testing [see Ch. 26, p. 507] is part of the neurologic examination, in practice you should do it at this point while you have the tuning fork in hand. The rest of the method described here, however, is concerned only with hearing.)

3. As the fork continues to vibrate, ask the patient, "Do you *hear* anything?" If he says, "No," have him close his eyes and question him again. (If he really cannot hear the fork in either ear, then he cannot have a conduction defect and must have a complete bilateral neural defect. But in that case, how could he hear your second question, with his eyes closed? Keep trying.)

4. When he says, "Yes," ask him, "Which ear?" Most patients with normal hearing will say, "Both."

A normal Weber is recorded as "midline." A lateralizing Weber is recorded as the side on which it is heard (e.g., "lateralized to the left") (see Ch. 4, p. 68).

Some overly cooperative patients with normal hearing will attempt to please you by picking one side. In that case, you may have to "help" the patient by repositioning the fork, repeating the test, and saying, "Can you hear it in both ears now?" However, you should not say this initially as it is a form of "leading the witness." In any event, such false lateralizations might give some information about the patient's personality, if not his ears. Of course, one can only know if this is a false lateralization by checking whether the results are consistent with the Rinne test and the other parts of the examination.

•

Historical Note

The Weber test is often miscredited to F.E. Weber, a German otologist who lived from 1832 to 1891. However, the basic physiology underlying the test principle was elucidated when he (F.E.) was only 2 years old by E.F.W. Weber (1806–1871), who published with his physiologist brother, E.H. Weber (1795–1878) (see epigram above), as well as with another brother W.E. Weber (1804–1891), who was a physicist. One of these Webers also gets credit, according to the oral tradition, for the selection of the 512-Hz tuning fork, one that is in the midrange of the conversational voice.

Clinically, the Weber test was popularized by Edouard Schmalz, who also invented the test now known as the Schwabach test, which is presented on page 213 (Morton, 1983).

•

The Rinne Test

Self-Study

Convince yourself of the fact that normally air conduction is better than bone conduction. Strike the tuning fork and place the base over your right mastoid prominence. Listen to the sound fade. The moment it disappears, quickly move the fork from the mastoid, and place the vibrating tines as close to the right external canal as possible without damping them on your hair or auricle (you may need to use a mirror and/or to use your free hand to hold your hair back from the ear). The sound will reappear. Repeat the test on the left side. Now try the Rinne on your partner, using the instructions given below.

A Method

1. Place the vibrating fork on one of the patient's mastoid prominences. Ask, "Do you hear anything?" (If the patient does not hear anything, you have identified total sensorineural hearing loss on that side, and should proceed to the other side.)

2. When the patient answers, "Yes," say, "Tell me the very instant it goes away."

3. When he says that it is gone, immediately move the fork from the mastoid and place the vibrating tines as close as possible to the ipsilateral external canal. If the patient doesn't spontaneously volunteer something like, "It came back," or, "I hear it," ask, "Now?" Normally, he will nod "yes" or say words to the effect that he can again hear the sound.

A normal Rinne test would be recorded as follows: AC (for air conduction) > BC (bone conduction) bilaterally (see Ch. 4, p. 68).

Patients with conduction defects will not hear the sound return because for them bone conduction is greater than air conduction. On the other hand, with sensorineural impairment, the Rinne test remains normal: both air conduction and bone conduction are decreased, but the relative superiority of air conduction remains. When you test a patient with unilateral sensorineural loss, you will note that the examination is performed very quickly on the bad side; that is, the sound fades much more rapidly than on the normal side.

Accordingly, some investigators have suggested quantitating the difference by counting the number of seconds required for bone conduction to decay on the two sides. This presumes that you are able to strike the tuning fork with the same impetus every time you perform the test. Another modification for picking up bilateral partial sensorineural loss in a patient who has a normal Rinne and Weber is to see whether you can still hear the vibrating fork when the patient reports that air conduction has ceased. This presumes that the examiner has normal hearing.

False Positives

Some overly cooperative patients may wait to "be sure" that the sound has disappeared from the mastoid and so delay reporting its cessation for so long that almost all fork vibrations have ceased before they say, "It's gone." For them, you may need to repeat the test, strongly emphasizing the words "the very instant it's gone" in the instructions.

•

Historical Note

Some examiners ask the patient to listen to a watch ticking. Perhaps this is in tribute to Sir Astley Cooper (1768–1848), who anticipated the Rinne test by performing it with a pocket watch rather than a tuning fork. For this, he won the Copley medal, although he is better remembered as the first surgeon to ligate an abdominal aneurysm (Morton, 1983). Others will remember him as being the attending physician of the medical student John Keats (Laborde, 1986).

•

Synthesizing the Results

Remember to check both the Weber and the Rinne for each ear. This will enable you to determine whether there is a hearing loss, whether it is unilateral or bilateral, and whether it involves a conduction or sensorineural defect (see Table 11-1). For example, what would cause the following? Weber lateralizes to the left, AC > BC R, BC > AC L.

(The most common cause of a lateralizing conduction defect is the occlusion of the external canal by cerumen. That is why you should do the Weber and Rinne after doing inspection of the ear.)

It is quite amazing how many patients who are described as "peculiar" or who have a vague psychiatric "diagnosis," turn out to have hearing loss when examined according to the above scheme. Many of these have been reported to have normal hearing by whispering alone, wristwatch alone, or the ubiquitous "grossly intact" test.

The Schwabach Test

The Schwabach test compares the patient's bone conduction with that of the examiner (who has normal hearing). As with the Rinne,

the vibrating tuning fork is placed against the mastoid, and the patient is asked to report when the vibrations cease. Immediately, the examiner places the tuning fork against his own mastoid, and records the time (in seconds) until the sound ceases. If he cannot hear the sound, the order of the examination is reversed. The examiner listens until the sound ceases, then places the tuning fork against the patient's mastoid.

The Schwabach is normal when patient and examiner have approximately equal conduction times. The Schwabach is said to be diminished when the examiner can hear the tone long after the patient. That is a sign of sensorineural impairment. The Schwabach is said to be increased or prolonged when the patient's bone conduction is appreciably longer than the examiner's. This occurs in conductive hearing loss because the room noise masks the sound of the tuning fork in a normal ear, but not in one with a conduction defect. Thus, this test is the only examination that should not be conducted in a perfectly quiet room!

A New Test

Very advanced. Some patients who are overly cooperative and/or cerebrally insufficient may give a paradoxical Rinne test (i.e., bone conduction greater than air conduction on the side of a unilateral total sensorineural defect). Such patients have "learned" to perceive the vibration of the fork against the skull on the defective side, coupled with the experience of hearing the BC in the opposite ear, as "hearing." The Schwabach test should clarify the situation. But in the event that your own hearing is impaired, and you cannot do a Schwabach, you might try the following maneuver.

Repeat the Weber test (which lateralizes to the healthy side), slowly marching the tuning fork from the midline towards the mastoid on the affected side. The patient will continue to lateralize the Weber correctly back to the intact side. But sometimes you will reach a zone of demarcation close to the afflicted ear where the patient begins to "lateralize" to the afflicted side. If you then occlude the good ear, the "line of demarcation" for the Weber will not move at all, because the "cooperating" patient is still responding to the learned skull sensation of the tuning fork, and not to the sound.

In contrast, a patient who is responding to sound will hear better in the occluded ear, and the zone of demarcation will shift.

The Politzer Test

Perform the Politzer test for unilateral hearing loss (to be distinguished from the Politzer maneuver, see below), by placing the gently vibrating tuning fork in front of the nares, and ask the patient to swallow. During swallowing, when the eustachian tubes are open, the vibrations will be transmitted to the middle ear. Accord-

Table 11-1. Diagnosis of Hearing Loss

Diagnosis	Weber Test	Rinne Test		Schwabach Test	
		Right	Left	Right	Left
Normal	Midline	AC>BC, about 60 sec	AC>BC, about 60 sec	N	N
Right conduction loss	—> R	BC>AC	AC>BC	P[a]	N
Partial right sensorineural loss	—> L	AC>BC, about 10 sec	AC>BC, about 60 sec	D[b]	N
Total right sensorineural loss	—> L	Can't hear at all (BC, 0 sec)	AC>BC	Can't hear	N
Bilateral conduction loss	Midline	BC>AC	BC>AC	Not done	
Bilateral partial sensorineural loss	Midline	AC>BC, about 10 sec	AC>BC, about 10 sec	D	D

[a]P, prolonged.
[b]D, diminished.

ingly, the patient will be able to hear the tuning fork only on the unaffected side, and only during swallowing.

For additional methods to check hearing, see Chapter 26 (p. 460).

The Politzer Maneuver

1. Also called the fistula test, the Politzer maneuver can be used to check for the presence of a fistula through the horizontal semicircular canal, in cases of chronic suppuration of the middle ear. A Politzer bag fitted with an atomizer tip is used to compress the air in the external canal. If a fistula is present, the patient will develop vertigo, and usually nystagmus. (A false-negative test may occur if the labyrinth is dead.)

This test may be performed in all patients with chronic middle-ear infection, especially if there is a history of vertigo. If a fistula is present, infection may track from the middle ear and the mastoid into the inner ear, causing complete deafness, and eventually meningitis (Adams et al., 1978).

2. The Politzer maneuver was also used in the predecongestant era to clear the eustachian tubes, especially in the negative form (i.e., using negative pressure from the Politzer bag to suck the pus out).

Appendix 11-1. Earlobe Crease: Sensitivity, Specificity, and Predictive Value

Answers to questions on page 207:

If the numbers in the Pasternac and Sami study were diluted out with persons who had no coronary artery disease, sensitivity would not change. Sensitivity is only concerned with how good the sign is in a population of persons who actually have the disease.

Specificity would not change, because both true negatives and false positives would increase proportionately.

Thus, sensitivity and specificity may be said to be "prevalence-free" statistics. This is another way of saying that they can be misleading if the study population is not representative of the usual population.

Positive predictive value, in contrast to the other values, would go down. In the usual population, the positive predictive value of the earlobe crease is far less than 91%. Consider the formula for positive predictive value (true positives/(true positives + false positives). Of its terms, only the false positives would increase, as patients without the disease are added to the study population. That means that the denominator, but not the numerator, will increase, so the positive predictive value will decrease.

For the world literature review, the sensitivity of the earlobe crease for coronary artery disease was 61%, the specificity was 71%, and the positive predictive value was 62%. For Elliott's cases, the sensitivity was 73%, the specificity 84%, and the positive predictive value 74%. The predictive values of a negative test, defined as the true negatives/(true negatives + false negatives) were 70% and 84%, respectively.

Appendix 11-2. Testing the Diagnosis of a Blocked Eustachian Tube

The diagnosis on page 211 could have been tested by: 1) Valsalva maneuver, 2) Politzer maneuver, or 3) decongestants as a therapeutic-diagnostic trial.

Appendix 11-3. Answer to Question on Page 211

The score is from the final movement of Beethoven's Ninth Symphony.

References

Adams GL, Boies LR Jr, Paparella MM: *Boies's Fundamentals of Otolaryngology*, ed 5. WB Saunders, Philadelphia, 1978.

Brady PM, Zive MA, Goldberg RJ, Gore JM, Dalen JE: A new wrinkle to the earlobe crease. *Arch Intern Med* 147:65–66, 1987.

Elliott WJ: Ear lobe crease and coronary artery disease. *Am J Med* 75:1024–1032, 1983.

Frank STM: Aural sign of coronary artery disease. *N Engl J Med* 289:327–328, 1973.

Laborde RP: The poet-physician: Medicine's impact on the lives and works of John Keats and Robert Bridges. *The Pharos* 49 (winter): 8–11, 1986.

Michet CJ, McKenna CH, Luther HS, O'Fallon WM: Relapsing polychondritis: Survival and predictive role of early disease manifestations. *Ann Intern Med* 104:74–78, 1986.

Morton LT: *A Medical Biography (Garrison and Morton)*, ed 4. Gower Publishing, Hampshire, 1983.

Ordia JI, Mortara RW, Spatz EL: Audible cerebrospinal fluid flow through a ventriculoperitoneal shunt. *J Neurosurg* 67:460–462, 1987.

Pasternac A, Sami M: Predictive value of the ear-crease sign in coronary artery disease. *Can Med Assoc J* 126:645–649, 1982.

Petrakis NL: Diagonal earlobe creases, type A behavior, and the death of Emperor Hadrian. *West J Med* 132:878–91, 1980.

Randall RE, Spong FW: Calcification of the auricular cartilage in a patient with hypopituitarism. *N Engl J Med* 269:1135–1137, 1963.

12
The Nose

Self-assessment quiz:

Q: Who invented the joke about the doctor who specialized in the left nostril?

A: "I tell you, the old doctor who could cure you of every illness has all but vanished and you find nothing but specialists these days. They even advertise in the newspapers. If you have something the matter with your nose, for instance, they'll send you to Paris, where they have the greatest nose specialist in all Europe. So you go to Paris. The specialist looks inside your nose and announces: Well, all right, I'll take care of your right nostril, but I really don't handle left nostrils; for that you'll have to go to Vienna where there's a really great left-nostril specialist. He'll look into it when we've finished here."

See Appendix 12-1 for author and source.

External Appearance

The bulbous swollen nose of rhinophyma (a variant of acne rosacea) permits an "elevator diagnosis" (Fig. 12-1). The term comes from the Greek word *rhino*, which means nose, and *phyma*, which means growth. Rhinophyma has a statistical association with ingestion of alcohol and other vasoactive influences such as climate. However, the sign is of unknown specificity, and, since most patients with alcoholism do not have it, of low sensitivity. An association with basal cell carcinoma has been clearly established (Roenigk, 1987).

Saddle nose is caused by the erosion of the bony portion of the nose. It is seen in congenital syphilis. (See Fig. 12-2.)

An appearance similar to saddle nose, but actually due to destruction of the cartilaginous portion, is also seen in what disease? (If you are reading this work in sequence, you have already come across this disease in Ch. 11 (p. 209), with the advice that you learn to cross-reference readings in this work with those in your favorite medical textbook.)

1. The nostrils flare during normal respiration only in diseases of the chest or in those abdominal conditions touching upon the diaphragm (see "Cope," Silen, 1979).

2. Midline granuloma can completely destroy the nose and other central facial structures including bone. At that stage, it is not usually a diagnostic problem.

Leprosy, fungi, trauma, and tumors may also destroy the external nose, though they are less devastating to other structures than midline granuloma.

3. Nose piercing for decorative purposes may cause infection and swelling, particularly if the stud is retained within the tissues. If the stud penetrates the lateral nasal cartilages, there is the possibility of perichondritis and necrosis of the cartilage, leading to alar collapse. In most cases, simple removal of the retained stud leads to uneventful healing (Watson et al., 1987).

Internal Appearance

Methods of Examination

The internal examination of the nose may be performed with 1) the otoscope with the nasal speculum inserted in place of the ear speculum (this is probably the one in your black bag), 2) a handheld Vienna nasal speculum (the type that opens when you squeeze the handle), or 3) simply a light and one's fingers. Most nonspecialists do not use the Vienna speculum, with or without a head mirror, so they are not able to do as detailed an examination as the specialist. Students should seek opportunities to work in the ENT clinic and practice the use of a head mirror. (Mastering the technique requires a great deal of practice. Dr. Douglas Lindsey of Arizona suggests assembling model airplanes in the focal point of light from a head mirror.) Outside the clinic or office, a head mirror is impractical, and a penlight or otoscope with the nasal speculum must suffice.

Use of Otoscope with Nasal Attachment

1. Place the nasal speculum on the otoscope head and turn on the light.
2. With your nondominant hand, push up lightly on the tip of the nose so as to make it easier to introduce the nasal speculum into the nostril.
3. Observe the color of the nasal mucosa, and check for ulcerations.
4. Check the septum for deviation or perforation.
5. If possible, visualize the middle and inferior turbinates. Check the middle meatus for purulent discharge or polyps.
6. Repeat the examination for the other nostril.
7. Clean the nondisposable plastic nasal speculum with soap and water, then soak it in a 10% solution of sodium hypochlorite (bleach) for 15 to 20 minutes. (Alcohol has also been used for this purpose, but bleach is effective for killing

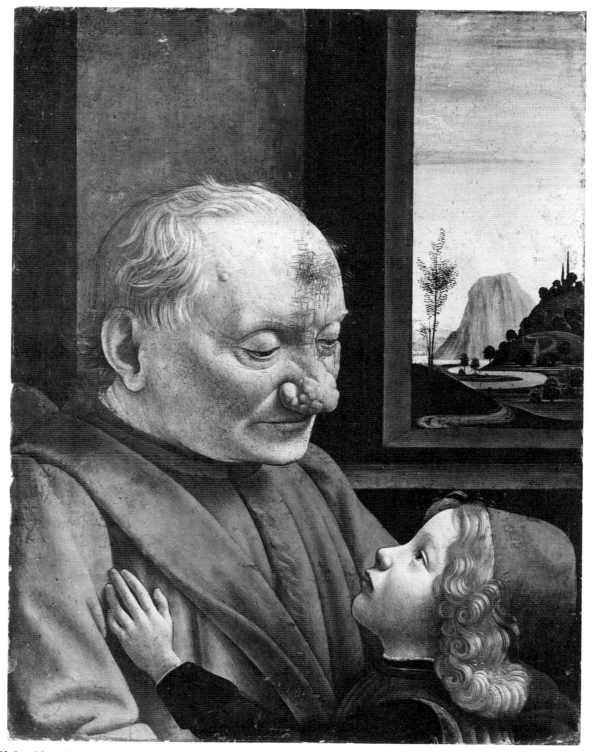

Figure 12-1. *Rhinophyma*. Portrait d'un vieillard et d'un jeune garcon *(Portrait of an old man and his grandson) by Ghirlandaio, the Louvre. Courtesy of the Réunion des Musées Nationaux.*

viruses, such as those of hepatitis and AIDS.* A disposable speculum is best of all.)

Use of Vienna Nasal Speculum

1. To expedite the examination, especially if a disease of the nose is suspected or if the membranes are swollen, use 0.5% phenylephrine (as a spray or applied with cotton) to shrink the membranes.

2. Hold the speculum in your nondominant hand. (The domi-

---

*Since the AIDS virus has been isolated from tears (CDC, 1985), and tears drain into the nose, it is presumably present in nasal secretions.

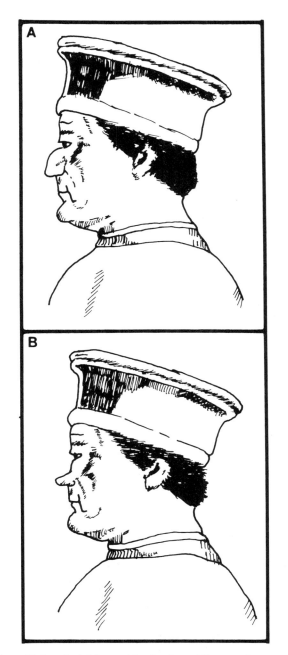

chlorite) for 20 minutes, or boil or autoclave for 15 to 20 minutes.

The Nasal Septum

A Method

If you are concerned about the possibility of a septal perforation, you may wish to perform the following special test:

1. In a darkened room, shine a light in one nostril (as with the otoscope and nasal speculum).

2. Look up the other nostril and see whether the beam of light shines through the septum. (This is not simply transillumination, which may occur normally if the light is sufficiently strong.)

3. Repeat from the other side.

Causes of Perforation

Septal perforation can result from trauma ("Major," Delp & Manning, 1975); chromium poisoning (Leopold, 1952); infection, including tuberculosis (DeGowin, 1965), infected intranasal hematoma, and syphilis (once the most common cause) (Adams et al., 1978); cocaine or heroin inhalation (Sapira & Cherubin, 1975); and a variety of connective tissue diseases, including Wegener's granulomatosis, midline granuloma, systemic lupus erythematosus, mixed cryoglobulinemia, rheumatoid arthritis, psoriatic arthritis, progressive systemic sclerosis, and mixed connective tissue disease (Wilkens et al., 1976).

Deviated Septum

A deviated septum is usually posttraumatic. As with most nasal findings, the history should have drawn your attention to it.

For the attending. The Latin word *saeptus* is from the perfect participle passive of the verb *saepire*, meaning to erect a fence or enclosure or hedgerow (Kidd, 1979). This masculine noun means "wall." For some reason, this has become septum in English, which would be a neuter noun were it Latin. The plural of septum would, were it Latin, be septa. However, the incorrect plural septa has been mistaken as the feminine singular by certain hepatologists, who created still another plural, septae. (Actually, since septum is an English word, the plural should be septums.) But, usage governs language, hence the "Latinically" incorrect title of this section.
The moral of the story is that once the masculine gender has been neutered, as with any castration, there is no going back.

Nasal Mucosa

Patients suffering from allergic rhinitis (or just recovering from an upper airway infection) may have a pale, boggy-looking nasal mucosa, or the mucosa may appear red and swollen, depending on the phase of the illness (Adams et al., 1978). A dry, red appearance is seen with overuse of decongestants. The mucus may be purulent in upper airway infections or sinusitis. Streaks of blood may be present after trauma, epistaxis, or repeated nose blowing.

Soft polyps are protrusions of the mucosa, which can be distinguished from the usual internal structures by the fact that they are not tender to palpation with the end of the speculum. They may be seen any time that allergic rhinitis becomes chronic, and may disappear with successful treatment. There is a triad of aspirin sensitivity, nasal polyposis, and asthma; the polyps may

Figure 12-2. *A, A false positive for the saddle nose of congenital syphilis. Redrawn from the portrait of the Duke of Urbino (Federigo Da Montefeltro) by Piero della Francesca in the Uffizi, Florence. B, How the Duke's nose would have looked if he truly had had congenital syphilis.*

nant hand is used to position the patient's head, manipulate instruments, or to hold the light if you don't have a head mirror.)

3. Insert the speculum so that it opens in an up-and-down direction, stabilizing it by placing your forefinger on the side of the patient's nose.
4. Inspect the intranasal structures in turn, as described above.
5. Clean the metal speculum with soap and water, then soak in a disinfectant solution (preferably 10% sodium hypo-

result from a chronic allergic rhinitis, which can be the first manifestation of this syndrome (Adams et al., 1978).

Other Findings in Internal Nose

In the older patient, the examination of the nose might reveal tumors. In the very young, foreign bodies such as peas, beans, and nuts are common and should be sought when there is a purulent discharge, particularly a unilateral one.

Cerebrospinal Fluid Rhinorrhea

A clear liquid dripping from the nose, especially in patients who have experienced trauma, suggests the diagnosis of cerebrospinal fluid (CSF) rhinorrhea (Anderson et al., 1961; Roberts, 1958). The connection between the subarachnoid space and the nose predisposes the patient to meningitis, and requires surgical intervention.

Trauma victims with a fracture of the cribriform plate may have CSF leaking from the nose or mouth. This is often mixed with blood, which does not clot. Such nasal secretions should be evaluated by placing a drop on a piece of filter paper (or paper towel) to see whether it separates into a central red spot with a clear, straw-colored outer ring or "halo." (The halo is due to cerebrospinal fluid.) Never place a nasogastric tube in a patient with this sign, because it may end up in the cranial vault (Timberlake, 1986).

Rhinorrhea with very high glucose levels, >30 mg/dl, approximating those in the CSF (40 to 80 mg/dl), would tend to support the diagnosis of CSF rhinorrhea. Unfortunately, glucose oxidase test tape, once recommended, is too sensitive for a bedside test, producing frequent false positives (Kirsch, 1967) due to the reducing substances found in tears. (Tears are relatively rich in glucose and may enter the nose through the nasolacrimal duct.) A glucose as high as 17 mg/dl was found in one case proven at surgery not to have CSF rhinorrhea (Crow et al., 1956). However, the trick may yet work using the new Chemstrip *blood* glucose strips (Ackerman et al., 1989).

Special Maneuvers: Sense of Smell

Although the examination of the first cranial nerve might also be considered part of the neurologic examination, it is included here because the cause of impairments in smell might be found on inspecting the nose.

The use of the *doctor's* sense of smell as a diagnostic tool is discussed in Chapter 13 (p. 228).

$$ Testing smell requires the use of a substance that is not irritating. Pepper and alcohol, for example, are not acceptable (especially as pure alcohol is odorless). My examining bag contains two plastic containers, one of ground cloves, and one of cinnamon, both reasonably fresh. Other good test substances would be nutmeg, allspice, or coffee.

A Method

1. Have the patient close his eyes and occlude one nostril, while you uncap one of the plastic containers and hold it near the other nostril. Instruct the patient to take a deep breath.

2. Ask the patient whether he can smell anything, and if so, ask him to identify the substance.

3. As a control, leave the cap on the vial, and ask whether he can smell the substance.

4. Repeat the test with the other substance (uncapped) and the other nostril. Also ask the patient whether the second odor was different from the first.

Interpretation

Most patients will not be able to identify the specific odors, and some may not be able to distinguish the two odors; what you are really trying to determine is whether they are aware of the odor at all. Thus, exclamations of partial recognition and frustration at being unable to name the specific substance are also evidence of intact olfactory function.

In patients who might be malingering or for some other reason trying to fool the examiner, watch for nostril flaring. Flaring of the nostrils is evidence that a bona attempt is being made, although it is more likely to be seen if the patient holds the object being sniffed than if the doctor does. The absence of nostril flaring tells you nothing.

Causes of Loss of Smell

Bilateral loss of smell always accompanies hypogonadotropic hypogonadism (Kallmann's syndrome). Impairment or loss of smell may be seen in zinc deficiency, head trauma, multiple sclerosis, sarcoid, Parkinson's disease, chronic renal failure, hepatic cirrhosis, pernicious anemia, Cushing's syndrome, hypothyroidism, diabetes mellitus, Turner's syndrome, primary amenorrhea (which might have been due to Turner's syndrome), pseudohypoparathyroidism, cystic fibrosis, laryngectomy, acute viral hepatitis, bronchial asthma, toxin exposure, and certain drugs (Delaney, 1983; Schiffman, 1983).

Local afflictions that produce bilateral loss of smell include Sjögren's syndrome, adenoid hypertrophy, allergic rhinitis, nasal polyposis, sinusitis, leprosy, ozena, and influenza-like infections (Delaney, 1983; Schiffman, 1983; Wechsler, 1963). Inflammatory nasal disease and post-viral disease were the most common causes in a series of 63 patients (Davidson et al., 1987).

Unilateral anosmia is very rare and is most often found in local afflictions, such as inflamed nasal mucosa, when the latter is worse on one side than the other. It can, however, be an excellent sign drawing attention to a frontal lobe tumor (Liddell, 1976). It is rare for trauma to affect the olfactory nerve on only one side.

For years, it was believed that the urinary odor produced after eating asparagus (due to unusual methyl thioesters) (White, 1975) was an inherited polymorphism since some subjects claimed not to excrete such odoriferous substances. However, it now develops that all persons excrete the substances, but the ability to smell the odors is polymorphous (Lison et al., 1980). The student should keep this sequence of theories in mind when considering less trivial researches.

Appendix 12-1. Answer to Question in the Epigram

The epigram is from Dostoevsky: *The Brothers Karamazov*, Part Four, Book Eleven, Chapter 9.

References

Ackerman WE, Juneja MM, Kaczorowski DM: A simple test for detecting CSF. *South Med J* 82:94, 1989.

Adams GL, Boies LR, Paparella MM: *Boies's Fundamentals of Otolaryngology*, ed 5. WB Saunders, Philadelphia, 1978.

Anderson WM, Schwarz GA, Gammon GD: Chronic spontaneous cerebrospinal rhinorrhea. *Arch Intern Med* 107:723–731, 1961.

CDC: Recommendations for preventing transmission of infection with human T-lymphotropic virus type III/lymphadenopathy-associated virus in the workplace. *MMWR* 34:682–695, 1985.

Crow HJ, Keogh C, Northfield DWC: The localisation of cerebrospinal fluid fistulae. *Lancet* 325–327, 1956.

Davidson TM, Jalowayski A, Murphy C, Jacobs RD: Evaluation and treatment of smell dysfunction. *West J Med* 146:434–436, 1987.

De Gowin EL: *Bedside Diagnostic Examination*. Macmillan, New York, 1965.

Delaney P: Taste and smell in disease. *N Engl J Med* 309:1062, 1983.

Delp MH, Manning RT (eds): *Major's Physical Diagnosis*. WB Saunders, Philadelphia, 1975.

Kidd DA: *Collins Gem Dictionary: Latin-English, English-Latin*. William Collins Sons, London, 1979.

Kirsch A: Diagnosis of cerebrospinal fluid rhinorrhea: Lack of specificity of the glucose oxidase testtape. *J Pediatr* 71:718–719, 1967.

Leopold SS: The Principles and Methods of Physical Diagnosis. WB Saunders, Philadelphia, 1952.

Liddell K: Smell as a diagnostic marker. *Postgrad Med J* 52:136–138, 1976.

Lison M, Blondheim SH, Melmed RN: A polymorphism of the ability to smell urinary metabolites of asparagus. *Br Med J* 281:1676–1678, 1980.

Roberts HJ: *Difficult Diagnosis: A Guide to the Interpretation of Obscure Illness*. WB Saunders, Philadelphia, 1958.

Roenigk RK: CO_2 laser vaporization for treatment of rhinophyma. *Mayo Clin Proc* 62:676–680, 1987.

Sapira JD, Cherubin CE: *Drug Abuse*. American Elsevier, New York, 1975.

Schiffman SS: Taste and smell in disease. *N Engl J Med* 308:1275–1279, 1983.

Silen W (ed): *Cope's Early Diagnosis of the Acute Abdomen*, ed 15. Oxford University Press, New York, 1979.

Timberlake GA: Trauma: In the Golden Hour. *Emerg Med* 19(Nov 30):79–95, 1986.

Watson MG, Campbell JB, Pahor AL: Complications of nose piercing. *Br Med J* 294:1262, 1987.

Wechsler IS: *Clinical Neurology*, ed 9. WB Saunders, Philadelphia, 1963.

White RH: Occurrence of S-methyl thioesters in urines of humans after they have eaten asparagus. *Science* 189:810, 1975.

Wilkens RF, Roth GJ, Novak A, Walike JW: Perforation of nasal septum in rheumatic diseases. *Arthritis Rheum* 19(1):119–121, 1976.

13
The Oropharynx

"Look to thy mouth; diseases enter there."
George Herbert (1593–1632), *The Church Porch*, Stanza 22

Order of Examination

Inspection

The patient should sit up straight, facing the examiner, at a height such that the physician can comfortably look in the mouth. A flashlight or the otoscope may be used as a light source at the bedside, although the head mirror of the ENT specialist provides superior illumination.

A Method

1. Inspect the lips (for findings see p. 222). Ask the patient to open his mouth, and inspect the oral aperture (see p. 222), then all the structures inside the mouth (with the dentures removed), including the dorsal surface of the tongue (see p. 223).

Check for fibrillations and fasciculations of the tongue (for significance, see Ch. 26, p. 493). This must be done with the tongue at rest and the patient breathing through his mouth. Most normal persons have "contraction fasciculations" when the tongue is held in forced extension. The method that involves the least amount of effort for the patient is to pull out his cheek by hooking your finger in the angle of the mouth, and then have the patient open his mouth slightly to permit inspection of the tongue at repose.

2. Use the tongue blade to retract the cheek and lips for complete inspection of the buccal mucosa (see p. 225), the opening of Stensen's and Wharton's ducts (see Ch. 14, p. 237), the teeth, and the gums (see p. 224).

3. Ask the patient to place the tongue on the roof of his mouth to permit inspection of its under surface and the floor of the mouth (all common sites for carcinoma, especially in older smokers).

4. Next inspect the palate (for findings, see p. 225).

5. Ask the patient to relax his tongue. (Do not ask him to protrude it for this part of the examination.) If you can't see well, depress the middle third of the tongue with the tongue blade in your nondominant hand, and if you still can't see well, pull the tongue forward. Do not touch the posterior portion of the tongue; you don't want him to gag until you are ready to test the gag reflex (see Ch. 26, p. 462). The tonsils, tonsillar fossa, the anterior and posterior pillars, the posterior and lateral phar-

yngeal walls, a portion of the base of the tongue, and occasionally the tip of the epiglottis (p. 228), can now be seen.

An Alternate Method

Stand behind the seated patient and have him extend his neck, open his mouth fully, and hold his breath in deep inspiration. The tongue and floor of the mouth drop with gravity; a tongue blade is seldom needed (Greally, 1988; Sprackling, 1988).

Palpation

Palpate all symptomatic or unusual-appearing areas in the mouth and pharynx. (The examiner should wear disposable gloves.) In persons at high risk for carcinoma, the tongue and floor of the mouth should also be palpated because moderate-sized tumors and cysts lying deep within the oral tissues may be found only in this way. Calculi in the submaxillary ducts can be felt. (The salivary glands are discussed in Ch. 14, p. 236.) The temporomandibular joints can be palpated by placing your fingertips in the external ear canals and having the patient open and close his mouth.

Percussion

The tongue may be examined for myotonia by placing a tongue blade across the mandibular teeth, having the patient place his tongue on top of the tongue blade, and tapping on the relaxed tongue with a reflex hammer. The reflex hammer may be wrapped in a disposable material if there is concern about a transmissible disease. (See Ch. 24, p. 416 for a description of myotonia as manifested in the hand.)

Olfaction

A Method

Ask the patient to count aloud from 1 to 10, while you put your nose in the stream of exhaled air. If you have reason to suspect a noxious odor, it is possible to turn your face away from the patient and still keep your nose in the stream.

Some patients have poor oral hygiene, or have been vomiting, so that the breath odors are masked by those coming from the mouth. In that case, have the patient rinse his mouth with a non-fragrant solution. With sufficient mouth care, one can reduce the odor sufficiently to be able to smell the breath that is actually emanating from the lungs.

Another method is to have the patient close his mouth. Place your nose where the steam would be if the patient were nose breathing on a cold day, and smell the air as it exits from his nostrils. (To demonstrate to yourself that nose-breathing decreases communication with the oral cavity, place a drop of peppermint oil on the tongue of a nose-breathing subject, and see how well you can smell the peppermint with the subject's mouth closed and then open.)

Specific findings are given on page 228.

Sialometry

A Method (Sreebny & Valdini, 1987)

In patients complaining of xerostomia (dry mouth), saliva flow can be quantitated by the following method:

1. Gather the equipment: 1) two measuring cylinders ($\geq$ 12 ml) calibrated to at least 0.1 ml; 2) two funnels; 3) a timer; and 4) salivary stimulants: paraffin wax (about 1.5 g) or 2% citric acid solution. The latter may be prepared by placing 1 g of crystalline citric acid, available from many chemical supply houses, in 20 ml of water, or by adding 8 ml of ReaLemon Concentrate (Borden Company) to 12 ml of water. A citric acid solution of the appropriate concentration is also available from the Interstate Drug Exchange, Inc., 1500 New Horizons Blvd., Amityville, NY 11701.

2. Instruct the patient not to brush his teeth, eat, drink, or smoke before the test. Samples should be collected after an overnight fast or at least 2 hours after a meal.

3. Perform the test in a quiet area.

4. Collection of unstimulated ("resting") saliva: Ask the patient not to move his tongue or lips and to collect and expectorate passively accumulated secretions into the funnel (thence into the cylinder) every 2 minutes for a period of 6 minutes. Swallowing is only permitted immediately after each expectoration.

5. Collection of stimulated saliva: 1) *Paraffin method*: Ask the patient to hold a piece of wax in his mouth until it becomes soft (30 seconds to 1 minute). Have him swallow saliva that has accumulated during this period. Then ask the patient to chew the wax and spit stimulated saliva into the funnel and cylinder every 2 minutes for a period of 6 minutes. 2) *Citric acid method*: Have the patient hold 20 ml of citric acid solution in his mouth for 1 minute, then expectorate it. Next have the patient spit the stimulated saliva into the cylinder every 2 minutes for a period of 6 minutes.

Interpretation

The normal flow rate for unstimulated, "resting" saliva is 0.3 to 0.5 ml/min; for stimulated saliva, 1 to 2 ml/min. A resting level of less than 0.1 ml/min can be considered xerostomic. Such a value implies a 60% to 75% loss in salivary gland function. Causes of dry mouth are described on page 225 and the salivary glands are considered in Chapter 14 (p. 236).

The Oral Aperture

Normally the mouth should open sufficiently to permit the introduction of the tips of the patient's own three middle fingers, vertically aligned, without the fingers touching the lips. Three conditions in which the oral aperture is smaller are: 1) tetanus (not usually a diagnostic problem); 2) various mechanical diseases of the jaw, especially disease of the temporomandibular joint; 3) progressive systemic sclerosis. Dr. Gerry Rodnan of Pennsylvania charted the progress of systemic sclerosis by recording the patient's MOA (maximum oral aperture). The patient's mouth,

opened as far as possible, was pressed against a piece of paper, such as a progress note sheet. Lipstick facilitated the measurement.

Lips

The most common deformity of the lips is seen in the cleft palate syndrome. Because of the resemblance to the lip of a rabbit, this was sometimes called hare lip, which has been absurdly transmogrified to "hair" lip. ("Hair-brained" has gone the opposite road [Burton, 1621].)

A hard lesion on the lip with a discrete edge could be molluscum contagiosum or a malignant epidermoid carcinoma. The distinction usually requires biopsy, although about 95% of labial epidermoid carcinomas occur on the *lower* lip.

A luetic chancre (a moist-centered ulceration) may occur on the lip. Such lesions are incorrectly stated to be confined to the upper lip. (If you suspect a luetic chancre, wear gloves, or at least wash your hands carefully after touching it, because the lesion is teeming with live spirochetes as can be seen by darkfield examination.)

Leukoplakia (literally "white plate") is often a precancerous lesion on the lips as on other mucosal surfaces.

Fever blisters ("cold sores") are caused by the *Herpes simplex* virus, usually type I. After the first inoculation, the virus inhabits the neural tissue in latent form and recrudesces on the skin, usually at the vermilion border, sometimes triggered by another illness such as a pulmonary or upper respiratory infection. At first, there is a vesicle or vesicles containing clear fluid. In a few days, the vesicles rupture, leaving a sore, inflamed, and infectious ulcer, which forms a crust, then heals without a scar. Primary herpes stomatitis (see p. 226) involving the oral mucosa, especially the gingiva and tongue, is common in children, but less common in adults. It may be quite severe.

Cheilitis is inflammation of the lips characterized by vertical fissures.

It may occur with regional enteritis; acrodermatitis enteropathica; alcoholism; deficiency of pyridoxine, riboflavin, or folate; sprue; kwashiorkor; viral illness; hypervitaminosis A; and iron-deficiency anemia, with or without the Plummer-Vinson syndrome (Beitman et al., 1981). The last may be associated with abnormalities of the nails (see Ch. 7, p. 133).

Angular stomatitis, the reddening and cracking of the lateral corners of the mouth, may be seen as a benign condition in patients who drool.

In children, it is given the specific name of perleche. Although the condition has been stated to be diagnostic for riboflavin deficiency, the most common cause is monilia. Angular stomatitis also occurs with anemia and lipstick allergy. I have seen it during upper respiratory viral syndromes in cold climates, and following the same regardless of climate.

Angular stomatitis must be differentiated from syphilitic rhagades (literally "cracks") in that the latter are not just reddened and inflamed but are fully epithelialized cracks, furrows, or ridges, radiating from the corners of the mouth, especially laterally. Rhagades, unlike angular stomatitis, are permanent. Formerly a medical student could bet against rhagades and for angular stomatitis, but as we eat more wisely and love less so, rhagades may make a comeback.

In Peutz-Jeghers' disease, adenomatous polyps of the intestine are associated with 10 to 20 pigmented macules around the mouth and lips. The lesions are about 1 mm in size, and like apple jelly in color. If the small, round, circumscribed lesions were red, like senile hemangiomas or cherry spots, one would better diagnose Osler-Weber-Rendu's disease (hereditary hemorrhagic telangiectasis).

Tongue

Macroglossia

A great deal has been written about macroglossia, which simply means a large tongue. However, the diagnosis of macroglossia is a matter of opinion, because no normal values are available for tongue size. The macroglossia reported in 22% of patients with primary systemic amyloidosis may also be associated with visible changes and palpable stiffness (Kyle & Greipp, 1983), but in Down's syndrome and myxedema, it is difficult to be sure how much is macroglossia and how much is simple protrusion.

Some authors have suggested that lateral teeth indentations upon the tongue are presumptive evidence of macroglossia. However, I have seen that finding in a number of patients thought to have neither a disease of the tongue, nor any of the known causes of macroglossia, which additionally include neonatal hypoglycemia syndrome (Combs et al., 1966), gargoylism, generalized gangliosidosis, glycogen storage disease, Wiedemann-Beckwith syndrome, acromegaly, and pemphigus vulgaris (Milgraum et al., 1985).

Glossitis

Glossitis means inflammation of the tongue. It can be confusing because the appearance of the tongue is different at different stages of the disease (Beitman et al., 1981). First there is papillary hypertrophy, then flattening, followed by granular fusion and finally atrophy. At first, the color may be rubric, "beefy," or magenta, but when atrophy occurs, the tongue will become pale and smooth and shiny.

Causes of glossitis (some of which overlap) include regional enteritis; alcoholism; sprue; kwashiorkor; pernicious anemia; malabsorption syndromes, deficiencies of pyridoxine, niacin, or riboflavin; amyloidosis; and (rarely) the carcinoid syndrome. In one study of patients with iron-deficiency anemia, who had an average hemoglobin of 8.7 g/dl, glossitis was seen in 17% (Kalra et al., 1986).

In geographic tongue, also called migratory glossitis, areas of denuded epithelium appear and are restored to normal, with the pattern changing over periods of a few days. The patient may suffer considerable anxiety from this otherwise harmless condition.

Black Tongue

A hairy black tongue secondary to broad spectrum antibiotic administration is usually attributed to Aspergillus niger, a customarily harmless organism that quietly vacates this ecologic niche after antibiotic administration is stopped.

White Patches

Monilia spots, which look something like flecks of cottage cheese, can be scraped off, although that often leaves a denuded bleeding undersurface. Leukoplakia cannot be scraped off with a tongue blade, because it is intrinsic.

Hairy leukoplakia is a distinctive lesion that occurs in persons seropositive for the acquired immunodeficiency syndrome (AIDS), who are at increased risk of developing frank AIDS (Centers for Disease Control, 1985, Hollander et al., 1986). It consists of white warty projections, particularly on the lateral aspects of the tongue and cheeks (Mindel, 1987).

Other Lesions

1. A smooth, round, red mass at the base of the tongue may be a lingual thyroid.

2. The tongue can become so red and inflamed that it resembles a strawberry. This appearance, due to the desquamation of the filiform papillae, may result from the erythrogenic toxin of scarlet fever or from other febrile illnesses, particularly in toxic shock and in Kawasaki's disease in children.

3. Absence of the fungiform papillae has been associated with familial dysautonomia.

4. Mucosal neuromas, which may occur in Sipple's syndrome (type IIβ or III multiple endocrine neoplasia or adenomatosis syndrome), are illustrated in Figure 13-1.

5. The location of indurated ulcers of the tongue can be diagnostically helpful. If they occur at the tip, in the midline, one should consider primary lues. Any midline indurated ulcer, whether or not it is at the tip, could also be tuberculosis. Histoplasmosis is a rare cause of indurated midline tongue ulcers. An indurated ulcer located laterally is suggestive of cancer, but cancer almost never appears as a midline lesion. A ragged, painful lesion on the undersurface of the tongue suggests Behçet's syndrome, although the

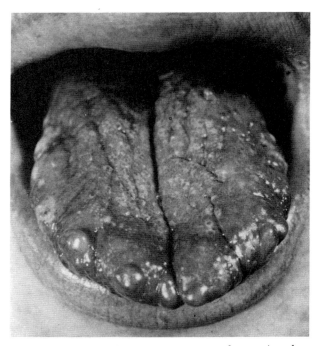

Figure 13-1. *Mucosal neuromas are seen at the anterior edges of the tongue. Do not look for them at the base, as the fungiform papillae might confuse you.*

lesions of this disease may also occur on the dorsal surface. Any collection of multiple indurated ulcers should suggest tuberculosis.

6. There are two types of tongue fissures, congenital and syphilitic. In the congenital case, most of the fissures are transverse. (They are of no clinical significance.) In syphilis, most of the fissures are longitudinal.

7. Blanching of the tongue because of arterial insufficiency due to giant cell arteritis occurred for 5 to 10 minutes at a time in one unusual patient (Grahame et al., 1968). Emboli from bacterial endocarditis can cause portions of the tongue to blanch. The Liebermeister syndrome is blanching of half of the tongue, as may occur in air embolism.

8. Caviar lesions, resembling little globs of purple-black caviar (as from the sturgeon, not orange caviar from the salmon) or perhaps buckshot, occur under the tongue. These are varicosities in the superficial sublingual veins, and their only importance is that they may frighten patients who notice them in the mirror (Bean, 1958).

9. The tongue may also show the lesions of aphthous stomatitis (see p. 226), lichen planus (p. 226), Peutz-Jeghers' disease, and Osler-Weber-Rendu's disease (hereditary hemorrhagic telangiectasia).

Other Findings

Examination of the sense of taste and of the motor function of the tongue is described in Chapter 26. Examination of the sublingual veins is covered in Chapter 19 (p. 357).

Teeth

Color

Children who have had neonatal jaundice may have biliverdin green teeth later in life. Tetracycline administration (during pregnancy or infancy) may cause smoker's brown teeth. Fluorosis may cause brown-and-black pits. Red teeth are seen in erythropoietic porphyria, but not in the more common acute intermittent porphyria. Dead teeth become slightly darker than the others.

Number

The teeth should be counted in any case in which a mysterious lesion appears in the jaw, as it may be an odontoma. Dr. Phil Bromberg of North Carolina first taught me the value of counting teeth in a patient with lung abscess—before the tooth is found on the chest film.

Loose Teeth

Most cases result from tooth-and-gum disease, but can result from jaw tumors or mercurialism. Periodontal disease is characterized by gingival pyorrhea and gum recession, the latter being the origin of the term "long in the tooth," since such gum disease especially afflicts the senescent.

Other Findings

1. Lipstick adhering to the teeth suggests dry mucous membranes, for example, in the sicca syndrome.

2. Erosion of the enamel on the lingual, palatal, and posterior surfaces of the teeth, due to frequent contact with gastric acid, is a sign of bulimia (Mitchell et al., 1987).

3. Increased interdental spaces may be congenital or acquired, as in acromegaly.

4. Transverse ridging of the teeth may be seen in children with previous episodes of bone growth arrest due to deficiency of vitamin C or D.

5. Teeth seen in congenital syphilis include the best-known Hutchinson's teeth. Hutchinson, an ophthalmologist, described the incisors as follows (Hutchinson, 1859):

> On looking at his teeth, all doubt as to the real nature of the case was dispelled. The lower incisors, just cut, were large, but presented singularly irregular edges, being thin and unequally serrate. The upper incisors were all deeply notched.

These teeth are sometimes called the notched teeth of congenital syphilis. Sometimes there is no notching of the incisors, but the teeth are still short and thin and tapered like the tip of a screwdriver: hence, they are called "screwdriver teeth." The molars may also be involved in congenital syphilis. The crown may consist of an agglomerate of unusual enamel globules resembling a mulberry, hence the name "mulberry molars." Moon's turreted molars are domed-shaped first molars.

6. Probing at the area where the third molar should be can often detect an impacted wisdom tooth, which can be the source of a low-grade fever of inapparent origin. The tooth is usually covered with a layer of gum under which trapped food particles feed bacteria.

7. Fever of inapparent origin can also be due to an apical abscess. One may be able to find a single tooth that is sensitive to direct percussion. Alternately, one can screen all such patients with the Panorex, but the finding of tooth sensitivity is bound to increase the predictive value of this test if selectively ordered.

Gums

Hypertrophy of the gums in dentulous patients may be seen in chronic administration of phenytoin (diphenylhydantoin), leukemic infiltration (particularly monomyelocytic leukemia), scurvy, or (rarely) lues.

All ulcerations of the mucosa (see p. 226) may also affect the gums.

Bleeding of the dentulous gums frequently results from periodontal disease. It also occurs in a variety of platelet defects, but it does not usually occur spontaneously with coagulation factor defects. Bleeding gums are seen in up to 93% of patients with scurvy, but never in scorbutic patients who are edentulous (Vilter et al., 1946).

Conditions that cause pigmentation of the mucosa (see p. 225) may also affect the gums. Acatalasemia causes black gingiva, with extensive ulceration. A linear pigmentation of the gums may occur in dentulous patients with lead poisoning (see Fig. 13-2). Look closely, and you will see that this early lead "line" is actually a series of stippled spots. To make a lead line more apparent, slip a small piece of white paper between the tooth and gum to serve as a background.

Lead lines were frequently seen in Birmingham, Alabama, when unbonded whiskey was cheaply made from sugar, which was then quite inexpensive. Revenue agents used hatchets to destroy the expensive copper tubing of illegal stills. To keep costs down, the moonshiners began to purchase inexpensive junked automobile radiators as a substitute for copper condenser coils. However, the radiators were soldered with lead, which adulterated the alcohol. When the price of sugar rose in the 1970s, the cost of moonshine escalated to a point at which some bonded alcoholic beverages became competitive. Lead lines became rare.

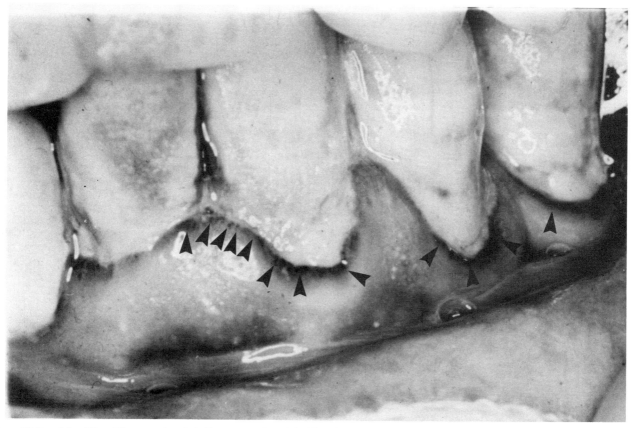

Figure 13-2. *A lead line. The arrowheads indicate a portion of the "line," which is actually a series of dots. Photograph reprinted courtesy of Cliggott Publications.*

False positives occur with prior medical or industrial exposure to bismuth or mercury, or with thallium intoxication (Grunfeld & Hinostroza, 1964).

Palate

The palate appears to be high and arched in Marfan's syndrome and in certain Marfanoid disorders such as homocystinuria and Sipple's syndrome (multiple endocrine adenomatosis type IIβ or III).

It is less widely appreciated that the palate of Down's syndrome is characteristically short and narrow, the latter aspect giving it the appearance of being high (Shapiro et al., 1967).

The torus palatinus is a congenital but not familial bony overgrowth of the midline suture of the hard palate, which protrudes down from the ceiling of the mouth. It is important to recognize this perfectly benign finding, so as not to biopsy it in search of cancer.

Midline granulomas can involve the palate, due either to the usual cryptogenic etiology or to syphilis, lymphoma, or exotic microorganisms.

Palatal defects can be a residual of unsuccessful surgery for cleft palate, radiotherapy for tumors, syphilitic gumma, or other necrotizing or infectious lesions. Tumors occasionally occur on the palate.

Dentures should always be removed so that the physician can inspect all of the mouth, but specifically the upper plates should be removed as a quick test of capillary integrity and platelet function.

The trauma caused by inserting the dentures and then removing them may result in petechiae of the hard palate, an early sign of thrombocytopenia or platelet abnormality.

Palate edema is seen in γ heavy-chain disease. (Also see "The Uvula," p. 226.)

The evaluation of motion of the soft palate is considered in Chapter 26 (p. 462).

Buccal Mucosa

Pigmentation

In patients with primary chronic adrenocortical insufficiency, the mucosa can develop spots of melanin, as if someone had sprinkled black fountain pen ink on the buccal mucosa. However, highly pigmented persons will often have large patches of buccal melanosis, especially opposite the molars. These are *not* the spots of chronic primary adrenocortical insufficiency.

Pallor

In one study, mucosal pallor was found in 30% of a group of patients with iron-deficiency anemia and an average hemoglobin of 8.7 g/dl (Kalra, 1986), but was found in only 4% of another group of patients with non-iron-deficiency anemia whose average hemoglobin was 10.32 g/dl.

Xerostomia

In patients with xerostomia, the buccal mucosa will appear pale and dry due to epithelial atrophy and the loss of the mucous coating. Erythematous areas may be present. The tongue blade sticking to the oral mucosa is a crude but probably valid indicator of oral dryness, which can be quantitated by the method on page 000. Associated findings in the oral cavity include: fissuring and atrophy of the filiform papillae of the tongue, cheilitis, oral ulcers, candidiasis, dental caries, and an inability to express saliva from the ducts of the parotid and submandibular/sublingual glands.

Causes of xerostomia include: radiation damage to the salivary glands from treatment of head and neck cancers, Sjögren's syndrome, drugs, pancreatic insufficiency, and type V hyperlipoproteinemia (Sreebny & Valdini, 1987).

The Dry Gingival-Labial Fold and Other Signs of Hypovolemia

Absence of saliva in the gingival-labial fold is positive evidence of dehydration, even in the patient who is mouth breathing. This is a more reliable sign than inspection of the buccal mucosa and tongue, which may become acutely dry due to mouth breathing, a frequent result of hyperventilation due to any cause.

■ Volume depletion is an emergent condition, and a number of other clinical methods, all of which are imperfect, have been proposed for detecting it:

1. Loss of the normal venous pressure, as seen in the jugular veins (see Ch. 19, p. 355) is suggestive, but is limited; i.e. that is, the cervical venous pressure cannot be visualized in some persons, such as those with a short neck, a fat neck, or veins that are inapparent for another reason. So in practice the jugular venous pressure is useful only as an exclusionary sign for hypovolemia (i.e., when it is abnormally increased).

2. Orthostatic hypotension (see Ch. 6) is useful, but it presupposes the absence of neural problems, including those that result from drugs and drug withdrawal (especially from alcohol or other sedative-hypnotics). In addition, it requires that the patient be able to stand, or that a tilt table be available.

3. Skin turgor assessment is discussed on page 120.

4. It is said that dehydrated patients do not have axillary sweat.

The assessment is especially difficult if the patient has signs of excessive salt and water, leading one to assume that the patient is volume expanded. These signs include pulmonary edema, ventricular diastolic gallops, ascites, and edema. However, a patient with chronic ascites and pedal edema due to cirrhotic hypoalbuminemia might bleed and become hypovolemic without mobilizing all his "third-space" fluid. In this instance, the absence of saliva in the labial-gingival fold is of great diagnostic utility; signs 2 and 4 may also be helpful.

Koplik's Spots

These white spots, the size and color of grains of salt, each on an erythematous background, are seen on the buccal mucosa, especially around the orifice of Stensen's duct and the lower labia. They are said to be pathognomonic for measles. However, ECHO 9 and Coxsackie A-16 infections may have oral mucosal spots just like Koplik's spots (Artenstein & Demis, 1964; Hoeprich, 1972).

Vesicles, Bullae, and Ulcerations

Bullae appearing in the buccal mucosa in the presence of a diffuse bullous skin lesion in an elderly male should suggest the diagnosis of pemphigus, which is customarily and erroneously thought of as "just" a skin disorder. In fact, it may be a general medical emergency, requiring steroid therapy to prevent severe shock and hypoalbuminemia. Some of the bullous mucosal lesions appearing in the presence of bullous skin lesions turn out to be pemphigoid, Stevens-Johnson syndrome (erythema multiforme bullosum), Snear-Usher syndrome, erosive lichen planus, and so on. But since a patient with pemphigus can become so ill so fast, it is the one mucosal lesion that everyone should think about.

Primary herpetic gingivostomatitis, which produces numerous oral vesicles that rapidly ulcerate, is accompanied by systemic signs and symptoms. The differential diagnosis includes hand-foot-and-mouth disease; herpangina (due to Coxsackie A virus), allergic stomatitis; and acute necrotizing ulcerative gingivitis.

Aphthous stomatitis is the most common cause of oral ulcers, aside from trauma. The benign but painful lesions have a grayish appearance on an erythematous base. They affect freely movable mucous membranes, such as found on the tongue, the soft palate, the buccal mucosa, and the floor of the mouth. They have regular, smooth borders, and are round to ovoid in shape. Ulcers of similar appearance may be associated with one quarter of cases of systemic lupus erythematous (Urman et al., 1978), Reiter's syndrome, ankylosing spondylitis, inflammatory bowel disease, Behçet's syndrome, cyclic neutropenia, and vitamin B_{12} deficiency (Burns & Davis, 1985); the first four tend to be oddly painless.

Aphthous ulcers must be differentiated from those of recurrent *Herpes simplex* (Balciunas & Overholser, 1987). The latter generally involves the lip-skin junction, but may affect circumscribed areas of the hard palate and gingiva, where the mucosa is firmly bound to the underlying periosteum. Herpetic lesions begin as vesicles and tend to occur in clusters. They are variable in shape and have somewhat irregular borders. In contrast, aphthous ulcers never begin as vesicles and do not occur in clusters, although they may be multiple.

Alone of all the fungi, histoplasmosis produces shallow ulcers on the mucous membranes.

White Lesions

1. Leukoplakia (see p. 222) may be associated with chronic irritation, as from cheek biting or smoking.

2. Lichen planus is the most common dermatologic disease with oral lesions. They are present in 30% to 40% of cases and are the only lesions in about 25% (Adams et al., 1978). The skin lesions are violaceous plaques with a fine scale, primarily on the flexor surfaces of the arms and legs. The oral lesions vary from well-defined white lesions to diffuse erythematous lesions to ulcerations. A fine network of radiating white lines called Wickham's striae is diagnostic when present (Balciunas & Overholser, 1987).

Noma

Noma (from the Greek *nome*, "spreading ulcer") is a gangrenous stomatitis due to synergistic aerobic and anaerobic bacteria. It may begin in a herpetic ulcer or other mucosal break and then spread to become a putrid fetid exudative round ulcer with a necrotic middle. If untreated, it may actually eat a hole in the cheek and can then spread across the face and kill. Although often a disease of malnourished and weakened children, it may also occur in adults and has even been a cause of death in a primate colony during an outbreak of simian AIDS (Schiødt et al., 1988).

The Throat

The Uvula

Abnormalities of the uvula itself are rare, except for the congenitally bifid uvula, which should suggest submucosal cleft palate, especially if there is a history of recurrent otitis media. Otherwise, it is only of aesthetic interest.

Displacement of the uvula is a sign of peritonsillar abscess or neurologic disease (see Ch. 26, p. 463).

Mueller's sign is uvular pulsation synchronous with systole; it occurs in aortic insufficiency and other conditions that produce a wide pulse pressure and high stroke volume. Sometimes, the uvula does not pulsate but merely flushes and pales in time with the heartbeat (Stone, 1986). The sign is insensitive since most patients with aortic insufficiency do not have it.

Swelling of the uvula has been reported in association with pharyngitis, either primary (due to viral or bacterial infection) or secondary and iatrogenic (as in hospitalized patients receiving strong medicaments by inhaler). Uvular swelling is also seen in the sleep apnea syndrome (Fig. 13-3) and in about one quarter of the patients with γ (but not α) heavy-chain disease (Seligman et al., 1979).

Pharynx and Tonsils

Pharyngeal erythema is commonly seen in viral infections such as the common cold, the exanthems, and influenza.

An exudative pharyngitis, which may show white or yellow follicles on the tonsils, suggests a bacterial infection due to streptococci, but also can be seen in viral infections, especially infectious mononucleosis.

Ulcerative pharyngeal lesions may be the presenting sign of leukemia or agranulocytosis.

White spots on the posterior pharyngeal wall are usually either patches of monilia (which are not easily dislodged by the tongue blade and which leave bleeding patches when they are) or residual curds of cottage cheese or ricotta (which are easily dis-

lodged by the tongue blade and which do not leave bleeding patches).

•

A patient with Hodgkin's disease and symptoms of an upper respiratory infection was admitted to determine if there was another cause for his fever. White patches seen on the posterior pharyngeal wall led to an ophthalmologic consultation to look for fungal endophthalmitis (not present) and plans for a bone marrow aspiration for material to culture for fungi. The latter was cancelled when it was discovered that the white patches appeared after a meal of cottage cheese and disappeared after the subsequent meal.

•

Membrane formation characteristically accompanies diphtheria.

Abscess formation is fortunately much less common in the antibiotic era. A patient with a peritonsillar abscess may have such severe dysphagia that he spits out his saliva. Even opening the mouth may be painful.

Retropharyngeal Swelling

Retropharyngeal abscess causes a retropharyngeal swelling which, unfortunately, is not always perfectly apparent.

In cases of a retropharyngeal swelling thought to be due to a goiter, exert upward pressure upon the thyroid while examining the pharynx directly or with a mirror, to determine if there is a continuity

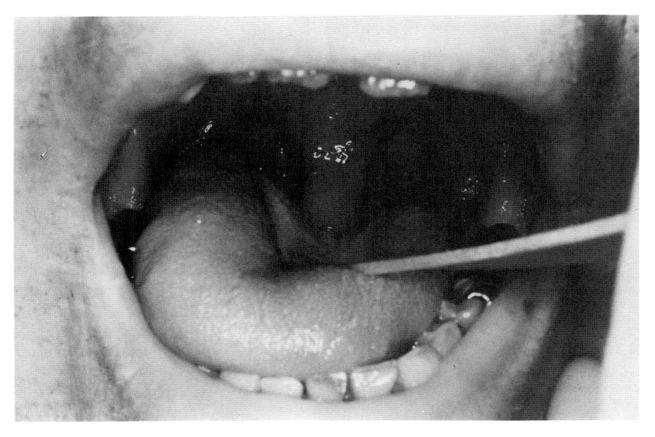

Figure 13-3. *A large uvula in a patient with obstructure sleep apnea. Photograph courtesy of Dr. John Shepard, Jr. of Minnesota.*

between the goiter and the retropharyngeal swelling (Crile, 1960). This is known as Stein's maneuver.

A small oropharynx is noted in patients with the nocturnal obstructive pulmonary disease variant of the sleep apnea syndrome (Shepard, 1987). This correlates perfectly with the cross-sectional area of the upper oropharynx as measured from the CAT scan.

The Epiglottis

🕩 A red, edematous epiglottis is seen in acute epiglottitis, a medical emergency.

The Larynx

Examination of the larynx is essential in patients complaining of persistent hoarseness. However, indirect laryngoscopy, using a head mirror and a laryngeal mirror, is beyond the scope of this book. If you wish to learn the technique, repeated, supervised practice in the ENT clinic is mandatory. (Otherwise, even if one does glimpse the larynx, one cannot be confident of recognizing the findings.)

A Bouquet of Odors*

The usefulness of the doctor's nose as a diagnostic tool was recognized over 2,000 years ago by Hippocrates and later by the Ayurvedic Sushruta in his Samhita (collected works) (Majno, 1975). Many of the odors are on the exhaled breath (see Table 13-1); some are due to the skin, perspiration, or other body secretions (Tables 13-2 and 13-3 and Appendix 13-1).

Acetone

The odor of acetone is the shibboleth of diabetic ketoacidosis. Theoretically, it could also be smelled in starvation ketoacidosis, but such patients probably do not burn enough fat for sufficiently long to exhale easily detectable amounts of acetone.

The ketoacidotic diabetic's breath is also described as "fruity," whereas pure acetone (nail polish remover) is not fruity. To me the ketoacidotic diabetic's breath smells like the chemistry laboratory in which one made longer ketones—like ripe bananas or like the breath after chewing fruit-flavored chewing gum.

I have seen diabetic ketoacidosis missed because the clinician *would not* smell the breath of a patient with poor dental hygiene; and in a second case because the physician could not smell the acetone through the odors from the unrinsed mouth.

The breath of alcoholic "ketoacidosis" does not smell like fruit because the predominant acid, β-hydroxybutyric, is not actually a keto acid; it's a hydroxy acid.

Ammonia

Both chronic renal failure and hepatic failure give rise to an ammoniacal odor, but the breath of the two may still be frequently distinguished.

*This is just one aspect of what Dr. Faith Fitzgerald of California refers to as "extracorporeal diagnosis" (Fitzgerald, 1989).

Table 13-1. Other Unusual Breath Odors in Diseases and Ingestions

General Category	Description	Disease or Substance
Sweet	Fruitlike: decomposing apples; acetone-like	Ketoacidosis; lacquer; chloroform; salicylates; phenol
Fishy	Fishy, rancid butter, boiled cabbage	Hypermethioninemia
Other	Burned oregano (or burned hemp)	Marijuana
	Camphor	Naphthalene (mothball or eucalyptus pica)
	Coal gas	Carbon monoxide (odorless but associated with coal gas)
	Garlic	Yellow phosphorus, arsenic, tellurium, parathion, malathion
	Metallic	Iodine
	Rotten eggs	Hydrogen sulfide, mercaptans
	Shoe polish	Nitrobenzene
	Disinfectant	Phenol, creosote
	Hydrocarbon	Various hydrocarbons

Source: *Hayden (1980).*

In renal failure, there is a second, fishy component of dimethylamine and trimethylamine (Simenhoff et al., 1977). Additionally, the breath of chronic renal failure often smells uriniferous.

Fetor hepaticus, on the other hand, has a musty component due to mercaptans, dimethylsulfide, and dimethyldisulfide (Tangerman et al., 1983).

Sewer Breath

The odor of sewage is caused by anaerobes, which may reside in the mouth or anywhere in the respiratory or gastrointestinal tract. Sewer breath may occur in periodontal disease, dental ab-

Table 13-2. Historical Use of Odors in Diagnosis

Description of Odor	Disease
Butcher shop	Yellow fever
Freshly baked brown bread	Typhoid
Freshly plucked feathers	Rubella
Putrid	Scurvy
Rotten straw	"Miliary fever"
Sour or musty bread	Pellagra
Stale beer	Scrofula
Sweetish	Diphtheria

Source: *Hayden (1980).*

scess, tonsillar infection, pulmonary abscess, bronchiectasis gastroparesis, esophageal diverticulum, and intestinal obstruction (in those still capable of belching).

Alcohol

Because pure ethanol is odorless, it is not possible to smell it on the breath. "Alcohol on the breath" is a misnomer now epidemic in emergency rooms. What one actually smells is the juniper berry in gin, fusel oil in whiskey, the bouquet of the fermented grape in wine, the hops (a kind of flower) in beer, or the acetaldehyde metabolite of alcohol.

Bitter Almonds

A smell of bitter almonds can be noticed on the breath of a victim of cyanide poisoning. This is due to hydrogen cyanide gas, which is intensely toxic. (Vomitus from such patients must be handled with care, lest medical personnel also be affected by the cyanide.) I have not yet detected this odor on the breath of a patient who has been overtreated with nitroprusside.

Pseudomonas

The characteristic sweet smell noted in cultures of *Pseudomonas* occurs in surface infections and may also be noted on the breath in *some* cases of *Pseudomonas* pneumonia.

Chemical Breath

Pharmaceutical breath refers to breath odors due to the ingestion of pharmaceutical materials, especially in suicide attempts. Paraldehyde, chloral hydrate, ethchlorvynol, and other drugs have characteristic odors. Solvent breath is due to such drugs or to halogenated straight-chain hydrocarbons, chloroform, or carbon tetrachloride (Teschke, 1984). A standard battery of such materials may be kept in the emergency room in capsules or vials that can be opened one at a time until the physician finds the odor that matches the patient's. In this way, the doctor's nose can serve as nature's own gas-liquid chromatograph, which is faster than the one in the chemistry laboratory.

Odors Due to Errors in Metabolism

Abnormal handling of methionine can produce an odor like that of boiled cabbage. An enzymatic block in leucine metabolism may produce an odor like that of sweaty feet or cheese, due to the accumulation of isovaleric acid (Liddell, 1976).

For the attending. It would be a simple matter to set up a teaching lab with concoctions of various materials, so that the students could learn to diagnose with their noses, just as radiology residents are taught to identify diagnostic patterns with their eyes. Alas, I do not know of a single school where this is done.

The remaining odors in this chapter would not lend themselves to this approach, because their specific components are either unknown or unavailable.

Miscellaneous

The common complaint of "halitosis" may result from a variety of conditions: food remnants; odoriferous foods; peridontal disorders; necrotic soft tissue lesions (e.g., Vincent's angina);

Table 13-3. Other Diseases and Ingestions Associated with Unusual Odors

Source of Odor	Description of Odor	Disease or Offending Substance
Inborn Errors of Metabolism		
Urine; sweat; sebum; cerumen	Maple syrup; caramel-like; burnt sugar	Maple syrup urine disease (branched-chain ketonuria)
Urine	Musty	Tyrosinemia
Urine	Like tomcat urine	β-Methylcrotonyl-glycinuria
Other Causes		
Urine	Ammoniacal	Urinary infection with urea-splitting bacteria (e.g., *Proteus* species)
Urine	Medicinal	Penicillin and derivatives
Urine, vomitus	Violets	Turpentine
Skin	Foul, unpleasant	Skin disease with protein breakdown, (e.g., pemphigus); hidradenitis suppurativa(?)
Vomitus	Garlic	Arsenic, phosphorus
Stool	Vile; foul	Malabsorption (e.g., cystic fibrosis, celiac 870)
Stool	Rancid	Shigellosis
Vaginal	Foul	Vaginitis; foreign body; sloughing fibroid; malignancy
Vaginal	Semen	Semen (especially in cases of suspected rape)
Pus	Nauseatingly sweet, like rotting apples	Gas gangrene
Pus	Fecal; like over-ripe Camembert cheese	Proteolytic bacteria

Sources: *Burton and Nadler (1978) and Hayden (1980).*

heavy smoking; or decreased salivary flow, due to Sjögren's syndrome, antihistamine use, astringent mouthwashes, radiation-induced sialadenitis, or amphetamine abuse.

Characteristic odors have been claimed for a great variety of diseases (Table 13-2), ranging from the nonspecific such as chronic sinusitis, through abnormal digestion of fat, through more specific entities such as streptococcal tonsillitis and diphtheria. The odor of typhoid has been likened to that of freshly baked bread.

•

I am reminded of the story that Dr. Rene Wegria tells of the golden days at Mount Sinai in New York City. One morning a great physician arrived for attending rounds, sniffed the air, and said to the resident, "Ah, I can smell that you have a case of typhoid. Let's see that patient first."

"I'm sorry, Professor," said the resident, "we can't see him. That patient was moved upstairs yesterday."

•

Appendix 13-1: Use of Body Odors in Diagnosis

Schizophrenia

To help doctors assess doubtful cases, a mental hospital in Australia, in the 1920s, provided a special room that was freshly whitewashed after use. Only in 1960 was it demonstrated that rats could distinguish some schizophrenic from nonschizophrenic sweat. *Trans*-3-methyl-2-hexenoic acid was found to be the only differing component (Liddell, 1976).

New-Mown Hay
(and Other Odors due to Metabolic Errors)

This musty smell is supposedly characteristic of phenylketonuria (PKU). The odor of PKU has also been described as like that of stale, sweaty locker-room towels, or as wolflike or barny (Liddell, 1976). The apocrypha of my student days taught that the mother of the first child diagnosed to have phenylketonuria took the child from pediatrician to pediatrician, complaining that the child smelled "musty, like a mouse." Each dismissed her as unbalanced, until Dr. Følling finally agreed to smell the child before laughing at its mother. To his surprise, the child indeed smelled musty, like a mouse. Because of the train of events that he set in motion, the mandatory testing of our day makes it unlikely that anyone will learn to smell that particular odor again.

Oasthouse urine disease is thought to be due to methionine malabsorption. An oasthouse in Great Britain is a shed in which hops and malt are stored. A physician might be able to experience the odor by taking a brewery tour, which usually includes the refrigerator where the hops are kept.

Other odors in urine and body fluids are listed in Table 13-3. Sweat odors are also discussed in Chapter 7 (p. 123).

References

Adams GL, Boies LR Jr, Paparella MM: *Boies's Fundamentals of Otolaryngology*, ed 5. WB Saunders, Philadelphia, 1978.

Artenstein MS, Demis DJ: Recent advances in the diagnosis and treatment of viral diseases of the skin. *N Engl J Med* 270:1101–1111, 1964.

Balciunas BA, Overholser CD: Diagnosis and treatment of common oral lesions. *Am Fam Physician* 35(5):206–220, 1987.

Bean WB: *Vascular Spiders and Related Lesions of the Skin*. Charles C Thomas, Springfield, IL, 1958. [The definitive study of vascular spiders and other skin lesions, written by a Chairman of Internal Medicine. This remains a model of clinical investigation.]

Beitman RG, Frost SS, Roth, JLA: Oral manifestations of gastrointestinal disease. *Dig Dis Sci* 26:741–747, 1981.

Burns RA, Davis WJ: Recurrent aphthous stomatitis. *Am Fam Physician* 32(2):99–104, 1985.

Burton BK, Nadler HL: Clinical diagnosis of the inborn errors of metabolism in the neonatal period. *Pediatrics* 61:398–405, 1978.

Burton R: *The Anatomy of Melancholy*. Oxford, 1621.

Centers for Disease Control: Oral viral lesion (hairy leukoplakia) associated with acquired immunodeficiency syndrome. *MMWR* 34:549–550, 1985.

Combs JT, Grunt JA, Brandt IK: New syndrome of neonatal hypoglycemia: Association with visceromegaly, macroglossia, microcephaly, and abnormal umbilicus. *N Engl J Med* 275:236243, 1966.

Crile G Jr: Recognition of a pathognomonic sign for the retropharyngeal goiter. *Am J Surg* 99:949–950, 1960.

Fitzgerald FT: Learning to emulate Sherlock Holmes. *Consultant*, April: 63–66, 69–72, 74, 1989.

Grahame R, Bluestone R, Holt PJL: Recurrent blanching of the tongue due to giant cell arteritis. *Ann Intern Med* 69:781–782, 1968.

Greally JM: Alternative to "Aaah." *Lancet* 1:539, 1988.

Grunfeld O, Hinostroza G: Thallium poisoning. *Arch Intern Med* 114:132–138, 1964.

Hayden GF: Olfactory diagnosis in medicine. *Postgrad Med* 67(April):110–118, 1980.

Hoeprich PD, ed: *Infectious Diseases*. Harper & Row, New York, 1972.

Hollander H, Greenspan D, Stringari S, Greenspan J: Hairy leukoplakia and the acquired immunodeficiency syndrome. *Ann Intern Med* 104:892, 1986.

Hutchinson J: On the different forms of inflammation of the eye consequent on inherited syphilis. *Ophthalmol Hosp Rep* 2:54–105, 1859

Kalra L, Hamlyn AN, Jones BJM: Blue sclerae: A common sign of iron deficiency. *Lancet* 2:1267–1268, 1986.

Kyle RA, Greipp PR: Amyloidosis (AL): Clinical and laboratory features in 229 cases. *Mayo Clin Proc* 58:665683, 1983.

Liddell K: Smell as a diagnostic marker. *Postgrad Med J* 52:136–138, 1976.

Majno G: *The Healing Hand: Man and Wound in the Ancient World*. Harvard University Press, Cambridge, MA, 1975.

Milgraum SS, Kanzler MH, Waldinger TP, Wong RC: Macroglossia: an unusual presentation of pemphigus vulgaris. *Arch Dermatol* 121:1328–1329, 1985.

Mindel A: Management of early HIV infection. *Br Med J* 294:1214–1218, 1987.

Mitchell JE, Seim HC, Colon E, Pomeroy C: Medical complications and medical management of bulimia. *Ann Intern Med* 107:71–77, 1987.

Schiødt M, Lackner A, Armitage G, Lerche N, Greenspan JS, Lowenstine, L: Oral lesions in rhesus monkeys associated with infection by simian AIDS retrovirus, serotype-I (SRV-1). *Oral Surg Oral Med Oral Pathol* 65:5055, 1988.

Seligman M, Mihaesco E, Preud'homme JL, Danon F, Brovet JC: Heavy chain diseases: Current findings and concepts. *Immunol Rev* 48:145–167, 1979.

Shapiro BL, Gorlin RJ, Redman RS, Bruhl, HH: The palate and Down's syndrome. *N Engl J Med* 276:1460–1463, 1967.

Shepard J Jr.: Grand Rounds. St. Louis University Medical Center, September 4, 1987.

Simenhoff ML, Burke JF, Saukkonen JJ, Ordinario AT, Doty, R: Biochemical profile of uremic breath. *N Engl J Med* 297:132–135, 1977.

Sprackling PD: Alternative to "Aaah." *Lancet* 1:769, 1988.

Sreebny LM, Valdini A: Xerostomia: A neglected symptom. *Arch Intern Med* 147:1333–1337, 1987.

Stone J: Sir Dominic John Corrigan. *Clin Cardiol* 9:403–406, 1986.

Tangerman A, Neuwese-Arends MT, van Tongeren JHM: A new sensitive assay for measuring volatile sulphur compounds in human breath by tenax trapping and gas chromatography and its application in liver cirrhosis. *Clin Chim Acta* 130:103–110, 1983.

Teschke R: Diagnostik akuter Vergiftungen durch halogenierte aliphatische Kohlenwasserstoffe. *Dtsch Med Wochenschr* 109:541–543, 1984.

Urman JD, Lowenstein MB, Abeles M, Weinstein A: Oral mucosal ulceration in systemic lupus erythematosus. *Arthritis Rheum* 21:58–61, 1978.

Vilter RW, Woolford RM, Spies TD: Severe scurvy: A clinical and hematologic study. *J Lab Clin Med* 31:609–630, 1946.

14
The Neck

"Cervicium dolores butyro aut adipe ursino prefricentur, rigores bubulo sebo, quod strumis prodest cum oleo. Dolorem inflexibilem—opisthotonum vocant—levat urina caprae auribus. . . . "

("Pains in the neck should be massaged with butter or bear grease, stiffness with beef wax, which latter is good for scrofula if mixed with oil. The painful rigidity—called opisthotonos—is relieved by pouring nanny-goat urine into the ears. . . . ")

Pliny the Elder: *Natural History*, Book 28, 52:192

The examination of the neck veins is described in Chapter 19, skin findings in Chapter 7 (p. 113), and the musculoskeletal examination in Chapter 24 (pp. 415 and 420).

Contour

A webbed neck (pterygium coli or winged neck) with a low posterior hairline should suggest the diagnosis of Turner's syndrome in a patient who is less than 5 feet tall and phenotypically female, or Noonan's syndrome* in either phenotypic males or females (Mendez & Opitz, 1985). Pterygium coli is also seen in the Bonnevie-Ulrich variant. A short neck is seen in the Klippel-Feil syndrome (see Fig. 14-1). A buffalo hump may occur in endogenous or exogenous Cushing's syndrome. Patients with obstructive sleep apnea tend to have short, stocky necks (a fact that was first pointed out to me by Dr. Ted Woodward of Maryland). Many of these patients wear unusually large-collared shirts (greater than size 17), and still leave them unbuttoned.

A lateral swelling in the neck, which appears during the Valsalva maneuver, is probably a laryngocele. This is a benign condition. It may occur bilaterally. The most pronounced example I ever saw was in the well-known trumpet player, John Birks (Dizzy) Gillespie. Glassblowers and patients with chronic obstructive airway disease are also prone to these diverticular outpouchings.

There are also other benign congenital cysts of the neck, related to embryonic structures, which may first appear in the second or third decade. These include branchial cleft cysts, cystic hygroma, and thyroglossal duct cysts (vide infra).

The Thyroid

Inspection

It is often possible to see thyromegaly in cases of thyroiditis, hypothyroid goiter, and hyperthyroidism, especially the last be-

*Noonan's syndrome has been erroneously referred to as the "male Turner syndrome."

cause weight loss has often thinned out the tissues that normally obscure the borders of the thyroid.

Lingual thyroids can be seen at the base of the tongue.

Maroni's sign is redness of the skin, occasionally with itching, over the anterior neck in the topographic projection of the thyroid gland. It is seen in hyperthyroidism.

Palpation

Most normal thyroid glands are palpable. (Sometimes a Valsalva maneuver will bring a retrosternal goiter up into the neck, where it can be felt.)

A Method

1. Ask the patient to sit in a comfortable position.

2. Hand the patient a large glass of water, saying, "In a moment, I am going to ask you to take some of the water. Hold it in your mouth, then swallow it when I tell you. That will help me to feel your thyroid gland."

3. Walk around to the patient's back, saying, "I won't hurt you," as you place your hands on the patient's neck.

4. Find the Adam's apple by palpation. (The first dozen times you do this you may have to look.) Although this is called the thyroid cartilage, the thyroid is actually inferior to this structure. (Thinking that the thyroid is located at the level of the thyroid cartilage is the reason that many untutored persons are unable to find the lateral lobes.)

5. Place your right index finger on the right lateral aspect of the thyroid cartilage, and your left index finger on the left lateral aspect. Next, move your two index fingers down to the cricoid cartilage; your index and third fingers are probably now at the level of the middle and upper thirds of the lateral lobes of the thyroid. (This varies with the anatomy of the patient and the examiner.)

6. Have the patient hold some water in his mouth and stare at the ceiling. (This will cause him to extend his neck.)

7. Instruct the patient to swallow. As he does so, the isthmus will ride up under your fingers, in the midline, then

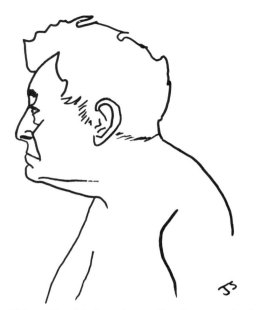

Figure 14-1.   Klippel-Feil syndrome. Note low posterior hair-line and short neck displacing the head anteriorly and inferiorly. Drawing of a patient of Dr. L. Mermel of Wisconsin.

back down again. The normal isthmus is of a soft consistency, and will be missed if you press too hard. (Palpation of the thyroid is a learned skill, and you should not be too concerned with what you miss on the first dozen attempts, but if you are consistently unable to feel the isthmus after about 20 palpations, you need to have a more experienced person demonstrate for you on a live patient—see "A Note to the Sophomore".)

8.   Now slip your fingers laterally and try to feel under the two sternocleidomastoids. Sometimes, all you will be able to do is to get a feeling for the fullness and consistency of those tissues. (In this way, palpation of the lateral lobes of the thyroid is akin to palpation of the ovaries on pelvic exam. Interpretation of the fullness encountered by your fingers requires considerable experience.)

9.   With your fingers at the anterior edges of the sternocleidomastoids, pull them laterally just a little. Have the patient maintain his head in some extension, but not so completely that the sternocleidomastoids are tensed. Ask him to swallow again. You should feel the upper parts of the lateral lobes ride up under your fingers, then down again. (Try this on yourself.) During your first dozen palpations of normal glands, you may not feel anything discrete.

An Alternate Method

Approach the patient from the front, and feel each lateral lobe in turn by using the fingers of one hand to retract the sternocleidomastoid muscle posteriorly, and the other to feel the underlying thyroid. Once the lateral lobes are located, the position of the isthmus can be predicted, and palpated during swallowing, also with the examiner in front of the patient.

Size

Try to estimate the size of the patient's thyroid: "normal," "twice normal," "one-and-a-half times normal," and so on. Large glands may be found in iodine-deficiency states, in which the gland attempts to compensate by hypertrophy and hyperplasia,

even though the patient tends to remain hypometabolic or eumetabolic. More often, however, a diffusely enlarged gland signifies Graves' disease (or Plummer-Vinson syndrome if nodular), and such patients are likely to be hypermetabolic. Enlargement of the thyroid is the most sensitive sign of Graves' disease, being found in from 81% to 98% of such patients, with the higher sensitivity in younger age groups (Nordyke et al., 1988). The external ocular signs of Graves' disease are described in Chapter 10 (see Table 10-2), and additional signs in Chapter 7 (pp. 108, 119, 126, 127, and 133) and Chapter 25 (p. 443). (Note that exophthalmos and pretibial myxedema do not occur in Plummer-Vinson syndrome.)

Small glands are felt in pituitary hypothyroidism and some cases of primary hypothyroidism. *No* gland is felt in athyreotic hypothyroidism.

Nodules

Describe the size and location of any nodules. A single nodule requires further evaluation. Many lumps or nodules in a hypermetabolic person may indicate toxic multinodular goiter (Plummer's syndrome), one of the most common forms of hyperthyroidism in the elderly patient.

Consistency

The consistency of the gland should be noted, but its importance should not be overstated until you have done a few dozen examinations, including a few glands of known abnormal consistency.

A firm rubbery gland is felt in some Hashimoto's thyroiditis, and also in de Quervain's thyroiditis. A hard gland is felt in cancer and in Riedel's thyroiditis.

Berry's Sign

Berry's sign of malignant thyromegaly is absence of the carotid pulsation (i.e., a malignant tumor tends to encase the carotid so that the pulsation is not detectable). Benign thyromegaly, on the other hand, does not encase the vessel ("Bailey," Clain, 1973).

A Note to the Sophomore

Don't get discouraged. After decades of palpating thyroid glands, I am still learning. The availability of mannikins in my student days would have helped. The only covariable available at that time was the [131]-I thyroidal uptake scan, which was usually ordered only in hyperthyroidism, when the gland was already sufficiently enlarged for even a junior medical student to recognize. At present, the technetium scan, a nonfunctional imager, is available, as are thyroidal ultrasounds and CAT scans. These offer an unusual opportunity in physical diagnosis: the use of independent covariables to accelerate the acquisition of skills. However, when comparing your findings with the independent covariable, remember that therapeutic intervention *may* have changed the size of the thyroid gland since the radionuclide image was recorded, so it is wise to seek the guidance of a faculty member or senior resident. If your institution has a thyroid clinic, you should attend it and practice there.

A Linguistic Diversion

Is Fig. 14-2 actually an illustration of the differential diagnosis of hyperthyroidism? The physician's right hand is obviously palpating the thyroid, while the left hand is apparently searching for ectopic thyroid hormone production from a struma ovarii (although this is not the best method of detecting struma ovarii). Or could this be factitious (exogenous) hyperthyroidism? Notice the decanter in

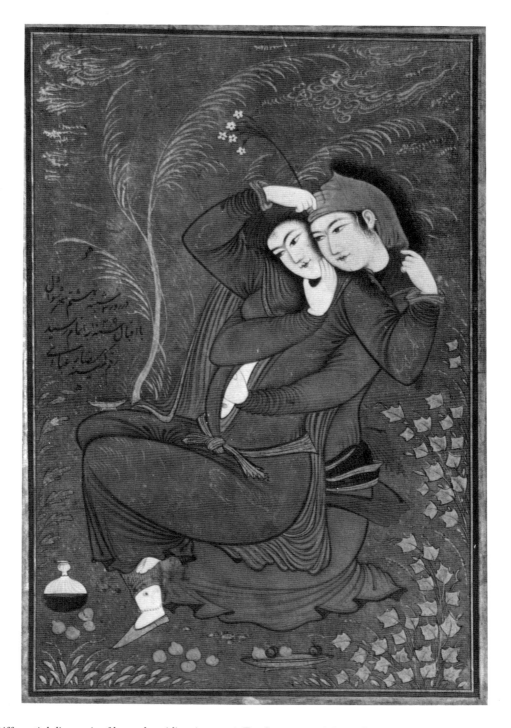

Figure 14-2. *Differential diagnosis of hyperthyroidism (see text).* Two Lovers, *a miniature by Riza-i-Abbasi of 17th century Persia, courtesy of the Metropolitan Museum of Art, New York, Francis M. Weld Fund, 1950 (50.164).*

the lower left, which might contain desiccated thyroid once used as an over-the-counter weight-loss medicament. What's wrong with this last idea?

Struma ovarii is an unfortunate phrase that we could do without. The original Latin *struma* did not mean goiter, but rather scrofula or "sore."* Struma (according to the story given by Bailey) came to be

used as a word for goiter because the Struma River (or Stryma) in Bulgaria was an area of endemic goiter—that is, the patients were actually *hypo*thyroid, not *hyper*thyroid. (This river was known to the Latins as Stryma, but the ancient Romans did not recognize the condition of hypothyroidism.) Thus, from its semantic derivation, struma ovarii is a Bulgarian ovary that produces an insufficient supply of thyroid hormone. Since even Bulgarian ovaries do not normally produce any thyroid hormone at all, struma ovarii would seem to be a "nonoxymoronquitur" (a chimera of a non-se-

*See any translation of the lines of Pliny in this chapter's epigram.

quitur and an oxymoron). In its present usage, struma ovarii is a tumor, located in an ovary, that produces thyroid hormone.

To those who would consider this concern for the precision of language to be an impractical affectation, I address this question: Why don't the Chinese rule the earth? They had pharmacopoieas, paper, a system of writing, moveable type, pi to four decimal places, and gunpowder long before anyone else. My explanation is the corruption of their language at the end of the Chou Dynasty. (See the epigram to the preface.)

Now, have you formulated idea(s) about why the decanter does not contain desiccated thyroid for use as a weight reduction medicament? The answer is in Appendix 14-1.

Auscultation

A systolic bruit over the thyroid gland, if present, may help to distinguish hyperthyroidism from other high output states. False-positive systolic thyroid bruits may be caused by aortic stenosis or aortic sclerosis. These radiating murmurs may be easily misinterpreted by regional specialists who do not routinely examine the whole patient.

The thyroid bruit of hyperthyroidism may be continuous when it is due to the arteriovenous communications that open up inside the highly vascular gland. The prevalence of thyroid continuous bruits (heard best over one of the lateral lobes) is from 20% to 36% in hyperthyroidism (Graf et al., 1947). False-positive continuous "thyroid bruits," which are actually venous hums, can be abolished by compressing the ipsilateral jugular veins (see Ch. 19, p. 366).

Cervical arterial flow murmurs of anemia or fever, in the absence of hyperthyroidism, may also mimic the finding of a thyroid bruit. The differential diagnosis of such a finding, as so often is the case, is elucidated by the company that it keeps.

Dr. Susan Ashbee of Alabama once had a patient who had no apparent thyroid disease but a short, harsh, diamond-shaped murmur heard easily over one lobe of the thyroid. The sound was clearly not a hyperthyroid bruit. The diagnosis of atherosclerotic stenosis of a thyroidal artery was never proved.

A bruit is unusual in Plummer-Vinson syndrome. In Graves' hyperthyroidism, a precordial Means-Lerman scratch may be heard (see Ch. 17, p. 306).

An Historical Interlude: "Dr. Jod" and Other Early Thyroidologists

In 1786, Parry saw his first case of hyperthyroidism, but he did not publish it until 1825, 4 years after Coindet published his cases in France (Coindet, 1821). Yet neither of these men have been granted eponymic immortality. Instead the disease is known in the English speaking world as Graves' disease (1835) or in the German-speaking world as von Basedow's disease (1840).

Coindet's cases were a complication of administering large doses of iodine to susceptible persons. Such iodide-induced hyperthyroidism later came to be called iodide-Basedow, which in German is Jod-Basedow, German nouns being capitalized.

Thus, not only has Coindet been deprived of credit for describing hyperthyroidism, but even the variant of hyperthyroidism that he specifically described has been credited by some to Dr. Jod— who does not exist!

Special Maneuvers

Thyroglossal Cyst

A method:

1. Grasp the suspected thyroglossal cyst between your thumb and forefinger.

2. Instruct the patient to stick out his tongue as far as possible. For example, say, "Please try to put your tongue on your chin."

Interpretation.   If the lump moves under your fingers as the patient extends his tongue, it is a thyroglossal duct cyst. This test is 100% sensitive and pathognomonic.

Pemberton's Sign*

A method.   Have the patient hold his arms extended above his head, touching his ears (see Fig. 14-3). The test is over after 3 minutes (negative Pemberton sign) or as soon as a positive occurs. A positive sign is a reported sensation of stuffiness, dizziness, congestion, or "funny feeling" in the head. It is caused by impeded venous outflow. Sometimes the face will become dusky.

Significance.   Although Pemberton's sign may be positive with thyromegaly, it is not diagnostic of diseases of the thyroid. It may also be a sign of thoracic outlet obstruction (see Ch. 18, p. 344) or of superior caval syndrome (see Ch. 19, p. 366).

What do you think is the diagnosis in the patient depicted in Figure 14-3?

Hints: The patient's mouth is open, and the tongue seems to be enlarged. There is some periorbital puffiness, a broad flat nose, and rather dull-looking facies. Prior impairment of linear growth is suggested by the fact that the subject's trunk is longer than his legs. Hypothermia may be inferred from the fact that warm clothing is being worn in the subtropical Mexican Gulf Coast region. Also, the patient is having a little difficulty keeping his arms perfectly apposed to the sides of his head; this might be due to a myopathy.

Beginning with the puffy face, one could diagnose either nephrotic syndrome or hypothyroidism. Since the face is red (on the original figurine), one might think of the malar flush (not rash) seen in mitral stenosis (see Ch. 17, p. 321), but the face could be red simply from of a positive Pemberton sign. Thyroid enlargement is the first entity to think of as an explanation for a positive Pemberton sign, and if that sign is positive, nephrotic syndrome and mitral stenosis can be dropped from the list of possibilities. Furthermore, there are a number of other findings, such as cold intolerance and macroglossia, which are explained by hypothyroidism but not by mitral stenosis or nephrotic syndrome.

Proceeding further with the diagnosis of hypothyroidism, the impairment of linear growth suggests that the patient has cretinism. The next step is the differential diagnosis of goitrous cretinism.

There are three possibilities:

1. Dietary iodine deficiency. (This would be rather unlikely, given the high iodine content of the usual diet of Gulf Coast fishing tribes.)
2. A dietary goitrogen. (This could be present in a diet containing rutabagas and white turnips, although one would have to postulate that the ingestion was chronic.)
3. One of the six known inherited defects in thyroid hormone synthesis.

I favor the second diagnosis in this patient. Unfortunately, the issue cannot be resolved, due to our inability to take a dietary history.

A note on cretins.   The word "cretin" is a shortened version of the French word for Christian, *chretien*. One story is that an early

---

*This is the H.S. Pemberton (1891–1956) of Liverpool cited by Bailey; not J.J. Pemberton, the early 20th century Mayo Clinic thyroidologist.

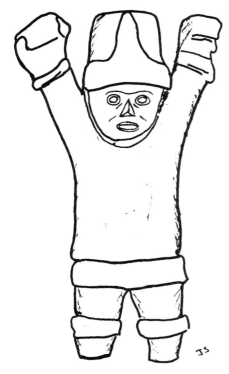

Figure 14-3. *Pemberton's sign. Drawing of a Huastec statue of the god Quetzlcoatl, depicted as an adolescent. The original figurine, which has a red face, is in the National Museum of Anthropology in Mexico City.*

band of Christians fled to the Pyrenees to escape religious persecution. There, they were protected from their pagan neighbors, but suffered an iodine-deficient diet. The whole community came to look like cretins, and when one strayed down to a pagan village, he was instantly noticeable as a Christian (*chretien*). A less opprobrious story is set years later in the Alps, where the name Christian was applied by Christian villagers to any imbecilic or malformed unfortunate, so as to remind the speaker that we are all God's creatures.

Parathyroid Glands

There are no specific physical maneuvers for the diagnosis of hyperparathyroidism. If you find a lump in the thyroid of a hypercalcemic patient, you should not jump to the conclusion that it is an enlarged parathyroid gland.

Analysis. About 90% of parathyroid adenomas and carcinomas are in the lower poles of the thyroid (and so impalpable). More than 90% are on the posterior surface of the thyroid (and so impalpable). On the other hand, hyperthyroidism is a more common disease that can be both nodular and, on occasion, hypercalcemic (see Christian's dictum, Ch. 7, p. 117).

In the usual nonmalignant case of hyperparathyroidism, the parathyroid glands are not palpable until they have reached individual weights of around 5 grams, by which time there should be obvious bone disease.

For the diagnosis of hypoparathyroidism, see the tetanic equivalents discussed in Chapter 26 (p. 488).

The Trachea

Inspection

Rarely, one can see a significant tracheal deviation due to a chronic condition such as an aortic aneurysm or, even more rarely, the scarring of old tuberculosis. But in acute situations, tracheal deviation is one of the spectrum of physical findings that permits the correct elucidation of intrapulmonary or intrapleural pathology, and is therefore discussed in Chapter 16 (p. 249) (as is the determination of tracheal position by palpation.)

Palpation

Tracheal Tug: Oliver's Sign

A method (as described by the discoverer):

Place the patient in the erect position and direct him to close his mouth and elevate his chin to the fullest extent, then grasp the cricoid cartilage between the finger and thumb, and use gentle upward pressure on it, when, if dilatation or aneurism exists, the pulsation of the aorta will be distinctly felt transmitted through the trachea to the hand. The act of examination will increase laryngeal distress should this accompany the disease. (Oliver, 1878)

Semiophysiology. The *aorta normally passes over the left bronchus*, which is part of a rigid system that extends up to the trachea. Thus, a bulging outward of the aneurysm depresses the left bronchus with each heartbeat. Each systolic movement is perceived by the examiner's fingers as a tug. Given these anatomic relationships, one can understand the wisdom of Cabot's warning that a tracheal tug felt only during inspiration has *no* pathologic significance and is frequently present in health. Cabot's second caveat was that the true aneurysmal tug will make the tissues move up and down, not in and out in the manner of the normal transmitted pulsations from the neck vessels.

Other Tracheal Tugs

1. If you press on the thyroid cartilage so as to displace it from the patient's right to his left, you also push the larynx laterally and the left bronchus more firmly against the aorta (see the section on Oliver's sign for a description of the anatomy.) If this maneuver produces transverse pulsations of the trachea, Cardarelli's sign is said to be positive. This sign has been erroneously equated with Oliver's sign as the "Oliver-Cardarelli sign."

2. Campbell's sign is a downward motion of the trachea during inspiration. It has been described as a physical finding of chronic airway obstruction (Godfrey et al., 1969).

It is best felt by resting the tip of the index finger on the thyroid cartilage. This sign is sometimes said to be present in any patient with respiratory distress, and anaesthetists associate it with deep anesthesia or carbon dioxide retention. However, I think the sign is more typical of chronic airways obstruction and is probably produced by the downward pull of the depressed diaphragm (Campbell, 1969)

This sign was subsequently found to correlate very well with both the 1-second forced expiratory volume and the specific airway conductance (Godfrey et al., 1970). Campbell has continued to use this sign for a quarter of a century (Stubbing et al., 1982). Although some workers require the tracheal descent on inspiration to be at least 2½ inches before it is accepted as a sign of pulmonary disease, Campbell and his coworkers describe three different grades whose increasing clinical intensity correlates with a worsening of the 1-second forced expiratory volume.

Percussion

There is no point in percussing the trachea.

•

In only one instance that I am aware of was the technique of percussion useful in making a laryngotracheal diagnosis.

A junior medical student on the wards of the Presbyterian-University Hospital in Pittsburgh was assigned to an attractive 23-year-old white woman admitted from the Pulmonary Clinic. She was found to have experienced the acute onset of aphonia in the absence of prior fever. Oddly enough, there were no significant physical findings and consultation for laryngoscopy was ordered.

In the course of interviewing the patient (who could only whisper), the student learned that the aphonia had its acute onset the Monday morning after the patient had experienced the unintended termination of an intense homosexual relationship. This sexual preference was less socially tolerated at that time, and the student was instructed by the Chief Resident to remove that portion of the history from the patient's chart. Since the patient had sworn the student to secrecy and would not whisper (literally) a word of this to anyone else, the student had no data with which to substantiate his diagnosis of conversion.

At laryngoscopy, no tumors, inflammations, or other lesions could be found, and a neurologic consult was ordered. By now, the patient's hospital bill was almost $90, incredibly high for the time, a month's income for an intern.

To make his diagnosis in the absence of the historical data, the student had to resort to determining the posttussive percussion note and recording it in the chart. At first his resident thought that the student was deranged, but the previous week the student had been the only person to correctly diagnose a case of tuberous sclerosis in a patient with cryptogenic seizures (having seen adenoma sebaceum in H.J. Robert's *Difficult Diagnosis*), so his bizarre physical diagnostic maneuvers were accordingly extended the minimal courtesy of an inquiry.

The student agreed that there was nothing about posttussive percussion notes anywhere in the medical literature and that there could be nothing of any significance in such a percussion note. But, he pointed out, when the patient coughed, she made sounds. That meant that she could control her larynx at times when she made no connection between such motor behavior and the social phenomena of speaking, crying, or making other sounds of emotional distress.

Full credit must be given to the resident, who was willing to listen to the reasoning of a medical student, accept it, and discharge the patient to his own clinic. At follow-up, she was completely asymptomatic.

•

Auscultation

Tracheal auscultation is helpful in diagnosing tracheal stenosis or other high-grade tracheal obstruction.

This diagnosis is suggested by the presence of a total pattern: a patient with tachypnea; great straining, especially with expiration; use of accessory expiratory muscles; normal tracheal position; the absence of local or lateralizing signs; breath sounds that are disproportionately soft for the amount of apparent distress; and

wheezes (actually stridor, see Ch. 16, p. 261), better heard over the center of the chest than on either side. In combination with this picture, tracheal breath sounds that are more prolonged, more harmonic, more high pitched, more squeaky, and/or more musical than usual make the working diagnosis of tracheal obstruction.

◗ If the patient's face is red, the diagnosis can be confirmed by airflow loop analysis and/or direct visualization. If the situation is acute, and the patient is beginning to turn blue, assume that the obstruction is at the level of the vocal cords and perform an emergency tracheostomy.

Tracheal obstruction and stridor heard with the neck flexed, but not with the neck extended, should suggested a congenital cardiovascular ring anomaly compressing the trachea and the esophagus. The patient is likely to have dysphagia, which is aggravated under similar circumstances, leading someone to christen this syndrome with the macabre title *dysphagia lusoria* or "dysphagia from a joke," the congenital anomaly being thought of as a joke of nature (a more misanthropic attribution than an error of nature).

Special Maneuvers: Kocher's Test*

Compress the lateral lobes of the thyroid. If this produces stridor audible without the stethoscope, the patient has either carcinoma of the thyroid, a goiter, or thyroiditis ("Bailey," Clain, 1973).

Self-Test

If you are reading this work in sequence, and you have followed the advice of looking up words and phrases with which you are not familiar, it will not surprise you to learn that relapsing polychondritis can affect the trachea, producing signs and symptoms.

Salivary Glands

Location

The salivary glands include the parotid glands, the submaxillary glands, and the sublingual glands.

The parotid glands are palpable just posterior to the angles of the mandible. The cervical portion of the submaxillary glands are medial and just anterior to the angle of the mandible; the buccal portion is above the myohyoid and is not usually examined. Thus, the name submaxillary, while not totally incorrect, is somewhat misleading. Actually, in young persons with firm tissues, the submaxillary glands may be difficult to palpate. A helpful trick is to have the patient swallow during palpation.

---

*Kocher was the Swiss physician who won the Nobel Prize for Medicine and Physiology in 1909 for his work on the thyroid gland. He was not the only Nobelist who was also a physical diagnostician. The Austrian, Robert Barany, won the same prize in 1914 for research on the physiology of the vestibular system, but is better known to us as the inventor of caloric testing (see Ch. 26, p. 480). Barany was the last clinician both to win the Nobel Prize and also to have a physical maneuver named after him. Philip Hench, who was co-winner of the Prize for work on adrenal corticosteroids, had a test named jointly for him (for mercury in the saliva) and a clinical phenomenon named solely for him (the amelioration of rheumatoid arthritis during obstructive jaundice), but I have not heard of a sign or a maneuver named for him.

Then one can often easily appreciate the glands, which are walnut-like in both size and shape.

The sublingual glands are the inferior glands of Blandin and Nühn on the undersurface of the tongue, and the larger ones that are palpable beneath the tongue in the floor of the mouth. They are described as not customarily being palpable, when it is more accurate to say that they are not customarily palpated.

As none of these glands have migrated since anatomy class, it is somewhat surprising that there is so much confusion in the literature about them. Some textbooks refer to the parotids when they must really be talking about the submaxillary glands. Perhaps the confusion may be partly explained by the next sentence.

Swellings

The submaxillary and parotid glands are often heir to the same afflictions. Accordingly, in the following differential diagnosis of parotid swellings, it must be understood that except for the obvious situations, such as a ductal calculus, anything that can cause swelling of the parotid can also cause swelling of the submaxillary glands, and vice versa.

Unilateral Swelling

A painful unilateral swelling may be due to bacterial parotitis, commonly from *Staphylococcus* or *Streptococcus viridans* infections, or from an obstruction in the duct. A calculus in Stensen's duct or Wharton's duct could produce painful unilateral swelling of the parotid or submaxillary gland, respectively (Federman, 1962). In one case, Wharton's duct was obstructed by a blade of grass on which a soldier was sucking (Talman, 1963).

Such obstructions can be diagnosed by inspection of the orifices: of Wharton's duct, just under the tongue about 5 mm lateral to the frenulum, and of Stensen's duct*, directly opposite the second upper molar. Sometimes the stone can be seen, or pus may be noted. If neither of these findings is present, compare the amount of saliva on the two sides; the obstructed side will be much drier. Giving a patient a slice of lemon to suck on will make the difference in wetness much more obvious, and may also quickly produce swelling of the submaxillary gland in cases of ductal occlusion, often accompanied by great pain.

One caveat is to avoid performing the lemon test in patients whose saliva may be infectious. If the tongue is held up, the saliva may shoot out of the mouth, traveling a foot or more.

A false positive: a unilateral swelling mimicking infectious parotitis is seen in actinomycosis.

Parotid tumors tend to be unilateral, but not painful.

Bilateral Swelling

Bilateral infectious parotitis is most commonly due to mumps, but may be seen with other viruses such as choriomeningitis virus.

Drug reactions can cause bilateral parotid swelling, either with or without pain. Such drugs include, but are not limited to, iodide, lead, propylthiouracil, mercury, isoproterenol, sulfonamides, and oxyphenbutazone.

---

*Stensen's duct is sometimes called Steno's duct. It is not only the same duct, but the same person, a Danish theologian (1636–1686). But he is not remembered for being the first to explain the functions of the ovary, to distinguish between stratified and volcanic rocks, or to understand the correct origins of fossils.

Leukemic infiltrates and lymphomas, both Hodgkin's and others, may involve the salivary glands bilaterally.

Mikulicz's disease, which is synonymous with Sjögren's syndrome, may cause bilateral enlargement of the salivary glands. This may be accompanied by xerostomia (see Ch. 13, p. 222).

Mikulicz's syndrome, which consists of the signs and symptoms of Mikulicz's disease occurring as a consequence of some disease other than Sjögren's, may be associated with tuberculosis, Waldenström's macroglobulinemia, systemic lupus erythematosus, or sarcoidosis. With the last disease, one may have Heerfordt's syndrome if there is uveitis or if cranial nerve VII is involved.

A collection of metabolic diseases, which may overlap to some degree, may also cause painless bilateral swelling. These include cirrhosis, pellagra, malnutrition, kwashiorkor, bulimarexia (Harris, 1983), vitamin A deficiency, excess starch ingestion (Silverman & Perkins, 1966), diabetes mellitus, poststarvation refeeding, obesity, and perhaps thyrotoxicosis.

Others have reported bilateral painless swelling due to periodic sialorrhea, pregnancy, lactation, stress, allergy, or heredity.

There is increasing evidence in the literature for a parotid abnormality associated with alcoholism, with or without liver disease (Barnett & Wilson, 1986).

Bilateral painless swelling of the submaxillary glands is also seen in sober male veterans over the age of 50. Some skeptics have challenged the veracity of the negative alcohol history claimed for these patients, but this phenomenon turns out to have been noted years ago by others (Kelemen & Montgomery, 1958).

The Frey syndrome, also called the auriculotemporal syndrome or gustatory sweating, occurs in patients who have had parotid surgery. When the patient is eating, the ipsilateral forehead becomes drenched with sweat, apparently because some remaining salivary nerve fibers connect with autonomic efferents.

Appendix 14-1. Answer to the Question on Page 233

Desiccated thyroid is not a liquid, and the Persians did not have it in any event.

References

Barnett JL, Wilson JAP: Alcoholic pancreatitis and parotitis: Utility of lipase and urinary amylase clearance determinations. *South Med J* 79:832–835, 1986.

Campbell EJM: Physical signs of diffuse airways obstruction and lung distention. *Thorax* 24:1–3, 1969.

Clain A (ed): *Hamilton Bailey's Demonstrations of Physical Signs in Clinical Surgery*, ed 15. Williams & Wilkins, Baltimore, 1973.

Coindet "Dr": Nouvelles recherches sur les effets de l'iode, et sur les précautions à suivre dans le traitement du doite par ce nouveau remède [New researches on the effects of iodide and on the precautions to be taken during the treatment of goitre with this new remedy]. *Ann Chimie Physique* 16:252–266, 1821.

Federman DD: Case records of the Massachusetts General Hospital 86–1962. *N Engl J Med* 267:1364–1367, 1962.

Godfrey S, Edwards RHT, Campbell EJM, Armitage P, Oppenheimer EA: Repeatability of physical signs in airways obstruction. *Thorax* 24:4–9, 1969.

Godfrey S, Edwards RHT, Campbell EJM, Newton-Howes J: Clinical and physiological associations of some physical signs observed in patients with chronic airways obstruction. *Thorax* 25:285–287, 1970.

Graf W, Moller T, Mannheimer E: The continuous murmur: Incidence and characteristics in different parts of the human body. *Acta Med Scan* 196 (suppl):167–191, 1947.

Harris RT: Bulimarexia and related serious eating disorders with medical complications. *Ann Intern Med* 99:820–827, 1983.

Kelemen G, Montgomery WW: Symmetrical, asymptomatic, submaxillary gland enlargement in older age groups. *N Engl J Med* 258:188–189, 1958.

Mendez HMM, Opitz JM: Noonan syndrome: A review. *Am J Med Genet* 21:493–506, 1985.

Nordyke RA, Gilbert FI Jr, Harada ASM: Graves' disease: Influence of age on clinical findings. *Arch Intern Med* 148:626–631, 1988.

Oliver WS: Physical diagnosis of thoracic aneurism. *Lancet* 2:406, 1878.

Silverman M, Perkins RL: Bilateral parotid enlargement and starch ingestion. *Ann Intern Med* 64:842–846, 1966.

Stubbing DG, Mathur PN, Roberts RS, Campbell EJM: Some physical signs in patients with chronic airflow obstruction. *Am Rev Respir Dis* 125:549–552, 1982.

Talman A: Unusual submaxillary "tumor": Report of a case. *N Engl J Med* 268:547–548, 1963.

15
The Breast

"To a virgin give nine pellets of rabbit droppings to keep her breasts always hard."
Translated from Pliny the Elder, *Natural History*, Book 28, 77:249

The examination of the breasts is an extremely important part of the physical examination in women, largely because breast cancer is such a common disease, the leading cause of death in women age 35 to 54. The examination should also not be neglected in men, although cancer of the male breast is rare.

Draping the Female Patient

Adequate exposure, of course, is essential, but many women will be uncomfortable if their modesty is not protected. Gynecologists often have the patient wear a gown that opens in the front, and place a sheet on the patient's lap. The gown can be opened to examine the breasts, then closed to cover them during the rest of the examination. The sheet can be used to cover the pubic area while the abdomen is inspected, then raised to cover the abdomen when the genitalia are examined. From the viewpoint of the internist or general physician, it is inconvenient to have the gown open in the front for purposes of the rest of the examination, especially the chest examination. (It cannot be easily raised because the patient will be sitting on it.) Therefore, some prefer to have the opening in back. To examine the breasts and auscult the heart, the physician can either lower the gown from the shoulders (when the patient is sitting) or raise it (when the patient is supine), keeping the lower part of the body covered with a sheet.

Inspection

A Method

Patients should be examined both seated and supine. While the patient is seated, disrobed to the waist, the breasts should be inspected. Look for asymmetry (a certain amount is normal); a change in contour or visible swelling; retraction, edema, erythema, or dimpling of the skin; or an increased prominence of the venous pattern. Skin retraction is usually a sign of carcinoma, although it can result from fat necrosis. If a tumor blocks the lymphatic drainage, an area of lymphedema, which often looks like an orange peel (peau d'orange, pronounced poe-der-awnj), may result. Local areas of redness indicate underly-

ing inflammation; this can occur in inflammatory carcinoma, or infection.

Changes induced by pregnancy are summarized in Table 22-2.

Traditionally, the inspection of the breasts has included the following maneuvers described by Haagensen: First, the patient's arms should be in her lap, so that the pectoral muscles are relaxed. Second, she should be asked to press her hands firmly on her hips to contract the pectoral muscles. Third, she should raise her arms above her head. If the patient has pendulous breasts, it may also be helpful to have her stand and lean forward, supported by the back of a chair or the examiner's hands.

These time-honored but time-consuming maneuvers seldom reveal changes suggesting a cancer in patients not having a palpable lump, and are often deleted from a screening examination.

Nipples

Particular attention should be paid to the nipples. An inverted nipple, unless long-standing, suggests carcinoma. Scaling or ulceration of the skin surrounding the nipple suggests Paget's disease of the breast, a malignant condition in which a lump may not be palpable.

Supernumerary Nipples

Supernumerary nipples or breasts (polythelia and polymastia) are rather frequent minor errors in development, having an incidence varying from 0.22% to 2.5%. They are more common in males, and in blacks. They are usually located in the mammary line on the thorax and abdomen, most commonly just below the normal left breast, but they may occur in the axilla, on the shoulder, flank, groin, thigh, or face. They may be mistaken for a pigmented mole, but close inspection generally reveals a miniature nipple and areola.

Although supernumerary nipples have been considered clues to the diagnosis of congenital heart disease, they are of very low sensitivity and diagnosticity. Other associations have been suggested (Pellegrini & Wagner, 1983) but not proved. In fact, the only statistically significant associations are with duplicate renal arteries and renal adenocarcinomas (Goedert et al., 1981). However, black infants with supernumerary nipples do not need to be investigated for renal anomalies (Robertson et al., 1986).

Absent Nipples

Absence of a nipple on only one side with an absent pectoralis major on the same side, sometimes in association with brachydactyly or a small hand, is known as *Poland's syndrome*. In children, it has been associated with leukemia (Hicsonmez & Ozsoylu, 1982), but it is also seen in adults with prolapsed mitral valve and no other associated abnormality.

Bilateral absence of nipples is a completely different syndrome. Sometimes it is associated with other congenital abnormalities.

Adrenocortical Insufficiency

I only examine the nipples of males intentionally when I am trying to make the diagnosis of chronic primary adrenocortical insufficiency. Because ACTH and its precursors have the melanocyte-stimulating hormone (MSH) peptide sequence, patients with primary adrenocortical insufficiency may eventually develop pigmentation of scars and nipples. However, the absence of pigmentation (light-pink nipples) is far more helpful in excluding the diagnosis than its presence is for establishing it. Just as the Indonesian connection altered the Dutch gene pool sufficiently to make pigmentation misleading (as Snapper and Kahn [1967] noted), the blue-eyed blond gene pool in the United States is so mixed with DNA from Mediterraneans and other swarthy people that pigmentation in any individual is worse than useless. Especially in black Americans, the "classic" skin signs of chronic primary adrenocortical insufficiency (including dark palms, dark elbows, and mucosal blue spots) are frequently encountered in those whose hypothalamic-pituitary-adrenocortical axes are paragons of adequate homeostasis.

Palpation

A Method

1. If the patient has large breasts, they may be palpated bimanually while she is still sitting up. Support the breast from below with one hand, and gently compress it from above with the other. It may be helpful to roll the tissue back and forth between the two hands.

2. In all patients, palpation is performed with the patient supine, with the arm on the side to be examined placed behind the head. Other methods of getting the breast to lie squarely on the chest wall are to prop up the shoulder and upper back on a pillow, or to hold the breast on the chest wall with one hand while examining it with the other (Scanlon, 1987).

3. An orderly examination is necessary to assure that no areas are missed. Some physicians use a pattern resembling the spokes of a wheel, starting with the tail of the breast in the axilla, and moving from the outer boundary of the breast toward the nipple until the entire circumference has been covered. Some use a spiral pattern, moving from the periareolar area to the periphery of the breast (Scanlon, 1987).

4. Use a gentle, rolling motion, pressing the breast tissue between your fingertips and the chest wall. Very small lumps are most easily felt with the tips of the finger, but lumps larger than about 1 cm can best be evaluated by bobbing them back and forth between the thumb and index or third finger. The texture of the tissue around the lump is best appreciated by passing the fingers over it lightly (Scanlon, 1987).

5. While performing the examination, explain to the patient what you are doing, and encourage her to do the examination herself once a month, preferably just after her menstrual period.

Remember that the word "doctor" comes from the Latin *docere*, which means to teach. Point out that 85% of solid lumps turn out to be benign (Mahoney & Csima, 1982). After fear, the biggest impediment to breast self-examination is that the patients have not been taught how to do it. Be sure to explain that the normal breast has many lumps and bumps, which enlarge and subside with the menstrual cycle. Frequent examinations, preferably starting at a young age, are needed so that the patient will learn to recognize what is normal.

The patient could perform the examination lying down, or while in the bath. Many breast lesions are discovered accidentally while bathing, and it has been suggested that a mass can be more easily detected under a slippery film of soap.

6. If the patient has come to you with a complaint of a mass in the breast, be sure to have her point it out to you, after you have completed your examination. It is not unheard of for the patient to find a mass that the doctor has missed.

7. Be sure to check the lymph nodes that drain the breast: axillary, supraclavicular, and infraclavicular (see Ch. 8).

8. Finally, palpate the nipple for a mass or induration, and with a vigorous pressure or stripping action, see whether a discharge can be expressed (see p. 241 and Fig. 15-1).

Findings

Normal Breast Tissue

The normal consistency of breast tissue is quite variable from one individual to another and at different times in the menstrual cycle. "Like a bean bag" is one good description that patients readily understand. The milk glands feel like radiating strands of firm tissue having a variable degree of granularity. Swelling, tenderness, and greater prominence of the glandular elements may be noted in the week before and during the menses. The normal inframammary ridge, a firm transverse ridge of tissue along the lower edge of the breast, most prominent in large breasts, should not be confused with a tumor. Checking for symmetry may help to ascertain what is normal in an individual patient.

Describing the Dimensions of Breast Nodules

If a nodule is found, you should describe the following dimensions:

1. *Size.* Plastic calipers are suggested (see Ch. 7, p. 121).
2. *Location.* The breast may be divided into four quadrants, with the axes passing through the nipple, but radial coordinates are more precise. Describe the mass in terms of distance from the nipple and hours on a clock. Sketch a diagram in the patient's record.
3. *Tenderness.*
4. *Consistency or firmness.*
5. *Shape.* Is the mass regular, irregular, discoid, round, nodular?
6. *Relation to surrounding tissues.* Is it freely mobile, or is it fixed to the fascia or the skin? The maneuvers described by Haagensen (p. 239) may be helpful. To demonstrate "tethering" of the skin above a carcinoma, elevate the breast gently with the hand, and look for an area of dimpling. Is the border between the lump and the normal tissue distinct, or difficult to discern?

Characteristics of Benign and Malignant Lumps

Benign lesions, such as areas of mastitis or fibrocystic nodules, are often tender, but the presence of tenderness does not rule out a malignancy. Benign lesions, such as cysts or fibroadenomas, tend to be well circumscribed, whereas the borders of a carcinoma may be indistinct. Carcinomas often feel hard. A mass that is fixed to surrounding tissues is likely to be cancerous.

However, the physical examination cannot be relied upon to distinguish benign from malignant lesions. Four of 10 cancers feel well circumscribed; 4 of 10 feel soft or cystic; and 6 of 10 are freely moveable (Mushlin, 1985).

Interobserver Variability

There can be considerable interobserver variability in the individual findings of the breast examination. In a study of 242 women presenting with a complaint of a lump in the breast, two observers disagreed about the consistency of the mass in 33%, about the presence of a clear boundary in 35%, and about the presence of homolateral axillary nodes in 45% (Yorkshire Breast Cancer Group, 1977).

There is also considerable variability in the synthesis of the findings. A study in which four surgeons specializing in breast disease each examined 100 patients (41 of whom had been admitted for breast biopsy and the remainder for other operations) showed that experts often differed in their opinions, especially about patients who did not have cancer. The examiners noted a mass in 32 to 42 cases, but in only 16 patients did all four surgeons agree as to whether biopsy should be performed. All four surgeons recommended biopsy in 11 of the 15 patients who turned out to have a malignancy (Boyd et al., 1981).

Sensitivity of the Physical Examination

The sensitivity of the examination of models to detect lumps is 17% to 83%, increasing with greater duration of search, but *not* with level of experience (Fletcher et al., 1985).

The sensitivity of breast palpation for detecting cancer has variously been reported as 24% (Hicks et al., 1979), 38% (Moskowitz, 1983), and 62% (Egan et al., 1977). Many early lesions are missed. Thus, it is now widely recommended that mammography be used to supplement the physical examination as a screening technique, because it has a higher sensitivity (62%, 72%, and 87%, respectively) in the studies cited above. However, the physical examination should not be omitted. In 7% of the cancers detected by physical examination, findings on mammography were benign, and 25% of the cancers were diagnosed between screenings because of self-discovered abnormalities (Hicks et al., 1979).

Auscultation

A mammary souffle may be heard over the engorged breasts of a pregnant woman. This may be either systolic or continuous. Its origin may be either arterial or venous (Perloff, 1980). The systolic form is easily distinguished, by location, from the systolic pulmonic flow murmur that is heard in about 50% of pregnant women. This, in turn, is distinguished from hemodynamically significant pulmonic stenosis, by attending to S2 as described in Chapter 17 (p. 321).

Discharge from the Breast

A discharge from the nipples is very common in premenopausal women. In an ambulatory population, it was found in 13% of nulligravida and 22% of parous women between the ages of 16 and 50. Prolonged lactation was the most common cause (29% of cases). No definite cause was found in 43% of 586 cases (Newman et al., 1983). Nipple discharge alone is a rare presenting symptom for carcinoma, occurring in less than 3% of pa-

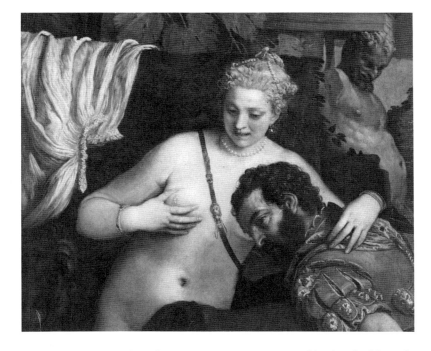

Figure 15-1. *After completing breast palpation, don't forget to attempt to express any blood or fluid from the nipple. (Detail from: Mars and Venus United by Love, by Veronese. Courtesy of the Metropolitan Museum of Art, John Stewart Kennedy Fund, 1910.)*

tients (Chaudary et al., 1982). Conversely, of patients with a nipple discharge, 5.9% (Chaudary et al., 1982) to 13.3% (Leis et al., 1988) have carcinoma.

Serous, Bloody, or Watery Discharge

A serous or bloody discharge from the nipple can result from a wide variety of causes (Atkins & Wolff 1964; Barnes, 1966). Benign causes include fibrocystic disease, duct papilloma, papillary cystadenoma, chronic infective mastitis, fibroadenoma, duct ectasia, hematoma, varicocele, fat necrosis, tuberculosis, toxoplasmosis, eczema of nipple, and breast abscess. Malignant causes include malignant melanoma, fibrosarcoma, carcinoma, Paget's disease of the breast, and neurosarcoma.

Watery discharge is rare, occurring in 2.2% of 503 patients with surgically significant nipple discharge, but 45.4% of such patients had carcinoma (Leis et al., 1988).

It is useful to test the discharge for occult blood. In a study of patients undergoing microdochectomy for a discharge that could be localized to a single duct, all 16 patients with an occult cancer had a positive test for occult blood. Of the 268 benign lesions, 69 produced a discharge that was negative for blood and 199 a discharge that was positive. The discharge was not tested in 8 cases (Chaudary et al., 1982). In an earlier study, all 27 cases that tested negative for blood had a benign cause (Atkins & Wolff, 1964). What is the sensitivity of occult blood for carcinoma, in patients presenting with only a discharge? What is the predictive value of a negative test? What was the specificity (in the study of 268 benign lesions)? What does this say about observation versus immediate surgery? Write your answers down before looking at Appendix 15-1.

Milky Discharges (Galactorrhea)

Abnormal milky discharge may occur in either sex at any age. Both intramammary and neurohumoral mechanisms must be considered. In theory, local etiologies should cause a unilateral discharge, and neurohumoral mechanisms, a bilateral one. However, the rule has many exceptions. Cystic disease may be bilateral, and one breast may initially be more responsive than the other to hormonal stimulation.

Mechanical stimulation has long been known to be a way to induce lactation. Eliciting the history may require some tact, as well as knowledge of the possibility. Lactation may also follow trauma or surgery to the breast or chest wall or an outbreak of herpes zoster, presumably through stimulation of the thoracic nerves.

Attenuation of the hypothalamic-pituitary suppression of prolactin production is another mechanism, which may result postpartum from pituitary necrosis (Sheehan's syndrome) or the Chiari-Frommel syndrome. Additional causes of lactation include other pituitary disorders, such as tumors, thyroid disorders, chorioepithelioma of the testis, hysterectomy, encephalitis, and ingestion of certain drugs, including oral contraceptives, phenothiazines, reserpine, and methyldopa (Barnes, 1966).

Gynecomastia

"Gynecomastia" means "a woman's breasts," and is therefore an abnormality only in men.

Prevalence

It has been said that breast tissue cannot be palpated in normal adult men. However, studies have shown that some palpable gynecomastia is quite common, about 36% in normal young adult men (Nuttall, 1979). It occurs commonly at the time of puberty, and may be more pronounced unilaterally. Between the ages of 14 and 14½, 65% of healthy Boy Scouts had some gynecomastia (Nydick et al., 1961). In a study of 214 hospitalized adult men (Niewoehner & Nuttall, 1984), gynecomastia was found to be related to age, the prevalence being highest (72%) in men aged 50 to 69 years, and increasing with body mass index (weight divided by the square of the height). An autopsy study revealed gynecomastia in 40% of an unselected series of 447 men, although the breasts were grossly enlarged in only four of these (Williams, 1963).

From the above, we can see that how one searches determines what one finds. Because so many of the negative gynecomastia evaluations are performed on men whose breast tissue is grasped from the side (and may in fact be only fat and not glandular tissue), I have modified my approach as follows: I place my finger in the nipple and invert it. If my finger does not encounter a bud of glandular tissue (not fat), I do not describe the patient as having gynecomastia no matter what the external contour. While it is impossible to correlate this technique with any of the above methods (or they with each other), I have not gone on any wild-goose chases since adopting it, while still adhering to the rules listed below under "Significance."

Etiology

Gynecomastia is believed to result in some cases from a decrease in the ratio of testosterone to estrogen. Thus, gynecomastia is a common finding in male neonates, due to the effect of maternal estrogens. As adipose tissue increases, more androstenedione is converted to estrone, explaining the relationship to body mass index.

Drugs associated with an increased prevalence of gynecomastia include beta blockers, spironolactone, quinidine, nitrates, cimetidine, antacids, steroids, and heparin, but all of these except cimetidine were associated with an elevated body mass index (Niewoehner & Nuttall, 1984). In an autopsy series, gynecomastia was significantly associated with certain prostatic and testicular abnormalities (including untreated prostatic carcinoma), adrenocortical hyperplasia, thyroid changes, pancreatic islet and pancreatic duct hyperplasia, cirrhosis of the liver, and diabetes mellitus (Williams, 1963).

Significance

Because gynecomastia is such a common finding, the issue is not whether it is present, but whether it requires a workup. Symptoms or signs that point to a need to investigate gynecomastia include pain, rapid breast enlargement, an eccentric or hard irregular breast mass, or a testicular mass (Niewoehner & Nuttall, 1984).

Appendix 15-1. Results of Testing Nipple Discharge for Occult Blood

Based on the finding of a 100% sensitivity of the test for occult blood (16/16 in the study by Chaudary et al.) and the 100% predictive value of a negative test (in the Atkins and Wolff study), patients with a negative test (and no lump) might be observed although at least one developed Paget's disease of the breast several years later (Chaudary et al., 1982), again illustrating the point that no test is perfect in medicine.

The test is not highly specific [TN/(TN + FP) = 69/(69 + 199) = .26].

References

Atkins H, Wolff B: Discharges from the nipple. *Br J Surg* 51:602–606, 1964.

Barnes AB: Diagnosis and treatment of abnormal breast secretions. *N Engl J Med* 275:1184, 1966.

Boyd NF, Sutherland HJ, Fish ED, Hiraki GY, Lickley HLA, Maurer VE: Prospective evaluation of physical examination of the breast. *Am J Surg* 142:307–426, 1981.

Chaudary MA, Millis RR, Davies GC, Hayward JL: Nipple discharge: The diagnostic value of testing for occult blood. *Ann Surg* 196:651–655, 1982.

Egan RL, Goldstein GT, McSweeney MM: Conventional mammography, physical examination, thermography, and xeroradiography in the detection of breast cancer. *Cancer* 39:1984–1992, 1977.

Fletcher SW, O'Malley MS, Bunce LA: Physicians' abilities to detect lumps in silicone breast models. *JAMA* 253:2224–2228, 1985.

Goedert JJ, McKeen EA, Fraumeni JF: Polymastia and renal adenocarcinoma. *Ann Intern Med* 95:182–184, 1981.

Hicks MJ, Davis JR, Layton JM, Present AJ: Sensitivity of mammography and physical examination of the breast for detecting breast cancer. *JAMA* 242:2080–2083, 1979.

Hicsonmez G, Ozsoylu S: Poland's syndrome and leukemia. *Am J Dis Child* 136:1098–1099, 1982.

Leis HP Jr, Greene FL, Cammarata A, Hilfer SE: Nipple discharge: Surgical significance. *South Med J* 81:20–26, 1988.

Mahoney L, Csima A: Clinical screening for breast cancer. *N Engl J Med* 306:546, 1982.

Moskowitz M: Screening for breast cancer: How effective are our tests? A critical review. *CA* 33:26–37, 1983.

Mushlin AI: Diagnostic tests in breast cancer: Clinical strategies based on diagnostic probabilities. *Ann Intern Med* 103:79–85, 1985.

Newman HF, Klein M, Northrup JD, Ray BF, Drucker M: Nipple discharge: Frequency and pathogenesis in an ambulatory population. *NY State J Med* 83:928–933, 1983.

Niewoehner KB, Nuttall FQ: Gynecomastia in a hospitalized male population. *Am J Med* 77:633–638, 1984.

Nuttall FQ: Gynecomastia as a physical finding in normal men. *J Clin Endocrinol Metab* 48:338–340, 1979.

Nydick M, Bustos J, Dale JH, Rawson RW: Gynecomastia in adolescent boys. *JAMA* 178:449–454, 1961.

Pellegrini JR, Wagner RF Jr: Polythelia and associated conditions. *Am Fam Physician* 28:129–132, 1983.

Perloff, JK: Cardiac auscultation. *DM* 26(9):1–47, 1980.

Robertson A, Sale P, Sathyanarayan: Lack of association of supernumerary nipples with renal anomalies in black infants. *J Pediatr* 109:502–503, 1986.

Scanlon E: A photo checklist for better breast palpation. *Primary Care Cancer* 7(9):13–20, 1987.

Snapper I, Kahn AI: Bedside Medicine, ed 2. Grune & Stratton, New York, 1967.

Yorkshire Breast Cancer Group: Observer variation in recording clinical data from women presenting with breast lesions. *Br Med J* 2:1196–1199, 1977.

Williams MJ: Gynecomastia: Its incidence, recognition and host characterization in 447 autopsy cases. *Am J Med* 34:103–112, 1963.

16
The Chest

"When the army was leaving Sardis, he met with an unhappy accident: a dog ran under his horse's feet, and the horse, taken by surprise, reared and threw its rider. As a result of the fall Pharnuches began to spit blood; and his sickness finally turned to consumption."

Herodotus, *The Histories*, Book Seven

The physical principles underlying some of the material in this chapter are summarized in the introduction to the synthesis section (p. 273) and in the discussion of pitch (p. 260).

Inspection

Posture and the Use of Accessory Muscles of Respiration

Certain observations, such as what position the patient assumes for most comfortable breathing, are generally made while noting the patient's general appearance (see Ch. 5). The posture assumed by patient with chronic obstructive lung disease to improve respiratory mechanics is shown in Figure 7-1.

Look at the sternocleidomastoid and other accessory muscles (especially in a bed-bound patient who cannot brace himself by leaning forward). In general, their use appears to signify that the forced expiratory volume in 1 second (FEV1) is decreased to 30% of normal or less. In one study of asthmatic patients, sternocleidomastoid muscle retraction was the only sign that correlated with pulmonary function results, appearing at a FEV1 between 1.0 and 1.5 liters (McFadden et al., 1973). With chronic compensatory use, the sternocleidomastoid muscles may develop noticeable hypertrophy (i.e., they will be thicker than the patient's own thumb).

Shape of the Thorax

"Increased AP Diameter"

An apparent increase in anteroposterior (AP) diameter is also referred to as a barrel chest or pulmonary kyphosis (Fig. 16-1). It occurs in pulmonary emphysema (or in patients with "senile kyphosis"). Interrater reliability for this sign is about 70% (Fletcher, 1952).

In point of fact, the AP diameter is not increased. In a study of 25 patients with emphysema, 22 patients with other diseases, and 16 normal subjects (Kilburn & Asmundsson, 1969), two physicians agreed that the 25 emphysema patients had an increased AP diameter. However, measurement of the actual inspiratory and ex-

piratory AP diameters by chest film and by direct measurement with calipers revealed no significant differences between the three groups. Because the emphysema patients weighed about 30 pounds less than normal subjects, the "increased" AP diameter may be an illusory, albeit constant, field/image effect due to a decreased abdominal AP diameter.

Deformities of the Thoracic Cage

Pectus carinatum ("pigeon breast"). In this deformity, the sternum protrudes from the narrowed thorax. Although it is thought of as a benign sign, in one study 45% of the patients with pectus carinatum had associated abnormalities on chest roentgenogram (Pena et al., 1981).

The deformity may be isolated, or familial, or associated with a specific disease such as acromegaly (Robicsek et al., 1979), childhood rickets, Noonan's syndrome (Mendez & Opitz, 1985), Marfan's syndrome, or anomalies of the diaphragm.

Pectus excavatum. The vulgar term for this deformity is "funnel chest." The inferior sternum and xiphoid are retracted toward the spine, producing either an oval pit near the infrasternal notch or a more extensive distortion. In one series, associated chest roentgenogram abnormalities were present in 72% of cases of pectus excavatum (Pena et al., 1981).

It has been associated with Noonan's syndrome, Marfan's syndrome, rickets, tracheomalacia (Lane et al., 1984), bronchomalacia (Godfrey, 1980), and congenital heart disease (Godfrey, 1980; Robinson, 1970), including prolapse of the mitral valve (see Ch. 17, p. 317).

Kyphosis, scoliosis, and lordosis. These deformities of the spine (see Ch. 24, p. 421) may cause serious distortions in respiratory mechanics.

Respiratory Motions

Signs of Small Airways Disease

Dyspneic and tachypneic persons with small airways disease breathe in a pattern that is observably different from that ex-

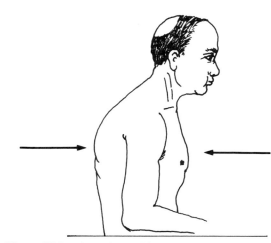

Figure 16-1. *A patient with an apparent increase in AP diameter.*

hibited by other dyspneic and tachypneic persons.

To acquaint yourself with the normal pattern of tachypneic breathing, exercise to the point of breathlessness, then observe yourself in the mirror with your chest nude. Notice that your entire chest is moving, and that you are taking deep breaths.

Patients with small airway disease, in contrast, tend to "breathe off the top." (The accessory muscles help them to do this.) They take many small breaths from a position of relative inspiration, but never seem to take very deep ones. If they do start to take deep breaths, they develop air trapping during expiration.

At end-expiration, the high transbronchial pressure can collapse the diseased terminal bronchioles, causing air trapping (and perhaps producing audible signs, see p. 261).

These patients tend to exhale with pursed lips. In this way, they increase expiratory airway resistance and thus the pressure in the small collapsible airways, preventing collapse. Since the airways are not at risk of collapse during inspiration, many patients who do purse their lips do it, quite unconsciously, only during expiration.

Also see Figure 7-1.

Chest Expansion

Asymmetric expansion: A method:

1. To compare the expansion of the two sides of the thorax in inspiration, stand behind the patient, whose head is facing directly forward, touching the *lateral* thorax with your hands. Do *not* place your hands posteriorly as instructed in most textbooks, for if you do, you will miss about half the cases of unilateral restrictions (and additionally will miss many patients with bilateral restriction.)

2. Watch your hands as the patient inhales. Do not press or offer resistance to the thorax.

Asymmetric chest expansion is a useful sign that may be more easily detected by palpation (see p. 250). Laennec noted the importance of this "volume sign" as evidence of restriction, and even had an illustration of it (Plate VII, Laennec, 1821). He used it to figure out which side had the "pleurisy."

Symmetric expansion: A method. Restricted symmetric expansion may be quantitated by measuring the difference in cir-

cumference of the chest between end-expiration and end-inspiration with a tape measure (preferably a spring-loaded one) placed at the nipple line.

The normal value has been stated (without citing data) to be 5 cm (about 2 inches) in the absence of emphysema (regardless of chest size!) (Fries, 1985). An expansion of 1.5 inches or less is considered definitely impaired (Fletcher, 1952). However, using a less stringent standard of 2 inches, one would probably detect all of the individuals with impaired expansion, at the cost of garnering a few false positives. Unfortunately, the error on repeated examination is usually at least 1 inch (Fletcher, 1952). So as a general rule, a single measurement of less than 1 inch is definitely abnormal, and a measurement of more than 3 inches is normal.

Symmetrically impaired chest expansion (less than 2.5 cm) can be an early sign of ankylosing spondylitis, and should be sought in young men presenting with low back pain (Fries, 1985).

Intercostal Spaces

Normally, the intercostal spaces bulge inward during inspiration and outward with expiration. This may be easily observed in a thin classmate.

An exaggeration of the inspiratory retraction occurs in patients with obstructive or restrictive lung disease, because there is an imbalance between the ability of the respiratory muscles to create a negative intrapleural pressure, and the impaired ability of the lungs to expand.

Focal exaggeration of inspiratory retraction indicates a regional imbalance in the two opposing forces discussed above. There might be a local obstruction with increased airway resistance, say in one of the bronchi. Or there might be a flail chest. In the latter, the affected ribs are separated from the rest of the chest, either by fracture or separation of the cartilages, and thus become a passive indicator of the underlying negative intrapleural pressure by their heightened inspiratory retraction.

Focally exaggerated retraction of the cardiac interspaces, concordant with ventricular systole, is Broadbent's sign of constrictive pericarditis.

Unilateral or focal loss of inspiratory retraction suggests an underlying consolidation, tension pneumothorax, or pleural effusion. In fact, even the small pleural effusion within the hydropneumothorax shown in Figure 16-10 produced this sign.

Exaggerated expiratory bulging of the interspaces results from a mechanism similar to that of heightened inspiratory retraction. Diffuse expiratory bulging suggests that a positive intrapleural pressure is being effectively transmitted through the chest wall, but the lungs are not being emptied. This is a sign of increased expiratory airway resistance, either chronic (as in emphysema) or acute (as in asthma).

Focal expiratory bulging may be seen on the side of a tension pneumothorax or over the area of a flail chest.

Constant focal bulging throughout all the phases of respiration can be caused by massive amounts of pleural fluid, or very rarely by underlying pulmonary consolidation.

Focal systolic bulging over the precordium is discussed in connection with the palpation of the point of maximum impulse (PMI) (Ch. 17, p. 285). Focal systolic bulging anywhere else is a sign of an arterial aneurysm.

Respiratory Paradox

Normally, the abdominal wall moves passively outward during inspiration, as the descending diaphragm squeezes the peritoneal contents down and out. Then the abdominal wall retracts during expiration as the diaphragmatic piston returns to its resting position.

■ In weakness or paralysis of the diaphragm, most commonly due to overwork in severe chronic obstructive lung disease, inspiration finds the helpless diaphragm being passively sucked upwards as the intercostal muscles do the work of inspiration. Now the abdominal wall retracts during inspiration. This is called respiratory paradox (Macklem, 1982). The sophomore who observes this sign of diaphragmatic fatigue should immediately ask his resident to see the patient, because the patient may be in need of mechanical ventilation.

False positives may be seen in vain persons wearing swimsuits who hope to be observed. Such persons voluntarily contract the abdominal muscles during inspiration, as may be detected by palpation.

Respiratory Alternans

When the diaphragm is mildly impaired, it may work for a few inspirations and then fatigue for a few. When this happens, the abdominal wall may move out normally for a few inspirations and then paradoxically move inward for a few inspirations, until the diaphragm is again rested. This sequence of events is called respiratory alternans (Macklem, 1982).

There are some marginal patients in whom respiratory paradox or alternans can only be seen in the perfectly erect position, because when they lean forward (or rarely when they are supine), the increased intraabdominal pressure can increase the dome of the flattened diaphragmatic leaves. This may improve efficiency to a degree that, in these marginal cases, allows the disappearance of the signs (Sharp, 1986).

Subcostal Angles and Hoover's Chest Sign

The subcostal angle is the angle between the xiphoid process and the right or left costal margin, as shown in Figure 16-2A.

A second, less strict definition is the angle between the right and left costal margins, viewed from the patient's feet. This more than

doubles the size of the angle, allowing for easier appreciation of the changes. Also, the xiphoid process may be difficult to observe in obese patients. Finally, this second definition alleviates the problem of deciding which portion of the curved costal angle should be chosen for the chord or tangent that defines the angle; one simply takes any segment available and matches it to the facing side.

However, several of the variations on Hoover's sign to be discussed below depend upon comparing the right and left subcostal angles, so this second definition will not be useful in that context.

A method:

1. With the patient supine, sit or stand at his side, and lean over towards his midline.

2. Lightly rest your right hand on the patient's left hypochondrium, with your thumb on the medial costal margins (higher than is shown in Fig. 16-2B), and the remaining fingers superiorly (toward the patient's head).

3. Lightly place your left hand on the patient's right costal margin, symmetric to your right hand.

4. Instruct the patient to take a deep breath. Normally, both hands will swing out symmetrically during inspiration and the thumbs will form a more obtuse angle, returning to a more acute angle with expiration.

The hands are not to offer resistance, but only to increase your appreciation of the change in angle. With practice, you can observe this sign without using your hands.

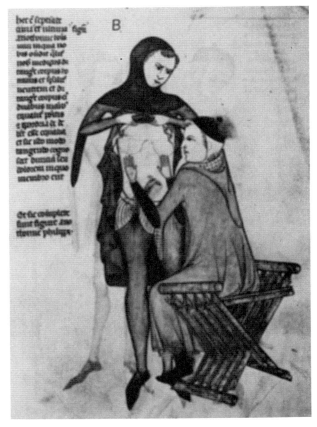

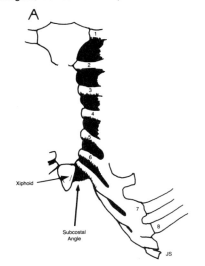

Figure 16-2. A, *The subcostal angle. B, The physician is checking the inspiratory movement of the subcostal angles. (I would move my hands higher up, see text.) Illustration from the* Anatéomia *of Guido da Vingevano (1345), from the Museum Conde, Chantilly. Photograph courtesy of Art Resource, New York.*

Interpretation. The subcostal angle during normal inspiration is determined by the balance between two forces: the lateral pull on the costal margins due to the intercostals, and the contrary action of the diaphragm normally exerted only at end-expiration when the diaphragm is flat. If the diaphragm is sufficiently flattened in early inspiration, as in emphysema, its fibers pull horizontally (coronally) rather than vertically (like a longitudinal piston), and might overcome the action of the intercostals, causing the costal margin to move *medially* during inspiration, and the angle to become more acute (Hoover's sign).

This sign has also been called "Hoover's groove" because one can sometimes see a groove as the flattened diaphragm pulls inward. In rachitic children, this becomes a constant groove called "Harrison's groove."

The most common cause of Hoover's sign is severe obstructive lung disease. " . . . When pulmonary emphysema is responsible for severe air hunger and dyspnea, the entire phrenic leaf on both sides is sufficiently flattened so that both costal margins in their entire extent are drawn toward the median line during inspiration" (Hoover, 1920a).

Patients with pure, severe restrictive pulmonary disease (who do not have flattened diaphragms) do *not* have Hoover's sign. Although they may have very little thoracic expansion, their subcostal angles will move in the correct way, in so far as they move at all.

Hoover's sign, if due to emphysema, may be lost in marginal cases if the patient leans forward (or sometimes if he simply is recumbent), because the increased abdominal pressure causes the diaphragmatic fibers to take a more convex orientation (Sharp, 1986).

Globular enlargement of the heart, as in dilated cardiomyopathy or rheumatic mitral valve disease with supervening right heart failure, could also flatten the diaphragm sufficiently to cause Hoover's sign (Hoover, 1920b). Or paralysis of the intercostal muscles can cause the balance of forces to shift in favor of the diaphragm (Hoover, 1920a).

However, this sign seems to be more valuable in pulmonary diseases than in heart disease or neurologic disease, because there are other ways (palpation and percussion) to estimate heart size and muscle strength, but fewer bedside techniques to show what the diaphragm is doing.

Variations on Hoover's sign. Hoover also described a number of variations of this sign, all based on the same principle (Hoover, 1920b).

Paralysis of the diaphragm, as in muscular dystrophy, or a rare case of poliomyelitis, will lead to an exaggeration of the normal symmetrical outward movement of the costal margin. An asymmetrical outward movement of the costal margins may be caused by several etiologies.

1. The side that moves more (*laterally*) may have had an increase in its hemidiaphragmatic curvature due to something pushing up from below, or from massive atelectasis of the lung pulling up from above. Hoover found the sign especially useful in cases of subphrenic abscess, in which the abscess pushed the hemidiaphragm up into a dome of greater curvature, thus allowing the intercostals on that side to win the tug-of-war. *Beware*: one case of a subphrenic abscess was reported in which the hemidiaphragm was scarred against the chest wall, and the adhesions caused the diaphragm to exert a direct horizontal pull that moved the costal margin medially during inspiration. Another patient with a subphrenic abscess had an ipsilateral pyopneumothorax, which tended to push the hemidiaphragm down, so that the two abnormalities canceled each other out, resulting in no observable abnormality of the costal margins during inspiration.

2. Unilateral *medial* movement will occur on the side that has a greatly depressed hemidiaphragm or paralysis of the intercostal muscles. The former may occur with tension pneumothorax or pleural effusion.

3. Inspiratory narrowing of the costal angle with relatively normal movement of the more lateral costal margins may occur if the heart or pericardial sac is just enlarged enough to depress the subcardial portion of the diaphragm. Hoover believed that he could thus determine the cause of dyspnea in some patients with both emphysema and heart disease. If only the medial portion of the costal border moved medially (making the angle more acute) during inspiration, but the lateral borders continued to move laterally, he attributed the dyspnea to the cardiac disease rather than the emphysema.

4. Asymmetry in the movement of the subcostal angle, when the lower and outer portions of the margins move laterally during inspiration, could result (left moving less) from left ventricular enlargement in the absence of right ventricular enlargement (as in aortic insufficiency) or (right moving less) right ventricular enlargement alone (as in pulmonary edema from phosgene poisoning, as Hoover learned during World War I). This refinement may seem like gilding the lily to the modern reader, who must keep in mind that the cardiac lesions seen in the first quarter of the century tended to be quite severe, since they had to be diagnostically obvious, and there was no such thing as cardiac surgery.

Potential usefulness of Hoover's sign. Hoover's meticulous observations were confirmed by fluoroscopy. This later invention seemed to be more precise than inference from inspection; required less individual instruction, skill, and experience; and produced an external image judged to be more "objective" in the Cartesian sense. Thus, Hoover's signs became a redundancy during the era when many physicians had fluoroscopy in their offices. With heightened concern about radiation doses and changes in remuneration, fluoroscopy disappeared from offices, and it may be worthwhile to resurrect these inspiratory signs. They give dynamic information not available from any type of static single image.

Litten's Phenomenon and Sign

A method. Have the (skinny) patient lie on his back on an examining table, with his head towards the window or other light source so that the lateral chest walls are illuminated brightly but obliquely. As you observe the interspaces in the lower portion of the chest on one side, have the patient take a deep breath. A rippling shadow may be seen moving down the intercostal spaces with each deep inspiration. (Rarely, a reverse ripple can be seen with expiration.) This shadow may be produced by the diaphragm itself, or some diaphragmatic-pleural interaction.

Litten's phenomenon may also be seen with a single strong overhead light if the thin patient is seated with his arms back away from the lateral aspects of the thorax, or with his arms positioned above his head as for Pemberton's maneuver (see Ch. 14, p. 234).

This test is less useful nowadays because it works only for asthenic individuals with prominent rib interspaces. We should remember that in the last century, the great physical diagnosticians of central Europe practiced on clinic patients, many of whom were extremely emaciated, whereas 20th century U.S. patients tend to be better fed.

Interpretation. Litten's sign is positive when the diaphragmatic movement is seen on one side but not the other. It may result from any cause of unilateral phrenic nerve palsy, or may indicate unilateral lower lobe disease (or subdiaphragmatic disease) severe enough to interfere with diaphragmatic excursion. Since the latter causes are usually readily apparent from the remainder of the physical examination, an isolated positive Litten's sign is usually equated with hemidiaphragmatic paralysis.

The Trachea

The trachea will shift from the midline only in cases of severe pathology.

A Method

With the patient sitting erect, visualize a line running from the symphysis mentis to the midpoint of the sternal notch. Ordinarily, the trachea will be on this line, or slightly (less than 4 mm) to the (patient's) right of this line. Your findings can be verified by palpation (vide infra).

Note that tracheal deviations may be missed if they are sought with the patient lying in bed, for reasons that elude me.

Significance

With lobar or segmental atelectasis of almost any etiology, the trachea is pulled *toward* the side of the atelectasis. On the other hand, it will be pulled to the side opposite that of a pneumothorax, especially during inspiration (Light, 1983).

The location of the trachea is one way to distinguish between pleural effusion and consolidation with bronchial obstruction, on the basis of the physical examination. In massive pleural effusion, the trachea is pushed away from the side that has the auscultatory findings; in massive consolidation with bronchial obstruction, the trachea may be pulled (by atelectasis) toward the side with the auscultatory findings.

False negatives comprising uncomplicated pleural thickening, as well as *minor* degrees of effusion, atelectasis, or consolidation without bronchial obstruction, may show no tracheal shift.

The trachea may be pushed away from a goiter. This can be a useful clue to the presence of a retrosternal goiter.

A confusing picture may be found in situs inversus, in which the trachea may "normally" be slightly to the left.

Pleural thickening with parenchymal scarring may be distinguished from pleural effusion because in the former the trachea may be pulled *toward* the diseased side.

In some cases of severe unilateral pleural scarring or severe unilateral parenchymal fibrosis, the trachea appears to be midline, but shifts toward the side of the lesion during a deep inspiration.

Venous Signs of Intrathoracic Disease

Although visible venous collaterals (comparable to those seen with portal hypertension and inferior vena caval syndrome) may not always appear in superior vena caval syndrome (due to the size of the thoracic wall and the frequently acute nature of the condition), it is still possible to make the diagnosis at the bedside, by methods described in Chapter 19 (p. 366).

When pulmonary tumors obstruct venous segments, one can see large anastomotic veins, as well as distended smaller veins, unilaterally over the chest wall ipsilateral to the tumor. One such patient with unilateral venous distention over his chest "tumor" turned out to have a retrosternal goiter. Another had an unusual pattern of chest wall venous distention bilaterally at the second interspace, with the patient in the standing position. This led the physician to seek and find egophony (vide infra) over an oat cell car-

cinoma. The ability to see such veins is enhanced by the use of red goggles (see Ch. 19, p. 366).

The signs of corona radiata and venous stars have already been discussed in Chapter 7 (p. 108).

Palpation

Palpation of the Chest Wall

A mass in the chest wall might be a tumor, although it is rare to find one that was not already known to the patient. A mass might also be an abscess, from a pointing empyema, tuberculosis of a rib, actinomycosis, or nocardiosis.

When an empyema is suspected, one should palpate the temperature of the overlying skin. A warm spot is a sign of empyema. The ancients used this fact by applying a slurry of wet clay over the thorax; the heat from the empyema would visibly dry the clay first over the area of empyema.

When the history is suggestive (trauma or a severe cough), palpate the ribs for acute fracture. You might find an area of point tenderness. If you support the patient's back with one hand, and press on the sternum with another, pain can sometimes be elicited at the untouched fracture site.

Other causes of localized tenderness include Tietze's syndrome (costochondritis). The pain can be produced by pressing over the involved costal cartilage, sometimes only one of them. Local anesthesia at this point relieves the pain (but is ineffective at points where pressure does not reproduce the pain.) Similarly, once the trigger point is located, corticosteroid injection can be used as part of a therapeutic-diagnostic test (Ausubel et al., 1959).

The pain of costochondritis is different from the chest wall pain produced by pressing the intercostal muscles or that discomfort produced in the fragile bones of the psychologically exhausted elderly by pressure directly on the sternum. The latter maneuver can also provoke pain in persons with leukemia and other marrow diseases. Tenderness at the junction of the manubrium and the body of the sternum or in the sternalis muscle overlying the sternum may be due to the sternalis syndrome (Semble & Wise, 1988).

Pressure over the xiphoid reproduces the pain of xiphoidalgia, along with its radiation, which may include the shoulder, back, epigastrium, or deep in the chest.

Sharp pain associated with hypermobility of the anterior end of a costal cartilage, most often the 10th rib, has been called the rib-tip syndrome. Pain and a snapping sensation may be elicited by the "hooking maneuver." Hook your curved fingers under the ribs at the costal margin and gently pull anteriorly (Semble & Wise, 1988).

Chest wall syndromes such as those described above were found (unassociated with coronary artery disease) in 13% of patients admitted to a medical department complaining of chest pain (Bechgaard, 1981).

Crepitus (literally, "crackling") due to small bubbles of air moving through the tissues (subcutaneous emphysema) in response to pressure may result from trauma to the trachea or the chest wall. Subcutaneous emphysema feels like plastic packing material that contains air cells. You can actually feel the air bubbles move under your fingers during palpation. (See the discussion of mediastinal crunch, [Ch. 17, p. 307], although it is possible to have one of these signs without the other, depending upon the distribution of the air.) Iatrogenic trauma (e.g., tracheostomy or chest tube placement) is a common cause of this finding. A fractured rib puncturing the pleura is an important consideration in a patient with a history of community-acquired trauma.

Palpation of the Trachea

The significance of tracheal deviation is explained in the section on inspection (vide supra).

A Method

Put your second and third fingers in the suprasternal notch and slide each as far laterally as possible, to the heads of the clavicles. Is the distance from the lateral tracheal wall to the clavicular head the same on both sides? If so, the trachea is midline.

The various tracheal tug signs are discussed in Chapter 14 (p. 235).

Palpation of Costal Expansion

After assessing the inspiratory expansion of the thorax by watching the motion of your hands (p. 246), pay attention to feeling the excursion:

> Every experienced examiner must often have perceived how much more distinctly he could palpate than see a disparity in excursion in symmetrical chest regions. This disparity is not due to a more delicate perception of the hand of differences in time or distance of excursion but to the perception of the comparative force of excursion. If one directs his attention to the comparative force of excursion, evidence will be got for disturbances in pulmonary ventilation that quite escape inspection. . . . There may be considerable stenosis of the main bronchus to a lung that will yield no other physical sign than diminished force of costal excursion on the affected side. (Hoover, 1926)

Hoover also states:

> Further observations on [the excursion of the costal borders] lead to the conviction that the comparative vigor of excursion . . . is a more delicate test than the comparative extent of excursion. The delicacy of this test is shown by the fact that in normal subjects the subcostal angle widens symmetrically with inspiration, but the left costal margin moves normally with less vigor than the right. The reason for this is the fact that the subcardial diaphragm to the left of the median line is slightly less convex than to the right. The difference in convexity under normal conditions is not sufficient to cause asymmetry in extent of excursion of the two inner halves of the costal margins, but the less vigorous excursion on the left is clearly perceived if the two borders are alternately restrained. It will be perceived that the left moves with less vigor under the restraining hand than the right. . . . (Hoover, 1926)

Tactile Fremitus

This term is a redundancy in the same sense as "palpable thrill," or my favorite, "physical disease."* Nevertheless, since some students and textbooks use "fremitus" to refer to, variously, bronchophony, egophony, whispered pectoriloquy, and spoken pectoriloquy, it is necessary to state that within this text fremitus means vibrations that are perceived in a tactile, nonacoustic manner.

A Method

1. Standing behind the patient, instruct him to say, "Toy boat," each time you touch him.

○   It has been pointed out (Dock, 1973) that the custom of having the patient say "99" during the palpation of the chest was due to a misunderstanding of our medical ancestors, who during a postgraduate year in Germany observed patients being told to say "99"

---

*If a thrill is not palpable, how can it be perceived (Dock, 1973)? If a disease is not physical, how can it manifest itself (Graham, 1967)?

in German (i.e., *neun und neunzig*, the "eu" diphthong being pronounced as in our words "boy" or "toy"). The direct translation into English eliminates the diphthong and changes the spectral characteristic of the sound so that less energy is expressed below 80 Hz. (If the German speakers had wanted our "nine" sound, they could have asked the patient to say *"nein"* [no].) To best approximate the German, we should use the words "toy" or "boy." Some prefer "blue moon" or "boogie-woogie," but these have not been studied.

This error has been perpetuated in textbooks for generations. Yet even a broken clock gives the correct time twice a day. In a comparative study of "toy boat" versus "99," there were a few cases in which the relatively weak vibratory signals from "99" were just perfect to distinguish a small lesion whose presence was masked by the strong signal of the diphthong. Yet for screening a large area of a thick chest, the diphthong was usually superior to the rarely more sensitive "99"; the latter also gave some false positives (Sapira, unpublished observations).

Perhaps one could have the best of both worlds by asking the patient to say "nine boys."

2. Pressing the palmar aspect of your hands and fingertips *firmly* against the patient's chest, note the intensity of the vibrations over the apices, in the interscapular area, down the paravertebral areas, across the supradiaphragmatic areas, laterally up to the axillary areas (having the patient raise his arms at this point), and then anterior to the areas of the right middle lobe and the lingula. The last are the only two places where the vibrations may normally be asymmetric. (Wiener and Nathanson would add the interscapular areas, see p. 251).

Vibratory Threshold in the Hands

It is said that low-frequency vibrations, such as those produced during the testing of vocal fremitus or by the cardiac impulse are equivalent to a 128-Hz tuning fork and that the latter can be better felt by the "palmar base of the fingers" (the volar distal metacarpal heads) than by the tips of the fingers (DeGowin, 1965). Assuming for the moment that an increased sensitivity would be desirable for a task that involves appreciating the local loss or diminution of a sensation, let us note that it is not always possible to replicate the DeGowin experiment with a 128-Hz tuning fork, especially in men (Orient, personal communication, 1988). In the lone scientific study that compared the fingertips to the "palmar base" across a wide variety of frequencies in healthy young persons of both sexes, the fingertips were *more* sensitive (Lofvenberg & Johansson, 1984).

This is an important finding because the method offered above produces a wide spectrum of frequencies, and it is not clear which frequency is altered when tactile fremitus is "decreased." In fact, 128 Hz would not be the best frequency to test for optimal function, since that has been reported variously as 150 to 200 Hz (Goff et al., 1965) or 200 to 300 Hz (Lofvenberg & Johansson, 1984). The variability may be due to studying groups of differing age and sex composition since older persons have poorer vibratory sensation than younger persons (Goff et al., 1965; Roland & Nielsen, 1980), but the frequencies at which threshold increases with age differ between men and women (Goff et al., 1965). The latter may explain why some report better vibratory discrimination for women (Roland & Nielsen, 1980) and others for men (Goff et al., 1965).

There are situations in which the palmar base, the fingertips, or even the hypothenar surface of the hands seem to work better, and these are usually replicable between observers for any given patient. The more important issue is to avoid missing a positive physical finding. I am unaware of anyone who has ever missed a lesion because of using the method given above.

Another Method

Wiener and Nathanson (1976–77) have difficulty comparing tactile fremitus from hands applied simultaneously to both sides of the chest. If you share this difficulty, you can use one hand applied sequentially, in the same manner as one uses a stethoscope (see p. 258).

Caveats

A common mistake is failure to attend to the pressure exerted by the hand, when checking for tactile fremitus in fat people. If one does not compress the fat equally on both sides, one can get very peculiar results. This is most likely to happen when checking with only one hand at a time and alternating from side to side. Of course, this is not a problem with thin people, who were the major subjects of the great European physical diagnosticians of the late 19th and early 20th century, and that may explain why this caveat does not appear in the ancient tomes.

If you do not examine for tactile fremitus precisely in the manner described, you will probably do no better than the 25% agreement reported in a study of 24 British physicians (Spitieri et al., 1988).

Wiener and Nathanson (1976–77) repeat the caveat of Norris and Landis (1938) that fremitus is normally increased in the right interscapular area; that is, it is comparatively decreased in the left interscapular area. The explanation is originally from the textbook of Norris and Landis (1,000 pages on the examination of the chest alone), which was cannibalized by Leopold (1952):

> Fremitus is normally more intense over the right upper lobe than over the left because the trachea lies in immediate contact with the apex of the right lung, whereas in the left side it is separated by a distance of 3 cm by the interposition of the aorta, internal carotid artery, esophagus, lymphatic and areolar tissue. . . . Fremitus is normally increased in intensity in the second right intercostal space because of the proximity of the bronchial bifurcation and posteriorly between the scapulae because of the proximity to large bronchi.

I have not found the asymmetries noted in the previous paragraph, but I do not use "99." I do use both hands simultaneously, ignoring all but the obvious differences between the two sides.

A Beginner's Interpretation of Tactile Fremitus

The beginner is advised to rate his findings of lateral disparity as definite or possible, and initially not to use any of the latter in composing the differential diagnosis. Depending upon the number of chest examinations performed, the prevalence of pathology, and the quality of supervision, most students will require months to years to achieve a useful (i.e., better than radiographic) expertise.

A few general rules apply:

1. First pick the abnormal side, if you can.
   a. Any side that shows generalized inspiratory restriction to inspection may be assumed to be the abnormal side.
   b. The abnormal side can also sometimes be determined by the sign of tracheal deviation. (Unfortunately, there is usually no shifting if there was no restriction on inspection.)
   c. If all else fails, the abnormal side is assumed to be the one that shows a posterior or lateral palpatory *segmental* abnormality. (Anteriorly, the heart may confound the decision.)

2. a. An increase in tactile fremitus over the abnormal side means that there is a direct solid communication from the bronchus, through the lung, out to the chest wall.
   b. A decrease means that there is obstruction in the bronchial system or that the lung is displaced away from the chest wall by air, fluid, or solid material (such as fibrous scar) in the pleural space.

3. Pleural effusion can cause findings that may confuse the unwary. Sometimes pleural effusion at the base of the lung will push the lung up and compress it in a firm atelectatic band. While tactile fremitus will be decreased (compared with the normal side) at the base due to the pleural effusion, the compressed (and therefore consolidated) lung at the top of the effusion may actually cause tactile fremitus to be locally increased. This phenomenon of a thin band of signs of consolidation above an effusion is discussed later, in connection with tubular breathing (p. 259) and egophony (p. 269).

4. If you are still having difficulty with your interpretation, don't worry. Just record your findings, and proceed with the rest of the examination. A large number of nondiagnostic findings is more useful than a very small number of more highly diagnostic findings (Sapira, 1981). The interpretation of all the findings in context is discussed at the end of this chapter.

Percussion

Learning How to Percuss

There are two basic types of percussion: 1) the more common indirect (mediate) method, in which the examiner strikes his own finger, and 2) the direct (immediate) method, in which the examiner strikes the chest wall with the percussing finger(s).

The four-finger immediate method was first demonstrated to me by Dr. John De Groote of Mississippi. While it is useful for covering large thoracic areas quickly, I find myself reverting to the one-finger mediate method, with which I have more experience, for the apices, the interscapular areas, and diaphragmatic descent.

Hoover championed another technique of percussion of the direct type. Since this method was designed for percussing the heart border, it is discussed in Ch. 17 (p. 287).

A Method

Place the third finger (pleximeter) of your left hand firmly against the surface to be percussed and then rap a pair of drum strokes on its distal phalanx, using the tip of your right third finger as a mallet (the plexor). The first beat of the pair is strong; the second softer. The excursion of the plexor is up to 4 inches for the first stroke and less than 2 inches for the second stroke, but this varies widely with the percussor and the tissue that is being percussed. (This is really not a rule, but only a general description of what beginners should try.) Some percussors strike only once (see Ch. 17, p. 287).

Obviously, medical students with long fingernails are advised to clip them close, especially on the plexor hand.

Developing Your Skill

Some people use the second finger, and some the third finger as the pleximeter. Some strike over the fingertip and some over the distal interphalangeal joint. Some strike with their third finger, some with the second, some with two or three fingers, and I have even seen descriptions of percussion by persons who use a tiny hammer as a plexor. This leads to the Student's Rule of Percussion: There is not one correct way to percuss. Do whatever works best for you. To facilitate each student developing that percussion note that is best for him, I suggest finding someone who already knows how to percuss and have him teach you (and your partner) in the following manner:

1. Have the more experienced person percuss some portion of your partner's body.

2. Then, with his pleximeter finger still in place, *you* produce the note—one-handed—by striking the more experienced person's finger. You should attempt to produce the same note. Are you hitting the same spot? Just as hard?

3. Put your finger as the pleximeter on your partner's body, and let the more experienced person percuss it. At this point, your partner may wish to comment on how firmly you are pressing in comparison to the proficient person.

4. Switch fingers back and forth several times until you feel ready to do the percussion yourself (two-handed). You should continue to strive to produce the same note that you heard the more experienced person produce. However, do not be discouraged if you are unable to do this at the beginning of the first learning session. It takes some people hours or even weeks before they can reliably reproduce the percussion note on demand. But once you have it, you will never lose it.

The question of whether the percussionist accomplishes his purpose by noting changes in sound or by feeling changes in vibratory quality was once debated enthusiastically. Probably both answers are correct at times. There are some situations in which one can continue to percuss accurately through the noise now so frequently encountered in teaching hospitals. But with other patients and other tissues, one is completely dependent upon the acoustic part of percussion, and so requires a silent room. Whatever the contribution of fingertip sonar to the percussionist's ability to delineate underlying structures, it should be preserved in full since each of us needs all the help he can get. Accordingly, students who play steel-stringed guitars or who for other reasons have fingertip calluses on their left hand are advised to percuss with their hands reversed. Thus, the noncalloused, sensitive right fingertip is the pleximeter, struck by the left hand's plexor.

A Musical Interlude and Pedagogic Instruction

Dr. Leopold Auenbrugger was the inventor of percussion. Supposedly, he got the idea by observing a wine merchant percussing out a half-full barrel. Later, he began to practice this technique on his patients. Although there are no photographic records, history tells us that he percussed immediately with one hand, using all four fingertips. The fingers didn't strike the chest directly, but through a silk cloth or a piece of clothing stretched tightly against it. (It was a modest age.) Although we find that startling today, it was probably an easier task to percuss through clothing on a malnourished clinic patient than to percuss the nude body surface of a contemporary patient, which may contain several extra centimeters of adipose tissue.

Auenbrugger meticulously checked his percussion results at autopsy and finally published his work in Latin, the language of scholars, in 1761. The medical community reacted to his "*novum inventum*" with the same initial indifference that has greeted most of the other major advances in our profession.

Auenbrugger, a wise man, left his position in a teaching hospital and went into private practice that afforded him the opportunity to indulge in the Viennese court life. The two great musicians of the court were Mozart and Salieri. Of the two, it was Salieri who was considered the greater musician by his contemporaries, Mozart dying a pauper. And it was with Salieri that Auenbrugger wrote the opera "The Chimney Sweep." Allusion to this opera has been used to strengthen the myth that percussion could only have been invented by a musician. Unfortunately for the myth, Auenbrugger wrote only the words.

The final musical aspect of percussion derives from the story about the young stranger in New York who approached an old man on the street asking, "How do you get to the Metropolitan Opera House"?

"Practice," said the old man. "Practice."

One must actually practice percussion in one's spare moments so as to obtain that minimal number of mindless physical repetitions requisite to a graceful and facile production, on demand, of the percussion note one wishes. You should practice before and after meals, before and after lectures, and during transportation. You can practice on furniture, or on your own body.

The best furniture for a novice to practice upon is a tabletop with a free-hanging edge, or a table with an armrest supported in only one position, like the one-armed chairs in lecture halls. Obviously, the free-hanging edge will give a more resonant percussion note than the surface right above a supporting piece of wood. When you have mastered the percussion of such surfaces, whose relatively dull portions can be visually inspected from below, you are ready to advance to percussing plasterboard walls, knowing that the vertical studs are usually placed 18 inches apart (see Ch. 17, p. 286).

It is also useful to practice upon one's own body. Percussion over the shin produces a flat sound; percussion centered over the liver or the heart produces a dull sound (or flat, see Ch. 17, pp. 323–324); percussion over the lung produces a resonant sound; and percussion over a stomach recently distended with a carbonated beverage will produce a hyperresonant sound. Another way to produce a hyperresonant sound is to percuss one's own distended cheeks. You can alter the musical tone of the percussion note by opening and closing the mouth. When you can play a musical scale by percussing on your cheek, you are ready for the chest.

Percussing the Chest

A first principle of chest percussion is that posteriorly nature has graciously provided us with a normal control hemithorax contralateral to the hemithorax with the lesion. Of course, this is not true anteriorly with the right middle lobe, so one must specifically examine the anterior surface of the patient's chest on the right, as described below.

Positioning the Patient

Never percuss the chest with the patient lying in the lateral recumbent position. For that matter, you should likewise never inspect, palpate, or auscult with the patient positioned as in Figure 16-3.

This precept is based upon the fact that the dependent side may have false-positive signs produced by the acoustical damping and restricting properties of the bed or examining table that is touching the hemithorax.

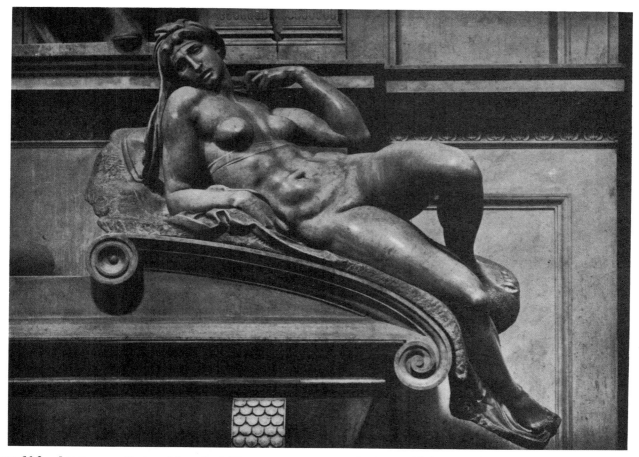

Figure 16-3.   *Improper positioning of the patient. (Do not attempt to percuss the thorax with the patient lying on her side like this.) "Dawn" on Lorenzo de Medici's tomb, by Michelangelo.*

In difficult circumstances, one could conceivably examine the chest by rolling the patient from side to side, examining each hemithorax when it is superior. This would require a great deal of prior experience on the examiner's part because he would have to "remember" what the other side sounded like, if he were to use the information provided by nature's control (the contralateral thorax).

If the patient is unable to sit up either because of stupor, muscular weakness or other inability to comply with the request, get someone else to hold him in a sitting position. This can be done by two persons standing by the sides of the bed, supporting the patient at the axillae, or sometimes by only one person standing at the foot of the bed holding the patient's extended arms. The latter is especially useful in otherwise cooperative patients who are simply weak. Please note that this is exactly what we do when we need to have a portable chest film taken. We do not accept the patient's inability to sit or stand alone as an excuse for a poor chest film, so why should we accept it as an excuse for a poor physical examination?

A note for the senior medical student.   When looking for internships, make rounds and observe the faculty at prospective hospitals. Do they examine only the anterior chest of a bed-bound patient, or do they examine the patient properly, with the house staff holding the patient up? This tells you what kind of data acquisition techniques you would learn in their programs.

A Method

1.   With the patient sitting, begin by comparing the right and left sides posteriorly, working your way down the interscapular paraspinal areas. Do not percuss over the vertebral column (see Ch. 24, p. 422 for direct percussion of the vertebrae).

When you get inferior to the scapulae, percuss the bases very carefully, alternating right and left, equidistant from the midline.

2.   Next, instruct the patient to raise his arms above his head, and percuss in the midaxillary line from the diaphragm up toward the axilla on one side, not switching sides until the percussion note changes. That is, do not switch from the right to the left lateral thorax with each pair of percussion notes, but mentally "collect" all the percussion notes of similar tone on the one side before going up the midaxillary line of the other side.

3.   Finally, percuss the axillae on both sides. These are the second most commonly missed portions of the lungs.

4.   Next, move anteriorly and percuss over the right middle lobe, the area in which findings are most commonly missed due to failure to examine it. Since the percussion note over its contralateral control is altered by the heart, you may use the anterior segments of the right upper lobe for comparison.

5.   Kronig's isthmi are two hyperresonant bands passing over the shoulders like tank-top straps, between the areas of dullness on the lateral neck and over the shoulder. They are easily percussed when one knows where they are. They may be examined either at the beginning of the chest percussion, or at the end, when one has again moved behind the patient in order to examine the diaphragms. The absence of Kronig's isthmus on one side is strong evidence of consolidation or pleural disease in the apical segment of that lung.

There are times when it is possible to detect slight differences between the percussion notes over the two apices. Invariably, the apex on the side with the duller note (not flat, just duller than the other side) has shown old pleural capping from prior tuberculosis on the roentgenogram. Acoustically, this makes no sense and is one reason to believe there may be a tactile sensation that contributes to the perceived percussion note, although one seems to be "hearing" a difference.

Although the above method moves from above to below posteriorly, you might be just as well advised to learn to percuss from below to above—if you have not already developed a method—for reasons to be given in the next paragraph. However, whichever starting point you use, the important issue is to compare one side with the other.

A Cautionary Note (Mea Culpa)

The great physical diagnosticians of yesteryear would be dismayed by the instruction (p. 253) to begin percussion at the top and work your way down. They taught, even in the United States, that one should begin inferiorly and proceed superiorly (Byfield, 1921; Strouse, 1919). Their reasoning was as follows: First, it was felt to be easier to detect a border between dullness and resonance if one started from the area of dullness. (This principle was even extended to the percussion of the heart borders by some examiners.) Second, and more relevant to the present situation, one might miss a resonant zone caudad to the dullness (see Fig. 16-4) if one stopped as soon as the dullness was reached. If you are not sufficiently thorough to be sure that you won't make this last mistake, percuss from below to above.

Significance of Dullness to Percussion

Dullness to percussion may signify consolidation of the underlying lung parenchyma, or it may be due to pleural disease: ei-

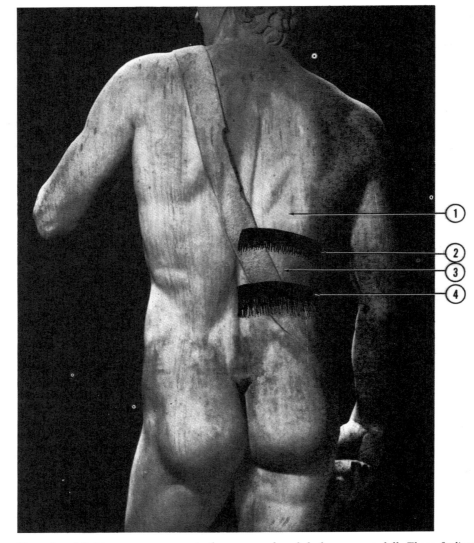

Figure 16-4. *The odd-numbered light zones are resonant; the even numbered dark zones are dull. These findings may occur in subdiaphragmatic abscess or in intrapulmonary consolidation. (Advanced: How would you make the distinction? Write your answer down before referring to the explanation in the text, p. 258.) David, by Michelangelo.*

ther fluid in the pleural space, or less commonly fibrous scarring and thickening of the pleura. To distinguish parenchymal from pleural disease requires integration with other findings on the examination, as was discussed for tracheal position. (See the advanced section below and the synthesis section, p. 280.)

Having found dullness over an area of the chest, you should immediately begin to think physiologically. The most likely cause of dullness is consolidation of the lung parenchyma, and this is most frequently due to pneumonia and/or neoplasia. In either case, the dullness will be ipsilateral to the side on which you have already found restriction on inspiration (by palpation). As a rule, you will already have noticed that the trachea is deviated toward the side of dullness, *if* the bronchus leading to the consolidated area is *closed*. However, if the bronchus is *open* or if the involved area is small in volume, the trachea may be in the midline. You may already have noticed changes in tactile fremitus over the area of dullness. If the bronchus serving the area of consolidation is open, tactile fremitus may be increased. But if the bronchus is obstructed by a tumor or by a glob of mucus, tactile fremitus could be decreased.

On the other hand, if dullness is not due to parenchymal disease, but rather to pleural fluid, you may obtain a constellation of physical findings exactly imitating those given above for consolidation with a closed bronchus, except that the trachea will be pushed away from the afflicted side. (Sometimes the distinction between consolidation with a closed bronchus and pleural effusion can also be made by noting the location of the auscultatory finding of egophony—see below).

Finally, dullness may exist over any area of pleural thickening. This would be ipsilateral to any volume sign found on inspection or palpation. The trachea might be pulled to the afflicted side, and tactile fremitus might be decreased on the afflicted side, depending on the specific disease that caused the pleural thickening and its extent.

When a patient is suspected of having a pleural effusion, an old trick is to reexamine him in a lateral decubitus position (this despite the previous advice that this position is normally not acceptable for an examination). You may wish to mark out the line of dullness with washable ink before the second examination.

Have the patient put his "bad side" up, for two reasons: 1) One never examines the inferior side if one examines a patient in the lateral decubitus position (p. 253), and 2) The point of the test is that the pleural fluid, under the influence of gravity, will fall toward the mediastinum (see Fig. 16-5). Then areas that were previously dull to percussion may, after up to ½ hour of the decubitus position, become resonant. On the other hand, dullness due to consolidation with bronchial obstruction will not shift in this way.

In modern times, this distinction is more precisely made by the lateral decubitus chest film, but at greater cost to the patient.

Very advanced. Thompson is able to distinguish three levels of dullness to percussion, which he utilizes in combination with auscultatory findings to make rather specific diagnoses (Thompson, 1979).

Red Herrings in the Percussion of the Chest

There are four situations in which percussion might lead you to diagnose a lung disease where there is actually none.

Pneumothorax

In a pneumothorax, the alveolar tissue beneath the percussed finger is replaced by air that has leaked into the pleural space. Since there are no alveoli to act as tiny sound baffles, the percussion note over the pneumothorax is even more resonant than usual. It sounds more like the percussion note over the gastric air bubble than like normal lung. However, since we are comparing right to

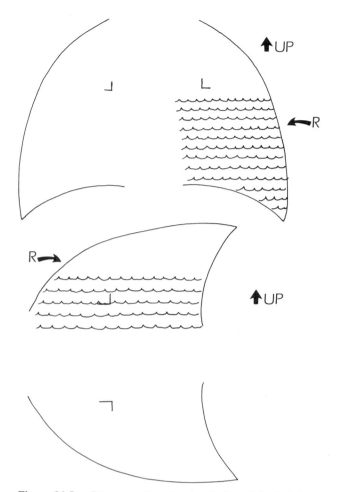

Figure 16-5. *Diagram of nonloculated pleural fluid shifting from the right lower axillary line, under the influence of gravity. Posterior view.*

left as we percuss the lung fields, the neophyte might assume the duller side to be the abnormal one. In the absence of changes to inspection, or knowledge of the coin test (see p. 272), this assumption would lead one exactly in the wrong direction. The error should be immediately recognized when the breath sounds are found to be absent or decreased on the hyperresonant side.

Recently, it has been suggested that the best place to check for the hyperresonance of pneumothorax is over the midclavicle, with the patient sitting or standing erect (Orriols, 1987).

Grocco's Triangle

Grocco's triangle (Leopold, 1952) is a paravertebral triangle of dullness (relative, not absolute) whose right angle is formed by the spine and the normal diaphragm (Fig. 16-6). It is found contralateral to a pleural effusion, but not to pleural thickening, and so may be used, if present, for the differentiation of the two processes. Note that it is a sign of relative dullness affecting the *normal* side.

Other conditions that can produce a Grocco triangle (false positives) result from conditions that produce upward pressure upon the ipsilateral hemidiaphragm (ascites, gaseous distention, tumor, pregnancy, etc.), very large ipsilateral pericardial effusions, and massive contralateral pneumonia. If the patient has had a right pneumonectomy with an elevated right diaphragm (and liver), there may be a false positive on the left. This suggests that the mechanism has nothing to do with the "truly" normal lung, but rather is an effect of acoustic muffling produced by the diseased side upon the "normal" side of the Grocco's triangle.

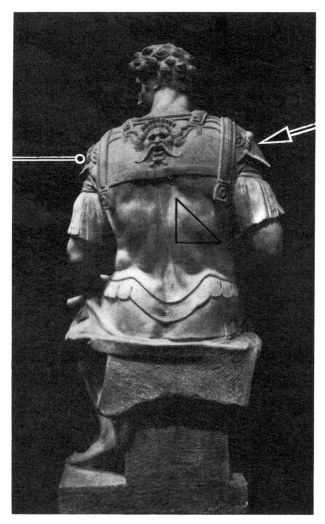

Figure 16-6. *Grocco's triangle. Guiliano de Medici, by Michelangelo. (Shaft with circle, abnormal side; shaft with arrowhead, "normal" side.)*

Any bilateral basal pulmonary process may confound the Grocco triangle, thus giving a false negative (Byfield, 1921).

Very advanced. One can sometimes find a spot of egophony (p. 269) within Grocco's triangle. Again, this happens in pleural effusion, but not in pleural thickening.

Skodaic Resonance

Skoda, the Czech physician (Sakula, 1981), described an area of hyperresonance above a pleural effusion (Fig. 16-7):

> That the lungs, partly deprived of air, should yield a tympanic sound—and a nontympanic sound when the quantity of air in them is increased—seems contrary to the laws of physics. The fact is certain, however, and is supported both by experiments on the cadaver . . . and also by this constant phenomenon, viz: when the lower portion of the lung is entirely compressed by any pleuritic effusion, and its upper portion reduced in volume, the percussion sound at the upper part of the thorax is distinctly tympanitic. (Skoda, 1839).

The mechanism for skodaic resonance is unknown.

Now, if the dullness over an area of pleural effusion were incorrectly attributed to the diaphragm, then the skodaic hyperresonance above it might be misinterpreted as normal and the reso-

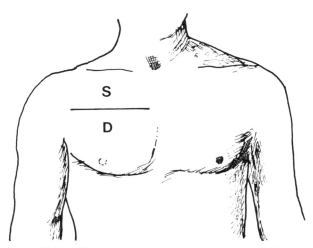

Figure 16-7. *The area of skodaic resonance (actually hyperresonance) is above the area of dullness due to pleural effusion. S = skodaic resonance; D = dullness. This is customarily and more easily determined posteriorly.*

nant, but duller, contralateral side incorrectly thought to be the site of pathology.

Ewart's Sign

Ewart's sign is dullness to percussion in the posterior lower left hemithorax, usually just under the tip of the scapula (Fig. 16-8). Since it is due to a massive pericardial effusion distending the pericardial sac backwards and compressing the lung (the fluid-filled mass will not by itself produce the findings), it is obvious that all the physical signs of consolidation may be present.

The requirements for Ewart's sign include a distensible pericardial sac that has not been previously scarred, and a massive chronic pericardial effusion that slowly stretches and distends it. Because patients now seldom go without medical intervention for sufficient time, the sign is found less frequently than in former years.

Other percussive signs for pericardial effusion are discussed in Ch. 17 (p. 323).

It is not widely appreciated that massive pericardial effusion can also produce a right-sided Ewart's sign, which should be called Conner's sign (Conner, 1926) (p. 324).

Percussing the Hemidiaphragms

Although this examination is discussed separately for pedagogic reasons, it can be performed at the same time as percussion of the chest fields.

A Beginner's Method

1. Preferably with the patient standing, percuss the posterior inferior right lung field at least a hand's width from the midline, beginning over the resonant lung and moving inferiorly to the area of dullness, remembering the sounds.

2. Percuss on the left side for comparison, looking for the same resonant tone over the lung and the same dullness beneath the diaphragm.

3. Go back to the right, with the patient breathing very quietly or, preferably, holding his breath in expiration. Mark the point at which resonance changes to dullness.

4. Have the patient hold the deepest possible inspiration, and again moving in the same line from superior to inferior, find and mark the point at which the resonance changes to dullness.

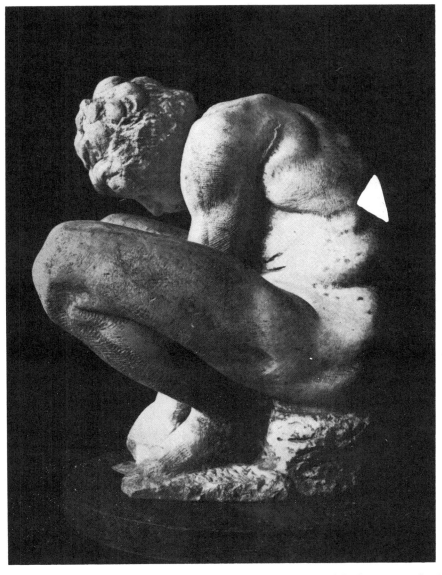

Figure 16-8. *The white triangle indicates the area in which Ewart's sign would be found. While shown in its classical (left infrascapular) location, it should be noted that Ewart's sign is of variable size, although it is always left and posterior (see text). Squatting boy, by Michelangelo.*

(Don't forget to tell the patient to exhale as soon as you are finished.)

5. Repeat for the left side. (You may have to switch back to the right, to be sure you have remembered the tones correctly.)

6. Compare the diaphragmatic descent on the two sides.

Note that this is not an exact technique. One is more concerned with the relative positions of the right and left hemidiaphragms in expiration and deep inspiration.

When you become proficient, you will shorten this technique to just one pass on each side.

Actually, the hemidiaphragms cannot be percussed in their three-dimensional surface. Nor do the body-wall insertions of the hemidiaphragms change during percussion. Rather, we determine the amounts of aerated lung near the body surface allowed by the changing shape of the hemidiaphragms, and call these the "movement" of the "diaphragm" or of the "hemidiaphragms."

Interpretation

Normally, the percussed resting positions of the two hemidiaphragms are equally high, or the right hemidiaphragm is a little higher than the left. Usually, both of them appear to move the same distance. Evidence for bilateral movement may be lost in extremely fat persons, persons who normally breathe from a position of relative inspiration (the emphysematous), or individuals with severe restrictive disease who are unable to take a deep breath. It is possible in normals for the left hemidiaphragm to move a bit more than the right, but it is still an indication to search for disease on the right.

If the resting position of the left hemidiaphragm is higher, this is definitely abnormal. There are several possible explanations: 1) The left hemidiaphragm may be paralyzed. In this case, the right hemidiaphragm will move down with inspiration, but the left will move paradoxically: up with inspiration, down with expiration. 2) There may be a left lower lobe lesion, causing an area of dullness that is indistinguishable from the left hemidiaphragm. 3) Rarely, a giant pericardial effusion will give a false-positive sign for an elevated left hemidiaphragm (Ewart's sign, see p. 256). 4) There may be a left upper quadrant abdominal mass, such as an enlarged kidney or spleen. In the last three conditions (2–4), the left hemidiaphragm, besides being higher, may seem to move only slightly, if at all, with respiration. 5) Very rarely, the patient may have situs inversus abdominalis.

If the right diaphragm is higher than the left, one might dismiss it as a normal variant. But all of the phenomena that can cause the left hemidiaphragm to be higher than the right, and that can impede the respiratory excursions, can also afflict the right side, *mutatis mutandis*. Because the right hemidiaphragm in normal persons is sometimes perceived to move less than the left, one cannot be dogmatic about the presence of pathology on the right side unless there is clear evidence of paralysis or of paradoxical motion.

Other Opinions on Diaphragmatic Percussion

Wiener and Nathanson (1976–77) state that the hemidiaphragms normally move 5 to 7 cm by percussion, and that the right hemidiaphragm is normally percussed 1 or 2 cm above the left. Most will usually agree with these figures, but percussion yields sufficient interobserver variability, especially among young examiners, that one should not diagnose an abnormality based solely upon the violation of either of these putative ranges of normality.

Macklem has pointed out that a better way to detect failure of descent of the hemidiaphragm on one side may be palpation of the abdomen. The side that fails to descend will generate noticeably less abdominal pressure on that side (Macklem, 1986).

The mediastinum will also shift away from the side of poor diaphragmatic descent, but most do not percuss the mediastinum in both full inspiration and expiration.

Reliability of Diaphragmatic Percussion

Two observers, one of whom was clearly the clinical superior of the other, determined diaphragmatic excursion by percussion in 29 patients (Williams et al., 1981). The authors were disappointed that they only agreed with each other (within 2 cm) about 60% of the time.

There are, of course, times when percussion of the diaphragm is, for one reason or another, as indeterminate as percussion of the heart size and contour may be. But there are other times when a disparity between the two sides is clearly detectable.

I agree that some persons are unable to percuss out diaphragmatic descent—my Aunt Minnie, for example.

Subphrenic Abscess

Before reading on, answer the study question in the legend to Figure 16-4.

Bailey (Clain, 1973) could find four zones of percussion in a patient with subphrenic abscess. The diaphragm lies between zone 1 and zone 3. Zone 1 is normal lung, zone 2 is compression atelectasis, zone 3 is gas in the abscess, and zone 4 is the normal dullness of the liver.

An internist would find this pattern of percussion more commonly in a right lower lobe pulmonary consolidation that afflicts a superior posterior portion of the right lower lobe (viz., zone 1 is again the normal lung, zone 2 is atelectatic or consolidated lung, zone 3 is the most inferior portion of the right lower lobe, and zone 4 is again liver dullness). Here the diaphragm is located between zone 3 and zone 4.

To distinguish the two situations, simply listen over zone 3. If you hear breath sounds, you know that you are listening to lung, that

the diaphragm is between zones 3 and 4, and that the dullness to percussion in zone 2 must be due to intrapulmonary consolidation not afflicting the most basal segments of the right lower lobe. If, on the other hand, there are no breath sounds in the resonant zone 3, you could assume that you are listening over the gas in a very large subphrenic abscess. (If the gas were in a pulmonary abscess, you might hear amphoric breathing, see p. 265).

Note that Bailey could never have made this distinction, because the apparatus used for diagnostic purposes in his book (his Fig. 1) does not include a stethoscope, nor is the word "stethoscope" to be found in the index. (Conversely, the methods outlined in the present text would be all but useless for attempting to diagnose pericardial calcification. This teaches us that our diagnostic experience is totally dependent upon the tools we use to search for disease.)

Auscultation

Use of the Stethoscope

It is assumed that you have purchased a stethoscope (see Ch. 1, p. 2), and have familiarized yourself with it for the purpose of taking blood pressures (Ch. 6, p. 87).

A Method

1. Make sure that the room is quiet. There is no substitute for this step.

2. Be sure that the patient is properly positioned.

3. Always show the patient the courtesy of warming up a cold stethoscope chest piece before placing it on his naked body. (Obviously, you would not try to listen through clothing.) A simple way to accomplish this is by rubbing the chest piece in your hands. (Carrying the stethoscope in your pocket until you are ready to use it works even better.)

4. Ask the patient to take deep breaths with his mouth open. You may need to allow him to rest during the examination to avoid hyperventilation.

5. Most of the examination of the chest is for relatively high-pitched sounds and is performed with the firmly applied diaphragm. Make certain that you are not hearing artifactual sounds due to such things as hair rubbing against the diaphragm or air rushing through an incomplete seal formed by the bell.

Sometimes, in thin patients with especially bony chests, a rubber-rimmed bell may work better. Apply the bell tightly, making a complete seal and also stretching the skin so as to form a diaphragm. If the stethoscope still does not fit perfectly, the edges may be sealed with damp cotton (Laennec, 1821).

6. Listen systematically to all parts of the lung fields, beginning at the apices, comparing the sound on one side with "nature's control," the corresponding spot on the other side of the chest. Proceed posteriorly down through the interscapular areas to the bases. Do not neglect the lateral aspects of the thorax, still comparing the two sides. Then listen to the patient anteriorly. If a woman's breast is in the way, move it gently aside, or ask the patient to hold it up for you.

Dimensions

You will be listening for: 1) the intensity of breath sounds, 2) the type of breath sounds, 3) the duration of the inspiratory and expiratory phases, 4) pitch and timbre, and 5) adventitious sounds.

You may find it helpful to review Chapter 4 (p. 69) for help in recording your observations.

Intensity

For the first 10 or 20 chests you examine, just describe the breath sounds as *present*; or if they are locally *absent*, so describe them. If you happen to *notice* breath sounds as *locally decreased*, you may note that also, provided that the decrease is as compared with nature's own control and that you can convince yourself of this on two different passes.

After this time, you may begin to *search* for locally decreased breath sounds, always being careful not to overread slight differences.

Some people have *diffusely decreased breath sounds*, but this statement on your part would mean that you are comparing them, not from one side to the control side, but to the remembered normal distribution of your total clinical experience. Thus, this statement is beyond your competence until you have examined the chests of several dozen people. Diffusely decreased breath sounds may be due to restrictive disease, airflow obstruction, or lung distention.

Locally decreased breath sounds result from local airway obstruction, or from interposition of mass between the aerated lung and the stethoscope, such as consolidation or pneumothorax or thickening of the pleural space due to fluid or fibrosis.

Breath Sounds Audible Without a Stethoscope

Normally, breath sounds become audible without a stethoscope at a distance of 3 feet, when the maximum flow rate measured at the mouth exceeds 110 liters/minute in expiration and 160 liters/minute in inspiration. However, some patients' breathing can be heard at the same distance with flow rates as low as 20 liters/minute and 55 liters/minute, respectively. This latter phenomenon may be due to localized stenosis or diffuse narrowing of the large airways, as in chronic bronchitis, asthma, or emphysema. Emphysema may be distinguished from the others in that the inspiratory phase is relatively quiet at the airway (Forgacs, 1969, and 1978). Also see the discussion of stridor (p. 261).

Breath Sound Intensity Score

The breath sound intensity (BSI) score (Bohadana et al., 1978) was derived as a clinical measure of airflow obstruction, although it may be confounded in subjects with associated restrictive disorders. The BSI is the sum of the scores derived from auscultation in six zones (upper anterior, midaxillary, and posterior basal chest regions on both sides). Sound intensity is graded as follows: 0 = absent breath sounds; 1 = barely audible; 2 = faint but definitely audible; 3 = normal; and 4 = louder than normal. Two independent observers achieved a correlation of +0.966 in scores from examining 20 unknown patients at 5-minute intervals ($p < .05$) Although the BSI correlates closely with various indices of airflow obstruction (or their logarithms) such as specific conductance, maximal expiratory flow at 50% of vital capacity, and forced expiratory volume at 1 second (FEV1) as a percentage of vital capacity, it seems to have been consigned to an ill-deserved obscurity.

Regional breath sounds in emphysema correlate with regional ventilation (Ploysongsang et al., 1982).

When a patient has been intubated, one must listen immediately for symmetrical aeration of both lungs to be sure that the endotracheal tube is properly positioned, and not in the esophagus or the right mainstem bronchus. However, keep in mind that air in the esophagus may mimic breath sounds in 62% of the cases of unintentional and unrecognized esophageal intubation. It is also helpful to listen over the *epigastrium* to hear the swish of air that occurs in 90% of cases of such accidental esophageal intubation (Adriani et al., 1988).

Types of Breath Sounds

Vesicular breath sounds and tubular breath sounds are considered in this section. Amphoric breath sounds are really a type of adventitious sound, and therefore are considered later (see p. 265).

Vesicular Breath Sounds

Vesicular breath sounds (called "alveolar" by some) are the normal sounds heard over the periphery of the lung fields, both anteriorly and posteriorly. You should listen to your own vesicular breath sounds right now.

Vesicular breath sounds are most important when they are not present. Pathologic processes may cause the normal (i.e., vesicular) breath sounds to be replaced by tubular breath sounds, or they may cause the intensity of the breath sounds to decrease or disappear. The specifics of these changes are discussed later. But for now, just remember that there are *no* pathologic processes that cause vesicular breath sounds to appear where they are normally not present. You need simply attend to their normal presence or their pathologic absence or diminution.

I do not use any of the fine gradations of vesicular breath sounds [such as bronchovesicular sounds] that you may see in some books, especially old ones. That does not mean that they might not be useful; it just means I have never mastered the technique to that degree.

Tubular Breath Sounds

Tubular breath sounds are also called tracheal breath sounds because you can practice hearing them in a normal person by ausculting over the trachea. Some texts call them bronchial breath sounds.

A self-study. When you were listening to the vesicular breath sounds, did you notice that the inspiratory phase is relatively long and pronounced while the expiratory phase is shorter and almost inaudible? Compare this with the tubular breath sounds over your own trachea, in which both phases of respiration are audible. Repeat the comparison until the difference is very clear in your mind. Have your study partner randomly move the stethoscope head between his trachea and his peripheral chest fields while you listen with closed eyes. Can you reliably hear the difference?

Significance. Tubular breath sounds at the periphery of the lung tell you that there is a solid connection between the lung tissue under your stethoscope all the way to the trachea, a bronchus, or a very large bronchiole. Stated another way, the usual acoustic baffles, the air-filled alveoli, have been replaced by solid matter.

The solid material may be intrinsic consolidation such as tumor or pneumonia, or more extrinsic consolidation such as abnormal lymph nodes. Compressed lung may also conduct sound relatively well. Such compression may result from extrinsic factors such as pleural fluid. There is generally a band of tubular breathing immediately above a pleural effusion (Fig. 16-9A). Very rarely, a thick fibrous scar extending from an air tube out to the periphery can cause a peripheral spot of tubular breathing.

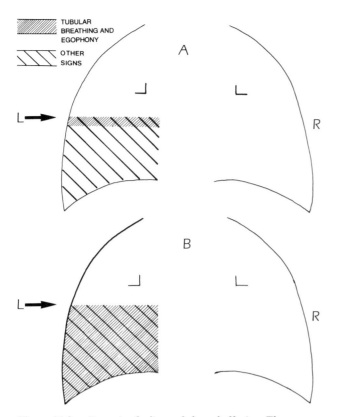

TUBULAR
BREATHING AND
EGOPHONY

OTHER
SIGNS

Figure 16-9. *Posterior findings of pleural effusion. The arrows indicate the upper limit of the pleural effusion. A, Tubular breathing and egophony (see p. 269) are heard only at the top of the effusion. If not, this could exactly mimic the findings in left lower lobe pulmonary consolidation with an obstructed bronchus. The other signs include inspiratory restriction, decreased tactile fremitus, dullness to percussion, and decreased breath sounds. B, A less common pattern. The other signs are as above except that tubular breathing and egophony are heard over the entire effusion.*

Tubular breathing is mostly white noise originating in the airways. The normal lung acts as a 200-Hz bypass filter, so that when the white noise travels through the lung to the chest wall, the sound has been changed into what we call vesicular breath sounds (Forgacs, 1969). Consolidated lung does not act as a filter, but permits all the frequencies to pass (Forgacs, 1969).

Pleural effusions can also produce tubular breath sounds over the entire area of the effusion, not just in a thin band at the top (Fig. 16-9B). In this case, the effusion does not simply float the lung up, but compresses it from without to within, as if by a cortex or peel at the periphery. This finding appears in the 11th edition of Cabot (1934), but for some reason dropped out of the textbooks and is unknown to many otherwise well-seasoned clinicians. Cabot noted it especially in thin persons, children, and asthmatics.

One of the d'Espine's signs is the only form of tubular breathing intentionally sought not over the periphery of the lung, but over a bony structure (see p. 267).

Inspiratory/Expiratory Ratio

There is no doubt that in obstructive lung disease the expiratory phase of respiration can increase relative to the inspiratory phase. But the normal ratio varies with what portion of the lung one is listening to. Accordingly, before one can be taught a scientific usage of this ratio, one needs to auscult enough lungs so as to accrue a

sufficient normal experience. And by that time one does not need to be taught by anyone. That is the reason that I do not teach this specific ratio.

Pitch, Tonality, and Timbre

Definition

Pitch refers to the predominant note of a musical sound. The physical unit for expressing pitch is cycles/per second (cps) or hertz (Hz). The higher the frequency, the higher the sound.

Sounds of only one tone, such as those emitted by an oboe, are said to be monotonal. Polytonal sounds may be either musical, as in a harmonica chord (e.g., the sounds made by the several apertures of the mouth organ) or nonmusical (e.g., the breaking of glass). Most lung sounds are actually polytonal but are named for the tone that has the greatest perceived amplitude, such as a "high-pitched wheeze." When the various tones are all of approximately the same amplitude, as in a wheeze or rhonchus, the modal tone is used as a descriptor.

The pitch is not the timbre. Timbre refers to the purity of the sound. An oboe has a pure timbre; a crashing cymbal does not. Some "musical" wheezes have a pure timbre; a pleural rub usually does not.

In the musical score in Figure 11-3, the pitch is indicated by the note, the timbre by the instrument for which the note is scored.

Semiophysiology

To produce a musical sound of a certain frequency, one must vibrate a violin string, or a membrane, or a column of air at that frequency. Think of the higher pitched sounds that tend to come from trumpets and lower pitched sounds that tend to come from tubas. Some auditors do not realize that a crucial issue in producing a given tone with a brass instrument is the diameter of the mouthpiece, which helps determine the frequency with which the lip will vibrate, the latter determining the pitch of the tone. Thus, it is hard to use your lip to produce an extremely low tone on the trumpet because the relatively small mouthpiece does not permit sufficient excursion of the lip to vibrate at a lower frequency. Conversely, it is very difficult to produce high tones on the tuba because the relatively large mouthpiece provides an insufficient support for the lip to vibrate through the small, rapid excursions needed to produce a high-frequency, high-pitched tone. This is different from the situation with other instruments in which the length of the tube determines the pitch of the sound, such as some woodwinds and the pipe organ.

In almost all biologic systems, including the lungs and the heart, the pitch of a sound is related to the frequency of the vibrations at the point of origin of the sound and is specifically not related to the length of the column of air or blood. For instance, the tone of some low-pitched wheezes would require a pipe organ 4 to 8 feet long—obviously a column of air longer than could exist in the human lung (Forgacs, 1978).

Very advanced. In his classic article "Crackles and Wheezes," Forgacs (1967) suggested that the pitch of the sounds was related to the mass moved, but that the linear velocity of the air stream was more important. The degree to which this latter function is independent of diameter remains unclear to me. Just think of the wind whistling through a cracked window. (Unfortunately, the data were not directly presented, though interested persons were offered an opportunity to listen to tapes of the sounds, at the Regional Respiratory Laboratory in London.) But later, in his 1978 paper, Forgacs related the velocity of flow to the intensity of the sound, and less so to the pitch.

Adventitious Sounds

Wheezes

Wheezes are continuous adventitious lung sounds that indicate airway obstruction. Wheezes should be described in terms of four dimensions: 1) timing, 2) location and place of maximum intensity, 3) pitch, and 4) tonality.

Timing. Wheezes generated within the thorax are more commonly heard in expiration, whereas those generated from the extrathoracic airway may also be heard in inspiration (see stridor, vide infra).

Expiratory wheezes may be divided into end-expiratory wheezes and holoexpiratory wheezes. End-expiratory wheezes signify bronchiolar disease, either primary (due to structural change) or secondary (as in *air trapping*). If you exhale with maximum vigor, you may even be able to hear such end-expiratory wheezes in yourself if you generate an intrathoracic end-expiratory pressure that is sufficiently high.

In general, expiratory wheezes appear at a peak expiratory flow rate under 50% of the predicted normal; however, holoexpiratory wheezes are associated with a lower peak expiratory flow rate than those that are end-expiratory (Shim & Williams, 1982).

If you hear an expiratory wheeze that continues uninterrupted into apparent inspiration, you can say that ventilation in one part of the lung is out of synchrony with that in another part (Forgacs, 1969).

The expiratory wheezes of asthma have the following specific characteristics: If an asthmatic patient reports wheezing, there is a 95% chance that you will be able to hear it. If the patient does not report wheezing, there is still a 30% chance that you will be able to hear it. Expiratory wheezes are less ominous than biphasic (expiratory plus inspiratory) wheezes (Shim & Williams, 1982). The disappearance of wheezes does not necessarily mean that the patient is improving; it may mean that respiratory failure has progressed sufficiently to lower the linear velocity of the air stream below the minimum required for sound production.

Inspiratory wheezes may be divided into holoinspiratory wheezes and end-inspiratory wheezes. Holoinspiratory wheezing, especially of the monotonal type in conjunction with expiratory monotonal wheezing (i.e., biphasic monotonal wheezing) is a sign of rigid stenosis, usually due to a foreign body, tumor, or fixed scar (Forgacs, 1969), especially when it emanates from high up in the tracheobronchial system (see also stridor).

A repetitive end-inspiratory wheeze immediately following some end-inspiratory crackles is almost diagnostic of delayed opening of small airways in deflated territories of the lungs.

See Table 16-1 for further specific examples of wheezes.

Location. It seems obvious that the location of the wheeze will be diagnostically useful, in that diffuse airway disease will produce wheezes of the same amplitude anteriorly and posteriorly, on the right and the left. This is the situation in asthma, pulmonary emphysema, and any other condition that involves diffuse obstructive airway disease. Conversely, focal obstruction will produce noises radiating from the point of origin (e.g., a peanut aspirated into the left lower lobe bronchus will make whistles or wheezes loudest on the left, but tracheal stenosis [see p. 236] will make a wheeze that is heard better in the upper center of the chest than peripherally).

A patient was reported to have "diffuse bilateral" wheezing. There were no adventitious sounds other than the wheezes, which were truly bilateral, but three times louder at the left base than the right. As the stethoscope was moved cephalad, the lessened amplitude of the wheeze became approximately the same on both sides. What is your diagnosis? (You might want to make a diagram.)

The correct diagnosis was partial obstruction of the left lower lobe bronchus. This illustrates that wheezes that are "bilateral" in distribution can still be focal in origin, from a point of maximal intensity, and so not truly "diffuse."

Tracheal auscultation: In a study of 181 asthmatic patients, wheezes could be better heard by tracheal than by chest auscultation in 48% of the patients, of whom wheezes could be heard *only* over the trachea in 48% (Waring et al., 1985). (Also see Table 16-1.)

Pitch. According to Forgacs, no definite conclusion can be drawn about the size of the obstructed airway from the pitch of the wheeze because the velocity of the airflow across the stenosis is of overriding importance (see p. 260).

However, the high-pitched wheeze is likely to be due to a fast vibration of air through a relatively narrow orifice (in the same way that the fast vibration is easiest through the narrower orifice of the trumpet mouthpiece than the wider one of the tuba mouthpiece), and is thus likely to signify bronchiolar and smaller airway disease. Diseases of the wider bronchi will tend to give a lower pitched wheeze, and also cause less decrease in the peak expiratory flow rate.

Tonality (monotonal versus polytonal). In the rare circumstance when a monotonal wheeze is truly a single note at its origin, it can be attributed to a single airway brought to the point of closure by stenosis, or by expiratory collapse of a single bronchus.

Forgacs' expiratory polytonal wheeze is probably the sound that some people call a sustained harmonic rhonchus. This is a sign of expiratory collapse of the lobar bronchi in diffuse airway obstruction.

But note that any polytonal wheeze may be filtered by the lung so that only one of its tones reaches the chest wall, and it is heard as monotonal.

Special Types of Wheezes

Stridor. The term stridor comes from the Latin, meaning a hiss, grating, creaking, whistle, or shriek. Thus, bruxism was formerly known as dental stridor, although this term has become obsolescent. Stridor now refers exclusively to pulmonary stridor, which is more like a hiss, whistle, or shriek.

If you have not heard stridor, you can imitate it by putting your mouth, lips, and tongue in position to pronounce "ee" as in "see," and then inhaling sharply through your nose to make a loud, high-pitched sound with your larynx or soft palate.

1. *Expiratory stridor* alone suggests an obstruction in the lower airways or in a bronchus, as with aspiration of a foreign body (such as the fabled pediatric peanut). In the latter, the obstruction occurs when the airflow is maximal and lumen diameter minimal.

2. *Inspiratory stridor* strongly suggests palatal, tracheal, laryngeal, or epiglottic obstruction (see Ch. 13, p. 228), and so is a medical emergency.

If there is no one available who is capable of performing a tracheostomy rapidly, be prepared to do a cricothyroidotomy. (For this purpose, you should have a number 20 scalpel and an endotracheal tube in your black bag, or at least a large bore needle or

Table 16-1.   Classification of Wheezes (Continuous Adventitious Lung Sounds)

Type	Single	Polytonal Sync	Async	Insp	Exp	Trachea or mouth	Chest	Presumed Cause and Site[a]	Specific Diseases
		Tonality		Timing		Location: Audible at			
1a	+ + +			+ +	+	+ +	+	Laryngeal or extrathoracic tracheal obstruction; *stridor*	Croup, whooping cough, neoplasms, polyps, hemangioma, laryngeal web, tracheal stenosis, laryngomalacia, psychogenic stridor
1b	+ + +			+	+ +	+ +	+	Functional laryngeal expiratory obstruction	Emotional laryngeal wheezing, factitious asthma
2	+ + +			+	+ +	+ +	+	Intrathoracic or lobar bronchial obstruction; *fixed monophonic wheeze*	Foreign body, tuberculosis, airway stenosis, tracheomalacia or bronchomalacia, airway compression (vascular enlargement or malformation, lymphadenopathy, cysts, neoplasms, dilated esophagus)
3a		+ + +	0		+ +	+ +	+	Dynamic compression of lobar bronchi in normals; *expiratory polyphonic wheeze*	Forced expiration in normals, organophosphate poisoning
3b		+ +	+		+ +	+ +	+	Dynamic compression of lobar and segmental bronchi in bronchitics; *expiratory polyphonic wheeze*	Asthma
4		0	+ + +	+	+ +	+ +	+	Nonuniform obstruction of several large airways; *random monophonic wheezes*	Asthma
5	+	0	+ + +	+ +	+	+	+ +	Variable airway obstruction in bronchorrheal states; *random "secretory" wheezes*	Organophosphate poisoning, chronic bronchitis, bronchiectasis, cystic fibrosis
6a		0	+ + +	+ + +		+	+ +	Fixed obstruction of peripheral large airways; *sequential inspiratory wheeze*	Interstitial fibrosis
6b	+	0	+ + +	+ + +		+	+ +	Fixed obstruction of peripheral large airways; *inspiratory "squawk"*	Interstitial fibrosis, hypersensitivity pneumonitis

Source: *Waring et al. (1985).*

Sync, synchronous; asyn, asynchronous; Insp, inspiration; Exp, expiration.

+ + +, almost always; + +, to a greater degree; +, to a lesser degree; 0, almost never.

[a]Italics indicate indicate terms that Forgacs and others have applied to these sounds.

two for delivering forced oxygen flow through the cricothyroid membrane.)

3. A patient with neoplastic obstruction at the tracheal bifurcation will have inspiratory and expiratory wheezing long before he develops true stridor. He will also retain any emphysematous air-trapping sounds in end-expiration if such were present previously. Only when the obstruction is so severe as to maintain increased end-expiratory airway pressure will the air-trapping sounds be lost. At the same time, the wheezes will become the high-pitched inspiratory and expiratory stridor of severe obstruction.

Wheezes in sleep apnea (Shepard's sign). Sleep apnea syndrome and other upper airway soft-tissue obstructive syndromes may cause a low-pitched wheeze or vibratory sound (usually expiratory) heard best over the neck. In a series of patients referred for sleep apnea, the sign was found in 50% (Shepard, 1986).

Of the sleep apnea patients who had the sign, 85% had it in the supine position while breathing through their noses. However, some had it in other positions or with mouth breathing. (To determine whether the sounds are dependent upon nose breathing, occlude the nostrils forcing the patient to mouth breathe. Do not simply ask the patient to mouth breathe as some will open their mouths but continue to nose breathe.)

False positives: Shepard's sign was heard once in a patient with unilateral vocal cord paralysis due to lung cancer. It has also been heard in thin asthmatics. In such patients, it may be a learned response to obstructive disease (i.e., expiratory snoring may serve as an "auto-PEEP").

Râles (Crackles or Discontinuous Adventitious Lung Sounds)

Introduction. Râles were originally described by Hippocrates, who likened them to the sound of boiling vinegar. Note that his definition was more restrictive than the one we use now (vide infra).

Terminology. When Laennec invented the stethoscope, he redescribed râles. (Laennec admitted that he had read the Hippocratic corpus but stated that he had forgotten about râles. This is undoubtedly an example of what Freud referred to as cryptogenic* memory.) Laennec now needed to invent a language to communicate his auscultatory findings. He used the generic French term *râles* to refer to any of the abnormal, adventitious chest sounds that he could identify in the first 3 years after he invented the stethoscope. This would be equivalent to the English word "rattle," with its connotation of "death rattle." Since so many of Laennec's patients (and in fact Laennec himself) were dying from pulmonary tuberculosis, it was considered unseemly to refer to râles in the patient's presence. Laennec, therefore, translated râles into the Latin *rhonchus* (a word that can actually be traced all the way back to a Greek word that meant snoring). In the process of translating Laennec's French and Latin into English, râles began to take on a more restricted meaning, as indicated in the "late 19th century" column of Table 16-2. Notice that in this scheme the Latin synonym, *rhonchus*, also took on a different, restricted meaning. Although this was not what Laennec intended, custom has power.

Recently, British auscultors have produced some new terms that seem more physiologically accurate. Forgacs refers to all discontinuous adventitious lung sounds as crackles. These are usually caused by the popping open of air spaces. Table 16-2 should permit physicians of all ages to communicate with each other.

A note on pronunciation. The inverted "v" over the "a" in the French word means that the "a" is pronounced as in the English word "palm." Please do not call these sounds "rails." Precision is a useful trait; sloppiness metastasizes.

Self-teaching (Majno, 1975) *

1. Obtain some very strong vinegar, or glacial acetic acid. (Vinegars diluted to 2.5% or 5% will not do.)
2. Heat it in an open pot.
3. Just as it begins to boil, you will hear the sound of râles.

Alternate teaching method. Place a lock of hair close to your ear, and rub the hairs together. The fine crackling sound is like that of inspiratory râles.

Dimensions and their significance. Râles may be described as to 1) timing, 2) location, 3) pitch, 4) amplitude, and 5) repeatability.

1. The *timing* is stated to be inspiratory, expiratory, or both. Wiener and Nathanson (1976–77) suggested that inspiratory râles be further divided into early and late.

Early inspiratory râles are said to correlate best with bronchoobstructive disease, while the late inspiratory râles are associated with "alveolar" (i.e., restrictive) disease (Forgacs, 1978; Nath & Capel, 1974).

Early inspiratory râles occurring in chronic bronchitis, asthma, and emphysema, generally mean that the 1-second forced expiratory volume as a percentage of vital capacity (FEV1/VC) is less than 44% (Nath & Capel, 1974).

Midinspiratory râles are thought to indicate bronchiectasis (Murphy, 1985).

Late inspiratory râles occur in fibrosing alveolitis, asbestosis, pneumonia, congestive heart failure, ("left-side") pulmonary sarcoid, scleroderma, rheumatoid lung, and idiopathic pulmonary fibrosis.

2. The *location* of the râles tells you where the abnormality is. Although an area of consolidation with an open bronchus may have inspiratory râles at the top, at the bottom, or all over the area of consolidation, or no râles at all. The râles due to a fixed lesion like pneumonia or interstitial pulmonary fibrosis stay in one place.

If râles "migrate" to the dependent portion of the lung as the patient changes position, the diagnosis is probably congestive heart failure. Here, the râles are usually *not* due to intraalveolar fluid as was once thought, but to the stiffening of the airways (which now audibly "pop open") from interstitial fluid. The latter is subject to gravity, hence explaining the "migration" (Forgacs, 1967, 1969). Such râles of "hydrostatic" origin, as those of left heart failure, come and go with varying wedge pressure. They tend to appear when the pressure rises above 20 to 25 mm Hg.

Changes in the râles' location are important for following the patient's progress. If a sitting patient is admitted in acute conges-

*Cryptogenic memory (meaning "coming from a secret or hidden place") refers to something remembered out of consciousness. Hence one is not aware that it is a memory, although it is accessible to recall given the right stimulus.

*Majno's masterwork is recommended for what Osler described as night-table reading. Read it for a few moments of pleasure before you drop off to sleep.

Table 16-2.   Terminology of Adventitious Sounds

Laennec's French	Late 19th Century English	Usual Timing	Late 20th Century English (?)	Robertson's, Coope's & Forgacs' English
Râle humide ou cre-pitation	Wet râles, fine crackling râles	Inspir.	Interrupted, high-pitched	Crackles
Râle muqueux ou gargouillement (mucoid, gargling)	Gurgling râles ("Rhonchi?")	Inspir.	Interrupted, medium-pitched	Crackles
Râle sec sonore ou ronflement (snoring)	Low-pitched wheeze (musi-cal) "rhonchus"? (stridor?)	Expir.	Continuous, low-pitched Continuous, medium-pitched	Wheezes
Râle sibilant sec ou sifflement (hissing)	High-pitched wheeze	Either	Continuous, high-pitched	Wheezes

Sources: *Forgacs (1967) and Robertson and Coope (1957).*

tive heart failure, with râles heard all over the posterior thoracic surface, and treatment causes the râles subsequently to be present only one third of the way up from the bases, we can presume improvement.

3. The empiric rule is that the higher the *pitch*, the more peripheral the lesion producing the râles tends to be.

a. The significance of high-pitched (*fine*, as opposed to low-pitched or coarse) inspiratory râles, the most common type, depends partly upon their intrinsic characteristics, and partly upon other findings on the chest examination.

If there are no other findings, isolated fine inspiratory râles usually indicate interstitial edema or pulmonary fibrosis. Bilateral fine crackles were heard in 10% to 12% of patients with chronic obstructive pulmonary disease, 20% of those with sarcoid and other granulomatous diseases, and 60% of patients with interstitial fibrosis and asbestosis (Epler et al., 1978). (In asbestosis, the râles may even appear before the radiographic changes (Shirai et al., 1981).) I am personally unable to structure a differential diagnosis based solely upon the nature of the fine crackles, although others believe this is possible (Kraman, 1986).

b. Chronic pulmonary fibrosis sometimes produces a distinct type of lower pitched crackle called "*Velcro*" râles, from the coarse sound made by the Velcro mesh on contemporary sphygmomanometer cuffs. These are not necessarily heard in the Hamman-Rich syndrome, whose authors only mentioned "fine and coarse moist râles," but no "Velcro" râles (Hamman & Rich, 1944).

4. The amplitude of râles is often given as a courtesy to other examiners so as to indicate the care required to find the râles. Sometimes amplitude implies the putative significance of the râles (i.e., loud râles are supposedly more important than soft râles). Yet I could find no scientific data in the literature on significance as a function of amplitude.

5. Further, râles may be described in terms of their *repeatability* (i.e., is the pattern of sounds recurrent or random?). *Random* inspiratory or expiratory râles, crackles, or gurgles may be due to liquid in large airways (Nath & Capel, 1974). Recurrent crackles have a visually monotonous pattern of recurrence (as determined by oscilloscopic playback) and are usually auditorily identified by experienced examiners as râles. In fact, this repeatability has been used as evidence for the theory that the sounds come from airways popping open, since it would be unlikely for bubbles to form and reform in the same manner on successive breaths (Forgacs, 1969).

Air bubbling through fluid, though it might seem to explain the

râles of congestive heart failure, could hardly explain the râles that occur in pure lung disease. Many lung diseases (including congestive heart failure) can cause stiffening of the lung tissue, so that some of the basal alveoli close at the end of expiration (unlike in normal persons) and thus need to snap open during inspiration. In this instance, the alveoli are said to have a change in their closing volume (i.e., the lung volume at which the contrasting pressures on the alveolus will cause it to close).

Coughing. "Posttussive" râles are râles that persist after cough or voluntary hyperventilation. They are heard in parenchymal infiltrations such as tuberculosis, or in interstitial pulmonary edema, such as that due to congestive heart failure, and so on.

Râles that disappear after cough or intentional hyperventilation may be due to a temporary luminal bolus of mucus or to "stasis" (i.e., hypoventilation of the base of the lung). This may be caused by chest splinting or loss of the sighing reflex. Such râles are by themselves of no great significance. However, one might still need to explain the cause of the stasis. For example, if splinting is due to pleuritic pain, one is obligated to explain why the patient is having pain. Sometimes, the explanation is simply abdominal compression of the lower lung fields during sleep, accounting for atelectatic râles present on first awakening.

False positives. Râles are sometimes a "false positive" finding in that they have been reported in 0%, 2%, 4.2%, 4.5%, and 14.5% of normal populations (Murphy, 1986; Shirai et al., 1981), in addition to the figures in Table 16-3. Such false positives are usually *not* as numerous (per unit time) as the plethora of crackles occurring almost continuously in pathologic conditions. For instance, these false positives might have but two or three crackles per inspiration. False positives are rarely found when the subject is ausculted posteriorly during normal tidal breathing from the functional residual capacity (FRC), but are more easily found on the anterior basal chest when the subject is breathing slowly and deeply from residual volume (Table 16-3). This no doubt explains the râles heard while rehydrating patients with diabetic ketoacidosis; their hyper-

Table 16-3.   Prevalence of Râles in Demonstrably Normal Subjects

	Anterior	Posterior
Tidal breathing from FRC	0%–2%	0%
Deep breathing from residual volume	43%–50%	0%–7%

Source: *Thacker and Kraman (1982) and Workum et al., (1982).*

ventilation causes them to breathe more from their residual volume.

Observer variability. The interobserver agreement for the presence of râles was 92% in one study, in which there was also close agreement between auscultatory findings and sound recordings (Shirai et al., 1981). However, another study showed rather poor agreement (kappa value 0.41, indicating that the agreement was about 41% of the way from the level expected by chance to that of perfect agreement). The results were felt to reflect the fact that basic skills of clinical examination were being poorly taught (Spitieri et al., 1988).

Amphoric Breathing

Amphoric breathing ("jar breathing") is also named cavernous breathing because of its diagnostic significance (vide infra). Amphoric breathing resembles tracheal breathing in that the two phases (inspiratory and expiratory) are much closer to each other in amplitude and duration than is the case with normal vesicular breathing. However, amphoric breathing has a more resonant and harmonious timbre than tracheal breathing, and its dominant tones tend to be about an octave lower. Further, amphoric breathing is heard where vesicular breath sounds are expected.

A self-experiment. Obtain a round-bottom Italian wine bottle of the type that comes wrapped in straw (e.g., a 1956 Orvieto). (Of course, you will need to empty it.) Alternately, a jug or a very large glass or ceramic container with a wide mouth will do. (Remember that *amphora* is the Greek word for a wide-mouthed, round-bottom jug or vase.) A large pickle jar, a 1-quart orange juice jar, or even a large peanut butter jar may be satisfactory; a flat-bottomed, narrow-mouthed wine jug is not, because the opening is too small and will tend to produce sounds resembling tubular, not amphoric breathing. The diameter of the opening should be about half the diameter of the base; the container should be two times as tall as it is wide. Preferably, the bottom should be convex, not flat. These specifications are important for producing the proper sound.

Remove the lid, and hold the container straight up and down. Bring the proximal lip of the container up against your lower lip and breathe in and out deeply through your own mouth, angling your breath into the jar, rather like playing a flute. As you breathe, listen to the resonance produced inside the container. This is the sound of amphoric breathing.

Next, take some newspaper, old writing paper, fiberglass insulation, or cotton balls and put them in the jar. These represent normal alveoli. Like the normal alveoli, they act as sound baffles.

Repeat the experiment, breathing across the top of the filled container. Note that the amphoric quality of the sounds has disappeared. This illustrates that amphoric breathing is *never* heard in the presence of alveoli or baffles. Thus, amphoric breathing—heard in an area of the lung that is expected to produce vesicular sounds—must be truly cavernous; the sound is of air rushing into and out of a cavity.

Leopold (1952) states that amphoric or cavernous breathing is normally heard over the occiput, when the subject's mouth is closed, but sometimes a better imitation is produced by having the subject open his mouth. Leopold also states that cavernous breathing may best be imitated by the whispered word "who." Others prefer the whispered word "war."

Significance. Amphoric breathing always signifies a cavern, hole, cyst, bleb, or other air-containing space in the lung, which

is in communication with the bronchial system. While the sensitivity of the sign is unknown, it is 100% diagnostic. Fig. 16-10 shows a lesion that produced this sign.

Cavities with relatively rigid and inflexible walls produce the best amphoric breath sounds. A perfectly resilient and deformable cavity, if such a thing could exist, would produce no amphoric (or other) sounds, since there would be no way to set up vibrations.

Once a cavity appears, and produces amphoric breathing, it should be permanent. Disappearance of a previously noted area of amphoric breathing should suggest that something has now filled the cavity, such as blood, pus, or an aspergilloma.

Pleural Rubs

A pleural rub is a creaky sound, reminiscent of unoiled leather. Classically, it has inspiratory and expiratory components, as one might infer from the fact that it is caused by inflamed visceral and parietal pleural surfaces rubbing against each other.

The pleural rub is one of the rare pathognomonic findings in medicine. It always means the presence of pleural inflammation adjacent to the area of the finding. However, it does not tell you whether that inflammation is caused by an adjacent pneumonia, tuberculous pleurisy, a pulmonary infarct, a tumor, a rheumatic pleural effusion (as in systemic lupus erythematosus), or some other specific etiology.

Pliny the Elder tells us that the artist Apelles did a new line drawing every day of his life ("Nulla die sine linea": no day without its line) and would hang each up in his window, lying out of sight so that he could hear passersby give their honest opinions. One day a shoemaker criticized a drawing because the sandals were rendered badly. The next day, Apelles corrected the error of the sandals and was lying out of sight when the same shoemaker came by. This time, the shoemaker approved of the sandals, but now thought the knee, which he had not previously remarked upon, to be awkwardly drawn. This so infuriated Apelles that he leaped up from his hiding place and shouted *"Ne supra crepidam, sutor judicaret!"* ("Not above the leather should the shoemaker judge it!")

This phrase is often mistranslated as "Let the shoemaker stick to his last," even by Robert Burton. It is given here to show that *crepidam* means leather and that a leathery pleural friction rub would be described as crepi*d*ant ("creaking like leather"). But râles, which are crackling, are described as crepi*t*ant (e.g., see "Crepitus," p. 249). To avoid confusion, let's abandon "crepi*t*ant" and "crepi*d*ant" and stick with "crackling" and "creaking."

Further, I suggest retaining the "creaking leathery" sound descriptor of the pleural friction rub, rather than switching to Forgacs's system, in which he refers to it as "crackling intermittent repetitive sounds" (Forgacs, 1969). He objects to the phrase "pleural friction rub" because it involves attributing an etiology to the sound. But the creaking intermittent rub of pleuritis usually sounds quite different from the inspiratory and expiratory sounds produced by a small airway opening, which Forgacs also describes with the above phrase.

Sometimes a more difficult distinction is between the pleural friction rub, which is usually inspiratory and expiratory (but not always, see p. 266), and the polyphonic, medium- to low-pitched wheeze.* If the respiration-associated sound occurs only in expiration, or is loudest then, it is probably a polyphonic wheeze (although some wheezes may be heard in inspiration.) As a general rule, if the sound is heard only in inspiration, it is probably a rub.

---

*The term "rhonchus," a more apt onomatopoeia for this type of sound, is falling out of favor. Note that this more modern usage of "rhonchus" is not the same as Laennec's (see p. 263).

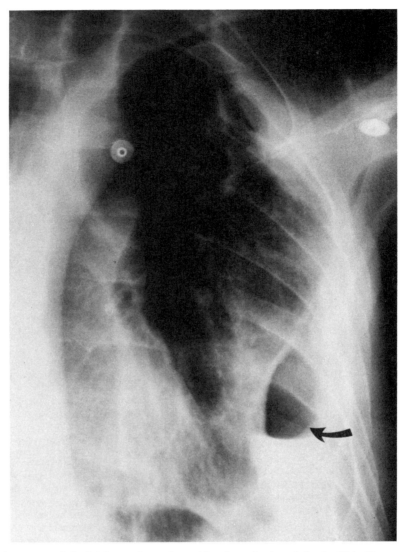

Figure 16-10.   *Apical lordotic view of the left lung of a patient with a bronchopleural fistula. This film was ordered to investigate the possibility of bilateral apical bullae, which were evidenced by amphoric breathing although they were not seen on two previous PA chest films. The hydropneumothorax (arrow) resulting from the bronchopleural fistula (which, oddly enough, was also not seen on the first two films) produced a succussion splash.*

Rubs can be heard in both phases, but may seem louder in inspiration if the movement of the opposing surfaces is faster.

Another way to distinguish between this wheeze and a rub is to note that the former tends to be transmitted more widely through the chest, whereas the latter is usually more localized. However, some wheezes originating from mucus plugs in terminal bronchioles can be quite localized; and pleural disease can, sometimes, involve large areas.

A third distinguishing characteristic is that the polyphonic wheeze may clear or change with deep breaths and/or vigorous coughing. The rub will almost always persist. Thus, evanescence, if present, diagnoses a wheeze.

Fourth, a clue that can be used by doctors with musical training is the fact that a "descending glissando" tone is diagnostic of a polyphonic wheeze. The musical tones that make up the sound chord may decrease in pitch as the expiratory sound is made, all of the tones descending as a harmonic chord. This change in sound frequency can result from a change in airflow velocity resulting from the difference in pressure generated in the bronchi during the different phases of expiration. Obviously, the phase of respiration will not affect the musical characteristics of the opposed inflamed pleural surfaces in the case of a pleural rub, so even if the rub had a musical chord, it would not glissando down the scale.

Other Adventitious Sounds

A peculiar series of "pops" can be heard during inspiration over a fractured rib. Sometimes the series of pops can also be heard in expiration. A grating or grinding sound is not always heard, despite one's expectation.

Laennec noted that one could diagnose an intestinal diaphragmatic hernia by ausculting borborygmi above the diaphragm. Nowadays that finding is more useful for the preoperative diagnosis of diaphragmatic rupture due to trauma (even though the sensitivity is only 7%) (Holm et al., 1988).

Left apical pneumothorax causes the mediastinal crunch (p. 307) (Semple & Lancaster, 1961).

d'Espine's Sign: Part One

Introduction

I was taught this d'Espine's sign at the bedside by Dr. Eugene D. Robin of California.

A Method

Compare the intensity of the breath sounds as heard over the vertebral column with the intensity of the sounds at the same level as heard to the right and left of the vertebral column. Normally, the vesicular breath sounds coming from the right and left lung are louder than the sounds heard over the vertebral body at the same level (Fig. 16-11A).

If the sounds over the vertebral body are louder, and actually tubular in quality, d'Espine's sign is positive (Fig. 16-11B).

d'Espine considered the sign to be positive if heard over the seventh cervical vertebra (C7) or more caudad. C7 is called the vertebra prominens (see Fig. 8-3) because of its relatively long and easily felt nonbifid spine. It is the first clearly palpable spine on running one's fingers down along the vertebral crests, although the spine of T1, immediately below it, is actually the most prominent one. However, d'Espine originally described his sign in children, whose anatomy is somewhat different from that of the adult. In adults, one should listen for the sign much lower, down around T4 and the region where the trachea bifurcates. The further caudad, the more likely a positive sign is to be significant. The more cephalad one listens, the more likely the sign is to appear as a false positive, probably for reasons similar to those that can produce egophony near the neck of many normal persons (vide infra). (Being "too cephalad," by the way, does not explain the false positives to be given below.)

Interpretation

○ A positive d'Espine's sign implies that the posterior mediastinum, a roentgenographically silent portion of the chest on the PA film, contains a solid lesion connecting the tracheobronchial system with the vertebral body. At the present time, the most common causes of the solid lesions are lymph nodes (lymphoma; sarcoid; metastatic malignancy; and the historical prototype, tuberculosis, much less common now) or tumor, with or without supplementary auscultatory conduction from lymph node metastases. The most common tumor is bronchogenic carcinoma.

The story of d'Espine's signs will be continued on page 270. The same diagrams (Fig. 16-11) will suffice for the pathophysiology of all. (Although shown for the trachea, the same phenomenon could occur with the bronchi or even very large bronchioles, provided that some tumor mass or other solid material provided contiguity between the tubes and the vertebral body.)

False Positives

A false-positive d'Espine's sign occurred in a patient with kyphoscoliosis. Tubular breath sounds were heard over the vertebral column. This patient also had a lung tumor (not in the posterior mediastinum), pleural effusion, and an ectatic aorta. But there were no tumor or lymph nodes in the posterior mediastinum, according to the CT scan. Part of his tracheobronchial system was applied to the aorta, which was tightly pressed against the kyphoscoliotic vertebral column.

This case was very puzzling. Although one can blame the kyphoscoliosis for producing an abnormal contiguity of the trachea, aortic arch, and vertebral body (above T5), normally d'Espine's sign is not present below T5, where the left mainstem bronchus lies against the aorta, which in turn seems to be sufficiently close to the vertebral body (Ledley et al., 1977) to produce a false positive. Perhaps the key lies in the word "sufficiently." In any event, this is an example of the interesting kind of puzzle that disrupts tedium for the thoughtful practicing physician, and involves available technology (the stethoscope).

A unilateral false-positive d'Espine's sign occurred in a patient with intrathoracic tracheal deviation. Tubular breath sounds were heard in the interscapular space on the side of the vertebral column containing the trachea. The sounds were heard less well over the vertebral column, but better there than over the contralateral side of the chest. On examination of the CT scan, it became apparent that the cause was simply tracheal malposition.

A peculiar false positive occurred in expiration only in a patient who swallowed air and maintained an air esophogram on his lateral chest film. It is assumed that the air in the esophagus was squeezed into motion during expiration, thus producing the tubular breath sound.

Special Maneuvers

A Note on Definitions

These definitions (Table 16-4) may sometimes differ from those in other texts. But they are precise and etymologically satisfying.

Bronchophony

Bronchophony literally means "bronchus sound" as it would be heard over the patient's bronchus. Of course, we do not search for bronchophony over the bronchus or trachea. It only becomes a sign (as was the case with tubular breathing, p. 259) when it is heard in an unusual place.

Both bronchophony and tubular breathing are signs of consolidation with an open bronchus, and so both may be heard over the same area of a diseased lung. However, they are different findings (i.e., the sound in bronchophony is actually produced by the patient's larynx). Bronchial breathing can be detected in a mute, whereas bronchophony cannot.

A Method for Eliciting Bronchophony: Teaching Exercise

1. Have your partner say, "Don't overuse the laboratory."*
2. Listen over the trachea, then over periphery of the lungs.

Normally, the voice sounds over the lungs are distant and muffled. In a patient with bronchophony, the voice sounds are heard as clearly as when you auscult over your partner's larynx.

Pectoriloquy

Pectoriloquy literally means "chest-speaking." That is, one ausculs the chest and hears speech (i.e., identifiable words, not just sounds [as in bronchophony]).

In order to understand words, one must recognize vowels, whose distinction depends upon being able to identify the high-pitched components known as formants. Normally aerated lung,

---

*Any sentence can be used.

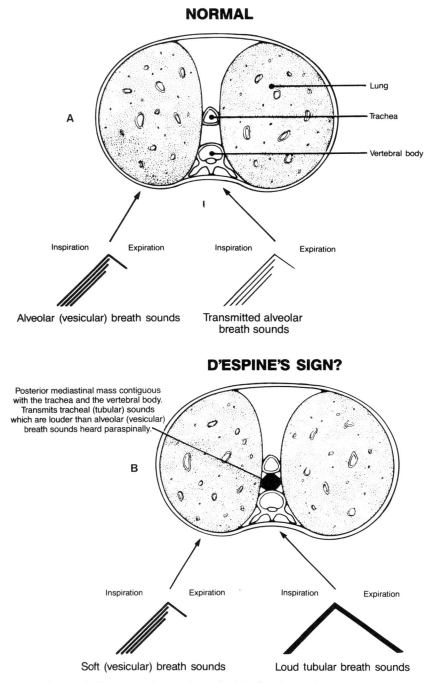

Figure 16-11. *A, Normal auscultatory findings over chest and vertebral bodies. In a quiet room, one can sometimes hear alveolar breath sounds of the juxtavertebral lung softly radiating to the vertebral body. B, d'Espine's sign? In the presence of a posterior mediastinal mass contiguous with the trachea and vertebral body, auscultation over the vertebral body reveals transmitted tracheal (tubular) breath sounds, which are louder than the vesicular breath sounds radiating from the lung on either side. The question mark indicates that there are actually two other d'Espine's signs. But the others (see text) are so overly sensitive that they generate too many false positives. Thus, perhaps the tubular breathing d'Espine's sign shown here should be the only sign of that name.*

acting as a 200-Hz bypass filter, screens out the formants. But solids such as solid lung, compressed lung, tumor, or lymph node do not. Most examiners check only for whispered pectoriloquy, not for spoken pectoriloquy.

Whispered pectoriloquy is probably the second most sensitive physical finding for consolidation, next to egophony, and in some individual cases may even be more useful than egophony.

A Method for Whispered Pectoriloquy

1. Have the patient whisper, "Sixty-six whiskeys, please," over and over (see pearl, p. 270 for an explanation for the choice of this phrase).

2. Listen over the trachea.

Table 16-4.   Definitions of Some Signs of Consolidation

Bronchophony	While ausculting remote from the bronchi and larynx, the examiner can hear the speaking patient's laryngeal ("bronchial") sounds, while not being able to distinguish the words.
Pectoriloquy	The examiner can clearly distinguish the word that the patient 1) speaks or 2) whispers.
Egophony	The spoken sound "ee" as in "bee" is heard by the auscultor as the "a" in "bay."

3. Now listen over the lung fields and see if you can find anything that sounds like what you heard over the trachea. (With experience, you can skip step 2.)

4. Call this sign positive only if you are sure about it. One way of testing yourself is to ask the patient to whisper a different number (e.g., his social security number) and see whether you can identify it.

Egophony ("E to A")

Egophony resembles pectoriloquy in that it also consists of loud resonance of the voice beneath the stethoscope. . . . The voice is higher pitched and sharper than the patient's natural voice, and has, so to speak, a silvery tone; it produces the illusion that someone is speaking in the patient's chest. It possesses, moreover, one constant characteristic from which it has seemed to me suitable to name the phenomenon; it is quavering and jerky, like the bleating of a goat and, as may be judged from the foregoing description, it is also similar in timbre to the noise made by that animal. This characteristic is subject to only slight variations, which the reader may picture to himself exactly if he calls to mind the effect produced by a chip placed between the teeth and lips of a person speaking, the sound of the voice when transmitted through a cracked reed, or the stammering nasal tone of a Punch and Judy showman. (Laennec, 1821)

Thus, egophony means "goat sound"; in this case, "ego" comes from the Greek root for "goat," not the Latin for "self." This technique competes with whispered pectoriloquy for the position of most sensitive physical finding for consolidation—if the bronchus is open.

A Method

1. Instruct the patient, "Say the word 'bee' each time I touch you with my stethoscope."

2. Auscult over the patient's chest with your stethoscope.

3. If you find a place that sounds like an "a" (as in "ate"), remove your earpieces to be sure that the patient is saying "e."

4. Then plug them back in to verify that you are hearing "a."

Teaching Devices

When listening for egophony, one is listening for a change in timbre, not for a change in pitch. Many students do not initially realize this, and so miss examples of egophony. An analogy is a trumpet note played with and without a wah-wah mute, or a guitar played with a wah-wah pedal. The pitch and amplitude remain the same, but the timbre of the sound is changed.

If you are unable to appreciate egophony in a situation in which someone else can, try the following:

1. Have the other person mark the patient's chest, indicating the area of egophony.

2. Place the diaphragm of your stethoscope over that area and have the patient hold it in place.

3. Instruct the patient, "Say the letter 'ee,' as in 'busy bee,' each time I nod" (or "at the same rate I am tapping your arm" if you are behind the patient.)

4. Place the stethoscope earpieces in your ears, but keep your hands on them.

5. Start nodding to the patient.

6. After you have heard a number of sounds, quickly pull the earpieces out of your ears on alternate vocalizations. Listen to the differences in the timbre of the sounds, not to the other similarities.

7. Now listen to two vocalizations with the earpieces in your canals and two with the earpieces removed.

8. Once you have identified the goatlike quality of the sound, take the stethoscope head back from the patient, and as he continues to say "ee" auscult over the area marked for egophony and then over a normal area, comparing the timbre of the sounds. (Over the normal area, the sound is not so different with the earpieces in or out of the ears.)

An alternate method. If you don't have a patient with egophony, try listening over the posterior neck or the top of a skull of a normal subject as he says "ee." You may have to look for this artifact in different locations (clavicle, lateral neck, etc.) in different subjects. The sound needs to traverse a path of solid tissue, without interposed alveoli.

After many years of listening for egophony, you will be able to detect deviations from the "e" that are not quite "a," but still clearly abnormal, although not so to neophytes.

Mechanism

What is the mechanism for egophony? I do not know. One hypothesis is that the "ee" sound also has high- and low-frequency harmonics,* including an "a" as in "hay." Like all harmonics, they are weaker than the parent tone. However, it happens that solid tissue preferentially absorbs some of the strong primary sound, but conducts the harmonics better, thus unmasking them. (This works only in the special case of "e" to "a." In the converse case, if the patient says "a," it will *not* sound like "e.")

One might object to this mechanism because the solid tissue of the chest wall obviously does not have the effect of converting an "e" to a goat sound. The difference is that the chest wall is not directly connected to the resonator (the vocal cords), while the neck tissue and the consolidated lung are so connected. While this explanation may be invalid, the observation certainly holds: no matter how fat the body wall, it does not convert "e" to "a," whereas if a little underlying lung is compressed by a pleural effusion, the goat sound appears.

---

*These "harmonics" may not be of pitch, but rather the Fourier waves other than frequency. The postulated "absorption" of the primary wave forms by solid tissue may be a sympathetic resonance, explaining why fluid never produces egophony until it *compresses* lung tissue.

Occurrence (with a Note on Epistemology)

Texts on physical diagnosis agree that egophony may be present at the top of a pleural effusion. However, it is not commonly appreciated that in addition to this thin disk of egophony at the top of a pleural effusion (supposedly due to upward compression of lung parenchyma by the underlying fluid), thin persons and young persons with massive pleural effusion may even have egophony over the entire area, as first noted by Laennec. Presumably, this is due to circumferential lung compression (Cabot, 1934).

Texts are uncertain as to whether egophony is also present over an area of consolidation! Some vote in the affirmative, some in the negative, and some are in the cloakroom. The latter two conclusions stem from lack of awareness that the patency of the bronchus and bronchioles leading to the area of consolidation will influence the outcome of the test. If the bronchus is patent (and thus connected to the resonator), egophony will appear. If the bronchus is obstructed (and the area of consolidation is disconnected from the resonator), there will not be egophony.

This issue should already have been unanimously decided by experience and thus illustrates the importance of enlightened skepticism in the thinking of the excellent physician. You should not trust every book wholeheartedly. You should read them, of course, because it would be impossible to recreate the entire medical experience by yourself, as Hippocrates implied when he wrote: "The art is long, but life is short." However, you should remember the less-quoted phrase that Hippocrates added to that aphorism: "Experience is deceiving." To believe everything you read with no qualifications is to indulge in the Myth of Infallibility. All physicians make mistakes; the excellent physician is the one who is corrigible.

Papers on laboratory medicine begin with a section entitled "Materials and Methods," which is intended to permit any other member of the scientific brotherhood to replicate the experiments, were any so inclined. The beauty of physical diagnosis is that the tools for replicating the statements of others are not those of an arcane exotic technology, accessible only to a well-funded few, but are the contents of your little black bag. Thus, physical diagnosis should be the most scientific of the disciplines. Alas, it usually is not.

False Positives

An important "false-positive" cause of egophony is fibrosis of the lung parenchyma in the absence of pleural effusion or parenchymal consolidation. This fibrosis may appear on chest radiograph as fibrous "stranding," especially the kind radiating out from the hilum as in patients with chronic obstructive and restrictive disease. Here the egophony seems to result from the selective conduction of harmonics through the fibrous tissue. The physical findings may enable one to predict the chest radiography when the egophony is bilateral and spotty, but so extensive that parenchymal consolidation cannot be the explanation because the patient would in that case be more breathless. Furthermore, other signs of parenchymal consolidation (except, rarely, tubular breathing) do not occur over such areas of egophony.

A spot of isolated egophony (i.e., unaccompanied by other signs of parenchymal consolidation) was once found over what I thought to be an azygos vein on the chest radiography. A CT scan showed this to be a tortuous brachiocephalic (innominate) artery, which apparently was compressing some lung tissue.

A True Negative

On one occasion, it was possible to diagnose what the radiologist had called a pleural effusion as actually being pleural thickening (fibrosis)—even though the trachea was not shifted. How? There was absolutely no egophony anywhere near the area of percussive dullness and decreased breath sounds.

As it was impossible to get the "fluid" to shift, no matter what position the radiologist put the patient in, further expensive procedures were planned to obtain a sample of the "fluid." This was

due to the fact that the diagnosis of pleural thickening was not accepted at first because of the difficulty of explaining how the patient's prior upper thoracic stab wounds could have produced a lower thoracic pleural fibrosis. However, an interview revealed that a chest tube had been placed in the lower thorax in the exact area of the pleural fibrosis.

The moral of that story is not that the interview should precede the physical examination (of course, it should), but that pleural effusion and pleural fibrosis can sometimes be distinguished by the fact that the former should compress lung somewhere and so produce an area of egophony, while pleural fibrosis and thickening *may* well not compress any lung tissue, and therefore will show no egophony.

Two Additional d'Espine's Signs

The first d'Espine's sign, tubular breathing heard over the vertebral column (see p. 267), was handed down by oral tradition at the University of Pittsburgh about 1960. The pathophysiology of this finding should suggest that other acoustic phenomena, which are based on the transmission of sound through a solid, might also be manifested over the vertebral column in case of a solid lesion in the posterior mediastinum. Unfortunately, it never occurred to me, and I was surprised on getting d'Espine's original papers to learn that he had described several signs heard over the vertebral bodies (whispered bronchophony, bronchophony, and tubular breathing), of which tubular breathing was the least sensitive. His own description follows:

The best signs of bronchial adenopathy are exclusively furnished by auscultation of the voice sounds and are almost always found in the immediate vicinity of the vertebral column between the seventh cervical vertebra and the uppermost thoracic vertebrae . . . There is a change given to the voice which is called whispering* in the first stage and bronchophony in the more advanced stage.

To these signs there is added [as discussed on p. 267], when the lesion is more obvious, the bronchial murmur [bronchial or tubular breathing] which extends through both phases of respiration, the intensity varying accordingly in these cases (d'Espine, 1904).

Following the advice of Professor Lasegue, we have them say, as distinctly as possible, the number *trois cent trente-trois* (333). . . . (d'Espine, 1907).

Caveats

1. Call these other signs positive only if you are sure.

2. As was the case with the words "99" in searching for tactile fremitus (see p. 250), Lasegue's instructions should not be translated literally. The number "333" in French contains a whispering sound. So this is simply Lasegue's clever trick of getting spoken words and sibilant whispers into the same signal so as to be able to do bronchophony and whispered and spoken pectoriloquy at the same time. To get the same effect in English, have the patient say "66 whiskies, please," not "333."

For the attending. In preparing this, I originally wrote that I could not find d'Espine's sign in any book. Later, I found all the signs mentioned in my medical school textbook of pediatrics, the seventh edition of Nelson. My notes show that I read the passage on at least three different occasions, but apparently ignored it, perhaps because the author of the passage described the signs as "not discriminating," or because pediatricians seemed to be less impressive physical diagnosticians than the internists I had observed. (Or perhaps because the index of this edition of Nelson

---

*d'Espine's *chuchotement*.

contains the entry, "Birds, for the," followed by the book's inclusive pagination, apparently a Parthian shot* fired by the indexer, who was rumored to be Nelson's son-in-law dragooned into a noxious service.) Whatever the cause, there are two principles elucidated: First, scholarship must be thorough because memory is faulty; and second, one good bedside demonstration is worth three readings of a textbook.

Auscultatory Percussion

Auscultatory percussion was originally described by Laennec, and was used to outline various solid organs (Norris & Landis, 1938). The stethoscope was placed upon the part to be investigated, and the examiner listened while percussing from the periphery toward the chest piece. The sounds became distinctly louder when the boundary of the organ was reached.

The principle of auscultatory percussion was developed for the detection of heart size, liver size, spleen size, kidney size, bone fractures, ascites, and pleural effusion (Cammann & Clark, 1840), but seems to have been lost. There seems to be no recognition of the common history by authors who appear to have rediscovered the technique on their own (for instance, see Webb's 1927 utilization of the technique for pleural effusion in Appendix 16-1; the various "scratch" tests for cardiac and hepatic size (see Ch. 17, p. 309 and Ch. 20, p. 384); the "puddle sign" of ascites (Ch. 20, p. 381); and Gairdner's coin test (p. 272).

In the modern era, credit goes to Guarino for developing auscultatory percussion first as a device for detecting pulmonary parenchymal lesions (Guarino, 1974). Using polyurethane models of the thorax, he found that the technique could locate small deep

---

*The Parthian cavalry were known for suddenly wheeling and shooting arrows back at the adversary from whom they had been pretending to flee.

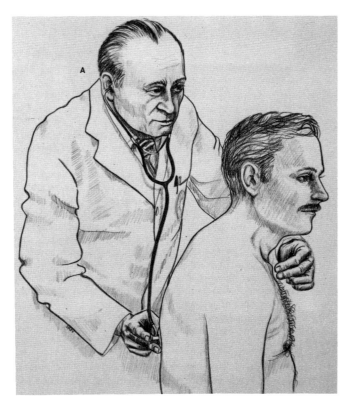

masses (Guarino, personal communication, 1988). (Recall that Guarino also developed auscultatory percussion of the skull [p. 152], bladder [p. 388], and ascites [p. 381].)

A Method

1. With the patient sitting or standing, percuss directly over the manubrium by tapping lightly with a fingertip. (Striking the manubrium avoids the interfering effects of the left ventricle, especially when the latter is enlarged [Guarino, personal communication, 1987].)

2. Auscult the tapping sound by placing the stethoscope diaphragm on the posterior thorax, and comparing the sounds on the two sides, moving from top to bottom, no more than the diameter of the diaphragm each time (Fig. 16-12A.)

3. A lesion will cause an area of dullness, like casting a shadow (Fig. 16-12B).

Interpretation

False positives. Thoracic deformities may cause false positives. Retained secretions may also cause areas of dullness that disappear quickly after coughing and may be the result of secretions in the bronchial or bronchiolar lumen, or other causes of transient atelectasis.

False negatives. The prevalence of false negatives in the original series (Guarino, 1980) was the same as for radiographic false negatives! Specific false negatives are lesions of the inferior or anterior pleura or lung, which are out of the apparent range of the sound transmissions. False negatives may also be produced by faulty technique (see "Comments" below).

Comments. This is an extremely sensitive method, claimed to be able to detect smaller lesions (e.g., 1.5 cm) than can be detected by conventional physical examination (Guarino, 1980).

Musicians who play percussion instruments must be particularly careful to have their finger strike through an excursion of the same distance and force each time. (Many percussion instrument players adjust their hand stroke to produce a constant sound intensity without being aware of it! Also see the note to the attending below.)

The manubrium is struck as a sounding board only to send a tone (anteriorly to posteriorly) to your stethoscope. It is not used to vibrate the entire thoracic skeleton. Accordingly, do not strike the chest too hard, or you may "shunt" the sound through the bony

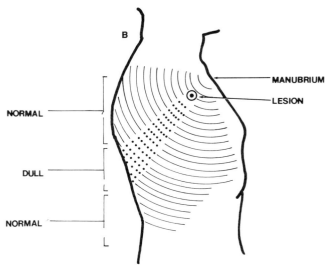

Figure 16-12. *A, Auscultatory percussion of the chest. B, Lateral view. Courtesy of Dr. J. Guarino of Idaho.*

skeleton rather than sending it through the lung parenchyma and so miss an intraparenchymal lesion.

Dr. Guarino reminds us to complete the examination by placing the diaphragm piece on opposite sides of the spinal column to detect hilar and mediastinal lesions (personal communication, 1984).

Take care not to overread the changes.

For the attending. When learning and teaching auscultatory percussion, I strongly recommend that the maneuver be subjected to the most critical scientific scrutiny. I do this by having the student auscult posteriorly, while I tap on the chest anteriorly with my eyes closed so that I cannot know which side of the chest the student is auscultating. It is very easy to unconsciously modify the intensity of the blow; in fact, it is very difficult to strike exactly the same blow every time. Accordingly, one must be especially aware of the observer effect (the unconscious tendency for the observer to produce the effect he desires.)

○ *The Coin Test*

This variant of percussive auscultation is diagnostic of pneumothorax or a giant bulla.

A Method

1. The patient holds a silver dollar (pure or alloyed) flat against the anterior hemithorax, under the clavicle, around the third interspace in the midclavicular line.

2. Auscult with your stethoscope posteriorly while striking the flat silver dollar with the edge of another silver dollar.

3. Repeat the test with the coin and stethoscope placed on the other hemithorax.

Normally, the auscultated sound is dull and tapping. Over the side of the pneumothorax, one hears a distinctly different sound that seems louder, more clicking, and more ringing, apparently due to the loss of sound muffling from the intervening lung, whose alveoli no longer act as anechoic baffles. This finding should, of course, be on the same side as the other physical findings, although the coin test works even with pneumothoraces so small as to give no difference even to percussion.

A caveat. Unfortunately, the coin test does not work with pennies, nickels, dimes, or quarters since they are too small to make enough of a "ringing" noise. A pair of Mexican 20-peso coins is a satisfactory substitute for silver dollars, but both are increasingly difficult to find.

A Self-Study

It is fairly easy to hear the normal sound of the coin test by practicing on one's partner. However, therapy for pneumothorax is instituted so quickly nowadays that most medical students do not have the opportunity to practice on a patient. The closest one can come to the sound of the coin test on the side with pneumothorax is by puffing out one's cheeks with the mouth closed and the jaws open, and then having one's partner hold the stethoscope over one cheek, while one percusses the coins over the other cheek. Compare this "pneumothorax" sound to the sound of the coin-striking when performed over the student's (presumably normal) lung.

To pick up very small pneumothoraces it is necessary to auscult over the supraclavicular fossae while percussing posteriorly high in the interscapular spaces. The smallest pneumothorax I have

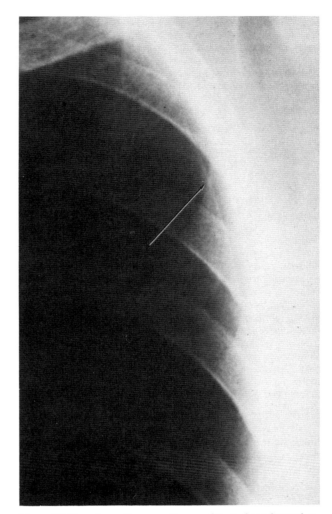

Figure 16-13. *A small pneumothorax, detected on physical examination by the coin test.*

ever detected is shown in Figure 16-13. Using this test for the first time, a naive medical student was also able to demonstrate this pneumothorax.

False positives may rarely occur over an area of subcutaneous emphysema. Air in the esophagus, as in achalasia, may cause a peculiar false-positive test only in the sternal region.

False negatives may occur. Normally, a pneumothorax results in a circumferential replacement of lung tissue by air. Thus, when we look at the pneumothorax in Figure 16-13 we are looking at a part of it, at a lateral tangent or chord through the rind that actually extends in front of and behind the central lung, which is still inflated. It is through this rind or outer corridor of air that the ringing coin sounds, not directly from front to back. Thus, if the pneumothorax is loculated by prior pleural adhesions, it might, if it is in the mid-axillary line, be easily visible on X ray, but not be detectable by the coin test, since there would be no peripheral semicircular corridor of air to carry the ringing sound. Recently, such a patient with a hydropneumothorax approximately 10 cm in height and 3 cm in transverse dimension was seen (Fig. 16-10). The hydropneumothorax was in the left axillary line only, and so was negative by the coin test.

Another false negative was found in a patient with bilateral apical pneumothoraces, who had known bilateral apical bullae. Here, the ringing sound was attributed to the bullae, there being no "normal" side for comparison. The fact that the radiologists had just as much trouble (three of them sequentially reading the same films as "bilateral bullae; no pneumothorax," "bilateral apical pneumothoraces," and "left pneumothorax") holds no consolation other than in illustration of the principle that the chest films are best interpreted by the person who has examined the patient.

False negatives may result from improper examining technique. As noted previously, one should never examine the chest for acoustic phenomena with the patient recumbent on the bed or examining table. With this test, the bedding may muffle the ringing of the coin sufficiently to make the distinction between the two sides too subtle for confident diagnosis.

Very advanced.   While auscultatory percussion works with the thumping of chests, the ringing of coins, the flicking of flanks (see Ch. 20, p. 381), and even the scratching of tissue (see Ch. 17, p. 309 and Ch. 20, p. 384), it does not work with a tuning fork. Michelson reviews the trials of the latter technique, some arguably successful (Michelson, 1926).

The Succussion Splash

Whenever there is a large body of fluid contained beneath a gas, there is a surface that can be made to splash by shaking the container. This is called the succussion splash, and it potentially can detect any cavity that contains an air-fluid level.

A Method

Originally, Hippocrates tested for the succussion splash by placing his ear up against the patient's body and shaking him. Now, we have the aesthetically superior device of the stethoscope, but we still must vigorously shake the patient's body to produce the splash. This can be difficult because one needs one hand to hold the stethoscope to the chest (or abdomen) and two more hands to shake the patient. Thus, if you cannot get someone to assist you by holding your stethoscope in place, you may have to revert to the Hippocratic method of placing your ear against the part of the patient's body that you are shaking.

Teaching Trick

Cabot used the following teaching trick to make the point that there must be a gas/liquid border to produce a succussion splash. He had the students fill a hot water bottle full to the top so that there was no air. One could shake it very vigorously and still not produce a splash. He then had the students empty the hot water bottle halfway and allow air to fill the remainder of the chamber before re-stoppering it. Shaking the bottle would now produce an excellent imitation of the succussion splash.

This exercise can also be used to illustrate how hard one must shake the bottle (and hence the patient) to produce the splash.

Significance

In the chest, a succussion splash is found in hydropneumothorax (Fig. 16-10) or rarely in hemopneumothorax. It might be thought that a lung abscess could produce a succussion splash, but it almost never does, probably because the pus is so thick that it won't splash; or perhaps because the gas/liquid phase border is too far from the ear or the stethoscope.

The succussion splash is also used to identify air-fluid levels in the abdomen as in gastric outlet obstruction (see p. 379).

The succussion splash was abandoned for a time because Hippocrates stated it to be useful in empyema, although it most decidedly is not unless the empyema is due to gas-forming bacteria. It was revived as a test of hydropneumothorax by Laennec.

Forced Expiratory Time

A Method

A simple test for airway obstruction is the clinical forced expiratory time (Lal et al., 1964):

1.   Place the bell of the stethoscope over the trachea in the suprasternal notch and set your stopwatch to zero.

2.   Instruct the patient to take in the deepest breath possible and then blow it all out, "as fast as you can."

3.   As the patient begins to exhale, start the stopwatch.

4.   As soon as you no longer hear audible expiration, turn the stopwatch off.

Interpretation

A value greater than 6 seconds suggests airway obstruction. The clinical forced expiratory time correlated extremely well with the forced expiratory time measured by spirometry, the latter being almost 1 second greater, on the average (Lal et al., 1964).

Comment

The original authors suggested three trials, and averaging the results.

Breath-holding prior to expiration is not obligatory, but rather a convenience for those examiners who use sweep secondhand wristwatches, instead of stopwatches. Such examiners must often wait for the second hand to reach a starting point.

Alternate Method

I have also seen this test performed by listening over the posterior superior thorax. If expiratory sounds were heard for more than 3 seconds after the beginning of visible expiration, the test was considered positive as a screen for obstructive pulmonary disease.

Also see the match test (p. 276).

Synthesis

Review of Principles

The Two Principles of Chest Inspection

1.   The chest normally expands with inspiration. This principle will help to identify the diseased side, in cases of unilateral disease.

2.   The negative inspiratory intrapleural pressure on each side is like two hands tugging equally on a wishbone. It keeps the trachea in the midline. Therefore, loss of the inspiratory negative intrapleural pressure on one side, as in pneumothorax, will permit the healthy side to win the tug-of-war. Similarly, an effusion will push the trachea to the healthy side. But scarring and atelectasis will pull the trachea toward the afflicted side.

The Two Principles of Chest Palpation

1.   Solid substances (like consolidated lung) transmit sound vibrations better than substances filled with air (like normal lung).

2.   If you want to feel the loudspeaker vibrate when you put your hand on the radio, don't wear insulated mittens. (Tactile fremitus is decreased by anything that acoustically insulates your hand, such as pleural effusion or thickening.)

The Two Principles of Chest Percussion

1.   Drums boom, but thighs thud. This means that the normal resonant lung will boom when it is percussed. But consolidation produces the same dullness or flatness as does percussion of the thigh.

2. There is no other principle of percussion.

The Two Principles of Chest Auscultation

1. If you plug up the loudspeaker or wear earmuffs, you won't hear the radio across the room. (Bronchial obstruction is like the first, and pleural disease like the second.)

2. Compressed lung cries like a goat. (Compressed or consolidated lung produces egophony.)

A Caveat: Observer Variation

In this chapter, the pioneering studies of observer variability done in Great Britain are cited. More recently, similar findings have been reviewed from this side of the Atlantic (Koran, 1975).

One's individual physical findings must be correct, because they are the bricks that comprise the wall of diagnosis. However, physical diagnosis can only be learned with experience. Accordingly, for the first few years, the student should use only those findings of which he is highly certain, remembering that the subjects in the papers on observer variability were all more experienced than he.

Self-Study

At this point, construct a 5 × 7 table for the following five diagnoses and seven techniques:

Diagnoses

1. Consolidation with the bronchus open
2. Consolidation with the bronchus closed
3. Pleural fluid
4. Pleural thickening
5. Pneumothorax

Techniques

1. Inspection of the tracheal position
2. Inspection of thoracic expansion
3. Palpation for fremitus
4. Percussion note
5. Auscultation of breath sounds
6. Auscultation for egophony or its equivalent (such as whispered pectoriloquy)
7. Other maneuvers

Of course, you may wish to try this exercise for other diagnoses and other diagnostic maneuvers.

See how much of the table you can fill in without turning to the answers (Table 16-5 in Appendix 16-2, p. 280). It is all right to struggle a bit. Ask yourself questions such as these: In which of these diseases would the trachea be pulled toward the side of the lesions, in which would it be pushed away, and in which would there be no change? If you get stuck, reread the pertinent parts of the text.

If you did not reason out perfectly the findings for each of the chest syndromes, review and try it again. You will probably get it nearly perfect the second time, and then you will never forget it. And you will have learned how to determine what you know and what you do not know.

A Pedagogic Note

There are many different styles of learning. Some persons learn best by reading textual material, understanding individual points, then building to higher levels of complexity. For such learners, there is expository material throughout the early portions of this chapter.

Other students learn best by learning principles, or by looking at tables. The preceding sections are for them.

Still others learn by problem solving when presented with a visual puzzle. For them, the illustrative diagrams that follow can be used as the entry point for understanding the physical examination of the chest.

However, regardless of your preferred style, at some point you should return to the beginning of the chapter and attempt to extend your understanding through the use of the other formats as well. In addition, you should be aware that not everyone will understand everything in this chapter on the first reading, but will understand it later, especially when the work is used in consultation while actually examining patients' chests in the 3rd and 4th years of medical school.

A Self-Test

As a further test of your understanding, look at the chest diagrams in Figures 16-14 through 16-19. How many of these conditions can you diagnose correctly? Write all your answers down before looking at the answers in Appendix 16-2.

In each diagram, the arrows external to the outline of the chest indicate the degree of expansion with inspiration. An "E" indicates the presence of egophony, or an equivalent such as whispered pectoriloquy. A "T" stands for tubular breathing. Other findings are as indicated in the individual legends.

Obviously, the lesions pictured are large. In reality, small lesions might have missing data, perhaps only tubular breath sounds or

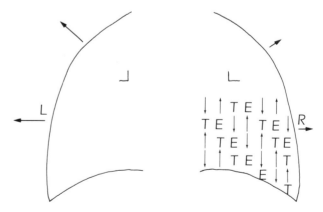

Figure 16-14. Posterior view. The patient obviously has restriction on the right side, which is presumed to be the abnormal one. The upward arrows indicate that tactile fremitus is increased (one might just as well say that tactile fremitus was decreased in all other fields; however, it is preferable to put all the findings in one area, and it would be unlikely for the right lower lobe to be the only normal portion of the lungs). The downward arrows denote a flat percussion note, T stands for tubular breathing, and E for egophony. Râles, in this condition, might not be found, or might be found anywhere in the marked area.

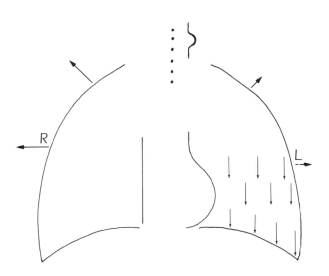
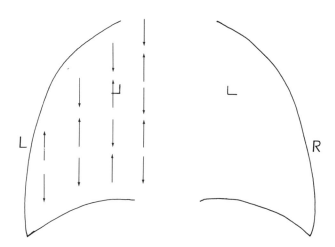

Figure 16-15. *Anterior view, to show the tracheal deviation. The downward arrows mark an area in which the tactile fremitus is decreased, the percussion note is flat, and the breath sounds are decreased or missing.*

only egophony or its equivalents. There might be only a spot that had râles.

○ *Diagnosis Based on the Location of Findings*

Consolidation

It is possible to make an educated guess about the etiology of various localized consolidations, based on the segment of the lung in which they occur (Johnson & Bauer, 1961):

I. Upper lobes
   A. Apical segment: Pancoast's syndrome or tuberculosis
   B. Anterior segment: Carcinoma or pneumonia, especially that due to aspiration
   C. Posterior segment: Pneumonia, especially aspiration, or tuberculosis

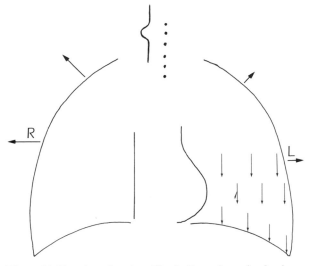

Figure 16-16. *Anterior view. The findings shown by the downward arrows are as in Figure 16-15. Egophony might also be found in the affected zone or in a thin band across its top.*

Figure 16-17. *Posterior view. The downward arrows indicate an area of decreased tactile fremitus and decreased breath sounds. The upward arrows show a zone of a more resonant percussion note.*

II. Middle lobe and lingula: Individually (unilaterally) pneumonia; Bilaterally, carcinoma, bacterial pneumonia, or disease involving the lymph nodes (especially tuberculosis)
III. Lower lobes
   A. Superior segment: Anything
   B. Basilar segments: Pneumonia or infarcts

A caveat. True consolidated lobar pneumonia is rarely encountered today, modern therapeutics having made the lobar heparization* state of pneumococcal pneumonia a rarity. The major cause of lung consolidation at present seems to be malignancy, either primary or metastatic to the lung.

For the attending. The assistant professor's snare is the right interscapular area, a rich source of false positive findings. The runner-up is the area overlying either scapula. Be very careful to compare both sides before calling a unilateral lesion under the scapula.

Pleural Effusion

For pleural effusions, laterality can be a clue. In congestive heart failure, effusions are usually bilateral or right sided. If the effusion is purely left-sided, consider pulmonary infarct, pericarditis, pancreatitis, or the "sympathetic effusion" of ascites (Weiss & Spodick, 1984; Wood & Wolferth, 1937).

Diffuse Lung Diseases

In previous sections, the value of the contralateral side (nature's own control) in the diagnosis of unilateral lesions is emphasized. However, physical examination can also be useful in the diagnosis of diffuse pulmonary abnormalities, such as chronic obstructive lung disease.

Physical Findings in Emphysema

In his classic study of patients with the "pink puffer" form of chronic obstructive lung disease, Fletcher noted: "Presumably

---

*Heparization, from the Latin *hepar* (liver), refers to the alveolar influx of red cells so massive that the lung at the autopsy table looks very much like a beefy red liver. This is to be distinguished from the therapeutic maneuver of heparinization, which uses a drug first derived from dog liver.

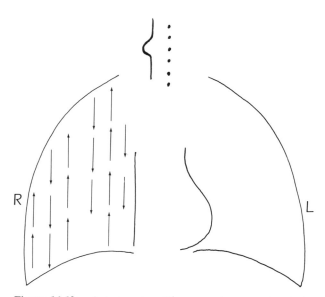

Figure 16-18. *Anterior view. The upward arrows denote increased intensity of tactile fremitus and breath sounds; the downward arrows denote a dull percussion note. There are no râles, egophony, or whispered pectoriloquy.*

so little attention has been given by clinicians to the problem of error in assessing physical signs because they seldom hunt in couples of equal seniority" (Fletcher, 1952). Fletcher had eight observers examine the same patients, and so was able to calculate the percentage disagreement for a number of the classical signs of emphysema.

Inspection. The signs were impaired expansion (19% disagreement); movement *en bloc* (23%); kyphosis (27%); barrel chest (29%); wide subcostal angle (31%); and my own favorite, use of accessory muscles (41% each). Please note that no criteria were defined for use by the examiners in this study.

Palpation. The only palpatory sign of emphysema given by Fletcher was absent apical impulse. In patients with emphysema who do not have an apical impulse in the expected place (i.e., an "absent" apical impulse), it can usually be found in the subxiphoid region. I cannot explain Fletcher's 26% disagreement rate.

Percussion. The percussive signs studied by Fletcher were impaired cardiac dullness (29% disagreement), impaired liver dullness (32% disagreement), and generalized hyperresonance (33% disagreement).

Auscultation. The auscultatory sign was impaired breath sounds, for which there was a surprising 29% disagreement.

Summary. Given the above, it is not surprising that there was a 29% disagreement rate for the global evaluation of "emphysema" (Fletcher, 1952).

The signs studied by Fletcher are not the only ones that are useful in diagnosing emphysema. On inspection, one will notice intercostal retraction, and various of Hoover's diaphragmatic signs (see p. 247). Tactile fremitus seems to be decreased, but since this is a generalized phenomenon it is difficult to quantitate. On percussion, the heart is vertical. This finding is sometimes referred to as a

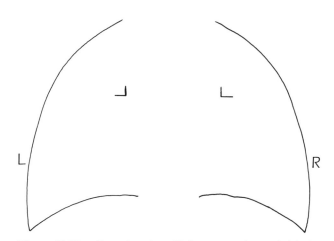

Figure 16-19. *Posterior view. Hydropneumothorax (pick the side). Pencil in your own illustration. Check your entries with the text.*

"drop heart" (shaped like a teardrop) or as microcardia, because of its resemblance to the small heart of adrenocortical insufficiency.

On auscultation, one also notes distant heart sounds and a prolonged expiratory phase of the breath sounds, which correlates with a prolonged clinical forced expiratory time (see p. 273).

A special maneuver that is rediscovered about every 10 years is the match test. The patient is asked to huff (not puff) a match out. Huffing is performed with the mouth and lips as wide open as possible, to prevent the direction of a jet of air. The normal individual can huff a match out at 6 to 8 inches on the first try. Patients with sufficient obstructive (or restrictive) disease have great difficulty with this test. Some require multiple trials to huff out the match at 6 inches, and some with severe disease are simply unable to accomplish this feat at all. For purposes of standardization, the match should be lit and allowed to burn down for a few seconds, then be held still, directly in front of the mouth.

For the attending. One can become very proficient at predicting the spirometric values from the results of the clinical examination; however, frequent practice is required to maintain this skill. More important than a display of roundsmanship is to convince young physicians that it can be done. An insistence on precision is heuristically and clinically useful because it leads to the ability to classify the majority of patients as obviously normal or obviously impaired.

Unilateral hyperlucent lung syndrome: Very advanced. There is only one type of emphysema in which one can use the contralateral side as a control for unilateral disease. That is the unilateral hyperlucent lung syndrome, or Swyer-James syndrome of unilateral emphysema.

One such patient had, to inspection, a restrictive pattern of breathing on the affected side. Palpation and percussion were unremarkable. The breath sounds were decreased on the affected side.

One could conclude from this that the shibboleth of "increased" or hyperresonant percussion note in emphysema is actually a reflection of the thin chest wall in these patients, and like the famous "increased AP diameter" (see p. 245), is an artifact of weight loss, and not a reflection of lung pathology.

Unfortunately for this hypothesis, some other patients with this syndrome are stated to have decreased tactile fremitus and an increased (hyperresonant) percussion note only on the affected side (Figueroa-Cases & Jenkins, 1968; Swyer & James, 1953).

Were my hypothesis correct about the increased percussion note coming from the thin chest wall, then there should not be unilateral increase in the Swyer-James syndrome. But in a second personal patient, the percussion note was also not changed on the affected side. Could others have described what they thought they should hear, after they saw the chest film?

A Statistical Interlude: The "Two Types" of Chronic Obstructive Lung Disease

Two forms of chronic obstructive lung disease, each supposedly antipodal to the other, have been popularized. Ectomorphs with emphysema were called "pink puffers" because they were able to maintain oxygenation, and also puffed against pursed lips to keep their intrabronchial expiratory airway pressure high. The group with chronic bronchitis were often cyanotic, and tended to be mesomorphic or endomorphic and edematous, hence the term "blue bloaters." While the pink puffers had small hearts, the blue bloaters were often suffering from right heart failure.

Although these two names call to mind the characteristic clinical appearance, emphysema is now a pathologic diagnosis, and chronic bronchitis a historical one, based on the production of at least 2 teaspoons of sputum every morning for at least 3 months out of at least 2 consecutive years.

Both types of chronic obstructive lung disease may be associated with the downward tracheal tug of inspiration, described on p. 249. This suggests to me that both involve some degree of pulmonary fibrosis.

When one actually tries to categorize each patient into one or the other of these two stereotypes, it is discovered that the largest single group is a third consisting of patients who do not clearly fit into either category.

Why then has the effort at dichotomization persisted?

Figure 16-20 shows two camels, or at least the part we are interested in, the humps. The one-humped camel is a dromedary, which inhabits North Africa and Western Asia. This Arabian camel is known to scientists as *Camelus dromedarius* (var. *gaussianus*?). The two-humped camel is an Indian or bactrian camel, known to scientists as *Camelus bactrianus* (var. *bimodalus*?). This two-humped camel has been hiding within the pages of all works concerned with the concept of disease.

To think of disease as a qualitative (therefore also quantitative)

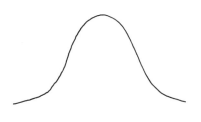

Figure 16-20.   *The one- and two-humped camels.*

difference from something called "health" or "normality," we act as though we believe that persons can be assigned to one or the other hump of the bimodal camel. One hump is "healthy" and the other hump is the disease we are studying. Just as Aristotle could not tolerate an undistributed middle (an act is either good or evil, but not both), the bimodal way of medical thought cannot easily tolerate an undistributed middle. The patient must either have the disease, or not. There are two humps and nothing in between but the camel's spine.

For example, a patient either has the malaria parasite in his body, and has malaria, or he does not have the parasite, and does not have malaria. There are no borderline, near-normal, or high-normal amounts of the parasite. The situation is dichotomous or bimodal, black and white.

Unfortunately, the bimodal camel is not as common as we might like. Obesity is clearly a disease when the subject is 100% overweight. But what about the subject who is 1%, or 10%, or 20.01% overweight? The frequency distribution of body weight is Gaussian, not bimodal. Similarly, blood pressures have a unimodal distribution, and the definition of high blood pressure must be arbitrary. (At present, the demarcation seems to be a diastolic varying, with author, between 90 and 100 mm Hg.) With a laboratory test, one might wish to use a standard probability parameter for defining the line of demarcation, such as the mean plus or minus so many standard deviations. (Such statements are often called "probabilistic statements.") But with a disease, we are forced to make a judgment about whether a disease is or is not present. For the individual patient, a probabilistic statement of affliction is not helpful.

Thus, the effort to dichotomize patients persists. Unimodal distributions with probabilistic cutoffs are intellectually unsatisfying. The bimodal camel is much more appealing. Once there is a variable that can be measured, one can obtain the correct answer, and is left only with the problem of effective therapy. Dichotomies, even when incorrect, "feel better" to the doctor.

For the attending. One might be inclined to conceive of chronic obstructive lung diseases in the elderly as a spectrum with pink puffers at one hump and blue bloaters at the other. (Of course, in this situation, we are speaking of two disease states, not a healthy and an unhealthy state.) Also, the situation is more complicated because there is more than one variable involved in the definitions (lung tissue destruction, sputum production, oxygen saturation, etc.).

It is important to recognize the problem of bimodal thinking, as it may inhibit the recognition of new clinical entities. For example, in Conn's syndrome the bimodal concept holds that either a patient has an adrenal tumor, which secretes clearly abnormal amounts of aldosterone, and which cannot be suppressed by certain standardized physiologic maneuvers, or he does not have the tumor. In the latter case, he does not have elevated levels of aldosterone, and the normal levels present can be clearly suppressed by the standard maneuvers. In this scheme, there is no middle ground. For instance, there can be no admission of adenomas without hyperaldosteronism. This may be one reason why it took so long to appreciate the relative frequency of hyperaldosteronism due to bilateral adrenal cortical hyperplasia (as opposed to an adenoma).

Clinical Examination in Perspective

Pulmonary Embolism With or Without Infarction: The Limitations of Clinical Examination

Pulmonary embolism clearly reveals the limitations of the history and physical examination as a test of hypotheses, as contrasted with their usefulness as generators of hypotheses. That is, the history and physical are quite helpful in suggesting the diagnosis of pulmonary embolism, but not very precise in confirming or excluding that diagnosis.

There are 12 signs that may occur when the pulmonary embolus is massive (Gorham, 1961):

1. Pulsation in the second or third left interspace at the sternal margin
2. P2 greater than A2
3. A pleural (or pleuropericardial?) rub near the pulmonic area
4. A systolic murmur at the pulmonic area (first described by Dr. Litten, frequently mentioned in these pages)
5. A diastolic murmur in the same place
6. An interscapular bruit
7. Unilateral decreased inspiratory expansion
8. Increased dullness to the right on percussion of the cardiac silhouette
9. Distended neck veins (with the patient sitting)
10. A gallop
11. Hepatomegaly
12. Die rote Blutwelle (the red blood wave—a red arterial wave that passes over the cyanotic face whenever a piece of the obstructing embolus becomes dislodged, permitting some additional oxygenated blood to pass into the systemic circulation)

These signs were collected by a pathologist, all of whose cases were autopsied. Thus, they are signs of a massive pulmonary embolism, severe enough to kill the patient. Even in such a severe case, the signs (especially 8 through 11) are not pathognomonic, and sign 12 has only been reported once (and seen in one other case of which I am aware.) The absence of all of these signs does not assure the absence of a pulmonary embolus.

Physical Examination and Role of Chest Radiograph

Historical perspective. In the days of liberal third-party payments for in-hospital tests, it became customary to obtain an admission chest film on all patients to "rule out pathology," even in the absence of clinical findings. The yield of this screening test was low.

Recently, Blue Cross-Blue Shield commissioned a study of the utility of routine chest radiographs, which concluded that the routine admission and preoperative chest film should be abandoned, since patients in whom chest films are likely to improve outcome are best identified by a careful history and physical examination (Tape & Mushlin, 1986)!

Another study found that the absence of some pulmonary auscultatory findings (wheezes, rhonchi, râles, diminished breath sounds) excluded pneumonia on a chest film with a greater than 95% certainty (Heckerling, 1986). Of course, one would prefer 100% certainty in a screening test, which should be highly sensitive. But inspection, palpation, percussion, and special vocal maneuvers were not even performed!

Another recent study revealed that only 3% of the radiographs taken in 75 febrile neutropenic patients with no signs or symptoms of pneumonia showed what might have been a pneumonic infiltrate (Jochelson et al., 1986).

Clearly, these studies, although they provide some estimate of the sensitivity of the clinical examination, were not designed to obtain maximum diagnostic information from the physical examination, but to exclude some statistical portion of the population from having a chest radiograph. However, the purpose of a physician is not the same as the purpose of an insurance company. The physician performs a physical examination in order to generate hypotheses about what is wrong with the patient, not to spare the cathode-ray tube.

Circumstances in which physical examination is superior to radiography. Although clinical examination is often used simply to infer findings that the chest radiograph can demonstrate in replicable form, the clinical examination is actually superior to the chest radiograph in certain circumstances. For one thing, certain findings are accessible to the stethoscope or to the observer's sight and touch, that are hidden from the X-ray beam. As Dr. Gerry Rodnan of Pennsylvania used to say, "You can't hear râles on a chest X ray."

For example, there is a roentgenologically silent portion of the chest behind the heart silhouette. To explore this area, one must order a lateral chest film. Unfortunately, it is almost impossible to get a lateral film on a bed-bound patient. However, you can always go over the patient with your stethoscope.

Another example is the circumstance of widespread pleural scarring (white-out), which leaves the chest roentgenographically silent, but not necessarily acoustically so. Sometimes the stethoscope can detect changes occurring in the residual lung when the radiograph cannot.

The clinical examination can also point to the correct diagnosis of findings that have been erroneously attributed to pleural effusion on the basis of the radiograph, for example, pleural thickening (see p. 255).

In addition, physical examination has the advantage that it is dynamic rather than static. In some patients, inspection of the subcostal angle movement can show that the correct diagnosis is an elevated diaphragm. (See p. 248.)

If the diaphragm is elevated due to paralysis, this can be detected (e.g., during inspection or percussion for diaphragmatic movement). If the diaphragm is elevated due to previous pneumonectomy (whose scar appears on physical examination but not on the radiograph), the absence of egophony can be the important clue. Alas, nothing is perfect. If the elevated diaphragm is due to atelectasis, the latter may itself produce egophony, thus suggesting the wrong diagnosis of pleural effusion. But in that case, inspection for tracheal deviation may make the distinction.

The distinction between a fat person with a high hemidiaphragm and a person with a lower lobe infiltrate is one of the most difficult in all of physical diagnosis. This is also a situation in which the chest film may not be as helpful as one might wish. Inspection, palpation, and percussion may all be equivocal. On auscultation, breath sounds are diminished over the dull area in both situations. However, the presence of tubular breathing, egophony, bronchophony, or whispered pectoriloquy, individually or combined, shows that one is dealing with a pathologic condition within the lung, not just a high hemidiaphragm (without underlying atelectasis), although the latter might be detected by Hoover's sign.

In the last decades, one hears erudite discussions of a chest film revolving around the controversy as to whether or not a finding represented a right middle lobe silhouette sign, or a right lower lobe lesion, or both. This could have been easily resolved by physical examination, had the examiner remembered to include the anterior lung fields in his percussion and auscultation.

Limitations of portable chest films. Probably the best known problem with the portable chest film is that most of the basal lung fields are not well visualized. Thus, a false sense of security can be generated by "normal portable AP." In fact, portable films are technically compromised in 6% to 37% of cases (Sherrier & McAdams, 1986). In one study using CT scans as the "gold standard," 17% of cases had an empyema that was missed by the portable film, 13% had large pleural effusions that were missed by the portable, and 15% of cases had malpositioned thoracostomy tubes that were not picked up on a portable film (Mirvis et al., 1987). In all, 70% of the CT scans added useful information not available from the portable film. Of course, things are probably worse than the above figures show because CT itself had an overall diagnostic accuracy of only 72% for empyema and 95% for lung abscess in another study from the same institution (Mirvis et al., 1985).

The physician with clinical examination skills is not totally dependent upon a picture of a shadow—a chest radiograph—for his total understanding of the patient's chest, or of the patient.

Further, the sophomore should appreciate that there is a lot more diagnostic inaccuracy in the reading of the chest film than has previously been published (Kuritzky et al., 1987). Considering the relative emphasis in contemporary medical education given to the reading of the portable chest film versus the performance of an accurate physical examination, it might even be that the physical is inherently more accurate—if only it were taught as vigorously! For more in this line, see Ch. 17, page 325).

Conclusions.   In summary, the chest roentgenogram is often useful as an independent covariable in physically assessing the patient's chest. However, it is not a perfect covariable and can therefore never substitute completely for the examination of the patient's chest by a thoughtful and skilled physician. Conversely, while there is enough overlap between the physical examination and the chest film to provide a good game of "predict the chest film," there are certain findings on the chest film that, by their nature, will always come as a surprise.

The chest film has also had an important impact of an epistemologic nature. In the 19th century, physical diagnosticians correlated their findings with autopsy. Thus, the findings defined diseases of such magnitude as to be usually fatal. With the chest film, the concept of a disease such as pneumococcal pneumonia could be extended to small nonlobar lesions, insufficient to kill but sufficient to make a roentgen shadow. In many of these latter cases, physical findings are subtle or absent.

Appendix 16-1. Auscultatory Percussion for the Detection of Pleural Effusion

For the resident.   The text of Webb's 1927 article follows:

Refinements in diagnosis are useful, and in the recognition of pleurisy with effusion, roentgen-ray facilities are not always at hand. For several years, I have found a method of auscultation with percussion of great service in detecting effusion.

The bell of the stethoscope is placed in the lower axilla, when the patient is seated, and the spinous process of the vertebrae are tapped gently from above downward with the percussion finger. If an effusion is present, a change to a note of higher and shorter pitch is detected at a spinous process which, in the case of the affected side, is above that of the normal side. In many instances, this change of tone accords with the apex of the Grocco triangle, and it does not in general coincide with the upper edge of the fluid content. The method should be practiced on normal persons, with the eyes closed, and it will be determined that the change of note is at the same spinous process on each side, about at the twelfth dorsal.

With thickened pleura, and with advanced tuberculous processes in the base of one lung, the tone related to this side may be changed throughout the range of percussion as compared with that of the opposite side, but there is no sudden change of note as there is in the presence of fluid. Should the effusion completely fill one pleura, no sudden change of note will be observed, but in such a case palpation of the trachea yields an important clue, as indeed it does in all cases of pleural effusion. The same procedure may be followed with the patient leaning a little forward, and gentle percussion made downward over the sternum. With a bed patient who is unable to sit up, the stethoscopic bell can be applied in the median axilla and gentle percussion made from the sternum toward the stethoscope; a distinct change of note will be observed before the bell is reached on the side containing the effusion, whereas on the normal side no such change will be observed.

This method of auscultatory percussion has been carried out in a large number of patients with and without pleuritic effusion, and the results have been carefully checked with aspiration and roentgen-ray examination. (Webb, 1927)

Personal experience.   This technique seems to work best with massive pleural effusion. Smaller effusions that produce only blunting of the costophrenic angle on the PA chest film do not have this sign in my experience, although they are sufficiently large to be detected by other techniques of physical examination.

Appendix 16-2.   Answers to Self-Test on Page 274

Figure	Diagnosis
16-14	Right lower lobe consolidation without bronchial obstruction
16-15	Left lower lobe consolidation with a closed bronchus (or left lower lobe with severe pleural thickening, scarring, and retraction)
16-16	Left pleural effusion
16-17	Left pneumothorax
16-18	The front view of Figure 16-17.* The trick, as in real life, is not to be fooled by the side that seems to be abnormal. Here, that is actually the normal side. The clue to solving the puzzle comes from tracheal inspection. If the trachea is shifted to the right, one sees from Table 16-5 that there are only three possibilities: left pneumothorax, left pleural effusion or thickening, and right consolidation with a closed bronchus. The second possibility is excluded by the relatively hyperresonant percussion note on the left, and the third is excluded by the relative increase in tactile fremitus and breath sound intensity on the right.
16-19	On the bottom are the physical signs of pleural effusion, and on the top of those of a pneumothorax. In addition, there should be a succussion splash.

*This frustrating piece of trickery was inserted to emphasize two points: 1) One can still reason out the diagnosis *and* the location in the absence of any focal finding (such as egophony, whispered pectoriloquy, decreased excursion, etc.) and in the absence of information about a diagnostic sign (here, the coin test); 2) Tracheal position, which I have noticed to be the first chest physical sign to be jettisoned by the jejune, is

Table 16-5. Textbook Findings in Unilateral Chest Syndromes[a]

	Consolidation with open bronchus	Consolidation (with atelectasis) with closed bronchus	Pleural effusion	Pleural thickening	Pneumothorax
Trachea shifted	−	Ipsilateral	Contralateral	Ipsilateral	Contralateral
Thoracic expansion	↓ Ipsilateral	↓ Ipsilateral	↓ Ipsilateral	↓ Ipsilateral	Not helpful[b]
Fremitus	↑ Ipsilateral	↓ Ipsilateral	↓ Ipsilateral	↓ Ipsilateral	↓ Ipsilateral
Percussion resonance	↓ Ipsilateral	↓ Ipsilateral	↓ Ipsilateral	↓ Ipsilateral	↑ Ipsilateral
Breath sounds	T Ipsilateral	↓ Ipsilateral	T or ↓ ipsilat	↓ Ipsilateral	↓ Ipsilateral
Egophony	+ Ipsilateral	− Ipsilateral	− or +	−	−
Other maneuvers	+ Whispered pectoriloquy	−	−	−	+ Coin test

+, present; −, absent or deceptive; ↓, decreased; ↑, increased; T, tubular.

[a] Note that small lesions may not cause any of these findings.

[b] A pneumothorax, if small, might produce no change in chest expansion at a time when all other signs are present. Or, the diaphragm on that side might be paralyzed (depending on the cause of the pneumothorax), so that the costal margins would flare out more, making the expansion appear greater. On the other hand, with enough damage to the intercostal muscles, as in traumatic pneumothorax, there might be less expansion on the affected side.

References

Adriani J, Narachi M, Ward M: Complications of endotracheal intubation. *South Med J* 81:739–744, 1988.

Ausubel H, Cohen, BD, LaDue JS: Tietze's disease of eight years duration. *N Engl J Med* 261:190, 1959.

Bechgaard P: Segmental thoracic pain in patients admitted to a medical department and a coronary unit. *Acta Med Scand* 644(Suppl): 87–89, 1981.

Bohadana AB, Peslin R, Uffholtz H: Breath sounds in the clinical assessment of airflow obstruction. *Thorax* 33:345–351, 1978.

Byfield AF: Aids in physical diagnosis. *Med Clin North Am* 5:143–155, 1921.

Cabot RC: *Physical Diagnosis*, ed 11. William Wood & Co, Baltimore, 1934.

Cammann P, Clark A: A new mode of ascertaining the dimensions, form, and condition of internal organs by percussion. *NY J Med Sur* 3:62–96, 1840.

Clain A, ed: *Hamilton Bailey's Demonstration of Physical Signs in Clinical Surgery*, ed 15. Williams & Wilkins, Baltimore, 1973.

Conner LA: On the diagnosis of pericardial effusion: With special reference to physical signs on the posterior aspect of the thorax. *Am Heart J* 1:421–433, 1926.

DeGowin EL: *Bedside Diagnostic Examination*. Macmillan, New York, 1965.

d'Espine MA: [The sea cure for scrofula at the Dollfus Asylum in Cannes.] *Bull Acad Med* (Paris) 42:400–420, 1904.

d'Espine MA: [The early diagnosis of tuberculosis of the mediastinal lymph nodes.] *Bull Acad Med* (Paris) 57:167–174, 1907.

Dock W: Examination of the chest: Advantages of conducting and reporting it in English. *Bull NY Acad Med* 49:575–582, 1973.

Epler GR, Carrington CB, Gaensler EA: Crackles (râles) in the interstitial pulmonary diseases. *Chest* 73:333–339, 1978.

Figueroa-Cases JC, Jenkins DE: Unilateral hyperlucency of the lung (Swyer and James syndrome): Case report with fourteen years' observation. *Am J Med* 44:301–309, 1968.

Fletcher CM: The clinical diagnosis of pulmonary emphysema—an experimental study. *Proc R Soc Med* 45:577–584, 1952.

Forgacs P: Crackles and wheezes. *Lancet* 2:203–205, 1967.

Forgacs P: Lung sounds. *Br J Dis Chest* 63:1–12, 1969.

Forgacs P: Functional basis of pulmonary sounds. *Chest* 73:399–405, 1978.

Fries JF: The reactive enthesiopathies. *DM* 31:1–46, 1985.

Godfrey S: Association between pectus excavatum and segmental bronchomalacia. *J Pediatrics* 96:649–652, 1980.

Goff GD, Rosner BS, Detre T, Kennard D: Vibration perception in normal man and medical patients. *J Neurol Neurosurg Psychiatry* 28:503–509, 1965.

Gorham LW: A study of pulmonary embolism. Part I. A clinicopathological investigation of 100 cases of massive embolism of the pulmonary artery: Diagnosis by physical signs and differentiation from acute myocardial infarction. *Arch Intern Med* 108:8–22, 1961.

Graham DT: Health, disease, and the mind-body problem: Linguistic parallelism. *Psychosom Med* 29:52–71, 1967.

Guarino JR: Auscultatory percussion: A new aid in the examination of the chest. *J Kansas Med Soc* 75:193–194, 1974.

Guarino JR: Auscultatory percussion of the chest. *Lancet* 1:1332–1334, 1980.

Hamman L: Spontaneous mediastinal emphysema. *Bull Johns Hopkins Hosp* 64:1–21, 1939.

Hamman L, Rich AR: Acute diffuse interstitial fibrosis of the lungs. *Bull Johns Hopkins Hosp* 74:177–204, 1944.

Heckerling PS: The need for chest roentgenograms in adults with acute respiratory illness: Clinical predictors. *Arch Intern Med* 146:1321–1324, 1986.

Holm A, Bessey PQ, Aldrete JS: Diaphragmatic rupture due to blunt trauma: Morbidity and mortality in 42 cases. *South Med J* 81:956–962, 1988.

Hoover CF: The diagnostic significance of inspiratory movements of the costal margins. *Am J Med Sci* 159:633–646, 1920a.

Hoover CF: Definitive percussion and inspection in estimating size and contour of the heart. *JAMA* 75:1626–1630, 1920b.

Hoover CF: The diagnostic aid in evaluating the vigor of inspiratory costal excursion. *Arch Intern Med* 37:773–779, 1926.

Jochelson MS, Altschuler J, Stomper PC: The yield of chest radiography in febrile and neutropenic patients. *Ann Intern Med* 105:708–709, 1986.

Johnson JR, Bauer LE: Segmental consolidation of the lung. *Am J Med* 30:147–156, 1961.

Kilburn KH, Asmundsson T: Anteroposterior chest diameter in emphysema: From maxim to measurement. *Arch Intern Med* 123:379–382, 1969.

Koran LM: The reliability of clinical methods, data, and judgments. *N Engl J Med* 293:642–646, 1975.

actually one of the most valuable, when used in conjunction with the other findings.

Kraman SS: Lung sounds for the clinician. *Arch Intern Med* 146:1411–2, 1986.

Kuritzky L, Haddy RI, Curry RW Sr: Interpretation of chest roentgenograms by primary care physicians. *South Med J* 80:1347–1351, 1987.

Laennec RTH: *Treatise on the Diseases of the Chest, in which They Are Described According to Their Anatomical Characters and Their Diagnosis, Established on a New Principle by Means of Acoustick Instruments*, translated by JT Forbes and C Underwood, London, 1821. [Republished under the auspices of the Library of the New York Academy of Medicine, Hafner Publishing Co, New York, 1962.]

Lal S, Ferguson AD, Campbell EJM: Forced expiratory time: A simple test for airway obstruction. *Br Med J* 1:814–817, 1964.

Lane RW, Weider DJ, Steinem C, Marin-Padilla M: Laryngomalacia: A review and case report of surgical treatment with resolution of pectus excavatum. *Arch Otolaryngol* 110:546–551, 1984.

Ledley RS, Whuang HK, Mazziotta JC: *Cross Sectional Anatomy: An Atlas for Computerized Tomography.* Williams & Wilkins, Baltimore, 1977.

Leopold SS: *The Principles and Methods of Physical Diagnosis.* WB Saunders, Philadelphia, 1952.

Light RW: *Pleural Diseases.* Lea & Febiger, Philadelphia, 1983.

Lofvenberg J, Johansson RS: Regional differences and interindividual variability in sensitivity to vibration in the glabrous skin of the human hand. *Brain Res* 301:65–72, 1984.

Macklem PT: The diaphragm in health and disease. *J Lab Clin Med* 99:601–610, 1982.

Macklem PT: Respiratory muscle dysfunction. *Hosp Pract* 21:83–95, 1986.

Majno G: *The Healing Hand: Man and Wound in the Ancient World.* Harvard University Press, Cambridge, MA, 1975.

McFadden ER Jr, Kiser R, deGroot WJ: Acute bronchial asthma: relations between clinical and physiologic manifestations. *N Engl J Med* 288:221–225, 1973.

Mendez HMM, Opitz JM: Noonan syndrome: A review. *Am J Med Genet* 21:493–506, 1985.

Michelson N: The limitations of the tuning fork in the diagnosis of pulmonary disease. *Am J Med Sci* 172:713–717, 1926.

Mirvis SE, Rodriguez A, Whitley NO, Tarr RJ: CT evaluation of thoracic infections after major trauma. *AJR* 144:1183–1187, 1985.

Mirvis SE, Tobin KD, Kostrubiak I, Belzberg H: Thoracic CT in detecting occult disease in critically ill patients. *AJR* 148:685–689, 1987.

Murphy RLH Jr.: Discontinuous adventitious lung sounds. *Semin Respir Med* 6:210–219, 1985.

Murphy RLH: Chest auscultation in occupational lung disease. *Semin Respir Med* 7:289–296, 1986.

Nath AR, Capel LH: Inspiratory crackles—early and late. *Thorax* 29:223–227, 1974.

Norris G, Landis HRM: *Diseases of the Chest*, ed 6. WB Saunders, Philadelphia, 1938.

Orriols R: A new physical sign in pneumothorax. *Ann Intern Med* 107:255, 1987.

Pena A, Perez L, Nurko S, Dorenbaum D: Pectus carinatum and pectus excavatum: Are they the same disease? *Am Surg* 47:215–218, 1981.

Ploysongsang Y, Paré JAP, Macklem PT: Correlation of regional breath sounds with regional ventilation in emphysema. *Am Rev Respir Dis* 126:526–529, 1982.

Robertson AJ, Coope R: Râles, rhonchi, and Laennec. *Lancet* 2:417–423, 1957.

Robicsek F, Cook JW, Daugherty HK, Selle JG: Pectus carinatum. *J Thorac Cardiovasc Surg* 78:52–61, 1979.

Robinson SJ: Diagnosis of congenital heart disease: Clues from the history and physical examination. *Cardiovasc Clin* 2:77–95, 1970.

Roland E, Nielsen VK: Vibratory thresholds in the hands. *Arch Neurol* 37:775–779, 1980.

Sakula A: Joseph Skoda 1805–1881: A centenary tribute to a pioneer of thoracic medicine. *Thorax* 36:404–411, 1981.

Sapira JD: Diagnostic strategies. *South Med J* 74:582–584, 1981.

Semble EL. Wise CM: Chest pain: A rheumatologist's perspective. *South Med J* 81:64–68, 1988.

Semple T, Lancaster WM: Noisy pneumothorax: Observations based on 24 cases. *Br Med J* 1:1342–1346, 1961.

Sharp JT: The respiratory muscles in chronic obstructive pulmonary disease. *Am Rev Respir Dis* 134:1089–1091, 1986.

Shepard J Jr: *Medical Grand Rounds.* St. Louis Veterans Administration Medical Center, St. Louis, October 22, 1986.

Sherrier RH, McAdams HP: Digital processing of portable films can reduce need for repeat studies. *Diagn Imag Clin Med* 8:117–118, 1986.

Shim CS, Williams H Jr: Relationship of wheezing to the severity of obstruction in asthma. *Arch Intern Med* 143:890–892, 1982.

Shirai F, Kudoh S, Shibuya A, Sada K, Mikami R: Crackles in asbestos workers: Auscultation and lung sound analysis. *Br J Dis Chest* 75:386–396, 1981.

Skoda J: [*Treatise on Percussion and Auscultation*]. J.G. Ritter, Vienna, 1839.

Spitieri MA, Cook DG, Clarke SW: Reliability of eliciting physical signs in examination of the chest. *Lancet* 1:873–875, 1988.

Strouse S: Pulmonary tuberculosis in association with other diseases in the general hospital. *Med Clin North Am* 5:143–155, 1919.

Swyer PR, James GCW: A case of unilateral pulmonary emphysema. *Thorax* 8:133–136, 1953.

Tape TG, Mushlin AI: The utility of routine chest radiographs. *Ann Intern Med* 104:663–670, 1986.

Thacker RE, Kraman SS: The prevalence of auscultatory crackles in subjects without lung disease. *Chest* 81:672–674, 1982.

Thompson DT: Examination of the chest: Is all the evidence obtained? *Practitioner* 222:99–104, 1979.

Waring WW, Beckerman RC, Hopkins RL: Continuous adventitious lung sounds: Site and method of production and significance. *Semin Respir Med* 6:201–209, 1985.

Webb GB: Auscultatory percussion in the diagnosis of pleural effusion. *JAMA* 88:99, 1927.

Weiss JM, Spodick DH: Laterality of pleural effusions in chronic congestive heart failure. *Am J Cardiol* 53:951, 1984.

Wiener SL, Nathanson M: *Med Times*, 1976–1977. [See reference in Chapter 29.]

Williams TJ, Ahmad D, Morgan WK: A clinical and roentgenographic correlation of diaphragmatic movement. *Arch Intern Med* 141:879–880, 1981.

Wood FC, Wolferth CC: The tolerance of certain cardiac patients for various recumbent positions (trepopnea). *Am J Med Sci* 191:354–378, 1937.

Workum P, Holford SK, Delbono EA, Murphy RLH. The prevalence and character of crackles (râles) in young women without significant lung disease. *Am Rev Respir Dis* 126:921–923, 1982.

17
The Heart

"We insist on the same regimen plus the use of chicken soup."*
Barron Larrey (Napoleon's surgeon), *Surgical Clinics from Military Camps and Hospitals Between 1792 and 1829,* vol. 10, Chez Gabon, Paris, 1829.

Inspection

The PMI (point of maximum impulse) is usually the only pulsation that can be seen. Normally it occurs during systole at the apex of the heart. Some normal persons do not have a visible PMI, especially if they have a thick body wall. Theoretically, if there is no visible systolic apical impulse, but there is a visible pulsation elsewhere (as rarely occurs), that pulsation would have to be considered the PMI. (If there is no visible pulsation, the PMI may still be found by palpation—see p. 284).

A Method

Look for the PMI with the patient standing erect, lying recumbent, or sometimes simply sitting.

Not surprisingly, persons who examine for the PMI with the patient in the left lateral decubitus position find the PMI to be laterally displaced. There would be no objection to the teaching of this method, were normal values available.

There are four questions to be answered by inspection of the precordium.

1. Can You See a PMI?

Obviously, if you cannot see a PMI, you do not need to answer the other questions, but instead can proceed to palpation. About 75% of patients seen for a routine checkup will not have a visible PMI.

However, you should be aware that after you have palpated the precordium and found the palpable PMI, it is often possible to go back and find a visible PMI by specifically looking at the area of the palpable PMI.

2. Is the PMI Systolic?

Normally the PMI is systolic.

One reported sign of constrictive pericarditis is a diastolic PMI (Stapleton & Groves, 1971). However, in constrictive pericarditis a systolic retraction of the PMI (Broadbent's sign) may occur, and this might look like a diastolic PMI in a patient with a fast heart rate. (Also see pp. 285–286 for other causes of palpable systolic refraction.) Broadbent's sign has also been reported in cases of right ventricular hypertrophy.

Perloff advises marking the skin with ink and illuminating obliquely with the beam of a pocket flashlight. Precordial retraction (not pulsation) is thus more readily seen than felt, especially when viewed across the chest or from the patient's feet.

3. Where Is the PMI Located?

Normally, a visible PMI is located at the apex. The apex is normally located in the fifth intercostal space at (or medial to) the midclavicular line. An old rule states that if the PMI is in the sixth intercostal space or below, or is lateral to the midclavicular line, it is abnormal, irrespective of the other features of the cardiac examination. Such displacement is usually from left ventricular enlargement (vide infra), but sometimes is due to leftward mediastinal shift. (The distinction is based upon the fact that only the latter will have a leftward tracheal shift.)

Why the midclavicular line?   A few precise physicians and at least one of the better physical diagnosis textbooks recommend describing the PMI in terms of its horizontal distance from the midsternal line. But the midclavicular line is preferred as a reference, for the following reasons:

   1.   When reading the case record, it is impossible to know the meaning of a PMI located *x* centimeters from the midsternal line, since we do not have a value for the "correcting" denominator (i.e., the transverse thoracic diameter at the same level).

   2.   There is no one normal value for the location of the PMI in terms of distance from the midsternal line. While 6 cm from the midsternal line might represent PMI displacement in a neonate with congenital heart disease, it could be evidence of microcardia in a Sumo wrestler.

---

*This quotation concerns the first removal of pericardial fluid from a patient with apparent tamponade. Pericardiocentesis was not technically performed, as the patient had a sword wound entering the pericardium, and a catheter was simply passed through the wound track.

This is not the first reference to chicken soup as a medicine. Credit for that discovery goes to an informant of Pliny the Elder, in *Natural History Book* 29,25:78: "Parthians prefer to put chicken brain on the wound. The soup made from the chicken is an excellent medicine for this and also miraculous in many other conditions."

The single "normal" value available to the literate proponents of the midsternal line ("less than 10 cm") is based on a total experience of 12 men and 6 women of unknown body size (Beilin & Mounsey, 1962).

3. The left midclavicular line is very convenient, because displacement of the PMI lateral to this line is abnormal, whether resulting from a mediastinal shift or inherent cardiac disease.

4. The objection voiced against the midclavicular line, that it is "subjective," is silly, as shown by the following method.

A method:

1. Locate the medial head of the left clavicle (collar bone) where it articulates with the first rib, and mark it at its most medial point.

2. Mark the clavicle at its lateral extreme, which is just above the acromium of the scapula, between the lateral edge of the trapezius (behind) and the superior deltoid muscle (in front).

3. Find the midpoint of the line connecting the above two points.

4. From Dorland's dictionary (1913), the midclavicular line is "a perpendicular line let fall from the center of the clavicle" (the midpoint you have just identified). DaCosta stated in 1909 that "this line, although commonly termed 'mammillary,' rarely passes through the nipple" (Rytand, 1968).

Determinations of the position of the midclavicular line by this method correlated well with radiographs, whereas persons who simply guess at its position miss it by up to 4 to 6.5 cm (lateral and medial misplacement, respectively) (Naylor et al., 1987).

Hypertrophy and dilatation. In left ventricular hypertrophy, the PMI and the apex might still be in the usual place if the patient has no accompanying left ventricular dilatation (enlargement). If the patient does have chamber dilatation (enlargement), the apex may be displaced laterally. Note that hypertrophy refers to the wall thickness, as learned in pathology and measured by echocardiography. Dilatation (enlargement) refers to the size of the *cavity* that the ventricle surrounds, manifested by the size of the silhouette as determined by percussion or radiography. ("Ventricle" comes from the Latin word for "sack." Sometimes we are talking about the thickness of the material walls of the sack ["hypertrophy"] and sometimes about the internal dimensions [the cavity proper] or the size of the total ["enlargement"].)

Other abnormalities. In right ventricular hypertrophy, the PMI can be seen in the subxiphoid region of the epigastrium. In dextrocardia, the PMI will be on the right side of the chest.

Teaching hint. You may wish to mark the patient's chest (with his permission) with a water-soluble marker, after you have found the PMI. This will help you to learn percussion of the heart border (see p. 286) without having to send the patient to fluoroscopy (rarely available these days) or for a radiograph. The heart border should be located just outside the PMI.

A massive pericardial effusion is an exception to the last statement (see p. 323), although most of the time such patients will not have a visible PMI. Why not? (Write down your answer before looking at Appendix 17-1.)

4. Is the PMI a Single Impulse?

Sometimes the PMI has a double impulse (in time). (Usually this is more easily felt than seen.) This can be a valuable sign of idiopathic hypertrophic subaortic stenosis (IHSS) (see p. 314) or bundle branch block (BBB) with asynchronous contraction of the ventricles.

It has been pointed out (Basta & Bettinger, 1979) that double systolic apical impulses are encountered in other conditions, including fixed aortic stenosis, ischemic heart disease with anterior wall dyskinesia, and a variety of myocardial diseases.

A triple apical impulse was found in 17 of 24 patients with subaortic stenosis.

Teaching trick. If the PMI is in an intercostal space, a tongue depressor held against the rib, with the end on the PMI, may be used as a lever to magnify the PMI for your careful scrutiny.

Palpation

A Method

Some palpate for wide-area, low-frequency events (such as right ventricular heaves) with the hypothenar surface. For restricted-area events such as the PMI, some palpate only with the fingertips. And some persons are best able to detect vibrations with the area of the palm at the base of the fingers (see Ch. 16, p. 250). See what works best for you.

The PMI

As indicated above, palpation is a more sensitive technique for assessing the PMI than is inspection. If you can't see the PMI, but you can feel it, then you will have to use palpation alone to answers questions 2 through 4 above. Even if you can inspect the PMI, you should always use palpation to check the answers. In addition, palpation can give some information that is very difficult or impossible to obtain from inspection.

Size

If the diameter of the PMI in its longest axis is larger than 2.3 cm (the diameter of a quarter), it is clearly abnormal. If it is 2.0 cm, the size of a nickel or larger, it is probably abnormal; however, many sophomores will think their own PMI is the size of a nickel, if they don't hold a nickel in their hand before palpation. With experience, you can appreciate more subtle distinctions. A PMI of 1.7 cm (the size of a penny) or smaller is normal.

One study (Eilen et al., 1983) showed no correlation between the left ventricular volume and the location of the PMI with the patient rolled into a 45-degree left decubitus position. However, in that position, an apical diameter of greater than 3 cm (the diameter of most stethoscope bells) was an indicator of left ventricular enlargement (see Table 17-1). The sensitivity was 92% and the negative predictive value 95%.

Duration

The neophyte should feel his own PMI to observe normal duration. In fact, that sensation could be used as a temporal standard during the palpation of the PMI in one's first 100 patients.

For the resident. The PMI normally occupies two thirds of systole or less. Accordingly, one can detect a prolonged duration by noting the PMI to reach or exceed the second heart sound. In one study, such a prolonged PMI was found in 13 of 13 patients with left ventricular hypertrophy (as judged by electrocardiographic voltage criteria). This compares with only 8 of the 13 detected by an increased forcefulness (Beilin & Mounsey, 1962).

Location

As noted above, the PMI should not be lateral to the left midclavicular line, nor below the fifth intercostal space. *Either* is abnormal.

Displacement in the absence of mediastinal shift requires chamber enlargement, not just wall hypertrophy. Only 8 of 13 patients with electrocardiographic evidence of left ventricular hypertrophy had a displaced PMI (Beilin & Mounsey, 1962).

Predictive values. As a general rule, if one diagnoses cardiac enlargement from a displaced PMI, one expects to find an enlarged heart shadow on the PA chest film, according to the Ungerleider-Gubner or Ungerleider-Clark criteria (Ungerleider & Clark, 1939; Ungerleider & Gubner, 1942). In 14 of 16 cases, there was perfect concordance between the presence (or absence) of a displaced PMI and the presence (or absence) of severe left ventricular enlargement on the chest film (Beilin & Mounsey, 1962).

The positive predictive value of a PMI lateral to the midclavicular line with the patient supine is stated to be a bit over 50% for detecting an echocardiographically enlarged left ventricular end-diastolic volume (Eilen et al., 1983). However, this study was possibly flawed because a single upper limit of normal for left ventricular end-diastolic volume was applied to all 41 subjects regardless of body size; such a procrustean judgment is at variance with biologic measurement.

Synthesis

Combining information about location and duration is of value in differential diagnosis, as shown in Table 17-1.

○   Some patients erroneously thought to be in congestive heart failure will have a normal sized heart by any method of mensuration. This set comprises constrictive pericarditis, tricuspid stenosis, inferior vena cava obstruction, pulmonary vein thrombosis, mitral stenosis, diastolic filling dysfunction, and ischemic (coronary artery) heart disease.

Right Ventricular Taps

The *left* parasternal border should be palpated for a *right* ventricular tap. This is also called a right ventricular bulge, lift, or heave. It is different from the subxyphoid point of maximal impulse found in patients with chronic obstructive lung disease, although it may be found concurrently if such patients also have acquired right ventricular hypertrophy. It is nondiagnostic in

that it may result from any etiology of right ventricular hypertrophy.

A Method

Place the ulnar edge of your right hand at the patient's *left* parasternal border, touching the third, fourth, and fifth interspaces. A systolic tap (moving your hand) is never felt in normal persons. Its presence implies severe right ventricular hypertrophy.

For the attending: A rounding ploy. Sometimes a right ventricular tap can be evoked by the same trick used for bringing out an evanescent right-sided gallop: ask the team to elevate the patient's legs (passively) so as to abruptly increase right ventricular inflow.

Ventricular Dyskinesia and Ventricular Aneurysms

Anterior ventricular dyskinesia may occasionally present as a palpable paradoxical (systolic) outward bulge. Previously, these were all thought to be ventricular aneurysms, but it is now realized that most of them are actually dyskinetic segments, indicative of locally impaired cardiac function, usually subsequent to ischemic heart disease. The pulsations resemble the apical PMI, but are usually much more medial. Additionally, they are usually larger than the normal PMI and usually more sustained, not having the acute tapping or "kicking" quality of the normal impulse.

Ventricular aneurysms, when palpable, may produce a systolic impulse, or they may cause a diastolic bulge. In the latter instance, the blood enters the heart during early or late rapid filling and causes the thin-walled, nonmuscular aneurysm to bulge, striking the chest wall. This finding may mimic a palpable S3 or S4, except there is no audible gallop (see pp. 286 and 296).

Thrills

A thrill is a continuous (i.e., noninstantaneous) palpable vibration. (A thrill lasts longer than the most prolonged PMI.)

Thrills accompany murmurs, and are the palpable counterpart of turbulence. One might put it, "A thrill is a murmur you can also hear with your fingers."

Innocent murmurs do not have thrills. Additionally, the thrill distinguishes grade 4 and above murmurs (which have thrills) from grade 3 murmurs (which do not) in the intensity scoring system that is presented later (see p. 303).

Other Palpatory Findings

1.   A systolic pulsation at the second or third interspace at the left sternal border suggests *pulmonary* hypertension, either primary or secondary, as in atrial septal defect, valvular pulmonic stenosis with poststenotic dilatation, dissecting aneurysm, or partial anomalous pulmonary venous return, in that order. Sometimes there is also a palpable valve closure or a diastolic thrill in the case of dissection.

Table 17-1. Most Likely Diagnosis Based on Palpation of the PMI

PMI	PMI Displaced?		
	Yes, But Only Laterally	Yes, But Not Just Laterally	No
Not prolonged or enlarged	Mediastinal shift (Leftward) or Left ventricular enlargement	Primary or secondary dilated cardiomyopathy	Normal
Prolonged and/or enlarged	Left ventricular hypertrophy combined with left ventricular enlargement		Left ventricular hypertrophy[a]

[a]For example, early aortic stenosis.

2. If there is a systolic impulse at the first or second right interspace at the sternal border, one should consider an aneurysm of the ascending aorta, aortic insufficiency (because of the large stroke volume being ejected into the dilated aortic root), aortic stenosis with poststenotic dilatation, a right-sided aortic arch, or simply a senescent and tortuous innominate artery (Hurst & Schlant, 1972).

3. If there is a systolic pulsation in the retrosternal notch, think of an aortic aneurysm.

4. An impulse occurring immediately *after* S1 may be due to systolic expansion of the dilated atria in mitral or tricuspid insufficiency. It is felt higher (more toward the base) than the apical PMI.

5. Patients with tricuspid insufficiency, restrictive cardiomyopathy, or constrictive pericarditis occasionally show a marked apical systolic retraction. (The last two may also have an abrupt early diastolic rebound, which can be misidentified as an abnormal systolic pulsation (Stapleton & Groves, 1971).

6. Occasionally a hyperkinetic but otherwise normal heart may show an early diastolic left parasternal rebound, which can be mistaken for a right ventricular tap if not timed correctly.

7. Some S3s are palpable, but S3s are significant even if only audible.

8. A palpable S4 over the ventricle (which is more significant than an audible but impalpable S4, see pp. 298–299) will occur just *before* S1. It signifies decreased compliance of the ventricle of origin, as from ischemic heart disease or increased afterload (due to arterial or pulmonary hypertension, or aortic or pulmonic stenosis). Methods for distinguishing right- and left-sided S4s are discussed on p. 298.

9. About 23% of pericardial friction rubs are palpable (see p. 305).

Percussion

A Pedagogic Note

The suggestion that medical students can learn to accurately percuss the cardiac border is met with general incredulity these days. (By "accurately," I mean with reasonable confidence in their ability to distinguish patients who clearly do not have an enlarged heart from those who do, before looking at the chest film.)

(This excludes the morbidly obese patient, who in essence is percussed while wearing an overcoat of cellular triglyceride.)

Admittedly, there is a body of experience, some published, indicating that there are persons who cannot percuss the cardiac border accurately. Similarly, there are persons who cannot play the violin. But that does not mean the violin cannot be played. Scientific studies have shown that in the hands of competent clinicians, the average error of percussion is about 1 cm (Kurtz & White, 1928; Mainland et al., 1938).

•

A cardiologist overheard me talking to a salesman about putting in some shelves for stereo equipment. When he asked about stud placement for putting up the shelf brackets, I told him I would locate them by percussion. The cardiologist made fun of percussion, saying that there was an error of 1 cm.

"You're right," I said, thinking he meant the heart borders.

"Well," he said, "you'd better drill a hole to be sure."

"Oh, I thought you meant the heart borders. I'll get the middle of the studs exactly right."

He said it couldn't be done, but I have done all my shelf brackets that way.

•

For the attending. The heart contains no gas and is surrounded by the most resonant part of the body. If it were not possible to percuss the outline of such a structure, then we should also abandon percussion of the lungs for infiltrates and of the acoustically less contrasted organs such as the liver. By direct count over a decade, the number of errors I made in percussing the heart borders was fewer than the number of chest films that had been misplaced by the radiology file room. Accordingly, I encourage the teaching of this technique, which after an initial investment is quick, accessible, and reasonably accurate.

A Method

The percussion note is produced in the same manner as described for the lung fields (Ch. 16, p. 251).

For the beginning student, probably the simplest method is to percuss in the interspaces, following the interspace from its lateral (resonant) area to the medial (dull) area. Begin with the patient's left apical heart border, proceeding superiorly and then repeating the procedure for the right border.

Some excellent examiners percuss in lines or strips perpendicular to the longitudinal axis of the body, moving across interspaces and ribs. They are experienced and can adjust for the changing percussion note of the rib and the intercostal muscle, but this technique is not suggested for the sophomore. Other experienced examiners percuss along lines perpendicular to the anticipated heart borders, but such anticipation is based upon experience and is also not recommended for the novice.

When you percuss, you may wish to back up over the border, percussing in reverse from dullness back to resonance as a double check.

Dullness is the first detectable tone of impaired resonance obtained when moving from the resonant lung to the cardiac border (or from the resonant lung to the hepatic border). Flatness is the tone of maximally impaired resonance, usually but not always located in the middle of the cardiac silhouette (or in the middle of the liver, again, usually but not always.) To hear true flatness, percuss your tibia.

Notice that many times the experienced percussor will strike two blows, a hard one and a soft one. They seem to learn to do this unconsciously, and I have never seen the exact reason written down, but suspect there must be some sensory information obtained from the difference in the vibrations between the strong and the soft note.

Probably any system works if it is used consistently. One must gain sufficient experience with the method, frequently correlating the observations with the PA chest film.

All normal radiologic values for heart size are based upon a PA (posterior to anterior) projection, which is made by placing the front of the chest against the plate with the beam generator behind the patient. The advantage of this technique is that the heart size is not much magnified. But when a patient is too ill to travel to the radiology department, one must obtain an AP (anterior to posterior) film, wherein the plate is held behind the patient, who is held up in bed, the beam coming from the portable beam generator at the foot of the bed. (Or if the patient is restrained in bed, one might place the plate underneath him and direct the beam downward.) On the AP film, the apparent heart size is artifactually enlarged. (Worse, in some hospitals it is not possible to tell which technique was used.)

Although we now use indirect (mediate) percussion, there were formerly several schools of direct (immediate) percussion. Direct percussion is sometimes better than indirect percussion when it comes to outlining the frontal projection of cardiac dullness, especially in thick-chested patients.

One method is as follows:

1. Use the same routes as for indirect percussion.
2. Using only the fleshy pulp of the middle finger of the right hand, slap the chest wall. Maximal excursion is required to produce a resonant sound.
3. After striking the chest, keep the flesh of the finger applied to the chest wall. For some reason this seems to improve the technique, possibly because part of percussion involves the appreciation of vibratory dampening.

A second technique:

Use the same method as above, but stroke the chest wall for a short distance after striking it. The original description and rationale follows:

There is no sharp boundary between the heart and surrounding lung. From the upper and left borders the lung encroaches over the precordial area as a wedge-shaped body. If the examiner is to define the border of the heart, he must employ the smallest pleximeter area and at the same time he must be able to penetrate the overlying lung to detect the resistant heart which lies beneath. Direct or immediate percussion best serves these purposes. The stroke should be made with the palmar surface of the terminal phalanx of the extended middle finger or ring finger. The blow should be made by firmly stroking the heart as if the examiner was seeking to penetrate the underlying tongue of the lung. One should not imitate the stroke of a piano hammer, which is made with a quick recoil to prevent damping of the string. The object of the firmly applied stroke is to damp the thoracic wall and so far as possible eliminate it from sharing in the pleximeter. (Hoover, 1920)

When using direct percussion, one only strikes the chest a single blow.

Locating the Apex

The lower portion of the left border of cardiac dullness is called the apex. This border shifts laterally in left ventricular enlargement and pericardial effusion (if massive).

False Positives

Rarely, the left border may be shifted because of disease of the right ventricle, but only if the right ventricle has undergone massive hypertrophy and enlargement. This may be caused by a condition of systolic overload (e.g., pulmonary hypertension or pulmonic stenosis) or of diastolic overload (e.g., chronic severe tricuspid insufficiency), resulting in a conversion of the right ventricle, which is normally a flow ventricle, into a pressure ventricle. Or it may be shifted from atelectasis of the left lung (see Ch. 16, p. 249).

Left Ventricular Enlargement
Versus Massive Pericardial Effusion

In the former, the PMI will be palpated just within the border of cardiac dullness (partly because the PMI is palpated in systole,

and the heart border is percussed in diastole, the longer phase of the cycle). In the case of pericardial effusion, the PMI stays where it was, the area of dullness alone being shifted leftward due to the fluid. Accordingly, the PMI if palpable will either be well within the border of cardiac dullness, or it will be obscured by the fluid, and hence not palpable.

A Digression on Pericardiocentesis*

Pericardiocentesis was first performed by the Viennese surgeon Franz Schuh in 1840, via the apical approach, before the roentgenogram was invented (Spodick, 1985). In Schuh's method, the needle is inserted 1 cm medial to the apex and aimed at the right sternoclavicular joint. Since there are no large vessels at the apex, there is no danger of rupturing them via this approach.

In 1896, the subxiphoid approach was introduced by Marfan, supplanting Schuh's method. Marfan's approach carries a grave risk of perforating the coronary arteries and veins. The customary procedure of clamping the needle to the exploring electrode of a running electrocardiograph machine does not warn of impending laceration of the vessels, but only retrospects the injury currents due to hitting the myocardium or the Q wave seen after accidentally entering the ventricular cavity. Monitoring the procedure with ultrasound still does not protect the blood vessels. Medical house staff have thus become reluctant to perform such a pericardiocentesis without the cardiac surgeons available for backup, and surgeons have begun to take over the procedure entirely.

Schuh's method is still available to those who are able to locate the cardiac apex by percussion. In case of doubt, one could also obtain a chest film with a paper clip taped to the patient's chest at the percussed apical dullness, near the intended insertion point. Roentgenography was unavailable during the first five decades in which pericardiocentesis was performed; this demonstrates the accuracy of percussion in the hands of some.

Upper Left Cardiac Border

The upper portion of the patient's left cardiac border of dullness includes the pulmonic outflow tract. In some cases of severe pulmonary hypertension, one can, *with practice*, find an out-bulging of the cardiac dullness silhouette at the second and/or third left interspace parasternally, unaccompanied by any alteration in the lower left border. (Associated palpatory findings are discussed on p. 285.)

The finding of a percussible (and/or palpable) pulmonary artery is not very sensitive. However, there are few false positives (lung tumor contiguous to the heart border, aneurysm of a right-sided aorta, etc.), so a positive test implies one of a limited number of pathologic explanations.

Right Cardiac Border

Boring as it may seem, it is necessary to percuss this border to estimate width. If the left border is percussed well inside the usual area (which one can identify because of having percussed the border in many normals), one might not know how to interpret the finding without also percussing out the right border. One could be dealing with the vertical or "drop" heart (so named because it resembles a water drop in shape) or with a shift of the mediastinum to the right (usually due to atelectasis of the right lung, in which case the trachea will usually be shifted—see Ch.

---

*Also see the epigram to this chapter for a French claim to the first pericardiocentesis.

16, p. 249). This is an important differential because the former usually signifies pulmonary emphysema (or rarely hypovolemia, especially of the chronic variety as in Addison's disease), while the latter points to other disease of the lung.

Other Uses of Percussion

The right cardiac contour, unfortunately, is not the right ventricle, which has no representation in the frontal projection, either of cardiac dullness or the chest film. However, right ventricular enlargement causes a flat percussion note, replacing the usual dull sternal percussion note beginning about 3 cm above the xiphoid. (Below that, flatness might be caused by the liver.) The higher that the flatness extends, the more likely that its cause may be a pericardial effusion rather than right ventricular enlargment (Moschcowitz, 1933).

For another method of outlining the cardiac profile, see the scratch test (p. 309).

Dullness from the manubrium over to the third costal cartilage on the right is seen in aneurysm of the arch of the aorta, and is called Potain's sign.

Very advanced. Perloff suggests locating gastric tympany prior to cardiac percussion, for the purpose of determining visceral situs inversus. If there is not sufficient air in the stomach to permit distinction of liver dullness from gastric tympany, Perloff suggests that the patient be instructed to inhale and swallow a few times, in order to induce aerophagia. Alternately, he could drink a carbonated beverage.

In failure of full diaphragmatic descent either due to paralysis or to atelectasis of the ipsilateral lung, the inspiratory intrapleural pressure on the impaired side will be higher (less negative) than on the other side. Thus, during inspiration, the mediastinum will move away from the affected side (Macklem, 1986). I have no experience with this method and suspect that it would be easier to first detect impaired diaphragmatic descent by Hoover's sign, and then to percuss the hemidiaphragms individually to see if either had paradoxical motion.

Auscultation

Question: *Why could Laennec detect the sounds of the heart better with his rolled-up quire of paper (see Ch. 1, p. 2) than with the application of his hand?*

Answer: *See Appendix 17-2 (and Fig. 17-14).*

In cardiac auscultation, even more than in other aspects of clinical examination, *die Methode ist alles.**

Auscultation is like a front-end-loaded mutual fund. It initially takes a great deal of time to master the technique, even in the present era, when heart sound simulators and cardiac sound recordings can provide a medical student with a lifetime of experience in just a few months. Unfortunately, most modern medical "educators" place less emphasis on the rudiments of the physical examination than on learning to prescribe for diseases that the students cannot even spell let alone diagnose. Yet in 30 years spent both in the trenches and rear headquarters, I have seen the treatment of disease change more often than a pedes-

---

*"The method is everything." This was supposedly the watchword of Emil Fisher and the other great fin de siecle *German organic chemists. Now that polypeptide synthesis has been automated, I suggest appropriating their motto for clinical examination.*

trian crossing sign, while the semiophysiology is as constant as taxation. Therefore, remember that once you know the correct diagnosis, you can always look up the treatment in a current textbook; but if you do not have the correct diagnosis, a chain of drugstores will be needed to provide enough medication to cover all the possibilities.

A reminder for sophomores. Again, be sure that the stethoscope earpieces are comfortable and are pointing *forward* when you place them in your auditory canals. Before you begin listening, tap the chest piece with your finger to be sure that it is "on line." If you do not, you could have an experience like the following:

•

Many years ago at a prize-winning New York university, the medical students learned auscultation by practicing with the inhabitants of a home for youngsters with rheumatic heart disease. One very serious and shy sophomore medical student was assigned a precocious and well-endowed teenage girl who had many interesting murmurs. The student spent an hour diligently moving the diaphragm and the bell back and forth around the girl's prominent mammae. Each murmur was to be tracked into all of its radiations by the technique of inching—moving the stethoscope head 1 inch at a time from the point where it was loudest to its quietest radiation. The student seriously stared at the mental picture of the murmurs, apparently oblivious to the girl's breasts just a few inches from his face. All of this provided great entertainment for his classmates, who could see that he had failed to put the earpieces, now hanging around his neck, into his auditory canals.

•

Dr. Campbell Moses of New York taught me that at the beginning of the auscultation of the heart, the patient should be told: "I may listen to your heart for a long time. That doesn't mean I'm hearing anything bad." Remember that the patient will be observing your facial expressions, but that you will not be attending to his responses, as you concentrate on what you are ausculting.

Much has been written about the technique of "inching" (see p. 290), the type of stethoscope that should be used, the importance of phonocardiography, ancillary aids such as amyl nitrite, and the various phases of the Valsalva maneuver. However, there are, in my view, only two issues that are critical to learning cardiac auscultation:

○ **Rule 1.** You must listen in a completely quiet* room. The reason should be clear from Table 17-2. In practice, this means turning off the television, turning off the radio, closing the door, closing the windows, removing all visitors from the room, and in some cases silencing thoughtless colleagues and superiors whose mumbling will interfere with your auscultation. There is *no substitute* for quiet.

A self-study. Have your partner stand 4 feet away and whisper a number, (e.g., his Social Security number). According to Table 17-2, that is 20 decibels. It is also much easier to hear than the average murmur of aortic or pulmonic insufficiency.

---

*Auscult bony chests by placing a 150-ml plastic infusion bag on the chest and a stethoscope on the bag (Perry et al., 1984).

Table 17-2. Levels of Noise from Common Sources

Source of Noise	Distance from Source (feet)	Noise Level	
		Decibels	Amplitude Ratios
Ordinary conversation	3	65	1778
Average office		47	223.9
Average whisper	4	20	10.0
Threshold of hearing		0	1.0

Source: *Rappaport and Sprague (1941).*

Now go into a nurse's station ("an average office") and repeat the experiment. Can you still identify a whispered nine-digit number (different from the first one)? About how many decibels were ambient?

Repeat the experiment 3 feet from an ordinary conversation. Can you still hear all the numbers? How many decibels were ambient?

At what location could you no longer pick up the whispered signal of 20 decibels? Is the average ward in your hospital louder or softer than that? How then could you possibly hear aortic or pulmonic insufficiency, which are even softer than 20 decibels?

Question: *What can you do when the room is completely quiet, but you still cannot hear well because the patient has his own noise generator, say the coarse rhonchi of obstructive pulmonary disease, or loud wheezes that obscure both the heart sounds and any murmur less than grade 4?*

Answer: *State the absence of meaningful data by noting in the record that you were unable to auscult the heart sounds. However, once the patient is quiet, you are obliged to return and complete the physical examination, even if it was begun several days earlier.*

○ **Rule 2.** Listen to one time at a time. That is, listen to only one part of the cardiac cycle at a time. You must first make sure you have identified systole and diastole (vide infra), but just this is not sufficient. Remember the rule of two diastoles (Ch. 4, p. 69).

The murmurs of pulmonic insufficiency and aortic insufficiency can only be heard by concentrating one's attention in the early portion of diastole. Other auscultatory phenomenon (e.g., a ventricular gallop, an opening snap) are also heard *only* in this brief time period. To hear this portion of diastole, *you must learn to listen to the space just after the second heart sound to the exclusion of all else.*

Other auscultatory phenomena (e.g., atrial gallops) are heard specifically in late diastole, just before the first heart sound. To hear them, concentrate only on the first heart sound and then when you know it's coming, listen only to the space just before it. (This is like catching the brass ring on the merry-go-round.)

If you do not systematically search through the three time periods (systole, early diastole, and late diastole), excluding your attention from the other two periods in turn, you will miss many important findings. If you miss a murmur, because of not listening to one phase at a time, it is not appropriate to say, "Some people can hear it and some people can't." Murmurs are either present or absent. The murmur is not a Zen koan about a tree falling in an uninhabited forest. It is a finding accessible to competent examiners, if they are listening in a quiet room, and if

they know what they are listening *for*. (Admittedly, some findings are present intermittently. And, there are some people who say they heard something they thought they were supposed to hear, even though they did not actually hear it. Intellectual honesty is always required.)

For the attending. With the heart sound simulator, first play a soft murmur or sound that the student cannot hear. Next play a loud version of the same thing; then decrease the gain successively. Finally, present the same murmur at different places in the cardiac cycle. In this way, the student learns to hear murmurs that "other persons can't."

Timing the Cardiac Cycle

Do not assume that the timing of the cardiac cycle is obvious. You must make a positive identification of the first heart sound, by palpating the PMI, or ausculting at the apex where S1 will usually be the loudest sound. Unfortunately, many patients will not have a palpable PMI, and in some conditions (e.g., first-degree heart block) S1 will be diminished, even at the apex (see p. 292). In cases like these, use the carotid upstroke, which occurs very quickly after the beginning of systole. (See Ch. 18, p. 331 for a detailed discussion of the carotid artery pulse.) This is especially helpful when ausculting a patient with a highly chaotic rhythm (e.g., atrial fibrillation with an irregular ventricular response).

For the attending. Any student may be publicly chastised if he permits himself to be entrapped into attempting to identify a simulated murmur (see p. 303) as systolic or diastolic without requiring of the tester the simultaneous presentation of an independent nonacoustic event akin to the carotid artery pulse. It is for this reason that I believe all cardiac sound simulators should be viewed from the beginning with the simultaneous phonocardiograph and electrocardiograph displayed, not to teach electrocardiography, but to act as an external cue to time sequencing, thus getting the student into the indispensable habit of determining systole from the very beginning.

Any teacher of physical diagnosis who considers this issue to be overemphasized is invited to begin his lecture by playing recordings or heart-sound simulations of several diastolic murmurs. After the students have drawn the murmur shapes, turn off the sound and then ask them to state retrospectively whether each murmur occurred in systole or diastole.

Alternately, ask a seasoned cardiologist what kinds of valvular lesions have been missed at his institution. Aortic insufficiency and to a lesser degree mitral stenosis are frequently signed out as inexplicable cardiomyopathy. Review of the old records may reveal that murmurs ("systolic") have occasionally been recorded, even when the patient had no systolic murmur, but did have a diastolic one.

Traditional Areas of Auscultation

Certain of the precordial areas have, by tradition, been associated with certain cardiac sounds and certain murmurs. (The murmurs themselves are be discussed in greater detail on pp. 299–303.) The definitions to be used in this work are as follows:

The *aortic area* is the second right interspace at the sternal border. Aortic stenosis murmurs *should* be loudest here, or at the right midclavicle.

Formerly, clinicians auscicled in this area for the second heart sound, believing (incorrectly) that the intensity of the entire second sound here was a perfect measure of aortic valve closure. This condemnable practice has been shown phonocardiographically to be unsound (Weisse et al., 1967), and only created confusion about the meaning of the term "A2" (see Ch. 4, p. 69 and "advanced" section below).

The *pulmonic area* is the second left interspace at the sternal border. Pulmonic murmurs and murmurs of patent ductus arteriosus should be loudest here.

Formerly, clinicians auscicled for the second heart sound in this area in the erroneous belief that they were listening only to the pulmonic component. They incorrectly labeled this sound "P2" (see Ch. 4, p. 69) and inferred that by comparing it with the intensity of the second sound in the aortic area that they could make some sort of statement about the relative pressure relationships of the right and left circulations. They were often wrong. If one wants to make a statement about these relationships (see p. 295), one must compare the two components of the second sound *at the same place*, usually the pulmonic area, sometimes at the third left interspace along the sternal border, or rarely even at the aortic area.

Together, the aortic and pulmonic areas are referred to as the *base*. This is supposed to be the base of a triangle whose apex is the PMI.

The *tricuspid area* is in the fifth intercostal space at the *left* sternal border. This surprises some sophomores who believe that right heart valves should be to the right of the sternum. Well-localized tricuspid murmurs and some murmurs of IHSS are heard here.

The *mitral area* is just medial to the apex, which is located by palpation and percussion. (Normally it should be in the fifth intercostal space at the left midclavicular line.) S1 is best heard in this location. Also, one expects to hear mitral murmurs here.

In wide open mitral insufficiency, the left side of the heart enlarges and the apex and the mitral valve (in terms of their topical acoustic representations) move laterally, sometimes to the anterior axillary line or beyond. By some books' definitions, the mitral area is supposed to be fixed. *Nondimeno, esso muovo.**

Worse, in severe pulmonary hypertension with the right ventricle converted into a pressure chamber, the right ventricle enlarges, moving slightly leftward. The tricuspid valve, in terms of its topographic representation, moves with it and might eventually move

---

*"Nevertheless it moves" was Galileo's whispered comment after being forced to recant his theory that the earth moves around the sun. We clinicians honor Galileo, the medical school dropout, not only for his scientific devotion to truth but because he invented the thermometer, which led to Sanctorius and the clinical thermometer; the barometer, which led to Riva-Rocci and the sphygmomanometer; and the pendulum, which led to Huygens' clock and the rest of the vital signs.

---

to the original mitral area. Such tricuspid insufficiency can produce a loud holosystolic murmur at the so-called mitral area.

Accordingly, I think of the mitral area less as a constant point and more as a metaphysical concept.

The description of these areas should not be taken to mean that you should listen *only* at those points, as some books have suggested. Inching* along the sternum and the precordium is also important, especially for determining radiation and the loudest point of a murmur. This technique is also useful for distinguishing two murmurs that occur in the same time frame, as with the murmur of mitral insufficiency and the coexistent murmur of aortic stenosis. As one inches along, one notes that what was initially thought to be one murmur now displays different pitch and timbre (see "Dimensions," p. 299) in different parts of the chest.

Heart Sounds (S1 and S2)

A Self-Study

Figure 17-1 contains some heart sound illustrations. However, they are not marked according to the portion of the text to which they refer. Conversely, the text contains no indication of what narrative portion matches any of those illustrations. Your job is to label the illustrations correctly, write the legends, and indicate in the text which passages are illustrated by each illustration. You should be able to get some of them on the first reading and the remainder on the second reading. If you cannot, ask for help from a more experienced person.

First Heart Sound (S1)

After ausculting the first heart sound, you should be able to answer three questions: 1) Is the heart sound single or doubled (i.e., split or duplicated)? 2) What is the intensity? 3) Is it always of the same intensity?

Doubled S1. (a) A widely split or doubled S1 might be due to a delay in closure of the tricuspid valve due to right bundle branch block. In that case the second heart sound should also be abnormal with a wide fixed split.

A wider apparent split of S1 could in reality be (b) an S1 followed by an early systolic click S1 (S1-ESC), or (c) an S4 followed by an S1 (S4-S1). To distinguish reliably between these two possibilities requires a phonocardiograph with simultaneous ECG recording. There is no reliable bedside method (Shaver et al., 1985), although there are clues.

The sequence S1-ESC is known by the company it keeps, or rather by the company the ejection click keeps (i.e., one may diagnose S1-ESC by finding evidence of mitral valve prolapse, either a midsystolic murmur, or if one were very lucky the characteristic whoop or honk). Sometimes the first component is so high-pitched that one can immediately diagnose S1-ESC because the S4 of S4-S1 could not be so snapping.

The suspicion of S1-ESC due to mitral valve prolapse can be confirmed, even in the absence of a murmur, whoop, or honk, by reexamining the patient in the standing versus the recumbent positions. If the second component of the sequence moves earlier in systole (closer to the first sound) when the patient stands, it is highly likely that the two sounds represent S1-ESC. (If the suspected click does not move appreciably, then the maneuver is of no help.)

The other sequence, S4-S1, can sometimes be suggested by the brief, low-pitched rumbling vibrations of the S4. Sometimes,

---

*The technique of inching was named by Dr. Sam Levine.

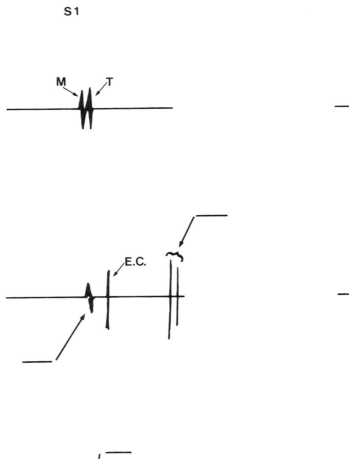

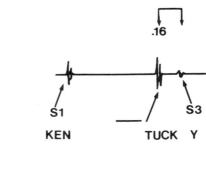

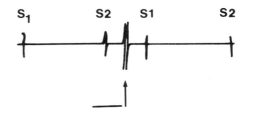

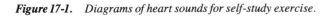

Figure 17-1.   *Diagrams of heart sounds for self-study exercise.*

one can palpate a low-frequency vibration (S4) occurring before the second component (S1). To so diagnose the S4 by palpation requires a large experience with thin patients. S4 may also change according to the maneuvers on page 299.

Listening with the bell, with alternate application of light and heavier pressure, might be helpful. If the extra sound is an S4, it may be more apparent with light pressure because of its low frequency. If it is an ESC, which is of higher pitch, it may be better appreciated as pressure turns the bell into a diaphragm.

Intensity of first heart sound.   Having determined whether the first heart sound is single, one next needs to listen for its intensity, which is usually best appreciated during auscultation near the apex, where S1 is normally louder than S2. If S2 is louder there, one has evidence for either an increase in the amplitude of the second heart sound (usually from an increase in P2, see pp. 294–295) or decreased amplitude of S1.

The intensity of S1 is primarily related to the degree of separation of the mitral valve leaflets at the onset of left ventricular systole (Shaver et al., 1985). An acoustic physicist could say that the intensity of S1 is due to the abruptness of valvular deceleration at closure. A musician could say that the intensity of S1 is due to the vigor with which the mitral valve and tricuspid valve beat shut. But a cardiologist might say that the intensity of S1 is due to the distance moved by the mitral and tricuspid valves before they are being slammed shut.

For convenience of discussion, we will subsequently confine ourselves to the mitral valve, which contributes most of the sound in S1. However, all statements also apply to the tricuspid valve.

(a) In first-degree heart block, the PR interval is prolonged, so that the mitral valve leaflets have to "wait" an extra few hundredths of a second before the (delayed) ventricular conduction slams them shut. During this delay, they float back toward the closed position, so that when the ventricular conduction finally occurs, they do not have quite so far to go. Thus, they produce a softer than usual S1, although S2 will continue to be of its usual intensity. (You might describe the resulting sounds as "lp dub," rather than the normal "lub dub.")

A muffled first heart sound does not always mean first-degree atrioventricular (AV) block.

(b) If a failing left ventricle cannot generate much pressure change per unit time, S1 may be muffled even though the sequence of AV conduction is of normal timing. You may already have made this diagnosis by looking at the neck veins, percussing the heart borders, and hearing a ventricular gallop. However, the left ventricular failure—possibly due to damage from ischemia, infarction, or aneurysm—is not always florid enough to have produced those other signs.

Other causes of a decrease in amplitude of S1 include: (c) left ventricular hypertrophy (Luisada & Portaluppi, 1983), (d) left bundle branch block (Luisada & Puppala, 1979), and (e) impaired apposition of the valves, as in mitral insufficiency. These may be distinguished by the PMI (see p. 285), paradoxical splitting of S2 (p. 295), and the characteristic murmur, respectively. (f) A muffled S1 due to asynergy of closure of the mitral and tricuspid valves need not result from a bundle branch block; an intraventricular conduction delay may suffice. This demonstrates the value of the electrocardiogram. (g) Hypertensive patients with normal PR intervals often have a soft S1 (Shaver et al., 1985).

An abnormal *increase* in the amplitude of S1 may occur in (a) mitral stenosis (which is associated with a characteristic murmur) or (b) hyperkinesis (as after vigorous exercise, excitement, exposure to a stressor, or high-output failure, see p. 310). (c) A booming S1 with aftervibrations has been noted in one patient with a left atrial myxoma (Shaver et al., 1985). (d) A recent study found that a loud S1 heard over the apex in patients with nonrheumatic mitral regurgitation is indicative of holosystolic mitral prolapse. Patients with the more common middle-to-late systolic prolapse have a normal S1 (Shaver et al., 1985).

Variable intensity of first heart sound.   Besides comparing the intensity of the normally louder apical S1 with the normally softer apical S2, it is important to listen for beat-to-beat variations in S1, again best done at the apex in most cases.

Second-degree heart block of Mobitz type I (but not of Mobitz type II) and third-degree heart block cause such a beat-to-beat variation.

In Mobitz type 1 heart block (see Ch. 6, p. 95), each successive PR interval is increased, until the skipped beat occurs. This causes a gradual diminution of intensity of the first, but not the second, heart sound. It may therefore be possible to diagnose second degree AV block from the missed beat, and to specify that the block is of Mobitz type 1 from the decreasing intensity of S1. The sound may be described like this: LUB-dub, lub-dub, lp-dub, pause, LUB-dub, lub-dub, lp-dub, pause, LUB-dub, lub-dub, lp-dub, pause, . . . It is easy to note the missed beat of second-degree AV block, but the change in intensity of the first heart sound with Mobitz type 1 is much more difficult to appreciate.

Musicians may wish to play the score in Figure 17-2A on a percussion instrument of their choice. The second heart sound is not shown for clarity of expression and because it does not change in intensity. The *ritardo* notation indicates a slight slowing, assuming the atrial rate to be the metronome. The decrescendo mark indicates the increasing softness of the S1 in each series.

The score for the first heart sound in Mobitz type II (see Ch. 6, p. 95) is musically much simpler (Fig. 17-2B), but clinically much more ominous. Since there is no prolongation of the PR interval before the dropped beat, there is no change in intensity of S1, and the sounds might be described thus: lub-dub, lub-dub, lub-dub, lub-dub, pause, lub-dub, lub-dub, lub-dub, lub-dub, pause, . . .

In third-degree heart block, none of the atrial impulses reach the ventricles. The atria beat regularly at their own rate, and the ventricles beat regularly at their own rate determined by the "escape" pacemaker (located in the AV node or lower). The atrial contraction (assuming that the atria are not fibrillating) continues to open widely the mitral (and tricuspid) valves. The ventricular contraction, occurring at an unrelated rate, closes the valves. But this random contraction may catch the AV valves at maximum excursion and slam them shut, producing a very loud sound. Or randomly, at minimal excursion, there will be a very soft sound. The variable intensity of S1, with normal S2, might thus be described: lub-dub, lp-dub, LUB-dub, Lub-dub, LUB-dub, lp-dub, Lub-dub, . . .

Musicians may wish to play "third-degree heart block" (Fig. 17-2C), which is scored for both heart sounds. However, S2 is of the same intensity throughout and may be ignored while ausculting for S1. S1 varies across the dynamic register. Note that the score is marked *largo*, to be played very slowly.

In fact, the only bradycardia with a variable S1 is third-degree heart block. Of course, a variable S1 may be heard in other forms of atrioventricular dissociation, but these will not produce a regular bradycardia.

While one might argue that third-degree heart block is best diagnosed with an electrocardiogram, there is still a place for bedside diagnosis, even in patients who are being electrocardiographically monitored; namely, some of the intensivists' unique and novel precordial leads are placed near the acromioclavicular joints and are not truly precordial exploring leads, but rather modified versions of lead I. If these are arranged so as to be perpendicular to the long axis of the P vector loop, the scalar P waves may be difficult to detect. On at least one occasion, it was possible to diagnose third-degree heart block by ausculting the patient while the beard-scratchers were puzzling over just such an afflictive tracing, and debating rearrangement of the leads.

Very advanced.   For pedagogic purposes, we have been speaking as if the heart sounds were produced by the valves clanging shut. However, Luisada believes that the heart sounds are really due to accelerations and decelerations of the "cardiohemic" system (the column of blood moving in relationship to the heart and vessels (Luisada & Portaluppi, 1983). Ordinarily, the

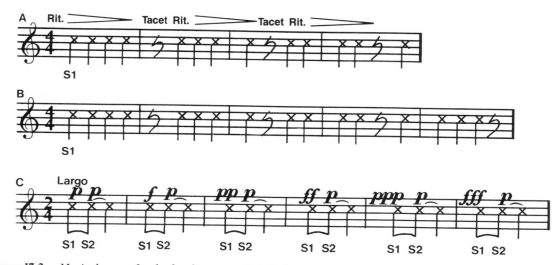

Figure 17-2. *Musical scores for the first heart sounds in Mobitz type I second-degree AV block (A) and Mobitz type II second-degree AV block (B) and for both heart sounds in third-degree heart block (C).*

accelerations and decelerations correlate in time with the valve events (although this is not always the case). Although the cardiohemic theory does agree with the empiric observations, there is a scientific rebuttal available (Dock, 1980).

Second Heart Sound (S2)

Amplitude of second heart sound. At the base, the collective S2 (A2 and P2 together) should be louder than S1. If it is not, something is different from normal.

Splitting of second heart sound. Normally, S2 is "split" during inspiration, and less so during expiration; this is known as "normal splitting." However, this phenomenon is not detectable in many normal persons. (*Historical note*: The normal inspiratory splitting of S2 was first described in 1866 by Potain [Leatham, 1954].)

The various types of splitting are diagrammed in Figure 17-3, to which you should refer while reading the discussions that follow.

The splitting is most likely to be found in the second or third left intercostal space, so these are the best places to *start* your search. Contrary to expert opinion, the splitting is not *always* most apparent there (Sainani et al., 1967).

Auscultation for splitting of S2 is useful for two reasons. First, if the splitting is not normal, this is a free clue to the existence of a small number of pathologic explanations (see p. 295). Second, even if the splitting is normal, the comparative intensities of the aortic (A2) and pulmonic (P2) components may often be useful information (see pp. 294–295).

The novice needs to be aware that initially S2 will not seem to have two distinct components but rather just a prolongation. One can learn this best with a heart sound simulator, which allows the A2-P2 interval to be mechanically varied. Alternately, or additionally, one can practice by tapping one's index and third finger on a hard surface, first simultaneously, then with one finger slightly after the other. In the latter situation, one can appreciate that two disparate events (the fingers tapping the desk) are felt as separate, but initially heard as one sound. With increasing intervals between the two taps, the sound becomes "longer" in duration; only when very wide temporal intervals are attained does

one actually hear a splitting into two distinct components. The latter is itself a sign of pathology in an adult (not in a child); if initially you can easily hear S2 split into two distinct sounds, you are probably hearing an abnormally wide split (.06 second or more) or a second heart sound followed either by a third heart sound or an opening snap.

A further problem with this psychoacoustic event is that the second component (P2) is often softer than the first component. Unfortunately, a soft sound following a loud sound is more difficult to appreciate as a separate event than is a loud sound following a soft sound with the same interval of separation. (This too can best be learned with a heart sound simulator.)

Failure of the beginner to realize that the "split" is at first a learned perception, not an easily apparent auscultatory event, is partly responsible for failure to utilize the convenient information that can thus be obtained.

Semiophysiology. The relatively negative intrathoracic pressure produced during inspiration sucks the blood into the right (but not the left) heart in excess of that which arrives during the expiratory phase. This extra blood results in a slightly increased right (but not left) ventricular ejection time. (It takes longer to empty an overcrowded elevator than one that is simply full.) The slight delay in the subsequent pulmonic closure sound produces splitting.

A second explanation for the normal delay in pulmonic closure during inspiration is that the capacitance of the pulmonary vasculature (but not of the systemic vasculature) is increased during inspiration. Thus there is less left ventricular filling. This in turn shortens the left ventricular ejection time (vis-à-vis that of the right) and so the A2 sound comes even earlier than usual, thus widening the split, as compared with the split in expiration (Curtiss et al., 1975). Note that the two explanations are not mutually exclusive, and may both be operational.

A method. Since the splitting is produced by the dynamic events in the chest, one cannot listen for splitting in held inspiration or held expiration (cf. pulsus paradoxus, p. 91). Those maneuvers will simply abolish the change. Rather, the patient must continue to breathe while one listens.

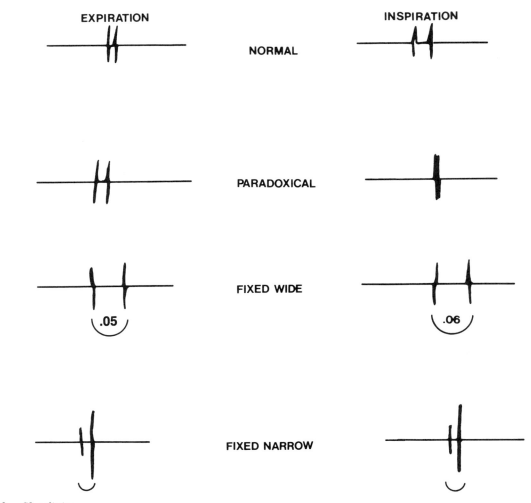

Figure 17-3. S2 splitting.

1. First listen only to those S2s that occur during expiration. Ignore anything that you hear during inspiration until you have a clear mental picture of the (baseline) S2 in expiration again. This will not be a mental picture of two discrete events as pictured in most textbooks, unless there is an abnormality; rather it is a sound image whose important dimension (at this point) is duration.

If you do perceive a split in expiration, then the patient either has fixed splitting of S2, paradoxical splitting of S2, or a normal S2 followed by an extra sound. The differential diagnosis of all of these is discussed beginning on page 295.

2. After you have a clear mental image of the expiratory S2, switch your acoustic attention to S2 in mid-to-end inspiration. It may be necessary to listen through several respiratory cycles. When you are first learning this technique, it may take so many respiratory cycles to develop a mental image of the inspiratory S2 that you have forgotten what the expiratory baseline (S2) sounded like. In that case, switch back to the expiratory phase and listen again. The question you must finally answer is this: Are the inspiratory S2s longer than the expiratory ones? If so, S2 is said to be normally split (proceed to "Relative intensity of A2 and P2".) If not, go to "Paradoxical splitting" on page 295.

Further considerations on the second heart sound:

1. It is easier to hear the normally split second heart sound in the upright position, since upright posture exaggerates most respiratory effects (unless there has been considerable cardiac failure). (Contributed by Dr. David Spodick of Massachusetts.)

2. As the student becomes more experienced, he will begin to readily identify longer and shorter second heart sounds. Next, he will find that he can actually begin to hear the inspiratory split. That is, he can actually hear two components to the split second sound, whereas before he could only hear a "long" sound, but could not clearly identify the two components. When this happens to the student, he will begin to appreciate for the first time that there are many perfectly normal persons with *distinctly* split second heart sounds, though the interval is normal. This is not a sign of increased prevalence of disease in one's classmates, but of improved skills.

Relative intensity of A2 and P2.   Once you have determined that S2 is normally split, you should compare the two components. This can usually be done most easily in inspiration, when the splitting is maximal. Normally, the aortic component (A2) is louder than the pulmonic component (P2), even over the pulmonic area. This produces a sound that musicians call diminuendo. You may familiarize yourself with this sound by returning to the finger-tapping exercise, this time striking the first finger much harder than the last. (It may take a little practice to produce the sound you desire.)

Accentuation of the aortic second sound may result from increased back pressure on the aortic valve leaflets, as in arterial hypertension. Sometimes this sound is said to have a tambour quality (like that of a tambourine without the metal discs in the rim). Other causes of an accentuated second sound include aortic insufficiency, coarctation, aneurysm of the ascending aorta, and rarely aortic stenosis (DeGowin, 1965).

At other times, the two components of S2 are equal. This can be pathologic, or it may simply mean that your stethoscope is closer to the origin of P2 than to the origin of A2. This finding needs to be recorded as A2 = P2, but it does not require an immediate explanation.

However, sometimes P2 is clearly louder than A2. The sound here is crescendo. Again, you can practice hearing this sound with the finger-tapping exercise, this time striking the first finger more vigorously. (For those who have played the drums, this will be remembered as the sound of a flam.) If P2 is louder than A2, an explanation is required. Either P2 is abnormally increased (as in pulmonary hypertension), or A2 is decreased (as in calcific or rheumatic aortic stenoses, which decrease the recursion of the aortic valve.)

In situations in which it is not possible to distinguish A2 from P2 on the basis of a recognizable type of splitting of S2, try inching down the left sternal border. The aortic component normally radiates further than the pulmonic component, so the latter will drop out first in the course of inching away. (This does not work with severe pulmonary hypertension.)

Single S2. Any condition that delays A2 may produce a "single S2," that is, one in which the splitting interval is less than 0.03 second. Also, conditions in which one component of S2 is either absent or inaudible will produce a single S2 (e.g., severe tetralogy of Fallot, severe semilunar valve stenosis, pulmonic valve atresia, most cases of tricuspid valve atresia, and other complex forms of congenital heart disease). But the most common cause of a single S2 in the general population is age greater than 50 years.

This finding has been attributed to a delayed A2, although a decreased inspiratory delay in P2 has also been reported (Shaver et al., 1985).

Paradoxical splitting. If S2 is "longer" i.e., more split) during expiration than inspiration, the splitting is called paradoxical. In this instance, A2 and P2 have reversed their sequence: P2 is now first. (*Self-test:* Can you recall the normal order of closure of the heart valves? If you have trouble, the mnemonic is "*many things are possible.*")

Paradoxical splitting may be due to anything that causes premature closure of the pulmonic valve, either by selectively shortening the right ventricular ejection time (patent ductus arteriosus with a left-to-right shunt through the ductus or rare cases of tricuspid insufficiency), or more commonly by selectively lengthening left ventricular ejection time. The last may result from electrical (such as left bundle branch block) or mechanical causes. Examples of the latter include ischemic heart disease and aortic stenosis (and possibly systemic hyperten-

sion). Although relatively minor aortic valve deformities may produce a murmur, paradoxical splitting implies that the stenosis is hemodynamically significant.

1. An additional cause for paradoxic splitting is early electrical activation of the right ventricle in Wolff-Parkinson-White syndrome, type B (Shaver et al., 1985).

2. A patient with left ventricular hypertrophy secondary to aortic stenosis had the latter repaired with a Bjork-Shiley valve, after which the patient still had a paradoxically split S2. Possibly, his left ventricular ejection time was still mechanically prolonged through some combination of fatigued myocardium and the slightly increased afterload caused by the prosthetic valve.

3. Paradoxical splitting is a rare finding in uncomplicated hypertension. The original teaching was that paradoxical splitting of S2 could occur in "systolic" hypertension. I agree that very rarely one can find a paradoxical splitting of S2 in diastolic hypertension. But since this may be due to a prolonged left ventricular ejection time (due to the high resistance systemic circulation into which the stroke volume must be driven), it should relate to increased peripheral vascular resistance, not just the systolic blood pressure. All things being equal, the systemic vascular resistance will be proportional to the mean arterial blood pressure, which in turn will be closer to the diastolic blood pressure than to the systolic (see the formula on p. 90). Thus, the hypertension that causes a paradoxical splitting of S2 should be best described as "systemic" (since it is selective for the greater circulation) rather than "systolic."

Another potential explanation for paradoxical splitting of S2 in systemic hypertension is the cardiomyopathy produced by the chronic hypertension. At first glance, this seems unlikely because cardiomyopathies are usually not accompanied by this finding. However, most cardiomyopathies make the right and left ventricles equally sluggish, whereas hypertensive cardiomyopathy could selectively increase left ventricular ejection time, since the precapillary pulmonary vascular resistance is normal, while the systemic vascular resistance is increased.

Pseudoparadoxical splitting:

1. Pseudoparadoxical splitting of S2 is due to the loss of P2 with inspiration due to the increasing distance of the heart from the stethoscope head, producing the "narrow" S2 of aortic valve-only closure during inspiration, and a normal S2 (A2 plus P2) during expiration. This is especially likely to occur in patients with severe chronic obstructive lung disease, who have a widely split S2 due to delayed closure of the pulmonic valve (so that the split is well heard during expiration) (Shaver et al., 1985).

2. Pseudoparadoxical splitting may also occur in some cases of constrictive pericarditis, where there is a peculiar splitting of the second heart sound, which is heard only at the beginning of inspiration (Beck et al., 1962).

Wide fixed splitting. If the second heart sound is split both during inspiration and expiration, it is said to have a fixed split. A fixed wide split of S2 can be due to delayed closure of the pulmonic valve, or to premature closure of the aortic valve. Delayed closure of the pulmonic valve can be electrical, as in right bundle branch block, or mechanical, from a selectively prolonged right ventricular ejection time. The latter can be from valvular pulmonic stenosis or from selective volume overload of the right heart as in atrial septal defect or partial anomalous pulmonary venous return. (Also see decreased pulmonary vascular impedance in Table 17-3.) Early closure of the aortic valve may result from a decreased left ventricular ejection time from either

Table 17-3.   Causes of Wide Splitting of the Second Heart Sound

Delayed Pulmonic Closure
  Delayed electrical activation of the right ventricle
    Complete RBBB (proximal type)
    Left ventricular paced beats
    Left ventricular ectopic beats
  Prolonged right ventricular ejection time
    Acute massive pulmonary embolus
    Pulmonary hypertension with right heart failure
    Pulmonic stenosis with intact septum (moderate to severe)
  Decreased impedance of the pulmonary vascular bed
    Normotensive atrial septal defect
    Idiopathic dilatation of the pulmonary artery
    Pulmonic stenosis
    Atrial septal defect, postoperative (70%)
Early Aortic Closure
  Shortened left ventricular mechanical systole (LVET)
    Mitral insufficiency
    Ventricular septal defect

Source: *Shaver et al. (1985).*

mitral insufficiency or a ventricular septal defect with a left to right shunt. (The latter also produces volume overload of the right ventricle.)

This sort of split is not always fixed, in the sense of being, say, 0.073 second in both inspiration and expiration. But because the split is very wide, the pulmonic and aortic components never get close enough together to make the normal mushy slurred single sound in expiration that is customarily and easily compared to the more prolonged split in inspiration. Hence the components of S2 are acoustically "fixed" in a (variably) split position.

The wide split S2 associated with delayed electrical activation of the right ventricle (right bundle branch block) is often accompanied by wide splitting of the first heart sound as well (see p. 290) (Shaver et al., 1985).

False-positive wide fixed splitting includes:
1. A normal S2 followed by the opening snap of mitral stenosis or tricuspid stenosis. The opening snap is discussed in detail later (see p. 319); for the present, it is sufficient to note that the interval between S2 and the opening snap is quite easily appreciated; the snap sounds exactly like a click or a snap; and the opening snap will become louder as one moves away from the base of the heart toward the mitral (or tricuspid) valve area, whereas the S2 will become softer.
2. The wide fixed split S2 must also be distinguished from a normal (single) S2 followed by a ventricular gallop (S3, vida infra). Again, the gallop can be heard better as one moves away from the pulmonic area down toward the responsible ventricle. Furthermore, the gallop is a low-pitched sound that can be better heard with the bell than with the diaphragm, in contrast to S2.
3. A pericardial knock of constrictive pericarditis can also imitate a wide fixed split S2 (see p. 306).

Once you are sure that the double sound is not one of the above, but a fixed split of S2, you must compare A2 and P2 (vide supra) and also assign an etiology to this abnormal finding.

Narrow fixed splitting.   It is apparent that wide fixed splitting of S2 is heard in many situations in which the right ventricular pressure and/or the pulmonary artery pressure are increased in the presence of a normal pulmonary vascular capacitance. However, when pulmonary hypertension occurs in the absence of volume overload, the second heart sound may have a narrow fixed split. Examples would be long-standing primary pulmonary hypertension and pulmonary hypertension due to repeated embolic epi-

sodes. Narrow fixed splitting is heard only by the experienced auscultor.

Some speculation.   If a wide fixed split of the second heart sound can be heard in atrial septal defect, partial anomalous pulmonary venous return, and ventricular septal defect (left to right shunt), why is it not found in pulmonic insufficiency, which can also be considered a form of volume overload of the right side of the heart? Conversely, if volume overload of the left side of the heart could delay left ventricular ejection time, why doesn't aortic insufficiency make the second heart sound paradoxically split?

Perhaps in these conditions the valvular insufficiency does not initially permit sufficient regurgitation to produce true volume overload. Ultimately, when the insufficiency is great enough to produce volume overload, an ejection murmur appears, mimicking aortic stenosis, due to the "functional" stenosis of high flow over a normal size valve (see p. 300). In that case, any paradoxical splitting that occurred would be falsely attributed to the supposed aortic stenosis (*mutatis mutandis* on the right side).

An accessible, reproducible, quantitative method for comparing regurgitant volume with stroke volume might help answer these questions.

A related question is why the second heart sound splits widely in volume overload pulmonary hypertension, and narrowly in vasculoprival pulmonary hypertension. In volume overload hypertension, of which atrial septal defect is the archetype, the large amount of right ventricular stroke volume is being delivered to a slack pulmonary vascular tree whose compliance is so high that one can fluoroscopically observe the pulmonary tree to move in systole (the "hilar dance"). Thus, it takes a long time for the pulmonary artery pressure to exceed right ventricular pressure and so to close the pulmonic valve. But in vasculoprival pulmonary hypertension due to the occlusion of the pulmonary vascular bed by clot, tumor, foreign body embolus, and so forth, there is not much compliance in the pulmonary vascular tree, and the pulmonary artery pressure rapidly rises in excess of the right ventricular pressure, closing the pulmonic valve more quickly (Shaver et al., 1985). (A small elevator fills faster than a large one.)

Self-Test.   Construct a logic tree for findings on auscultation of the second heart sound. One correct answer is found in Figure 17-4.

Note to sophomores.   At this point, you may be asking why so much detail? It would certainly be possible to acquire much of this inferential information in other ways. If the diagnosis can be arrived at through the use of shortcuts, why go through all this complexity?

One answer (which avoids the issue of cost) is that as a general principle of medicine, anyone who knows the mental geography of the problem is entitled to use shortcuts. But you can't know it is a shortcut until you know the whole neighborhood in detail. Many of the people who believe they are using shortcuts are, in fact, simply lost.

Gallops (S3 and S4)

Gallops are adventitious cardiac sounds that change the regular rhythm of "lub dub" into a triple rhythm resembling a horse's gallop, or more correctly, canter. Also, like a horse's hoof beat, these are low-pitched sounds, resembling a man's grunt, and are best heard with the bell of the stethoscope. Because they are lower pitched than the other heart sounds, the neophyte should specifically note the pitch of the gallop so as to help his auditors be sure that he is describing a gallop and not something else.

The other dimensions that should be described for a gallop are timing, location, and change with maneuvers.

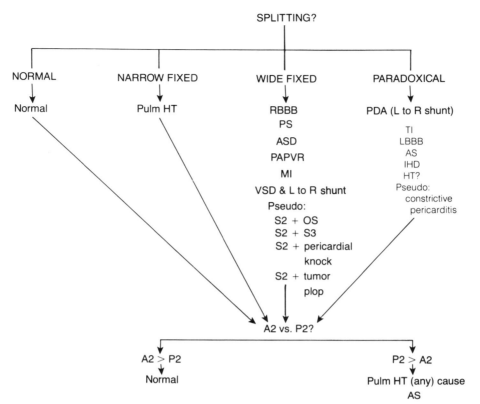

Figure 17-4. *Branching logic tree for S2 splitting. Pulm HT, pulmonary hypertension; RBBB, right bundle branch block; PS, pulmonic stenosis; ASD, atrial septal defect; PAPVR, partial anomalous pulmonary venous return; MI, mitral insufficiency; VSD, ventricular septal defect; L to R, left-to-right shunt; OS, opening snap; MS, mitral stenosis; TS, tricuspid stenosis; PDA, patent ductus arteriosus; TI, tricuspid insufficiency; LBBB, left bundle branch block; AS, aortic stenosis; IHD, ischemic heart disease; HT, hypertension.*

Note on Use of Bell and Diaphragm of Stethoscope

We speak of using the bell, *lightly* applied to the chest, for detecting low-pitched sounds, and the diaphragm for detecting high-pitched sounds. This has led some young persons to expect, erroneously, that a low-pitched sound such as a gallop would not be heard if ausculted with the diaphragm. In fact, the diaphragm is a superior auscultatory device for many sounds since the transmission is from solid to solid. The lightly applied bell detects high-pitched sounds, but *preferentially* detects low-pitched sounds. Thus, when there are many sound events across a wide frequency spectrum, the lightly applied bell directs one's attention more to those of lower pitch, but many of these are also discernible with the diaphragm.

Timing

The rule of listening specifically to one phase of the cycle at a time is especially important for finding subtle sounds like ventricular gallops.

○   A useful teaching trick to help you hear (as well as identify) a ventricular diastolic gallop (an S3) is to say the word "Kentucky" with the Southern pronunciation "Ken-TUCK-uh." The syllable "ken" stands for S1, "tuck" stands for S2, and "uh" is the S3. In normally spoken English, the interval between the last two syllables will approximate the interval between S2 and S3. Once you have identified S1 and S2, silently say the word "Kentuck(y)" as you listen. This helps to cue your ear to the portion of early diastole (*before* atrial contraction), which contains the gallop.

For the atrial diastolic gallop (S4), think of the word "(Ten)nessee," where the first syllable stands for the gallop. Again, the interval between the first two syllables will closely approximate the interval between S4 and S1. Unfortunately, the customary pronunciation of the word places the accent on the third syllable, whereas in auscultation at the apex, the stress should be on S1.

Remember, listen to one time at a time.

Gallops in Patients with a Tachycardia

Since S3 and S4 occur in different parts of diastole, it becomes obvious that one can sometimes hear what is called a quadruple rhythm: S4, S1, S2, S3. But if the heart rate speeds up, the S3 and S4 may occur at the same time, making a knocking sound called a summation gallop (Fig. 17-5).

○   If you have a patient with a very fast heart rate and a single loud gallop in diastole, slow the patient's heart rate briefly either by having the patient perform the Valsalva maneuver (see Ch. 6, p. 98) or by pressing on the carotid sinus (see Ch. 18, p. 336). If the sound in diastole is a summation gallop, you will be able to hear the quadruple rhythm appear during the relative slowing of the heart. It will disappear again as the S3 and S4 fuse together into the triple rhythm summation gallop with resumption of the tachycardia.

If the induced slowing of the heart does *not* produce a quadruple rhythm, then the diastolic sound is either S3 or S4; one must determine which one it is in the customary manner.

Since one will have only a few beats to make the distinction, one must have a prepared ear. This is why the beginning medical student should gain mastery of many physical maneuvers that are

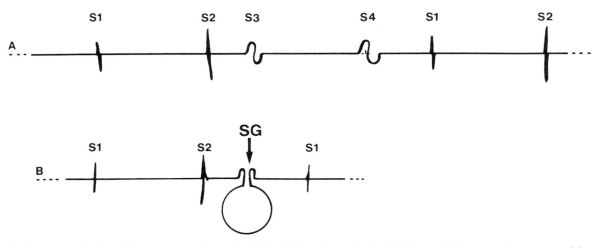

Figure 17-5. *A, Quadruple gallop; B, summation gallop (SG). With tachycardia, the R-R interval shortens at the expense of diastole, the distance between S2 and S1. The portion of diastole that shortens is that between S3 and S4. You can make a topologic model of this by putting a pencil or other cylinder on the page between S3 and S4 in Figure 17-5A, and bending the page so that S3 and S4 occur next to each other, or superimposed. (The page, viewed from the edge, would then look as shown in B.)*

infrequently used, but which must be applied in less than desirable circumstances that do not permit the examiner a leisure study.

If an S4 is palpable, it is easier to identify in the presence of a tachycardia. One need palpate only *two* impulses per cardiac cycle. These will be located close together in time, at the PMI, just as diastole changes to systole. With auscultation, on the other hand, one must identify a minimum of three events per cardiac cycle, and must also arrange them mentally so as to identify them.

Very advanced. Dr. Joe Ojile of Missouri heard a quintuple rhythm, the description of which was greeted with open skepticism by the full professors at morning report.* However, he was vindicated when he produced the patient's electrocardiogram. The patient was in a Mobitz type II block with 2:1 conduction. The "extra" gallop (fifth sound) was appearing coincident with the nonconducted atrial contraction. Thus, this patient had an S1, S2, S3, and two atrial gallops, one occurring with each atrial contraction.

Location

Both the S3 and the S4 are generally best heard over the left sternal border near the xiphoid, if originating from the right ventricle. If originating from the left ventricle, they are best heard toward the apex.

Response to Maneuvers

Exercise augments both third and fourth heart sounds. A few sit-ups may be all that is required (Perloff, 1980).

An S3 arising from the right ventricle (but *not* one from the left ventricle) *may* be evoked or augmented by maneuvers that increase flow to the right side of the heart, such as: 1) inspiration, 2) passive elevation of the patient's legs, or 3) pressure on the liver. If such maneuvers do *not* augment the gallop, one does not know whether it is left- or right-sided or both.

The same maneuvers may be used to attempt to differentiate right- and left-sided S4s.

---

*A nearly extinct practice, in which a chief of service who is a broadly based internist hears the presentation (by a doctor who has personally and thoroughly examined the patient) and offers a critical analysis of each such patient newly admitted.

Significance

Ventricular gallop (S3). An S3 usually indicates that ventricular compliance is subnormal. It is the only central (cardiac) sign of congestive heart failure, and is extremely important in the diagnosis of this entity. In fact, the presence of an audible S3 should ordinarily be considered diagnostic of congestive heart failure, until proven otherwise. It is the failing heart's way of saying: "I have such a low ejection fraction that as soon as the added blood from the atrium even *starts* to fill me (i.e., even before the atrial kick), it beats as a mallet against my tired, fatigued, completely noncompliant drumhead."

Patients with tricuspid insufficiency or mitral insufficiency are also stated to have ventricular diastolic gallops even without congestive heart failure. (Presumably the drumhead need not be of decreased compliance if the mallet is big enough, which it would be when the stroke volume is composed of both the venous inflow and a large regurgitant volume from the last systole.) This gallop is not heard with mild degrees of insufficiency.

Other causes of an S3 not due to congestive failure are hypertrophic cardiomyopathy, right ventricular infarct, or constrictive pericarditis (Reddy et al., 1985). The last *may* actually be a pericardial knock (see p. 306).

False positives: The most common false positive is a "physiologic S3," sometimes heard in a perfectly healthy young person, under the age of about 20, or some may say 40 (Reddy et al., 1985).

Although a stenotic mitral valve impedes ventricular filling and so may inhibit the appearance of a pathologic S3, it does not always prevent the occurrence of a left-sided physiologic S3 (Reddy et al., 1985).

Other sounds occurring around the same time as the S3 (see Table 17-7), which are thus potential false positives, include a widely split S2 (p. 296), an opening snap (p. 306), the tumor plop (p. 306), and the pericardial knock (p. 306).

Atrial gallop (S4). A pathologic S4 is due to the blood rushing into a ventricle with decreased compliance. The ventricular compliance has been "used up" by the blood that entered in early diastole. (It is as if the drumhead has been tightened.) The blood coming into the ventricle during atrial contraction acts as a mallet striking the noncompliant drumhead of the ventricle. (The name "atrial" refers not to the source of the noise, but to the late diastolic atrial contraction that usually propels the "mallet of blood.")

If the S4 is heard only some of the time, irrespective of the respiratory cycle, this can be a clue to the presence of complete AV dissociation. Why?
(Rarely, however, one can find an atrial gallop in situations in which there is no atrial "kick," e.g., in atrial fibrillation.)
False positives: Inexperienced examiners often believe an S4 to be present even when it is not recordable, perhaps confusing it with a split S1 (Jordan et al., 1987).

Until 1968, the differential diagnosis of an S4 was as follows: aortic stenosis and equivalents (such as IHSS), or hypertension (left-sided S4); pulmonic stenosis or pulmonary hypertension (right-sided S4); coronary artery disease (right- or left-sided S4).

It is also stated that situations of high stroke volume can produce an S4. In fact, a pathologic S4 can result anytime there is decreased left ventricular compliance from heart disease. Here, one should also hear an S3, although if the heart rate is fast, S3 and S4 might appear as a summation gallop (vide supra). However, specific etiologies of congestive heart failure (such as hyperthyroidism and anemia) do not in themselves cause an S4 unless heart failure has supervened, contrary to the implication in some textbooks of differential diagnosis.
Atrial flutter may also cause a pathologic S4 (Reddy et al., 1985).

In the 1970s, Spodick published an elegant series of doubleblind experiments that showed that many apparently normal men over age 50 had an audible (but not a palpable) S4, which could be recorded (Rectra et al., 1972; Spodick, 1977; Swistak et al., 1974). This phenomenon is much more common than the innocent S3 of healthy young persons.

The traditionalists did not give up without a rigorous defense, and the issue is still controversial (Abram, 1975; Fowler & Adolph, 1972; Jordan et al., 1987; Wayne, 1974).

Personal opinion: At the present one may ignore an isolated, impalpable S4 in an asymptomatic man over age 50. However, if the S4 is palpable, accord it the full respect of the pre-1968 differential diagnosis given above, irrespective of the patient's age (Reddy et al., 1985). (In practice, this works almost all the time, despite the controversy.)

Murmurs

Historical Perspective

Murmurs have traditionally been among the most valuable signs of structural heart disease. For years, the ability of a physician to auscult and interpret cardiac murmurs helped to make his reputation. For a number of reasons, this situation has changed. First, many of the people skilled in this area and its teaching have emigrated from the medical schools. Second, the prevalence of patients with murmurs has decreased because of the waning of rheumatic fever and, to a lesser extent, advances in

the surgical correction of congenital heart defects. Third, the whole manner in which patients were studied has increasingly involved sophisticated imaging technology. The current generation of Doppler echocardiographs promises to achieve the dream of accurate, noninvasive delineation of all murmur-producing cardiac structural defects, cashing the diagnostic promissory notes previously written (in varying degrees) for the techniques of electrocardiography, ballistocardiography, vectorcardiography, phonocardiography, external pulse recordings, kymocardiography, M-mode echocardiography, and probably a few others now mercifully forgotten. If one were skilled at Doppler echocardiography and had access to the machine for every patient, this section would mostly be of use to the historian of medicine. However, since financial, political, and economic constraints appear to make that eventuality increasingly remote, this section is provided on a portable diagnostic device used for detecting murmurs known as CANDID, for its acronym "*C*omputer-*A*ssisted *N*on-*D*oppler *I*nfra-ultrasound *D*evice." It is "computer assisted" by the portable computer that sits on top of your neck. It is "infra-ultrasound" because it operates at low sound frequencies (20 to 50,000 Hz), beneath the range of the ultrasound device, and the word "Doppler" is mentioned to be *á la mode*. Its inventor, Dr. Laennec, originally gave it a whimsical name ("stethoscope"), suggesting that it would enable the physician to see into the chest, and this no doubt has contributed to its unpopularity. In fact, this device is so arcane that no restrictive regulations yet govern its use.

An Epistemologic Note

In one study, five experts could agree as to whether a murmur was present or absent in only 53% of the cases (Dobrow et al., 1964). What does this mean?
The answer is that it is always possible to find someone who cannot do something (Butterworth & Reppert, 1960), but that this does not mean that the thing cannot be done. Another way of saying it, more kindly, is that there can be a problem of observer variability (Koran, 1975).

Dimensions

The dimensions that one should attempt to describe for every murmur are:

1. Timing
2. Shape
3. Location
4. Radiation
5. Pitch (tone)
6. Timbre (purity of pitch)
7. Intensity
8. Effects of special maneuvers, including change in patient position

Table 17-4 illustrates how the first six dimensions, when taken together, are diagnostically specific. The effects of special maneuvers are discussed on page 307.

Timing

The timing of a murmur places it into one of two mutually exclusive differential diagnoses: systolic murmurs and diastolic murmurs. Additionally, while some systolic murmurs are innocent, or at least not due to structural defects of the heart, few diastolic murmurs are without pathologic significance.

Table 17-4.   Customary (but Not Inviolate) Dimensions of the Valvular Murmurs

Lesion	Timing	Shape	Location	Radiation	Pitch	Timbre	Intensity
AS	Sys	Diamond	A	Carotids, RMClav	L to H	Coarse to pure	2–4
AI	Dias	Decrescendo	A	Sternal borders	H to M	Coarse to pure	1–2
MS	Dias	Decrescendo-crescendo	M	Almost none	L to M	Rumbling	1–4
MI	Sys	Holosystolic or diamond	M	Axilla	L to H	Pure to coarse	2–4
PS[a]	Sys	Diamond	P	Little	L to H	Coarse	2–4
PI	Dias	Same as AI	P	Left sternal border	H to M	Coarse	1–2
TS	Dias	Same as MS	T	Almost none	L to M	Rumbling	1–2
TI	Sys	Holosystolic or diamond	T	See text	L to H	Coarse to pure	1–2

A, aortic; M, mitral; P, pulmonic; T, tricuspid; I, insufficiency (regurgitation); S, stenosis; RMClav, right midclavicle; H, high; M, medium; L, low; Sys, systolic; Dias, diastolic.

[a]Most of the murmurs of most congenital heart defects that have a left-to-right shunt are actually due to relative pulmonic stenosis (i.e., to increase flow over a normal-sized pulmonic valve), not to flow through the defect(s). Patent ductus arteriosus is the constant exception to this rule.

A method.   Review the methods for identifying the first heart sound (p. 289). Once you have found S1, switch your attention away from the palpable PMI or the carotid upstroke and pay attention to the murmur. If it occurs after the first heart sound, then it *must* be in systole. If it is not in systole, it *must* be in diastole. Although this sounds simple, it takes about 10 practice trials to learn it. However, as with the rest of the clinical examination, once you have it, you will never lose it.

Shape

The shape of the murmur is what it would look like on an oscilloscope display or a phonocardiographic recording—see the schematic tracings illustrated in Figures 17-6 and 17-7.

Systolic murmurs.   For systolic murmurs, there are two basic possibilities: the murmur may be diamond shaped or holosystolic.

1. A diamond-shaped murmur may also be called kite shaped, or crescendo-decrescendo, referring to the electrocardiographic appearance (Fig. 17-7).

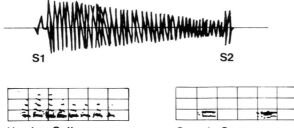

Figure 17-6.   *This holosystolic murmur used to be called a sea gull murmur, primarily because of the timbre. (Other causes of the sea gull timbre are given on p. 302.) The insets show Audubon Society recordings of the herring sea gull and the Canadian honking goose (Robbins et al., 1966). (Although traditionally shown and sounding as if it had the same amplitude throughout systole, the holosystolic murmur actually may have a slight decrease in amplitude. Notice that the "holosystolic" bird calls are also slightly decrescendo.)*

The term *ejection murmur* is often used, but is confusing because certain types of regurgitant (*nonejection*) murmurs (such as those due to tricuspid or mitral valve prolapse, papillary muscle dysfunction, or the midsystolic failure of coaption of the mitral valve leaflets that occurs in idiopathic hypertrophic subaortic stenosis) can also have this shape.

The diamond-shaped murmur results from systolic turbulent flow at any of the four valves, and is not as diagnostic as some of the other shapes (Table 17-4).

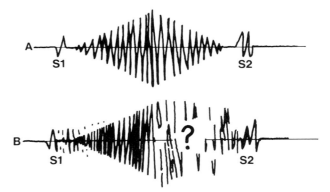

Figure 17-7.   *A, Diamond-shaped or kite-shaped murmur. A phonocardiographic recording is diagramatically represented here. In recent.years, the mirror-image vibrations beneath the baseline have not been shown in diagrams (e.g., Fig. 17-8, a point of confusion for the tyro, who now sees a pyramid and not a diamond). B, The diamond-shaped murmur as it may sound to a beginning student. For instance, preceding the ejection murmur the slight pause after S1 may (or may not) be perceived. Further, it may be initially difficult to distinguish the crescendo component. Then too, once the brain has adjusted its perceptive mechanism to the increasing amplitude, the subsequent decrescendo may be missed. (Remember that auscultation is a psychoacoustic event.) The shapes of murmurs were only appreciated after recordings became available, and are best learned with devices like a phonocardiogram or heart sound simulator that reinforce auscultation with simultaneous visual presentation.*

While it is traditional to think of the murmur as turbulence due to a normal amount of blood trying to get through a small hole, it should be obvious that a similar sound will be made by an increased amount of blood trying to get through a normal-sized hole. In other words, one can have a murmur of aortic stenosis, say, or pulmonic stenosis, when the actual aortic or pulmonic valves are completely normal, but the amount of blood flow is increased. These are called *flow murmurs* or murmurs of relative stenosis (also see p. 314). Pulmonic flow murmurs frequently occur during the last trimester of pregnancy or with congenital heart diseases that cause left-to-right shunts. Aortic flow murmurs may be heard in all conditions in which there is increased stroke volume, such as pregnancy, fever, anemia, thyrotoxicosis, and excitement with tachycardia.

If there is no underlying valvular disease, the pure flow murmur is usually heard better at the pulmonic area than at the aortic area for two reasons: 1) The aortic murmur is anatomically "pointed" away from the anterior chest (superiorly and posteriorly with the aorta), while the pulmonic murmur is "pointed" to the lungs and still heard at the left upper sternal border. 2) The pulmonic valve is normally a bit smaller than the aortic and so will sound the flow murmur better. But if there is so much as a little bit of aortic sclerosis, the flow murmur due to anemia, fever, and so forth will augment the basic underlying murmur and will be heard best at the aortic, not the pulmonic area.

2. A holosystolic murmur continues throughout systole, maintaining the same apparent amplitude and timbre. It comes from the Greek prefix meaning entire, or complete in the sense of being without blemish, variation, or change. If there is any *significant* change in intensity, timbre, or any other characteristic, the murmur is not holosystolic, even if it seems to fill all the time during systole (i.e., even if it is pansystolic, which simply means "across systole"). Holosystolic murmurs are due to mitral, or sometimes tricuspid, insufficiency.

Specifically, the holosystolic murmur results from *severe* mitral (or tricuspid) insufficiency, for example, that due to bacterial endocarditis or severe rheumatic heart disease, in which the mitral insufficiency is fixed and gaping.

Auscultors from the rheumatic fever era believed that such holosystolic murmurs started before the first heart sound (presumably during the phase of isometric contraction).

3. On the other hand, the *non*holosystolic murmur of aortic stenosis is preceded by a silent period after S1. Also, in cases of mitral insufficiency due not to rheumatic valvular disease but to, say, papillary muscle dysfunction, there is no murmur during that time (early systole) when the valve leaflets are still competent. (In practice, it can be hard to prove these differences without a phonocardiograph.)

The time that a diamond-shaped murmur ends, in relation to the two components of S2, is of diagnostic value (Fig. 17-8). For example, the murmur of aortic stenosis must end before A2. A murmur extending past A2 could be pulmonic stenosis, but not aortic stenosis. However, the ability to perceive whether a murmur goes through one or both components of the second heart sound requires some experience. Although these signs were formerly taught to medical students, perhaps in part as a way of testing their understanding of cardiac physiology, they are now very difficult for most to learn, given the new shortened clinical examination curricula.

Some workers refer to early systolic, midsystolic, and late systolic murmurs. I am not sure why this scheme is used, because almost all systolic murmurs begin sometime in early (the first half of) systole, as can be shown by recordings; all have sound extend-

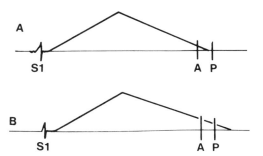

Figure 17-8. *A, A diamond-shaped murmur (with mirror-image subbaseline vibrations omitted) that passes through the first (aortic) component of S2. This systolic murmur must be due to mitral insufficiency, tricuspid insufficiency, or pulmonic stenosis. It cannot be due to aortic stenosis, either organic or relative, because the murmur continues after the closure of the aortic valve. B, A diamond-shaped murmur that continues through both components of S2. This murmur cannot be due to aortic stenosis or pulmonic stenosis as both those valves have already closed while the murmur still continues. Of course, if the murmur had ended before S2, no etiology could be excluded.*

ing through midsystole; and almost all have some sound in late (the last half of) systole. If these terms are being used to refer to the peak intensity of a diamond-shaped murmur, they might be useful for one phenomenon: in mitral valve prolapse, the peak moves to an earlier point in systole when the patient stands up (see p. 308).

Diastolic murmurs. Almost all diastolic murmurs begin in early diastole with a decrescendo sound. Those murmurs that have *only* this component are called decrescendo murmurs. These are due to insufficiency of the aortic, or sometimes the pulmonic valve.

Some murmurs also have a late diastolic crescendo component. These are called decrescendo-crescendo murmurs; 99% of them are due to relative or absolute stenosis of either the tricuspid or the mitral valve, usually the latter.

These last two are low-pitched. If high-pitched, one should diagnose coronary artery stenosis (Dock & Zoneraich, 1967).

A pedagogic note. If a diastolic murmur can be assigned to one of two valves, on the basis of its shape, and four more dimensions remain to be described, there is, diagnostically speaking, a redundancy of dimensions; that is, there are more dimensions available than are needed to diagnose the individual murmurs, according to Table 17-4. A corollary for the sophomore and junior medical student is to base the diagnosis of a murmur on those few dimensions of greatest certainty. This is a good habit that should generalize into other areas.

In some clinical situations, one cannot perfectly apprehend every dimension. Thus, a mastery of all dimensions is required to pick those that permit the most confident analysis in any given case. Because of the vast amount of ordered experience that will be later required to perform such a masterful analysis in a difficult case, the student should now discipline himself to *attempt* to describe all the dimensions of each murmur, even when its etiology is already known.

As with systolic murmurs, diastolic turbulence may be produced by either a normal amount of blood flowing across a valve lumen that is decreased in size (e.g., rheumatic mitral stenosis) or by an excessive volume of blood flowing across a normal size lumen (e.g., the relative tricuspid stenosis murmur of atrial septal defect, namely, the flow across the tricuspid valve consists not only of the normal systemic venous return, but also a portion of the pulmonary venous return that has passed from left atrium to right atrium across the atrial septal defect. Here, the tricuspid valve is anatomically normal but functionally small vis-à-vis the increased blood flow.) See also the Carey Coombs murmur (p. 321).

Location at Which the Murmur Is Loudest

Murmurs from specific valves are usually *best* heard in the traditional valve areas (see p. 290). However, some murmurs may be heard best in other areas. Always note the specific place where the murmur is loudest, even if it is not one of the usual areas.

Radiation

Aortic and pulmonic insufficiency murmurs tend to radiate from the base caudad. Aortic stenosis murmurs tend to radiate to the neck and right clavicle. Pulmonic stenosis murmurs do not radiate very far, probably because of a lower pressure in the right ventricle. Tricuspid and mitral stenosis murmurs tend not to radiate; sometimes they can only be heard in an area about the size of a thumbprint. Tricuspid insufficiency murmurs radiate backward through the venous system, rarely being audible in unusual places like the neck veins or the varicose veins of the leg (Becker & Dick, 1962). Mitral insufficiency murmurs tend to radiate laterally, sometimes all the way to the armpit ("axilla" in Latin) or even to the subscapular region in the back. (Do not confuse the axilla with the axillary line, as many do, thereby losing a valuable discriminant between mitral insufficiency and aortic stenosis.)

1.   For years, radiation of the murmur to the axilla (not the axillary lines) was used as a finding specific for mitral insufficiency. Murmurs of aortic stenosis rarely (i.e., in less than 5% of cases) radiate there, whereas murmurs of mitral insufficiency often (but not always) do so. I have heard patients with such a radiation in whom the murmur was coming from aortic sclerosis, as proven at catheterization. This may have been a manifestation of the Gallavardin phenomenon (discussed on p. 318). In any event, it demonstrates how tenuous are the footholds of clinical diagnosis.

2.   Before the era of cardiac surgery, one could still find patients with severe rheumatic aortic stenosis in whom the murmurs sometimes radiated to the top of the head, and in one case even to the right elbow. But at the present time, radiation to the right midclavicle, with amplification, as popularized by Spodick, is the maneuver I find myself relying upon most. (As far as simple radiation goes, I have heard the murmurs of both mitral insufficiency and tricuspid insufficiency radiate to the right midclavicle, but they were not amplified.)

3.   According to an old piece of bedside lore, there was a form of mitral insufficiency in which only the anterior leaflet of the valve was deformed or flail due to rupture of the chordae tendinae (Guiliani, 1967). This lesion, like some ventricular septal defects, was said to produce a murmur (and even a thrill) in the left subscapular area.

Recently, the paravertebral systolic murmur was offered as a sign of postmyocardial infarction ventricular septal rupture. This is not an unexpected location, since this is just the location in which the murmur may be heard in congenital ventricular septal defect. However, it was stated that a murmur in this area was *never* secondary to mitral insufficiency (Benson & Raj, 1982). But nothing is perfect. One such patient went to catheterization in 1987, where it

was proved beyond any doubt that the murmur that radiated posteriorly was due to mitral insufficiency and *not* to a ruptured septum.

Pitch

Pitch is the same as tone, and refers to a note being played upon a musical instrument. Since murmurs are not pure sound generators like the oboe, pitch is used, in cardiology, to refer to the predominant register of tones, when it can be identified. As a rule, a high-pitched murmur is due to a high pressure gradient, a narrow aperture, or both, like a strong wind passing through a cracked window, as in aortic or mitral insufficiency. Low-pitched murmurs are generally due to a low pressure gradient, a large orifice, or both, as in mitral stenosis or tricuspid stenosis. White noise has no pitch, and murmurs of impure timbre (vide infra) may not have a predominant pitch (e.g., *some* cases of aortic stenosis). If a murmur does not have a predominant pitch, don't assign one to it.

An alternate theory (Bruns, 1959) explains the pitch of murmurs in a different way.
The distinction between pitch and timbre is given on page 260.

Timbre

Timbre refers to the "color" of a musical tone. For instance, an oboe, a clarinet, and a trumpet could each play the same note (tone), say concert C, but an experienced listener could identify each instrument by its timbre. White noise has "poor" timbre, because it is harsh, coarse, and nonharmonic.

In cardiology, the timbre refers to the purity of the murmur (or the lack thereof). The semiophysiology of pure timbre involves the repeated vibration of something at a constant frequency with dominant harmonics. Thus, murmurs due simply to hemic turbulence do not usually have good timbre. But if there is something that can be vibrated, such as a valve (see p. 316), various degrees of musicality can result.

Murmurs described as "honks," "whoops," and "cooing like a dove" are more pure than those which are "harsh." The former may be described as "musical." A prolapsed mitral valve, which most resembles a single reed instrument, produces one of the most "musical" murmurs (i.e., one with pure ["good"] timbre). Aortic stenosis *can* produce the least musical murmur, a "harsh" murmur with impure timbre.   The timbre of the murmurs of tricuspid and mitral stenosis is somewhat like that of the male voice speaking the word "rub." Thus, some cases of mitral stenosis have a relatively pure timbre even though they are low-pitched rumbles. The murmur of ruptured chordae tendineae resembles someone humming through a kazoo (pure tone but impure timbre). (However, as with all diseases there are milder forms discovered with time, and some cases of ruptured chordae tendineae are nonemergent ambulatory ones presenting with only one chorda tendinea ruptured and a flail mitral leaflet that sounds just like everyday mitral regurgitation.) Most cases of aortic insufficiency have a poor timbre, sounding almost like the white noise of breath sounds, without a predominant pitch. However, some cases of aortic insufficiency will produce a diastolic cooing sea gull murmur (see Fig. 17-6 and p. 303), which has a very good timbre.

Such musical diastolic murmurs were once thought to be of ominous prognosis because of the association with syphilitic aortic leaflet retroversion. With the decreasing prevalence of cardiovascular syphilis, the same murmur is now heard more frequently with aortic insufficiency of the usual causes, and no longer has such a bad prognosis (Sheikh et al., 1984).

Some cases of aortic stenosis or rheumatic mitral insufficiency may also have a cooing dove or sea gull murmur.

Descriptive Phrases: A Caution

Many phrases, particularly the birdcalls,* used to describe murmurs actually describe shape, pitch, and timbre *simultaneously*. For instance, the "sea gull murmur," which resembles the musical call of a herring gull (*Larus argentatus*), has high tones, relatively pure timbre, and a pansystolic shape. Persons who do not understand this may misname a murmur based on only one or two dimensions, thus confusing others to whom these dramatic descriptive phrases have very complete and specific meanings. Worse, the former may never learn to identify the other dimensions.

Self-experiment: Ask five classmates to commit to writing their working definitions of "blowing murmur," "musical murmur," and "sea gull murmur." How much consistency is there?

If mitral regurgitation is due to prolapse, it may sound more like a Canadian goose (*Branta canadensis*), as may tricuspid prolapse. Aortic insufficiency, when birdlike, tends to sound somewhat like the great black-backed gull (*Larus marinus*), but higher pitched, like the common tern (*Sterna hirundo*). Aortic stenosis, when birdlike, sounds more like the laughing gull (*Larus atricilla*).

Intensity

By tradition, murmurs are graded on a scale of 1 to 6, which was initially a research tool in a study of systolic murmurs (Freeman & Levine, 1933; Levine & Harvey, 1949).

Grade 1. The murmur is heard, but not at first.
Grade 2. The faintest murmur that can be heard immediately upon placing the stethoscope on the precordium.
Grade 3. A murmur intermediate between grades 2 and 4. It is louder than a grade 2, but is not associated with a thrill.
Grade 4. A murmur that is associated with a thrill, but is not as loud as a grade 5.
Grade 5. A murmur that can be heard through the stethoscope if just the rim is held against the chest (i.e., with the chest piece tilted).
Grade 6. A murmur that can be heard with the stethoscope head held in front of the patient's chest without actually touching it.

The reason for grading intensity is that Freeman and Levine found that innocent systolic murmurs were almost never grade 3 or more. This was a useful piece of information in an era in which there was no cardiac catheterization and no surgical treatment, but a great deal of worry about innocent (or not-so-innocent) systolic murmurs.

Although most young clinicians use intensity as one of only

---

*If one examines the records of actual birdcalls, such as those available from the Audubon Society, one discovers that the different species of sea gulls, doves, etc. each have remarkably different calls, so the avian analogy could be quite confusing, as well as incorrect, if the species is not given with the genus.

Table 17-5. Innocent Systolic Murmurs

Murmur	Origin
Vibratory systolic murmur (Still's murmur)	Pulmonic leaflets
Pulmonic systolic murmur	Pulmonary trunk
Peripheral pulmonic murmur	Pulmonary branches
Supraclavicular or brachiocephalic murmur	Origins of brachiocephalic vessels
Systolic mammary souffle	Breast vessels during pregnancy
Aortic sclerosis	Fibrous thickening of aortic cusps

Source: *Perloff (1980).*

two or three dimensions in their descriptions of murmurs, it is placed at the end of this list because it is of *less use in diagnosis* than the other dimensions. While innocent systolic murmurs do indeed tend to be of grade 2 or less, many (noninnocent) structural abnormalities may also produce only a grade 2 murmur, including diastolic murmurs (which Freeman and Levine did not study) and right-sided murmurs.

Innocent Murmurs

Innocent murmurs are discussed last for clarity because they *lack* the characteristics and associated findings of the various pathologic murmurs that have just been described (Table 17-4).

Innocent murmurs are only grade 1 to 2, and more than 99% are systolic (Table 17-5).

One common form is the vibratory murmur originally described by Still. This is a short, buzzing murmur that probably originates from periodic vibrations of the pulmonic leaflets at their attachments. It is best heard at sites overlying the body of the right ventricle. A pulmonic midsystolic murmur occurring in young persons represents an exaggeration of normal ejection vibrations within the pulmonary trunk. These are the kinds heard in high-output states such as pregnancy, anemia, fever, and hyperthyroidism. (See p. 301 for reasons why such murmurs are "pulmonic," not "aortic.") Innocent supraclavicular systolic murmurs originate in the brachiocephalic arteries and are always louder above the clavicles. Perloff considers aortic sclerosis (see p. 314) to be one of the innocent murmurs (as it is when it is *mild*). The mammary souffle* is discussed in Chapter 15 (p. 241).

Imitating the Sound of Murmurs

For the attending.   Mitral or tricuspid insufficiency murmurs of the holosystolic type may best be imitated by whistling until the mouth is dry and the musicality is thus lost. Another method is to listen through the stethoscope while holding the diaphragm in your hand and quickly drawing a finger from the ulnar to the thenar side of the dorsum of the hand. (This is not completely satisfactory because the heart sounds are omitted.)

The murmur of aortic stenosis has been likened to the sound of a steam engine chugging up a hill. For prairie dwellers and young persons who have never heard a steam engine on an upgrade, the grunt made by older persons of Mediterranean stock as they settle their arthritic joints into a chair is a passable substitute. (This sound is sometimes called a *kretschmer*.)

---

*Here, souffle is pronounced "sue-full," not "sue-flay." The former means whisper or breath. The latter is an egg dish, inflated and inspired.

Another way to imitate the murmur of aortic or pulmonic stenosis is to place the bell in your hand, and draw a circle on the back of your hand. Start the circle by striking the back of your hand with your finger to generate as "S1." The sound will crescendo, and, if you end the circle at the starting point and do not raise your finger, you will have to slow down, producing the decrescendo part of the murmur. There will not be an "S2" with this technique, but in some cases of very severe aortic stenosis, the aortic valve opens so little that closure produces a very feeble aortic component of the second sound. In these cases, there are places on the chest where S2 is not audible, so this is a pretty good imitation.

A good approximation of the sound of aortic and pulmonic insufficiency can be generated by listening through the stethoscope with the diaphragm on your anterior neck while whispering the word "par," "peer," or "tare." The consonant, snapping from the lips, represents S2. The rest of the word is the decrescendo murmur. It should be of the same pitch and timbre as your breath sounds. (That is why the patient must always hold his breath during the search for this murmur.)

Another way to imitate the murmur of aortic insufficiency is to place your stethoscope in the palm of your hand as before, but this time, start the sound by striking the back of your hand (for S2) and draw your finger down your arm in the direction of your elbow. To decrease the volume of the murmur, you might even start at the wrist and stroke about halfway down toward the elbow.

Both of these techniques produce a murmur of too great a volume. Once you have "heard" this murmur, change your technique so as to produce a grade 2 murmur.

These murmurs are discussed in greater detail on page 309.

Continuous Versus To-and-Fro Murmurs

Murmurs occupying both systole and diastole are of two types, diagrammed in Figure 17-9. The first sounds like one (continuous) murmur in terms of pitch and timbre. The most common example if the patient is sitting or standing is the cervical venous hum (see Table 17-6 and Ch. 19, p. 366).

The other murmur occupying systole and diastole, the to-and-fro murmur, actually sounds like two different murmurs, as it is. It can be caused by any combination of lesions capable of producing a systolic and a diastolic murmur. The to-and-fro murmur is not always continuous. Usually, it has a late diastolic silence (if the diastolic component is due to aortic or pulmonic insufficiency), or a mid-diastolic silence (if the diastolic component is due to mitral or tricuspid stenosis), or an early or late systolic silence. There are also great pitch and timbre differences in the systolic and diastolic components. However, when first stumbled upon, the psychoacoustic event most closely resembles what is shown in the figure. It is only after careful timing and auscultation that the silent spots and pitch and timbre differences are detected. Then the auscultor knows not to do the differential diagnosis of Table 17-6, but rather the separate differential of (at least) one diastolic and one systolic murmur.

Table 17-6. Differential Diagnosis of Continuous Thoracic Murmurs (in Order of Decreasing Frequency)

Diagnosis	Key Findings
Cervical venous hum	Disappears on compression of the jugular vein
Hepatic venous hum (see Ch. 20, p. 378)	Often disappears with epigastric pressure (Rusconi et al., 1985)
Mammary souffle (see Ch. 15, p. 241)	Disappears upon pressing hard with stethoscope
Patent ductus arteriosus (Gibson's murmur)[a]	Loudest at 2nd left intercostal space
Coronary arteriovenous fistula	Loudest at lower sternal borders
98% of cases, ruptured aneurysm of sinus of Valsalva (Pan-Chih et al., 1981)	Loudest at upper right sternal border; sudden onset
Bronchial collaterals	Associated signs of congenital heart disease
High-grade coarctation	Brachial/pedal arterial pressure gradient
Anomalous left coronary artery arising from pulmonary artery	
Anomalous pulmonary artery arising from the aorta	
Pulmonary artery branch stenosis	Heard outside the area of cardiac dullness
Pulmonary AV fistula	Same as above
ASD with mitral stenosis or atresia	Altered by the Valsalva maneuver
88% of aortic-atrial fistulas (Hurley et al., 1986)	
Superior caval syndrome due to syphilitic aneurysmal dilatation of aortic root and mediastinitis	Systolic accentuation; 2nd & 3rd right interspaces (Lian, 1937)

Source: *Holmes et al. (1966).*

[a]*This was called the "machinery murmur" because it had the continuous harsh sound of the early 20th century machine shops whose devices were individually belt-driven by a single master rotor kept in continuous motion. Neither the machine shop nor the murmur are much extant. Those patients who do not have surgical care develop pulmonary diastolic hypertension and the murmur becomes purely systolic.*

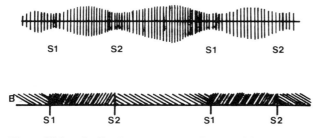

Figure 17-9.   *A, Continuous murmur; B, to-and-fro murmur.*

Venous hums as continuous murmurs and systolic murmurs.   The cervical continuous venous hum was first ausculted by Laennec (1819), who likened the sound to that of a seashell put to one's ear. The diagnosis of cervical venous hums is given in Chapter 19 (p. 366).

Mammary souffles, hyperthyroid eyeball bruits, and other potentially continuous murmurs of increased flow may all be considered examples of venous hums. However, the venous hums most likely to cause difficulty during the auscultation of the heart are those coming from the liver.

The latter was first reported by Pegot in 1833, and the autopsy was published by Cruveilhier in 1835. That patient had superficial abdominal varices which were ausculted as the source of the venous hum. The venous hum of cirrhosis in the absence of visible abdominal wall varices was explicated in 1868 by Trousseau (Bloom, 1950). (The diagnosis of hepatic venous hums is given in Ch. 20, p. 378.)

Hepatic venous hums are snares for the unwary cardiologist. It is not well appreciated that these venous hums may also be heard in alcoholic hepatitis, hepatoma, and a wide variety of other liver diseases (Clain et al., 1966). Nor is it appreciated that these venous hums may radiate from the liver to the precordial area (McFadzean & Gray, 1953) or even be heard *better* precordially than over the liver (Bloom, 1950). Finally, while usually continuous, these murmurs may be only systolic (Clain et al., 1966), in which case they are named "arterial murmurs," which does nothing to lessen the confusion of the auscultor who is not aware of their true meaning.

Pericardial Friction Rubs

Timbre

A pericardial friction rub sounds like creaky leather, or in some cases, a rhonchus beating in time with the heart.

Location

Pericardial rubs are often not heard over all parts of the precordial area. A rub may be audible only in an area about the size of a nickel (2 cm in diameter) and sometimes is heard only at the border of cardiac dullness. About 84% of rubs are best heard along the left sternal border (Spodick, 1975).

Phases

A three-component (triphasic) pericardial friction rub is pathognomonic for pericarditis (generally acute or subacute; rubs are absent in chronic, constrictive pericarditis). "Three component" means that there are three sounds for each cardiac contraction, or what a musician would call a triplet. Note that the middle note of the triplet is quite soft in many cases, so that one must listen carefully and repeatedly in a perfectly quiet room in order to detect this diagnostically perfect finding.

In a study of 100 patients with acute pericardial friction rubs, about 55% of the rubs were triphasic. One patient with pericarditis was even found to have a quadriphasic rub (Spodick, 1975).

If the rub has two components (biphasic), one can be reasonably certain that there is pericarditis.

In the same study (Spodick, 1975), about 33% of the rubs were biphasic; all of these had a systolic component plus either an early or late diastolic component. About 9% would have been triphasic if the heart rate had been slower, since these patients had a summation diastolic component similar to a summation gallop. Such biphasic "to-and-fro" rubs may also be due to absence of atrial systole. However, atrial or other arrhythmias are rare in acute pericarditis, unless it is accompanied by underlying myocardial or valvular disease (Spodick, 1983).

If the rub has only one component, it is still indicative of pericarditis; however, such a rub is likely to be misidentified as a murmur. In that situation, the optimum way to resolve the problem is not to order an echocardiogram, but to reexamine the patient until one "catches" the rub demonstrating its other components. Rubs, like gallops, tend to be evanescent in borderline situations.

The etiology of pericardial rubs is discussed on page 324.

About 10% of the patients with pericardial rubs have pericardial effusion, thus demonstrating that a rub does *not* rule out an effusion (Spodick, 1975).

The Pleuropericardial Rub

It is often hard to tell what is meant by this phrase. What we will mean is that the clinician has heard a pericardial rub synchronous with the cardiac cycle and accentuated according to respiratory phase. Actually, this is the case with most pericardial rubs (Harvey, 1961; Spodick, 1975). We will not use this word to refer to the concept that both the pleural surface and its facing parietal pericardial surface are inflamed, because this has not always been directly proved in any case and may not be relevant in most. Even in patients with known pulmonary disease, a rub does not necessarily originate from the pleura. Patients with viral pneumonia could also have a viral pericarditis (Levine & Harvey, 1949). However, in one patient who had a pulmonary infarction, the pleural friction rub heard near the heart border did appear at one point to have a superimposed cardiac cycle accentuation (a pericardiopleural rub?). How can one tell the difference?

The traditional advice has been to distinguish between pleural and pericardial etiologies by having the patient hold his breath in a given phase of respiration. However, it is quite possible that a rub of pericardial origin might not be heard during one phase of respiration (vide supra), and if one were to pick that phase, one might erroneously conclude that the rub was pleural. Accordingly, if one wishes to try this maneuver, one should have the patient hold his breath both in full inspiration and later in full expiration.

Other Systolic Adventitious Heart Sounds

Systolic Clicks (Prolapse Clicks Versus Ejection Clicks)

In general, early- to mid-systolic clicks result from 1) mitral or tricuspid valve prolapse (these are *not* ejection clicks); 2) high-pressure valve opening; 3) nonstenotic congenital bicuspid aortic valves and the entire spectrum of mild to severe stenosis of the aortic valve (Shaver et al., 1985); 4) dilatation of the great vessels (poststenotic or aneurysmal); 5) systemic hypertension, in the setting of a tortuous sclerotic aortic root (a tight, noncompliant arterial tree and forceful left ventricular ejection) (Shaver et al., 1985); or 6) a prosthetic valve (see p. 306).

False positives: As mentioned earlier, an early systolic click must be distinguished from a doubled S1 and from an S4-S-1 complex (see p. 290).

An ejection click in the presence of aortic stenosis implies that the stenosis is valvular, and not supravalvular or subvalvular (idiopathic hypertropic subaortic stenosis). Similarly, pulmonic ejection clicks occur in pulmonic valvular stenosis, but not in subvalvular stenosis. They may also occur in other conditions of pulmonic valve dilatation such as hyperthyroidism and idiopathic dilatation of the pulmonary artery, of which latter 80% will also have a pulmonic insufficiency murmur (Ramsey et al., 1967).

Both aortic and pulmonic ejection clicks occur very early in systole, right after the first heart sound. They may be distinguished from each other by the fact that they are best heard in their respective valvular areas and do not radiate well (Shaver et al., 1985).

A more important distinction is that between both of these ejection clicks and the "nonejection" prolapse clicks of mitral valve and tricuspid valve prolapse. These latter clicks are best heard over their respective valve areas and usually occur later in systole. If the patient stands up, the prolapse click may then occur earlier in systole. Such positional movement does not occur with the ejection clicks (see p. 290).

○   Any early systolic click almost guarantees that an accompanying murmur is *not* innocent.

Means-Lerman Scratch of Hyperthyroidism

A peculiar systolic scratchy sound, halfway between a murmur and a friction rub, was first reported in 6% of male and 12% of female patients with hyperthyroidism. All of the patients with this sound were in the subgroup that had no other cardiac symptoms or signs (Lerman & Means, 1932).

> . . . We have noted an unusual noise in the moderate and severe cases of hyperthyroidism. It consists of a rough grating systolic murmur which has some of the characteristics of a friction rub, heard best over the sternum in the region of the second interspace. It is superficial, heard best at the end of full expiration and obscured by full inspiration. Its intensity subsides as the metabolism and heart rate drop under the influence of (treatment) and usually disappears after (thyroidectomy). On several occasions the diagnosis of pericarditis was suspected by members of the hospital staff on the basis of this friction rub. We are not certain as to its causation . . . It may have some relationship to the dilated pulmonary conus often seen in the roentgen ray pictures in this condition. (Lerman & Means, 1932)

Over 30 years later, this sound was shown to be due to a combination of early pulmonic ejection sounds superimposed upon a short scratchy ejection murmur, in turn due to the increased velocity of ejection in this disorder (Leonard et al., 1963).

A Means-Lerman scratch can also be heard in patients with fever and anemia, but normal thyroid status.

Other Diastolic Adventitious Heart Sounds

Timing the Early Diastolic Sounds

Before Bell Telephone Company was split up, it was easy to teach the unit of 0.04 second because that was the interval between picking up the receiver (releasing the depressed receiver rest) and hearing the dial tone. Now, this interval must be learned phonocardiographically or from some heart sound simulators. For those who wish to take the trouble, the early diastolic intervals are given in Table 17-7.

Early Diastolic Tumor Plops

Atrial myxomas often grow on pedunculated stalks that permit considerable mobility. They not only produce changing or positional diastolic (and sometimes systolic) murmurs, but in early diastole they may plop into the ventricle. The early diastolic sound so produced is called a "tumor plop."

Table 17-7.   Early Diastolic Intervals

S2 (normal expiration)	< 0.03 sec
S2 (inspiration, young persons)[a]	0.04–0.05 sec
S2 (widely split)	0.06–0.08 sec
S2 opening snap (Reddy et al., 1985)	0.03–0.15 sec
S2 pericardial knock	0.10–0.12 sec
S2-S3	0.14–0.16 sec
S2-S3 in normal children (Reddy et al., 1985)	0.12–0.20 sec

[a]*This value decreases with age, such that a single S2 during both phases of respiration may be perceived in normal subjects older than 40 years (Reddy et al., 1985).*

Early Diastolic Pericardial Knock

Constrictive pericarditis produces an early diastolic "pericardial knock" at approximately the same time as S3. (The incoming blood strikes a "pretightened" drumhead.) It may be accentuated by having the patient squat (Nicholson et al., 1980).

Early Diastolic Opening Snap

The opening snap of mitral or tricuspid stenosis, discussed further on page 319, needs to be distinguished from a widely split S2 (see p. 296). Opening sounds or clicks can also be heard with 1) prosthetic mitral valves, 2) mitral regurgitation, 3) ventricular septal defect, 4) thyrotoxicosis, 5) tricuspid atresia with a large atrial septal defect, and 6) second- or third-degree AV block (Reddy et al., 1985).

Early Diastolic Click

An early diastolic click may be heard in 5% to 15% of patients with mitral valve prolapse (Cheng, 1987), due to reverse ballooning of the prolapsed mitral leaflet.

Late Diastolic Pacemaker Sound

Rarely, a right ventricular pacemaker produces a late diastolic (presystolic) sound called the "pacemaker sound," which occurs immediately after the onset of the pacing stimulus. Its high-pitched and clicking characteristics differentiate it from an S4. The sound is believed to be caused by contraction of chest wall muscles, which are stimulated by the electrical impulse from the pacemaker. This does not necessarily imply perforation of the right ventricle (Perloff, 1980).

Other Adventitious Heart Sounds that May Be Systolic and/or Diastolic

Prosthetic Valve Sounds

The auscultatory findings depend upon the type of valve that was implanted. The acoustic characteristics of various prosthetic devices have been reviewed (Smith et al., 1981). Ball valves produce opening and closing clicks. Disk valves produce closing clicks. Tissue (porcine) valves usually produce closing sounds in both aortic and mitral positions. These sounds are crisp and high-pitched, but much less prominent than those of mechanical devices. A pericardial xenograft or a porcine mitral valve may also have an opening sound (Smith et al., 1981; Szkopiec et al., 1983).

Prosthetic valves typically produce a systolic murmur. Disk or porcine mitral valves also may have a diastolic rumble (Smith et al., 1981). However, aortic diastolic murmurs, ball valve diastolic murmurs, and new diastolic murmurs are due to prosthetic valve dysfunction until proven otherwise (Reeves, 1982).

Mill Wheel Sound of Air Embolism

■   There is one very unusual type of almost continuous sound that does not deserve to be called a murmur because it is more like a splashing sound, resembling that of a water wheel at a grist mill. In fact, it is called a mill wheel or a mill pond murmur. The splashing is due to intracardiac blood, and the diagnosis is air embolism. You should immediately roll the patient onto his left side, to decrease the chance of embolism to the brain.

Mediastinal Crunch

There is little* to add to the story of spontaneous mediastinal emphysema and its auscultatory hallmark, the mediastinal crunch, as it was originally told (Hamman, 1939):

> **Case 1.**   On February 12th, 1933, Dr. W. Cabell Moore invited me to come to Washington to see a physician, fifty-one

---

*See page 266.

years of age, who had symptoms strongly suggesting the occurrence of coronary occlusion. Theretofore he had always been a robust, healthy man busily engaged in carrying on an exacting practice. On the morning of February 8, while shaving, he was suddenly seized with intense pain under the sternum radiating to the left shoulder . . .

. . . I examined the heart and the lungs with the greatest care and could detect nothing that was to the least degree abnormal. When I expressed chagrin at my lack of skill, the patient laughingly said that he could easily bring on the sound which excited so much interest. He turned on his left side and after shifting about for a few moments said, 'There it is, I hear it now.' I put my stethoscope over the apex of the heart and with each impulse there occurred the most extraordinary crunching, bubbling sound . . .

Case 2. . . . On the previous afternoon while sitting quietly in a chair, he suddenly had a feeling of pressure under the sternum as though a lump were forming. Soon swelling actually appeared above the clavicles and he had severe pain on breathing deeply, on swallowing and on turning the head . . . There was subcutaneous crepitation over the front of the neck which extended backward to the trapezius muscle on both sides and downward over the clavicles to about the second rib on the left and to the nipple on the right. When I put my stethoscope over the heart, there was the same systolic crunching sound which had so perplexed me when I heard it over the heart of the Washington physician . . .

Case 3. . . . A young physician, twenty-five years of age, an interne at the Emergency Hospital, Washington was admitted as a patient, February 21, 1934, complaining of pain in the left side of the chest and peculiar crackling noises in the region of the heart. He had had a slight cold for two or three weeks with a little cough and mucoid expectoration. On the day before entering the hospital he had had rather sharp pain over the heart increased by deep breathing and by coughing. A few hours later as he was leaning on his desk, he suddenly heard a curious crackling noise, apparently coming from that part of the chest where the pain was located. He listened with interest and observed that the crackling sound came synchronously with the heartbeat. When he sat up straight the sound immediately vanished . . .

. . . When the patient turned upon his left side a curious moist crepitant, or crackling, noise was heard with each contraction of the heart, so loud that through the stethoscope it was almost painful to the ear. It could be heard by the bare ear held a foot from the chest wall. When the patient turned upon his back these peculiar sounds at once disappeared . . .

Case 4. . . . As he got out of the car he was taken suddenly with a very severe pain under the lower end of the sternum and a sensation of pressure or choking . . .

. . . While the patient was lying on his back, just inside the apex beat, could be heard a queer crackling, bubbling sound with each systole. When he turned upon his side, the sound disappeared . . .

Case 5. . . . At about 5:45 o'clock on the afternoon of January 11, while walking from work, he was seized suddenly with a severe, sharp, stabbing pain over the lower part of the left chest . . .

. . . Over the left axillary area were found the physical signs of a partial pneumothorax. The area of cardiac dullness was much diminished in extent.

. . . Over the lower portion of the sternum and to the left of it, in the fourth and fifth interspaces, there were curious crunching, clicking sounds varying in intensity with each systole . . .

Case 6. . . . At about three o'clock the following morning the mother was awakened by hearing the boy cry out with pain. When she went to him he complained of severe pain over the right lower chest . . .

. . . The evening before, subcutaneous emphysema had been noted above both clavicles. On this morning it was more pronounced and extended up the neck on both sides to the ears. Over the whole sternum, and louder still over the heart, numerous crackling, popping sounds could be heard greatly accentuated with each contraction of the heart . . .

Case 7. Dr. L., 25 years of age, resident obstetrician at Sinai Hospital, is a short, stockily built man of vigorous appearance . . . On September 6, 1937, while eating lunch, he began to notice pain in the lower left axillary area . . .

. . . When he shifted to the left side loud bubbling, crackling sounds occurred synchronously with the slow beating of the heart, louder with systole than with diastole . . .

In order to mark clearly the essential clinical features of spontaneous interstitial emphysema of the lungs and mediastinum I shall summarize the important symptoms.

Interstitial emphysema of the lung may occur without the least effort, when the patient is quietly standing, sitting or lying down . . .

In many instances a peculiar and distinctive sound is heard over the heart synchronous with its contractions. Usually the sound is heard only during systole but at times it may be heard also during diastole.

The area of cardiac dullness is diminished or completely obliterated, the dullness being replaced by a hyperresonant percussion note . . .

When air appears in the subcutaneous tissues of the neck the diagnosis is at once assured.

A more recent case was reported by Dr. David Rosen of Minnesota. A patient presented to the emergency room with a stab wound to the chest and a mediastinal crunch, which the surgeon did not believe to be significant. When the wound was probed with a gloved finger, the patient developed third-degree heart block and required an emergency pacemaker.

Also see Chapter 16, page 280.

Special Maneuvers

Maneuvers that Affect the Intensity of Murmurs

Listening to the patient during various maneuvers and changes in position may be necessary to hear certain murmurs, and may also help in the differential diagnosis (Cochran, 1978; Nellen et al., 1967; Rothman & Goldberger, 1983), particularly when the maneuvers are used as excluders.

Position

1. Before you can legitimately say that a patient does not have a murmur of aortic insufficiency, you must listen to him in a sitting position, leaning forward, with his breath held, preferably in expiration (also see p. 309).

2. Listen for the murmur of mitral stenosis with the patient in the left lateral decubitus position. The best time to listen is immediately after the patient has rolled into that position. First, place the stethoscope bell just a bit inside the PMI or the percussed apex, and then have the patient roll into position. I adopted this idea from Dr. Sam Levine, who believed that much of the augmentation of the murmur in the left lateral decubitus position was due to the exercise (and increased flow) of moving into that posture. (Other methods of bringing out the mitral stenosis murmur—having the patient inhale amyl nitrite or hop up and down 25 times so as to cause a tachycardia—work by a similar mechanism (Levine, 1945).)

3. Standing decreases ventricular filling and so increases only two murmurs, that of IHSS and 74% of cases of mitral valve prolapse (Popp & Winkle, 1976; Rothman & Goldberger, 1983). (In some instances, it may just make the prolapse murmur longer, so that it seems louder.) Standing decreases all other valvular murmurs, including aortic stenosis, pulmonic stenosis, valvular mitral insufficiency, or tricuspid insufficiency (Cochran, 1978; Rothman & Goldberger, 1983).

4. Squatting increases ventricular filling and increases afterload.* It decreases the murmur in 89% of IHSS but usually does not decrease the murmurs of valvular aortic stenosis, valvular mitral insufficiency, or pulmonic stenosis. Squatting can increase the murmur of mitral insufficiency. It increases the pulmonary flow murmur and the ventricular defect murmur of a ventricular septal defect forcing more of the blood through the defect into the right heart (Lembo et al., 1986; Rothman & Goldberger, 1983).

Because of the effects on afterload, squatting also increases the murmur of aortic insufficiency. (In fact, squatting is the second best way to elicit the murmur of aortic insufficiency [Vogelpoel et al., 1969]. The best way is transient arterial occlusion [p. 309].)

Except for the case of ventricular septal defect, all of the statements in this section have published exceptions (Lembo et al., 1986).

Inspiration

Inspiration may increase the murmur of the right-sided lesions' pulmonic stenosis, pulmonic insufficiency, tricuspid stenosis, and especially tricuspid insufficiency (see p. 322). It has been suggested that left-sided murmurs can be identified by their tendency to *decrease* in intensity with inspiration; but this sign is valid only if the heart tones remain of constant intensity, because otherwise the decrease may simply be due to the increased distance between the heart and the stethoscope caused by the inflated lungs.

In one study, an increase in the murmur with inspiration had a 100% sensitivity for a right-sided origin. The specificity was 88%, and the predictive value of a positive test was 67% (Lembo et al., 1988).

Cycle Length

As a general rule, the cycle length affects ventricular filling and will therefore specifically alter those murmurs produced by an obstruction to the normal outflow. Thus, the murmurs of aortic stenosis (and probably of pulmonic stenosis) increase after a longer diastole, while the murmur of mitral insufficiency (and probably of tricuspid insufficiency) do not (Rothman & Goldberger, 1983). It is believed that the murmur of IHSS also changes with cycle length, but this can be extremely confusing at the bedside, and should be used only within the strict limitations explained on page 315.

Amyl Nitrite

A method. Crack open an ampule and have the patient inhale deeply as you listen. The amyl nitrite will induce a tachycardia. Make your judgment about the murmur when you hear the increase in rate. The biggest change occurs first, so you should try to make a quick decision. To be able to make a good decision on the basis of small evanescent auditory samples requires a great

deal of experience. This method was probably more useful in earlier days when phonocardiograms were widely available.

To diminish the odor in the room, you may wish to dispose of the ampule in a closed container, preferably one filled with potassium hydroxide. Because the amyl nitrite causes a vascular headache in a large percentage of people, you need to inquire about that before leaving your patient.

Mechanism. The inhalation of amyl nitrite causes a decrease in afterload, or at least the portion due to systemic vascular resistance. It can be thought of as a "reverse handgrip" (vide infra), as it generally causes opposite effects.

Effect on systolic murmurs. Amyl nitrite intensified the murmur of 84% of cases of aortic stenosis and 89% of cases of IHSS, but only 0, 6, 13, and less than 22% of series of cases of mitral insufficiency. However, because of the increased flow and increased venous return, the murmur of 84% to 89% of cases of tricuspid insufficiency also increased (Rothman & Goldberger, 1983). The murmur usually decreases in small ventricular septal defects (Lembo et al., 1986; Rothman & Goldberger, 1983).

The murmur of isolated valvular pulmonic stenosis increased in 88% of cases. However, if the stenosis was subvalvular, the murmur paradoxically decreased if the ventricular hypertrophy was sufficiently severe. And if the pulmonic stenosis was part of the tetralogy of Fallot, the murmur definitely decreased (Rothman & Goldberger, 1983).

A decrease in a systolic murmur with amyl nitrite was 80% sensitive for a diagnosis of mitral regurgitation or ventricular septal defect, with a specificity of 90% and a positive predictive value of 84% (Lembo et al., 1988).

Effect on diastolic murmurs. In 60% to 82% of cases of mitral stenosis and tricuspid stenosis, the murmurs increased. However, 86% of the Flint murmurs (see p. 325) decreased (Rothman & Goldberger, 1983).

Amyl nitrite decreased 80% to 93% of the murmurs of aortic insufficiency, but none of the murmurs of pulmonic insufficiency (Lembo et al., 1986; Rothman & Goldberger, 1983).

Handgrip

This isometric exercise increases systemic vascular resistance (or afterload). Thus, it may be thought of as a "nonpharmacologic" phenylephrine infusion.

A method. Place the patient in the position in which the murmur is best heard. Auscult the murmur at rest and then during 1 minute of sustained maximal handgrip. Although the studies of this maneuver used a handgrip dynamometer (McCraw et al., 1972), it is said that a typical response can be elicited by squeezing a rolled-up face cloth or merely by clenching the fist forcefully (Fowler, 1980).

The expected increase in systemic vascular resistance does not always occur, and the murmur does not always change in the expected direction. In a few patients with aortic insufficiency, mitral insufficiency, mitral stenosis, and ventricular septal defect, the measured change was in an opposite direction from that predicted (Lembo et al., 1986), so the result of the handgrip should be used only as a weak excluder. For example, an increase in a systolic murmur almost always excludes aortic stenosis or IHSS (Rothman & Goldberger, 1983). A decrease in the intensity of a systolic murmur almost excludes ventricular septal defect and mitral insufficiency. A decrease in the intensity of a diastolic murmur with handgrip would tend to exclude the diagnoses of aortic insufficiency and mitral stenosis.

An increase in the murmur with handgrip was 68% sensitive for mitral insufficiency or ventricular septal defect, with a specificity of 92% and a positive predictive value of 84% (Lembo et al., 1988). A decrease in the murmur with handgrip was 85% sensitive for IHSS, with a specificity of 75% and a positive predictive value of 46% (Lembo et al., 1988).

---

*Afterload is aortic valve resistance plus systemic vascular resistance. If there is no aortic valve lesion, then afterload is the same as the peripheral vascular resistance, which is now called systemic vascular resistance by some. If there is an aortic valve lesion then its resistance is fixed and the change in afterload will be due to the change in systemic vascular resistance.

Transient Arterial Occlusion

Just as Duroziez increased the diastolic murmur of aortic insufficiency heard at the femoral artery by increasing the downstream resistance (see p. 310), so may all murmurs of left-sided insufficiency (also including mitral insufficiency and ventricular septal defect) be augmented by transiently occluding the brachial arteries with blood pressure cuffs inflated 20 to 40 mm Hg above systolic pressure for 20 seconds (Lembo et al., 1986).

An increase in a left-sided insufficiency murmur with transient arterial occlusion was 75% sensitive for aortic insufficiency and 80% sensitive for mitral insufficiency or ventricular septal defect, with positive predictive values of 100% (Lembo et al., 1986, 1988). Although not perfectly sensitive (sometimes there is no change), none of these murmurs decreased with the maneuver, so a decrease in intensity would be a useful excluder.

Valsalva Maneuver

For the attending. Phonocardiologists discovered that the response of murmurs to various phases of the Valsalva maneuver (see Ch. 6, p. 98) could be diagnostically useful. However, many of these experts did not indicate which phase of the Valsalva maneuver they were referring to in their charts. Because the different phases may have different effects on the same murmur, the resulting literature is confused and confusing.

Worse, some of the phases of the Valsalva maneuver are passed through in just a few heartbeats. It seems optimistic at best to suggest that a neophyte can identify the phase from changes in the R-R interval without an external recording device such as an electrocardiograph machine. Furthermore, it is not clear how the physician can be expected to learn to identify a change in intensity that lasts for but a few beats, now that the phonocardiograph is in a pecuniary, insalubrious, and ill-deserved eclipse.

For all these reasons, I personally do not teach the Valsalva maneuver. However, the fortunate few whose "bedside" equipment includes intraarterial recording devices can consult a comprehensive review (Nishimura & Tajik, 1986).

The Scratch Test

The frontal cardiac silhouette has been outlined by what is now known as the scratch test. The original description (Burton-Opitz, 1925) cannot be improved upon:

> I should like to call attention to a simple method of auscultatory stroking which has given excellent results as proved by means of the fluoroscope and Roentgen photographs. While I have used this procedure principally in mapping out the heart, it may be applied with equal accuracy to other organs, such as the liver and kidneys.
>
> The bell of the stethophone is placed over the sternum at the second interspace. By means of a blunt colored pencil, short vertical strokes are then made from without inward, beginning about three inches to the right of the sternum. As the pencil is moved inward, a line will eventually be reached when the sound suddenly increases in its intensity. This point is marked with the pencil. The stethophone is then lowered about an inch each time and this process repeated, until the entire right border of the heart has been charted in this manner.
>
> The stethophone is now raised to its former level at the second intercostal space, while stroking movements are made with the pencil beginning at a point three inches to the left of the sternum. The point at which a sudden increase in the intensity of the sound is noted is again marked. The stethophone is then moved downward and this process repeated. At about the fourth rib, the stethophone is shifted towards the left so that it comes to lie over the main mass of the ventricles. Sweeping oblique strokes are then made, beginning about four inches above the bell of the stethophone. This process is repeated in

successive radial lines until the entire left border of the heart has been outlined.

> The accuracy of this method may be tested in the following manner. A paste made of mucilage and barium sulphate is applied with a camel's hair brush in such a way that the different colored marks are joined with one another in the form of a line about three millimeters in width. The patient is then fluoroscoped. If the outlining has been correctly done, the barium line cannot be differentiated from the dark borders of the heart. Furthermore, if the patient moves the tip of his index finger along the barium line, it can readily be noted whether this line corresponds with the fluoroscopic findings. Additional proof of the accuracy of this method has been obtained by the taking of numerous X-ray plates showing the barium line superimposed upon the boundary of the heart shadow.

Synthesis

> The rest of my account will be concerned with the hidden membranes of the heart—a piece of craftsmanship deserving description above all others. There are membranes in the cavities, and fibres as well, spread out like cobwebs through the chambers of the heart and surrounding the orifices on all sides and emplanting filaments into the solid wall of the heart. In my opinion these serve as the guy-ropes and stays of the heart and its vessels, and as foundation to the arteries. Now there is a pair of these arteries, and on the entrance of each, three membranes have been contrived, with their edges rounded to the approximate extent of a semicircle. When they come together it is wonderful to see how precisely they close off the entrance to the arteries. *(The Hippocratic Writings*, edited by G.E.R. Lloyd and translated by Iain M. Lonie)

This section might equally well be called cogitation, after Osler's famous fifth maneuver (i.e., inspection, palpation, percussion, auscultation, and cogitation).

Aortic Insufficiency*

Detecting the Murmur

Listening for the Murmur

In order to hear an aortic insufficiency murmur, you must specifically listen for it with the patient properly positioned (see p. 308). It is worth reemphasizing that the breath must be held; the timbre of the aortic insufficiency murmur is similar to that of the normal breath sounds over the precordium.

The murmur may be augmented by squatting (see p. 308) or transient arterial occlusion (vide supra).

Sensitivity

The sensitivity of auscultation for the diagnosis of aortic insufficiency is 73% (Grayburn et al., 1986; Meyers et al., 1982). The sensitivity of the diastolic murmur for some examiners has also been determined for each degree of aortic insufficiency (Cohn et al., 1967): it was 32% for trivial lesions, 69% for mild lesions, 65% for moderate lesions, and 95% (Cohn et al., 1967) to 100% (Bland & Wheeler, 1957; Segal et al., 1956) for severe lesions. In grade 1 lesions accompanied by aortic stenosis, the sensitivity of the murmur was only 40%, and in grade 1 lesions accompanied by mitral stenosis, the sensitivity was 25% (Linhart, 1971).

To give a perspective on the relative worth of technology, the sensitivity of auscultation of the murmur for the diagnosis of aortic

---

*In reference to a valve, insufficiency and regurgitation are synonymous.

insufficiency is still superior to the sensitivity of magnetic resonance imaging for the diagnosis of multiple sclerosis (Stewart et al., 1987).

Does Length of Murmur Predict Severity of Insufficiency?

One would predict that the degree of aortic insufficiency could be estimated from the (inverse) length of the murmur, based upon the Wiggers diagram of simultaneous pressure curves versus time (i.e., with a small degree of aortic insufficiency, it would take more time for the pressure in the left ventricle to rise up to the aortic pressure than if there were a huge leak). With the latter, the pressure would presumably equilibrate rather quickly and so retrograde flow would diminish quickly, producing a short-lived murmur. Unfortunately, I have not been able to find a single paper in which this hypothesis has been tested by actually measuring the duration of the murmur. Given the present unwarranted underuse of phonocardiography, it is unlikely that this situation will improve in the near future. Other than Hill's sign (p. 311), I know of no reliable predictor of the degree of the murmur, including the pulse pressure (see p. 311).

Peripheral Signs

In addition to helping to distinguish the aortic insufficiency murmur from that of pulmonic insufficiency, some peripheral signs of aortic insufficiency can be helpful when the patient is unable to sit up and hold his breath for auscultation, or when ventilatory sounds or the noises of a busy hospital unit confound serious precordial auscultation.

Duroziez's Sign

A method.   In a quiet room, place the diaphragm of the stethoscope over the femoral artery. *Gradually* compress the artery. At first, a systolic murmur will be heard. (This occurs in everyone.)

Continue *slowly* to increase the pressure on the artery. In aortic insufficiency, a very early diastolic decrescendo murmur will also be heard at a critical point: a pressure equivalent to the diastolic plus ¾ of the pulse pressure (Luisada, 1943). If the pressure of the stethoscope is too great or too little, the murmur will not be heard.

In patients with unilateral atherosclerosis, it may be possible to elicit a Duroziez's sign over one femoral artery but not the (obstructed) other.

Sensitivity.   The sensitivity of a properly performed Duroziez's sign is 58% to 100% (Sapira, 1981).

False negatives.   Causes of false negatives include very mild aortic insufficiency, superimposed mitral valvular disease (due to decreased left ventricular stroke volume—mitral stenosis decreasing left ventricular filling and mitral insufficiency decreasing left ventricular forward ejection), superimposed aortic stenosis, and any other situation that interferes with pulse-wave propagation from the heart to the femoral artery (such as coarctation of the aorta or occlusive iliofemoral arterial disease).

False positives.   Double murmurs may also be heard in high-output states such as thyrotoxicosis, patent ductus arteriosus, fever, severe anemia, and an arteriovenous fistula in the leg being examined. All of these high-output double murmurs (except patent ductus arteriosus) are forward-flow murmurs, as opposed to the double murmur of aortic insufficiency, whose diastolic component is a reversed-flow murmur due to the blood actually moving backward toward the incompetent valve. The forward-flow diastolic components may be distinguished from the reversed-flow diastolic components of aortic insufficiency (and patent ductus arteriosus) by a technique originally described in the 19th century by Potain as a modification of the method of Duroziez, and later (in English) by Blumgart and Ernstene, as follows.

While listening to the diastolic murmur, tilt the stethoscope so that the cephalad rim is compressing the femoral artery (Fig. 17-10A). With a forward-flow diastolic murmur, the sound-gener-

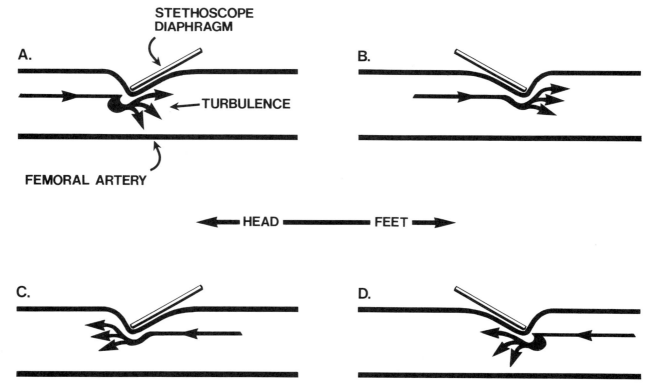

Figure 17-10.   *Duroziez's sign. Distinguishing a forward flow (A and B) from a reverse flow (C and D) diastolic component (see text).*

ating turbulence will now be under the stethoscope and will be well heard. Now tilt the stethoscope so that the caudad edge is compressing the femoral artery (Fig. 17-10B). The forward-flow sound-generating turbulence will now be occurring downstream from the stethoscope, and the diastolic component will become softer or disappear (Blumgart & Ernstene, 1933).

With a reversed-flow diastolic component, the opposite occurs. Pressing in with the cephalad rim of the stethoscope will cause the reversed-flow murmurs to be softer, while pressing with the caudad rim accentuates the sound (Fig. 17-10,C and D).

Using this modification, the positive predictive value of the Duroziez murmur approaches 100%, the degree of imprecision reflecting exactly the prevalence of patent ductus arteriosus in one's clinical population (Sapira, 1981), although patent ductus is easily diagnosed on separate clinical grounds (see footnote to Table 17-6).

Another use of the Duroziez sign is simply to make the diagnosis of aortic insufficiency in those cases in which the precordial diastolic murmur is not heard. At first this seems paradoxical, since both murmurs result from the diastolic reversal of flow in the aorta. But consider that Duroziez's murmur is produced right under your stethoscope, by your stethoscope, while the aortic whiff must be ausculted remote from its origin under a blanket of bone and muscle. Furthermore, adventitious lung sounds and ventilators interfere less with femoral than with precordial auscultation.

Hill's Sign

This sign, although useful for estimating severity of the regurgitation (or other high stroke volume conditions), is so little used that you could become an instant expert, just as anyone who takes up croquet in the United States can immediately be ranked.

A method. With the patient in the horizontal position, compare the brachial artery systolic pressure with the popliteal (or dorsalis pedal) artery systolic pressure, indirectly determined by palpation or auscultation.

Normally, the two indirectly determined pressures will be the same, or the apparent systolic pressure in the lower extremity will be up to 20 mm Hg higher (see Ch. 6, p. 89).

Although high stroke volume due to any cause (such as hyperthyroidism, arteriovenous fistula, pregnancy, beriberi, or strenuous muscular exertion) may cause the indirect systolic pressure to be more than 20 mm Hg *higher* in the *lower* extremity than in the upper, aortic insufficiency is the most important cause. Unfortunately, mild ("one plus") aortic insufficiency generates brachial-pedal gradients of less than 20 mm Hg. But above 20 mm Hg, a positive Hill's sign is highly significant, and the degree of the systolic pressure gradient is directly proportional to the degree of aortic insufficiency determined at cardiac catheterization (Sapira, 1981), if you have already independently determined that aortic regurgitation is the cause of the increased stroke volume.

Caveat. Because the dependent variable is the systolic blood pressure, the test cannot be performed in patients whose systolic blood pressure varies from beat to beat, for example, those with atrial fibrillation and highly irregular R-R intervals (see Ch. 6, p. 91).

Semiophysiology. The pathophysiology of Hill's sign is still uncertain. Some experts believe that in conditions of high stroke volume, a rebound wave returns from the periphery. The summation of the rebound wave and the aortic pressure pulse wave is believed to produce Hill's sign. This would certainly explain why Hill's sign is lost with direct intraarterial recordings, and why it is seen in so many conditions with high stroke volume. It would also explain why the degree of the artifact predicts the severity of the valve lesion, since greater insufficiency should result in a larger stroke volume. It would even explain how the sign can be lost in aortic stenosis

(which decreases stroke volume) and mitral stenosis (through interfering with ventricular filling, thus reducing the stroke volume), should either of these conditions appear in association with the aortic insufficiency (Sapira, 1981). But it does not explain why the summation wave should be present in the popliteal or dorsalis pedis vessels and not in the brachial vessels.

So, another idea is that with large stroke volume there is also a pressure wave at right angles to the forward wave, like dinner moving through a boa constrictor. The two waves sum only in the lower extremities because the upper extremity vessels exit the aorta at right angles.

Remember, this is an artifact of indirect blood pressure measurement. This sign is not useful when making direct measurements from the aorta and femoral artery (Sapira, 1981).

False positives. Severe, selective atherosclerosis in the upper extremity (i.e., Takayasu's disease) can cause a false-positive Hill's sign.

False negatives. Hill's sign (like Duroziez's sign) requires a high stroke volume and no interference to propagation of the pulse wave. Thus, mitral stenosis (see p. 319), aortic valvular stenosis, and aortic internal obstruction will each make the sign disappear.

There is an interesting situation in which the Duroziez murmur is maintained but Hill's sign disappears: the supervention of low-output cardiac failure, replacing the previous high-output cardiac failure. In this case, there is no longer sufficient stroke volume to produce the Hill's sign. This is an extremely important clue that tells you the time for surgical intervention has passed, a conclusion that can soon be ratified by expert opinion, supported by a quire of expensive studies.

Another instance in which Hill's sign may be lost before Duroziez's sign is atherosclerosis or other obstructive disease occurring between the femoral artery (where Duroziez's sign is sought) and the popliteal (or dorsalis pedis) where the measurement is made for Hill's sign.

Other Occasionally Useful Peripheral Signs of Aortic Insufficiency

Carotid shudder. In a patient with a basal diastolic murmur in whom it is not possible to perform the tests for Duroziez's sign or Hill's sign because of atrial fibrillation or iliofemoral thrombosis, evidence for aortic insufficiency may be adduced by finding the carotid shudder, discussed in Chapter 18 (p. 333).

De Musset's sign. De Musset's head-bobbing sign, best seen in patients who are sitting or standing quietly, consists of a bobbing or brief forward shaking of the head in time with the heartbeat. It is the only sign that will spontaneously attract one's attention, but it is not very sensitive and also has false positives (Sapira, 1981).

Very advanced. De Musset (who was not a physician) was considered one of the greatest French poets of the 19th century. He is now remembered only as a lover of George Sand and as the discoverer of this sign, a reflection of his own luetic aortic insufficiency (Sapira, 1981). As Osler once remarked about Jean Astruc, "It is strange how the memory of a man may float to posterity on what he would have himself regarded as the most trifling of all his works" (Osler, 1987).

Corrigan's pulse. Corrigan's pulse (see Ch. 18, p. 332), also known as Watson's water hammer pulse, was first described by de Vieussens in 1715 (Stone, 1986). This sign, rarely felt today, is a palpable manifestation of wide pulse pressure. It is of imperfect sensitivity and specificity for the diagnosis of aortic insufficiency and can even be felt in patent ductus arteriosus.

Pulse pressure. Despite the conventional wisdom, the pulse pressure is of little use in assessing the degree of aortic insufficiency present in any given patient (Bloomfield & Sinclair-Smith, 1973), even when the pulse pressure is constant from time to time.

Nor does it matter whether the gold standard for the degree of aortic insufficiency is that observed at surgery of the mitral valve (Cohn et al., 1967) or the angiogram taken preoperatively (Cohn et al., 1967; Frank et al., 1965.)

Nor does the pulse pressure correlate with prognosis, despite repeated statements to the contrary. When used as part of a triad, abnormal blood pressures could predict a group with lower mean survival, but there was no statistical evidence that blood pressure alone so correlated (Spagnuolo et al., 1971). In another study, the blood pressure measurements failed to predict death, including that occurring perioperatively (Smith et al., 1976). In a third, there was no significant prediction of myocardial death versus an excellent surgical outcome, although the latter group tended to have the lower diastolic and wider pulse pressure (Samuels et al., 1979). A fourth study similarly found no predictive value for the pulse pressure regarding perioperative mortality (Louagie et al., 1984). All of these papers were found in a review claiming just the opposite of what they showed.

The diastolic blood pressure was also of little use (Cohn et al., 1967). Admittedly, the combination of a diastolic pressure of at least 70 mm Hg and a pulse pressure of less than 40 mm Hg excluded the presence of moderate or severe aortic insufficiency, but the contrary was not true (Cohn et al., 1967).

Rosenbach's sign.   In one series of aortic insufficiency patients (Tice, 1911), 14% had hepatic pulsation (see Ch. 20, p. 383). This sign is rarely seen today, because patients are usually operated upon before their lesion becomes severe enough to produce it.

Gerhard's sign.   The sign is pulsation of the spleen, which can be detected only if the spleen is enlarged for another reason.

Becker's sign.   Visible pulsations of the retinal arterioles are called Becker's sign.

Mueller's sign.   A pulsating uvula is called Mueller's sign (see Ch. 13, p. 227).

"Pistol shot" sounds.   A "pistol shot" sound is heard at the femoral artery in 45% of cases of very severe aortic insufficiency (Tice, 1911). It is nondiagnostic, also being found in other high stroke volume states such as anemia and hyperthyroidism (Levine & Harvey, 1949).

Traube's sounds.   Traube's femoral double sound eludes most examiners because they do not perform the requisite maneuver. As repeatedly pointed out (Laubry et al., 1931; Traube, 1872), if one simply applies the stethoscope lightly to the femoral artery one will almost never hear the double tone. But if one compresses the femoral artery distal to the stethoscope head with just the correct amount of pressure, one will be able to find the double tone, likened by Traube to heart tones.

The sensitivity of the double tone was 24% in a series of 124 patients with aortic insufficiency (Tice, 1911). A few of these patients had triple tones.

A historical interlude.   The Franco-Prussian War may have had an influence on the diagnosis of aortic insufficiency in the United States. In the second half of the 19th century, the German medical tradition seems to have had greater influence on medical education and practice in the United States than the French, possibly because the United States was less well-positioned to import medical traditions earlier when the French tradition was ascendant.

In the first paper describing the double tones (Fraentzel, 1867), it is stated by Fraentzel that Traube had recently made this discovery. It is noteworthy that Traube was the *Geheim Rath* and Fraentzel was his assistant.

(A *Geheim Rath*, literally a "secret advisor," was an extra-academic appointment, not limited to the medical or academic world. Persons of eminence could be appointed by and to the king or baron. Because of their political power, many of these *Geheim Rath* personages found that they could attract to themselves ambitious, more energetic young workers, especially in academia. In time, a *Geheim Rath* came to mean an academic entrepreneur whose time had passed, but who continued to put his name on the original work of his assistants, who were free to leave if they objected. They didn't, of course, because they hoped one day also to become a *Geheim Rath*. Predictably, the Queen of Medicine soon left Germany. We are indeed fortunate to live in a time and place in which older academicians do not exploit their fiduciary relationship with their younger colleagues.)

Traube obviously discovered his sign by pressing on the femoral artery distally, while following Duroziez's instructions on how to produce the sign bearing the latter's name. How else can one explain what Traube was doing (i.e., listening to a patient with aortic insufficiency at the femoral artery with his finger compressing the artery distally)?

In the second paper (Traube, 1872), published right after the Franco-Prussian war, Traube himself noted a very few cases in which the double tone could be heard *without* the Duroziez maneuver ("*so erscheint auch in dem Ausnahmefall der Doppelton ohne dass die Arterie comprimirt zu werden braucht*") (Traube, 1872).

This second Traube sign, performed without distal arterial compression (which further distanced him psychologically from the Frenchman Duroziez) was very rare and was found only in cases of severe aortic insufficiency with massive left ventricular dilatation. Traube himself heard it only five times (Traube, 1872) in 5 years. This second Traube sign (the one attempted in the United States) will usually be absent in aortic insufficiency.

In contrast, Duroziez's sign is encountered frequently, yet has been unpopular in this country. Most American texts mention it only to denigrate its usefulness, despite the fact that most such authors do not seem to have read Duroziez's papers and do not give correct instructions on how to produce the sign (Sapira, 1981). Further, most of the criticisms leveled against Duroziez's sign were answered in his original papers, which oddly enough have yet to be translated into English in their entirety.

Has the vigorous promotion of a rare sign of aortic insufficiency in preference to a more useful Gallic maneuver been nothing more than the residual influence of the Franco-Prussian War and a *Geheim Rath*?

Useless "signs"

Two signs of aortic insufficiency that are usually presented in textbooks of physical diagnosis are actually useless.

Quincke's sign.   Quincke's pulse can be seen by exerting, on the edge of the nail, a pressure that is greater than the diastolic but less than the systolic. Quincke described it thus:

> . . . a clear (whitish) zone in the nails can be produced by an even pressure, . . . in the area between the whitish, clear, zone and the red, injected, zone of the capillary system of the nail-bed, in the majority of persons examined there is with each heart beat a forward and backward movement of the margin between the red (zone) and the clear (white) zone, and one can convince himself that the increase of the redness follows a moment later than the apex beat and is still clearly systolic and rather rapid; while the backward movement of the edge of the redness seems to take place more slowly. (Major, 1945; Quincke, 1868)

This is a normal phenomenon present in everyone, not a pathognomonic sign of aortic insufficiency or anything else (Sapira, 1981). The first person to notice that the Quincke pulse was present in normal persons was Quincke himself!

Mayne's sign.   Another useless "sign" erroneously thought to indicate aortic insufficiency is Mayne's sign (Abbas & Sapira,

1987). This is a decrease in the indirect diastolic blood pressure of 15 mm of mercury when the arm is held above the head, as compared with the baseline diastolic blood pressure taken with the arm at the level of the heart (Mayne, 1953). This sign occurs in 65% of normal persons (Abbas & Sapira, 1987).

Etiologies

1. It is a rule of thumb (Harvey et al., 1963) that rheumatic lesions of the aortic valve and syphilitic *valvular* disease (i.e., luetic* involvement of the leaflets without valve-ring dilatation) produce a diastolic decrescendo murmur that radiates best to the third or fourth *left* (not right) intercostal space, while aortic insufficiency murmurs due to bacterial endocarditis or aortic root (nonvalvular) causes usually radiate more loudly to the *right* sternal border. So, if the murmur radiates best to the right, be alert for endocarditis or other entities associated with aortic root disease (such as aortic aneurysm, dilatation of the aortic root, aortic dissection, aneurysm of the sinus of Valsalva, Marfan's syndrome, traumatic valve deformity, osteogenesis imperfecta, rheumatoid spondylitis, Behçet's syndrome, and syphilis (Harvey et al., 1963).) But if it is loudest on the left, you should search for coexistent disease of another valve, a common finding in rheumatic disease.

2. The murmur of aortic insufficiency can result from hypertension with diastolic pressures above 130 mm Hg. If the patient is given a ganglionic blocker (such as hexamethonium) that causes orthostatic hypotension, the murmur goes away when the patient is tilted upright (Leonard & Allensworth, 1963). When the patient is placed recumbent, the blood pressure rises, and the murmur will return.

Some older hypertensives may also have AI murmurs at diastolic pressures as low as 90 to 100 mm Hg. Perhaps there is also some underlying structural abnormality, but the murmur disappears when the diastolic pressure is lowered to 80 to 90 mm Hg (Leonard & Allensworth, 1963).

3. Aortic valve fenestration (Friedman & Hathaway, 1958), which is usually not hemodynamically significant, may produce an audible aortic insufficiency murmur. This lesion is hard to find by echocardiography, but is more frequent than expected at careful autopsy.

4. For years, students were taught about an early diastolic decrescendo blow heard in chronic renal failure and putatively due to aortic insufficiency. Yet there were no associated peripheral signs of aortic insufficiency, and the murmur quickly disappeared with treatment. Attempts to find the aortic insufficiency at catheterization were so unsuccessful that some concluded this sound was actually a pericardial rub. We now know that this sound is due to volume overload pulmonic insufficiency (Perez et al., 1985) (see p. 321).

Epistemology

The signs of aortic insufficiency in the present section were derived predominantly from studies of chronic aortic insufficiency. The semiophysiology of acute aortic insufficiency remains a terra incognita despite the statements (unreferenced) of many experts that the semiophysiology is different, based upon the "fact" that the ventricle has not had time to enlarge and so produce a large stroke volume. From personal experience, I know that some high stroke volume signs *are* sometimes evident in acute aortic insufficiency, although I do not know how often, because of insufficient experi-

*"Syphilis" was the name of the afflicted hero in Frascatorius' 1530 poem. "Lues" is Latin for misfortune and became a euphemistic synonym for syphilis during considerate bedside presentations prior to penicillin. We retain and practice it today for similar reasons.

ence. I also know that some of the expert statements about the semiophysiology of acute aortic insufficiency are written by the same people that believe that Quincke's sign is a sign of aortic insufficiency and do not realize that it is a normal finding. How much of modern clinical scholarship is based upon perceptive clinical experience and how much of it is simply sequential copying thus remains unknown. This teaches us that medical history repeats itself and medical professors repeat each other.

Aortic Stenosis

Clinical Findings

If you have been reading this text sequentially, you already know almost everything that you need to know about valvular aortic stenosis. First, you know that aortic valvular stenosis is manifested clinically by the presence of the characteristic murmur in a patient with left ventricular hypertrophy. Second, you are aware of the utility of the right midclavicular amplification of this murmur (Spodick et al., 1976) (see p. 302). Third, severe cases produce paradoxical splitting of S2 (see p. 295). (The carotid shudder and the parvus-et-tardus carotid upstroke are discussed in Ch. 18, pp. 333 and 331, respectively.)

Remember, aortic stenosis produces a murmur that can be heard in any of the anterior areas covered by General Patton's sash (as portrayed in the motion picture starring George C. Scott). This red sash passed, anteriorly, from the right midclavicular area down over the aortic valve area, further down to the apex, and to the fifth and sixth intercostal spaces in the anterior and midaxillary lines, but *not* into the axilla.

An increase in the murmur with handgrip almost always excludes aortic stenosis (see p. 308). The murmur tends to increase in intensity after a long diastole (see p. 308) or amyl nitrite (see p. 308).

O   *An additional bedside method for evaluating the degree of stenosis*: Estimate the interval between the peak PMI (felt with the right hand) and the peak of the carotid artery upstroke (felt with the left hand). Ordinarily, these are very close together, but they become separated in time in proportion to the severity of the stenosis (Chun & Dunn, 1982). While the effective use of this estimate requires a lot of experience with aortic stenosis patients, it also requires an appreciation of normal, something that one can begin accruing immediately.

A narrow pulse pressure, once cited as a characteristic feature of aortic stenosis, no longer seems to be of diagnostic value in the present population of patients with aortic stenosis (Lombard & Selzer, 1987), although in individual cases it could be helpful *if present*.

Etiologies

The etiology of aortic stenosis depends upon the location of one's practice. Where there is still rheumatic fever, most cases in younger persons (under age 50) are rheumatic. Where rheumatic fever becomes rare and the population lives long enough to get the degenerative diseases, half the cases under 50 will be due to bicuspid valves and half over 50 will be due to degenerative calcification of tricuspid valves (Passik et al., 1987).

Differential Diagnosis: When Is Aortic Stenosis Not Aortic Stenosis?

One problem for the auscultor is to recognize when the murmur of aortic stenosis is not from valvular aortic stenosis. Can you name a condition in which that is the case? Write your answer down. After reading the next section, you should be able to list several.

1. Relative Aortic Stenosis

Relative aortic stenosis from aortic insufficiency is not absolute aortic stenosis. (If you gave a different answer, it might still be right—read on.) In aortic insufficiency, the left ventricle is filled not only from the left atrium but also by the regurgitant blood passing back through the defective aortic valve (both events occurring in diastole). Thus, on the next systole, there is an increased stroke volume across the aortic valve, which (although leaky) is normal in area. The increased flow over the normal valve produces the same turbulence as a normal stroke volume flowing over a decreased valve area (see p. 300). This relative flow murmur may be misinterpreted as an absolute valvular murmur. (The words we use to communicate clinical findings, like language in general, are quite treacherous, unforgiving, persistent in their obfuscation, and concealing of their misdirection, as Count Korzybski pointed out in *General Semantics*.)

2. Aortic Sclerosis

Aortic sclerosis is a roughening of the valve that may not initially cause obstruction or a systolic gradient, but that can produce a murmur identical to that of aortic stenosis. Mild aortic sclerosis does not in and of itself produce a delay in left ventricular ejection time, and so, unlike severe valvular aortic stenosis, will not produce a paradoxical split of S2. Unfortunately, cases of aortic stenosis too mild to produce a paradoxical split of S2 can be very difficult to distinguish from aortic sclerosis.

Worse, in some cases of aortic sclerosis (proven by catheterization), the murmur radiated to the right midclavicle, and was grade 3/6. This is especially likely with concurrent severe anemia. After transfusion, the murmur may diminish to grade 1/6, although the radiation and amplification persist. Although intellectually it seems obvious that the synergistic effects of turbulence and high flow could produce such a mimicking of the murmur of significant valvular aortic stenosis, it can be quite startling to hear in real life.

A caveat. We are speaking here of the difference between severe valvular aortic stenosis (as epitomized say by rheumatic valvular disease) and very mild degrees of degenerative sclerosis of the aortic valve, which cause roughening and a murmur but no obstruction. It should be pointed out that with the passage of much time the sclerotic process can itself evolve into an obstructive process, and the distinction can no longer be made by physical examination or much else short of direct inspection of the valve.

3. Aortic Stenosis Mimicked by Mitral Insufficiency

When the systolic regurgitant jet squirts back into the left atrium, and vibrates the aorta opposite the enlarged left atrium, these vibrations may be heard at the aortic root area as a diamond-shaped systolic murmur, as documented by intracardiac phonocardiography (Antman et al., 1978).

4. Nonvalvular Lesions

Obstruction to the aortic outflow tract may also occur above the valve (supravalvular aortic stenosis) or below (subvalvular aortic stenosis, generally known as idiopathic hypertrophic subaortic stenosis or IHSS, vide infra).

Depending upon the location of the supravalvular stenosis, these rare patients may have a coarctation-like picture. Sometimes the blood pressures in the two arms are unequal. Many of these congenital anomalies can be traced to bouts of maternal hypercalcemia. As infants and children, these patients are thought to show elfin facies and a "machine-like" sound to the speaking voice, but this stereotype should not be relied upon for diagnosis in an adult.

Idiopathic* Hypertrophic Subaortic Stenosis

An Overview

In the Platonic (ideal) form of IHSS, there is a ring of cardiac muscle just beneath the valve that contracts in systole, so that the wall of the ventricle forms an obstruction to its own outflow (Fig. 17-11).

IHSS receives more attention in this chapter than it deserves from the standpoint of its prevalence because it is so epistemologically useful when contrasted to valvular aortic stenosis of either the rheumatic (now waning) or the bicuspid (now waxing) type.

In point of fact, the question of IHSS is much more complicated and evolving than suggested here. Related issues include the morphology of the muscle wall, the condition of the coronary circulation, and the diastolic filling abnormalities. And it is in-

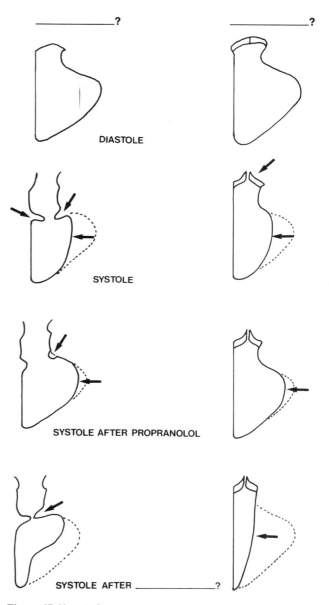

Figure 17-11. *A diagrammatic representation of two lesions. Can you fill in the blanks? (Answer in Appendix 17-3.)*

---

*You should pardon the expression (see Appendix 7-2, p. 135).

creasingly being recognized that in many cases of IHSS, the obstruction is not due to a ring of muscle, but to contact between the septal leaflet of the mitral valve and the outflow tract (Wigle, 1987). (The midsystolic diamond-shaped ejection murmur occurs in both types.) However, the entity was first appreciated in terms of the dramatic physical findings of IHSS, and is considered here from that viewpoint. The reader interested in learning more is advised to read almost anything by S.E. Epstein, including his most recent review (Maron et al., 1987.)

Very advanced. The symmetrical ring of muscle that produces obstruction should probably be referred to as subaortic muscular stenosis. This should be distinguished from hypertrophic obstructive cardiomyopathy, in which the entire left ventricular wall is hypertrophied (Goodwin, 1972). Although there are overlaps, both of these may be different from the entity asymmetric septal hypertrophy, in which there is no apparent involvement of the free wall of the left ventricle. A partial outflow obstruction can occur in patients with an asymmetric hypertrophy of the muscle on the septal side of the outflow track. However, in some cases, asymmetric septal hypertrophy may apparently progress to subaortic stenosis. In other cases, it occurs in families, in which the abnormal genotype may manifest either as asymmetric septal hypertrophy or as subaortic stenosis in different individuals (Maron & Epstein, 1979).

For the attending. Whatever you do, you must not begin every sentence with "I can remember when I was a student . . . " Therefore, I would not dare tell the following story to anyone under the age of 40.

•

When I was a student, Drs. Jack Myers, Eddie Fisher, et al., published one of the first cases of IHSS. I can still recall the debate that transpired in the student lab (where we did the routine hemoglobin, hematocrit, white blood cell count, differential, and urinalysis) as to whether or not it was worth learning about this entity, which appeared in none of our texts. The nay-sayers won the day, arguing that if it took such luminaries so much time to find a single case, it could not be a very important disease. While this story seems to me to be of value to younger persons, it only bores them. As Dr. David Oldach of Maryland once said to me, "Please don't tell us such things. Let us learn them for ourselves." Still, like Ovid, sometimes I cannot take my own advice and so apologize with La Rochefoucauld's *"Peu de gens savent etre vieux"* (few of us know how to be old).

•

Importance of Establishing the Diagnosis

Distinguishing valvular aortic stenosis from IHSS has important therapeutic implications, which might be predicted from the response of the murmurs to various maneuvers. A patient with IHSS would do worse on digitalis because of the increased contraction of the subaortic muscle ring. A patient with aortic stenosis would not get worse on digitalis, although his condition might not be improved. Conversely, the administration of propranolol to a patient with aortic stenosis might decrease inotropy sufficiently to cause congestive heart failure, whereas beta blockers are a desirable therapy for IHSS, as they decrease the degree of dynamic obstruction.

Clinical Findings

One way to distinguish valvular aortic stenosis from IHSS on the physical examination is by the carotid upstroke (see Ch. 18, p. 332). Another way is to note the intensity of the second heart sound. It is usually louder in IHSS than in true valvular aortic stenosis.

Third, the murmur of aortic stenosis decreases with standing whereas that of IHSS increases, as noted above (p. 308), due to the decrease in filling pressure. In IHSS, there is more of a gradient across the obstruction when the ventricle is less expanded. This effect is partly related to a change in contractility, but is conveniently remembered by thinking that the stenosing lips of the muscle have less distance to travel and therefore create a more effective stenosis if the ventricular chamber is small (Fig. 17-11).

Fourth, as expected from the fact that standing and squatting have opposite effects on ventricular filling, the murmur of IHSS may get softer with the patient squatting (Rothman & Goldberger, 1983), while that of aortic stenosis usually does not.

Fifth, the murmur of IHSS gets softer during the post-Valsalva release (see Fig. 6-7), while the murmur of valvular aortic stenosis gets louder. This effect may also be comprehended in terms of ventricular filling and an increased end diastolic volume. (With respect to the caveats about the Valsalva maneuver on p. 309, note that we have specified the phase.)

Sixth, the murmur of aortic stenosis is loudest over the aortic valve area, but the murmur of IHSS may actually be loudest at the left sternal border.

Seventh, if an ejection click is present, valvular aortic stenosis is likely.

Eighth, if you are able to hear the heart during a spontaneous extrasystole (or, rarely, an extrasystole induced by rapping on the chest), it will be noted that the murmur of IHSS gets louder during the extrasystole, while the murmur of aortic stenosis gets softer. However, the murmur of valvular aortic stenosis will be louder during the immediate post-extrasystolic beat. You would expect the murmur of IHSS to become softer during the post-extrasystolic beat, but this finding is unreliable because the murmur is also longer (as shown by recordings) and some auscultors perceive the "longer" to be louder. During the post-extrasystolic beat, the pulse pressure regularly becomes less in IHSS. This (the Brockenbrough sign) can sometimes be felt as a diminished pulse at the bedside (Kramer et al., 1986).

False Positives

Be aware of the "detection" of this "lesion" by echocardiography in many persons who do not have it, due to the phenomenon of the angled septum (Fowles et al., 1980). Such patients do not have the murmur either, but it is difficult to impress house staff who "heard" the murmur because they first read the echo report. This is analogous to hearing the nonexistent S4 (Jordan et al., 1987).

In this connection, I have noticed the Credibility Hierarchy, a ranking of diagnosers of valvular heart disease, arranged in order of decreasing credibility:

1. A visiting professor (that is, a stranger in town who carries a slide case)
2. "Cardiology" (not the discipline, but a piece of paper typed by a secretary who may or may not have understood the dictation correctly)
3. The cardiology fellow (who started last month and has not yet been found to have hearing loss)
4. Student Schwein (whose sister dated the cardiology fellow from St. Hellebore, last year)
5. The attending physician (who has not yet developed a reputation but who did go to the bedside and personally examine the patient with all present).

This is mentioned not only because I have occupied roles 1 and 5 within the same week, but because the hierarchy is in exact inverse order of ease and accessibility for testing the accuracy of the findings by means of direct comparison tête-à-tête.

Mitral Insufficiency

Clinical Findings

The clinical findings in mitral insufficiency will vary somewhat with the etiology (vide infra). The characteristics of the murmur are described on page 301. The most helpful differentiating feature is that the mitral insufficiency murmur tends to radiate to the axilla.

A comatose patient with a history of hypertension and a previous myocardial infarction had a systolic murmur, thought by house staff to be that of aortic stenosis. On auscultation, a grade 3/6 coarse ("white noise") holosystolic murmur could be heard over the apex. It radiated weakly to the left axilla (where it was grade 2/6) and to the back (grade 1/6), but not to the right midclavicular area. What is your diagnosis? (Write it down.)

Because the murmur was holosystolic and was not heard at the right midclavicular area, it was not consistent with aortic stenosis. The apical location and the radiation to the axilla were not suggestive of tricuspid insufficiency. One did not diagnose ruptured ventricular septum because the murmur was louder in the axilla than posteriorly, and because Friedberg (1956) and others have encountered proved mitral insufficiency murmurs that radiated to the back. One diagnosed mitral insufficiency, correctly, as it turned out.

More commonly in this situation, the murmur is a diamond-shaped murmur, rather than a holosystolic one. Could you then recapitulate the above reasoning? Try it. (Check your answer with Appendix 17-4).

Etiology

An Overview

Mitral insufficiency can either be primary (usually with a holosystolic murmur), or secondary to some other process that leads to a failure of perfect coaption of the leaflets of the mitral valve.

Primary mitral insufficiency was formerly a common manifestation of the then-common disease, rheumatic fever. At the present time, the most common single cause is probably mitral valve prolapse. Other causes include infective endocarditis, trauma, carcinoid syndrome with either an atrial septal defect or pulmonary involvement, systemic lupus erythematosus, rheumatoid arthritis, ankylosing spondylitis, Marfan's syndrome, Ehlers-Danlos, pseudoxanthoma elasticum, and various congenital malformations of the mitral valve.

Secondary mitral insufficiency is most frequently caused by either papillary muscle dysfunction or cardiomyopathy (or other types of congestive heart failure), wherein the heart (including the mitral annulus) enlarges beyond the competence of the mitral valve (which cannot enlarge concordantly). Papillary muscle dysfunction may ultimately be due to acute ischemia or infarction, or even chronic infarction of the papillary muscles. Besides dilated, hypertrophic, or restrictive cardiomyopathy, causes of a dilated mitral annulus include mitral annular calcification and radiation therapy.

Other etiologies that are not unanimously classified as to type include mucocutaneous lymph node syndrome (Kawasaki's disease), osteogenesis imperfecta, some of the mucopolysaccharidoses, and Fabry's disease (Olson et al., 1987).

Very advanced. Rupture of the chordae tendineae may sometimes be the mechanism for the mitral insufficiency in several of the conditions listed above, including the connective tissue disorders and infective endocarditis, although chordal rupture is usually "spontaneous" (i.e., of unknown etiology).

Originally, it was believed that this disease presented with a dramatic acute onset, a "whirring" systolic murmur due to the ruptured chordae being spun in the regurgitant jet of blood, and pulmonary edema leading to death if surgical intervention was not undertaken. We now know that the disease is usually less dramatic in onset, does not always produce the whirring holosystolic murmur, and is usually a progressive disease rather than an acutely fatal one (Oliveira et al., 1983).

This disease thus illustrates an important principle of medicine: when new diseases are constructed and described, inevitably the very worst cases are reported first. After the picture of a flagrant disease with high mortality and morbidity is set in the literature, later series note less severe cases. But by then it is difficult to convince people that the original descriptions were only one part of the spectrum of disease.

The corollary to this is that relatively rare diseases, of which the average physician is unlikely to see many cases, will have their original noxious image persist in the medical public's mind much longer than that of more common diseases. The latter will more likely permit consensual validation of the existence of a class of patients whose state is more benign than the original description.

A second corollary, more subtle but more important, is that in the study of the therapy of a disease, one should not use historical controls. If one does not have a concurrent control group, but instead gives all current patients a new remedy and compares their outcome to the outcome of patients studied before the remedy became available, it is easy to be misled. Current patients are probably less severely afflicted than those diagnosed when the disease was first described, and will seem to "do somewhat better" on any equivalent new therapy.

A subcorollary is that for relatively rare diseases, for which the average physician is most dependent upon the literature reports of others, this shift in the description of the natural history is least likely to be appreciated. Thus, if remedies for a very rare disease are compared using historical controls, the new remedy is likely to appear much better than the old therapy, even if both are actually of equal efficacy.

Mitral Valve Prolapse

> The regurgitation in some such cases might depend on no actual valvular lesion. Relaxation of the walls of the ventricle or of the papillary muscles might allow some slight regurgitation during a portion of the systolic period. (Griffith, 1892)

Variability of the murmur. The honk or whoop or coo of mitral valve prolapse may vary from beat to beat, this variability being one of the factors that led early auscultors to doubt a cardiac origin. The variability, when it is present, results from the fact that the prolapsed mitral valve is like a clarinet reed and can only be sounded when the dP/dT is perfect for that reed. Because there is a slight beat-to-beat variation in the amount of blood flow and the dP/dt across the valve (in systole), there may be wide variation in the resulting sound. With some honks, the variation in dP/dt causes a variation in timbre, so that one may hear a goose on one beat and a pigeon on the next. In some patients, the honk is heard only during premature ventricular contractions. At other times the overriding influence is the venous return to the left side of the heart, so the variability is a function of respiration, and one hears the sound only with one phase of respiration. Thus, it is easy to see how the honk was once thought to be of pulmonary origin.

In addition to mitral valve prolapse and tricuspid valve prolapse, a honk has also been detected in cases of infectious endocarditis of the mitral and tricuspid valves, and in presumed mitral annulus dysfunction secondary to primary myocardial disease or ischemic heart disease (Sheikh et al., 1984). It is interesting that while the honk is more pronounced (or appears exclusively) with standing in the case of prolapsed mitral valve, in the other causes of "honking" on standing, the honk actually disappeared or decreased in intensity, but never appeared or became louder.

○ *Caveat.* However, most prolapsed valves cause murmurs of the usual type and not bird songs.

Systolic clicks.   Mitral valve prolapse may be associated with a systolic click, by a mechanism illustrated in Figure 17-12.

The click precedes the murmur. (Thus, the murmur, if accompanied by the click, cannot be holosystolic, as the portion of systole between the first heart sound and the click is silent.)

One should always auscult for mitral valve prolapse with the patient in the *standing position*, because the murmur may become louder and/or longer (Rothman & Goldberger, 1983) (see p. 308). Also, with standing, the ejection click may occur earlier in systole (see p. 290), or appear if it was previously absent (Popp & Winkle, 1976).

There are patients who have only the early systolic click, and no murmur. There have even been patients with prolapse seen on echocardiography who have no murmur and no click, and some patients will have one set of findings at one point and another when studied later in the same position. (Forget this while you solve the problem given in the next paragraph.) (Note, however, that it is possible to produce "echocardiographic MVP" by an abnormal inferiorly directed orientation of the transducer [Cheng, 1987].)

Epidemiology.   With the irruption of echocardiographers, mitral valve prolapse could be diagnosed in the absence of a click or a murmur. In fact, only 9% of patients with mitral valve prolapse found in the Framingham study (Savage et al., 1983) had clicks and 9% had murmurs. Only 2% had both findings. Conversely, this study revealed that only 50% of people with clicks alone had echocardiographic mitral valve prolapse, although the additional presence of the murmur made the diagnosis more certain. In the free-living population without recognizable mitral valve prolapse, 1% had clicks and 3.53% had murmurs (Savage et al., 1983).

Self-Test: If the prevalence of mitral valve prolapse in Framingham was 7.11%, and the number of subjects was 2,925, calculate the murmur's positive predictive value for mitral valve prolapse and the negative predictive value of no murmur. Answers are in Appendix 17-5 (p. 327).

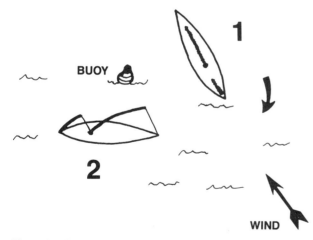

Figure 17-12.   *Mechanism for the systolic click in mitral valve prolapse. Look at sailboat 1, which is just coming around the mark (buoy). The wind is out of its sails. Soon it will turn into the position of sailboat 2, the sails of which are completely filled by the wind. If the sails on the first boat abruptly catch the wind as it turns into position, there will be a snapping or popping sound. This is analogous to the click heard in mitral valve prolapse. Obviously, if the sailboat rounds the mark very slowly, and the sails fill out gradually, the same excursion will not necessarily produce a snap or a pop, just as mitral valve prolapse is not always accompanied by a click. This should also explain why the presence or absence of a click is unrelated to the presence or absence of a murmur.*

History.   For the neophyte who believes that diseases are fixed and easily discoverable entities, the story of mitral valve prolapse may substitute for that sad sense of history possessed by the quinquagenarians who have lived long enough to see their investigative techniques tarnished, their specialty transformed in the maelstrom of time, and their pet "diseases" as prevalent as the schottische.

Mitral valve prolapse, currently the most common of mitral valve diseases, said to afflict 4% of the population, did not appear in any of the pathology, medicine, or cardiology textbooks of my school days!

For many years, it was known that tall, thin, ectomorphic, asthenic, apparently healthy patients who had a very straight thoracic vertebral column, an anterior-posterior/transverse thoracic diameter less than expected, and sometimes pectus excavatum, might also have a systolic murmur over the mitral valve area. These patients were said to have the "straight-back syndrome." It was assumed that their apical systolic murmur was due to the heart being squeezed between the sternum and the straight back. The straightness of the back was easily demonstrated by observing it from the side when the patient raised his arms, or by a lateral chest film. From the days when grand rounds were still grand and rounds, I can remember learned cardiologists demonstrating the bedside diagnosis of this syndrome in patients about to be freed from the onerous burden of the diagnosis of heart disease. The learned discussors would point out the lack of historical evidence of heart disease (such as cyanosis or rheumatic fever); the absence of physical findings other than the systolic murmur; the total absence of electrocardiographic findings (except for "clockwise rotation of the heart," a diagnosis that is now as obsolete as the pterodactyl); and the altered cardiac borders on the posterior-anterior (PA) chest film (further evidence that the heart was "trapped" between the sternum and the straight back).

At the same time, there was another entity that was also believed to be artifactual in nature. Ausculting the hearts of some patients, one could hear a "whoop" or a "honk." These sounds were described as short musical cries, but were not believed to be cardiac in origin, as they were not present during every cardiac cycle. The noises were sometimes preceded by a systolic click, a phenomenon that had also been noticed in patients with a straight-back syndrome. (However, in the latter case the click was considered to be an innocent aortic sound demonstrating the good function of the heart, and in no way related to the murmur that was considered nonpathologic albeit cardiac in origin.)

As the reader has already guessed, the "honk" or "whoop" was definitely of cardiac origin (Behar et al., 1967). This was demonstrated by intracardiac phonocardiography, angiography, and (very rarely) by autopsy, which revealed the same lesion ("ballooned mitral valve") seen in patients with Marfan's syndrome and mitral insufficiency. Eventually, it was noted that patients with such "parachute" mitral valves (later included in the set of mitral valve prolapse) could have the systolic click and murmur without a honk or a whoop. Then it was observed that many of these patients, while not having Marfan's syndrome, did have a marfanoid appearance; that is, their skeletons resembled those of patients with the presumably benign straight-back syndrome. At the same time, other workers, building up the other side of the corbelled arch, showed that thoracic cage abnormalities were frequently accompanied by mitral valve prolapse. Finally, we began to realize that the patients with the so-called innocent straight-back syndrome actually had no such "syndrome," but merely manifested the thoracic skeletal signs of the same connective tissue disease diathesis as their mitral valve prolapse (Bon Tempo et al., 1975; Salomon et al., 1975).

Associated findings.   In addition to pectus excavatum, scoliosis, and the habital signs of the straight-back syndrome (vide supra), women with mitral valve prolapse will have an increased prevalence of small breasts, and vice versa (Rosenberg et al., 1983).

Associated diseases.   Mitral valve prolapse may also occur in association with the Marfan syndrome, Ehlers-Danlos syndrome, von Willebrand syndrome, pseudoxanthoma elasticum, osteogenesis imperfecta, adult polycystic renal disease, some cardiomyopathies, and several types of congenital heart disease (Olson et al., 1987), including secundum atrial septal defect (Cheng, 1987).

Associated neuroses.   The newest finding seen as part of the mitral valve prolapse syndrome is agoraphobia; this might be related to the tachyarrhythmias to which patients with mitral valve prolapse are subject (Kantor et al., 1980). However, this association between agoraphobia and other neuroses in mitral valve prolapse has been questioned (Hickey et al., 1983). Who is correct?

As a general rule, we follow Claude Bernard in asserting that both are correct, the difference between the two results being due to unstated differences in the experiments that were done. Here, the disparate origins of the populations sampled represent a fertile source of unstated differences.

In other studies, patients with various psychiatric disorders, such as anorexia-bulimia (Johnson et al., 1986), have been found to have a greater prevalence of mitral valve prolapse than a control group. The most interesting paper of this type finds that the incidence of mitral valve prolapse in anorexia nervosa varies inversely with the weight of the subjects. The authors reasoned that as the subject lost weight and the left ventricular end diastolic dimensions decreased, the mitral valve, not shrinking comparably, became redundant. When the subject gained weight, those cardiac dimensions also increased and took up the slack in the prolapsed valve (Meyers et al., 1986). To the degree that this finding can be replicated and extended, we are faced with the novel proposition that mitral valve prolapse is a state, not a trait. This raises another of those philosophical questions so plentiful in medicine: if something is a state, not a trait, is it truly a disease, or is it a diathesis?

When Is a Mitral Insufficiency Murmur Not Mitral Insufficiency? (The Gallavardin Phenomenon)

Calcific aortic stenosis is most likely to produce the Gallavardin phenomenon. The Gallavardin phenomenon is a change in the pitch and timbre (but not shape) of an aortic valvular stenosis murmur with location, so as to imitate coexistent mitral regurgitation. That is, at the aortic area, the murmur is heard as harsh and dirty, but as one inches down to the apex, the timbre and tone become more pure, musical, and high pitched, imitating mitral insufficiency. The rough murmur originates from the turbulent blood flow at the aortic root, whereas the high-pitched musical murmur at the apex must come from the harmonic echoes from the symmetrical fibrocalcific cusps (Fig. 17-13). It is important to know of this phenomenon because otherwise the auscultor might falsely believe that the two different murmurs (differing in pitch and timbre) represent two different lesions, and so incorrectly diagnose mitral insufficiency in addition to the true aortic stenosis (or, uncommonly, sclerosis).

For the attending:

a. The pathophysiology of the Gallavardin phenomenon may not be quite so simple as I have just implied. Gallavardin believed that it was due to the preferential transmission of the harmonic high-pitched components to the apex through solid tissue, while the lower components were transmitted to the neck via the flow of blood (Gallavardin & Ravault, 1925). To my knowledge, this testable hypothesis has been neither refuted nor further examined. Gallavardin's own belief is close to the theory of Bruns, which is both general and exact (Bruns, 1959). But, it would not necessarily explain why the Gallavardin phenomenon is always associated with aortic valve calcification.

There is evidence in at least one case that the murmur was actually due to the mitral insufficiency of papillary muscle dysfunction (Giles et al., 1974). Yet this cannot be the explanation in all cases. I have had patients with the Gallavardin phenomenon who had no papillary muscle dysfunction (i.e., no mitral insufficiency) when ex-

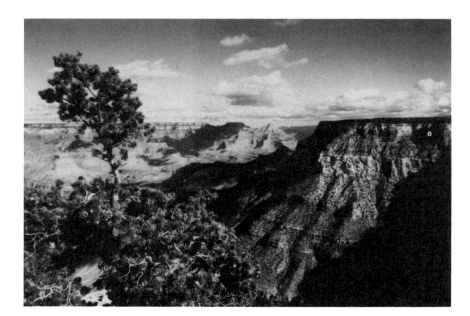

Figure 17-13.   *The Grand Canyon of Arizona. The high-pitched murmur heard at the apex in calcific aortic stenosis may be thought of as nothing more than the high-pitched echoes (as of a human voice or yodel) reverberating back to, and beyond, the point of origin. However, in this situation, the sound generator is the murmur, not the human voice; and the sounding board that reflects the high-pitched components is the calcific valve, not the wall of the canyon. Please note that this is a hypothesis, not a fact, and remember that an analogy is not a proof. Photograph courtesy of Dianne Dietrich Leis Photography, San Diego.*

amined by Doppler ultrasound (vide infra). Perhaps there is more than one Gallavardin phenomenon.

b. A 64-year-old white man with known coronary artery disease and angina was noted to have the "murmur of mitral insufficiency" on one of many admissions. In fact, the patient had a diamond-shaped murmur heard at the apex, but he also (when auscultated in a quiet room) had a coarse basal systolic murmur with right midclavicular amplification. The diagnosis of Gallavardin phenomenon was considered so bizarre by the house staff that they actually wagered on the Doppler studies, and gave odds to boot.

The predicted calcification of the aortic valve is shown in Figure 17-14A. The gradient across the valve can be calculated from the Doppler envelope shown in Figure 17-14B (see legend), revealing a moderate degree of aortic stenosis.

Does this prove that the patient did not also have mitral insufficiency? It does not. And the peak Doppler velocity overestimates the aortic gradient as determined at catheterization (Krafchek et al., 1985). So a special search was instituted for mitral insufficiency, and it was not seen on echo. A special Doppler study did show "mitral insufficiency" as demonstrated in Figure 17-14C (see legend), but the "gradient" of 4 mm Hg is not significant. (Such "physiologic" mitral and tricuspid "insufficiency" is often found by Doppler in the absence of any physical signs or other evidence of valvular disease [see Table 17-9, p. 326].)

Mitral Stenosis

Clinical Findings

Auscultation

Mitral stenosis has traditionally been associated with four auscultatory findings: a cracking, loud S1; a loud S2 (from an increased P2 supposedly reflecting pulmonic hypertension); an opening snap; and the classic diastolic murmur.

In point of fact, no correlation has been demonstrated between the amplitude of the pulmonic valve closure sound and the pulmonary artery pressure. Rather, the amplitude of P2 correlated with the degree of the patient's skinniness. There was also no significant correlation between the amplitude of S1 at the apex and the severity of the mitral stenosis. In fact, S1 could be soft or inaudible with mitral valve calcification (Surawicz et al., 1966). The opening snap was present in 90% of the patients with pure mitral stenosis and noncalcified mitral valves, but this finding was lost with increasing calcification and so was more likely to be present in milder cases (Surawicz et al., 1966). Thus, Tavel detected an opening snap in only 75% of all his cases (Reddy et al., 1985). There were only 2 of 141 patients with mitral stenosis who did not have the diastolic murmur, which is, therefore, the "best" sign (Surawicz et al., 1966). However, the presystolic component may be inaudible when atrial fibrillation supervenes.

Methods of augmenting the mitral stenosis murmur are discussed on page 308.

The phonocardiographic findings of mitral stenosis are diagrammed in Figure 17-15. The auscultatory findings were imitated by Duroziez with the phrase "*fout ta-ta rou*" (say it out loud, please). By this, he meant that the presystolic late diastolic crescendo murmur ending in a cracking S1 could be represented by the word "*fout*." The "*ta-ta*" represented the loud S2 followed by the opening snap. Finally, the "*rou*" coming off the opening snap is the early diastolic decrescendo murmur. Those who have heard the murmur of mitral stenosis can appreciate that Duroziez's phrase is a wonderful verbal mimicking of the sound. However, it does not seem to have caught on in the English-speaking United States. Accordingly, I propose an English language equivalent:

The owner of the now-defunct Stork Club in sophisticated New

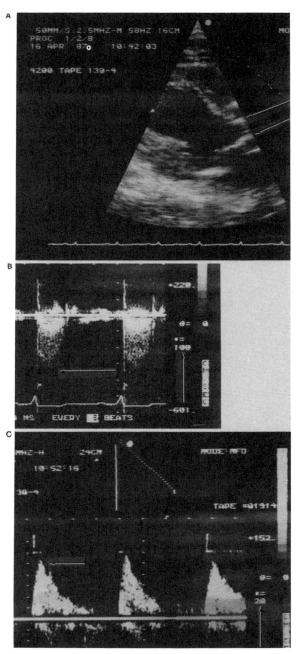

Figure 17-14. *A, Echo cardiogram. Arrows point to calcification in the aortic valve. B. Calculating the gradient from the Doppler envelope: the paired arrows point to the number "100" in the lower right-hand corner and to the Doppler envelope, displayed negatively. The "100" is the scale setting, and means that each mark is 100 cm/sec velocity or 1 m/sec. The modified Bernoulli equation states that the maximum velocity in m/sec, squared, times 4 equals the gradient in mm Hg. Now look at the horizontal arrow. The peak velocity is 320 cm/sec or 3.2 m/sec, so the gradient = (3.2)(3.2) × 4 = 41 mm Hg, a moderate degree of aortic stenosis. C, A special Doppler study of the mitral valve. The vertical arrow shows that the scale has been adjusted to 20 cm/sec. Five marks tells us that the maximum velocity is 100 cm/sec or 1 m/sec. Therefore, the "gradient" is (1)(1) × 4 = 4 mm Hg (i.e., no gradient to speak of). This is an example of physiologic or "false-positive" mitral insufficiency by Doppler (see Table 17-9).*

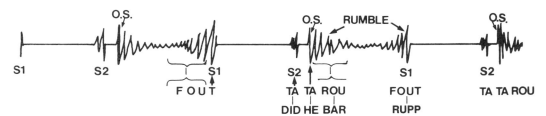

Figure 17-15. *Phonocardiographic findings in pure mitral stenosis (see text).*

York was notorious for barring certain persons from entering. We might wonder what would have happened if the University of Kentucky's bucolic basketball coach, Aldolph Rupp, had attempted to get in. About the owner, we would have asked: "Did he bar Rupp?"

Here, the first two words substitute for the *"ta-ta,"* being the S2 and the opening snap, respectively. "Bar" refers to the early decrescendo component of the diastolic murmur, while "Rupp" is the late diastolic component crescendoing to the cracking S1.

So far, we have been discussing mitral stenosis with normal sinus rhythm. In that instance, the sound sequence of mitral stenosis can be reasoned out. But when atrial fibrillation supervenes, the delirium cordis produces auscultatory phenomena so chaotic that the neophyte cannot possibly hope to reason them out. Accordingly, this is the only auscultatory phenomenon that one must memorize. Obtain a tape recording or phonograph record of mitral stenosis in the presence of atrial fibrillation, and memorize the sound.

A verbal imitation might be obtained by quickly repeating several times the following phrase, with its odd unpredictable sequence of rumblings and snappings: "In Walla Walla, Washington, my pocket was picked as I watched the Walla Walla cricketers rub wickets."

Evaluating the Severity of Mitral Stenosis

For the cardiology fellow.   After World War II, a dissemination of cardiac catheterization gave clinicians the opportunity to correlate the physiology of individual cases of mitral stenosis with the clinical features. At that time, cardiologists knew that the degree of mitral stenosis correlated inversely (albeit imperfectly) with the duration of the 2-OS (the interval between S2 and the opening snap) (Reddy et al., 1985). At the same time, the prevalence of mitral stenosis in those portions of the world most likely to have cardiac catheterization laboratories began decreasing, not only because of surgical correction but because the prevalence of rheumatic fever was dropping.

Subsequently, the persons referred to by I.S. Snapper (Snapper & Kahn, 1967) as "wizards" began to deprecate the 2-OS interval to audiences whose membership had increasingly rare opportunity to test mitral stenotic pronouncements at the bedside. The wizards correctly pointed out that there were a variety of factors not related to stenosis of the mitral valve, which affected the second heart sound, as well as some that might affect the timing of the opening snap. As phonocardiography was replaced by echocardiography, the 2-OS interval was pedagogued to oblivion.

Contemporary thinking further holds that the intensity and duration of the rumble in diastole does correlate with the severity of the stenosis. The following patient permits the testing of both these ideas.

●

Examination of a patient with pure mitral stenosis revealed a very soft murmur. The decrescendo portion ended well before mid-diastole, and the late diastolic crescendo was so short as to be almost inaudible. Accordingly, she was thought to have quite mild

mitral stenosis, and was being catheterized to search for other lesions (apparently thought to be inaccessible to clinical examination). But the 2-OS was extremely short.

The catheterization showed isolated mitral stenosis, with a high gradient (35 mm), a finding unexpected by some, and the patient was scheduled for surgery.

In this one patient, the 2-OS interval and the duration and intensity of the mitral rumble gave discrepant predictions, but the 2-OS was the accurate one. This should not be surprising because, without gainsaying the other factors that can have an influence on the 2-OS, the basic determinant is still the diastolic pressure gradient across the valve. High left atrial pressure in early diastole will snap the valve open faster than a low pressure head. On the other hand, the duration and intensity of the rumble are more dependent upon flow, that is, cardiac output. A decreasing cardiac output in the presence of a great degree of mitral stenosis might actually make a murmur softer than expected.

●

At this point, one is singed by his own petard because the biophysics of mitral stenosis is oversimplified in the above passages, hidden behind phrases such as the "basic determinant," "more dependent upon flow," and "more accurate [prediction]." Actually, the relationships are given by the Gorlin formula:

$$\text{valve area} = \frac{\text{blood flow}}{K \times 44.5 \times \sqrt{\text{pressure gradient}}}$$

The formula may be rearranged by multiplying both sides of the equation by the denominator on the right side of the original equation:

$$K \times 44.5 \times \sqrt{\text{pressure gradient}} \times \text{valve area} = \text{blood flow}$$

Removing the constants for simplification, the equal sign is replaced by an "is proportional to" sign:

$$\sqrt{\text{pressure gradient}} \times \text{valve area} \; \alpha \; \text{cardiac output}.$$

Finally, we recall that in pure mitral stenosis, flow is equal to cardiac output. Thus, *for an anatomically fixed degree of mitral stenosis (i.e., a given valve area), the pressure gradient will change with the cardiac output,* which in turn will change with the pulse rate. Thus, pressure gradient and cardiac output are not independent entities as implied.

$$\sqrt{\text{pressure gradient}} \times \text{valve area} \; \alpha \; \text{stroke volume} \times \text{heart rate}$$

The valve area is the only remaining constant in the patient.

As you might have guessed from this demurrer, the 2-OS is not infallible (also shown by Rackley et al., 1968). Nevertheless, in some individuals (such as the patient above) it can be very useful. A large experience and thorough review of both sides of this issue have been presented (Surawicz et al., 1966).

Associated Findings

Although much has been written of the malar flush (Fig. 9-6A) in mitral stenosis, this was seen only in very severe cases, which nowadays have been detected and surgically treated prior to that clue's appearance. (The malar flush can also be seen in pulmonic stenosis, without mitral stenosis.)

In my experience, patients with mitral stenosis tend to be short, mesomorphic women with square faces and square jaws who seem to prefer their hair short or brushed away from their faces.

Etiology

Although mitral stenosis was probably of rheumatic origin in 99% of patients in a surgical series, other causes have been reported. These include massive annular calcification, infective endocarditis with large obstructing vegetations, systemic lupus erythematosus, rheumatoid arthritis, gout, amyloidosis, Whipple's disease, methysergide therapy, carcinoid syndrome with associated atrial septal defect or pulmonary involvement, mucopolysaccharidoses, Fabry's disease, pseudoxanthoma elasticum, and congenital mitral stenosis (Olson et al., 1987).

Differential Diagnosis: When Is the Mitral Stenosis Murmur Not From Valvular Mitral Stenosis?

1. The Flint* murmur is a presystolic (that is, late diastolic) murmur sounding just like the presystolic rumble of mitral stenosis in a patient who has aortic insufficiency but no anatomical stenosis of the mitral valve. In diastole, the regurgitant jet of blood coming back into the left ventricle through the incompetent aortic valve keeps the anterior mitral leaflet from its full diastolic excursion. In mechanistic terms, this regurgitant jet holds the anterior mitral leaflet in a relatively "closed" (stenotic) position throughout diastole. At the end of diastole when the atria contract, the blood expelled from the left atrium into the ventricle is obstructed by this anterior mitral leaflet, and turbulence and a murmur are created, just as if the anterior leaflet of the mitral valve were being held in a closed ("stenotic") position from actual rheumatic scarring. Thus, mitral stenosis is not mitral stenosis when it is due to the effects of the regurgitant jet of aortic insufficiency. (To distinguish the Flint murmur from valvular mitral stenosis at the bedside, see p. 325.)

Yes, there can be a right-sided Flint murmur (Kambe et al., 1979).

2. Between 1958 and 1971, I saw Dr. Jack Myers of Pennsylvania make only four or five diagnostic errors, one of which was to diagnose mitral stenosis on the basis of a rumbling diastolic murmur in a case of pure mitral insufficiency. He was so sure of his diagnosis that he accused the pathologist of missing the lesion. The pathologist retorted that he had noticed that all examiners had heard the classic rumble, but a careful search of both mitral and tricuspid valves had revealed only mitral insufficiency.

We now know that relative mitral stenosis can occur in a situation in which there is no structural mitral stenosis (Fortuin & Craige, 1973). Just as the increased stroke volume produced by aortic insufficiency can cause an aortic stenosis murmur, the increased left atrial stroke volume due to mitral insufficiency can cause turbulent blood flow and a rumble.

A few years later, Dr. Myers himself was teaching about the relative mitral stenosis of increased flow.

This story illustrates two points: 1) The really good diagnosticians are the ones who can reprogram their brains. 2) The rumble of mitral stenosis must be extremely specific if it took such an adept clinician so long to learn the exception to the rule.

Very advanced. The diastolic flow murmur of relative mitral stenosis occurring in acute rheumatic fever is specifically called the Carey Coombs murmur after the one doctor who described it. (Right, there was no doctor Carey!)

---

*Not Austin-Flint. There was no Dr. Austin anymore than there was a Dr. Jod (see Ch. 14). Austin was his first name. We will meet two more nonexistent cardiologists shortly.

Pulmonic Insufficiency

Clinical Findings

The murmur of pulmonic insufficiency, heard best in the second left interspace, tends to have a brief crescendo in the very beginning of diastole before it becomes decrescendo. However, the shape of the Steell* murmur (pulmonic insufficiency secondary to pulmonary hypertension) may be indistinguishable from that of aortic insufficiency. The Graham Steell murmur can be high pitched like that of aortic insufficiency, or it can be of a lower pitch.

The differential diagnosis of aortic from pulmonic insufficiency is given on page 325.

Etiology

Pulmonic insufficiency, like other valvular abnormalities, may be considered to be either primary or secondary. Primary pulmonic insufficiency would be seen in a few cases of rheumatic heart disease and in some rare cases of infective endocarditis of the pulmonic valve. Since a major risk factor for infective endocarditis is now intravenous drug abuse, we should note that the endocarditis of the drug abuser usually (99% of cases) spares the pulmonic valve (Sapira & Cherubin, 1975). Syphilis also spares the pulmonic valve.

Secondary pulmonic insufficiency is known by the company it keeps. It may be the Steell murmur of pulmonary hypertension (which occurred in 12% of cases of mitral stenosis [Linhart, 1971]), or it may result from idiopathic dilatation of the pulmonary artery or from the transient volume overload seen in patients with chronic renal failure (Perez et al., 1985).

Pulmonic Stenosis

Clinical Findings

There may be a right ventricular tap. S2 may sound widely split (see p. 296) or single when P2 is softened to nothingness. The systolic murmur of pulmonic stenosis is maximal at the pulmonic area, but otherwise sounds similar to that of aortic stenosis. It may even radiate into the carotids, the left more than the right.

The response to amyl nitrite may help to differentiate isolated valvular pulmonic stenosis, infundibular pulmonic stenosis, and tetralogy of Fallot (see p. 308).

Etiology and a Consideration of Congenital Heart Disease

Pulmonic stenosis also may be either primary or secondary (relative). The primary form may be either congenital (with the murmur heard before age 5) or rheumatic (murmur first heard after the age of 5, in the presence of other valvular abnormalities because rheumatic fever rarely strikes only the pulmonic valve and infective endocarditis does not cause stenosis of this valve).

Secondary or relative pulmonic stenosis occurs in atrial septal defect, and ventricular septal defect, as long as the flow is from left to right. With ventricular septal defect, there may be a second systolic murmur due to the blood passing through the septal defect. One wishes to diagnose ventricular septal defect quickly, before the shunt reverses, not only because it is easier to do so then (before there can be confusion with tetralogy of Fallot), but also because surgical correction is most useful before the ominous supervention of pulmonary hypertension. The diagnosis of tetralogy of

---

*Also called the "Graham-Steell" murmur. As you have correctly guessed, there was no Dr. Graham; it was Steell's first name.

Fallot is suggested by the picture of a cyanotic patient with a ventricular septal defect and a single or very soft S2.

Atrial septal defect is characterized by a widely "fixed" split S2. It is different from probe-patent foramen ovale, in which an anatomic seal has not occurred. Probe-patent foramen ovale has no murmur or other physical findings, but, like atrial septal defect, it can be associated with paradoxical embolism (a venous embolus reaching the systemic circulation by passing through the foramen ovale). This happens if the foramen ovale opens, as it can whenever the right atrial pressure exceeds the left atrial pressure (e.g., in pulmonary hypertension with right-sided "backward" heart failure). This possibility is worth remembering because the prevalence of probe-patent foramen ovale is 34% during the first 3 decades of life, decreasing to 20% through the 9th and 10th decades (Hagen et al., 1984).

This differential has covered all the major congenital defects, except two that you have already diagnosed: coarctation of the aorta (by taking the blood pressure in the leg) and patent ductus arteriosus (from Gibson's murmur, p. 304).

Tricuspid Insufficiency

Clinical Findings

The Murmur

Tricuspid insufficiency causes a systolic murmur at the *left* sternal border in the fourth and fifth intercostal spaces, which usually does *not* radiate to the axilla.

Dr. George Massing of Alabama taught me an important exception to the rule that radiation into the left axilla excludes the tricuspid valve as a source for the insufficiency murmur. In cases of severe pulmonary hypertension, in which the right ventricle changes from a volume chamber to a pressure chamber, it is possible for the murmur of mitral insufficiency to be mimicked by tricuspid insufficiency in every respect.

In 1946, Carvallo described a highly diagnostic sign of tricuspid insufficiency: inspiratory augmentation (or appearance) of a systolic murmur at the lower left sternal border, due to increased filling of the right heart. The sensitivity is at least 61% (Gooch et al., 1983; Rothman & Goldberger, 1983), being higher in severe cases (Maisel et al., 1984). Unfortunately, inspiration tends to move the heart away from the examiner, counterbalancing the murmur's intracardiac increase. But on those occasions when the sign is positive, it is highly significant (although there has been a documented false positive, i.e., a patient who had the sign but no tricuspid insufficiency [Leon et al., 1965].)

Once you have detected inspiratory augmentation of the murmur of tricuspid insufficiency, its subsequent loss should suggest the possible supervention of right ventricular failure or some impediment to right ventricular inflow. The same probably holds for all the augmentatory signs given in this section.

As previously noted, right-sided acoustical events may also be augmented or produced by increasing venous return, as by having an assistant rapidly lift the patient's legs into the air.

Another trick is Vitums's sign, taught to me by Dr. Dan Cabaniss of Alabama. The appearance or increase in intensity of the typical murmur when squeezing down on the liver is presumptive evidence of tricuspid insufficiency. As with Carvallo's sign, this is probably highly diagnostic, although only 56% sensitive (Gooch et al., 1983).

Peripheral Venous Signs

1. Tricuspid insufficiency causes prominent systolic waves in the jugular venous pulse (CV merger, see Ch. 19, p. 363).

2. Sometimes the murmur of tricuspid insufficiency, but not that of mitral insufficiency, can be detected over peripheral veins.

Unfortunately, this sign has not caught on because of an apparent tendency for the neophyte to overdiagnose innocent cervical hums as being due to tricuspid insufficiency. There are three ways to avoid this problem:

a. Listen over a varicose vein in the leg. Unfortunately, this works only in patients who have varicose veins, and the test is helpful only when it is positive (Becker & Dick, 1962).

b. Note the timing of the murmur. If it is continuous, it is a hum and cannot be due to tricuspid insufficiency. On the other hand, if the murmur has the same timing and shape as the murmur you hear over the precordium, it is unlikely to be a venous hum.

c. Occlude the venous system *distal* to the point at which you are listening. This will abolish a venous hum because the venous return can no longer rush past the point of obliteration and past your stethoscope on its way back to the right atrium. If the murmur persists, you know it must be due to tricuspid insufficiency. This is true even if the intensity decreases somewhat, due to the fact that the *distal* obliteration decreases venous deformability and so acts as an acoustic baffle. (Remember that in tricuspid insufficiency the murmur runs backwards, from the systolic pressure head in the right ventricle back through the insufficient tricuspid valve into the right atrium and thence into the venous system.)

Expansile Liver

This sign is also based upon the backwards transmission of the pressure generated in the right ventricle during systole.

So as not to be fooled by the aortic pulsations, try to get your fingers under the inferior edge of the liver. If the liver is truly expansile, it should move caudally during systole, in the same axis as the one in which the aorta lies. On the other hand, if you are merely feeling a transmitted aortic pulsation, the liver will not move down toward your fingers but rather will bound outward from the midline.

Better yet, if you can do it, surround as much of the circumference of the liver as possible with the spread fingers of two hands, with the hands as opposite to each other as possible. The center of the liver should be equidistant from each of the fingers, in so far as is possible. If the liver is truly expansile, your hands will be moved apart from each other during each systole. If, as is usually the case, the liver is *not* expansile, but rather the aortic pulsations are being transmitted, the liver will merely jerk in one direction during systole, rather than expanding.

The hepatic expansion of tricuspid insufficiency is only 17% sensitive (Cha & Gooch, 1983). First, it requires severe insufficiency in combination with a high right ventricular systolic pressure. Second, if the insufficiency is chronic, the patient may have developed cardiac cirrhosis, which inhibits the ability of the liver to expand.

Two important false positives are Rosenbach's sign of aortic insufficiency (see p. 312) and presystolic A waves, which can be felt in the liver and misidentified as systolic (see Ch. 19, p. 364).

Murmur of Relative Tricuspid Stenosis

Once again, an increased amount of blood flowing over a normal valve produces the same type of sound as a normal amount of blood flowing across a valve of decreased area. This murmur of relative tricuspid stenosis is also augmented or elicited by hepatic pressure.

This sign confounds more often than it is diagnostically helpful, probably because cases of tricuspid insufficiency that regurgitate a sufficient amount of blood to produce the sign are easily diagnosed by other means.

Paul Wood's Winking Earlobe Sign

This really excellent sign was taught to me by Dr. Dan Cabaniss of Alabama. The right earlobe blinks in time with the heartbeat, because of retrograde cardiac ejection into the venous system (which also causes the venous distention of CV merger, see Ch. 19, p. 363).

The winking earlobe sign may be present even in those patients in whom there is no apparent CV merger (Byrd, 1984) or in whom the external and internal jugular veins are themselves inapparent. While its sensitivity is not 100% (it is more like 80% in chronic moderate tricuspid insufficiency), the finding is very dramatic when present.

False positives. In conditions of high stroke volume, the earlobes can be moved by the arterial pulse pressure. The diagnostic difference is not only the company kept but also the following three characteristics: 1) With true positives, the right earlobe tends to be preferentially affected, probably because there is a straighter path from the right jugular vein down into the right ventricle. The carotid pulsations tend to shake both earlobes equally. 2) With false positives, only the part of the earlobe closest to the carotid artery shakes, whereas most or all of the earlobe winks with a true positive. 3) A true positive wink can be abolished by obliterating the jugular venous system from below, as by compressing the lateral neck without compressing the carotids, whereas this maneuver will not affect a cardioarterial shaking.

Very advanced. It was possible to correctly diagnose second-degree heart block by carefully observing the regularly missing earlobe pulsation in a patient with tricuspid insufficiency.

Hepatojugular Reflux

This sign was first described by William Pasteur as being diagnostic (supposedly) for tricuspid insufficiency (Pasteur, 1885). While it is a sensitive (66%) sign (Maisel et al., 1984) of tricuspid insufficiency, hepatojugular reflux (not reflex) is obviously not as diagnostic as Pasteur suggested. See Chapter 19 (p. 361) for his entire article.

Lateral Head Bobbing

This sign is discussed in Chapter 9 (p. 147).

A Difficult Differential

For the attending. A patient with biventricular cardiomyopathy was admitted with a coarse, high-pitched, diamond-shaped murmur that radiated all the way to the left axilla, but not to the right midclavicle. Mitral insufficiency secondary to dilatation of the left ventricle was diagnosed. After his ventricular failure was treated, others diagnosed tricuspid—not mitral—insufficiency. On reauscultation, the murmur was now only heard at the tricuspid area, and it no longer radiated to the axilla. No positive evidence for tricuspid insufficiency could be produced from the neck veins, Vitums's sign, the winking earlobe, and so on. Because of other problems related to his cardiomyopathy, he was eventually catheterized and found to have both tricuspid and mitral insufficiency.

○　　This explicates how the absence of a large number of signs of high-positive predictive value but imperfect sensitivity does not rule out a diagnosis. Note that a systolic murmur itself was of high sensitivity for each lesion, but of little value in distinguishing one from the other or from the concurrence of both. This also indicates that "inching" (see p. 290) is not always effective in distinguishing two murmurs in the same time frame. Finally, this case illustrates the deficiency of Occam's razor.

Etiology

As with mitral insufficiency, tricuspid insufficiency can be due to primary direct disease of the valve (as in infectious endocarditis or rheumatic valvulitis), or it can be secondary to dilation of the ventricle. If the signs wax and wane with increasing severity and with treatment of the ventricular problem, one may diagnose secondary tricuspid insufficiency.

However, one is often dependent upon the case record for the results of past physical examinations. Thus, all examiners contributing to the care of the patient and the charting must be competent before one can use the appearance and disappearance of severe signs as evidence of secondary (versus primary) tricuspid insufficiency.

Tricuspid Stenosis

Clinical Signs

Clinically, tricuspid stenosis perfectly mimics mitral stenosis except in never developing secondary left atrial hypertrophy, right ventricular hypertrophy, and then pulmonary hypertension.

Conversely, tricuspid stenosis has four findings of its own that are lacking in isolated mitral stenosis: 1) giant A waves and impaired Y descent in the venous pulse (see Ch. 19, p. 364); 2) inspiratory augmentation of the diastolic rumble in up to 80% of cases of tricuspid stenosis (Rothman & Goldberger, 1983)*; 3) Kussmaul's sign (Ch. 19, p. 360); and 4) a jugular or clavicular presystolic click (see Ch. 19, p. 366).

False positives. If mitral stenosis leads to severe pulmonary hypertension, then secondary tricuspid regurgitation can lead to relative tricuspid stenosis, hence giant A waves and a diastolic rumble that increases with inspiration despite an anatomically normal tricuspid valve. Fortunately, this is a very rare cause of false positives.

Pericardial Effusion†

Inspection

The best inspection clue is the absence of an observable PMI in situations in which, because of the very enlarged cardiac profile to percussion, one would be expected.

Auenbrugger's sign, an epicardial bulging due to massive pericardial effusion, is rarely seen these days. Why? (Write down your answers before turning to the Appendix 17-6.)

Palpation

Similarly, a PMI may not be palpable at the apex of the percussed silhouette. Instead, it may be palpable inside the borders of cardiac dullness.

Percussion

Of course, a large effusion will cause an enlargement of the percussed silhouette. Rotch's sign refers to a lateral displacement of the right cardiac border. (Although some say with great confidence that this sign must be nonexistent due to the impossibility of percussing the right border of the heart, Dr. Rotch would be surprised to hear this news, were he alive.)

Pericardial effusion can also be diagnosed from the obliteration of the cardiophrenic angles, as detected by percussion. A blunting of the angle on the right (the cardiac hepatic angle) is known as Ebstein's sign.

Moschcowitz described a triad of signs that although individually inconclusive were together "thoroughly reliable as confirmed by roentgenogram examination or at autopsy" (Moschcowitz, 1933). These were: 1) widening of the area of cardiac *flatness* to

---

*It is not 100% since inspiration may decrease the murmur by increasing the distance between the sound point source and the stethoscope.

†For tamponade or constrictive pericarditis, see Table 19-2.

percussion; 2) widening of the area of cardiac *dullness* in the second intercostal space; and 3) an abrupt transition from pulmonary resonance to cardiac flatness. Moschcowitz noted that only the last had not yet been described in 1933.

Dressler's sign is a flat sound over the lower half of the sternum. Disregarding intermediate degrees of dullness and focusing his attention only on areas of absolutely flat percussion notes, percussion gave the correct diagnosis in 58% of Dressler's cases, as compared with only 13% for the chest film (Dressler, 1960).

Very advanced. Dr. H.B. Weiss reports on experiments done in the 1920s at the University of Cincinnati with Dr. Roger Morris:

> We side-tracked patients on the way to the morgue and passed them through the x-ray department. After careful percussion, we used lead strips on the patients' chests as markers [for the boundaries found by percussion] and made an AP film, following which we would start with an injection of 100 cc of ascitic fluid into the pericardial sac. We found that after injecting 250 cc there was a change in the cardiac silhouette principally at the mediastinum. This location may have been influenced by the fact that the cadaver was recumbent. Larger amounts of fluid produced more enlargement, including the body of the heart. (I do not remember that this was ever published.)

Signs of Consolidation (by Percussion and Auscultation)

Ewart described signs of consolidation of the left lower posterior lung fields due to massive pericardial effusion extending posteriorly (see p. 256).

Right posterior thorax signs of consolidation (Conner's sign) also occur in cases of pericardial effusion. In addition to dullness to percussion, the auscultatory signs of consolidation, such as tubular breathing, may be detected in the same area. Conner found posterior thoracic signs to be absent in only 18% of the pericardial effusions he studied. But in any patient who had an Ewart's sign, right-sided findings were always present, although usually less extensive than those on the left (Conner, 1926).

An Ewart's or Conner's sign that disappears when the patient leans forward is Bamberger's sign of pericardial effusion.

Auscultation

Although the softness of the heart sounds in cases of pericardial effusion has received a great deal of emphasis, this best known of the findings is of limited usefulness. 1) It does not occur with very small degrees of pericardial effusion. 2) Even with large pericardial effusions detected by other techniques, this sign may be absent. 3) False positives exist, for example, in many older patients or emphysematous patients.

In cases of pericardial effusion, the presence of a rub tells you nothing about the volume of fluid present. However, it does tell you that the etiology is more likely to be viral, bacterial, postirradiation, or post myocardial infarction (Markiewicz et al., 1980). Rubs are also heard in 25% of rheumatoid effusions, 14% to 83% of uremic effusions, but only 7% of neoplastic effusions (Markiewicz et al., 1980; Rutsky & Rostand 1987). Rubs are usually not heard in effusions due to myxedema or congestive failure.

Other Tests

The ice water test is described in Chapter 28 (p. 555). Pulsus paradoxus, a sign of tamponade, is discussed in Chapter 6 (p. 91). The loss of the Y descent in the cervical veins is described in Chapter 19 (p. 365).

When Is (Apparent) Congestive Heart Failure Not Congestive Heart Failure?

From the inclusion of this question at this point, the astute student may guess that one answer is, when it is pericardial tamponade (see Ch. 19, Table 19-2). But can you think of three others? Write your answers down before consulting Appendix 17-7.

Apparent Combination Lesions

Murmur of Aortic Insufficiency Plus Murmur of Aortic Stenosis

The differential is between *relative* aortic stenosis in severe aortic insufficiency, due to the large stroke volume, and valvular aortic stenosis. This absolute aortic stenosis may be distinguished from relative aortic stenosis by the former's paradoxical splitting of S2, a slow rise of the carotid artery pulse wave, and a delay in time between the PMI at the apex and the peak carotid pulse rise (Chun & Dunn, 1982).

If other valves are involved, as in rheumatic heart disease, there is a greater statistical likelihood of structural aortic valvular stenosis. Conversely, if the aortic insufficiency is known to be luetic, or is thought to be due to aortic root disease (because the murmur radiates down the right side of the sternum), structural aortic valvular stenosis is unlikely, from Occam's razor (i.e., there would have to be a second disease to explain the structural aortic valvular stenosis).

Murmur of Aortic Stenosis Plus Murmur of Mitral Insufficiency

This combination occurs with increasing frequency. In most of the situations to be described, there actually is a functional obstruction to aortic outflow, although the aortic valve itself is normal. There are five possible etiologies:

1. Idiopathic Hypertrophic Subaortic Stenosis

IHSS may cause changes in the anatomy and positioning of the papillary muscles so that there is poor coaption of the mitral valve (Kramer et al., 1986).

2. Mitral Valve Prolapse

If the floppy valve leaflet is sufficiently flail, it may not only fail to coapt, but may even flutter back into the left ventricular outflow tract, producing a systolic murmur. The best way to detect a prolapsed mitral valve as a cause of this combination is to find a midsystolic click. Some workers have suggested that such prolapse can be diagnosed by changing the patient's position and noticing the murmur occupying earlier portions of systole. However, IHSS murmurs may become louder on standing and so seem to be "earlier."

Alternately, to refute the hypothesis that a prolapsed mitral valve leaflet is responsible for an aortic outflow murmur, you could find evidence independent of the murmur for valvular aortic stenosis (e.g., delayed carotid upstroke, a paradoxically split S2, and prolonged apical-carotic impulse interval [see p. 313]). A prolapsing mitral valve alone does not cause sufficient obstruction to produce such signs.

Note that in the above two cases, we have not suggested ausculting at Spodick's point (the right midclavicle) for amplification of the murmur of aortic stenosis, since all forms of aortic stenosis discussed in this section will show such midclavicular amplification. However, Spodick's point can be used for refuting the existence of aortic stenosis in the next diagnosis.

3. Aortic Stenosis Mimicked by Mitral Insufficiency

When the systolic regurgitant jet squirts back into the left atrium and vibrates the aorta opposing the enlarged left atrium, the vibrations may be heard at the aortic root area as a diamond-shaped systolic murmur, as documented by intracardiac phonocardiography (Antman et al., 1978).

4. Gallavardin Phenomenon

See page 318.

5. True Aortic Stenosis and True Mitral Insufficiency

Primary disease of both valves is most frequently seen in rheumatic heart disease. The best support for this diagnosis will be the finding of additional valvular lesions.

A Diastolic Decrescendo Murmur Accompanying Mitral Valve Disease

The differential diagnosis is between (rheumatic) aortic insufficiency and pulmonic insufficiency (Steell's murmur, p. 321). Features that may help include the radiation of the murmur (see Table 17-4) and the response to amyl nitrite (which often diminishes the murmurs of aortic insufficiency, but not that of pulmonic insufficiency) or handgrip. A decrease in the intensity of the murmur with handgrip excludes aortic insufficiency (see p. 308).

A test of high diagnosticity but low sensitivity is to auscult in the left axilla for the Cole-Cecil murmur, first described by Foster in 1874, and resurrected in 1908 (Cole & Cecil, 1908). If one can hear the diastolic decrescendo murmur there, one is listening to aortic insufficiency, not pulmonic insufficiency. (If one cannot hear the murmur in the axilla, no conclusion can be drawn.)

In differentiating the two murmurs, one should also search for the associated peripheral signs of aortic insufficiency (see pp. 309–312), which are helpful only if present. Conversely, one should be cautious about diagnosing a Steell murmur (see p. 321) unless there is physical evidence of right ventricular hypertrophy (such as a right ventricular tap, see p. 285).

Murmur of Aortic Insufficiency Plus Murmur of Mitral Stenosis

The Flint murmur is the murmur of rheumatic mitral stenosis where such does not exist. It is due to relative mitral stenosis, the aortic regurgitant jet keeping the anterior mitral leaflet in a relatively closed position, obstructing diastolic filling of the left ventricle. The following discussion of the signs distinguishing the Flint murmur (see p. 321) from the murmur of true mitral stenosis is summarized in Table 17-8.

First, look for the other signs of true mitral stenosis, which are not seen accompanying the Flint murmur. Of these, the opening snap, if present, is best. When present, a loud first heart sound also strongly favors true mitral stenosis. This is due to the fact that the left atrial/left ventricular pressure gradient maintains the mitral valve leaflets in a relatively wide open position until the beginning of ventricular systole, at which point they are slammed shut through a wide excursion. With the Flint murmur, the regurgitant jet holds the anterior leaflet of the mitral valve in a relatively closed position, reducing the excursion and reducing the normal intensity of the sound of mitral valve closure by about half. Furthermore, with the Flint murmur mechanism there may be asynchrony to the closure of the two leaflets, also making the sound "mushy" or soft.

Next, attend to the pitch of the mitral murmur. The Flint murmur tends to be higher pitched and the true mitral stenosis murmur more rumbling, although these features do not permit a perfect distinction.

If you come upon that ancient instrument, the phonocardiograph, you may wish to use amyl nitrite (see p. 308) and observe

Table 17-8. Differential Diagnosis of Flint Murmur Versus True Mitral Stenosis Combined with Aortic Insufficiency

Finding	Mitral Stenosis	Flint Murmur
Opening snap	Maybe	Never
Loud S1	Often	Never
Increased P2	Often	Never
Diastolic thrill	Maybe	Never
High-pitched	Never	Maybe
Apical presystolic wave	Only with mild MS	Maybe
Effect on murmur of amyl nitrite	Usually louder (60%–82%) or no change	Often softer (86%)
Effect on murmur of pressor infusion	Usually not louder	Louder
Rhythm	Usually atrial fibrillation	Usually sinus
Duroziez's murmur	May be lost	May be present
Hill's sign	May be lost	May be present

its effect upon the diastolic rumble. A decrease in the lower pitched murmur with amyl nitrite supports the diagnosis of a Flint murmur. This is because the amyl nitrite decreases systemic vascular resistance (also called afterload), decreasing the amount of blood regurgitating back into the left ventricle in diastole, decreasing the degree of displacement of the anterior leaflet of the mitral valve in diastole, and so decreasing the murmur. But if the murmur gets louder, it suggests that the mitral rumble is due to mitral stenosis.

By an opposite mechanism, infusion of a pressor agent causes the murmur of mitral stenosis to become softer or to remain unchanged. The Flint murmur may get louder, or remain unchanged. The increased afterload increases the aortic/left ventricular diastolic gradient in aortic insufficiency, thus increasing the relative mitral stenosis that causes the Flint murmur. On the other hand, it tends to decrease the forward flow and possibly decrease the flow across the truly stenotic mitral valve. Squatting and isometric handgrip are two nonpharmacologic techniques producing the same distinctions (see p. 308).

A palpable presystolic wave at the apex would favor but not guarantee the diagnosis of a Flint murmur (Basta & Bettinger, 1979).

A final piece of evidence is based upon the fact that aortic insufficiency patients with mitral stenosis tend to lose their Duroziez's and Hill's signs. Unfortunately, Hill's sign requires a hemodynamically significant degree of aortic insufficiency. Also, the reliability of the absence of the Duroziez murmur requires that the auscultor be good enough to detect it consistently when present. So these two findings tend to be helpful only when present, suggesting that the Flint murmur is the correct diagnosis.

A Comparison of Clinical Examination with Doppler Echocardiography

In the proper hands, Doppler echocardiography represents an epochal advance in the diagnosis of valvular heart disease. However, it has produced two problems: First, it can detect very minor lesions that do not produce audible murmurs. Second, it can detect "lesions" where there are none demonstrable by other techniques. While echocardiographers are developing techniques for eliminating such false positives, the individual consultor has no way of knowing—for any given patient—whether the reading is a true positive or a false positive. The potential extent of such false positives is shown in Table 17-9.

Aortic stenosis is a lesion which illustrates some of the pitfalls of uncritical acceptance of the interpretations of the results of this wonderful device.

Echocardiography and clinical examination are both good ways to diagnose aortic stenosis, but the sensitivity and specificity of these methods are highly variable in different institutions.

As this work was being composed, continuous wave (and color) Doppler echocardiography appeared and swept all other imaging forms before it, so far as aortic stenosis is concerned. Since its adoption for this purpose should be a model for subsequent developments with other lesions, some comments about the technology might be appropriate in the way of providing protocriteria to be reviewed prior to burning one's stethoscope.

1. Not all studies are technically satisfactory. Unsatisfactory studies occurred in 3% to 7.4% of recently reported series (Krafchek et al., 1985, Oh et al., 1988; Richards et al., 1986; Yeager et al., 1986). Even among those recordings rated as fair, satisfactory, or good, the readers were, not surprisingly, more accurate with the good tracings than with the others (Currie et al., 1985).

2. Experienced readers are more accurate than less experienced readers (Currie et al., 1985; Panidis et al., 1986). Error is most likely when the junior reader misidentifies the gain setting, but such does not appear in the journals.

3. Moderate to severe concommitant aortic insufficiency decreases accuracy. So does atrial fibrillation (Panidis et al., 1986).

4. At the present time, a mean gradient of 30 to 50 mm can be operationally and prognostically confusing (Yeager et al., 1986). (Because the gradient changes with flow, several groups are trying to estimate valve area from the continuity equation, which is imperfect.)

5. Because catheterization laboratories traditionally report peak-to-peak gradients, Dopplerphiles have complained that the instantaneous mean gradient would be a more appropriate independent covariable to the calculated Doppler gradient. While this is often technically true, Krafchek et al. had the same correlation coefficient for both peak-to-peak and mean gradients (Krafchek et al., 1985).

6. Dopplerphiles have also noted that *simultaneous* catheterization and echo yield better correlations of gradients (as they should, since flow is essentially the same for both measures—see #4 above) (Currie et al., 1985). But that fact is irrelevant to the reality of practice, where we do not do both tests at the same time.

7. Finally, a mean correlation coefficient of 0.85 between the Doppler mean gradient and the catheterization mean gradient looks good. In fact, this result is obtained by averaging five papers quoted here (Currie et al., 1985; Krafchek et al., 1985; Oh et al., 1988; Panidis et al., 1986; Yeager et al., 1986). But this is essentially the same correlation coefficient obtained in a study in which the Doppler peak gradient overestimated the catheterization peak-to-peak gradient in individual cases by from 1 to 53 mm Hg (Krafchek et al., 1985), a not inconsequential error. The Doppler mean gradient revealed gradients for 18% of the study population in whom there was *no* gradient by catheterization! Conclusion: In individual patients, the errors of the technique are not unimportant.

Conclusions

Some workers believe that all auscultatory findings must be confirmed by Doppler. While this is fine for positive findings, it will not be practical for negative findings until every physician has a color-Doppler-echocardiogram-cum-technician in his little black bag.

Like all technologic aids, echocardiography can be used in a highly ineffective way. These errors are made all too often:

1. Providing the consultant with insufficient clinical information.
2. Making the consultant guess what you are looking for.
3. Failing to understand the limitations of the technology, particularly when you are substituting it for your own skills.
4. Interpreting the absence of evidence as evidence of absence.
5. Forgetting the basic law of consultation exemplified in the following story.

•

Many years ago, there was an actor on the Yiddish stage named Boris Tomashevsky. One night as he was removing his makeup after a performance, a beautiful young woman appeared at his dressing room door to tell him how wonderful he was. He listened and spoke, and one thing led to another.

The next morning he let her out of his dressing room, expecting never to see her again, but the following night she again appeared, this time with a baby in her arms and demanding money, which he refused.

"But you don't understand, Mr. Tomashevsky," she said. "I am a young widow. My husband died and left me with nothing but this baby whom I must support. My baby must have bread."

"I am Tomashevsky, the Actor," he replied in his most stentorian tones. "If it's bread you want, you should go to Tomashevsky the baker."

Moral: what you get depends upon whom you ask.

•

Appendix 17-1.
Massive Pericardial Effusion and the PMI

Why patients with a massive pericardial effusion usually do not have a visible PMI (see p. 284): With a massive pericardial effusion, the heart swings and contracts inside a bag of fluid that keeps it from striking the chest wall and making the PMI. This is the same reason that you do not bump the floor when you sit on a water bed.

Appendix 17-2. Why Laennec
Could Hear Better than He Could Palpate

Laennec could hear what he could not palpate because the threshold of hearing is lower than that for feeling, except at extremely low frequencies (see Fig. 17-16).

Table 17-9.   False-Positive Rates for Doppler Echocardiography in Some Reports

Lesion Reference	Percentage
Aortic stenosis	
Krafchek et al., 1985	18%
Nitta et al., 1988	12%
Aortic insufficiency	
Kostucki et al., 1985	32%
Mitral insufficiency	
Kostucki et al., 1985	36%
Pulmonic insufficiency	
Yock et al., 1984	40%
Takao et al., 1985	78%
Kostucki et al., 1985	92%
Tricuspid insufficiency	
Jacksch et al., 1985	21%
Kostucki et al., 1985	44%
Yock et al., 1984	96%

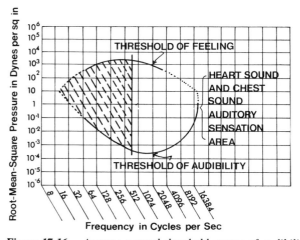

Figure 17-16. Average normal threshold curves of audibility and feeling. Reprinted from Rappaport and Sprague (1941) with the permission of the American Heart Association.

Appendix 17-3. Key to Figure 17-11

In Figure 17-11, the left column is IHSS, the right is valvular aortic stenosis. The bottom row represents volume depletion (or standing up). Now, can you draw the intensity of the murmur under each condition?

Appendix 17-4. Differential Diagnosis of a Murmur

The exclusions were based on the dimensions of location, radiation, and intensity; therefore the reasoning is the same.

Appendix 17-5. Self-Test on Mitral Valve Prolapse (see p. 317)

(a) The positive predictive value of a murmur = TP/(TP + FP). The number of persons with mitral valve prolapse was 208, and of these, 9% or 19 had a murmur (TP = 19). Of the 2,717 persons without mitral valve prolapse, 3.53% or 96 had a murmur (FP = 96). Therefore, the positive PV = 16.5%.

(b) The predictive value of a negative test = TN/(TN + FN). The number of true negatives is (2,717 − 96) or 2,621, and the number of false negatives is (208 − 19) or 189. Hence, the predictive value of a negative test is 93%.

Appendix 17-6. Auenbrugger's Sign

Auenbrugger's sign is rarely seen these days because: 1) it is rarely sought, 2) our patients have more fat than Auenbrugger's did, 3) effusion is diagnosed much earlier because of echocardiography, and 4) Auenbrugger's patients lived prior to pericardiocentesis.

Appendix 17-7. When Is Congestive Heart Failure Not Congestive Heart Failure?

Constrictive pericarditis, inferior vena cava thrombosis, and tricuspid stenosis.

References

Abbas F, Sapira JD: Mayne's sign is not pathognomonic of aortic insufficiency. *South Med J* 80:1051–1052, 1987.

Abram J: The fourth heart sound—a normal finding? *Am J Cardiol* 36:534–535, 1975.

Antman EM, Angoff GH, Sloss LJ: Demonstration of the mechanism by which mitral regurgitation mimics aortic stenosis. *Am J Cardiol* 42:1044–1048, 1978.

Basta LL, Bettinger JJ: The cardiac impulse: A new look at an old art. *Am Heart J* 97:96–111, 1979.

Beck W, Schrire V, Vogelpoel L: Splitting of the second heart sound in constrictive pericarditis, with observations on the mechanism of pulsus paradoxus. *Am Heart J* 64:765–778, 1962.

Becker DJ, Dick MM: Saphenous varix bruit in tricuspid valve incompetence. *N Engl J Med* 267:766–768, 1962.

Behar VS, Whalen RE, McIntosh HD: The ballooning mitral valve in patients with the "precordial honk" or "whoop." *Am J Cardiol* 20:789–795, 1967.

Beilin L, Mounsey P: The left ventricular impulse in hypertensive heart disease. *Br Heart J* 24:409–421, 1962.

Benson R, Raj MV: Paravertebral systolic murmur with septal rupture. *N Engl J Med* 307:1086, 1982.

Bland EF, Wheeler EO: Severe aortic regurgitation in young people. *N Engl J Med* 256:667–672, 1957.

Bloom HJG: Venous hums in hepatic cirrhosis. *Br Heart J* 12:343–350, 1950.

Bloomfield DA, Sinclair-Smith BC: Aortic insufficiency: A physiological and clinical appraisal. *South Med J* 66:55–65, 1973.

Blumgart HL, Ernstene HC: Two mechanisms in the production of Duroziez's sign: The diagnostic significance and a clinical test for differentiating between them. *JAMA* 100:173–177, 1933.

Bon Tempo CP, Ronan JA, de Leon A, Twigg H: Radiographic appearance of the thorax in systolic murmur syndrome. *Am J Cardiol* 36:27–31, 1975.

Bruns DL: A general theory of the causes of murmurs in the cardiovascular system. *Am J Med* 27:360–374, 1959.

Burton-Opitz R: A simple auscultatory method of physical diagnosis. *NY State J Med* 25:18–19, 1925.

Butterworth JS, Reppert EH: Auscultatory acumen in the general medical population. *JAMA* 164:114–116, 1960.

Byrd MD: Lateral systolic pulsation of the earlobe: A sign of tricuspid regurgitation. *Am J Cardiol* 54:244, 1984.

Cha SD, Gooch AS: Diagnosis of tricuspid regurgitation: Current status. *Arch Intern Med* 143:1763–1764, 1983.

Cheng TO: Mitral valve prolapse. *DM* 33:481–534, 1987.

Chun PK, Dunn BE: Clinical clue of severe aortic stenosis: Simultaneous palpation of the carotid and apical impulses. *Arch Intern Med* 142:2284–2288, 1982.

Clain D, Wartnaby K, Sherlock S: Abdominal arterial murmurs in liver disease. *Lancet* 2:516–519, 1966.

Cochran PT: Bedside aids to auscultation of the heart. *JAMA* 239:54–55, 1978.

Cohn LH, Mason DT, Ross J Jr, Morrow AG, Braunwald E: Preoperative assessment of aortic regurgitation in patients with mitral valve disease. *Am J Cardiol* 19:177–182, 1967.

Cole R, Cecil AB: The axillary diastolic murmur in aortic insufficiency. *Johns Hopkins Hosp Bull* 19:353–361, 1908.

Conner LA: On the diagnosis of pericardial effusion: With special reference to physical signs on the posterior aspect of the thorax. *Am Heart J* 1:421–433, 1926.

Currie PJ, Seward JB, Reeder GS, Vlietstra RE, Bresnahan DR, Bresnahan JF, Smith HC, Hagler DJ, Tajik AJ: Continuous-wave Doppler echocardiographic assessment of severity of calcific aortic stenosis: A simultaneous Doppler-catheter correlative study in 100 adult patients. *Circulation* 71:1162–1169, 1985.

Curtiss EI, Matthews RG, Shaver JA: Mechanism of normal splitting of the second heart sound. *Circulation* 51:157–164, 1975.

DaCosta JC Jr: *Principles and Practice of Physical Diagnosis*, ed 1. WB Saunders, Philadelphia, 1909.

De Gowin EL: *Beside Diagnostic Examination*. Macmillan, New York, 1965.

Dobrow RJ, Calatayud JB, Abraham S, Caceres CA: A study of physician variation and heart sound interpretation. *Med Ann District of Columbia* 33:305–308, 355–356, 1964.

Dock W: Korotkoff's sounds. *N Engl J Med* 302:1264–1267, 1980.

Dock W, Zoneraich S: A diastolic murmur arising in a stenosed coronary artery. *Am J Med* 42:617–619, 1967.

Dressler W: Percussion of the sternum: I. Aid to differentiation of pericardial effusion and cardiac dilatation. *JAMA* 173:761–764, 1960.

Eilen SD, Crawford MH, O'Rourke RA: Accuracy of precordial palpation for detecting increased left ventricular volume. *Ann Intern Med* 99:628–630, 1983.

Fortuin NJ, Craige E: Echocardiographic studies of genesis of mitral diastolic murmurs. *Br Heart J* 35:75–81, 1973.

Fowler NO: *Cardiac Diagnosis and Treatment*, ed 3. Harper & Row, New York, 1980.

Fowler NO, Adolph RJ: Fourth sound—gallop or split first sound? *Am J Cardiol* 30:441–444, 1972.

Fowles RE, Martin RP, Popp RL: Apparent asymmetric septal hypertrophy due to angled interventricular septum. *Am J Cardiol* 46:386–392, 1980.

Fraentzel: Report from the clinic of *Geheim Rath* Traube: About two cases demonstrating phenomena of aortic valve insufficiency. *Berl Klinische Wochenschrift* 4:455–458, 1867.

Frank MJ, Casanegra P, Migliori AJ, Levinson GE: The clinical evaluation of aortic regurgitation. *Arch Intern Med* 116:357–365, 1965.

Freeman AR, Levine SA: Clinical significance of systolic murmurs: Study of 1000 consecutive "noncardiac" cases. *Ann Intern Med* 6:1371–1379, 1933.

Friedberg CK: Diseases of the Heart, ed 2. WB Saunders, Philadelphia, 1956.

Friedman B, Hathaway B: Fenestration of the semilunar cusps, and "functional" aortic and pulmonic valve insufficiency. *Am J Med* 24:549–558, 1958. [Although the entity was originally described for the aortic valve by both Corrigan and Hope, this citation is more lucent.]

Gallavardin L, Ravault P: The murmur of aortic stenosis undergoes a change in timbre becoming musical when radiating to the apex. *Lyon Med* 135:523–529, 1925.

Giles TD, Martinez EC, Burch GE: Gallavardin phenomenon in aortic stenosis: A possible mechanism. *Arch Intern Med* 134:747–749, 1974.

Gooch AS, Cha SD, Maranhao V: The use of the hepatic pressure maneuver to identify the murmur of tricuspid regurgitation. *Clin Cardiol* 6(2):77–280, 1983.

Goodwin JF: Clarification of the cardiomyopathies. *Mod Concepts Cardiovasc Dis* 41:41–46, 1972.

Grayburn PA, Smith MD, Handshoe R, Friedman BJ, DeMaria AN: Detection of aortic insufficiency with standard echocardiography, pulsed Doppler echocardiography, and auscultation. *Ann Intern Med* 104:599–605, 1986.

Griffith JPC: Mid-systolic and late-systolic mitral murmurs. *Am J Med Sci* 104:285–294, 1892.

Guiliani ER: Mitral valve incompetence due to flail anterior leaflet: A new physical sign. *Am J Cardiol* 20:L784–788, 1967.

Hagen PT, Scholz DG, Edwards WD: Incidence and size of patent foramen ovale in the first ten decades of life: An autopsy study of 965 normal hearts. *Mayo Clin Proc* 59:17–20, 1984.

Hamman L: Spontaneous mediastinal emphysema. *Bull Johns Hopkins Hosp* 64:1–21, 1939.

Harvey WP: Auscultatory findings in diseases of the pericardium. *Am J Cardiol* 7:15–20, 1961.

Harvey WP, Corrado MA, Perloff JK: Right-sided murmurs of aortic insufficiency. *Am J Med Sci* 245:533–542, 1963.

Hickey AJ, Andrews G, Wilcken DE: Independence of mitral valve prolapse and neurosis. *Br Heart J* 50:333–336, 1983.

Holmes JC, Fowler NO, Helmsworth JA: Coronary arteriovenous fistula and aortic sinus aneurysm rupture. *Arch Intern Med* 118:43–54, 1966.

Hoover CF: Definitive percussion and inspection in estimating size and contour of the heart. *JAMA* 75:1626–1630, 1920.

Hurley DV, Nishimura RA, Schaff HV, Edwards WD: Aortic dissection with fistula to right atrium. *J Thorac Cardiovasc Surg* 92:953–957, 1986.

Hurst JW, Schlant RC: *Examination of the Heart: Part Three. Inspection and Palpation of the Anterior Chest*. American Heart Association, New York, 1972.

Jacksch R, Karsch KR, Seiple L: Accuracy in detection and quantification of tricuspid regurgitation by contrast and Doppler echocardiography. *J Coll Cardiol* 5:499, 1985.

Johnson GL, Humphries LL, Shirley PB, Mazzoleni A, Noonan JA: Mitral valve prolapse in patients with anorexia nervosa and bulimia. *Arch Intern Med* 146:1525–1529, 1986.

Jordan MD, Taylor CR, Nyhuis AW, Tavel ME: Audibility of the fourth heart sound. *Arch Intern Med* 147:721–726, 1987.

Kambe T, Hibi N, Fukui Y, Nishimura K, Ichimiya S, Toguchi M, Sakamoto N. Clinical study on the right-sided Austin Flint murmur using intracardiac phonocardiography. *Am Heart J* 98:701–707, 1979.

Kantor JS, Zitrin CM, Zeldis SM: Mitral valve prolapse syndrome in agoraphobic patients. *Am J Psychiatry* 137:467–469, 1980.

Koran LM: The reliability of clinical methods: Data and judgments. *N Engl J Med* 293:642–646, 1975.

Kostucki W, Vandenbossche JL, Friart A, Englert M: Psuedo regurgitant valvular flow patterns in normal individuals. *J Cardiovasc Ultrasonogr* 4:315, 1985.

Krafchek J, Robertson JH, Radford M, Adams D, Kisslo J: A reconsideration of Doppler assessed gradients in suspected aortic stenosis. *Am Heart J* 110:765–769, 1985.

Kramer DS, French WJ, Criley JM: The postextrasystolic murmur response to gradient in hypertrophic cardiomyopathy. *Ann Intern Med* 104:772–776, 1986.

Kurtz CM, White PD: The percussion of the heart borders and the roentgen ray shadow of the heart. *Am J Med Sci* 74:53–59, 1928.

Laubry C, Brosse T, van Bogaert A: Doubles tones et doubles souffles vasculaires au cours de l'insuffisance aortique [Vascular double tones and double murmurs in aortic insufficiency]. *Annal Med* 30:193–248, 1931.

Leatham A: Splitting of the first and second heart sounds. *Lancet* 2:602–613, 1954.

Lembo NJ, Dell'Italia LJ, Crawford MH, O'Rourke RA: Diagnosis of left-sided regurgitant murmurs by transient arterial occlusion: A new maneuver using blood pressure cuffs. *Ann Intern Med* 105:368–370, 1986.

Lembo NJ, Dell'Italia LJ, Crawford MH, O'Rourke RA: Bedside diagnosis of systolic murmurs. *N Engl J Med* 318:1572–1578, 1988.

Leon DF, Leonard JJ, Lancaster JF, Kroetz FW, Shaver JA: Effect of respiration on pansystolic regurgitant murmurs as studied by biatrial intracardiac phonocardiography. *Am J Med* 39:429–411, 1965.

Leonard JJ, Allensworth D: Differential diagnosis of the early diastolic murmur. In: Segal BL (ed), *The Theory and Practice of Auscultation*. FA Davis, Philadelphia, 1963.

Leonard JJ, Renfro NL, de Groot WJ, Page WL: The auscultatory diagnosis of the hyperkinetic state. In: Segal BL (ed), *The Theory and Practice of Auscultation*. FA Davis, Philadelphia, 1963.

Lerman J, Means JH: Cardiovascular symptomatology in exophthalmic goiter. *Am Heart J* 8:55–65, 1932.

Levine SA: *Clinical Heart Disease*, ed 3. WB Saunders, Philadelphia, 1945, 462 pp. [This book is still useful for teaching clinical auscultation with a phonocardiogram, which is probably the best way to teach it. Even for those using the American Heart Association classic by

Leonard and Kroetz, this work is useful for showing the actual phonocardiograms, thus indicating the sometimes "fuzzy" nature of the heart sounds. The concept of a heart sound as a psychoacoustic event is not always best served by diagrams that imply an ease of appreciation not consistent with the reality of auscultation.]

Levine SA, Harvey WP: *Clinical Auscultation of the Heart.* WB Saunders, Philadelphia, 1949.

Lian C: Le souffle continu cave superieur. *Bull Mem Soc Med Hopitaux Paris* 53:1088–1099, 1937.

Linhart JW: Aortic regurgitation: Clinical, hemodynamic, surgical, and angiographic correlations. *Ann Thorac Surg* 11:27–37, 1971.

Lombard JT, Selzer A: Valvular aortic stenosis: A clinical and hemodynamic profile of patients. *Ann Intern Med* 106:292–298, 1987.

Louagie Y, Brohet C, Robert A, Lopez E, Jaumin P, Schoevaerdts J-C, Chalant C-H: Factors influencing postoperative survival in aortic regurgitation: Analysis by Cox regression model. *J Thorac Cardiovasc Surg* 88:225–233, 1984.

Luisada AA: On the pathogenesis of the signs of Traube and Duroziez in aortic insufficiency: A graphic study. *Am Heart J* 26:721–736, 1943.

Luisada AA, Portaluppi F: The main heart sounds as vibrations of the cardiohemic system: Old controversy and new facts. *Am J Cardiol* 52:1136, 1983.

Luisada AA, Puppala BL: The first heart sound in left bundle branch block. *Cardiovasc Med* 4:217–226, 1979.

Macklem PT: Respiratory muscle dysfunction. *Hosp Pract* 21:83–95, 1986.

Mainland D, Stewart CB, Halifax NS: A comparison of percussion and radiography in locating the heart and superior mediastinal vessels. *Am Heart J* 15:515–527, 1938.

Maisel AS, Atwood JE, Goldberger AL: Hepatojugular reflux: Useful in the bedside diagnosis of tricuspid regurgitation. *Ann Intern Med* 101:781–782, 1984.

Major RH: *Classic Descriptions of Disease with Biographical Sketches of the Authors*, ed 3. Charles C Thomas, Springfield, IL, 1945.

Markiewicz W, Brik A, Brook G, Edoute Y, Monakier I, Markiewicz Y: Pericardial rub in pericardial effusion: Lack of correlation with amount of fluid. *Chest* 77:643–646, 1980.

Maron BJ, Bonow RO, Cannon RO, Leon MB, Epstein SE: Hypertrophic cardiomyopathy: Interrelations of clinical manifestations, pathophysiology, and therapy. *N Engl J Med* 316:780–789, 1987.

Maron BJ, Epstein SE: Hypertrophic cardiomyopathy: A discussion of nomenclature. *Am J Cardiol* 43:1242–1244, 1979.

Mayne B: On aortic regurgitation: A new physical sign. *Ir J Med Sci* 6:80–81, 1953.

McCraw DB, Siegel W, Stonecipher HK, Nutter DO, Schlant RC, Hurst JW: Response of heart murmur intensity to isometric (handgrip) exercise. *Br Heart J* 34:605–610, 1972.

McFadzean AJS, Gray J: Hepatic venous hum in cirrhosis of the liver. *Lancet* 2:1128–1130, 1953.

Meyers DG, Sagar KB, Ingram RF, Paulsen WJH, Romhilt DW: Diagnosis of aortic insufficiency: Comparison of auscultation and M-mode echocardiography to angiography. *South Med J* 75:1192–1194, 1982.

Meyers DG, Starke H, Pearson PH, Wilken MK: Mitral valve prolapse in anorexia nervosa. *Ann Intern Med* 105:384–385, 1986.

Moschcowitz E: A new sign of pericardial effusion. *JAMA* 100:1663–1664, 1933. [This was written 8 years after the author described Moschcowitz's disease, thrombotic thrombocytopenic purpura.]

Naylor CD, McCormack DG, Sullivan SN: The midclavicular line: A wandering landmark. *Can Med Assoc J* 136:48–50, 1987.

Nellen M, Gotsman M, Vogelpoel L, Beck W, Shire V: Effect of prompt squatting on the systolic murmur of idiopathic hypertrophic obstructive cardiomyopathy. *Br Med J* 3:140–143, 1967.

Nicholson WJ, Cobbs BW Jr, Franch RH, Crawley IS: Early diastolic sound of constrictive pericarditis. *Am J Cardiol* 45:378–382, 1980.

Nishimura RA, Tajik AJ: The Valsalva maneuver and response revisited. *Mayo Clin Proc* 61:211–217, 1986.

Nitta M, Takamoto T, Taniguchi K, Hultgren H: Diagnostic accuracy of continuous wave Doppler echocardiography in severe aortic stenosis in the elderly. *Jpn Heart J* 29:169–178, 1988.

Oh JK, Taliercio CP, Holmes DR Jr, Reeder GS, Bailey KR, Seward JB, Tajik AJ: Prediction of the severity of aortic stenosis by Doppler aortic valve area determination: Prospective Doppler-catheterization correlation in 100 patients. *J Am Coll Cardiol* 11:1227–1234, 1988.

Oliveira DBG, Dawkins KD, Kay PH, Paneth M: Chordal rupture: I. Aetiology and natural history. *Br Heart J* 50:312–317, 1983.

Olson LJ, Subramanian R, Ackermann DM, Orszulak TA, Edwards WD: Surgical pathology of the mitral valve: A study of 712 cases spanning 21 years. *Mayo Clin Proc* 62:22–34, 1987.

Osler W: *Men and Books* (EF Nation, ed). The Sacrum Press, Durham, 1987.

Pan-Chih, Ching-Heng T, Chen-Chun, Chieh-Fu L: Surgical treatment of the ruptured aneurysm of the aortic sinuses. *Ann Thorac Surg* 32:162–166, 1981.

Panidis IP, Mintz GS, Ross J: Value and limitations of Doppler ultrasound in the evaluation of aortic stenosis: A statistical analysis of 70 consecutive patients. *Am Heart J* 112:150–158, 1986.

Passik CS, Ackermann DW, Pluth JR, Edwards WD: Temporal changes in the causes of aortic stenosis: A surgical pathologic study of 646 cases. *Mayo Clin Proc* 62:119–123, 1987.

Pasteur W: Note on a new physical sign of tricuspid regurgitation. *Lancet* 2:524–525, 1885.

Perez JE, Smith CA, Meltzer VN: Pulmonic valve insufficiency: A common cause of transient diastolic murmurs in renal failure. *Ann Intern Med* 103:497–502, 1985.

Perloff JK: Cardiac auscultation. *DM* 26(9):1–47, 1980.

Perry GY, Pitlik S, Greenwald M, Rosenfeld JB. Cardiac auscultation of bony chests. *Isr J Med Sci* 20:260–261, 1984.

Popp RL, Winkle RA: Mitral-valve prolapse syndrome. *JAMA* 236:867, 1976.

Quincke H: II. Beobachtungen ber capillar- und venepuls. [Observations on capillary pulsations and venous pulsations.] *Klin Wochenschr* 5:357–359, 1868.

Rackley CE, Craig RJ, McIntosh HD, Orgain ES: Phonocardiographic discrepancies in the assessment of mitral stenosis. *Arch Intern Med* 121:50–53, 1968.

Ramsey HW, De la Torre A, Linhart JW, Krovetz LJ, Schiebler GL: Idiopathic dilatation of the pulmonary artery. *Am J Cardiol* 20:324–330, 1967.

Rappaport MB, Sprague HB: Physiologic and physical laws that govern auscultation. *Am Heart J* 21:258–318, 1941.

Rectra EH, Khan AH, Pigott VM, Spodick DH: Audibility of the fourth heart sound: A prospective, "blind" auscultatory and polygraphic investigation. *JAMA* 221:36–41, 1972.

Reddy PS, Salemi R, Shaver JA: Normal and abnormal heart sounds in cardiac diagnosis: Part II. Diastolic sounds. *Curr Probl Cardiol* 10(4):8–55, 1985.

Reeves WC: The normally functioning prosthetic valve. *Ann Intern Med* 97:144–145, 1982.

Richards KL, Cannon SR, Miller JF, Crawford MH: Calculation of aortic valve area by Doppler echocardiography: A direct application of the continuity equation. *Circulation* 73:964–969, 1986.

Robbins CS, Bruun B, Zim HS: *A Guide to Field Identification: Birds of North America.* Golden Press, New York, 1966.

Rosenberg CA, Derman GH, Grabb WC, Buda AJ: Hypomastia and mitral valve prolapse. *N Engl J Med* 309:1230–1232, 1983.

Rothman A, Goldberger AL: Aids to cardiac auscultation. *Ann Intern Med* 99:346–353, 1983.

Rusconi C, Salmi A, Faggiano P, Pavia L, Orlando G: Soffio continuo precordiale da sindrome di Cruveilhier-Baumgarten inapparente: Diagnosi al letto del paziente. *Minerva Cardioangiol* 33:519–524, 1985.

Rutsky EA, Rostand SG: Treatment of pericarditis and pericardial effusion. *Am J Kidney Dis* 10:2–8, 1987.

Rytand DA: The midclavicular line: Where is it? *Ann Intern Med* 69:329–330, 1968.

Sainani GS, Luisada AA, Gupta PD: Mapping the precordium: I. Heart sounds of normal subjects. *Am J Cardiol* 19:788–792, 1967.

Salomon J, Shah P, Heinle RA: Thoracic skeletal abnormalities in idiopathic mitral valve prolapse. *Am J Cardiol* 36:32–36, 1975.

Samuels DA, Curfman GD, Friedlich AL, Buckley MJ, Austen WG: Valve replacement for aortic regurgitation: Long-term follow-up with factors influencing the results. *Circulation* 60:647–654, 1979.

Sapira JD: Quincke, de Musset, Duroziez and Hill: Some aortic regurgitations. *South Med J* 74:459–467, 1981.

Sapira JD, Cherubin CE: *Drug Abuse.* American Elsevier, New York, 1975.

Savage DD, Devereux RB, Garrison RJ, Castelli WP, Anderson SJ, Levy D, Thomas HE, Kannel WB, Feinleib M: Mitral valve prolapse in the general population. 2. Clinical features: The Framingham study. *Am Heart J* 106:577–581, 1983.

Segal J, Harvey WP, Hufnagel C: A clinical study of one hundred cases of severe aortic insufficiency. *Am J Med* 21:200–210, 1956.

Shaver JA, Salerni R, Reddy PS: Normal and abnormal heart sounds in cardiac diagnosis: Part I. Systolic sounds. *Curr Probl Cardiol* 10(3):1–63, 1985.

Sheikh MU, Lee WR, Mills RJ, Dais K: Musical murmurs: Clinical implications, long-term prognosis, and echo-phonocardiographic features. *Am Heart J* 108:377–386, 1984.

Shimada R, Takeshita A, Nakamura M, Tokunaga K, Hirata T: Diagnosis of tricuspid stenosis by M-mode and two-dimensional echocardiography. *Am J Cardiol* 53:164–168, 1984.

Smith HJ, Neutze JM, Roche HG, Agnew TM, Barratt-Boyes BG. The natural history of rheumatic aortic regurgitation and the indications for surgery. *Br Heart J* 38:147–154, 1976.

Smith ND, Raizada V, Abrams J: Auscultation of the normally functioning prosthetic valve. *Ann Intern Med* 95:594–598, 1981.

Snapper I, Kahn AI: *Bedside Medicine*, ed 2. Grune & Stratton, New York, 1967.

Spagnuolo M, Kloth H, Taranta A, Doyle E, Pasternack B: Natural history of aortic regurgitation: Criteria predictive of death, congestive heart failure, and angina in young patients. *Circulation* 44:368–380, 1971.

Spodick DH: Pericardial rub: Prospective, multiple observer investigation of pericardial friction in 100 patients. *Am J Cardiol* 35:357–362, 1975.

Spodick DH: Perception of binary acoustic events associated with the first heart sound. *Am Heart J* 93:137–140, 1977.

Spodick DH: The normal and diseased pericardium: Current concepts of pericardial physiology, diagnosis, and treatment. *J Am Coll Cardiol* 1:240–251, 1983.

Spodick DH: The hairy hearts of hoary heroes and other tales: Medical history of the pericardium from antiquity through the twentieth century. In: Fowler NO (ed), *The Pericardium in Health and Disease.* Futura, Mt. Kisco, 1985.

Spodick DH, Kerigan AT, de la Paz LR, Shahamatpour A, Kino M: Preferential clavicular transmission and amplification of aortic valve murmurs. *Chest* 70:337–340, 1976.

Stapleton JF, Groves BM: Precordial palpation. *Am Heart J* 81:409–427, 1971.

Stewart JM, Houser OW, Baker HL Jr, O'Brien PC, Rodriguez M: Magnetic resonance imaging and clinical relationship in multiple sclerosis. *Mayo Clin Proc* 62:174–184, 1987.

Stone J: Sir Dominic John Corrigan. *Clin Cardiol* 9:403–406, 1986.

Surawicz B, Mercer C, Chlebus H, Reeves J, Spencer F: Role of the phonocardiogram in evaluation of the severity of mitral stenosis and detection of associated valvular lesions. *Circulation* 34:795–806, 1966.

Swistak M, Mushlin H, Spodick DH: Comparative prevalence of the fourth heart sound in hypertensive and matched normal persons. *Am J Cardiol* 33:614–616, 1974.

Szkopiec RL, Desser KB, Benchimol A, Sheasby C: Phonocardiographic findings in patients with normally functioning Ionescu-Shiley prostheses. *Am J Cardiol* 51:970–972, 1983.

Takao S, Miyatake K, Izumi S, Kineshita N, Sakakibara H, Nimura Y: Physiologic pulmonary regurgitation detected by the Doppler technique and its differential diagnosis. *J Am Coll Cardiol* 5:499, 1985.

Tavel ME: The fourth heart sound—a premature requiem? *Circulation* 49:4–6, 1974.

Tice F: The clinical determination and significance of some of the peripheral signs of aortic insufficiency. *IMJ* 20:271–287, 1911.

Traube L: Über den Doppelton in der Cruralis bei Insufficienze der Aortenklappen [On the femoral doubletone in valvular aortic insufficiency]. *Berl Klin Wochenschr* 9:573–574, 1872.

Ungerleider HE, Clark CP: A study of the transverse diameter of the heart silhouette with prediction table based on the teleoroentgenogram. *Am Heart J* 17:90–102, 1939.

Ungerleider HE, Gubner R: Evaluation of heart size measurements. *Am Heart J* 24:494–510, 1942.

Vogelpoel L, Nellen M, Beck W, Schrire V: The value of squatting in the diagnosis of mild aortic regurgitation. *Am Heart J* 77:709–710, 1969.

Wayne HH: Significance of the fourth sound. *Am Heart J* 88:126, 1974.

Weisse AB, Schwartz ML, Heinz A, Cyrsky FT, Webb NC Jr: Intensity of the normal second heart sound components in their traditional auscultatory areas. *Am J Med* 43:171–177, 1967.

Wigle ED: Hypertrophic cardiomyopathy: A 1987 viewpoint. *Circulation* 75:311–322, 1987.

Yeager M, Yock PG, Popp RL: Comparison of Doppler-derived pressure gradient to that determined at cardiac catheterization in adults with aortic valve stenosis: Implications for management. *Am J Cardiol* 54:644–648, 1986.

Yock PG, Naasz C, Schnittger I, Popp RL: Doppler tricuspid and pulmonic regurgitation in normals: Is it real? *Circulation* 70(Suppl II): 40, 1984.

18
Arteries

"Everywhere he feels his heart because its vessels run to all his limbs."
The Secret Book of the Physician (Egyptian c. 1550 BC)

Palpation, auscultation, and the special maneuver of taking the blood pressure are all oriented to the same purpose—determining occlusion and flow. Therefore, this chapter is organized by region (or by specific vessel) rather than in the usual manner by method of investigation.

○   There are five points to remember in examining the arteries:

1.   In patients with atrial fibrillation, or any other condition producing wide beat-to-beat variation in stroke volume, it is a good idea to palpate the arterial pulse in both sides at the same time. Thus, the relative strength of each side during the same stroke volume can be compared. Otherwise, one runs the risk of missing all but the most blatant degrees of decrease in arterial pulsation, especially as the arterial pressure is less useful (Ch. 6, p. 91). (This is also a good general rule of examination even if the patient is not in atrial fibrillation.)

2.   A bruit can be consistently produced over any vessel if one compresses it sufficiently with the stethoscope. (This misadventure is most likely to visit those who are not aware of its possibility.)

3.   *Meador's Rule*:* The worst thing you can do in a case of suspected arterial vascular disease is to fail to measure the blood pressures in all appropriate portions of the extremities. This may seem self-evident, but needs to be emphasized to the neophyte who believes that simple palpation will often suffice. Such neophytes should note that peripheral vascular surgeons with years of experience do not rely on palpation, but quantitate their observations with pressure measurements, often with the use of a Doppler, even though their diagnostic acumen may be the equal of the laboratory.

4.   Patients with palpably normal pulses may still have arterial insufficiency, which may be inferred from deficient capillary refill. This can be detected in any capillary bed that will blanch. The fingernails and toenails are used the most, but one can also use the fingertips and the hypothenar eminences in some persons. In fact,

one can produce a visible capillary bed in almost any part of the integument by applying $\frac{1}{2}$% to $\frac{1}{4}$% histamine in cold cream. But such pharmacologic dilation may confound the following tests, especially if homolateral controls are not available.

A method.   After finding a capillary bed, observe a pink portion of the bed and blanch it with finger pressure. When releasing the pressure, note how long (in seconds) it takes for the pink color to return (Fagan, 1988). Normally, this should occur quickly and smoothly, within 1 second. The crescendo (or time action curve) will be very similar to that of your own capillary beds.

There is one caveat: some vascular beds such as that on the volar surface of the forearm will normally fill more slowly than those of the fingertips, which have an abundant supply of dedicated vessels. Thus, one may compare one side with another, or patient area to doctor area, but one should not compare different areas of the patient.

5.   Toe temperature as an indicator of peripheral perfusion and prognosis in shock is discussed in Chapter 25 (p. 444).

Carotid (and Vertebral) Arteries

Inspection

Branches of the internal carotid artery are accessible to direct inspection in the fundus. The plaque of Hollenhorst is a sign of an ulcerated atheromatous plaque in the ipsilateral carotid system (see Ch. 10, p. 190).

Palpation: Pulse Wave Contour

Although all arteries have a recordable pulse wave contour, the carotid artery is the best artery for detecting it, in terms of cardiac assessment.

Examine Figure 18-1, and see whether you can tell the significance of each of the tracings. Then read on. Tracing A is a normal one for comparison.

Pulsus parvus et tardus*

This sign of aortic stenosis (see p. 313) may also be called the anacrotic pulse because of the anacrotic notch, indicated on the

---

*Named for Dr. Cliff Meador, a Tennessee endocrinologist. When he was Dean at the University of Alabama, he had the habit of asking, "What is the worst thing I could do here?" when others might have asked, "What is the best way of doing this?" This question initially seemed peculiar, but I later realized that it showed great insight.

---

*"Small and slow-rising." This phrase does *not* mean bradycardia.

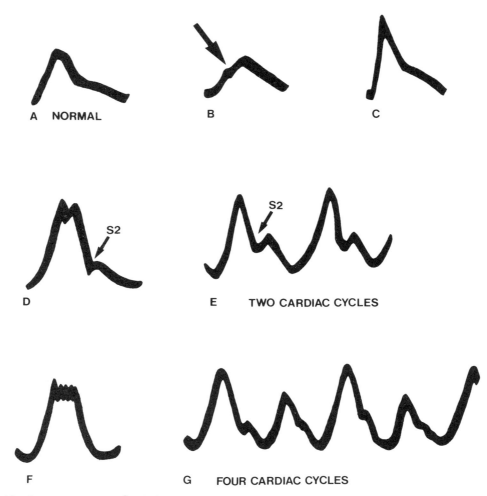

Figure 18-1.   *Carotid pulse wave contours. See text.*

pulse wave contour (Fig. 18-1B) by the arrow. I can almost never feel the notch. Also, the exact rate of rise of the carotid upstroke is poorly estimated by clinical examination (Spodick et al., 1982). However, in cases of *severe* aortic stenosis, the upstroke is so delayed that one can learn to detect it at the bedside.

A teaching trick (Fig. 18-2).   Take a Pasteur pipette with a bulb syringe at the proper end and a balloon tied around the distal end. With a glass file, make a nick where indicated by the cross-hatchings on the diagram. This will later permit you to remove the "aortic stenosis."

Fill the whole apparatus with water. Feeling the balloon (the vessel) with one hand, squeeze the bulb (the heart) with the other. You will note a delayed upstroke. Compare this to the sensation of brisk upstroke felt at your own carotid artery. Feel the balloon again.

Through the balloon, break off the tip of the Pasteur pipette at the file mark, taking care not to cut the balloon or your fingers. Now squeeze the bulb again and note the difference in the "carotid upstroke." Now that you have removed the "aortic stenosis" (the tapered end of the pipette), the "carotid upstroke" should be normal.

False positives.   Carotid upstroke may also be measurably decreased from any cause of left ventricular outflow obstruction (e.g., idiopathic hypertrophic subaortic stenosis, IHSS), any

significant vascular obstruction (e.g., atheroma between the left ventricle and the carotid artery), or any decrease in forward stroke volume (e.g., congestive heart failure, mitral insufficiency, or ventricular septal defect with a left-to-right shunt).

False negatives.   Unfortunately, carotid upstroke increases in the aged due to the changed compliance of their atherosclerotic vessels. Thus, in the elderly, the decreased carotid upstroke of aortic stenosis plus the increased upstroke due to age may yield an upstroke that seems to be within the range of normal values, albeit for a younger population (Flohr et al., 1981). This is not an artifact due to unskilled palpation, but can be demonstrated with external carotid pulse tracings.

Corrigan Pulse

The Corrigan, or Watson water hammer pulse (Fig. 18-1C), was first described by de Vieussens. One hundred years later, Corrigan and Hope, Irish clinicians, noted that many patients with aortic insufficiency had a de Vieussens's pulse. Later still, Watson described the pulse as feeling like a water hammer, a Victorian child's toy. This pulse can also be easily detected at the radial artery.

A teaching trick.   To make a water hammer, take a piece of thin-walled glass laboratory tubing and seal one end in a Bunsen burner. Add water about one third of the way up. Heat the open

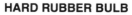

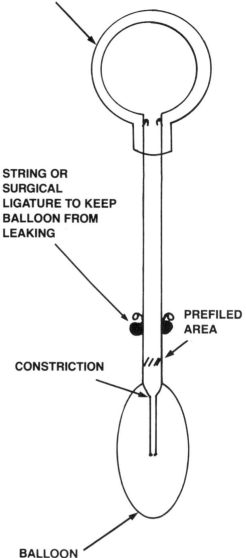

HARD RUBBER BULB

**STRING OR
SURGICAL
LIGATURE TO KEEP
BALLOON FROM
LEAKING**

**PREFILED
AREA**

CONSTRICTION

BALLOON

Figure 18-2. *Apparatus to demonstrate carotid upstroke in severe aortic stenosis.*

end so that you will be able to close it quickly, then boil the water to produce steam while the open end is still workable.

As the steam flows out the hot end of the tubing, seal it off quickly. Permit the tube to cool for a few minutes. After the steam condenses, the tube will contain water under a vacuum.

Holding the tube in your hand, turn it so that the water is at the top. The sensation caused by the water falling through the vacuum is what Watson felt in his patients' pulses.

False positives. Like many of the old signs of aortic insufficiency, this one is actually a sign of wide pulse pressure and/or a high stroke volume being ejected down a relatively lax vascular tree. Thus, *any condition* marked by high stroke volume/high flow/wide pulse pressure has been found to produce a water hammer pulse.

Additionally, mitral insufficiency may rarely have a Corrigan pulse.

False negatives. Mild cases of aortic insufficiency have insufficient flow to cause a water hammer pulse (see Ch. 17, p. 312).

Bisferiens Pulse

The first type of bisferiens pulse (Fig. 18-1D) is supposedly sensitive for the diagnosis of IHSS. However, it has been found in combined aortic stenosis and insufficiency (Wood, 1956). In aortic stenosis, it seems to indicate a good cardiac reserve (McAlpin & Kattus, 1965).

The other type of bisferiens pulse (Fig. 18-1E), also called a dicrotic pulse, is seen in conditions of low peripheral resistance and normal or increased cardiac output (stroke volume), such as fever or anxiety.

Auscultatory evidence of pulsus bisferiens may be sought as follows (McAlpin & Kattus, 1965): While ausculting over the brachial artery, gradually increase the pressure of the stethoscope bell, using the edge closest to the heart to indent the brachial artery. Eventually, one will hear the usual indentation systolic bruit, which, in cases of pulsus bisferiens will—at a critical pressure somewhere below systolic—split into two short bruits.

This technique detected bisferiens pulses that were otherwise detectable only by utilizing graphic recordings of the pulse wave.

Carotid Shudder

Evidence for a peculiar systolic tactile phenomenon called a carotid shudder was first presented in 1945 (Evans & Lewes, 1945). At the time, the sign was believed to occur only in conjoined aortic stenosis and aortic incompetence, and not in either lesion in the absence of the other. The carotid artery tracings (Fig. 18-1F) showed that the systolic peak was replaced by a number of rough undulations, which apparently produced the tactile sensation of "shuddering" or "shivering." Dr. Eugene D. Robin of California also taught a variation of this sign in which the systolic undulations were very fine, so that the tactile sensation was more like a cat purring. Whereas coarse shudders are invariably palpable, fine shudders are at times felt and at other times not perceived (Alpert et al., 1976).

This sign is useful, but insensitive (i.e., most patients with combined aortic insufficiency and stenosis do not have it). Further, the carotid shudder may be less diagnostic than originally thought (Table 18-1). In a study of the carotid pulse tracings of 73 patients with advanced aortic disease documented by cardiac catheterization, neither the fine nor coarse undulations had any significance other than indicating the presence of aortic valve disease, being found in isolated stenosis or insufficiency, as well as in combined lesions (Alpert et al., 1976).

Table 18-1. Incidence of Carotid Shudders in Patients with Proven Aortic Valve Disease

Patient Group	Coarse Shudder Present	Fine Shudder Present
Aortic stenosis (n = 30)	50%	17%
Aortic insufficiency (n = 29)	24%	24%
Combined aortic stenosis and insufficiency (n = 14)	43%	14%

Source: *Alpert et al. (1976).*

The carotid shudder does not guarantee the presence of a major lesion. I have detected this sign in patients with no aortic regurgitation and no aortic valve systolic gradient at cardiac catheterization. Others had no significant stenosis as judged by the Doppler velocity display. All had calcification of the aortic ring and the aortic valve by echocardiogram.

Other false positives result from carotid obstruction and kinking.

Palpation: Inequalities of Carotid Pulsations

Pulsus Alternans (Inequality Across Time)

Figure 18-1G does not represent bigeminy, since the beats occur at perfectly regular intervals.

Pulsus alternans is an important sign of myocardial failure, due either to a primary myocardial problem or to an overwhelming challenge to the myocardium, for example, from a greatly increased peripheral vascular resistance. It may also occur during tachycardias.

Inequality Between Sides

Obviously the weaker carotid pulse is on the side of the carotid stenosis.

Specific false positives for unequal carotid pulsations are aortic aneurysm, double aortic arch, atypical coarctation, and cervical rib syndromes (Silverstein, Lehrer, et al., 1960). However, if the carotid and superficial temporal pulses are both missing only on one side, then there is probably ipsilateral occlusion of the common carotid (Silverstein, Lehrer, et al., 1960).

Auscultation (Including the Vertebral Arteries)*

Systolic Neck Bruits†

A method.   Listen over the carotid artery high in the neck and inch downward toward the precordium in order to help distinguish a carotid bruit from a transmitted heart murmur. Be sure to listen with the bell of the stethoscope over the bifurcation of the common carotid at the level of the upper border of the thyroid cartilage (Gilroy & Meyer, 1962). Also listen in the subclavian fossa just posterior to the sternocleidomastoid, immediately above its clavicular origin, and over the posterior neck. (Remember that the subclavian artery is the origin of the vertebral artery.)

An important bruit is believed to be one that is high pitched or loud (Duncan et al., 1975). Furthermore, bruits at the top of the neck are thought to be more important than those at the base that do not radiate, especially if the latter can be altered by subclavian compression (David et al., 1973; Ziegler et al., 1971).

False negatives.   The absence of a bruit is not so helpful, as there may be total occlusion of the vessel (Matthews, 1961). Also, some significant lesions reportedly do not produce a bruit (Table 18-5).

False positives.   With carotid vessels, as with others, a systolic bruit can be produced in a completely normal vessel merely by pressing hard enough to indent the vessels with the stethoscope, thus causing stenosis with turbulence. In fact, failure to

produce a murmur under such circumstances could be considered evidence that the vessel is thrombosed.

Rationale.   The main reason for ausculting for cervical carotid bruits in symptomatic patients is to assess the likelihood that there is a surgically correctable lesion, whose repair will decrease morbidity. Numerous studies concerning the diagnosticity of carotid and subclavian bruits, with highly variable methodology and results, are cited in Tables 18-2 through 18-7.

An asymptomatic carotid bruit (even when not due to stethoscope indentation) may not be a marker for increased risk of stroke, as was formerly believed (Bergan et al., 1984). Some of the recent skepticism may result from heightened cognizance of the limitations of carotid endarterectomy; diagnostic enthusiasm could return when better therapy is available (Mohr, 1981).

Effect of contralateral carotid compression on murmur intensity.   A carotid murmur may be intensified by compression of the contralateral carotid providing the circle of Willis is intact. This test was 83% sensitive (Allen & Mustian, 1962). Furthermore, the test rules out a silent occlusion on the side being compressed. This test must be distinguished from one invented in the 17th century by Caleb Parry (Webster et al., 1958), in which the carotid artery is compressed, one side at a time, to see if seizures, syncope, or (later) EEG changes occur, indicating severely impaired collateral circulation through the anterior communicating artery. This test had a sensitivity of 92% and only a 14% false-positive rate, but has been abandoned in recent years because a screening test should have no morbidity and this one has caused hemiplegia (Silverstein, Doniger et al., 1960; Silverstein, Lehrer, et al., 1960) and even death (Webster et al., 1955).

Continuous Neck Bruits

A continuous murmur over a partially obstructed artery indicates that the gradient continues to exist in both systole and diastole. This situation is found with high-grade occlusion and insufficient collateralization. There are many conditions that produce a false positive (Table 18-7).

Ausculting for Heart Sounds in the Neck

Suppression of the heart sounds over the carotids on turning the head (Table 18-6) (Gilroy & Meyer, 1962) and softness of the heart sounds (determined both clinically or by phonocardiographic display) have been advocated as signs of obstructive disease of the carotids (Kartchner & McRae, 1969).

Factors Affecting the Intensity of Murmurs: the Phillips Equation

The variables that affect the intensity of bruits (e.g., due to carotid stenosis) are related by the Phillips equation (Allen & Mustian, 1962) (Fig. 18-3).

Variables related to position of stethoscope.   The angle Θ is the angle formed between the flow of blood in the vessel and the line of auditory inspection (angle of insonation) of the stethoscope. Thus, were the stethoscope in the direct line of flow of the blood in the vessel, the angle would be zero, so the cosine (and the cos²) would be unity. At a 45-degree angle, the cos² = 0.5. It becomes zero at a 90-degree angle, thus demonstrating that the stethoscope must be placed in a position distal to the occlusion and facing it. (This is also the biophysical explanation for the Ernstene-Blumgart modification of the Duroziez murmur test, which can distinguish forward flow from reversed flow; see Ch. 17, p. 311).

The distance (in cm) between the stethoscope and the occlusion is given by *r*. Like most radiation functions, it is an inverse

---

*Also see "Internal Carotid Artery" on page 342.

†"Bruit" is French for noise and is used in English as synonymous with murmur.

$$\text{Intensity of a murmur} = .037 \bullet (\text{Cos}\Theta)^2 \frac{\text{pId } V^6 S^2}{(145 \times 10^3 \text{ cm/sec})^3 r^2}$$

(Ergs/cm²sec)

Θ = *Angle between stethoscope sighting-origin of murmur and the direction of blood flow*

p = *1.055 Gm/cm³, density of the blood*

I = *circumference of the orifice, in cm*

d = *thickness of stenotic ring, in cm*

V = *blood velocity at the stenosis, ∼ 200 cm/sec, increasing to ∼ 230 cm/sec in some cases*

S = *0.19*

r = *Distance from stethoscope to origin of murmur, in cm*

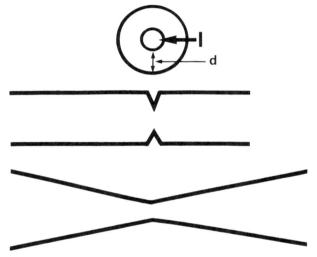

Figure 18-3. *The Phillips equation (after Allen & Mustian, 1962). See text.*

square law, teaching us that there will be a disproportionate decrease in the intensity of the murmur as one places the stethoscope further from its source. Since none of these two stethoscope placement factors were controlled in the studies reported in Tables 18-3 through 18-7, this becomes an obvious source of variability.

Other variables. The circumference of the stenotic orifice (in cm) is given by *I* (Fig. 18-3). As the circumference becomes smaller, the murmur becomes quieter. Thus, statements such as "an 86% reduction is required to produce a murmur" may be true for some stenoses, such as the aortic, but may not be true for vessels as small as 3 mm, which may be incapable of producing a murmur, regardless of the other factors (Allen & Mustian, 1962).

The thickness of the stenotic ring (in cm) is given by *d* (Fig. 18-3). Practically, a vessel with a long length of occlusion may reach a very narrow orifice, but so gradually that the thickness of the stenotic ring approaches zero (see bottom vessel). Such stenoses may not produce an audible murmur. This, in combination with the circumference factor, probably explains many of the false negatives in Tables 18-2 through 18-7, as well as the peculiar fact that kinking of the carotid artery causes a murmur in some cases but not in others (Allen & Mustian, 1962).

The density of the blood (in g/cm³, usually about 1.055) is given

by *p*. This variable decreases in anemia, but since anemia increases both the mechanical and the reflex flow of blood (and hence its velocity), the net effect is an increase in the murmur in that condition.

The velocity of the blood (in cm/sec) is given by *V*. Since *V* is raised to the sixth power, it is obviously one of the major factors producing an intense murmur. It is also the basis for the increase in murmur upon compression of the contralateral carotid artery, since that maneuver increases flow through the collateral, uncompressed artery. The measured increase in the volume of the murmur agrees very closely with that predicted from this formula (Allen & Mustian, 1962).

Very advanced. Where the thickness of the stenotic ring is 0.15 cm, the internal diameter of the artery is 0.8 cm, the distance to the stethoscope is 0.5 cm, the internal diameter of the orifice is 0.5 cm, the angle is zero (hence cos² = 1), and the velocity of blood *V* is 200 cm/sec, the calculated intensity of sound is 2.7×10^{-5} ergs/cm² sec. Most people have, at 300 hz, an auditory threshold around 10^{-8} ergs/cm² sec (Allen & Mustian, 1962).

Although Allen and Mustian use the "general equation of Phillips" (Phillips, 1956), that equation described the intensity of sound generated by fluid passing through cylinders. In the Phillips equation, *I* refers to the *length* of the cylinder, not the circumference. Thus, Allen and Mustian's analysis may work but still not be perfectly accurate. (J. Orient, personal communication, 1988).

The Phillips equation was also interpreted differently by Bruns, who developed a new theory concerning the causes and characteristics of murmurs (Bruns, 1959).

Maneuvers and Other Factors Affecting the Intensity and Duration of Murmurs

See Table 18.8.

Special Maneuvers

Carotid Artery Compression in Vascular Headache

Carotid artery pressure may be used as an aid in the diagnosis of migraine and migrainoid headaches (referred to collectively as "vascular headaches"). If the patient is seen early in the attack, while the cephalalgia still has its characteristic pulsatile quality, the patient is asked to rate his pain on a scale of 0 to 10. Damping of the pulse wave contour by ipsilateral carotid compression will, early in attacks of vascular headache, be accompanied by a diminution in the pain score. After the compression is released, the pain score tends to return toward the original higher score within just a few beats. This pain relief must be shown not to be replicated with placebo neck stimulation (i.e., rubbing the mastoid process, pinching the skin over the carotid artery without compressing it, etc). Furthermore, the test is useless once the headache has passed through the pulsatile pain phase and is in the steady pain phase.

This is one of the four criteria, of which three are required to diagnose vascular headache. The others are: 1) unilateral pain, 2) throbbing onset, and 3) relief by ergot alkaloids.

Carotid Sinus Reflex

Historical background. The carotid sinus reflex *qua* reflex was elucidated by Hering, who is probably best remembered for the Hering-Breuer* reflex.

---

*Breuer is also remembered as the partner of Sigmund Freud in the early studies of the technique that led to psychoanalysis.

Table 18-2.   Auscultation for Ipsilateral Systolic Bruits as a Sign of Stenosis in Symptomatic Patients

Citation	Population	Sensitivity[a]	False-Positive Rate[b]	"Gold Standard" (Independent Covariable)
Silverstein, 1959		13%	—	Angiography or autopsy
Peart & Rob, 1960		57%	1% from external carotid	Operation
Allen & Mustian, 1962	Patients with bruits	—	20% (3% from external carotid	Angiography or neurologic exam
Gilroy & Meyer, 1962		57%	6%	Angiography
Rennie et al., 1964	Includes subclavian lesions	48%	21%	Angiography
DeWeese et al., 1968		75%	—	Operation
Kartchner & McRae, 1969	Ausculted 3 places & used visual display	88%	15%	Angiography
Shapiro et al., 1970		87%	33%	Angiography
Ziegler et al., 1971		27%	10%	Angiography
David et al., 1973		73%	13%	Angiography
Gee et al., 1977	Consecutive patients with proved stenoses	58%		Angiography

[a]Hypothesis: *Any time the sensitivity of a sign varies by threefold, either the populations are not drawn from the same universe or there is a significant but unpublished variability in the way the sign was elicited.*

[b]*False-positive rate = false positives/(false positives + true positives).*

A method (after Lown & Levine, 1961):

1. Tilt the (recumbent) patient's head backward and to the side so that either one of the carotid sinuses is readily palpated. The sinus is usually situated just below the angle of the jaw at the level of the uppermost portion of the thyroid cartilage (Fig. 18-4).
2. Massage the carotid sinus with pressure directed medially and posteriorly, compressing the artery and the sinus against the vertebral spine.
3. Apply vigorous massage for not more than five seconds at a time. The procedure may be repeated after several seconds' rest.

4. *Never* massage both carotid bodies at the same time.

If this technique is carefully followed, adverse consequences are extremely uncommon. These primarily result from interference with cerebral blood flow. Accordingly, the maneuver should be avoided in patients with historical or physical evidence of cerebrovascular disease (e.g., a carotid bruit), and in patients over the age of 75. Patients with coronary insufficiency may develop asystole (Lown & Levine, 1961).

Customary response.   The carotid sinus reflex results in a variable effect on respiratory rate (Lown & Levine, 1961) plus two cardiovascular responses: 1) those of the heart, especially

Table 18-3.   Prevalence of Systolic Carotid Bruits in Normal and Asymptomatic Populations

Citation	Population	Prevalence	"Gold Standard" (Independent Covariable)
Allen & Mustian, 1962	Normals age 22–35	7%	None
Hammond & Eisinger, 1962	Normal persons	31% including children; 17% if older than 20	None
Wolf et al., 1981	Asymptomatic persons in community survey		Neurologic exam
	age 44–54	3.5%	
	age 65–79	7.0%	
Welch & Crowley, 1970	Asymptomatic pilots	Less than 1.0%	Neurologic exam, phonocardiogram, EEG, skull films
Ropper et al., 1982	Patients over 65 undergoing elective nonneurologic surgery	14%	Neurologic exam
Crevasse & Logue, 1958	Neurologically asymptomatic patients	6%–7%	Neurologic exam
	Nursing home patients	7%	
	Nursing home patients with no neurologic findings	2%	

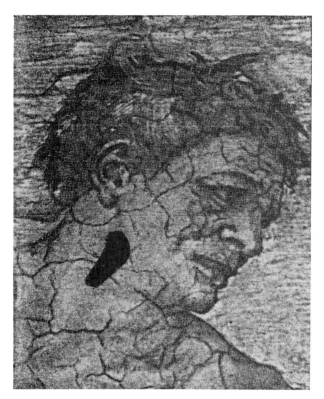

Figure 18-4. *The carotid sinus. Adam, by Michelangelo. Detail from the Temptation and Expulsion, Sistine Chapel.*

chronotropic and conductive (bradydromic)* and 2) some independent depressor responses.

It is well recognized that most subjects with cardiovascular disease have a brisk carotid sinus reflex but many normal subjects do not. Some type of cardiac response is elicited in 82% of persons over the age of 40, but in only 18% of those under 40, possibly because of the coexistence of cardiovascular disease in the older group.

Slowing of the sinus rhythm is seen in only 5% of normal subjects. A fall in the systolic blood pressure occurs in 60% of subjects. Again the figure is higher for older subjects and for those who have cardiovascular disease. Less hypotension is evoked in healthy soldiers.

---

*Bradydromic is derived from the Greek *brady* (slow) and *drome* (run); it refers to the slowing of AV conduction.

Some differential diagnoses of
arrhythmias made with the carotid sinus pressure:

1. Regular bradycardia. A sinus bradycardia gradually slows further during carotid sinus massage. In paroxysmn atrial tachycardia 3:1 AV block, as with many second-degree heart blocks, an effective carotid sinus reflex can cause an irregular or jerky slowing of the heartbeat with an irregular or jerky reacceleration when the pressure is removed.

A clue to 2:1 block specifically is paradoxic acceleration of the ventricular rate during the carotid sinus stimulation. The vagally induced slowing of atrial impulses permits the previously blocked alternate impulse (which had reached the AV node when it was refractory to conduction) to now pass through. Thus, conduction is now 1:1, and the ventricular rate is faster (Fig. 18-5).

(Complete heart block is not affected by carotid sinus pressure, but can be identified by observing the variability in the first heart sound [S1] [see Ch. 17, p. 292].)

2. Regular rhythm, with rate between 70 and 100. Such a rhythm is naturally assumed to result from a normal sinus mechanism. However, if carotid sinus pressure produces an abrupt slowing or halving of the rate, with a jerky return after the pressure is released, it should suggest to you that the mechanism is not sinus, but rather atrial flutter or paroxysmal atrial tachycardia with block.

3. Rapid regular rhythm. When the heart rate is regular and rapid (between 120 and 300/min), carotid sinus stimulation is useful even if you cannot study the patient with an electrocardiogram.

(a) If the carotid sinus stimulation abruptly stops the tachycardia, but the rhythm remains slow (<100/min) and regular after the release of pressure, one was probably dealing with paroxysmal atrial tachycardia.

(b) If carotid stimulation temporarily slows the ventricular rate, you can be sure that the arrhythmia is not ventricular tachycardia.

(c) If the slowing of the rate with carotid sinus pressure is smooth and gradual, with a similar smooth and gradual return to the original rate after release, it must be sinus tachycardia. This smooth deceleration and reacceleration has been likened to a train slowing down (without stopping) at a station to pick up a mailbag, and then speeding up to its original rate.

(d) If recovery from the temporary slowing is jerky, you must again think of atrial flutter or paroxysmal atrial tachycardia with block.

4. Rapid, irregular rhythm. If the original rate is rapid and irregular, but the slowed heart rate is regular, atrial fibrillation has been excluded. However, if the heart slows while maintaining an irregular rhythm, but exercise accelerates and regularizes it, the differential diagnosis includes atrial flutter, premature beats, or paroxysmal atrial tachycardia with block (Lown & Levine, 1961).

Table 18-4. Prevalence of Carotid and/or Subclavian (Vertebral) Systolic Bruits in Normal or Asymptomatic Patients

Citation	Population	Prevalence	"Gold Standard" (Independent Covariable)
Rennie et al., 1964	Normal persons	40%	None
	Asymptomatic patients	43%	Neurologic exam
Braun et al., 1966	Medical outpatients of four examiners	2%–12%; 20% in children; less if older, until age 80	None
Roederer et al., 1984	Asymptomatic patients referred to the vascular laboratory (?)	14%	Neurologic exam
Heyman et al., 1980	Asymptomatic patients (in a community survey), older than 45 yrs	4.4%	Neurologic exam
Welch & Crowley, 1970	Asymptomatic pilots Symptomatic pilots	Less than 1% Less than 1%	Neurologic exam, phonocardiogram, EEG, skull films

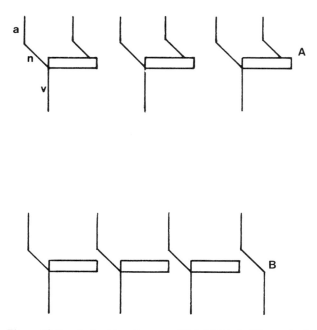

Figure 18-5. *A, Ladder diagram of 2:1 AV block. The vertical dashes in the row labeled "a" symbolize atrial depolarizations. The vertical dashes in the row labeled "v" symbolize ventricular depolarizations. The diagonals in the row labeled "n" represent nodal transmission. The rectangles indicate the refractory period in the nodal tissue, their breadth being proportional to duration. Note that alternate atrial impulses reach the node during the refractory period and so are not transmitted to the ventricle. Since there are twice as many atrial impulses as ventricular ones, the block is called 2:1. B, The effect of carotid sinus pressure. The atrial rate is slowed, but the ventricular rate is paradoxically increased because the atrial impulses arrive after the refractory period (itself unchanged) has passed. Whenever carotid sinus pressure causes an increase in ventricular rate, consider that this may be the mechanism.*

5. Digitalis intoxication. Since digitalization may sensitize the carotid sinus reflex, carotid sinus stimulation can be used as a nonpharmacologic test for the presence of digitalis intoxication, even before the characteristic arrhythmias occur spontaneously. If such stimulation produces advanced degrees of heart block, ectopic beats with fixed coupling, or the emergence of rapid and regular ventricular response in a patient with atrial fibrillation (representing conversion to a nodal ventricular rhythm while the atria continue to fibrillate), digitalis intoxication is highly likely, especially if carotid sinus stimulation did not previously cause these events in a particular patient.

Very advanced. There is no electrocardiographic way to distinguish 2:1 AV block from 2:1 sinus exit block, a distinction that can be significant in terms of both underlying diagnosis and, in the case of the former, the use of drugs that could further slow atrioventricular conduction. Should carotid sinus pressure increase the block (slow the pulse), the diagnosis of atrioventricular block would seem secure. Conversely, if there were no effect, the test would be suggestive of sinus exit block, although it would not be definitive.

It was formerly taught that the right carotid artery should be massaged to affect the sinus node and the left carotid massaged to affect the atrioventricular node. I know of no data to support this. Can you think of a good senior medical student project based upon the testing of such a hypothesis?

The Levine test. Carotid sinus massage sufficient to produce bradycardia may relieve chest pain due to angina pectoris. Although this test was first described by Wassermann, his eponym was already associated with a serologic test (for syphilis). The test is known today as the Levine test for the man who popularized it.

A method (after Lown & Levine, 1961):

1. Have an attendant (or the patient if no one else is available) hold the stethoscope over the precordium, so that you can listen for the bradycardia. Both your hands are now free, one to brace the patient's head and one to massage the carotid sinus by the method described on page 336.

2. Establish that the pain is still present.

3. Massage the right carotid first. If this does not produce appreciable cardiac slowing, massage the left.

4. Once slowing has occurred, ask the patient whether the pain has become *worse.*

Table 18-5.   Auscultation for Systolic Carotid Bruits in Asymptomatic Patients

Citation	Population	Sensitivity	False-Positive Rate[a]	"Gold Standard" (Independent Covariable)
David et al., 1973	Asymptomatic	90%	14%	Angiography
Hennerici et al., 1981	Asymptomatic (includes subclavian lesions)	36%	22%	Doppler (which had independently been shown to be 97% accurate for carotid and 90% accurate for subclavian lesions, compared with angiography)
Busuttil et al., 1981	Asymptomatic	—	38%	Oculopneumo-plethysmography[b]
Clauss et al., 1982	Uncertain	—	10% from external carotid	Not stated

[a]*Anytime the false-positive rate of a test varies more than threefold, there is probably a huge difference in the ways patients are examined, assuming that the patient populations are truly samples of the same universe.*

[b]*See text for various standardization studies; probably the accuracy is around 90%.*

Table 18-6. Examination of the Subclavian (Vertebral) System (also see Table 18-4)

Citation	Dependent Variable	Population	Objective Covariable	Sensitivity	False Positives
Hennerici et al., 1981	Systolic bruit, includes carotids	Asymptomatic patients	Doppler	28%	23%
Gilroy & Meyer, 1962	Systolic bruit	Symptomatic patients	Angiography	45%	60%
	Heart sounds suppressed with neck turning		—	—	42%
	Absence of heart sounds in all positions of head		—	—	25%

If the heart has been slowed, the patient with angina pectoris behaves in a characteristic fashion:

There is a pause before the answer is given, frequently with a look of uncertainty and puzzlement. "No doctor, the pain is all gone"; or "It is letting up." Disappearance or lessening of the pain occurs almost instantly within several seconds of the onset of slowing of the heart though the heart may promptly reaccelerate. Generally the pain does not recur.

Of importance in the proper performance of the test is the exact wording of the question. The objective is to mislead the patient by suggesting that this maneuver has aggravated the chest discomfort. If, despite this misdirection, the patient says the pain is lessened or disappeared, one can be certain that the subjective change is real and has not been suggested by the examiner. (Lown & Levine, 1961)

I prefer not to lead witnesses, especially overly cooperative ones, in any direction. Therefore, I have modified the test as follows: I ask for a baseline measurement of pain on a 0 to 10 scale. Then I ask what number the pain is, *during* the pressure. Unless the pain is gone, I repeat the baseline and experimental measure-

ments while performing placebo maneuvers: rubbing the mastoid, pinching the skin over the carotid sinus, and so forth. (Note that in a *scientific* study, the placebo should be first half of the time and second half of the time.)

This test is diagnostic of angina pectoris when positive, provided that the same pain relief scores were not obtained with the placebo maneuvers. (However, if negative, it does not rule out angina pectoris as the cause of the chest pain.)

Carotid sinus reflex in left bundle branch block. Slowing the ventricular rate with carotid sinus massage may sometimes eliminate left bundle branch block temporarily, permitting you to inspect the electrocardiogram for the signs of anterior myocardial infarction, which can be impossible to detect in the presence of left bundle branch block.

Therapeutic use of the carotid sinus reflex in pulmonary edema. Carotid sinus stimulation has been found effective in alleviating pulmonary edema in 80% of hypertensive or ischemic cases. Relief is immediate, and coincides with the onset of bradycardia. The episode may be completely reversed. Carotid sinus stimulation has been carried out intermittently (i.e., for no more than 5 minutes at a time) for as long as 30 minutes. If the reflex becomes extinguished on one side, a good response may be elicited by stimulating the other side. This technique has not been effective in the presence of atrial fibrillation or aortic valve disease (Lown & Levine, 1961).

Table 18-7. Continuous Carotid Bruits as a Sign of Carotid Stenosis (Including Evocation by Contralateral Carotid Compression)

Prevalence (Berry, 1965; Crevasse & Logue, 1958)	False Positives (Allen, 1965) (% of cases with continuous murmur that had this diagnosis)
1% of hospitalized patients 1% of nursing home patients	Aortic arch syndrome (Myers et al., 1956) Severe anemia and fever (8%) Allen & Mustian, 1962) Meningioma Glomus jugulare tumor Thyrotoxicosis Paget's disease Normal people (!) Carotid-cavernous sinus fistula or intracranial angioma (13%) (Allen & Mustian, 1962) Contralateral occlusive disease

Note: *Although these authors wrote of "Continuous murmurs" in practice, some of them are simply systolic murmurs with a diastolic murmur added and thus are "continuing" murmurs and not truly "continuous" as defined on page 304.*

Table 18-8. Factors Affecting the Intensity and Duration of Bruits

	Factors Increasing Bruit Intensity & Duration	Factors Decreasing Bruit Intensity & Duration
1. Side Branch	Diminished side branch flow due to manual compression	Augmented side branch flow due to pharmacologic agents
2. Collateral	No/poor collaterals	Abundant collaterals
3. Outflow	Augmented outflow Arteriolar dilatation due to pharmacologic agents or regional exercise	Diminished outflow Compression of artery manually or with BP cuff

Source: *Kurtz (1984).*

Carotid Sinus Syncope

When I was a medical student, I was told the following story.

●

Clinician Soma Weiss was once presented the case of a Boston streetcar conductor, who experienced syncope every morning at a certain corner, but at no other time. Apparently, at this particular corner the conductor had to turn the car and his head to the right. In those days, streetcar conductors wore wing collars (Fig. 18-6). Weiss hypothesized that the stiff starched collar was pressing into the patient's carotid sinus, causing a reflex bradycardia or asystole. He tested the hypothesis by pressing with his fingers on the supine patient's carotid sinus, reproducing the symptoms.

●

After hearing this story, I faithfully inquired about the tightness of the collar in all my patients admitted with syncope. However, by this time the wing collar had given way to the soft cloth collar of modern low cut, so my inquiries were diagnostically fruitless, as I would have known had I read the original paper instead of listening to stories:

This 65-year-old white streetcar motorman entered the hospital complaining of dizziness and fainting attacks. His symptoms began about 18 months previously when, one day while running his car, he suddenly felt very dizzy and lost consciousness. He started to fall, but was caught by a man standing behind him, and regained consciousness immediately. He had another similar attack some months later while running the streetcar. Quite frequently, while working, he noticed dizziness and diplopia. These were always brought on by turning his head from side to side watching traffic. Moreover, he had eight or ten fainting attacks while at home reading. It was always his custom to wear a celluloid collar which was quite loose. When he sat reading, his neck slipped down into the collar in such a fashion as to press against the right carotid sinus. This fact was not brought to light until we started our investigation. During the 18 months preceding that, he consulted several physicians, who were unable to find any cause for his fainting. Finally, he was examined by Dr. Walter Burrage at the Massachusetts General Hospital, who pressed on the right carotid sinus and immediately precipitated a fainting attack. The patient stated that this was entirely similar to his spontaneous attacks. He was referred to us for study.

Routine physical examination was negative except for slight enlargement of the heart and generalized arteriosclerosis. Blood counts and urine were normal. Blood pressure was 136/72. Kahn [serologic test for syphilis] was negative. Electrocardiogram was normal. Both carotid arteries were readily palpable. Pressure on either carotid sinus caused slowing of the pulse, fall in blood pressure, dizziness, fainting and convulsions. Pulse and blood pressure measurements were made with the patient turning his head from side to side while wearing one of his celluloid collars. These movements caused pressure on the carotid sinuses, and resulted in slight slowing of the heart rate, fall in blood pressure as much as 40 mm Hg systolic, sometimes dizziness, but not fainting. The patient was advised to wear a soft collar which he has done for the past month. In that time he has had no more attacks of dizziness or fainting. (Weiss & Baker, 1933)

As a Gallic footnote in the interest of truth, consider the following case report:

Last November 3, there presented in my consultation room a chief quarryman named Armand C. who was 53 years old and gave a history that before May of 1929 nothing particular had happened . . .

In May of 1929 the wife of our patient while helping him to put on a very tight collar slipped a finger between the rigid collar and his neck: Immediately her husband collapsed in a faint . . .

On the 3rd of November while in Liege on business he went to a barber. Here, when the razor went over his neck it provoked a sudden and prolonged syncope . . .

[This has been understood in English to mean a carotid sinus so sensitive that syncope occurred when the skin over the sinus was barely touched by a razor. It would not be possible to stimulate the carotid sinus in that way. No doubt what Armand remembered was the razor going over his neck. But when a barber shaves a customer's neck, the thumb that is not holding the razor is used to straighten the customer's skin, and this is done by pressing up the neck toward the angle of the jaw (i.e., over the carotid sinus), as the reader may observe by visiting a barber shop. Thus, I think the razor has been unjustly accused all these years, when the real culprit must have been the barber's thumb pressing on the carotid sinus.]

I systematically searched by strong compression in many places of the carotid and paracarotid regions of my patient carefully going over the left carotid and above the region of the left carotid sinus but not getting any noticeable reaction. I then approached the carotid sinus itself going at the level of the thyroid cartilage to the inferior angle of the jaw. Hardly had I begun to compress—I hesitate to say I even touched it—when Armand C. cried in a voice strangled with anguish, "I'm going." Immediately I ceased the compression which had been only an instant. Armand C. was pale as death, his lips without any color, his eyes dim, lying totally inert without consciousness, without movement, without pulse, without respiration. When the syncope went on more than 15 seconds after I had stopped pressing on him, I ausculted the precordial region with great attention: There was absolute silence. Finally, there supervened a grand mal seizure. . . . (Roskam, 1930) [The patient survived the episode, and went back into normal sinus rhythm.]

Notice that this report predates that of Soma Weiss.

We previously noted that the carotid sinus reflex could be useful, although it was missing in many normal persons. Now we have described a disease due to a hyperactive carotid sinus reflex. The question is at what point does a carotid sinus reflex merit the adjective "hyperactive"?

For screening purposes, a carotid sinus reflex is arbitrarily called hyperactive (Lown & Levine, 1961) if there is a greater than 50% slowing of the rate, or a greater than 40 mm Hg drop in the systolic blood pressure (during carotid sinus massage). Of all the persons who meet these criteria, only one third will have symptomatic carotid sinus syncope. Thus, if the patient does *not* meet these criteria, a hyperactive carotid sinus reflex is ruled out. However, if a patient with syncope does meet the criteria for hyperactive carotid sinus reflex, but the symptoms are not reproduced by carotid sinus massage, one still has not diagnosed carotid sinus syncope.

Carotid sinus syncope may be the mechanism for tussive (cough) syncope (Wenger et al., 1980), which is most likely to occur in patients with chronic obstructive pulmonary disease and well-developed thoracic musculature. Among the many other sug-

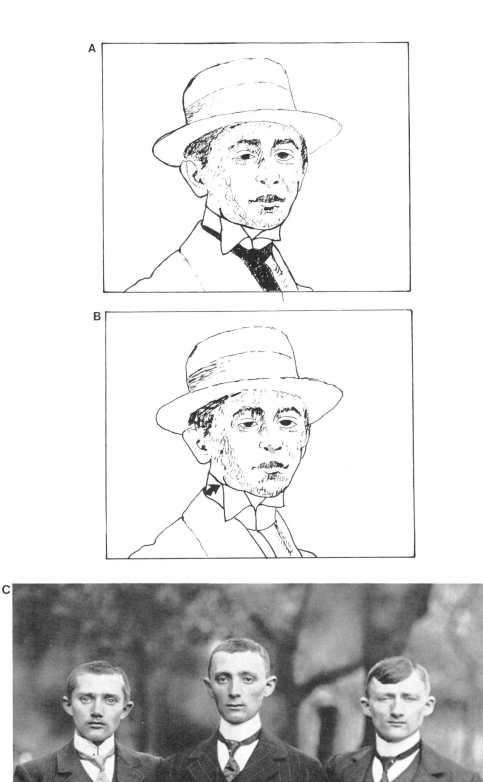

Figure 18-6. *A, A wing collar. B, The model's tie is removed to show how the stiff, starched, angled point of the wing collar might press the carotid sinus. C, A celluloid collar. This must be the type of collar that Armand's wife stuck her finger under (see text).*

gested mechanisms for tussive syncope are AV dissociation (Saito et al., 1982), reflex vasodilation (Chadda et al., 1986), or possibly decreased cerebral blood flow from increased venous pressure.

Subclavian Steal Syndrome

In patients complaining of neurologic or left upper extremity symptoms, especially if brought on by exercise, you should always compare the blood pressure and pulses of the left arm with those in the right, in order to identify patients with the surgically reversible subclavian steal syndrome. The word "steal" refers to the exercise-induced theft of blood from the vertebral artery due to occlusion of the subclavian artery proximal to the origin of the vertebral. Although at first it seems startling to consider, such occlusions actually lead to a reversal of flow (arteriographically demonstrated) in the ipsilateral, usually left, vertebral artery. In other words, the blood goes first to the brain, and then to the arm, bypassing the traffic jam in the subclavian.

In the old days, we made the diagnosis by history. Typically, a man (60% of cases occur in men) in his fifties (plus or minus 10 years) complained of sudden vertigo, ataxia, lightheadedness, confusion, headache, and/or visual disturbances, while brushing his crewcut with his left hand. In a third of the cases, there are hemispheric rather than vertebrobasilar symptoms, and these might include transient (or even completed) monoplegia, or hemiplegia, or, rarely, transient blindness. About 12% of patients have no neurologic symptoms, but rather upper extremity claudication,* easy fatiguability, and weakness of an intermittent and transient (i.e., not stroke-like) nature. Such symptoms can also accompany the neurologic symptoms in about half the patients experiencing the latter.

In over 85% of the patients, the syndrome is acquired (i.e., atherosclerotic) and left-sided. On physical examination, such patients have absence or diminution of the left radial pulse (compared with the right) and/or a left brachial systolic blood pressure that is 20 mm Hg less than that on the right. The remainder either have a congenital or traumatic cause, right subclavian steal syndrome, or bilateral disease confounding the comparative study of the upper extremity arterial circulation (Larrieu et al., 1979; Lawson et al., 1979).

Internal Carotid Artery

Direct Palpation

Some have recommended direct palpation of the internal carotid artery in the pharynx:

> The patient is placed in the supine position and requested to breathe through the mouth. The examining physician, wearing a rubber glove moistened with water to minimize the friction that initiates the gag reflex, gently palpates the posterior wall of the pharynx with the forefinger and very slowly draws the finger laterally as far as the pharyngopalatine muscle. When this muscle is relaxed, distinct pulsation of the artery can be felt more readily, while the thumb of the other hand is pressing externally in the carotid fossa. If, after repeated trials, no pulsation is detected, it would seem safe to assume that the lumen of the artery is very narrow or nonexistent. Palpation on both sides of the pharynx should always be carried out. Clonic contractions of the pharyngopalatine muscle may simulate the pulse. These contrac-

tions may be differentiated from the pulsation of the internal carotid by timing them with the usually visible common carotid pulsation in the neck. If repeated gagging occurs, the procedure should be terminated, because contraction of the pharyngopalatine muscle pushes the examining finger medially and covers the artery. The palpation must be light and gentle, as too much pressure causes gagging. In my experience it has not been necessary to block the gag reflex by injecting cocaine into the pharynx. (Dunning, 1953)

However, others say that pharyngeal palpation is of no diagnostic value; one study found the sensitivity (prospectively) to be 0% (Silverstein, Lehrer, et al., 1960).

Checking for Reversal of Flow in the Internal Carotid

There are two pairs of vessels in which reversal of direction of flow is a sign of internal carotid artery disease (Fig. 18-7). Not all these pairs of vessels are always palpable, and the signs to be given are of low sensitivity but presumably higher diagnosticity.

Palpate the supraorbital artery, then see whether its pulsations are dampened if you obliterate the preauricular pulsation (the temporal artery). This should not normally occur, because the temporal artery comes from the external carotid, and the supraorbital artery is a branch of the internal carotid. If digital pressure on the temporal artery does dampen or obliterate the supraorbital pulse, it suggests that there is reversal of flow in the supraorbital artery, which must be receiving anastomoses from the temporal artery branches. This implies internal carotid occlusion. However, when performed with a Doppler probe, this test has a sensitivity of as little as 50% and a false-positive rate up to 20% (Clauss et al., 1982).

The facial artery (formerly known as the external maxillary artery), a branch of the external carotid, may be similarly compressed where it passes through its notch on the lower edge of the mandible. Normally, this should not affect the angular (also called the supratrochlear or frontal) pulsation (if any) because the latter is derived from the internal carotid. If it does, it also implies reversal of flow and an internal carotid obstruction, as I learned from J. P. Mohr of New York.

Note that in both cases, initial absence of the internal carotid branch pulsations does not count. They must be present but lost with compression of the paired artery from the external carotid in order to have a positive sign.

Ocular Pressures

If I can find a cooperative ophthalmologist, I find ophthalmodynamometry or ocular plethysmography to be useful techniques for evaluating vessels I cannot palpate (the retinal branches of the internal carotid). The ophthalmologist determines the pressure in the retinal artery, while I simultaneously take the ipsilateral brachial artery blood pressure. If the systolic pressure by ocular study is less than 50% of that in the ipsilateral brachial artery, further investigation of the anterior circulation is warranted.

Be aware that ophthalmodynamometry interpretation was initially based upon a comparison between the readings in the right and left eye. A difference of 10 mm Hg was believed to indicate diminished or absent blood flow in the carotid artery on the side of the lower pressure (Hollenhorst, 1958). Other ophthalmodynamometers read in weight units, and differences more than 8 g were considered abnormal (Paulson, 1976). But with greater experience, it became apparent that both false-negative and false-positive results were obtained by comparing one eye with the other (Batko & Appen, 1979). Most obviously, bilateral disease could produce a false negative, if one had no idea as to what the absolute pressure value should be. In fact, I have wondered whether the occasional superior results of ocular pneumoplethysmography (McDonald et al., 1979) were due not so much to the gadget but to

---

*The word "claudication," meaning "limping," derives from Claudius, the limping Emperor of Rome. From a strict semantic viewpoint, one should not speak of claudication of the upper extremities, but the other manifestations of exercise-induced ischemia are analogous in the upper and lower limbs.

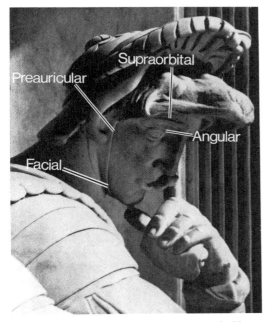

Figure 18-7. *The preauricular artery is easy to find because it passes in front of the ear, right under Lorenzo's chin strap. It is normally palpable. For purposes of testing, it is paired with the supraorbital, if the latter is palpable (it often is not, even in normal individuals). The facial artery passes beneath the mandible at the point where Lorenzo's chin strap crosses the mandible's lower border. The facial artery pulsation is often not detectable in normal persons. If it is, it is studied in conjunction with the angular at the nasal canthus (also called the supratrochlear artery or the frontal artery), if the latter is also palpable. Lorenzo de Medici, by Michelangelo.*

the use of an ophthalmic/brachial systolic pressure ratio of 0.66 as the normal cutoff.

Significance. Ophthalmodynamometry and, more recently, the various ocular plethysmography measurements are not perfect, especially when side-to-side comparisons must be made. Ophthalmodynamometry has reported sensitivities for the detection of internal carotid disease of 77% (Shapiro et al., 1970), 80% (Silverstein, Lehrer, et al., 1960), and 89% (DeWeese et al., 1968), using surgery and angiography as the independent covariables. Ocular pneumoplethysmography detected 92% of carotid stenoses greater than 75% using the criterion of an ophthalmic/brachial systolic blood pressure ratio less than 0.77 *or* an ophthalmic artery systolic pressure less than 110 mm Hg. In the same study, 90.2% of patients with stenoses no greater than 50% had pressures that did not meet this criterion (Gee et al., 1977). These methods compare favorably with palpation of the carotid pulses, which has a sensitivity of from 11% to 40% (Jacobsen & Skinhøj, 1957; Shapiro et al., 1970; Silverstein, Lehrer, et al., 1960) and false positive rates

varying from 7% to 60% (Shapiro et al., 1970; Silverstein, Lehrer, et al., 1960). Auscultation and palpation together detected only 93% of patients, but when the ophthalmodynamometry was added to the other two, the detection rate rose to 100% (Shapiro et al., 1970). The message is, again, to start with simpler and more general tests and proceed to more diagnostic and restricted tests.

Some use ophthalmodynamometry in the diagnosis of intracerebral postural hypotension (Hollenhorst & Kublin, 1963). Apparently, some individuals can have postural hypotension of the retinal arteries (and presumably of the cerebral circulation) with no significant detectable change in the brachial artery blood pressures upon assuming the erect posture.

Auscultation: Fisher's Contralateral Systolic Bruit

A sign of contralateral internal carotid artery *occlusion*, this murmur is heard at the carotid bifurcation, the eyeball, and over the skull (not necessarily in all three places in a given patient). The semiophysiology is total occlusion on the silent side and collateral increased flow producing the murmur on the normal side.

The sensitivity was initially reported to be 100%, although there was mention of a patient with the bruit only at the carotid bifurcation and not at the eyeball. Other patients had the murmur missing over the skull (Fisher, 1957). However, a later study found the sensitivity of the contralateral carotid murmur to be only 10% (Silverstein, Lehrer, et al., 1960) and the sensitivity of the contralateral murmur specifically over the eyeball to be only 5% (Edwards et al., 1960). .

False positives were not initially quantitated; Fisher described them as "a rarity." Later, no false positives were found for the eye or skull murmur (Welch & Crowley, 1970), although there was a 3% false-positive rate for the carotid murmur indicating the wrong side (Silverstein, Lehrer, et al., 1960) (i.e., being ipsilateral rather than contralateral to the lesion).

Other causes of bruits over the skull and eyeballs are discussed in Chapters 9 (p. 151) and 10 (p. 202).

Dynamic Auscultation: Distinguishing Internal and External Carotid Bruits

About 10% of carotid bruits actually originate in the external carotid arteries (Allen & Mustian, 1962; Kurtz, 1984; Peart & Rob, 1960). The effect of various maneuvers on bruits originating from the internal versus the external carotid is given in Table 18-9.

Vascular Tinnitus

Some patients who have tinnitus (especially when unaccompanied by other evidence of ear pathology) may have vascular tinnitus. This is especially likely when the symptom is unilateral and episodic. If you can examine such patients during an attack, they can often detect a phasic component to the tinnitus. Ask them to time it with hand movements, and take the patient's pulse in the other wrist. Simultaneity of the two phenomena supports a vascular etiology. If compression of the ipsilateral carotid artery abolishes the tinnitus, the diagnosis is clinched.

Table 18-9.   Distinguishing Internal from External Carotid Murmurs by Dynamic Auscultation

	Hyperventilation	Breath Holding	Compression of Ipsilateral Superficial Temporal and Facial Arteries
Internal Carotid	Decrease	Increase	Increase
External Carotid	Increase	Decrease	Decrease

Source: *Kurtz (1984).*

Temporal Arteries

The temporal arteries are first felt just anterior to the tragus. It is most important to palpate them in patients in whom temporal arteritis, giant cell aortitis, Takayasu's arteritis, or polymyalgia rheumatica is suspected, including patients with headache or unilateral visual problems. In temporal arteritis, the temporal arteries may be nodular, inflamed, or tender. Rarely, the temporal artery pulsation can be felt only on one side, a finding that is almost pathognomonic of temporal arteritis (on the side where the pulsation is absent).

Ideally, these arteries should be palpated in all patients as a guide to the general state of arterial sclerosis throughout the body. Furthermore, one must learn what they feel like in normal persons, so as not to equate the arterial sclerosis of aging with the findings of an inflamed artery.

Subclavian Artery

The subclavian artery is located in the anterior medial corner of the supraclavicular fossa in the angle of the posterior aspect of the clavicular insertion of the sternocleidomastoid. Normally, the pulsations are equal, and there usually are no bruits. (However, see Table 18-4.)

Patients undergoing hemodialysis typically have supraclavicular bruits on the same side as the dialysis access (Wheeler, 1982). These can be heard between dialyses in 72% to 93% and during dialysis in 38%. Transient (less than 5 seconds) brachial artery occlusion (by manually squeezing it) causes the murmur to disappear.

It is useful to auscult for bruits during the special maneuvers described for diagnosing thoracic outlet syndromes.

Thoracic Outlet Syndromes

A variety of symptoms in the upper extremity have been attributed to compression of the neural and vascular structures as they exit from the thorax. The history is the most important feature in making the diagnosis. Patients complain of pain in the neck, shoulder, and arm (82%) and numbness or tingling (82%). Less common are swelling (24%) and cyanosis (12%) (Heughan, 1984). Activities such as hair drying or hanging up clothes may bring on symptoms, but symptoms are often worse after, rather than during, the activity (Riddell & Smith, 1986).

A large number of maneuvers have been recommended to make this diagnosis (DeGowin, 1965; Spittell, 1983). In each of these, one palpates the ipsilateral radial artery while listening for a bruit over the subclavian artery. Disappearance or diminution of the radial pulse, and/or the appearance of a bruit over the subclavian artery, constitutes a positive test.

Adson's Maneuver for the Scalenus Anticus Syndrome

This is the best-known maneuver. The patient is asked to rotate his head toward the side being tested, with the neck maximally extended (chin raised). He then takes a deep breath and holds it in inspiration, so as to maximally squeeze the scalenus anticus muscle against the subclavian artery. (Also see Ch. 24, lateral rupture of the cervical intervertebral disc, p. 421.)

Hyperabduction Maneuver for Subclavian Artery Compression

Have the patient raise each arm in turn over his head in approximately the position assumed in sleeping (180 degrees of abduction at the shoulder, about 90 degrees of flexion at the elbow, volar surfaces of the arms forward, shoulder rotated as far posteriorly as possible). While in this position, have the patient squeeze a tennis ball 10 times, then perform the palpation and auscultation.

Costoclavicular Test for Costoclavicular Syndrome

This test can be performed either actively and/or passively. In the former method, the seated subject is asked to move both shoulders toward each other in the back, and then to move them both as far toward the floor as possible. This is the position occasioned by carrying heavy weights or marching with full pack (Stallworth & Horne, 1984). When the test is done passively, it must be performed on one side at a time.

Interpretation

These tests must be interpreted cautiously, because positive results can be obtained in asymptomatic patients. The radial pulse could be obliterated by hyperabducting the shoulder in 82% of asymptomatic army recruits (Wright, 1945). In one laboratory, approximately 50% of the subjects showed diminished pulsations during the hyperabduction and costoclavicular maneuver. Thus, those authors considered a test to be positive only if the maneuver reproduced the patient's neurologic or vascular symptoms (Stallworth & Horne, 1984).

Vascular Anomalies

The left subclavian artery may occasionally have an abnormal takeoff from a right aortic arch, passing in front of the trachea and esophagus. This may produce unexplained stridor or even dysphagia known as dysphagia lusoria ("dysphagia of a joke," the joke being one that nature performed upon the patient). Vascular ring anomalies may have the same effect.

Wrist Arteries

Palpation of Radial Artery

Both radial and ulnar arteries should be palpated routinely. I can still see and hear Dr. Jack Myers exclaiming, "Everyone takes the pulse but no one bothers to feel the vessel," as he proceeded by radial artery palpation to diagnose yet another case of Mönckeberg's sclerosis or perhaps simply arteriosclerosis as the cause of what is now called "pseudohypertension" (see Ch. 6, p. 93).

Perloff recommends using the thumb for radial arterial palpation because the artery will never roll. This is exactly the reason why I always palpate with my fingers. If there is a sclerosed artery (sclerosed, not stenosed) that rolls from my fingers, I have found an abnormality and informed myself of a potential difficulty in performing an arterial puncture. Also, using several fingers will help in determining how deformable the artery is, and in perceiving the pulse wave contour.

Although anacrotic notches, dicrotic notches, and bisferiens pulse can be detected at the radial artery, it makes more sense to feel for pulse contour at the carotid artery. However, the ability to detect and time the peak of the radial systolic pulsation enables one to compare it with that of the femoral artery pulse, simultaneously palpated with the other hand.

Normally, the peak of the arterial pulse waves occurs in the femoral artery before it occurs in the radial, because the radial artery is actually farther from the heart. This sequence is reversed when there is an obstruction in the aorta above the femoral artery. Most commonly, such an obstruction is caused by coarctation of the aorta in a young person, and severe aortic atherosclerosis in an older person. (Such severe obstruction is actually a rare event in atherosclerosis; however, patients with undiagnosed and untreated coarctation of the aorta do not usually live into the age groups that develop severe atherosclerosis.)

Palpation of Ulnar Artery

Many people have difficulty finding the ulnar pulsations, which are absent in only 3% of the population (Spittell, 1983). Be sure that you are far enough toward the ulnar side. Passively extend the wrist to move the artery closer to the surface. Use three fingers so that you are more likely to encounter the pulsation despite the vagaries of its location variation.

The Allen Test

My modification of the Allen test for patency of the deep palmar arch is performed as follows:

1. Compress the patient's right radial artery using at least three of your fingers or your thumb to obtain a secure purchase.
2. Have the patient vigorously clench and unclench his right hand three times to make it blanch. Observe the filling due to the ulnar artery. Release the radial artery pressure.
3. Repeat on the left. Did both palms show the same pink area? Did refilling occur over both with equal speed?
4. Repeat the above sequence, compressing the ulnar arteries.

Several students have shown me a modification of the Allen test, which they use to predict ulnar artery patency in a patient who is about to have a radial artery puncture for an arterial blood gas determination. This modification seems superior to my generation's technique of simply palpating the ulnar artery pulsation.

1. Compress both the radial and ulnar arteries as the patient clenches his fist until it blanches.
2. Release only the ulnar artery, to see if the hand will pink up. (If it does not, you might want to do a brachial artery stick.)

Very advanced. In the original paper, there are other tests described for the digital arteries (Allen, 1929):

1. Look for excessive pallor after 2 minutes of elevation in some but not all digits.
2. Look for abnormal rubor after 2 minutes of dependency in one or more but not all digits.
3. Squeeze the blood out of a digit for 5 seconds, with the patient's hand elevated. Normally, there should be a return to the normal red color as soon as the pressure is released.
4. Sometimes one can palpate the individual digital arteries at the base of the fingers by laterally grasping the volar digital tissue between your forefinger and thumb. (Another version is to grasp all the patient's fingers at the bases between the bases of one's own fingers, in the manner of the first grasp of professional wrestlers.)

Raynaud's Phenomenon

Historical Perspective

Medical student Maurice Raynaud's thesis for the doctorate of medicine, entitled "On the local asphyxia and symmetrical gangrene of the extremities," was published in 1862. In it, he described an initial "pallor" that was replaced in the more severe cases by a cyanotic color, and then a vermillion that finally gave way to the normal pink (Raynaud, 1862). The next year, he described the stage of pallor as being a "gray green pallor" and the cyanotic stage as being "black" (Raynaud, 1865), in a paper that was brought to my attention by Dr. Gerry Rodnan of Pennsylvania. Most authorities (such as the texts of Snapper and Bailey, see Ch. 29) describe the sequence as white followed by blue followed by red. However, blue followed by white followed by red has been seen (Delp & Manning, 1975), as well as only blue or only white (Sutton & Sutton, 1937). I believe that all these may occur, the actual shades being not so important if we keep the semiophysiology in mind.

Semiophysiology

The white (pallor) obviously represents blanching and ischemia, the vasospasm having squeezed all the blood out of the fingers, as it were. The final stage of red or vermillion is obviously the reactive hyperemia seen when the zenith of the attack is past and the (compensatory) increased blood flow to the hands is repairing the ravages of the prior oxygen famine. And the blue, whenever it appears, is obviously cyanotic blood, of the type of acrocyanosis you can imitate in yourself by placing a rubber band about your finger. Here the blood is held in prolonged contact with the tissues, and becomes blue as its oxygen is removed. This could occur early or late, through two different mechanisms: First, the venous capillaries could be in spasm at a time when there was still some arterial flow. In that case, the blood would pour into the fingers and become trapped, just as with the rubber band. Or, the venous capillaries could be completely normal, but the arterial side could let in a small amount of blood, still sufficient to color the fingers, but with such a slow transit that the tissues could remove enough oxygen to turn the fingers blue.

Criterion for Diagnosis

The diagnosis is made by inducing some form of the phenomenon in one hand by the immersion of the *other* hand in a bucket of ice water. Where the proclivity for the response has passed, and it is not possible to induce it, one is totally dependent upon the history of some triphasic color response, including a white phase (G. Rodnan, personal communication, 1977).

Significance

Please note that I have been referring to Raynaud's phenomenon, not Raynaud's disease. When the sign first appears, one does not know what condition it heralds (Table 18-10). I take the position that there is no such thing as Raynaud's disease, the phenomenon always being a sign of some underlying condition. Even if you were to follow a patient with only Raynaud's phenomenon for 30 years, I could still claim that such a patient would eventually develop other manifestations. (This is not a very sound position scientifically, is it? That is, the hypothesis is not falsifiable [see definition, p. 4].) If you wish to say that there is a Raynaud's disease, you will initially diagnose it in 20% to 30% of patients with Raynaud's phenomenon (Blunt & Porter, 1981).

Aorta

Dissecting Aneurysm (Dissecting Hematoma)

■ About 68% of the patients with an aortic dissection are hypertensive (McCloy et al., 1965), despite appearing clammy and restless, as if in shock. A sinus tachycardia is often present. A "double" pulse may result from sequential filling of the true and false lumen. The extremity blood pressures may be unequal (see Ch. 6, p. 89). A cold pulseless extremity suggests vascular occlusion at the aortic take-off. A warm pulseless extremity is a sign that the dissecting hematoma has performed an autosympathectomy (Glenn, 1983). An aortic insufficiency murmur may be heard if a proximal dissection has involved the aortic valve, or there may be murmurs over major branches such as the carotid or subclavian (Wheat & Palmer, 1971). In the rare instance of dissection with reentry, there may be a bruit over the abdominal aorta (Rivin, 1972).

Potain's sign is described in Ch. 17 (p. 288).

Saccular Aneurysms

The physical findings of a saccular aneurysm of the thoracic aorta might include a diminished blood pressure in the left arm, an aortic insufficiency murmur due to dilatation of the aortic root, an increase in retrosternal manubrial dullness, Potain's sign, and an aortic tracheal tug (see Ch. 14, p. 235).

A saccular abdominal aortic aneurysm is a pulsatile mass that usually is readily palpable on routine examination of the abdomen.

Two Methods

1. An aneurysm must be distinguished from a viscus that is simply transmitting a pulsation. Put your hands on both sides of the pulsation, and see whether it moves them apart. A viscus that is simply being knocked about by extrinsic forces does not expand, whereas an abdominal aortic aneurysm does.

2. Because it is fixed proximally and distally, an abdominal aneurysm cannot be moved cephalad or caudad in a longitudinal direction on bimanual palpation, but it can be moved laterally (Guarino, 1975).

Aneurysmal Size

By direct measurement (e.g., autopsy or ultrasound), a normal adult infrarenal aorta is 1.8 cm in diameter; most agree that a diameter greater than 3.5 cm is "aneurysmal" (Fortner & Johansen, 1984). But the normal width of the aorta in older patients is stated to be 4 to 5 cm, as judged by indirect means (Wiener & Nathanson, 1976–77).

Large aneurysms, and those increasing rapidly in size, are most prone to rupture (Bernstein et al., 1976; Crane, 1955). However, palpation is an unreliable method for judging the size. Once an aneurysm is detected, following the diameter by physical examination may be helpful if a clear increase is noted, but not very reassuring if an increase cannot be discerned.

The tension on the aortic wall follows the law of Laplace: tension (T) = intraluminal pressure (P) × aortic radius (r). The risk of rupture thus increases with diameter and systemic hypertension. In an autopsy series of 44 patients with abdominal aortic aneurysms, 82% of aneurysms larger than 7 cm had ruptured fatally, whereas only 4% of those under 6 cm had done so (Crane, 1955). The average growth rate is 0.4 cm per year (Bernstein et al., 1976).

Table 18-10.   Disorders Associated with Raynaud's Phenomenon

Connective Tissue Diseases
Progressive systemic sclerosis (17–28%) (+4)
Systemic lupus erythematosus (5–16%) (+3)
Mixed connective tissue disease (3–13%) (+4)
Dermatomyositis/polymyositis (1%) (+2)
Rheumatoid arthritis (1%)

Blood Abnormalities
Cryoglobulinemia (and overlap with arteritis cases) (2–24%)
Cryofibrinogenemia
Cold hemagglutinins
Monoclonal gammopathy
Polycythemia

Occupational
Percussion and vibratory tool workers (e.g., chainsaw) (1–2%)
Traumatic occlusive arterial disease
Vinyl chloride workers

Arterial Diseases (for vasculitis, see cryoglobulinemia)
Thromboangiitis obliterans
Thromboembolism
Arteriosclerosis (1–13%)
Fabry's disease
Pseudoxanthoma elasticum
Polyarteritis nodosa
Giant cell arteritis

Neurovascular Compression
Thoracic outlet syndromes (e.g., cervical rib, scalenus anticus syndrome)
Crutch pressure
Carpal tunnel syndrome

Drugs and Toxins
Ergot
Methysergide
Beta-adrenergic blocking drugs
Chemotherapy
Vinyl chloride
Methamphetamine

Miscellaneous
Reflex sympathetic dystrophy
Hypothyroidism
Pheochromocytoma
Neoplasm
Primary pulmonary hypertension
Variant angina
Addison's disease
Acromegaly

Source: *Blunt and Porter (1981), Rodnan (personal communication, 1977), and Spencer-Green (1983).*

Note: *The percentages are the prevalence of the given disease among all patients with Raynaud's phenomenon; the pluses are the sensitivity of the phenomenon among all patients with the disease (i.e., a "+4" sensitivity in progressive systemic sclerosis (PSS) means most patients with PSS will have Raynaud's phenomenon; but only 17% to 28% of patients with Raynaud's phenomenon will have PSS).*

Diagnosticity of Palpation

Sensitivity. Palpation is 28% to 69% sensitive, compared with 56% for conventional radiography (Lederle et al., 1988; Robicsek, 1981). Palpation is 100% sensitive in screening patients with an abdominal girth less than 100 cm, but otherwise is inferior to ultrasound and CT scan, which are 100% correct (Lederle et al., 1988; Robiscek, 1981).

False positives. Since a tortuous aorta may be mistaken for an aneurysm, it is not surprising that the predictive value of a positive test for a "definite" pulsatile mass or aneurysm has ranged from 100% (Robicsek, 1981) down to 50% (Lederle et al., 1988).

Auscultation

Systolic bruits are heard in 28% of abdominal aneurysms (Estes, 1950). The differential diagnosis of such a bruit includes renal vascular disease (vide infra). Other etiologies (and the incidence in normal persons) are discussed in Ch. 20 (p. 377).

Associated Clinical Findings

About 4% of patients with abdominal aortic aneurysms will also have another aneurysm. But more than 60% of patients with peripheral (e.g., femoral or popliteal) aneurysms also had a concomitant abdominal aortic aneurysm (of which 40% were overlooked on the physical examination) (Dent et al., 1972). (Can you deduce from the Laplace equation why peripheral aneurysms predict aortic aneurysms more than vice versa?) (Answer is in Appendix 18-1).

Findings with a Ruptured Aneurysm

A leaking abdominal aneurysm causes the diagnostic triad of back, flank, or abdominal pain; a pulsatile abdominal mass; and hypotension. Such patients should be taken to the operating room without delaying for diagnostic studies (Fortner & Johansen, 1984).

Synthesis of Coarctation

Legrand's periscapular pulsation of the collaterals works well in adults. Sir Thomas Lewis' femoral pulse delay is described on pages 344 and 349. Sir George Pickering first noted that the top of the body is warmer than the bottom. This is a reflection of blood flow to the two areas and may be visually demonstrated without a thermometer by scratching above the umbilicus (which turns red quickly) and below the umbilicus (which will be white). Potain's upper limb hypertension has already been described in Chapter 6 (p. 89). Finally, Gerbode's sign is useful in children (who may have femoral arteries that are difficult to palpate) as well as adults: The prone patient places a hand touching the ipsilateral foot (the knee flexed) behind the back. The physician squeezes the two together, squeezing the blood out. When the compression is released the hand will immediately pink up, but the foot will not. This test should also work well in other aortic obstructions (Gerbode, 1976).

The Leriche Syndrome

Patients with both exercised-induced ischemia and vasculogenic impotence are said to have the Leriche syndrome, which is due to aorto-iliac disease.

> As a rule, patients are young adults (the youngest of ours was 29); mostly males—but Delannoy reports a woman, aged 41. In general, . . . they come to the physician for one or the other of the following symptoms:
> *In the male: inability to keep a stable erection*, the blood flow being insufficient to fill the spongious processes. . . . If the disease is left to itself, sexual impotency will soon be permanent.
> *Extreme liability to fatigue of both lower limbs.* It is not the well-known "intermittent claudication," but an extreme weariness, which comes quickly on walking, sometimes even in ordinary standing position.

> *Usually a global atrophy of both lower limbs* which is difficult to appreciate as a normal limb lacks as a term of comparison. One must be on one's guard, not to overlook bilateral atrophy.
> *No trophic changes*, either of the skin, or of the nails. Toes look normal. It is difficult to believe that the circulation is severely impaired. . . .
> *Pallor of the legs and feet*, even when standing. At rest, the limb looks as if a Martin rubber bandage had just been released. When the legs are raised to the vertical, the pallor becomes striking, being like ivory or marble.
> The *clinical investigation* reveals, moreover: that no pulse can be found, either in the leg, or in the groin. The iliac pulse is not felt. That of the aorta will be perceived very high-up, above the umbilicus. . . .
> One should never diagnose a "neuritis" or a "polyneuritis" of the lower limbs, unless one has carefully examined the femoral pulses and the oscillometric curve. (Leriche & Morel, 1948)

Penile Artery

In patients with a history of impotence, the nocturnal tumescence (postage stamp) test (see Ch. 3, p. 42) may point to vascular insufficiency as a possible etiology.

The Doppler device may be used to measure penile artery pressures. A gradient of 40 mm Hg between the brachial and penile systolic blood pressures is evidence of vascular occlusive disease (Barry & Hodges, 1978). Others have used the penile-brachial systolic blood pressure ratio, stating that a ratio <0.6 is diagnostic of vasculogenic impotence, between 0.6 and 0.75 is compatible with vasculogenic impotence but not necessarily diagnostic, and >0.75 is compatible with normal pelvic hemodynamics (Goldstein et al., 1982).

Because measurements under resting conditions may be inadequate, a pelvic steal test (comparable to the DeWeese test, see p. 351), has been described (Goldstein et al., 1982). After the resting brachial and cavernosal pressures were determined, patients were asked to flex and extend their ankles against a resistance for a maximum of 3 minutes or to the point of claudication or extreme fatigue. A positive pelvic steal test was defined as being any decrease in penile-brachial systolic blood pressure ratio of 0.15 or more.

Renal Arteries

Renal artery bruits should be sought in all hypertensive patients.

Anterior Bruits

A method. Search above the umbilicus for anterior bruits (Fig. 18-8), pressing the bell of the stethoscope deep into the abdomen. As the skin of the anterior wall is stretched tightly over the bell, it is converted into a diaphragm, facilitating the recognition of high-pitched murmurs.

A useful trick for preventing pain in the examiner's ear while pressing the stethoscope deeply is to pull out one of the earpieces, so as to decompress the system. While still pressing into the abdominal wall, replace the earpiece.

About half (39% to 75%) of the patients with renal vascular disease have an abnormally high-pitched anterior systolic bruit, radiating laterally toward the flanks (Hocken, 1966; Shapiro et al., 1969). However, normotensive patients can have some sort of anterior abdominal bruit 0% to 16% of the time (Table 18-11).

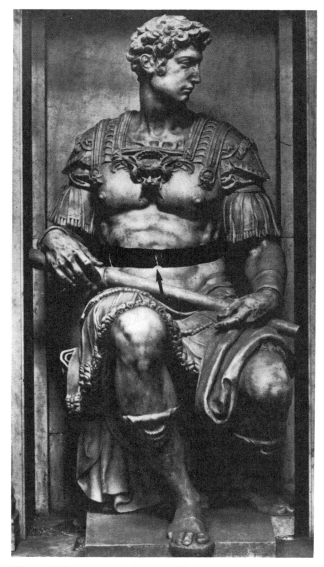

Figure 18-8. *Anterior abdominal bruits due to renal arterial hypertension may be heard in a band just above the umbilicus. Do not listen anteriorly while the patient is seated like this; have him lie down. Guiliano de Medici, by Michelangelo.*

In the essential hypertensive patients, the false-positive rate is 1% to 28%.

True positives due to renal vascular disease can usually be distinguished from false positives by radiation, pitch, and timing.

1.   True renal vascular bruits tend to be asymmetric in their "radiation" over the anterior abdominal surface, although again bilateral renal artery disease can produce a central abdominal murmur that "radiates" equally well into both flanks. But the point is that it does radiate into the flanks, whereas the "normal" aortic bruits tend not to radiate more than a hand's width from the midline on either side.

2.   Renal artery stenosis murmurs tend to be more high pitched and shrill than the rushing murmur produced by an atheromatous plaque in the aorta or stethoscopic compression of the aorta. Just as the trumpet makes higher notes than the wider-bored trombone, so does the renal artery stenosis murmur pro-

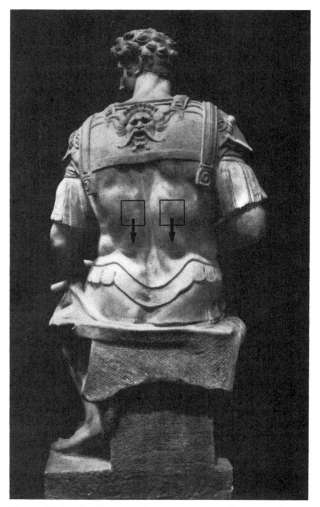

Figure 18-9. *In listening for posterior renal arterial bruits, start high and work your way down each side, in the region indicated. Guiliano de Medici, by Michelangelo.*

duce chords that are higher pitched (in the register of stethoscopic tonality) than does the wider-bored aorta.

3.   The true-positive bruit tends to last longer. Some extend into early diastole or even late diastole. The latter are sometimes referred to as continuation bruits. Sometimes the bruit is truly continuous.

Continuous Bruits

Continuous or systolic-diastolic continuation murmurs were initially reported to have a sensitivity of 90% (and later 80%) in the diagnosis of fibromuscular hyperplasia as a cause of renal vascular hypertension (Hunt et al., 1962). But for *all* causes of renal vascular hypertension, the sensitivity is only 39% to 63% (Grim et al., 1979, Hunt et al., 1969; Moser & Caldwell, 1962). The systolic-diastolic murmur was less common in a series of renal vascular hypertension patients than the continuous murmur (7% versus 56%). The former was more suggestive of renal artery atherosclerosis, and the latter of fibromuscular disease (Hunt et al., 1969).

The continuous bruit false-positive rate is 1% in essential hypertension and 0% to 7% in the normal population (Grim et al., 1979; Rivin, 1972), the higher figure including venous hums, which

Table 18-11. Prevalence of Anterior Abdominal Bruits

Citation	Normotensive	Hypertension (Not Renal Vascular)	Renal Vascular Hypertension Atherosclerotic	Renal Vascular Hypertension Fibromuscular
Hocken, 1966		7%		
Shapiro et al., 1969			43%[a]	
Julius & Stewart, 1967	16%	28%	64%[a]	
Grim et al., 1979	0%	1%	39%[a]	
Hunt et al., 1969			36%	80%
Simon et al., 1972				
Epigastric		6%	38%	55%
Flank		1%	8%	20%

[a]*Types not distinguished.*

should not entrap the thoughtful (see Ch. 19, p. 366). Other false positives include hepatic and splenic diseases (see Ch. 20, p. 378) and arteriovenous communications within the kidney (Hunt et al., 1969), either congenital, acquired (e.g., in a hypernephroma), or iatrogenic (e.g., after an unfortunate renal biopsy) (Clain et al., 1966).

The semiophysiology of these diastolic murmurs is uncertain. A possible explanation was offered by a very interesting patient.

A man who was said to have right-sided renovascular hypertension, as demonstrated by prior arteriography, was presented without benefit of old records (always a mistake). On physical examination in a noisy room (also a mistake), there was an anterior abdominal bruit that radiated to the "wrong" (left) side. Furthermore, this bruit had the high-pitched musical tones, which are highly specific for renal artery stenosis.

Because this abdominal bruit had not previously been noted, the next morning the patient was reexamined in a quiet room. The same murmur was heard on the left, but in addition, there was a softer systolic murmur, radiating to the right, with a diastolic component (on the right, but not on the left).

The explanation became apparent when the old records were finally recovered. The patient had a left renal artery stenosis, but also a complete occlusion of the right renal artery, possibly accounting for the discharge misdiagnosis of "right renal artery stenosis." Furthermore, the angiographer noted rich collateralization of the right, but not the left. Apparently, the flow in the collaterals produced the systolic-diastolic murmur.

Posterior Renal Artery Bruits

A Method

Using the diaphragm of the stethoscope, listen over the areas indicated in Fig. 18-9.

Interpretation

Posterior renal artery bruits are almost always systolic. Continuous posterior bruits, while rarely due to renal vascular hypertension, can also result from a number of other causes (see anterior continuous bruits, p. 348).

The sensitivity of any kind of posterior bruit for the diagnosis of renal vascular disease is 9% to 12% (Kaplan, 1986; Shapiro et al., 1969).

The false-positive rate is close to zero. I am personally unaware of any posterior murmur, systolic or continuous, that was truly "innocent." There is always an abnormal structural cause.

When there is a posterior bruit not due to renal vascular disease, it is often continuous (see differential diagnosis of anterior continuous bruits on p. 348); or it has diastolic continuation; or it is louder anteriorly; or it has an unusual location. Such tip-offs result in the predictive value of a positive test being close to 100%.

In summary, this sign is reliable if present but meaningless if absent.

This murmur becomes important in bilateral renal vascular diseases such as fibromuscular hyperplasia (in premenopausal women) or in atheromatous renal vascular disease (as in older men), especially when one is using screening tests, such as the rapid sequence IVP, which compares function between the two sides. Such tests are much less useful in bilateral renal vascular disease, in which there is no "control" side, but knowing that the patient has bilateral posterior bruits may permit the clinician to skip such screening tests and proceed directly to arteriography.

Arteries of the Lower Extremities

Femoral Artery

Palpation

1. With the patient lying supine, his legs perfectly extended at the hips, place your fingers above the inguinal ligament about halfway across the thigh where it joins the torso. Push down with the same force as used to insert a clove of garlic into a leg of lamb. The pulsation is the femoral artery.

Note that as with all arteries, there is some anatomic variation. In some persons, it may be easier to feel it below the inguinal ligament.

2. Sometimes the femoral arteries are more medial and sometimes more lateral, but they are normally symmetrical. To take advantage of this, try feeling for both at once. When you find one, you will know where the other should be. This method is particularly useful in older persons who may have inequality of the pulsation's intensity due to vascular disease.

3. The femoral artery is medial to the femoral nerve, but lateral to the vein. If an attempted femoral artery puncture has produced radiating pain or venous blood, the location of the stick mark can be a useful future guide.

As noted above, the peak of the femoral pulse contour should arrive before that of the radial pulse.

Auscultation and Dynamic Auscultation

Be sure to auscult for bruits. If aortic insufficiency is suspected, check for Duroziez's sign (see Ch. 17, p. 310).

Bruits over the femoral triangle or the anteromedial thigh may be augmented with exercise, and may develop a diastolic component. Carter's protocol for regional exercise involves ausculting with the patient supine, before and after full flexion and extension of the ankle at a rate of 1 cycle per second for 1 to 2 minutes (Kurtz, 1984).

The bruit-occlusion test is useful for localizing a stenosis when a bruit is heard over the common femoral artery in the inguinal region. After initial auscultation at rest, the examiner compresses the superficial femoral artery near the apex of the femoral triangle. If the observed bruit disappears or decreases in intensity, a stenosis is presumed to be present in the common femoral artery or proximal superficial femoral artery. In contrast, if the bruit does not change or becomes louder, the stenosis may reside in the profunda femoral artery or another branch vessel. In patients with a femoropopliteal bypass graft, impending occlusion can be suspected if compression causes the bruit to decrease or disappear, whereas an increase in bruit intensity suggests a lesion in the profunda femoral artery.

Complete disappearance of a distal bruit with proximal arterial compression almost always indicates stenosis in the compressed vessel (Kurtz, 1984).

Popliteal Artery

Palpation

A method:

1.   Lean over the supine patient and put your hands on the sides of the knee, tucking your fingers into the popliteal space.

2.   As you palpate for the vessel, lift the patient's knee, passively flexing it.

3.   Move the knee no more than 10 degrees at a time, stopping to palpate for the popliteal artery.

4.   If you get to 90 degrees of flexion and still cannot palpate the popliteal artery, stop and repeat on the other side.

Interpretation.   If both popliteal arteries are impalpable, and you have never examined the patient before, the findings are probably uninterpretable.

If the popliteal pulsation was previously symmetrical and is now asymmetrical or absent on one side, you have identified an occlusion of recent onset.

If only one popliteal artery pulsation is present in a patient not previously examined, you have identified an occlusion of unknown duration.

If both popliteal arteries are impalpable, and were present the last time you examined the patient, something has changed. The change may be as inconsequential as an alteration in pulse pressure, or as major as a saddle embolus (which will also cause a diminution in the other lower extremity pulses.)

Skin temperature

1.   When examining a patient with symptoms suggestive of ischemia, don't forget to feel the skin over the *symptomatic area.* (I use the dorsal surfaces of my fingers.) Coldness is a classic, but insensitive, sign of chronic arterial insufficiency. It

is more common in acute arterial insufficiency, a condition that will attract the clinician's attention in other, more dramatic ways.

○   **2.**   In *chronic* arterial insufficiency, with claudication, you should also compare the skin temperature of the *asymptomatic* knee. In unilateral popliteal disease, the *ipsilateral* knee may be *warmer*, not cooler. This paradox is explained by the fact that there are arterial anastomoses around the knee. In distinguishing femoral (high) from popliteal (low) obstruction, this test had a 55% sensitivity and 0% false positives (Zweifler, 1965).

Checking Blood Pressure at the Popliteal Artery

$$ If you wish to take the lower extremity blood pressure at the popliteal artery, you will need a thigh cuff. After attaching the thigh cuff, roll the patient into the prone position and passively flex the knee to 90 degrees. Place your stethoscope in the popliteal space over the area where the artery is or should be auscultable.

Posterior Tibial and Dorsalis Pedis Arteries

Palpation

A pair of methods:

1.   Using your right hand for the patient's right ankle, and left hand for the patient's left ankle, place your first two fingertips beneath and behind the medial malleolus to palpate the posterior tibial artery. "Beneath and behind" means in the posterior inferior quadrant, which is from 3 o'clock to 6 o'clock on the right ankle and from 6 o'clock to 9 o'clock on the left.

Question: *How far out does one need to go from the center of the malleolus to find the artery?*
Answer: *In most patients, the artery occurs at the point where one can begin to feel muscle above the bone.*

Some students find it easier to feel the pulse if they compress the tissues by pushing with the fingers of the other hand from the lateral side toward the palpating fingers.

2.   Palpating the dorsalis pedis can be difficult because it is not always located where it was in anatomy class. To find an aberrantly placed dorsalis pedis pulse, place all four fingers, held together in a transverse picket line, about halfway down the lateral dorsum of the foot. Press lightly at first, then more deeply. If you do not feel a pulsation, edge your way medially. If your picket line does not find the dorsalis pedis, move it one finger-breadth distally and repeat. Then if needed move it one finger-breadth proximally from the initial position, until all of the central portion of the dorsal foot has been covered.

Teaching trick.   Find a conscious patient whose pedal pulsations are inapparent to you, but apparent to someone else. Both of you should examine the patient at the same time, and ask the patient to describe the differences in palpatory technique. For example, are you both searching in the same spot? Are you pressing harder or softer than the other examiner?

○   Some students are deceived into thinking they are feeling the patient's pulse when they are in reality feeling the pulse in their own fingertips. Use your other hand to check your own radial pulse to assure that it is not simultaneous with the pulse you are attributing to the patient.

Congenital absence of pulses. A study of 1,000 children between the ages of 1 and 10, who had presumably not yet had the opportunity to develop obliterative atherosclerotic disease, revealed that all had posterior tibial pulses, but dorsalis pedis pulses were absent on the right in 3%, on the left in 3.7%, and bilaterally in 5.3%. One or both dorsalis pedis pulses were missing in 12.9% of whites, as compared with 3.8% of blacks (Barnhorst & Barner, 1968).

My (remembered) experience in adults suggests that the figure (0%) for the absence of posterior tibial pulses is a bit low, and that for the dorsalis pedis pulses is a bit high. (Testing this would make a nice student project.)

Some workers have tried to improve on the rules given above by feeling for the anterior tibial and the peroneal arteries. The former is located anteriorly, midway between the two malleoli, just above the ankle joint. The latter is 1 cm anterior and medial to the lateral malleolus. Either of these may substitute for the dorsalis pedis. However, the absence of the posterior tibial pulsations is still a problem.

Special Maneuvers for Diagnosing Arterial Insufficiency

DeWeese test. Following the lead of earlier investigators, DeWeese reported a series of 13 patients with claudication due to arterial atherosclerotic occlusive disease in the iliofemoral or popliteal region. All had palpable pedal pulses when examined at rest. However, if the patients exercised (such as by running in place) to the point of symptomatic claudication, all had disappearance of the pedal pulses.

Obstruction was demonstrated by aortography in 11 patients. Of these, five had thromboendarterectomy. Of these five, four had a good surgical result, with demonstrated maintenance of the pulses with moderate exercise postoperatively. The one patient left with continued distal narrowing of the femoral artery continued to have postexercise loss of the pedal pulses (De-Weese 1960).

One cannot rule out obstructive vascular disease as a cause of intermittent claudication unless the pulses are maintained after exercising to the point of symptoms. If they are maintained, it should be remembered that intermittent claudication may also reflect a cauda equina problem due to spinal stenosis (Hall, 1983). Pulses disappearing with exercise are an indication for angiography; otherwise, a CT scan of the spine may be the appropriate test.

Dorsalis pedis-to-brachial systolic blood pressure ratio. Patients with symptoms of exercise-induced ischemia in the thigh, hip, or buttocks, will have segmental hypotension, that is, blood pressure in the postobstructive arterial segment that is significantly lower than that obtained from the presumably non-obstructed brachial artery. (Note that indirectly determined blood pressures at the popliteal or dorsalis pedis are normally up to 10 mm higher than in the arm, see Ch. 6, p. 89).

In patients with exercise-induced ischemia (but no ischemia at rest), the dorsalis pedis-to-brachial systolic blood pressure ratio is usually 0.5 or higher, and the resting dorsalis pedis blood pressure is generally greater than 60 mm Hg (Mannick, 1983). In patients with rest ischemia, the ratio is 0.4 or less, and the dorsalis pedis blood pressure is generally less than 60 mm. Determining the dorsalis pedis-to-brachial systolic pressure index is more diagnostic than listening for bruits.

1. The ratio is also useful for predicting response to therapy. Limbs with a higher ratio (a mean of 0.6 or more as compared with a mean of 0.45) were more likely to improve with transluminal angioplasty (Rooke et al., 1987).

2. As with the simple DeWeese test described above, there is no reason why one cannot improve upon the test by inducing a stress on the system (i.e., a more significant gradient can be elicited by inducing segmental hypotension in the symptomatic region, using vigorous muscular exercise to create a demand for an increased blood flow).

Buerger's test. Another marker of arterial insufficiency is Buerger's test. Elevate the recumbent patient's legs above his head. If the veins collapse and the sole on the same side becomes pale, the test is positive. This is best seen when the disease is unilateral (the other side serving as a control) and in bright sunlight. Next, let the legs hang below the trunk, off the edge of the bed, for 3 minutes. The affected side will become ruddy, bluish, and plethoric.

Pedagogic Inspiration

In one study, attending vascular surgeons compared themselves with house staff and students in their ability to diagnose peripheral occlusive disease. Each was allowed to take a history and to palpate the abdominal aorta, the femoral, popliteal, dorsalis pedis, and posterior tibial pulses and to use an ordinary stethoscope. If after an examination at rest, there still was some question as to the patient's anatomic lesions, the patient was exercised to tolerance and the examination repeated. In 102 patients, the surgeons made an anatomically correct diagnosis (as verified by the vascular laboratory) in 96%, and were partly correct in the other 4%. Their younger colleagues were totally correct in 62%, partly correct in 35%, and were totally wrong in 3%. Noninvasive laboratory tests were much better than the younger physicians, but not quite as good as the attendings (Baker et al., 1978). These results suggest that performance improves with experience, a conclusion that will not be surprising to athletes and musicians. They may also explain the younger generation's rush to the laboratory.

Microvasculature

There are only two parts of the body where the microvasculature can be visualized at the bedside. One is in the nail fold (see Ch. 7, p. 134) and the other is in the fundus oculi (see Ch. 10).

Synthesis

Mycotic Aneurysms

First described and named by Osler, "mycotic" refers not to the infectious agent (since few are fungal; most are bacterial) but to the fact that the infected aneurysm appeared to Osler to be in the shape of a mushroom. The only good clue is petechial seeding of the area supplied by the infected vessel.

Dr. David Dobmeyer of Missouri once asked me to see a patient who was septic and thought to be suffering from endocarditis. His petechial rash was peculiar in that it afflicted one lower extremity almost exclusively. Knowing that the patient had previously received shrapnel wounds high in that extremity, I raised the possibility of an infected aneurysm. This produced much risibility in the direction of house staff elbows, until 6 days later, when the march of the imaging procedures suggested the very same diagnosis, which was indeed confirmed at curative surgery. There never was any endocarditis.

Arteriovenous Fistulas

If the arteriovenous fistula is observable, one can palpate the thrill and auscult the murmur. In some fistulas that are not accessible to direct inspection, palpation, or auscultation, Branham's sign may be performed (see Ch. 6, p. 94).

Suspect an arteriovenous fistula in patients with a high cardiac output state, a hypertrophied limb, or a pulsatile mass, especially if any of these occur posttrauma.

Appendix 18-1.   Answer to Question on Page 347

The aorta has a wider diameter than the peripheral vessels and both experience the same pressure. Therefore, aortic wall tension should be higher and aneurysms should form there first. By the time peripheral vessel aneurysms appear, the aorta has a good chance of one of its aneuryms already having grown to noticeable size.

References

Allen EV: Thromboangiitis obliterans: Methods of diagnosis of chronic occlusive arterial lesions distal to the wrist with illustrative cases. *Am J Med Sci* 178:237–244, 1929.

Allen N: The significance of vascular murmurs in the head and neck. *Geriatrics* 20:525–538, 1965.

Allen N, Mustian V: Origin and significance of vascular murmurs of the head and neck. *Medicine* 41:227–247, 1962.

Alpert JS, Vieweg WVR, Hagan AD: Incidence and morphology of carotid shudders in aortic valve disease. *Am Heart J* 92:435–440, 1976.

Baker WH, String T, Hayes AC, Turner D: Diagnosis of peripheral occlusive disease: Comparison of clinical evaluation and noninvasive laboratory. *Arch Surg* 113:1308–1310, 1978.

Barnhorst DA, Barner HB: Prevalence of congenitally absent pedal pulses. *N Engl J Med* 278:264–265, 1968.

Barry JM, Hodges CV: Impotence: A diagnostic approach. *J Urol* 119: 575–578, 1978.

Batko KA, Appen RE: Ophthalmodynamometry: A reappraisal. *Ann Ophthalmol* 11:1499–1508, 1979.

Bergan JJ, Yao JST, Flinn WR: Managing the asymptomatic carotid bruit. *Chest* 86:628–632, 1984.

Bernstein EF, Dilley RB, Goldberg LE, Gosink BB, Leopold GR: Growth rates of small abdominal aortic aneurysms. *Surgery* 80:765–773, 1976.

Berry JN: Benign intracranial and neck bruits in an adult. *Ann Intern Med* 63:661–663, 1965.

Blunt RJ, Porter JM: Raynaud syndrome. *Semin Arthritis Rheum* 10:282–308, 1981.

Braun HA, Reynolds WA, Diettert GA, McCarthy, CG: Auscultation of the neck: Incidence of cervical bruits in 4,296 consecutive patients. *Rocky Mountain Med J* 65:51–53, 1966.

Bruns DL: A general theory of the causes of murmurs in the cardiovascular system. *Am J Med* 27:360–374, 1959.

Busuttil RW, Baker JD, Davidson RK, Machleder HI: Carotid artery stenosis—hemodynamic significance and clinical course. *JAMA* 245:1438–1441, 1981.

Chadda KD, Peters R, Bloomfield B, Kops R: Cough syncope treated with a long-term vasoconstrictor. *JAMA* 255:1289–1291, 1986.

Clain D, Wartnaby K, Sherlock S: Abdominal arterial murmurs in liver disease. *Lancet* 2:516–519, 1966.

Clauss RH, Clauss P, Babu SC, Shah PM: Noninvasive testing for carotid disease. *Cardiovasc Rev Rep* 3:1372–1382, 1982.

Crane C: Arteriosclerotic aneurysms of the abdominal aorta: Some pathological and clinical correlates. *N Engl J Med* 253:954–958, 1955.

Crevasse LE, Logue RB: Carotid artery murmurs: Continuous murmur over carotid bulb—new sign of carotid artery insufficiency. *JAMA* 167:2177–2182, 1958.

David TE, Humphries AW, Young JR, Beven EG: A correlation of neck bruits and arteriosclerotic carotid arteries. *Arch Surg* 107:729–731, 1973.

DeGowin EL: *Bedside Diagnostic Examination*. Macmillan, New York, 1965.

Delp MH, Manning RT: *Major's Physical Diagnosis*. WB Saunders, Philadelphia, 1975.

Dent TL, Lindenauer SM, Ernst CB, Fry WJ: Multiple arteriosclerotic aneurysms. *Arch Surg* 105:339–344, 1972.

DeWeese JA: Pedal pulses disappearing with exercise: A test for intermittent claudication. *N Engl J Med* 262:1214–1217, 1960.

DeWeese JA, Rob CG, Satran R, Norris FH, Lipchik EO, Zehl DN, Long JM: Surgical treatment for occlusive disease of the carotid artery. *Ann Surg* 168:85–94, 1968.

Duncan GW, Gruber JO, Dewey CF Jr., Myers GO, Lees RS: Evaluation of carotid stenosis by phonoangiography. *N Engl J Med* 293:1124–1125, 1975.

Dunning HS: Detection of occlusion of the internal carotid by pharyngeal palpation. *JAMA* 152:321, 1953.

Edwards CH, Gordon NS, Rob C: The surgical treatment of internal carotid artery occlusion. *Q J Med* 29:67–84, 1960.

Estes JE: Abdominal aortic aneurysm: A study of one hundred two cases. *Circulation* 2:258–264, 1950.

Evans W, Lewes D: The carotid shudder. *Br Heart J* 7:171–172, 1945.

Fagan MJ: Relationship between nurses' assessments of perfusion and toe temperature in pediatric patients with cardiovascular disease. *Heart Lung* 17:157–165, 1988.

Fisher CM: Cranial bruit associated with occlusion of the internal carotid artery. *Neurology* 7:298–306, 1957.

Flohr KH, Weir EK, Chesler E: Diagnosis of aortic stenosis in older age groups using external carotid pulse recordings and phonocardiography. *Br Heart J* 45:577–582, 1981.

Fortner G, Johansen K: Abdominal aortic aneurysms. *West J Med* 140:50–59, 1984.

Gee W, Oller DW, Amundsen DG, Goodreau JJ: The asymptomatic carotid bruit and the ocular pneumoplethysmography. *Arch Surg* 112:1381–1388, 1977.

Gilroy J, Meyer JS: Auscultation of the neck in occlusive cerebrovascular disease. *Circulation* 25:300–310, 1962.

Glenn WWL, ed: *Thoracic and Cardiovascular Surgery*, ed 4. Appleton-Century-Crofts, Norwalk, CT, 1983.

Goldstein I, Siroky MB, Nath RI, McMillian TN, Menzoian JO, Krane RJ: Vasculogenic impotence: Role of the pelvic steal test. *J Urol* 128:300–306, 1982.

Grim CE, Luft FC, Weinberger MH, Grim CM: Sensitivity and specificity of screening tests for renal vascular hypertension. *Ann Intern Med* 91:617–622, 1979.

Guarino JR: Abdominal aortic aneurysm: A new diagnostic sign. *J Kansas Med Soc* 76:108, 1975.

Hall H: Examination of the patient with low back pain. *Bull Rheum Dis* 33(4):1–8, 1983.

Hammond JH, Eisinger RP: Carotid bruits in 1,000 normal subjects. *Arch Intern Med* 109:563–565, 1962.

Hennerici M, Aulich A, Sandmann W, Freund, J-J: Incidence of asymptomatic extracranial arterial disease. *Stroke* 12:750–758, 1981.

Heughan C: Thoracic outlet compression. *Can J Surg* 27:35–36, 1984.

Heyman A, Wilkinson WE, Heyden S, Helms MJ, Bartel AG, Karp HR, Tyroler HA, Hames CG: Risk of stroke in asymptomatic persons with cervical arterial bruits: A population study in Evans County, Georgia. *N Engl J Med* 302:838–841, 1980.

Hocken AG: Renovascular hypertension. *Arch Intern Med* 117:364–372, 1966.

Hollenhorst RW: Ophthalmodynamometry and intracranial vascular disease. *Med Clin North Am* 42:951–958, 1958.

Hollenhorst RW, Kublin JG: Ophthalmodynamometry in the diagnosis of intracerebral orthostatic hypotension. *Proc Staff Meetings Mayo Clin* 38:532–546, 1963.

Hunt JC, Harrison EG Jr, Kincaid OW, Bernatz PE, Davis GD: Idiopathic fibrous and fibromuscular stenoses of the renal arteries associated with hypertension. *Proc Staff Meetings Mayo Clin* 37:181–216, 1962.

Hunt JC, Strong CG, Sheps SG, Bernatz PE: Diagnosis and management of renovascular hypertension. *Am J Cardiol* 23:434–445, 1969.

Jacobsen H-H, Skinhøj E: Thrombosis of the internal carotid artery verified by arteriography. *Dan Med Bull* 4:240–248, 1957.

Julius S, Stewart BH: Diagnostic significance of abdominal murmurs. *N Engl J Med* 276:1175–1178, 1967.

Kaplan NM: *Clinical Hypertension*, ed 4. Williams & Wilkins, Baltimore, 1986.

Kartchner ME, McRae LP: Auscultation for carotid bruits in cerebrovascular insufficiency. *JAMA* 210:494–497, 1969.

Kurtz KJ: Dynamic vascular auscultation. *Am J Med* 76:1066–1074, 1984.

Larrieu AJ, Tyers FO, Williams FH, Morettin LB, Derrick JR: Subclavian steal syndrome: An update. *South Med J* 72:1374–1376, 1979.

Lawson JD, Peteracek MR, Buckspan GS, Dean RH: Subclavian steal: Review of the clinical manifestations. *South Med J* 72:1369–1373, 1979.

Lederle FA, Walker JM, Reinke DB: Selective screening for abdominal aortic aneurysms with physical examination and ultrasound. *Arch Intern Med* 148:1753–1756, 1988.

Leriche R, Morel A: The syndrome of thrombotic obliteration of the aortic bifurcation. *Ann Surg* 127:193–206, 1948.

Lown B, Levine SA: The carotid sinus: Clinical value of its stimulation. *Circulation* 23:766–789, 1961. [A classic]

Mannick JA: Evaluation of chronic lower-extremity ischemia. *N Engl J Med* 309:841–843, 1983.

Matthews WB: Observations on the carotid bruit. *J Neurol Neurosurg Psychiatry* 24:161–166, 1961.

McAlpin RN, Kattus AA: Brachial artery bruits in aortic valve disease and hypertrophic subaortic stenosis. *N Engl J Med* 273:1012–1018, 1965.

McCloy RM, Spittell JA Jr, McGoon DC: Dissecting aortic hematoma or aneurysm. *Circulation* 31:665–669, 1965.

McDonald PT, Collins GJ, Andersen CA: Ocular pneumoplethosmography: Detection of carotid occlusive disease. *Ann Surg* 189:44–48, 1979.

Mohr JP: Asymptomatic carotid artery disease. *Stroke* 13:431–433, 1981.

Moser RJ Jr, Caldwell JR: Abdominal murmurs, an aid in the diagnosis of renal artery disease in hypertension. *Ann Intern Med* 56:471–483, 1962.

Myers JD, Murdaugh HV, McIntosh HD, Blaisdell RK: Observations on continuous murmurs over partially occluded arteries. *Arch Intern Med* 97:726–739, 1956.

Paulson OB: Ophthalmodynamometry in internal carotid artery occlusion. *Stroke* 7:564–566, 1976.

Peart WS, Rob C: Arterial auscultation. *Lancet* 2:219–220, 1960.

Phillips OM: The intensity of aeolian tones. *J Fluid Mechanics* 1:607–624, 1956.

Raynaud AGM: *On the Local Asphyxia and Symmetrical Gangrene of the Extremities*. Rignoux, Paris, 1862.

Raynaud AGM: Cited as a personal communication. In: Horteloup P, *On Scleroderma*. Asselin, Paris, 1865.

Rennie L, Ejrup B, McDowell F: Arterial bruits in cerebrovascular disease. *Neurology* 14:751–756, 1964.

Riddell DH, Smith BM: Thoracic and vascular aspects of thoracic outlet syndrome: 1986 update. *Clin Orthop Related Res* 207:31–36 1986.

Rivin AU: Abdominal vascular sounds. *JAMA* 221:688–690, 1972.

Robicsek F: The diagnosis of abdominal aneurysms. *Surgery* 89:275–276, 1981.

Roederer GO, Langlois YE, Jager KA, Primozich JF, Beach KW, Phillips DJ, Strandness DE: The natural history of carotid arterial disease in asymptomatic patients with cervical bruits. *Stroke* 15:605–613, 1984.

Rooke RW, Stanson AW, Johnson CM, Sheedy PF II, Miller WE, Hollier LH, Osmundson PJ: Percutaneous transluminal angioplasty in the lower extremities: A 5-year experience. *Mayo Clin Proc* 62:85–91, 1987.

Ropper AH, Wechsler LR, Wilson SL: Carotid bruit and the risk of elective surgery. *N Engl J Med* 307:1388–1390, 1982.

Roskam J: A new syndrome—serious cardiac syncope and repeated syncope from a hypercarotid sinus. *Presse Medicale* 38:590–591, 1930.

Saito D, Matsuno S, Matsushita K, Takeda H, Hyodo T, Haraoka S, Watanabe A, Nagashima H: Cough syncope due to atrio-ventricular block. *Jpn Heart J* 23:1015–1020, 1982.

Schwartz SI, ed: *Principles of Surgery*. McGraw-Hill, New York, 1969.

Shapiro AP, Perez-Stable E, Scheib ET, Bron K, Moutsos SE, Berg G, Misage JR, Bahnson H, Fisher B, Drapanas T: Renal artery stenosis and hypertension. *Am J Med* 47:175–193, 1969.

Shapiro HM, Ng L, Mishkin M, Reivich M: Direct thermometry, ophthalmodynamometry, auscultation and palpation in extracranial cerebrovascular disease: An evaluation of rapid diagnostic methods. *Stroke* 1:205–218, 1970.

Silverstein A: Occlusive disease of the carotid arteries. *Circulation* 20:4–16, 1959.

Silverstein A, Doniger D, Bender MB: Manual compression of the carotid vessels, carotid sinus hypersensitivity, and carotid artery occlusions. *Ann Intern Med* 52:172–181, 1960.

Silverstein A, Lehrer GM, Mones R: Relation of certain diagnostic features of carotid occlusion to collateral circulation. *Neurology* 10:409–417, 1960.

Simon N, Franklin SS, Bleifer KH, Maxwell MH: Clinical characteristics of renovascular hypertension. *JAMA* 220:1209–1218, 1972.

Spencer-Green G: Raynaud's phenomenon. *Bull Rheum Dis* 33(5):3, 1983.

Spittell JA Jr: Some uncommon types of occlusive peripheral arterial disease. *Curr Probl Cardiol* 8:23–28, 1983.

Spodick DH, Sugiura T, Doi Y, Paladino D, Haffty B: Rate of rise of the carotid pulse: An investigation of observer error in a common clinical measurement. *Am J Cardiol* 49:159–162, 1982.

Stallworth S, Horne JB: Diagnosis and management of thoracic outlet syndrome. *Arch Surg* 119:1149–1151, 1984.

Sutton RL, Sutton RL Jr: *An Introduction to Dermatology*, ed 3. CV Mosby, St. Louis, 1937.

Webster JE, Gurdjian ES, Martin FA: Mechanism of syncope due to unilateral compression of carotid bifurcation. *Arch Neurol Psychiatry* 74:556–558, 1955.

Webster JE, Gurdjian E, Lindner DW, Hardy WG: Neurosurgical aspects of occlusive cerebral vascular disease. *Radiology* 70:825–830, 1958.

Weiner SL, Nathanson M: *Med Times*, 1976–1977. [See reference in Chapter 29.]

Weiss S, Baker JP: The carotid sinus reflex in health and disease: Its role in the causation of fainting and convulsions. *Medicine* 12:298–353, 1933. [Soma Weiss taught the author's teacher, Jack Myers. Since the author is now teaching you, you are Soma Weiss's medical great-grandchild. Probably, you could get back to any of the others in this bibliography, even to Hippocrates, through more circuitous genealogies, were records available. The point is that a great tradition is now presented to you in your turn.]

Welch LK, Crowley WJ Jr: Bruits of the head and neck. *Stroke* 1:245–247, 1970.

Wenger TL, Dohrmann ML, Strauss HC, Conley MJ, Wechsler AS, Wagner GS: Hypersensitive carotid sinus syndrome manifested as cough syncope. *PACE* 3:332–339, 1980.

Wheat MW Jr, Palmer RF: Dissecting aneurysms of the aorta. *Curr Probl Surg* 1–43, 1971.

Wheeler SD: Long-term hemodialysis and supraclavicular bruits: A method of examination. *JAMA* 247:1026, 1982.

Wolf PA, Kannel WB, Sorlie P, McNamara P: Asymptomatic carotid bruit and risk of stroke: The Framingham study. *JAMA* 245:1442–1445, 1981.

Wood P: *Diseases of the Heart and Circulation*, ed 2. JB Lippincott, Philadelphia, 1956.

Wright IS: The neurovascular syndrome produced by hyperabduction of the arms: Immediate changes produced in 150 normal controls and effects on some persons of prolonged hyperabduction of arms as in sleeping and in certain occupations. *Am Heart J* 29:1–19, 1945.

Ziegler DK, Zileli T, Dick A, Sebaugh JL: Correlation of bruits over the carotid with angiographically demonstrated lesions. *Neurology* 21:860–865, 1971.

Zweifler AJ: Significance of knee skin temperature in ischemic legs. *Arch Intern Med* 115:151–154, 1965.

19
Veins

"All the blood is under the jurisdiction of the heart. The twelve blood vessels are deeply hidden between the muscles and cannot be seen. Only those on the outer ankles are visible because there is nothing to cover them in these places. All other blood vessels that are on the surface of the body are veins. The harmful effects of wind and rain enter the system first through the skin, being then conveyed to the capillaries. When these are full, the blood goes to the veins and these in turn empty into the big vessels. The blood current flows continuously in a circle and never stops."

Chinese Classic of Internal Medicine, 2,000 years before William Harvey (Hume, 1930)

Venous Pressure

A Method: Inspecting the Neck Veins

1. Begin with the patient relaxing comfortably in bed with the head of the bed elevated between 30 and 45 degrees.

2. Look for the two different jugular* veins. The *internal* jugular vein may be seen posterior and superior to the medial fourth of the clavicle, running cephalad until it disappears under the sternocleidomastoid muscle. (Right above the clavicle, one is actually looking at the superior jugular bulb, which lies between the clavicular and sternal insertions of the sternocleidomastoid, where the latter muscle splits into the two heads.) The second vein is the *external* jugular, which crosses over the top of the sternocleidomastoid muscle. There are advantages to using each.

Perloff considers the internal jugular to be the better vein for pressure estimation and waveform (venous pulsation) analysis, but one cannot always see this vein well. Furthermore, with extremely high venous pressure, it may be difficult to move a sick patient to a position sufficiently erect to permit a clear view of the internal jugular vein collapse, which is how one determines the venous pressure (vide infra). The external jugular is less often inapparent than the internal jugular vein. Because the external jugular is seen for a longer distance, it is more often usable in a bed-bound patient in whom the pressure is extremely high, especially when the internal jugular vein is too short to permit stripping it to be sure there is reflux from below (vide infra). When both external and internal jugular veins are visible, the pulsations (see p. 363) should be more definitive in the internal jugular system.

I suggest that the neophyte try observing both veins. After you have examined 100 patients, you will know which method works for you.

3. If the jugular veins cannot be seen, lower the top half of the bed until they appear. Be sure to check that both the left and

---

*Same as cervical.

the right external jugular veins distend at approximately the same degree of elevation, during the same phase of respiration. If the left external jugular vein is selectively distended, this is a useful diagnostic clue to certain entities to be discussed below (see p. 363). Most use the right jugular veins to make measurements because they take a straighter path into the right atrium and yield less chance of interference with the waveform by ectatic arteries.

4. In some patients, the jugular veins are inapparent to the clinician even when actually full. To distinguish between inapparent veins and the absence of venous fullness ("distention") in a given patient, have the patient perform the Valsalva maneuver for about 10 seconds. This will temporarily increase venous pressure to an abnormal degree; if you still cannot see the jugular veins, then they are inapparent (see Fig. 19-1, Valsalva panel). You can make then no statement about venous pressure based on the neck veins in this patient, and will have to find another method of estimating it. See page 357.

5. If the veins appear to be spontaneously distended, you must next determine whether they represent the pressure from below or are simply prominent. To do this, strip the vein in the following manner:

    a. Place your adjacent forefingers over a distended segment of the external jugular vein. (The internal jugular vein or bulb does not usually have a visible segment sufficiently long to permit these manipulations.)

    b. Strip the vein of its blood by moving your fingers apart while maintaining firm pressure on the vein. The vein should now be flat as you maintain pressure on it with both fingers.

    c. To test for "filling from below" (from the heart back up into the veins), release only the finger closest to the heart. Maintain the other finger in its place.

    d. If the central venous pressure is high enough, the vein will fill in a retrograde fashion ("from below"). (See Fig. 19-1, stripping panel).

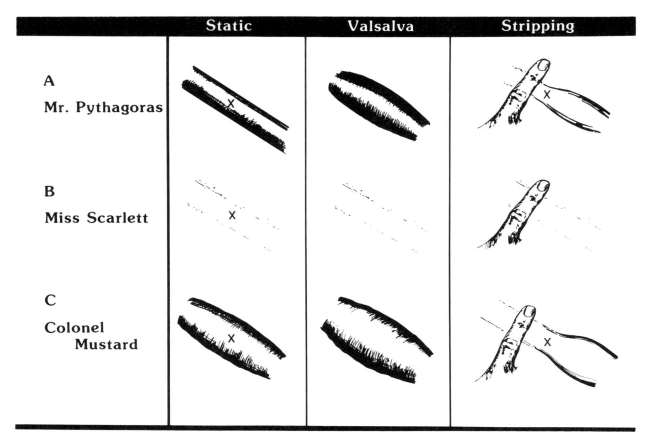

Figure 19-1. *A, At the top left is shown a segment of Mr. Pythagoras' external jugular vein as he is propped up at an angle in bed. Let "x" be a point on the vein that is 16 cm vertically above the center of the right atrium (see text, p. 357). If the jugular venous pulsations (the theoretical meniscus) are seen higher than this point, then Mr. Pythagoras would have an elevated venous pressure even if his veins did not appear to be "distended."* Valsalva panel: *This shows Mr. Pythagoras's right external jugular vein during the Valsalva maneuver. It is now distended. Based on this panel alone, one cannot determine whether or not Mr. Pythagoras has elevated venous pressure when he is not doing the Valsalva maneuver. The panel simply shows that his external jugular vein can be easily demonstrated.* Stripping panel: *If the pressure in the lower segment backfills the vein to a point "x" which is more than 16 cm vertically above the center of the right atrium, the venous pressure is increased. (Of course, the vein* above *the occluding finger will become distended [not shown], and if that finger is removed, the vein will be seen to fill from above, confirming that the blood in the veins flows from the head toward the heart, a fact that is already known. See chapter epigram.)*

B, Miss Scarlett is a refined princess who has done no physical work in her life and therefore has an underdeveloped venous system. Additionally, she has such a diminished cephalic blood flow that there is little need for venous return; thus, her external jugular vein is all but inapparent. "X" is a point about 16 cm vertically above the center of her right atrium, but by simple inspection of this point, it is not possible to determine whether her venous pressure is elevated or normal. Valsalva panel: *A sustained Valsalva maneuver can generate venous pressures greater than 30 cm of water, but even with this excess of intravenous pressure, no distention of Miss Scarlett's pristine jugular venous system is seen! Thus, in this particular patient, the absence of "jugular venous distention" means absolutely nothing! Specifically, it cannot be used as evidence against congestive heart failure or other causes of elevated systemic venous pressure.* Stripping panel: *The stripping maneuver shows no backfill because there is insufficient venous development. In fact, were the panel to illustrate release of the superior finger, it would look the same. Miss Scarlett's veins are simply inapparent no matter what the pressure.*

C, Colonel Mustard spent many years at physical labor in the colonies and has extremely well-developed jugular veins. But what is his true venous pressure? Valsalva panel: *The expected increase in the jugular distention which is already present helps not at all, and is shown only for completeness.* Stripping panel: *On stripping the vein and releasing the inferior finger, we can see backfill to the point of "x," where venous pulsations would also be seen. (The distention in the vein above the finger, which would eventually occur, is not shown and would not be searched for.) The flat segment of vein from the finger down to "x" is what guarantees that the correct venous pressure has been found. If "x" is less than 16 cm above the center of the right atrium, then the venous pressure is normal. Note that Colonel Mustard could have what is called "jugular venous distention" at rest (left-hand panel) even if his venous pressure were normal. Thus, the "finding" of "distention" means absolutely nothing.*

Of course, if the venous valves were perfectly competent, the vein would not fill in retrograde fashion, but the distention of any vein tends to impair coaption of the venous valves, so this is almost never a problem.

6. Take the venous pressure measurement.
   a. Look for the fluttering waves in inspiration or expiration. If you can see them, then you are looking at the top of the venous column, which is analogous to the meniscus in the venous pressure measurement manometer (vide infra). It is helpful to exaggerate the vein by shining a penlight on it obliquely, so as to cast a shadow posteriorly on the neck. (This is especially useful for detecting pulsations.)
   ❍ b. In order to find the top of the column, it may be necessary to have the head of the bed elevated and depressed several times, repeating the stripping motion each time.
   c. The venous pressure is estimated to be the *vertical distance* between the top of the blood column (the "fluttering") and the right atrium. (The angle of the patient and the distance along the vein do not matter.) With the patient supine, the right atrium (the zero reference point, i.e., the point at which the venous pressure is zero) is located in the fourth intercostal space about 35% to 50% of the distance from the sternum to the bed, along the anterior-posterior diameter. (To verify this, look at a CT scan, if you have not had the opportunity to look at about 25 cadavers, as we did years ago.) The upper limit of normal, by this method, is 16 cm. (For normal values obtained by using other zero reference points, see p. 360.)

Note. This is now a minority report, which differs from the current vulgar methods such as those using the angle of Louis as a zero reference point. The angle of Louis (the sternal angle) is supposed to be 5 cm above the center of the right atrium in all people and in all positions. I call this the Cardiologist's Constant.* This is obviously not the case (see Figs. 19-2 and 19-3), despite the fact that in many prestigious textbooks the Cardiologist's Constant seems to be as durable as Planck's Constant. Why argue over a few centimeters? The reason is that sloppy thinking and imprecise language are contagious.

Validity

It is stated that the examination of the jugular veins is the most reliable means of clinical estimation of (peripheral) venous pressure "and actually often exceeds in accuracy the measurement of venous pressure with the saline manometer [see p. 360] in inexpert hands" (Fowler, 1967). This statement is an interesting epistemologic pretzel knot: assuming it is true, how would one know it (i.e., what would be the independent covariable to the other two)? The key word in Fowler's statement may be "inexpert," which is undefined.

However, two other interested observers concluded that the *central* venous pressure *cannot* be reliably estimated by inspection of the jugular veins, based on a study involving independent and simultaneous measurement of the central venous pressure (Davison & Cannon, 1974). (Of course, the peripheral and central venous pressures cannot be exactly the same. Otherwise, the

blood would not flow.) Yet, 90% coincidence could be achieved in that study if one were willing to accept an error of up to 4 cm. Clinically, if one estimates a pressure of 24 cm of water, it does not matter very much whether it is truly 20 or 28. Similarly, if one estimates a pressure of 8 or 10 cm of water, one can be confident that the true value is not above 16 (the upper limit of normal). Thus, although not perfect, such an estimation becomes one more brick in the Great Wall of diagnosis.

Other Nonmanometric Methods

1. Wiener and Nathanson (1976–77) estimate the external jugular venous pressure with the patient supine. The vein is stripped and the meniscus observed after a *moderate inspiration*. They state that the meniscus in normal people is usually 3.5 cm *below* the angle of Louis. (Using the Cardiologist's Constant, this would give a "normal" pressure of 1.5 cm!) In a patient with very high venous pressure, it would not be possible to see the meniscus during inspiration. Thus, with this method, one could tell that the venous pressure was high, but would not know how high. Therefore, . . . do it right. (Elevate the head of the bed in such patients.)

2. In contemporary intensive care units, it is often difficult for the attending physician to get an unimpeded view of a jugular vein whose vascular connection to the right atrium has not been impeded by medical interventions. Accordingly, it is helpful to
❍ use a modification of the *Gärtner maneuver* (Dennison, 1969). This consists of raising and lowering the hand while stripping its veins until one finds a point of elevation at which they are no longer distended. One then slightly lowers the hand until the veins begin to distend, and the vertical distance from this point down to the right atrium is the estimated venous pressure.

A Self-Study

While seated or standing, place one hand as far above your head as possible and make a fist; leave your other hand hanging open at your side. After about 15 seconds, place both your hands in front of you and inspect them for color and vein distention. The hand that was elevated is paler, and the veins are not distended; the dependent hand is darker and the veins distended.

Repeat, reversing the hands.

Have your partner perform this while your eyes are closed. After both his hands are brought level, open your eyes and see if you can determine which one had been elevated.

Historical note. This is the basis of an old carnival confidence game. The con man is blindfolded or has his back turned, while the "mark" (victim) holds a gambled coin in the clenched hand. The con man keeps guessing wrong at two-to-one odds and pays off until the "mark" gets greedy and raises the stakes.

3. Another method is *von Recklinghausen's maneuver*, in which a supine patient has one hand resting on the bed and one resting upon the thigh. If the veins are swollen in *both* hands, elevated venous pressure is diagnosed, but if only the veins in the lower hand are swollen, the venous pressure is said to be normal.

Gärtner's method gives a continuously distributed measurement. But for those who like two-humped camels [see Ch. 16, p. 277], von Recklinghausen's method may be preferable.

4. If the *sublingual* veins are distended with the patient in the sitting position, one can be certain that the venous pressure in this segment of the venous tree is elevated. The most common

---

*It has also been given as 2.5, 8, and 10 cm!

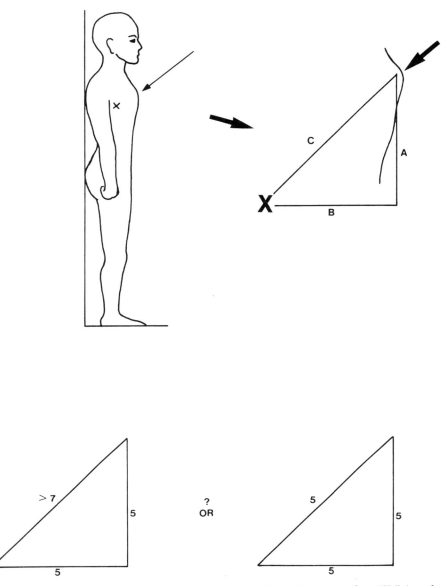

Figure 19-2. *Pythagoras's angle of Louis is marked with an arrow and the center of his right atrium with an "X." An enlarged version of the area of interest is shown at the top right. If it is true that the angle of Louis is always 5 cm above the center of the right atrium, then side A of the triangle would be 5 cm with Pythagoras erect. By the same statement, side B of the triangle would be 5 cm with Pythagoras recumbent (turn the book on its side to see this), and side C would be 5 cm with Pythagoras at a 45-degree angle. This leads to the triangle shown at the bottom right, contradicting the Theorem of Pythagoras ($A^2 + B^2 = C^2$), which would give the triangle at bottom left.*

cause of such an elevation is congestive heart failure. However, there is no reason that this sign could not be positive in superior vena caval syndrome, constrictive pericarditis, or pericardial tamponade. Dr. John DeGroote of Mississippi first persuaded me of the utility of this sign.

Manometric Determination of Peripheral Venous Pressure

History

In the 1950s, elevated venous pressure was sought by manometry in patients suspected of having congestive heart failure (see "A Method", p. 360). The requisite venipuncture also provided the opportunity to perform a circulation time, which could sepa-

rate high-output from low-output congestive failure (see p. 369), a distinction still useful although currently arrived at by other, more expensive, means.

In the 1960s, the peripheral venous pressure determination was abandoned since the central venous line was coming into widespread use. Cases of high-output cardiac failure were increasingly diagnosed at cardiac catheterization.

In the 1970s, the flow-directed balloon-tip (Swan-Ganz) catheter gave us the opportunity to determine left ventricular filling pressure. Despite the fact that this catheter had to be passed through all previously accessible venous compartments, potentially permitting measurement of central and peripheral venous pressures, such measures disappeared from medical center charts. Unfortunately for clinical examination, the left atrial fill-

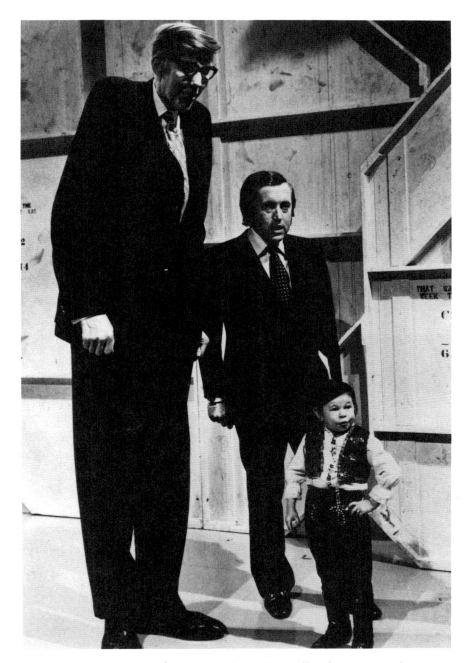

Figure 19-3. *Dan Koehler (98 inches tall), Mishu (32⁵/₈ inches), and David Frost (65 inches) represent the extremes and approximate mean of a Gaussian distribution. Would you expect the Cardiologist's Constant to be the same in all? Photograph from the* Guinness Book of World Records, *published by Sterling Publishing Co, Inc., New York, copyright 1987 by Guinness Superlatives Ltd. Reprinted with permission.*

ing pressure does not always correlate with the peripheral venous pressure as determined clinically. Although the external jugular venous pressure does correlate with the central venous pressure, this statistically significant correlation is felt by some to be clinically treacherous (Davison & Cannon, 1974). Thus, as our technology has become more sophisticated and much more expensive, it has become almost impossible for the medical student or house officer to determine the accuracy of his own clinical examination, which has usually deteriorated to the worse-than-useless statement that "the neck veins were (or were not) distended" (see legend to Fig. 19-1).

The final death knell for the direct determination of the pe-

ripheral venous pressure came in the 1970s when third-party payers, such as Blue Cross and Blue Shield, refused to pay the $10 or $15 fee for the peripheral venous pressure (with or without a circulation time). (Yet these same carriers pay for the much more expensive determination of ejection fraction by radionuclide cardiography, which appears to be used in clinical practice in exactly the same way as the venous pressure and the circulation time.)

Nevertheless, "hallowed techniques of physical diagnosis tend to rise Phoenix-like from their own ashes" (Snapper & Kahn, 1967). The expense of the radionuclide determinations may eventually be noticed by the bureaucrats who increasingly dictate the specifics of current medical care. The morbidity and mortality resulting from epidemic use of the flow-directed balloon-tip (Swan-Ganz) catheter may prove to outweigh its marginal benefits (Robin, 1985). And a much cheaper and noninvasive set of measurements obtainable at the bedside from the M-mode echocardiogram (Askenazi et al., 1981) may supplant the Swan-Ganz for measuring left atrial pressure. (This new technique uses the echocardiographic equivalent of the S2-opening snap interval once used by bedside clinicians to determine the severity of mitral stenosis. See Ch. 17, p. 320.)

A Method

1. Place the supine patient's right arm on a pillow or towels so that the antecubital vein will be at the zero reference point.

As noted above, the zero reference point used in this text is a point one third to one half the distance from the sternum down to the bed. Many other zero reference points have previously been offered; these are given in Table 19-1.

Which one should be selected? As elsewhere in medicine, one prefers those that take account of the variability in body size and that permit an easy determination. That said, probably any one is satisfactory if you use it consistently and become familiar with its inherent reliability.

2. Insert a needle attached to a three-way stopcock and a manometer (the same apparatus as is used for the Quincke puncture of the lumbar interspace for obtaining cerebrospinal fluid samples and pressures).

3. Via the third port of the stopcock, fill the manometer with sterile saline. Allow the saline to flow into the vein until the

Table 19-1. Zero Reference Points Previously Used for Venous Pressure Measurements

Authority	Normal Venous Pressure	Zero Reference Point
Moritz & Tabora, 1910	1–9 cm	Right atrium as remembered from anatomy class
Taylor et al., 1930	4–8 cm	5 cm below the horizontal plane of the anterior surface of the sternum at its 4th costochondral junction
Friedberg, 1956	3–10 cm	The point of Taylor et al. modified "depending on the approximate thickness of the chest wall"
Lyons et al., 1938	??	10 cm above the level of the skin on the subject's back when the subject is recumbent
Hussey, 1939	4–12 cm	The midaxillary line
Winsor & Burch, 1946	5–14 cm	Half the distance from the base of xiphoid to the table (if the patient is tilted up at an angle, the point is half the distance to the patient's back, along the 4th intercostal space

Source: *Friedberg (1956).*

pressure equilibrates. Alternately, use sterile 5% sodium citrate, an anticoagulant.

4. Read the equilibration point when the patient is not coughing, sneezing, or performing a Valsalva maneuver. Note that the pressure normally *drops* with inspiration. If it increases paradoxically, the patient has a positive Kussmaul's sign of constrictive pericarditis (vide infra).

5. You may wish to perform the test for hepatojugular reflux at this point (see p. 361). The advantage of doing this now is that the pressure is directly measured in the manometer, so if the hepatic compression causes an elevation of 3 cm in the venous pressure, it is easy to see irrespective of the patient's venous anatomy and position in bed (two factors that may complicate the inspection of the jugular veins).

6. Continue with the circulation time (see Appendix 19-1).

Significance

Use the normal values corresponding to the zero reference point that you chose.

In general, the pressure in congestive heart failure is greater than 16 cm, occasionally as high as 30 cm. The pressure may also be elevated with pericardial tamponade, tricuspid stenosis, superior vena caval syndrome, constrictive pericarditis, and restrictive cardiac disease.

False positives. The pressure may be elevated acutely if the patient is straining, or in obstructive lung disease if an elevated intrapleural pressure is maintained through most of the respiratory cycle.

False negatives. In *pure* acute left-sided ("backwards") heart failure (prior to renal retention of sodium), the pressure may be normal.

Kussmaul's Sign

Et spiritum tumore cohibente venarum.
[And his inspirations engorged his veins.] (Ammianus Marcellinus, XXV 3, 23)
(Death scene of Julian, who had been stabbed in the ribs by a Persian spear.)

Self-Test *(to be answered in Appendix 19-2): Could this be the first description of Kussmaul's sign in pericardial tamponade? (Be careful, this is a curve ball.)*

Kussmaul's sign is the inspiratory distention of the neck veins. It is probably one of the easiest of all physical signs to master, especially since it is the exact opposite of the normal expiratory distention of the cervical veins.

A Self-Study

Simply look at your recumbent partner's neck veins and notice how the pressure drops during a strong inspiration. The pulsations are no longer seen. In some persons even the vein's location may become inapparent.

Semiophysiology

Inspiration generates a negative intrapleural pressure, which sucks the venous blood into the heart. But with constrictive pericarditis and some other diseases, there is sufficient impairment of right heart filling that the blood sucked into the chest cannot enter the heart, and the venous pressure rises. In such patients, inspiration will cause a "paradoxical" rise in the venous pressure. At the bedside, this can be detected by inspection: the flutterings or vein filling are seen in inspiration, but disappear in expiration (the veins go flat), the exact opposite of what you saw in your partner.

Significance

Kussmaul's sign is seen in constrictive pericarditis, some cases of endomyocardial restrictive disease (such as endocardial fibroelastosis), myocardial restrictive disease (such as amyloidosis), tricuspid stenosis, congestive failure (especially that called right-sided), superior vena caval syndrome (see p. 366), and right ventricular infarction. But, contrary to what was formerly taught, it is never seen in uncomplicated pericardial tamponade. (See Table 19-2.) In fact, its appearance in the latter setting suggests the development of a constrictive or restrictive pericardial component and/or epimyocardial fibrosis.

Hepatojugular Reflux

History

William Pasteur first described what we now call hepatojugular reflux in 1885:

In several cases in which there was reason to suspect functional incompetence of the tricuspid valve which have recently come under my observation, a physical sign has been present to which I believe attention has not been drawn, and of which I have been unable to find any mention either in the standard textbooks or in the best known monographs on the subject of cardiac disease. This sign consists in a distension—with or without pulsation—of the superficial veins of the neck, occurring when firm pressure is exerted over the liver in the direction of the spinal column, and independent of the movements of respiration. A little consideration of the anatomical relations of the parts concerned will suggest the facility with which an impediment may be created to the flow of blood, in either direction, through the vena cava inferior by such a manoeuvre, especially when the liver is obviously enlarged. It seems to me that the state thus produced is virtually that which obtains as a chronic condition in long-standing and severe cases of tricuspid incompetence as far as regards the tension in the systemic venous system in the immediate vicinity of the heart. Assuming the existence of tricuspid regurgitation and of a source of compression of the vena cava inferior, it is obvious that with each systole an excessive reflux of blood must take place into the vena cava superior and its tributary veins. It may be noted that the question of pulsation, as compared with distension or undulation, is merely one of degree of morbid venous tension. Although the number

of cases in which I have observed this phenomenon is certainly limited, I have never failed to elicit it when there was indubitable evidence of tricuspid incompetence; on the other hand, I have hitherto invariably failed to obtain it in other forms of cardiac valvular disease, and in various cases of hepatic enlargement from causes other than passive congestion. I cannot but think that this sign may furnish an important aid to diagnosis in cases where the usual signs of tricuspid regurgitation are ill-developed or in abeyance, and that it may prove a valuable factor in the difficult general problem of prognosis in cases of cardiac disease.

My chief object in making this short communication is to draw attention to a point which I believe to be of some importance, with a view to stimulate observation, and it may be to elicit further facts. (Pasteur, 1885)

I cite this article for several reasons:

1. This is the entire article, requiring two paragraphs and occupying less than one quarter of one page.
2. Pasteur was unable to obtain this sign in other forms of cardiac valvular disease, so he believed it to be diagnostic of tricuspid insufficiency. (Could it be possible that none of his other patients had heart failure? We should realize that even one of our best colleagues was capable of such a miss, illustrating the truth of Jean de la Bruyere's statement: "The exact contrary of what is generally believed is often the truth.")

The foundation for the modern concept of the hepatojugular reflux was built by Rondot in three papers in 1898. Rondot's clinical acuity may be judged from the fact that he sometimes noticed a muffling of the first heart sound to occur during the performance of the hepatojugular reflux. Today, we would say that this maneuver causes an abnormal elevation in the right atrial pressure, decreasing the early systolic pressure gradient between the right ventricle and right atrium, and so decreasing dP/dT, thus making the sound of tricuspid closure softer than usual. In his day, Rondot could say only empirically that this change pointed toward disease of the tricuspid valve.

Rondot was the first to point out that the hepatojugular reflux was not pathognomonic for tricuspid insufficiency, but was found in a wide variety of conditions involving the heart. Since many of his remarks on the differential diagnosis are not available in the English literature, a translation of his conclusions follows:

1. The hepatojugular reflux is usually seen in states of low output cardiac failure (*etats asystolique*) of cardiac or aortic origin, with or without tricuspid insufficiency, when decompensation occurs. It should not be considered pathognomonic of tricuspid valve dysfunction since there is very little correlation with the signs of this latter lesion, particularly by its xiphoid murmur.

Its disappearance usually coincides with the disappearance of the symptoms of cardiac failure, but it can occasionally disappear in the terminal period of cardiac insufficiency or when the

Table 19-2. Findings in Some Diseases of the Right Heart and Pericardium

	RV Infarction (Cintron et al., 1981)	Pure Constrictive Pericarditis[a] (Shabetai et al., 1970; Spodick, 1983)	Pure Tamponade (Large, Acute Effusion) (Reddy et al., 1982)
Kussmaul's sign	30%–100% (Cintron et al., 1981; Dell 'Italia, 1983)	33% (late, severe)	NO
Pulsus paradoxus (see Ch. 6, p.91) (Reddy et al., 1982; Shabetai et al., 1970; Spodick, 1983)	71% (Lorell et al., 1979)	NO	>70%–100%
Y descent prominent	71%[b]	33%	NO

[a]Also see Broadbent's sign (p. 246).
[b]Or is it an X descent? (Goldstein, 1989).

latter is complicated by an abundant pericardial effusion. Its absence is usually the rule in valvular heart disease or diseases of the aorta or of the pulmonary artery while they are well compensated.

2. In cardiac dilatations, the hepatojugular reflux is only seen with the weakening of myocardial function:

   (a.) In acute illnesses of the bronchi and of the lungs and even more particularly in bronchopneumonia, pneumonia, and "splenopneumonia" [right heart failure with secondary tricuspid insufficiency];

   (b.) In acute illnesses of the digestive tract and of the liver where, however, one does not see it with the same frequency [inferior vena caval obstruction from ascites?];

   (c.) In nephritis, where its appearance . . . is rare even during the acute phases of Bright's disease specifically, and in the latter is more an indicator of periods of cardiac decompensation that are complications of the "renal heart" [hypertensive cardiomyopathy?]

3. During pericardial effusions, one does not find any reflux if the liquid is abundant enough to compress the right auricle, but the reflux is usually seen as soon as this compression ceases. Then the reflux disappears again when the auricular myocardium finally regains its normal function.

Thus, one explains the disappearance of the reflux during cardiac failure when pericardial effusion supervenes.

If the state of cardiac failure appears quite evident but is in contrast with heart sounds that are over a large surface; and if the outline of the percussion dullness exceeds inferiorly and laterally beyond the area of the apical impulse and thus reveals a concomitant effusion; the absence of the hepatojugular reflux should put one on guard for the possibility of a vast retrocardiac collection (i.e., pericardial effusion), either free or walled off.

The general conclusion to draw from these facts is that the hepatojugular reflux may be considered as a sign of weakening of the right auricular myocardium. Thus it corroborates signs that are diagnostic of right-sided cardiac insufficiency of either cardiovascular, reflex, or toxic-infectious origin; and the reflux is also able to demonstrate such cardiac failure when the latter's other manifestations are barely noticeable or even remain in a latent state. It thus permits one to institute a medical treatment aimed in a special manner at ameliorating the functions of the myocardium. (Rondot, 1898)

A Method (modified from Ducas et al., 1983)

1. Position the patient with his trunk initially around 45 degrees from the horizontal, and observe the jugular pulsations during quiet breathing. Alter the position as needed to identify the highest angle of elevation at which those pulsations can be seen. This is the baseline venous pressure. (You will be searching for a 3-cm rise in venous pressure. Accordingly, if the jugular vein is too short to demonstrate such a rise, you may have to crank up the head of the bed so that the vein rises 3 cm on the vertical.)

2. Apply your hand to the right upper quadrant or the middle of the abdomen. It is not necessary to press over the liver to produce the phenomenon. (In fact, if there is tenderness, you should not press in that area because you do not wish the patient to guard, perform a Valsalva maneuver, or interrupt his normal breathing pattern in any way.)

3. Press down, maintaining a pressure of 35 mm Hg. (You can practice over a semi-inflated blood pressure cuff or place the blood pressure cuff over the abdomen to be sure that sufficient pressure is applied.)

4. Instruct the patient to continue to breathe normally through his mouth. Do not attempt to measure the venous pres-

sure for at least 10 seconds, so that both respiratory artifacts and tensing of the abdominal muscles may subside. (Each alters jugular venous pressure.) The best time to take another venous pressure measurement is at 1 minute of pressure. This should be used as the gold standard in ambiguous cases for reasons given under "advanced."

5. A venous pressure *rise* of more than 3 cm is abnormal and hepatojugular reflux is said to be present (Ducas et al., 1983).

For the attending. You will note that performing abdominal compression for a whole minute in a normal subject who does not guard or perform the Valsalva maneuver will usually cause the venous pressure to decrease. The abdominal compression acts as a tourniquet, interfering with venous return to the right heart. It is true that in normals there may sometimes be an initial rise in pressure from the hydraulic effect, but the cumulative effect at 1 minute is a drop in pressure to normal (Hitzig, 1945; Hultgren, 1950).

Semiophysiology

One of the best theories advanced is that the mechanism of the hepatojugular reflux, at least in congestive heart failure, is systemic venous hypertension (Burch & Ray, 1954). This makes the venous system an inelastic, tight, noncompliant hydraulic system. In any such hydraulic system a unit of pressure exerted upon the smaller vessels (e.g., splanchnic veins) is transmitted to the larger vessels (e.g., cervical veins), just as you activate your four automobile brakes by foot pressure on one cylinder.

Significance

A positive hepatojugular reflux is seen in heart failure, including backward right heart failure, as well as early or incipient failure. It is also seen in constrictive pericarditis, pericardial tamponade, tricuspid insufficiency, inferior vena caval obstruction (Ducas et al., 1983; Fowler, 1967), and in the conditions noted by Rondot (see p. 361).

There is no hepatojugular reflux in pure left-sided backward heart failure (Hitzig, 1945; Hultgren, 1950).

One prospective study showed hepatojugular reflux to have a 66% sensitivity and a 100% specificity for distinguishing tricuspid from mitral insufficiency (Maisel et al., 1984). So Pasteur's original idea was good albeit restricted.

For the cardiology resident. This sign has long been used to distinguish the hepatomegaly of right heart failure (positive test) from other forms of hepatomegaly (negative test). However, inferior vena caval syndrome (see p. 366), which can produce hepatomegaly and mimic right heart failure in other ways, may be an especially treacherous positive test (i.e., it can lead the unwary to diagnose primary heart failure and to overlook the real problem).

Validity

Some authors have concluded that this test is not useful (Ducas et al., 1983). Curiously enough, even Fowler suggests that "the observation may be confirmed by measuring the pressure in an arm vein with a saline manometer" (Fowler, 1967), although in another context he called the latter method less reliable than inspection of the jugular veins (see p. 355). I find the test very useful when I know that it has been performed correctly by the method described above.

Correlative Signs of Congestive Heart Failure

Venous hypertension and hepatojugular reflux formerly correlated with the presence of an S3 gallop and edema, but nowadays loop diuretics and vasodilators are given so quickly and frequently that by the time the patient is "stabilized," only the peripheral edema may still be present.

Selective Distention of the Left External Jugular Vein

Selective distention of the left external jugular vein has been reported as a sign of persistent left superior vena cava, which is present in 3% to 4% of patients with congenital heart disease (Colman, 1967; Horwitz et al., 1973). However, increased left jugular vein distention may also be seen in selective compression of the left jugular venous system by aortic dissection or atherosclerotic aortic tortuosity, usually the latter, which additionally may involve the left internal jugular vein, due to left innominate vein compression (Sleight, 1962).

Jugular Venous Pulsations

Normal Venous Pulsations

If there is sufficient undamped distention of the jugular veins, then the venous pulse waves can be analyzed.

○ Undulations called the A, C, and V waves have been described (see Fig. 19-4), but often are not distinctly seen. It is much easier to look for the X and Y descents, two inflickerings of the venous column (each similar to the brief inflickering of the retinal venous diameters at the optic disc in that phenomenon misnamed retinal venous "pulsation" [see Ch. 10, p. 178]).

The A wave (Fig. 19-4) is due to *a*trial contraction.

It is possible to diagnose atrial fibrillation based on disappearance of the A waves. In 2:1 AV block, there will be two A waves in the jugular pulse wave contour for every heartbeat. But in atrial flutter with a 3:1 block, it is almost impossible to pick up three A waves per heartbeat.

The C wave (for *c*usp) is due to the bulging of the tricuspid cusps into the right atrium at the beginning of systole, according to Potain. The interval between the A and C waves is, in essence, the PR interval.

In Mobitz type I second-degree heart block, the experienced and astute observer will note a gradual prolongation of the interval between the A wave and the C wave in the jugular venous pulse. In fact, this is the way in which Wenckebach discovered his phenomenon, before the invention of the string galvanometer electrocardiograph machine. (He published jugular venous pulsation recordings.) In Mobitz type II second-degree heart block, the interval will not increase, but at the time of the dropped beat there will be an A wave that is *not* followed by the customary C wave.

The X descent is due to the relaxation of the atrium. The V wave is due to the *v*olume of blood entering the atrium during ventricular systole (atrial diastole), when the tricuspid valve is closed. The Y descent results from the blood flowing rapidly into the ventricle when the tricuspid valve opens.

Other wave forms are seen in special venous beds with special equipment, but not clinically.

A Method

1. Adjust the angle of the bed so that the venous oscillations can be easily seen in the shadow cast by the penlight.

2. With your hand on the PMI, or on the left carotid (as you are watching the right side of the neck), or with your stethoscope

auscultating the patient's heart, time the cardiac cycle. There should be two inflickerings during each cardiac cycle. The brief collapse seen *during* ventricular systole is the X descent. (As you hear S1, simultaneously say "down." The inflickering that occurs during that vocalization is the X descent.) The other collapse, seen during diastole, is the Y descent.

3. Our interest in the X descent is in ascertaining that it is present. (If it is not, that means that ventricular pressure is being transmitted into the right atrium during ventricular systole because of tricuspid insufficiency (vide infra).

4. Now turn your attention to the Y descent. (The Y descent will be blunted in conditions of impaired ventricular filling such as tricuspid stenosis.)

Teaching Tricks

○ Xerox or trace the normal jugular venous pulse shown in the upper left-hand corner of Fig. 19-4, and mark the area that represents systole. Carry this tracing on a card in your wallet, and place it on the pillow next to the patient while examining the jugular pulsations.

Beginners should remember the following caveats:

1. Do not try to learn jugular venous pulsation on any patient who has a pulse rate over 100 per minute.
2. Do not try to learn jugular venous pulsations on a patient with a highly chaotic rhythm, such as atrial fibrillation.
3. Note that the jugular venous pulsations are optimally seen only during one phase of respiration in many persons who are breathing deeply. A corollary is that in patients who are breathing deeply and quickly, it may be very hard to learn jugular venous pulsations.
4. The carotid impulse may produce movements that mimic venous pulsations, especially when the carotid pulse is dicrotic. Such false pulsations will continue after you occlude (with a finger) the jugular vein as low in the neck (proximal) as possible. Of course, true jugular venous pulsations will be obliterated by this maneuver and will only return on releasing the occlusion. (Also see "CV Merger.")

Abnormal Pulsations

CV Merger

In patients with tricuspid insufficiency (see Ch. 17, p. 322), the regurgitation of blood into the right atrium during systole eliminates the X descent (Fig. 19-4, lower left). The resulting bulge is sometimes called the "CV merger." You can quickly learn to identify this pulse wave contour because there is only one remaining collapse, the Y descent, which is present in diastole, not systole. This sign is not extremely sensitive; only 40% of patients with tricuspid insufficiency will manifest the CV merger (Cha and Gooch, 1983).

Because the X descent occurs during systole, there is an important *false positive*. A hyperdynamic circulation can cause the appearance of giant C waves, obliterating the X descent, in the absence of tricuspid insufficiency. This *apparent* CV merger is due simply to the hyperdynamic stroke of the carotid arteries transmitted through the cervical tissues, making the veins appear to bulge out during systole.

To distinguish this artifact from a true positive, try the following: 1) If you are inspecting the external jugular, try teaching trick #4. Simply compress the external jugular vein between the

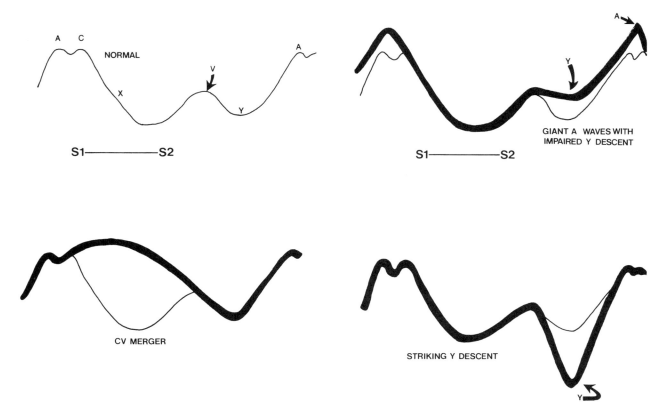

Figure 19-4.   *Jugular venous pulsations. Idealized normal (top left), and abnormal tracings superimposed on the normal. See text.*

site of inspection (the apparent CV merger pulsations) and the heart. If the giant C waves continue, they are presumably due to transmitted carotid pulsations. 2) Can you obliterate the giant C waves by compressing the ipsilateral carotid artery? If so, they are false positives, not true venous waves. 3) Is the venous pressure elevated? Dr. Mike Fisher of Maryland believes that CV merger should not be accepted in the absence of an increased venous pressure. 4) Do the pulsations change with the patient's position? Venous pulsations are present to absent, depending on position, whereas arterial pulsations are minimally changed. 5) Are the pulsations subject to respiratory variation? Venous pulsations are; arterial pulsations are not. 6) Does abdominal compression change the height or motion of the pulses? If so, they are venous (Ewy, 1987).

Laennec was not the first person to observe CV merger. But while others confused it with the carotid pulse from a hyperdynamic left ventricle, Laennec knew how to distinguish the two conditions, and stated that he had never seen CV merger without right ventricular "hypertrophy" (failure).

CV merger has also been reported in atrial fibrillation (Marriott, 1989).

Giant A Waves with Blunted Y Descent, and a Note on Cannon A Waves

Tricuspid stenosis results in a *blunted Y descent* and giant A waves (Fig. 19-4, upper right). The giant A wave is due to the atrium contracting against a stenotic tricuspid valve, pushing blood back up into the cervical veins. Similarly, the blunted Y descent in early diastole is due to impairment of blood flow into the right ventricle. The same type of pulse tracing may be seen with increased right ventricular end-diastolic pressure as in pul-

monic stenosis (infundibular or valvular), pulmonary vascular obstruction (primary pulmonary hypertension or pulmonary embolism), chronic pulmonary disease, large right atrial clots or tumors, and cardiomyopathies (congestive, hypertrophic, and restrictive) (Ewy, 1987).

This type of pulse wave tracing may appear to have only one venous collapse (the X descent), which occurs in systole.

I became convinced of the importance of the Y descent when I saw Dr. Frank Kroetz of Tennessee diagnose stenosis of the tricuspid valve on the basis of a blunted Y descent alone, in a patient who also had mitral stenosis, at a time when the textbooks said this was an impossible pair of diagnoses to make. Dr. Kroetz stated that his diagnosis was confirmed by the presence of two opening snaps. Cardiac catheterization proved him correct.

Giant A waves should not be confused with *cannon A waves*. Giant A waves occur on *every beat* (if the patient is in sinus rhythm), but cannon A waves, a specific sign of atrioventricular dissociation, occur *irregularly, on a minority of beats*. A cannon A wave is produced during AV dissociation if the atria happen to contract at a time when the (dissociated) ventricular contraction has just shut the tricuspid valve. The atrial systolic stroke volume, being denied egress to the right ventricle, has nowhere to go but back into the venous system, producing the cannon A wave. But since it is a rare coincidence for the dissociated atrial and ventricular contractions to occur in the requisite sequence, the cannon A waves occur irregularly (randomly) and on a minority of beats. In a sense they result from the same mechanism as the giant A waves; both are due to impaired right ventricular acceptance of the atrial systolic stroke volume, one relatively fixed and one intermittent.

Very advanced. Cannon A waves can also occur during premature ventricular contractions with retrograde conduction. Or, if a long PR interval is interrupted by a premature atrial contraction (PAC), so that the tricuspid valve leaflets have floated back almost to the closed position before the atrial contraction occurs, a single cannon A wave may result.

Some junctional (nodal) ectopic rhythms can produce cannon A waves. This is the only situation in which the cannon A wave can be seen on every beat, or at least every beat that involves retrograde conduction of the ectopic impulse to the atria.

Rapid Y Descent

A rapid Y descent (Fig. 19-4, lower right) occurs in about one third of patients with constrictive pericarditis. If the patient is not properly positioned, the jugular pulse may appear to have but one inflickering per cardiac cycle, occurring in diastole, not systole. That appearance could lead you to believe that you are really dealing with the CV merger of tricuspid insufficiency. To bring out the normal X descent of constrictive pericarditis, raise the head of the bed a little, and the X descent will appear. If the patient really has CV merger from severe tricuspid insufficiency, the X descent cannot be demonstrated, no matter how far you raise the bed. The prominent Y descent of the jugular veins was formerly known as Friederich's sign (Friedrich, 1864, 1865).

The rapid Y descent is a good sign of constrictive pericarditis and restrictive right ventricular disease. It may also be seen in right ventricular infarction (Table 19-2). Its absence is of no use. But, its presence *excludes* the diagnosis of pericardial tamponade.

A logical flow chart for venous pulsations is given in Figure 19-5.

Atrial Septal Defect Pattern

A characteristic jugular venous pulse has been noted in 41% of patients with atrial septal defect (Tavel et al., 1968). It is characterized by high-peaked V waves, which often exceed the A waves in height. This pattern indicates the presence of a large left-to-right shunt, and is lost when pulmonary hypertension supervenes. It is rarely seen in persons without atrial septal defects.

An Historical and Epistemologic Perspective: A Case of Vasovagal Syncope

To illustrate the current desuetude of clinical examination, note that in the classic report on vagovagal reflex causing complete heart block (Weiss & Ferris, 1934), the diagnosis was made during a spontaneous attack, when the patient was not connected to an electrocardiograph. The authors observed that "the venous pulsations over the neck were more rapid than the apical rate." They were sufficiently confident of this observation that they subsequently passed a small rubber balloon into the patient's esophageal diverticulum and inflated it to induce complete heart block. By this means, they reproduced the patient's symptoms, which had usually been precipitated by swallowing food, especially sticky food such as peanut butter and crackers.

Auscultation

Venous Hums

A more or less continuous murmur emanating from the cervical (jugular) veins is called a cervical venous hum. Its only significance is that it may be confused with pathologic murmurs, especially when the hum is louder either in systole or diastole.

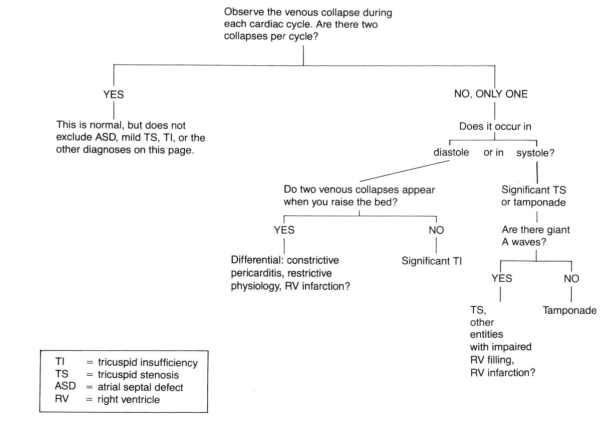

Figure 19-5. *Logical flow chart for venous pulsations. TI, tricuspid insufficiency; TS, tricuspid stenosis; ASD, atrial septal defect; RV, right ventricle.*

One can stumble upon the cervical venous hum in 2.3% to 27% of adult outpatients (Braun et al., 1966; Jones, 1962) and in 31% to 66% of normal children (Graf et al., 1947), regardless of any underlying disease, especially if the patient is examined in the sitting or erect position during quiet breathing. The hum can be heard anywhere in the lower neck and is abolished during: 1) the Valsalva maneuver, 2) recumbency, or 3) compression of the ipsilateral internal jugular vein distal to the point at which the venous hum is heard. The last can be achieved by pressing just lateral to the thyroid cartilage (Jones, 1962).

Venous hums are also discussed in Chapters 17 (p. 304) and 20 (p. 378).

Patients on renal dialysis have a very high incidence of cervical venous hums: 56% to 88% prevalence during hemodialysis and 34% between dialysis treatments (Wheeler, 1982). Although attributed to the increased blood flow due to their access fistulae, compression of the artery leading to the fistula does not decrease the hum (as opposed to the flow murmur discussed in Ch. 18, p. 344).

Other Findings

A mid-systolic jugular or clavicular venous pistol shot may be heard in tricuspid insufficiency. If the patient has varicose veins in the leg, it may be possible to hear the murmur of tricuspid insufficiency disease there (see Ch. 17, p. 322).

A jugular or clavicular presystolic click has been heard in tricuspid stenosis and other conditions of high central venous pressure (Fisher, 1984).

Venous Syndromes

Superior Vena Caval Syndrome

Obstruction of the superior vena cava by thrombosis or by external compression (e.g., from tumor) is called the superior vena caval syndrome. The first three venous signs to be discussed can all be demonstrated at the bedside, once one has mastered the determination of venous pressure and Kussmaul's sign. However, the beginner should use manometry (p. 360) to learn and to demonstrate these signs in a more replicative fashion. Note that manometry can be performed in any accessible lower extremity vein, most conveniently the long saphenous vein anterior to the medial malleolus.

○ The first sign, an elevation of venous pressure in the arms (or neck) in the presence of normal lower extremity venous pressures, is pathognomonic for superior vena caval syndrome. The second sign, also pathognomonic, is a further elevation of the upper extremity venous pressure following the placement of a tourniquet around the patient's *upper* thorax. Simply have the patient lie on the tourniquet before you measure the baseline venous pressure, and when you are ready to do this test pull the two ends of the tourniquet over the anterior chest where they may be tied snugly enough to prevent caudad flow through the chest wall venous collaterals. (This test works even when these venous collaterals are not visible.) Third, there is Kussmaul's sign, which is less specific in the diagnostic sense.

It should be clear that the cost of the radiologic procedures needed to replace the above diagnostic maneuvers (such as CT scan, nuclear magnetic resonance, and venography) is easily an order of magnitude beyond the money "saved" by third-party payers reluctant to reimburse for venous pressure determinations. Obviously these tests could also be used to monitor the results of therapy of the superior vena caval syndrome.

Additional signs occurring in *chronic* superior vena caval syndrome include visible anastomotic veins, and the reversal in the usual direction of drainage of the supraumbilical abdominal veins (Ch. 20, p. 372), which can be determined by stripping the vein in the manner shown in Figure 19-1.

In an earlier era, one could use red-tinted glasses, worn by fluoroscopists to speed accommodation to the darkness of the fluoroscopy suite, to enhance examination of such superficial veins (Fear & Muggia, 1962; Sprunt & Wolff, 1962). Alas, image intensifiers have made these goggles as exolete as the bromsulphthalein retention test.

Portal hypertension of otherwise unexplained etiology in the presence of the superior vena caval syndrome tells you that the obstruction is below the part of the superior vena cava that receives the azygos vein.

A 29-year-old patient of Dr. Bob Meyer of Indiana was admitted with a superior vena caval syndrome and esophageal varices. The etiology of the syndrome was demonstrated to be fibrosing mediastinitis. A venogram revealed bilateral cutoff at the level of the axillary veins, but the presence of portal hypertension led the antediluvian clinicians to insist upon the presence of an additional obstruction below the entrance of the azygos vein into the superior vena cava. This was later documented by this nuclear magnetic resonance scan (done in an attempt to delineate the anatomic relations sufficiently to permit a surgical procedure).

In this situation, the azygos vein shares the venous hypertension and acts as a decompressing collateral, reversing the flow through the esophageal veins (which become varices) and thence to the coronary veins and so into the portal circulation. This is the same route (but with a reversal of flow) as seen in the more usual primary portal hypertension. Conversely, if there is no portal hypertension, one can only say that the patient has not had the syndrome long enough, and/or that the obstruction is above the entrance of the azygos vein into the superior vena cava.

Inferior Vena Caval Syndrome

In the inferior vena caval syndrome, the venous pressure (measured by manometer) should be elevated in the lower extremity, but not in the upper. This lower extremity pressure should rise further with a tourniquet secured snugly around the waist of the patient, thus cutting off the decompressing cephalad flow in the collaterals. Dr. Laura Miketo of Ohio has noted an additional sign: the pressure in the upper manometer actually drops during the tying of the tourniquet, and then rises when the tourniquet is released, as the pressure in the lower extremity manometer is dropping.

The skin signs of inferior vena caval syndrome are further discussed in Ch. 20 (p. 372). See also Figure 20-3.

Deep-Vein Thrombosis

Upper Extremity Deep-Vein Thrombosis

Thrombosis of the axillary and/or subclavian vein is an excellent example of an entity that can be diagnosed clinically by the concatenation of individually nonspecific findings. Spontaneous thrombosis tends to affect the left, and posttraumatic thrombosis the right. The patient is usually a young active male. Pain and/or swelling of the affected side is the first symptom. There is always swelling (usually nonpitting) that can be quantitated by circumferential measurement. Dilated collateral veins are always seen in white patients and often in black patients. Arm discoloration is also reported in 70% of white patients. A palpable vein (often the axillary) is present in only about a third of the patients. Venous pressures are elevated on the affected side only (Adams & DeWeese, 1971; Prescott & Tikoff, 1979).

Lower Extremity Deep-Vein Thrombosis

In patients complaining of pain and swelling in the calf, the possibility of deep vein thrombosis is always a concern, and is difficult to rule out clinically. Although the signs to be given are not individually perfect (Table 19-3), they are suggestive of the diagnosis if they occur together, provided one has ruled out mimics such as the pseudothrombophlebitis syndrome (see Ch. 25, p. 443).

Inspection. Check the popliteal space, the saphenous vein in the thigh, and the superficial veins for visible inflammation.

Pratt's sign is the presence of three dilated veins, called sentinel veins, over the tibia. The dilation persists when the legs are elevated to 45 degrees. In fact, one, two, or four such veins would have the same significance, but do not yet have eponyms. You may want to stake a claim. (A patient admitted for the evaluation of a lung mass had dilation of three veins over his left shin when supine. The veins on the right side were not dilated, and there was no evidence of thrombophlebitis. However, the veins collapsed when the leg was elevated, so this was not Pratt's sign. The patient had pelvic vein compression due to prostatic carcinoma.)

Palpation. Palpate for cords in the greater saphenous vein and its branches. In a unilateral thrombophlebitis of the calf or the thigh, an increase in skin temperature may be found. When seeking this sign, ignore the knees. (Warmth over the knee may be due to arthritis, Paget's disease synovitis, or to the collateralization of arterial disease [see Ch. 18, p. 350].)

Also check for pitting edema. Before edema is apparent to inspection, it can thicken the skin enough to make it feel "stiff" (compared with the other side) when one pinches it (Rose's test).

Percussion. Lisker's sign is tenderness to percussion of the medial anterior tibial surface. Lisker's sign is said to be present in 65% of patients with thrombophlebitis (DeGowin, 1965) but, unlike Homan's sign, absent in lumbosacral disease.

Special maneuvers:

1. Localizing tenderness. Grasp the soleus muscle and pull it and the gastrocnemius muscle posteriorly and superiorly, away from the tibia. Now squeeze the muscles gently from the side. (Start at the bottom and inch up.)

If pain is produced by this maneuver (called Bancroft's sign or Moses's sign), the patient either has muscle pain or thrombosis of the veins of the soleus, but *not* necessarily thrombophlebitis of the (deep) posterior tibial vein.

Next, press the gastrocnemius forward against the tibia. If this produces pain, greater than before, one has found thrombophlebitis of the posterior tibial vein.

2. Quantitating tenderness. In Lowenberg's sign, the two calves are wrapped with cuffs to see if both can tolerate a pressure of 180 mm Hg and if both are equally sensitive. Because the sign involves two variables, and vague criteria, I prefer the modification taught to me by Dr. Jim Scheuer of New York: Wrap a blood pressure cuff around the extremity and pump it up, noting the pressure at which pain occurs. The sign is positive when pain occurs on the affected side at one half the pressure required on the normal side.

In yet another modification, Ramirez simply inflates the cuff to 4 mm Hg above the venous pressure and waits for the pain to appear. In thrombophlebitis, the pain is said to increase over 5 minutes of occlusion and to improve with the eventual release of the pressure. Unfortunately, the same thing may happen in a normal patient, so one should modify this test to include a comparison with the normal side.

3. Homan's sign. If passive dorsiflexion of the foot produces calf pain, the patient is said to have Homan's sign. False positives are seen in women who wear high heels ("Bailey", Clain, 1973), as well as with herniated intervertebral discs and other forms of lumbosacral disease (DeGowin, 1965).

4. Louvel's sign. This is venous pain induced by coughing, and prevented by pressing over the proximal end of the vein with your finger, to block the venous distention.

5. Quantitation of swelling. Quantitation of the swelling of the affected side is useful if the thrombophlebitis is unilateral. Both legs should be measured a given distance up and down from the patella or the tibial plateau, for instance, 10 cm down from the tibial plateau on both sides for the calf and 20 cm above the superior border of the patella for the thigh. (Obviously, an elastic tourniquet is not a suitable measuring device, although a graduate of a U.S. medical school was once observed to be using it as such.)

Based upon 95% confidence limits,* the circumferences of

Table 19-3. Clinical Signs in Thrombophlebitis

Sign	Sensitivity	False-Positive Rate[a]
Rubor (redness)	16%	13%
Venous dilatation	25%	11%
Calor (heat)	29%–50%	0%–23%
Tenderness	41%–60%	11%–61%
Tumor (swelling)	81%–83%	6%–55%
Homan's sign[b]	8%–10%[c]	11%–12%

Source: *McLachlin et al. (1962) and Vaccaro et al. (1987).*
[a]*Prevalence of the sign in suspects without the disease.*
[b]*Homan withdrew his own eponym (which he had never claimed), preferring "dorsiflexion sign" (McLachlin et al., 1962).*
[c]*DeGowin (1965) claims 35%.*

*A statistical note: The distributions have been recalculated from the original paper and expressed in 95% confidence limits, since that is the way the clinician thinks with an individual patient before him. The standard deviation is useful in animal experiments, but the standard deviation increases with an increasing sample size. To present a clinician with a standard deviation assumes: 1) his population size is the same as that in the published paper, and 2) with increasing experience, his population size will *not* increase. The latter is obviously unrealistic except for very rare conditions. The standard error of the mean improves the situation somewhat for the experimentalist who wishes to know if the difference between two groups is greater than could be expected by chance. What the clinician wishes to know is how his individual patient compares with a group of normal patients. For this, the 95% confidence limits give him the answer. As a rough rule, doubling the quotient of the standard deviation (divided by) the square root of the sample size gives the 95% confidence limit of that mean (e.g., mean = 100, SD = 24, n = 16, 95% confidence limits = 88-112).

the normal thighs are less than 1.5 cm different, and abnormal thighs (as judged by impedence plethysmography) are more than 1.9 cm different (Hull et al., 1985). (Unfortunately, there are still differences in shape, total body size, and distance above the tibial plateau that have not been addressed in the literature.)

Similarly, the calves are normally within 1.68 cm of each other. Abnormal calves (as judged by impedance plethysmography) tend to be at least 2.5 cm different in circumference (Hull et al., 1985).

False positive. One resident physician noted that she had a chronic calf asymmetry of more than 2 cm, but no history of venous disease or other disease of the lower extremity. She believed the asymmetry to be due to the fact that one of her legs was shorter than the other. When she leaned over to touch her toes, it was apparent that the thinner calf was, as expected, that of the longer leg. (The length of the leg can be measured using the method in Ch. 24 [p. 430]. In this case, the pelvis could be seen to be tilted ever so slightly, and the sacroiliac joint of the longer leg was a bit higher than the other.)

Also see pseudothrombophlebitis (see Ch. 25, p. 443).

Trousseau's Syndrome

I am lost; the phlebitis that has just appeared tonight leaves me no doubt about the nature of my illness. (A. Trousseau, quoted in Stolinsky, 1983)

Trousseau's syndrome is clinically apparent thrombophlebitis (either superficial or deep) in association with malignancy. It is often migratory, and may occur in somewhat unusual sites (e.g., arm veins). Although originally described in association with gastric carcinoma (the diagnosis Trousseau made in himself), that disease has become rarer since the original description. Pancreatic carcinoma, for which Trousseau's sign has a sensitivity of less than 14% (Pinzon et al., 1986), is now much more common. Other associations are with carcinoma of the lungs, breast, prostate, and even head and neck squamous cell carcinomas.

Varicose Veins

Varicose veins are tortuous, dilated, and lengthened veins. They are diagnosed by inspection, with the patient standing.

When occurring in combination with port wine staining of the skin, varicose veins are strongly suggestive of an arteriovenous fistula. Varicose veins may pulsate in tricuspid insufficiency, even if you cannot hear the murmur over the veins (Brickner et al., 1962).

Greater Saphenous Vein Tests

Trendelenburg-Brodie test. This test was first described by Brodie (Brodie, 1846), although usually attributed to Trendelenburg, who was 2 years old in 1846 and did not publish this paper until 1890.

A method:

1. Elevate the limb to be examined, thus draining it passively.

2. Compress the greater saphenous vein at mid-thigh with your fingers, a tourniquet, or a blood pressure cuff inflated above the venous pressure but below the arterial pressure.

3. Have the patient stand for a minute. If the arterial supply is normal, the greater saphenous vein will fill *slowly* over half a minute. Rapid filling indicates backfilling from incompetent communicating veins.

4. Release the tourniquet. Further backfilling at this point requires that the greater saphenous vein valves be incompetent (as they will be in a distended vein).

False positives are produced by failure to initially drain the vein (step 1), or by otherwise distending it (Trendelenburg, 1890). Arterial insufficiency will produce a false negative.

Trendelenburg described two other tests:

1. The first test makes use of the fact that in the supine patient, the blood column in the greater saphenous vein forms a sort of manometer attached to the abdominal cavity. If the leg is elevated slightly above the level of the heart, the fluid level in an incompetent saphenous vein rises with coughing, straining, or even with flicking a finger against the abdominal wall.

2. To check for the presence of communicating veins to the deep veins (before ligating the greater saphenous vein), Trendelenburg recommended compressing the greater saphenous vein with the patient horizontal and the varices filled, and then raising the leg high. If the greater saphenous vein is the only efferent channel, the varices remain filled, but if there are communicating channels, the varices empty, albeit slowly (Trendelenburg, 1890).

Perthes's test*

A method:

1. While the patient is standing, apply a tourniquet (or a blood pressure cuff inflated above the venous pressure and below the arterial) at midthigh.

2. Have the patient walk around the room for 5 minutes with the compression in place, and note the effect on the vein.

Interpretation: Normally the muscle compression will empty the greater saphenous vein through normal communicating veins, which will drain through normal deep veins. Thus, the normal greater saphenous vein will actually be smaller after the walk.

If the greater saphenous and communicating veins are *both* incompetent, there will be no emptying and no change in the size of the visible greater saphenous.

If the deep vein is obstructed, and the communicating veins incompetent, there will be a further increase in venous distention, often accompanied by pain.

Percussion test

A method:

1. Place the sensitive fingers of one hand on the greater saphenous vein below the knee.

2. Place the other hand at least a foot away, above the knee, and with the tips of the fingers rap the greater saphenous vein sharply (about 60 mm Hg/100 msec) so as to send a fluid wave through it.

Interpretation: If the greater saphenous vein valves are incompetent (as surely they will be if that vein has become so distended that it can be seen and palpated over the distance of a foot), then it may be possible to feel the venous impulse traveling backwards down the leg.

False positives may result from thrombosis of the vein, or a

---

*G.C. Perthes is today remembered only as one of the triumvirate who described in three different papers, in as many languages, Legg-Calvé-Perthes disease in 1910. But he was actually a pioneer in the radiation therapy of carcinoma (Perthes, 1903).

blow so hard that the leg muscles shake and are misinterpreted. False negatives may result from too light a blow or insufficiently sensitive palpating fingers.

Appendix 19-1. The Circulation Time

A Method

1. Continuing from the manometric determination of venous pressure (p. 360), switch the stopcock so that the manometer port is now disconnected from the vein and the injection port is now connected to your injector syringe, which has been filled with an indicator of your choice (Table 19-4).

2. Instruct the patient to begin searching for the subjective sensation, for those maneuvers utilizing such an end point. Review the agreed-upon signal for the detection of the subjective sensation, where relevant.

3. Start your stopwatch and rapidly inject the indicator substance.

4. Stop the stopwatch at the end point (Table 19-4).

Interpretation

Prolonged circulation times are found in low-output congestive heart failure. False positives occur in myxedema and polycythemia. False negatives (i.e., shortened circulation times, or in the case of congestive heart failure, shorter than expected circulation times) occur in right-to-left shunts and high-output states with or without supervening congestive heart failure. The latter

include hyperthyroidism, anemia, beriberi, arteriovenous fistula (including severe erythrodermatitis, pregnancy, and Paget's disease) and fever.

Some have argued for abandoning the circulation time because its correlation with cardiac output (index) was once "only" 0.64, $p < .05$ (Selzer et al., 1968), when both variables were treated as continuous. Yet, if one wished to use the test only as a means of diagnosing presence or absence of congestive heart failure based on a dichotomous classification of an abnormal or a normal circulation time, it would appear in an even more favorable light.

Appendix 19-2. Answer to Self-Test on Kussmaul's Sign

The epigram cannot be the first description of Kussmaul's sign in pericardial tamponade for the following reasons:

1. Julian was stabbed in the liver, not in the pericardium.
2. The translation is wrong. Actually, the *inspirations* are being choked off by the veins.
3. Finally, you don't get Kussmaul's sign in pericardial tamponade, but in constrictive pericarditis and right ventricular infarction. (See Table 19-2.)

References

Adams JT, DeWeese JA: "Effort" thrombosis of the axillary and subclavian veins. *J Trauma* 11:923–930, 1971.
Askenazi J, Koenigsberg DI, Ziegler J, Lesch M: Echocardiographic estimates of pulmonary artery wedge pressure. *N Engl J Med* 305: 1586–1588, 1981.

Table 19-4.   Indicators Used in Determining Circulation Time

Indicator	End Point	Normal Time	Advantages and Disadvantages
5 cc of 20% Decholin	Bitter taste	10–16 sec	Excellent end point but requires conscious, articulate patient; Decholin difficult to find; rare anaphylaxis
2 cc of 20% solution or 3 cc of 15% solution or 4 cc of a 10% solution of fluorescein (the last is used for fluorescein angiography in ophthalmology dept.)	Greenish fluorescence of the lips, tongue; histamine-wheal anywhere on body	10–16 sec	Requires Wood's light; does not require patient cooperation; correlation with Decholin circulation time (the gold standard) excellent (Knott & Barlow, 1964)
3–5 cc of 20% calcium gluconate	Hot sensation in the throat	10–16 sec	End point difficult for some patients to describe, offsetting ubiquity of calcium gluconate
10 cc of 10% magnesium sulfate	Same as calcium gluconate	7–17 sec	Same as calcium gluconate (the two can be mixed)
0.8 mg/kg body weight riboflavin	Fluorescence; see fluorescein above	10–16 sec	Injectable riboflavin may be difficult to find on the spur of the moment
2.5 cc of a solution prepared by dissolving 2.5 g of saccharin in 2 cc of warm, not boiling, water; sterilize by passing through a millipore filter	Sweet taste	9–16	
0.5 cc of 1% alpha lobeline	Cough, followed by hyperventilation	11–12 sec	
5 drops of ether in 10 drops of normal saline. Paraldehyde is safer to use	Characteristic odor	4–8 sec	

The arm-to-tongue (or other arterial target) circulation time is the total circulation time. The arm-to-lung circulation time (as determined with ether) is essentially the "right-sided" circulation time; if it is subtracted from the total circulation time, one obtains the "left-sided" circulation time. The left-sided circulation may also be directly measured since inhalation of 50% carbon dioxide produces hyperpnea and tachypnea when the bolus reaches the carotid sinus (normal = 5–10 sec). In cases of pure "backward" left- or right-sided failure, only the circulation time for the afflicted segment may be prolonged.

Braun HA, Reynolds WA, Diettert GA, McCarthy CG: Auscultation of the neck. *Rocky Mountain Med J* 65:51–53, 1966.

Brickner PW, Scudder WT, Weinrib M: Pulsating varicose veins in functional tricuspid insufficiency. *Circulation* 25:126–129, 1962.

Brodie BC: *Lectures Illustrative of Various Subjects in Pathology and Surgery.* Longman, London, 1846.

Burch GE, Ray CT: Mechanism of the hepatojugular reflux in congestive heart failure. *Am Heart J* 48:373–382, 1954.

Cha SD, Gooch AS: Diagnosis of tricuspid regurgitation: Current status. *Arch Intern Med* 143:1763–1764, 1983.

Cintron G, Hernandez E, Linares E, Aranda J: Bedside recognition, incidence and clinical course of right ventricular infarction. *Am J Cardiol* 47:224–227, 1981.

Clain A (ed): *Hamilton Bailey's Demonstrations of Physican Signs in Clinical Surgery,* ed 15. Williams & Wilkins, Baltimore, 1973.

Colman AL: Diagnosis of left superior vena cava by clinical inspection, a new physical sign. *Am Heart J* 73:115–120, 1967.

Davison R, Cannon R: Estimation of central venous pressure by examination of jugular veins. *Am Heart J* 87:279–282, 1974.

DeGowin EL: *Bedside Diagnostic Examination.* Macmillan, New York, 1965.

Dell'Italia LJ, Starling MR, O'Rourke RA: Physical examination for exclusion of hemodynamically important right ventricular infarction. *Ann Intern Med* 99:608–611, 1983.

Dennison D: Bedside diagnosis: Heart failure. *Emerg Med* March:10–15, 1969.

Ducas J, Magder S, McGregor M: Validity of hepatojugular reflux as a clinical test for congestive heart failure. *Am J Cardiol* 52:1299–1303, 1983.

Ewy GA: Evaluation of the neck veins. *Hosp Pract* 22(3A):72–80, 1987.

Fear RE, Muggia FM: Convenient visualization of venous patterns. *Arch Intern Med* 110:898–899, 1962.

Fisher J: Jugular venous valves and physical signs. *Chest* 85:685–686, 1984.

Fowler NO: *Examination of the Heart: Part II Inspection and Palpation of Venous and Arterial Pulses.* American Heart Association, Dallas, 1967.

Friedberg CK: *Diseases of the Heart*, ed 2. WB Saunders, Philadelphia, 1956.

Friedrich N: Zur Diagnose der Herzbeutelverwachsungen. *Virchows Arch [Pathol Anat]* 29:296–304, 1864.

Friedrich N: Ueber den Venenpuls. *Deutsches Arch Klin Med* 1:241–291, 1865.

Gerbode F: A simple test to identify coarctation of the aorta. *Ann Surg* 184:615–617, 1976.

Goldstein J: Medical Grand Rounds. St. Louis Veterans Administration Medical Center, St. Louis, September 6, 1989.

Graf W, Moller T, Mannheimer E: The continuous murmur: Incidence and characteristics in different parts of the human body. *Acta Med Scand* Suppl 196:167–191, 1947.

Hitzig WM: Venous pressure curves in normal and abnormal circulatory states. *J Mt Sinai Hosp* 12:309–334, 1945.

Horwitz S A JE, Attie F H, EL, Espino-Vela J: Clinical diagnosis of persistent left superior vena cava by observation of jugular pulses. *Am Heart J* 86:759–763, 1973.

Hull RD, Hirsh J, Carter CJ, Jay RM, Ockelford PA, Buller HR, Turpie AG, Powers P, Kinch D, Dodd PE, Gill GJ, Leclerc JR, Gent M: Diagnostic efficacy of impedance plethysmography for clinically suspected deep vein thrombosis: A randomized trial. *Ann Intern Med* 102:21–28, 1985.

Hultgren HN: The effect of increased venous return on the venous pressure in patients with congestive heart failure. *Am Heart J* 39:592–603, 1950.

Hume EH: Medicine in China, old and new. *Am Med Hist* 2:272–280, 1930.

Jones FL: Frequency, characteristics, and importance of the cervical venous hum in adults. *N Engl J Med* 267:658–660, 1962.

Knott DH, Barlow G: The comparison of fluorescein and Decholin circulation times. *Am J Med Sci* 247:304–306, 1964.

Lorell B, Leinbach R, Pohorst G, Gold HK, Dinsmore RE, Hutter AM, Pastore JO, DeSanctis RW: Right ventricular infarction. *Am J Cardiol* 43:465–471, 1979.

Maisel AS, Atwood JE, Goldberger AL: Hepatojugular reflux, useful in the bedside diagnosis of tricuspid regurgitation. *Ann Intern Med* 101:781–782, 1984.

Marriott HJJ: Bedside diagnosis of cardiac arrhythmia. *Arrhythmia Clinic* 6:11–19, 1989.

McLachlin J, Richards T, Paterson JC. An evaluation of clinical signs in the diagnosis of venous thrombosis. *Arch Surg* 85:738–744, 1962.

Pasteur W: New physical sign of tricuspid regurgitation. *Lancet* 2:524, 1885.

Perthes GC: [On the effects of roentgen-rays on epithelial cells, especially from cancer.] *Archiv Klin Chir* 71:9551000, 1903.

Pinzon R, Drewinko B, Trujillo JM, Guinee V, Giaco G: Pancreatic carcinoma and Trousseau's syndrome: experience at a large cancer center. *J Clin Oncol* 4:509–514, 1986.

Prescott SM, Tikoff G: Deep venous thrombosis of the upper extremity: A reappraisal. *Circulation* 59:923–930, 1979.

Reddy PS, Leon DF, Shaver JA (eds): *Pericardial Disease.* Raven Press, New York, 1982.

Robin ED: The cult of the Swan-Ganz catheter: Overuse and abuse of pulmonary flow catheters. *Ann Intern Med* 103:445449, 1985.

Rondot E: Le reflux hepato-jugulaire [The hepatojugular reflux]. *Gaz Hebdomadaire Sci Med Bordeaux* 19:567–571, 579–582, 590–592, 1898.

Selzer A, Dunlap RW, Wray JW, Russell J: A critical appraisal of the circulation time test. *Arch Intern Med* 122:491–495, 1968.

Shabetai R, Fowler NV, Gunteroth W: The hemodynamics of cardiac tamponade and constrictive pericarditis. *Am J Cardiol* 26:480–490, 1970.

Sleight P: Unilateral elevation of the internal jugular pulse. *Br Heart J* 24:726–730, 1962.

Snapper I, Kahn AI: *Bedside Medicine*, ed 2. Grune & Stratton, New York, 1967.

Spodick DH: The normal and diseased pericardium: Current concepts of pericardial physiology, diagnosis and treatment. *J Am Coll Cardiol* 1:240–251, 1983.

Sprunt WH, Wolff AD: The value of seeing red while needling veins. *N Engl J Med* 267:1196, 1962.

Stolinsky DC: Trousseau's phenomenon. *Blood* 62:1304, 1983.

Tavel ME, Bard RA, Franklin LC, Feigenbaum H, Fisch C: The jugular venous pulse in atrial septal defect. *Arch Intern Med* 121:524–529, 1968.

Trendelenburg F: [Ligation of the great saphenous vein in varicose veins of the leg]. *Beitr Klin Chir* 7:195–210, 1890. [This paper was reprinted, with a translation, in the short-lived journal *Medical Classics* 4:989–1023, 1940.]

Vaccaro P, Van Aman M, Miller S, Fachman J, Smead WL: Shortcomings of physical examination and impedance plethysmography in the diagnosis of lower extremity deep venous thrombosis. *Angiology* 38:232–235, 1987.

Weiss S, Ferris E: Adams-Stokes syndrome with transient complete heart block of vagovagal reflex origin: Mechanism and treatment. *Arch Intern Med* 54:931–951, 1934.

Wheeler SD: Long-term hemodialysis and supraclavicular bruits. *JAMA* 247:1026, 1982.

Wiener SL, Nathanson M: *Med Times,* 1976–77. [See reference in Chapter 29.]

20
The Abdomen

"Every month for three successive days they purge themselves, for their health's sake, with emetics and clysters, in the belief that all disease comes from the food a man eats."

Herodotus, *The Histories*, Book 2

Inspection

Contour

One should always take a moment to stand at the foot of the bed and look at the nude abdomen. This has been traditionally taught as a useful way to observe visible peristaltic waves in cases of intestinal obstruction. Dr. A.I. Mendeloff of Maryland points out that it is even better for noticing asymmetry due to hepatomegaly and splenomegaly. These organs are sometimes more obvious on inspection than on palpation. (Also see "Ascites," p. 379.)

Cope states that the ladder pattern of abdominal distention visualized on the anterior abdominal wall indicates obstruction of the lower ileum ("Cope," Silen, 1979). He also states that moderate distention of the large bowel can be seen on the anterior abdominal surface as an inverted U extending from the right lower quadrant to the right upper quadrant, across to the splenic flexure, and down to the left lower quadrant. (In both cases, the drawings that are presented really resemble the patterns of dilated bowel seen on flat plates of the abdomen in those conditions.) In recent experience, these patterns are uncommon and incomplete. I suspect that Cope's patients were much thinner.

Pseudocyst of the pancreas may produce a localized bulge.

When inspected from the side, patients with acute pancreatitis show a peculiar Cupid's bow profile (Fig. 20-1,A). The dimple in the Cupid's bow is approximately at the umbilicus. The absence of this sign in a patient with a known elevation in amylase has correctly suggested the diagnosis of macroamylasemia without pancreatitis. Conversely, the presence of this sign caused one (correctly) to switch the preferred diagnosis from aortic aneurysm to acute pancreatitis. (The Cupid's bow is not pathognomonic; it can be seen in other gastrointestinal conditions causing adynamic ileus.)

The epigastric bulge due to massive pericardial effusion is known as Auenbrugger's sign. This is the same Auenbrugger we met at the opera in Chapter 16 (p. 252).

The term "scaphoid" does not mean "unremarkable." It means "shaped like a skiff or dinghy," in that the sides of the boat are represented by the costal margins and the pubis and anterior iliac spines, while the bottom of the boat is represented by the abdominal wall sunken in under the effects of gravity, with the patient in the supine position. The significance of the scaphoid abdomen is that none of the above findings are seen, and, in contrast to the situation with an obese abdomen, they would be seen if present.

Abnormalities of the Umbilicus

Normally, the umbilicus is located within 1 cm of the midpoint between the xiphoid and the symphysis pubis, unless there are scars or a history of pregnancy carried to term. Deviation of more than 1 cm is often the clue that leads to extremely thorough palpation.

Dr. Frank Iber of Illinois notes that hepatomegaly of 1 or 2 years' duration will stretch the upper abdominal segment, so that the distance between the xiphoid and the umbilicus is 2 cm longer than the distance from the umbilicus to the symphysis pubis. Such a downward displacement of the umbilicus can also be caused by ascites. In this case it is known as *Tanyol's sign*.

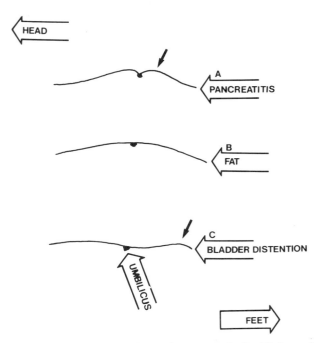

Figure 20-1. *Lateral abdominal contours. A, Cupid's bow of pancreatitis; B, fat; C, bladder distention.*

Upward displacement of the umbilicus occurs in pelvic tumors, the most common of which is still pregnancy.

Eversion or outward protrusion of a previously inverted umbilicus (Fig. 20-2) was thought to be a sign of chronic ascites, but there are false positives.

Respiratory Motion

The importance of examining the total abdominal surface for the phenomena of respiratory alternans and respiratory paradox (Macklem, 1986) is discussed in Chapter 16 (p. 246).

Additionally, Cope suggests looking for local limitations of respiratory movement of the abdominal wall in patients suspected of having an acute abdomen. For instance, in appendicitis with acute peritonitis, the right iliac region will very frequently remain selectively immobile during inspiration. In some cases of acute pancreatitis, the epigastric zone may be motionless. In generalized peritonitis, there is hardly any abdominal wall motion.

Markings

Ecchymoses

Subcutaneous blood from intraperitoneal or retroperitoneal hemorrhage may dissect to the skin overlying the flanks or to the anterior abdominal wall and cause a discoloration resembling a bruise or a subcutaneous injection site of heparin.

○ A periumbilical bruise is known as *Cullen's sign,* for the Baltimore doctor who described it in a case of ruptured ectopic pregnancy (Cullen, 1918). (This sign is to be distinguished from a green or jaundiced lesion at the umbilicus, which is Ransohoff's sign of a ruptured bile duct.) A similar discoloration in the flanks is called *Turner's sign* (not Grey-Turner's sign; there was no doctor Grey). This was described in a patient with acute pancreatitis by G. Grey Turner, 2 years after Cullen's report. In the same article, he described an earlier case of pancreatitis in which the bruising was periumbilical (Turner, 1920)!

Preservation of the two different eponyms has obscured the fact that these are the same sign. The topographic location of the ecchymosis does *not* point to the etiology. In fact, the same pancreatitic patient may have "both" signs (Dickson & Imrie, 1984). Other locations have been an appendectomy scar, a laparotomy scar, and umbilical and femoral hernias.

The sensitivity is less than 1% for ruptured ectopic pregnancy (Smith & Wright, 1935) and only 3% for acute pancreatitis, appearing late, between the 2nd and 6th hospital day (Dickson & Imrie, 1984). Further, it is not diagnostically specific, being also seen in ovarian cyst hemorrhage, strangulated umbilical hernia, bilateral acute salpingitis in the presence of intrauterine pregnancy, hemoperitoneum (not from ectopic pregnancy), hemorrhagic ascites from adenocarcinoma of the liver or renal sarcoma metastatic to the peritoneum (Smith & Wright, 1935), carcinoma of the liver (Mabin & Gelfand, 1974), strangulation of the ileum with hemorrhage, hypothyroid myopathy, and cirrhosis with portal hypertension (Kelley, 1961).

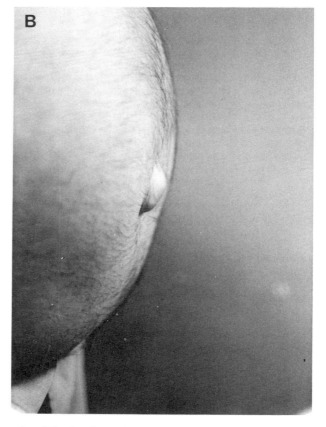

Figure 20-2. *A, The everted umbilicus sign of chronic ascites. Drawing of an Igbo female tutelary spirit on display in the Baltimore Museum of Art. B, A false-positive everted belly button seen in an obese patient possessing a lax abdominal wall. But there was no evidence of portal hypertension, hypoalbuminemia, liver disease, or ascites by any imaging procedure. Photograph courtesy of Dr. Tim Rice of Missouri. Another false positive is shown in Figure 20-4.*

Striae

Abdominal striae are the longitudinal stretch marks seen in pregnancy, Cushing's syndrome, and rapid gain and loss of weight. It has been taught that striae are usually red, but that they are purple in cases of idiopathic (noniatrogenic) Cushing's syndrome, because of the erythrocytosis resulting from the excess adrenal androgens.

Venous Pattern

Prominent venous patterns may be seen in portal hypertension or inferior vena caval syndrome (Fig. 20-3) or even in some aged normal persons (Snapper & Kahn, 1967). The clinician should note both the location of the veins and the direction of blood flow. In pure portal hypertension, the visible collateral veins tend to occur around the umbilicus. Those cephalad to the umbilicus drain in a cephalad direction, while those veins caudad to the umbilicus drain caudally. Thus, the direction of flow in pure portal hypertension is merely an exaggeration of the normal, but invisible, situation.

Perseus slew the Medusa by using his shield as a mirror, so that he did not have to look at her directly and thereby share the fate of others who had become transfixed by her horrible appearance.

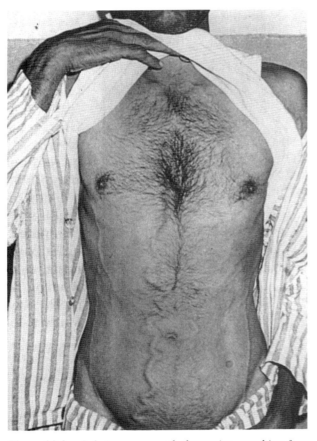

Figure 20-3. Inferior vena caval obstruction, resulting from carcinoma in the body of the pancreas. This is not a caput Medusa *of portal hypertension, even though the individual veins look snakelike. The* caput Medusa *radiates out from the umbilicus. The veins of inferior vena caval syndrome simply pass the umbilicus on their north-south route. Photograph courtesy of Dr. Syed A. Hoda of Louisiana and* Consultant *magazine.*

Her head (the *caput Medusa*) was surrounded by a bunch of snakes, in place of hair. Before the age of surgery for portal hypertension, a rare patient with severe chronic portal hypertension could develop such large periumbilical venous collaterals that the veins stuck out like a bunch of snakes, the *caput Medusa*. However, *caput Medusa* should not be diagnosed just because there is a visible vein or two somewhere on the abdomen; otherwise this rare sign loses its diagnostic significance.

In those rare cases of superior vena caval syndrome (see Ch. 19, p. 366) in which collaterals can be found in the upper abdomen, the normal direction of drainage is reversed, with the veins superior to the umbilicus actually draining caudally.

In cases of pure inferior vena caval syndrome, the collateral veins tend to appear more laterally in the flanks. They drain in a cephalad direction, regardless of whether they are above or below the umbilicus. In the inferior vena caval syndrome, it is more difficult to determine direction of flow by stripping the veins and seeing in which direction they fill than it is in portal hypertension (Missal et al., 1965).

(In chronic liver disease with portal hypertension and ascites compressing the inferior vena cava, there may be a mixed picture in which the veins are lateral and periumbilical. The venous flow is cephalad in the veins superior to the umbilicus, but may be indeterminate in the veins inferior to the umbilicus.)

In cases in which the direction of venous flow cannot be determined, the consultant should be prepared to discount the finding of flank veins as being indicative of inferior vena caval disease, especially if there are no other signs of such disease. However, if one has previously examined the patient, and that venous pattern has just recently appeared, it is in itself collaborative evidence of inferior vena caval disease.

Self-Assessment

Before reading the legends, write down your diagnosis for the patients pictured in Figures 20-4 and 20-5.

Palpation

The palpation of the abdomen should be done in an orderly sequence, beginning with the right upper quadrant, and proceeding to the left upper quadrant, the left lower quadrant, the right lower quadrant, and the periumbilical area, with particular attention to the aorta (see Ch. 18, p. 346). If the patient is complaining of pain, the order should be altered so that the painful area is examined last.

To help the patient relax the abdominal musculature, it is often helpful to have him flex his knees and hips, resting the soles on the bed.

The palpation of specific organs, such as the liver, gallbladder, spleen, and kidneys, is discussed in detail in their respective sections later in the chapter.

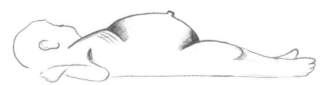

Figure 20-4. Drawing of the lateral profile autopsy photograph of Pepper's 1901 case of neuroblastoma metastatic to the liver. Notice that the tumorous liver is holding the abdomen up, whereas ascites alone would fall into the flanks in response to gravity with the patient supine. Note also the protuberant umbilicus.

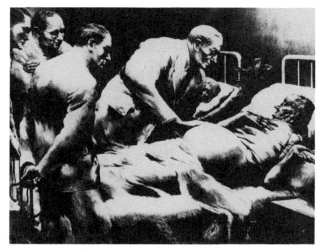

Figure 20-5. Ward Rounds, *lithograph by Robert Riggs. What is your diagnosis? Three that have been offered are pregnancy, ovarian cyst, and ascites. What do you think of each of these? (See Appendix 20-1.) What is the patient holding in her left hand? Photograph reproduced from* Medicine and the Artist (Ars Medica) *by permission of the Philadelphia Museum of Art.*

One also palpates for masses. Colonic carcinoma may present as a palpable mass in any one of the four abdominal quadrants. Pseudocolonic tumor or phantom tumor due to stool is frequent in the left lower quadrant, less frequent in the left upper quadrant. Wiener and Nathanson (1976–77) state that such phantom tumors may also occur in the right colon.

A giant phytobezoar in the left hypochondrium felt like a head of lettuce (iceberg or Boston, not Romaine).

Palpating the Abdomen in the Presence of Abdominal Pain

Local Rigidity (Local Guarding)
Local muscle rigidity over an area of peritonitis is frequently present (but by no means invariable). In the most extreme case, the particular section of the abdominal wall is persistently stiff and will not move with respiration. In lesser degree, the muscle stiffens almost as soon as the hand touches the skin. In the least degree, the rigidity occurs only when the fingers are pressed in more deeply. Take care to exclude the rigidity due to patient apprehension, or a rough or cold examining hand. Cope emphasizes that there are many false negatives, and that an appendix may be on the verge of rupturing into the peritoneal cavity even though the abdominal wall is flaccid ("Cope," Silen, 1979).

For the early diagnosis of the acute abdomen, Cope suggests the most likely (not the only) possibilities, as listed in Table 20-1.

Induced Guarding
One portion of the interview can be combined with a physical maneuver in the differential diagnosis of abdominal pain. Ask the patient to rate his abdominal pain on a scale of 1 to 10 (first baseline). Second, press over the area of tenderness to see how many points, if any, hand pressure will increase the pain. Then obtain a third, postpressure pain rating (second baseline). Finally, have the patient lift his head from the bed and put his chin on the chest, to induce voluntary guarding. Press again, and get a fourth rating.

Caveat. It is essential that the pressure be the same each time. This can be difficult to assure. One way is to allow one's fist to fall on the abdomen each time from the same height. Of course, one must apologize to the patient for inducing the pain, explaining that it is part of the examination. Alternately, one can place a blood pressure cuff and sphygomanometer on the abdomen with the cuff partly inflated and the manometer screw valve well sealed. Press to produce the same amount of pressure each time.

Interpretation. Pain of intraperitoneal origin will be lessened by the maneuver of voluntary guarding, which protects the peritoneal contents. In such patients, the fourth rating should be less than the second. Pain originating in the abdominal wall, peripheral nerves, or higher centers will not be ameliorated by this maneuver.

Alternate method. In a modification of this test, the guarding is induced by having the patient cross his arms while supine and then sit up. The abdomen is palpated as the patient reaches halfway between recumbent and sitting, the point of maximal abdominal musculature contraction and guarding.

This test was studied in a group of patients admitted to the emergency ward with localized abdominal pain (Thompson & Francis, 1977). (Patients with abdominal rigidity, in whom the test is useless and inappropriate, and those suspected of having an intraabdominal abscess, in whom the test is needless and possibly dangerous, were excluded.) A positive test was reduction of abdominal wall tenderness at midway palpation. A negative test was worsening of pain at this point.

The predictive value of a positive test and the sensitivity were both 99% for appendiceal abscess, cholecystitis, bowel obstruction, ruptured ovarian cyst, ureteral colic, urinary tract infection, and so forth.

The predictive value of a negative test for patients who were "undiagnosable" was 96%. (Almost half of the latter group went to a negative surgical exploration.)

Rebound and Referred Tests

Blumberg's sign (rebound tenderness). This is a general pain test for picking up early peritonitis in any area.

A method: Having palpated the tender areas as deeply as circumstances permit, the palpating hand is abruptly withdrawn. The previously stretched abdominal musculature will then spring back into place, carrying with it the peritoneum. If the peritoneum is inflamed, the patient will wince or cry out. This sign is often called *rebound tenderness.* (Bailey [Clain, 1973] correctly emphasizes that this test is quite unnecessary in patients with undoubted, involuntary rigidity.)

Referred rebound test. Cope does not recommend the rebound tenderness test (Blumberg's sign, first method) because he considers it cruel and not useful. But this modification may be useful with patients suspected of being not completely cooperative or precise in reporting their sensations.

A method:

1. If the patient has, for example, pain in the right upper quadrant, which was unconvincing to previous examiners, press slowly and deeply into a place where there is no pain, such as the left upper quadrant.

2. Then release the pressure suddenly, as if to test for rebound tenderness in the left upper quadrant, and ask, "Does that hurt?"

Interpretation: If the patient points to the right upper quadrant, at the same location as before, as the site of the pain, while denying any pain in the left upper quadrant, the test is positive. That means that the patient is reporting accurately, or else is an extremely clever and well-read dissembler.

The test is useful only if positive. A negative test does *not* prove that the patient has not been accurately reporting the original right upper quadrant pain.

Table 20-1. Differential Diagnoses of Abdominal Pain

Periumbilical pain without signs elsewhere

    Acute appendicitis
    Acute obstruction of the small bowel
    Acute gastritis
    Intestinal colic
    Acute pancreatitis

Severe abdominal pain with rigidity of the entire abdominal wall
and prostration

    Perforated peptic ulcer
    Other gut perforations
    Dissecting aneurysm

Tenderness and rigidity in the right upper quadrant

    Leaking duodenal ulcer
    Acute cholecystitis
    Appendicitis with a high appendix
    Pleurisy

Tenderness and rigidity in the left upper quadrant

    Pancreatitis
    Perforated gastric ulcer with a subphrenic abscess
    Leaking diverticulosis
    Ruptured spleen
    Leaking aneurysm of the splenic artery
    Acute perinephritis

Tenderness and rigidity in the right lower quadrant

    Appendicitis
    Leaking duodenal ulcer
    Acute pyelonephritis
    Regional ileitis
    Inflamed ileocecal glands
    Inflamed Meckel's diverticulum
    Cholecystitis with a low gallbladder
    Biliary peritonitis

Tenderness and rigidity in the left lower quadrant

    Diverticulitis
    Cancer of the colon
    Pelvic peritonitis spreading upward

Source: "Cope," Silen, 1979.

Cope's method.   It is useful to cross-palpate from the opposite side. For example, if you are evaluating pain in the left upper quadrant, press in the right upper quadrant and slowly move your palpating hand across the midline. If pressure in the right upper quadrant produces pain in the left upper quadrant before your hand crosses the midline, this tells you that the pain is coming from an abdominal condition and is not thoracic or referred. This also works well in the lower quadrants ("Cope," Silen, 1979).

A second method of Blumberg.   Blumberg also pressed in the left iliac fossa, and if the patient complained of pain anywhere in the lower abdomen (i.e., *referred* pain), he used this as evidence supporting the provisional diagnosis of acute appendicitis, although the sign is also positive in other acute abdominal conditions.

Rovsing's sign.   Rovsing also pressed on the left iliac fossa. If the direct pressure there produced referred pain in the right iliac fossa, the likelihood of appendicitis was increased. This is not a perfect test; there are both false positives and false negatives.

Note that the above assumes that the examiner is standing at the right side of the examining table and examining the patient with the right hand. This assumption is traditional in medicine, but not very important. If you feel more comfortable beginning on the left side and examining with the left hand (or with the right hand for that matter), then perform the examination that way. If you modify the text to accommodate your own preference, a knowledge of basic anatomy will permit you to alter the instructions mutatis mutandis.

Hyperesthesia

Hyperesthesia to light touch in the referred dermatomes may sometimes occur in acute abdominal conditions. Patients with appendicitis may have hyperesthesia in the anterior right lower quadrant.

Hyperesthesia in the region shown in Fig. 20-6 (Boas' sign) is a sign of gallbladder disease. This test is especially useful in patients who are schizophrenic or demented. They will grimace if the test is positive, even though they may not be able to report their experiences verbally. Few patients know about this test, so if it is positive, any suspicion of malingering should be discarded. Unfortunately, Boas' sign has a sensitivity of less than 7% (Gunn & Keddie, 1972).

In diabetic patients, thoracoabdominal neuropathy may mimic the symptoms of intraabdominal pathology such as gallbladder disease or appendicitis. There may be hyperesthesia in a dermatomal distribution (Harati & Niakan, 1986). Another consideration in the differential diagnosis of abdominal pain accompanied by hyperesthesia is herpes zoster. The characteristic skin eruption may not appear for several days.

Abdominal Wall

Sometimes one notices a different consistency to the abdominal wall on deep palpation. This consistency has been variously described as "doughy," "grainy," "stringy," and "glandular." The tissue

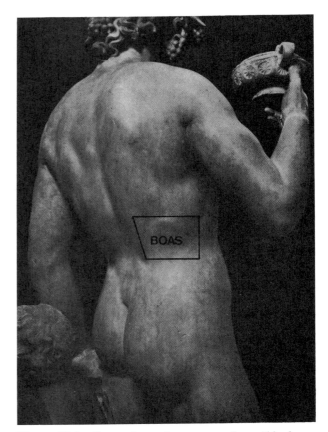

Figure 20-6. *Rectangle encloses area of possible hyperesthesia in gallbladder disease. Bacchus, by Michelangelo.*

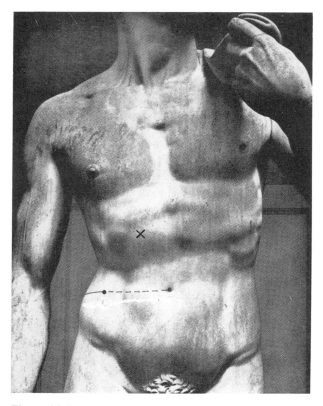

Figure 20-7. *McBurney's point (marked by the dot); area to check for Murphy's sign (p. 386) (marked by the X). David, by Michelangelo.*

feels a bit like postmenstrual breast tissue, which has lost some of its water content but is still glandular. The most benign cause of this sensation is the residual fat following a period of weight loss, but granulomatous peritonitis, especially that due to tuberculosis, may also cause this consistency, comparable to dough on a breadboard. And sometimes this sensation is due to peritoneal metastases, especially of malignant melanoma.

Peritoneal metastases may also feel discrete or lumpy. Plaques of "fatty" or glandular-feeling material are separated by areas of completely normal consistency a few centimeters in width. The mapped out sensation of this abnormal resistance to palpation would resemble an abstract expressionist painting (as by Jackson Pollock), in which paint had been thrown on the canvas and allowed to drip, with clear spaces in between.

A Note on McBurney's Point

Classically, the tenderness of acute appendicitis is localized over McBurney's point (see the dot in Fig. 20-7), until rupture and generalized peritonitis supervene. This valuable point has been misidentified in so many works that McBurney's own description is cited:

> And I believe that in every case the seat of the greatest pain, *determined by the pressure of one finger*, has been very exactly between an inch and a half and two inches from the anterior spinous process of the ilium on a straight line drawn from that process to the umbilicus. This may appear to be an affectation of accuracy, but, so far as my experience goes, the observation is correct. (McBurney, 1889)

Often, the patient with acute appendicitis may be able to localize his pain precisely with one finger, especially after a cough or the Valsalva maneuver.

With aberrant locations of the appendix (such as retrocecal), the tenderness will not be in the expected location.

Study question: *If the patient in Figure 20-7 actually has a perinephric abscess, what side is it on? (See Appendix 20-2.)*

Facial Expression

While palpating the abdomen, be sure to observe the patient's facial expression. Gentle pressure over an inflamed appendix is nauseatingly painful, and may elicit a characteristic facial expression (Fig. 20-8).

Not all patients with appendicitis have this expression, and it may also occur in intestinal strangulation and infective peritonitis due to any cause. However, it is conspicuously absent in salpingitis, mesenteric adenitis, and other conditions in the differential diagnosis of acute appendicitis (Odom, 1982).

Percussion

○ There should always be hepatic dullness in the right midaxillary line, except in the presence of free air under the diaphragm, which produces resonance ("Cope," Silen, 1979). The availability of upright films of the abdomen (Fig. 20-9) has made this a rare maneuver in the United States.

Subphrenic abscess, an intraabdominal disease, may be diagnosed by percussion of the chest (see Ch. 16, Fig. 16-4, p. 254).

The percussion of specific organs is discussed later (pp. 383 and 385).

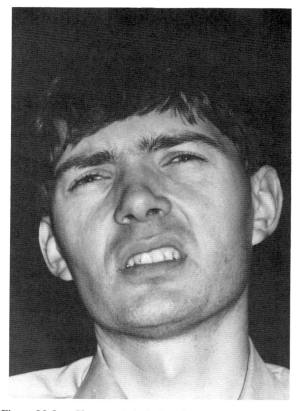

Figure 20-8. *Characteristic facies of acute appendicitis. Note the aura of malaise, and the upward curling of the upper lip. Photograph courtesy of Dr. Nicholas J. Odom of Newcastle upon Tyne, England.*

Auscultation

Bowel Sounds

At the present time, this is a surprisingly controversial subject. Some gastroenterologists see no point in listening for bowel sounds, whereas others with gray beards find it valuable. Both groups would undoubtedly agree with the following consensus statements:

○ **1.** If you wish to hear bowel sounds, you should apply your stethoscope to the abdomen *before* performing palpation or percussion, as these may disturb the peritoneal contents into silent pouting. (However, the auscultation should be recorded in the case record in the usual sequence, after percussion.)

2. As far as the routine screening physical examination is concerned, auscultation of the bowel sounds is of low yield.

A Method

1. Warm the chest piece of your stethoscope by rubbing it briskly in the palm of your hand.

2. Lightly rest the chest piece of the stethoscope in each of the four quadrants of the abdomen. Listen for bowel sounds. If no bowel sounds are heard, enter this fact in the case record, along with a note about the length of time that you listened. To hear the tinkles and rushes* of small bowel obstruction, which occur between periods of silence every 10 to 20 minutes (during episodes of cramping abdominal pain), you must listen for 20 minutes! Major (Delp & Manning, 1975) cleverly makes the suggestion that if there is anything to suggest the presence of a small bowel obstruction one should begin the auscultation of the abdomen during the interview. Remove one of the stethoscope earpieces from your ear to listen to the patient's words. When the patient interrupts his story because of abdominal pain, switch your attention to the ear that is connected to the stethoscope.

3. Feel free to modify this method according to the comments below.

Interpretation

No particular type of bowel sounds, or absence of same, is diagnostic of any one condition, except for the very high-pitched tinkles and rushes of small bowel obstruction.

The complete absence of sounds can be due to very advanced intestinal obstruction, secondary ileus, primary disease of the bowel, or as a normal acoustic occurrence between episodes of normal bowel motility.

Increased peristalsis can occur with any obstruction from the pylorus to the cecum, but similar sounds also occur during diarrhea of any etiology.

Murmurs

Murmurs due to renal vascular disease are discussed in Chapter 18 (p. 348).

---

*"Tinkles" are bowel sounds of musical timbre occurring one to two octaves higher than normal. Some require them to have a frequency above 512 Hz (high C) (Dennis, 1954). "Rushes" are bowel sounds accelerated to at least three times normal speed.

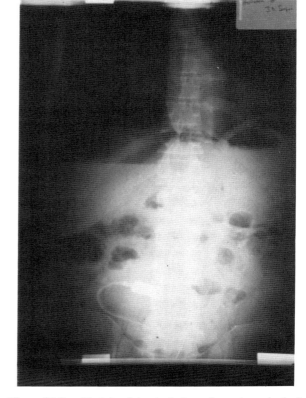

Figure 20-9. *Upright abdominal plate of a patient who had a hollow percussion note in his right midaxillary line where liver dullness would have been expected. Notice the air under the diaphragm.*

Systolic Murmurs

Epigastric murmurs. The prevalence of systolic epigastric murmurs (excluding radiating heart murmurs) in normal persons was found to be from 6.5% to 16% in three different series (Edwards et al., 1970; Julius & Stewart, 1967; Rivin, 1972). Conversely, of patients with abdominal systolic murmurs, 13% were found to have no explanatory lesion on angiography (McLaughlin et al., 1975).

Epigastric murmurs have been produced by increased blood flow in febrile adults (McSherry, 1979) or in children with acute infectious gastrointestinal disease (Lee, 1967).

Special populations have other prevalences: 21% of pregnant women (McSherry, 1979); 10% to 20% of "thin women of childbearing age" (Mohun, 1976); 25% to 26% of Canadian women of childbearing age (McSherry, 1979); 20% of females but only 3% of males, although higher in the younger ages for both groups (Julius & Stewart, 1967; McSherry, 1979); 27% of gastroenterology outpatients (Watson et al., 1973); and 31% of psychiatric inpatients (Watson et al., 1973). The figures for patients with essential hypertension but no renal vascular disease tend to run slightly higher than those for normals and are given in Chapter 18 (p. 349).

It is to be hoped that none of these figures are contaminated by including murmurs radiating from the heart or produced by the overly exuberant application of the stethoscope to a normal vessel.

Systolic epigastric bruits have been reported in disease of the aorta (Clain et al., 1966; Rivin, 1972). (See also aneurysms, Ch. 18, pp. 346 and 347.) They are also found in 90% of cases of stenosis of branches of the aorta such as the celiac axis and the superior mesenteric artery (Rob, 1966).

This raises the issue of the syndrome of external celiac axis compression, either by a fibrotic celiac ganglion or by the median arcuate ligament of the diaphragm, producing gastrointestinal pain that is relieved by surgery. (Some very experienced angiographers, such as Klaus Bron of Pennsylvania, do not believe that this syndrome exists because the same lesion may be seen in persons without symptoms.) Some believe the murmur characteristically extends into early diastole (although not continuous) (Watson et al., 1973). However, as many as 14% of patients in one series did not have this murmur (Ghosh et al., 1982), and a small proportion of normal persons (0% to 1%) may have such a diastolic continuation of their innocent systolic murmurs (Grim et al., 1979). Others believe that the murmur is characterized by its disappearance or diminution on inspiration (Ghosh et al., 1982), but this does not always occur. Also, some believe that such respiratory change is actually characteristic of an innocent murmur (Watson et al., 1973).

An epigastric systolic bruit that shifts downward in location when the patient assumes the standing position should suggest an aneurysm in the freely movable omentum, which in one case was found to be in the gastroepiploic artery (Hatano et al., 1980). (Also see "Examination of the Liver, Auscultation" on p. 383.)

Right upper quadrant systolic murmurs.   When not due to renal vascular disease, such murmurs are from the liver or its vessels.

Specifically, a systolic murmur is heard in 14% of hepatomas (Benner & Labby, 1961), other primary malignant tumors, metastatic liver tumors (Sherman & Hardison, 1979), occasionally a benign liver tumor such as an adult hemangioma or a childhood hemangioendothelioma (Smith et al., 1978), and cirrhosis either with alcoholic hepatitis (Clain et al., 1966) or portocaval shunt (Goldstein, 1968). Arteriovenous malformations and 80% of posttraumatic arterioportal fistulas also have systolic bruits in this location (Strodel et al., 1987). Tricuspid regurgitation may produce a bruit heard at the liver. For some discriminatory features of murmurs heard over the liver, see page 383.

Left upper quadrant systolic murmurs.   When not due to renal vascular disease, such murmurs are due to disease of the spleen or its vessels, especially the splenic artery.

A splenic murmur can be produced simply from massive (grade 4 or better) splenomegaly (Bjorkman, 1953). The splenic artery can have a murmur if there is dissection (Serebro, 1965) or tortuosity (Smythe & Gibson, 1963), or in the 39% of cases of carcinoma of the body or tail of the pancreas in which the tumor actually impinges on the splenic artery (Bauerlein & de la Vega, 1963; Serebro, 1965).

Continuous Murmurs

Epigastric continuous murmurs.   A high-pitched continuous "hepatic" venous hum (coming from the vena cava?) is heard in less than 4% of normal persons (Rivin, 1972). It is usually heard to the right of the umbilicus, and has the same physiology as the cervical venous hums discussed in Chapter 19 (p. 366). Specifically, it diminishes or disappears during the forced exhalation phase of the Valsalva maneuver (Hardison, 1977).

A similar high-pitched venous hum of more variable radiation is also heard in portal hypertension and in fact is considered diagnostic of that condition (Hardison, 1977). This hum has been called the Cruveilhier-Baumgarten *murmur.*

Cruveilhier-Baumgarten is certainly one eponym that has been overmarketed. A congenitally patent umbilical vein with portal hypertension (but not cirrhosis or other liver disease) is called Cruveilhier-Baumgarten *disease.* (This is extremely rare, less than a few dozen cases.) The Cruveilhier-Baumgarten *syndrome,* although defined differently by different authors, usually includes cirrhosis (or some other initiating liver disease), portal hypertension, and the paraumbilical anastamotic veins that are the source of the diagnostic Cruveilhier-Baumgarten *murmur.* (The umbilical vein is *not* recanalized in this syndrome (LaFortune et al., 1985), despite statements to the contrary.) Finally, Cruveilhier-Baumgarten *cirrhosis* is both obsolete and inaccurate in that there is nothing specific about the kind of cirrhosis that causes the syndrome.

The Cruveilhier-Baumgarten murmur (or hum) becomes *louder* during the forced expiratory phase of the Valsalva maneuver (Hardison, 1977). However, during normal respiration it becomes louder during early inspiration, but softer during later inspiration (Cheng et al., 1954). (Since there are those who believe that an increase in such a murmur during inspiration is due to compression of the splenic vein and signifies no more than the splenomegaly, it is hard to know the exact significance of these changes, especially considering that splenomegaly itself will be a frequent concomitant of portal hypertension.) Although any murmur that significantly diminishes or disappears with epigastric pressure is undoubtedly a Cruveilhier-Baumgarten murmur, not all Cruveilhier-Baumgarten murmurs will have this unique sign (Hardison, 1977). (Also see Ch. 17, p. 304.) One constant is that the murmur increases or appears 30 to 60 minutes after an oral glucose load (Cheng et al., 1954; Ramakrishnan, 1978).

How was this latter phenomenon discovered? In the old days, it was convenient to make the diagnosis of portal hypertension by comparing the paraumbilical vein's glucose content with that of a peripheral vein 30 to 60 minutes after a 50-g oral glucose load. The markedly higher values (20 to 50 mg/dl) in the paraumbilical vein showed convincingly that it was not simply a peripheral vein but an integral part of the portal venous system. During such a test, someone must have listened to the hum and made the observation. (There are still hundreds of such observations waiting to be made right now.)

Patients with chronic intestinal arterial insufficiency with ischemia may also have continuous bruits (Sarr et al., 1980).

The loudest continuous epigastric bruits are heard in aortovenous fistulas, such as those involving the renal veins (Celoria et al., 1987), the iliac veins, or the inferior vena cava (Magee & Mellick, 1977).

Right upper quadrant continuous murmurs.   Such bruits originate from the right renal artery, the kidney, or the liver.

Causes of hepatic bruits include cirrhosis (McFadzean & Gray, 1953), alcoholic hepatitis (Clain et al., 1966), 45% of hepatomas (Kingston et al., 1985), hepatic Hodgkin's disease (Jones et al., 1978), hepatic arteriovenous malformations and shunts (McFadzean & Gray, 1953; Shumacker & Waldhausen, 1961), and posttraumatic arterioportal fistulas (Strodel et al., 1987).

Left upper quadrant continuous murmurs.   Those that do not originate from the left renal artery or kidney may be caused by a splenic arteriovenous fistula (occurring in about one third of cases) (Bloom, 1950) or by grade 4 to 5 splenomegaly (Fig. 20-14) (Cassel et al., 1957; Williams et al., 1980).

Rubs

Friction rubs over the liver can be heard in hepatoma, cholangiocarcinoma, and 10% of cases of metastatic carcinoma

(Fenster & Klatskin, 1961). Rubs are less frequent in inflammatory conditions including pyogenic abscess, viral hepatitis, alcoholic hepatitis, cholecystitis, tuberculous peritonitis, and perihepatitis secondary to lupus erythematosus or the gonococcus. If a murmur coexists, diagnose neoplasia, not inflammation (Sherman & Hardison, 1979).

It should not be surprising that is also possible to auscult a rub over an inflamed gallbladder or a splenic infarct.

Special Maneuvers

Valsalva Maneuver

After a 20-second vigorous Valsalva maneuver, the patient with an acute abdomen will often be able to point to a specific area of tenderness. Identifying this area first allows one to plan a strategy that minimizes discomfort to the patient, permitting a more adequate (as well as more humane) examination.

Obturator Test

The purpose of this test is to move the obturator muscle passively, an action that normally produces no pain. However, if the obturator muscle is inflamed due to pathology of a neighboring viscus, pain is produced.

A Method

1. With the patient supine, flex the thigh and rotate it fully inward (Fig. 20-10).

2. Repeat on the opposite side.

Interpretation

This test is positive if the inward rotation produces pain, usually referred to the hypogastrium (i.e., the central inferior abdomen, where the bladder is located).

In appendicitis, the test is positive on the right but not the left. It can be positive on either side in pelvic abscess or pelvic hemorrhage. It can also be positive if there is pus in the pelvis, even if the pus came from above.

Reverse Psoas Maneuver

The reverse psoas maneuver, also called Cope's iliopsoas test, is useful in detecting psoas irritation from appendicitis, psoas abscess, or psoas hematoma.

A Method

1. Have the patient roll onto his left side. Hyperextend the right hip (away from the position that the patient would naturally assume with a right psoas sign—see the drawing of St. Sebastian, Fig. 5-2) to see whether pain can be elicited.

2. Repeat on the other side to check for nonappendiceal left psoas lesions.

Detecting a Ventral Hernia

If the supine patient places his chin on his chest, or attempts a sit-up with his hands folded on his chest, he will need to contract his rectus abdominis muscles, thereby making an abdominal ventral hernia more apparent to inspection and palpation.

A Valsalva maneuver may distend a hernia that can be seen more readily than felt.

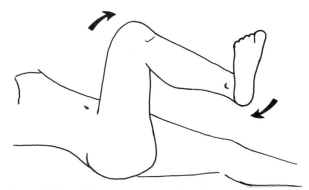

Figure 20-10. *The obturator test. Standing lateral to the leg, pull the ankle toward you and push the knee away from you.*

Auscultation After Tube Placement

After placing a feeding tube or other gastric tube, one can check the position by instilling air while listening distally, over the stomach, for a hissing or bubbling sound.

A caveat. Gary Albers of Missouri told of a comatose patient in whom a nurse passed a nasogastric tube and, hearing the expected bubbling sound near the stomach, began feedings. Soon the patient developed a left-sided pneumonia with empyema. Investigation revealed that the feeding tube had been passed into the left lower lobe of the lung and through the pleura into the subpleural space.

Conversely, one should listen over the stomach after an endotracheal tube has been placed.

The Succussion Splash

The same principles described in Chapter 16 (p. 273) apply to gastric outlet obstruction or any other abdominal condition in which a nonviscous liquid forms the lower portion of a gas-liquid interface. Note that there must be a large amount of the gas over the liquid phase. Also, the patient must be in a condition that permits him to be passively shaken, and the splash must be located sufficiently close to the abdominal wall that it can be detected with a stethoscope.

Flat and upright films are superior to the succussion splash for finding air-fluid levels. However, the succussion splash, while an insensitive maneuver, is cheap and quick. Since there are many normally occurring gas-fluid interfaces in the abdominal cavity, the succussion splash is less specific than in the chest, where it is always abnormal (Fig. 16-10, p. 266).

Hannington-Kiff Sign

The Hannington-Kiff sign for strangulated obturator hernia is given in Chapter 26 (p. 500).

Synthesis

Ascites

Inspection

Patients with ascites are said to have a protruding abdomen like the deity Buddha (as well as some umbilical signs, see p. 371).

Unfortunately, many persons who are obese or who have abdominal muscular hypotonia may have such an appearance.

Dr. Frank Iber of Illinois states: "Flank bulge in the supine patient is clearly distinguishable from the flab of fatness and indicates ascites often when other methods are equivocal. The fluid distends only as far back as the peritoneum goes; fat goes further back." See Figure 20-4. But less experienced examiners have reported difficulty (Table 20-2, "Bulging flanks").

Palpation

There are two basic techniques for palpating fluid in the flanks. The first of these is the well-known fluid wave (Fig. 20-11).

A method:

   1. With the patient supine, place one hand on the lateral aspect of the patient's abdomen (flanks) between the costal margin and the ilium in the anterior axillary line. (Because of the differences in human anatomy from subject to subject, I advise the beginner to pretend that the peritoneal cavity is one quarter full of water and that the water is to be sloshed with the right hand so that it ripples in a wave striking the left flank, where the left hand and fingers are prepared to sense the impact. The hands should be placed appropriately.)

   2. Have the patient or an assistant place the ulnar surface of one hand above the umbilicus in the craniocaudal dimension, wedging it into the abdomen. This procedure prevents false positives due to the percussing hand's thumping the body wall so hard that the shock wave ripples over the anterior abdominal wall to the opposite side.

   3. Thump with one hand and palpate with the other. You will sense a shock wave if sufficient ascites are present.

   4. As a check for artifacts or unilateral insensitivities of the examiner, let the palpating hand now percuss and vice versa.

When properly performed, this test is of high predictive value (> 70%) for ascites if positive. But obviously, it is of limited sensitivity, since it requires sufficient fluid in the peritoneal cavity to make a wave (Table 20-2).

A fluid wave can be detected in the erect position in some patients in whom it is inapparent in the supine position (Guarino, 1986).

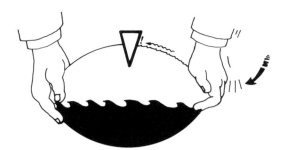

Figure 20-11. *Diagrammatic representation of the fluid wave. The wedge represents the hand of the patient or assistant, which intercepts any anterior wall vibrations.*

A second method. This method was learned by watching Dr. Jack Myers of Pennsylvania. It seems to have the same diagnostic outcome as checking for a fluid wave, but it has the advantage of not requiring an awake patient or an assistant.

   1. Place the patient supine.

   2. Lean over the patient and place your hands, with volar surfaces toward you, behind his presumably bulging flanks, with the dorsal surfaces touching the bed.

   3. Quickly flip up the flanks about 3 or 4 inches. Note whether you can feel fluid falling back into the bulging flanks.

Percussion

There are two percussive techniques.

Periumbilical hyperresonance. With the patient supine, percuss the abdomen, demonstrating that hyperresonance is present only around the umbilicus. Supposedly, with severe ascites, the gas-filled loops of bowel will all float to the top.

Shifting dullness
   A method:

   1. Have the patient lie supine.

   2. Percussing circumferentially from above to below, mark the point at which the percussion note becomes dull, *if* you can find one. (This is actually the test for flank dullness, see Table 20-2.) If this point of dullness is due to fluid, there should actu-

Table 20-2.   Detection of Ascites (Ultrasound as the gold standard)

Method	Sensitivity		Specificity[a]		% Accuracy
	Cummings et al. (1985)	Cattau et al. (1982)	Cummings et al. (1985)	Cattau et al. (1982)	Examiner 3 (Cattau et al., 1982)
Abdominal distention	72%	—	65%	—	—
Bulging flanks	72%	78%	70%	40%	62%
Flank dullness	—	94%	—	29%	50%
Fluid wave	53%	50%	90%	82%	81%
Shifting dullness	88%	83%	56%	56%	81%
Puddle sign	—	55%	—	51%	79%
Overall physical exam	—	—	—	—	89%
Roentgenogram	—	50%			
Paracentesis	—	67%			

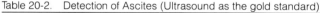

Note: [a]*False positives: Tests for ascites, being tests for free fluid in the peritoneum, could theoretically have false positives due to any cause of mobile fluid, such as blood, succus entericus (after a perforation), or fluid in an obstructed loop of intestine. But hemorrhage, perforation, or obstruction sufficient to cause enough such fluid to produce a false positive should be easily diagnosed on other grounds.*

ally be a series of such points (a line) of dullness, parallel to the floor. Mark this line. (See Fig. 20-12.)

3. Do the same thing on the other side. If you have correctly percussed out the surface of the ascitic fluid, this line should be in a position corresponding to the one on the other side.

4. Roll the patient over on the right side.

5. Percuss the left (superior) flank dorsal to the line you had marked. If this previously dull area is now resonant, you have produced evidence for the shifting dullness of ascites.

6. Confirm this by turning the patient over onto his left side, percussing now the right side mutatis mutandis.

Of the classic tests for ascites, this one is one of the most sensitive (Table 20-2). But the mesenteric fat of the obese patient generates many false positives, thus lowering the specificity. And Cope reported a false positive due to severe unilateral hydronephrosis ("Cope", Silen, 1979).

Auscultatory Percussion

The "puddle sign"
<u>A method:</u>

1. Have the patient lie on his belly for 5 minutes and then raise himself up to a position on "all fours." That is, he is to support himself on his knees and forearms so that the middle portion of the abdomen is the most dependent. (The expectation is that any ascites in the peritoneum will now follow gravity to the most dependent portion and form a puddle.)

2. Place the diaphragm of the stethoscope over the most dependent portion of the abdomen.

3. Perform auscultatory percussion by flicking one finger of the hand not holding the stethoscope at a constant light intensity at a constant location on the flank. Sound waves so generated must pass through any fluid that is present in order to reach the stethoscope.

4. Gradually move the stethoscope toward the *opposite* flank while continuing to percuss the flank.

5. A positive sign consists of an abrupt perceived increase in the intensity and clarity of the note just as the stethoscope moves beyond the edge of the pool of fluid. If such a change is heard, repeat the procedure, flicking the opposite flank *mutatis mutandis*. Having found the border of the puddle on both sides, ask the patient to sit up. With the stethoscope in the same position as before, the percussion note from both sides should become clear, if the fluid is free-flowing (and hence, in most cases, ascites), because the fluid will move inferiorly.

The interested reader is referred to the original work (Lawson & Weissbein, 1959), which includes phonocardiographic studies and dog experiments concerned with the exact acoustical components perceived by the ear. The originators were able to detect as little as 120 ml of ascites (Lawson & Weissbein, 1959), but this has not been a universal clinical experience (Cattau et al., 1982; McLean, 1987).

<u>An alternate method:</u> Simply place the stethoscope at the most dependent portion of the abdomen and flick with your finger, gradually moving it down the abdomen toward the stethoscope. It does not make much sound until it passes the ascitic fluid-intestine interface. Then with both the flicking finger and the stethoscope "under the puddle," the sound abruptly becomes noticeably louder.

An additional benefit of this method (which has not been stan-

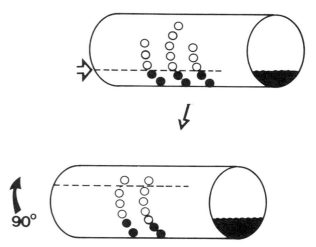

Figure 20-12. *The semiophysiology of shifting dullness can be best understood by likening the ascitic patient to a wine barrel that can be percussed and rolled. The open circles (○) represent a relatively resonant percussion note; the solid circles (●) a dull or flat note. The line of demarcation (arrow) between the resonant and the dull areas should correspond to the fluid level in the barrel.*

Of course, it would not be unusual to get dullness in a person as one neared the inferior surface of the body, which is lying supine in bed, because of the musculoskeletal structures on the dorsal surface of the body. (Furthermore, as was pointed out in Ch. 16, p. 252, the simple opposition of the body to the bed will cause dullness.) In order to demonstrate fluid, we need to show that the dullness shifts.

In the lower half of the figure, the barrel is rotated toward the right lateral decubitus position. Actually, the barrel has been rotated less than the 90-degree rotation noted, for ease of illustration. Note that the original line of dullness, marked on the barrel with a dashed line, has now rotated superiorly. The original percussion markings have been erased, and replaced with new ones obtained with the barrel in the rotated position.

It should be obvious from this illustration that it is very difficult to detect small amounts of fluid with this technique.

dardized) is that sometimes, with small amounts of ascites, one can flick hard enough to "splash" some of the fluid. This squishing sound, heard through the stethoscope, might be called an abdominoscopic succussion splash.

Unfortunately, the position required for this test is very uncomfortable for both patient and examiner. For that reason alone, Guarino's variation might be preferred.

Guarino's variation
<u>A method:</u>

1. Have the patient void, then sit or preferably stand for 3 minutes to allow free fluid to gravitate to the pelvis.

2. Hold the lower edge of the diaphragm piece of the stethoscope with one hand immediately above the pubic crest in the midline (Fig. 20-13).

3. Apply finger-flicking percussion with the other hand along three or more lines from the subcostal margin perpendicularly down toward the pelvis.

<u>Interpretation:</u> Normally, there is a sharp change from a dull note to a loud one along a horizontal line across the pelvic

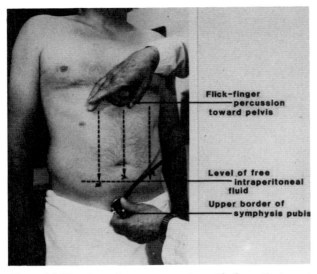

Figure 20-13. *Auscultatory percussion with the patient erect may turn out to be more sensitive than with the patient prone. Photograph courtesy of Dr. J.R. Guarino of Idaho.*

baseline (at the upper edge of the diaphragm piece, which has a diameter of 4.5 cm), due to compression of the abdominal viscera. A change in note occurring above the pelvic baseline is strongly suggestive of intraperitoneal fluid. The demarcation disappears when the patient lies down and the fluid gravitates back into the flanks, and reappears after 3 minutes of the upright posture (Guarino, 1986).

In a study of patients undergoing ambulatory peritoneal dialysis, 140 ml of fluid could be detected with good agreement between observers. A clearer end point was obtained with a hand-held ultrasound instrument than with a conventional stethoscope (McLean, 1987).

Blaxland's method. The differentiation of ascites from a massive ovarian cyst is given in Chapter 22 (p. 407). Fortunately, it is rarely needed, as most ovarian cysts do not become large enough to produce dullness in the flanks.

Sensitivity and Specificity of Various Signs of Ascites

The sensitivity and specificity for various physical maneuvers in the detection of ascites are shown in Table 20-2. Comparable (and generally lower) figures for paracentesis and the abdominal roentgenogram are also shown. Finally, the only superior examiner in the two papers was examiner 3 in Cattau et al., 1982; his results are given separately in terms of percentage accuracy. Note his 89% overall physical examination diagnostic accuracy despite the lower figures for the individual maneuvers.

Examination of the Liver

Inspection

Infrequently, a cirrhotic or cancerous liver may be observed during inspiration. Formerly, it was most often seen during inspection for Litten's sign (descent of the diaphragm observed in the axillary intercostal interspaces, see Ch. 16, p. 248).

Palpation

Hanger, a clinician who invented one of the first liver function tests (the cephalin flocculation test), used to say that as far as the

liver is concerned, one good feel is worth two good laboratory tests.

A method:

1. With the patient supine, and the physician at the patient's right, the examining hand is placed on the abdomen and moved downward and cephalad as the patient is instructed to take a deep breath. The deep inspiration flattens the diaphragm and moves the liver down against the examiner's exploring hand.

Some examiners (pokers) place the hand on the abdominal wall, parallel to the rectus muscle, with fingers pointing toward the patient's head, and poke for the edge of the liver. However, Dr. Frank Iber of Illinois is of the opinion that most contemporary hepatologists are hookers rather than pokers. By this he means that they palpate the liver with the fingers (pointing at the patient's feet) hooked gently into the abdomen. In this way, the more sensitive finger pads (rather than the finger tips) are facing the liver edge. A position that is *not* optimal is to place the fingers parallel to the ribs instead of to the rectus muscle, so that you are not feeling with all your fingers.

2. Some examiners use the left hand to push adipose and other redundant tissue out of the way of the palpating right hand.

3. There are two technical problems related to the abdominal musculature. First, some persons have difficulty relaxing their abdominal muscles, even with their knees and hips flexed. This is especially true when a strange, threatening person (the physician) is pushing on them. A better examination can be obtained in such subjects by the judicious administration of vocal anesthesia. For example, at the first sign of resistance, say slowly and softly : "Just take it easy . . . breathe comfortably . . . just pretend that my hand is going to fall down through your abdomen . . . all the way through your abdomen through your back . . . my hand is going all the way through your body to the bed, down to the floor." (Students have pointed out to me that when I do this, my voice assumes a dull, monotonous tone, and it sounds as though I am trying to induce a hypnotic trance.)

A second problem, which causes a false positive, is that in some cases the anterior abdominal muscles overlap as they insert into the inferior rib cage. One is occasionally fooled into thinking one is feeling the liver when one is really feeling well-developed muscles. Since such healthy persons tend to develop their muscles symmetrically, just palpate under the left costal margin. If another "liver" is felt there, of the same size, shape, and consistency as on the right, you have not yet palpated the true liver.

4. There are two technical reasons for missing the liver during palpation: 1) severe abdominal distention, as with ascites, so that the exploring hand can never get down to the liver; and 2) failure to begin the search far enough caudad, in a patient with massive hepatomegaly. If one begins cephalad to the liver edge, one might work all the way up to the right costal margin and never "catch the edge." This last is remediable!

The purposes of palpation are:

1. To evaluate consistency;
2. To feel the liver for nodules;
3. To find extremely large, clearly abnormal livers; and
4. To detect systolic pulsations.

1. A stony hard liver is usually due to tumor; a very hard liver with a sharp hard edge is usually cirrhotic; and a moderately firm liver may be due to acute passive congestion, which causes tension in Glisson's capsule. Soft "normal" livers may be felt in fatty infiltration of the liver, but are usually not massively enlarged.

2. When nodules are found by palpation, they are usually due to cancer rather than nodular cirrhosis.

Dr. Iber believes that he can discriminate nodular livers. Tumors are said to be reliably differentiated from cirrhosis in that the former are "mountains on a plateau," whereas cirrhosis feels like "rivers on a plain."

3. It is to be emphasized that the liver is *not* palpated for the purposes of determining its *exact* size. That requires percussion, the scratch test, or auscultatory percussion (see p. 384).

A palpable liver is not necessarily enlarged. Using palpability as a sign of enlargement has a 54% false-positive rate if liver size is judged by the hepatic scintiscan (Rosenfield et al., 1974). This fact seems to be rediscovered every few years (Ariel & Briceno, 1976; Meyhoff et al., 1979; Naftalis & Leevy, 1963; Peternel et al., 1966; Riemenschneider & Whalen, 1965), but is forgotten even more often (Halpern et al., 1974).

Aside from the variability in palpatory measurements (Meyhoff et al., 1979), the length of a line cannot be determined just by knowing where it ends with respect to the right costal margin; one must also know where it begins. Yet our most influential and popular medical journals publish clinical pathological conferences with liver measurements in "finger-breadths below the costal border" units, a meaningless measure, even if all examiners had uniform finger-breadths and took care to take the measurement at the same phase of respiration.

In measuring the craniocaudal dimension of the liver in the right midclavicular line, many workers use a combination of percussion of the upper border and palpation of the lower border. Unfortunately, the lower border is often not palpable. Additionally, there are no scientifically verified normal values for this procedure. Finally, with this technique the mean maximum variation between four clinicians was 8 cm (Blendis et al., 1970).

When I have simultaneously determined a liver size by percussion-to-palpation, and again by percussion-to-percussion (vide infra), the value obtained from the former is always greater than that obtained from the latter. The reason is that it is possible to get a hollow percussion sound over the inferior, thin edge of the liver and so underestimate its true size. This fact also explains why different techniques of liver percussion also yield different normal values (vide infra).

4. *Expansive systolic hepatic pulsations:* These are frequently discussed as a sign of tricuspid insufficiency (see Ch. 17, p. 322) or aortic insufficiency (see Ch. 17, p. 312). It is less well appreciated that most *true* hepatic expansile pulsations (as distinct from the false positives due to misinterpretation of aortic pulse transmission) are not of either of these etiologies, but are presystolic hepatic venous pulsations. The last generally have the same diagnostic significance as large A waves in the jugular venous pulse (see Ch. 19, p. 364). (See Ch. 17, p. 312, for the method of distinguishing expansile hepatic pulsations from hepatic bouncing due to transmitted aortic pulsations.)

Percussion

Some examiners recommend fist percussion over the liver to elicit the tenderness of hepatitis.

The remainder of this section is only concerned with determining hepatic size.

A method:

1. Have the supine patient breathe quietly.

2. Percuss in the right midclavicular line, going from resonance to dullness. Use a (hard) percussion note. (The tone should be easily audible to the examiner when standing upright.)

3. Determine the upper and lower borders of dullness, and measure the span between them.

Normal values are available for hepatic dullness from a nomogram (Castell et al., 1969), although this method severely underestimates the true size of the liver as determined by ultrasound (Homeida et al., 1976; Sapira & Williamson, 1979) or scintiscanning (Sullivan et al., 1976). This is because it is difficult to locate the dome of the liver by percussion, and because it is possible to obtain a resonant percussion note over a very thin lower edge of the liver.

In the benchmark study (Castell et al., 1969), liver dullness was determined in 116 normal subjects. No independent covariable (e.g., ultrasound) was used. The mean liver dullness in the right midclavicular line for males (in centimeters) was found to be 0.032 times the weight (in pounds), plus 0.18 times the height (in inches), minus 7.86. For females, the mean liver dullness in the right midclavicular line was given by 0.027 times the weight (in pounds), plus 0.22 times the height (in inches), minus 10.75. The 95% confidence limits were plus or minus 3 cm. A slide rule based on these calculations was developed by the Upjohn Company under the trade name Hepat-A-Rule.

Williamson's method:

1. Have the patient hold his breath in deep inspiration during percussion. (This flattens the diaphragmatic dome, thus decreasing the error of underestimation.)

2. Percuss in the right midclavicular line to determine upper and lower borders of hepatic dullness. Use an *extremely* soft percussion note (i.e., one that can be heard only if the examiner places his ear close to the patient).

This method gives measurements closer to those from ultrasound (Sapira & Williamson, 1979) and a formula for converting to the true (ultrasound) value: $U = (G - 4.44)/.603$, where U is the ultrasonically determined craniocaudal dimension of the liver in the right midclavicular line (in centimeters) and G (for gentle) is the same dimension (in centimeters) by Williamson's technique. However, since there are currently no normal values for adult liver size by ultrasound (no "gold standard"), the neophyte is advised to try both techniques: the former for the purpose of comparing the value with normal "dullness," and the latter against that future date when normal values for liver size have become available.

Any given technique of percussion will yield intraobserver and interobserver variations of a little more than 2 cm (Castell et al., 1969; Malchow-Moller et al., 1984). Thus, each examiner probably needs to record his method, his own data, and his impressions (normal, large, or indeterminate).

Auscultation

The etiologies of murmurs over the right upper quadrant are listed on page 378. If there is no hepatomegaly or if there is a friction rub, hepatic murmurs that do not change with position or respiration tend to be due to neoplasia.

Murmurs heard only over the left lobe of the liver, which decrease with standing or in the lateral decubitus position, are more properly called epigastric bruits. Although they may be found with cirrhosis or neoplastic disease, they are thought to actually represent aortic compression by an enlarged liver (Sherman & Hardison, 1979).

Special Maneuvers

Auscultatory percussion and the "scratch test" (see Ch. 17, p. 309) have also been used to estimate hepatic size as well as contour. The examiner places his stethoscope just beneath the xiphoid and percusses or scratches, moving from the lower abdomen toward the costal margin, noting the point at which the percussion blow or scratch sound becomes greatly increased (Kukowka, 1972). Obviously, the percussion blows or scratches must be of constant intensity.

Many persons have difficulty with the scratch test because they scratch too vigorously and thus tighten the skin, producing false positives. One should scratch lightly and in a direction parallel to that of the expected liver edge. If the skin is already tightly stretched, as in severe ascites, one may obtain a false positive.

The scratch test has been the subject of only one comparative study, in which it was found to be as good as (or as bad as) the techniques of palpation and (nonauscultatory) percussion for finding the lower edge of the liver, when compared with the results of a liver scintiscan. By almost any technique, the midclavicular dimension could be obtained in half the subjects within 3 cm of that obtained by scintiscan (Sullivan et al., 1976). Given that the accuracy of the hepatic scintiscan in that study is also unknown, I am not sure that the examiners were as imprecise as they thought themselves to be. (Three observers gave unanimous opinions about the normality or abnormality of liver size in only 50% to 55% of scintiscans [Meyhoff et al., 1979].)

Of course, both the scratch test and auscultatory percussion should be used only when the lower boundary of the liver extends beneath the right costal margin. Thus, these methods are not useful with small livers (or with advanced liver disease accompanied by ascites).

Examination of the Spleen

Inspection

Inspect the abdomen during inspiration, and see whether a left upper quadrant mass descends. (If it does, it *might* be the spleen.)

Palpation

The spleen, in contrast to other masses in the left upper quadrant, moves greatly with inspiration and *may* have a readily palpable notch (the splenic hilus).

Several methods:

1. With the patient supine, stand at the patient's right, and feel for the spleen with your right hand below the costal margin, pressing your fingers in deeply. (The examining fingertips will be felt to ride momentarily over the edge of the spleen at the zenith of inspiration.)

In cases of extreme splenomegaly, you may not catch the lower edge of the spleen, the palpating hand being above it. Thus, a general sensation of resistance in this position requires moving the palpating hand down into the lower left quadrant, and slowly inching up, so as to catch the lower edge of such elephantine spleens.

a. The above method may be improved upon by placing the left hand in the subcostovertebral area and (simultaneously with the right hand's palpation), pulling upwards with the left hand so as to provide a better definition of the spleen.

b. In very obese patients, it may be necessary to place the left hand more anteriorly so that it can press away intervening adiposity. However, in patients who are very fat, this trick seldom finds a spleen that is not apparent to percussion (vide infra).

c. Bailey (Clain, 1973) suggests placing the left hand over the lateral aspect of the costal margin and drawing the skin and subcutaneous tissues downward toward the right hand. This leaves a loose fold of skin under the costal margin.

d. To avoid pushing the spleen away, some suggest placing only the index finger lightly just below the left costal margin (Lipp et al., 1944).

2. Place the patient who is placed in a *modified* right lateral decubitus position; modified, in that the flexed right arm supports the dependent right rib cage, throwing the left subcostal area into aerial relief. Stand behind the patient and palpate with the right hand anterior to the left hand, the latter being at the posterior axillary line. The pulp of the fingers "hooks" over the costal margin and down to the spleen edge.

3. Have the patient sit in a chair while you lean over the patient's left shoulder from behind. Palpate with your left hand in the patient's left anterior axillary line, and your right hand medial to the left, covering the subcostal area from the left midclavicular line laterally. Both hands feel for the spleen.

4. Place the patient in the prone position, supporting himself on knees and elbows or knees and chest. Standing at his left, use your hand to try to catch a spleen tip.

I have not yet been able to palpate a spleen by the third or fourth method that was not apparent from examination by the first or second method.

In all positions, the patient should be instructed to breathe *deeply* so that the left hemidiaphragm will move the spleen down into the palpating range. Because many patients respond by tensing the abdominal muscles, give the instruction to breathe deeply *after* you have positioned your hands.

If you are not sure whether you have felt a spleen tip, ask the patient to report his sensations. He will often describe a "catching" sensation if indeed his spleen has touched your hand or fingers.

5. Place a pillow beneath the knees of the supine patient. Have the patient push the spleen forward by placing his left fist beneath his ribs. Stand on the left side of the patient's head and search with the fingers of both hands under the left costal margin ("Bailey," Clain, 1973).

6. A Russian method involves rotating the patient into the right lateral decubitus position and palpating with the right hand, with the examiner remaining on the right side of the bed (Povzhitov & Mironets, 1978). A detailed description is also available in English (Mitchell, 1973). Using the left hand to palpate, with the patient in the same position, makes this a Danish method (Videbaek et al., 1982).

7. A unique Danish method involves rotating the patient into the left lateral decubitus position (Videbaek et al., 1982).

8. It has been claimed that splenic palpation may be facilitated by having the patient jump up and down 20 to 25 times before palpation, which is carried out by having the patient stand in front of the examiner and bend slightly forward (Bremen, 1973).

9. Bimanual palpation, the right reinforcing the costovertebral space and the left feeling below the left costal margin, may be employed with the patient standing (Lipp et al., 1944).

Quantitating spleen size. A semiquantitative system for measuring spleen size (Hackett, 1944) is given in Fig. 20-14.

False positives:

1. *Pseudosplenomegaly,* in my experience, is most commonly due to colonic feces. In general, a very large mass will turn out to be the spleen, not feces. (The splenic notch has not proved to be helpful in making the distinction because it is not usually identifiable with absolute certainty.) The gold standard for distinguishing the two is reexamination after purgation or enema.

Renal cysts and tumors, the left lobe of the liver, and lower costal cartilages have also been misidentified as the spleen.

2. Many palpable spleens are neither pathologic nor enlarged (Dell & Klinefelter, 1946). Palpable but not pathologic spleens have been found in 2.3% to 3.8% of patients in an office practice (Lipp et al., 1944); 3% of presumably normal college freshmen (McIntyre & Ebaugh, 1967); 10.4% of hospitalized patients who were having liver scans (Sullivan & Williams, 1976); and 12% of women in the immediate postpartum period who had extreme relaxation of their abdominal musculature (Berris, 1966).

Sensitivity. The reported sensitivities for palpation of splenomegaly range from 28% (Halpern et al., 1974) to 100% (Aito, 1974).

Actually, the sensitivity increases with increasing size of the spleen on scintiscan, being 50% for moderately enlarged spleens (600 to 750 g) and 80% for greatly enlarged spleens (900 to 1,600 g), and approaching 100% with the largest spleens (>2,350 g) (Fischer, 1971; Fischer & Wolf, 1973).

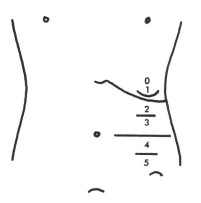

Figure 20-14. *Hackett's semiquantitative system for measuring spleen size. 0, normal or nonpalpated spleen ("negative" spleen); 1, spleen palpable only when the subject draws a deep breath; 2, spleens ranging from those at the costal margin palpable without assistance from the subject to those whose lower border reaches a point halfway to a horizontal line through the umbilicus; 3, spleens projecting more than halfway to the umbilical level but not beyond it; 4, spleens below the umbilical level but not more than halfway to the line of the symphysis pubis; 5, all spleens larger than those mentioned above.*

Interrater reliability. All four observers agreed on the presence or absence of splenomegaly by palpation in 88% of 32 patients (Blendis et al., 1970).

Hardness. Once you have palpated the spleen, it is important to attempt to determine whether it is hard like a Genoa or kosher salami or merely tense like an uncooked wiener. If hard ("firm"), the splenomegaly is fibrotic and thus chronic, as in 44% of patients with Laennec's cirrhosis (Ratnoff & Patek, 1942). If merely tense, the splenomegaly is acute.

Percussion

○ *A method.* Percuss over the lowest intercostal space in the left anterior axillary line, during expiration and deep inspiration (Castell, 1967; Castell & Frank, 1977). Enlarged but nonpalpable spleens will cause a dullness of the percussion note during deep inspiration, with resonance returning during expiration, when the diaphragm and spleen again move cephalad.

This technique is best learned upon a patient whose palpable splenomegaly is resolving. Daily examinations will determine a point at which the percussion sign is still positive although the examiner can no longer definitely feel the spleen tip. Resolving splenomegaly of this type is commonly found in infectious mononucleosis, viral hepatitis, and about 10% of patients with thyrotoxicosis who have just been definitively treated.

Another method. In a resurrection of a 19th century technique, splenomegaly has been evaluated by percussing the spleen outline with the patient in the right lateral decubitus position (Nixon, 1954). Normal values were not determined.

Significance. In the only study that directly compared Nixon's percussion method and Castell's percussion method on the same 48 normal and 17 enlarged spleens, using the spleen scintiscan as the independent covariable, Castell's technique was found to be more sensitive (82%) than palpation in two positions (70%), but also had a higher false-positive rate (17%). Conversely, Nixon's method was found to be less sensitive (59%) than palpation, but had a lower false-positive rate (6%) (Sullivan & Williams, 1976).

When using scintiscans as an independent covariable, remember their high rate of false positives when compared with the plain radiographic length of the spleen (Westin et al., 1972), a point often documented but rarely acknowledged (Aito, 1974). Although the scintiscan is considered to be an "objective" test, sanctified as revealed truth by virtue of being typed on a laboratory slip, in fact the interpretation is also quite subjective, especially in the absence of scientifically determined normal values for spleen size (Sapira, 1981).

Differential Diagnosis of Splenomegaly

While many books of differential diagnosis list dozens of entities under splenomegaly, it is possible to shorten the lists drastically by using combinations of findings or modifiers of findings. (The power of combinations of nonspecific findings are explained in Ch. 27, pp. 536–537). The specific lists were suggested by those in Major (Delp & Manning, 1975) and so are based upon the experiences of Dameshek, Welsch, Major, Delp, Manning, and Wilson. Two reminders are needed. First, all diagnostic medicine is playing the odds; thus, in any given case there is a small chance that through omission a listing (iterative) method may not initially include the correct diagnosis. Second, it is most efficient to place the lists in order of increasing length and hence decreasing utility, as in Table 20-3.

Table 20-3.   Differential Diagnosis of Splenomegaly

A. Splenomegaly in the presence of intense jaundice (i.e., total bilirubin greater than 10 mg/dl)
   1. Hepatic disease with portal hypertension
B. Splenomegaly and less-than-intense jaundice
   1. Hepatic disease with portal hypertension
   2. Hemolytic anemia
C. Splenomegaly and pallor
   1. Leukemia
   2. Lymphoma
   3. Hypersplenism of any cause
D. Splenomegaly and significant lymph node enlargement
   1. Lymphocytic leukemia
   2. Lymphoma
   3. Sarcoidosis
E. Splenomegaly and hepatomegaly
   1. Hepatic disease with portal hypertension
   2. Leukemia
   3. Polycythemia vera
   4. Hemolytic anemia
   5. Myeloid metaplasia
   6. Gaucher's disease
F. Massive splenomegaly (i.e., a spleen that is clearly below the umbilicus even during expiration, a "4" or "5" on the spleen-o-meter in Fig. 20-14)
   1. Chronic granulocytic leukemia
   2. Myeloid metaplasia
   3. Polycythemia vera
   4. Hodgkin's disease
   5. Malaria
   6. Kala-azar
   7. Gaucher's disease
G. Smaller spleens than in F
   1. Infections
   2. Pernicious anemia
   3. Hemolytic anemia
   4. Sarcoidosis
   5. Acute leukemia
   6. Hepatic disease with portal hypertension
   7. Chronic lymphocytic leukemia
   8. Other lymphomas
   9. Any of the entities in list F, during the time the spleen is enlarging to its maximum

Self-Study.   Combinations of lists may be used. Prove to yourself the power of lists and combinations by noting the diagnostic possibilities for a patient with hepatomegaly, massive splenomegaly, and a normal hematocrit. Write them down, now, before referring to Appendix 20-3.

Auscultation

Bruits and rubs over the spleen are discussed on page 378.

Splenic Rupture

■ Usually there is a history of abdominal trauma, which may be followed by a deceptive period of relative freedom from symptoms. At presentation, there may be tenderness in the left upper quadrant, abdominal rigidity (in about half the cases), and even shock.
   Special maneuvers helpful in the diagnosis include shifting dullness and referred pain or hyperesthesia in the shoulder (usually but not invariably the left, called Kehr's sign). The last is *not* made worse by movement of the joint or pressure over the site, but rather by having the patient lie supine for about 10 minutes with the foot of the bed raised 0.5 m. If the peritoneal cavity contains liquid blood,

this maneuver will cause it to gravitate toward the diaphragm, bringing on the symptoms and signs of diaphragmatic irritation ("Bailey," Clain, 1973).

Gallbladder

Murphy's Sign

A method.   A modification of Moynihan's method of eliciting Murphy's sign of acute cholecystitis is as follows:

   1. With the patient supine, place your left hand, with your fingers pointing toward the midline, on the patient's lowermost right anterior rib cage, so that your index finger is reposing on the most inferior rib. Although the exact location of the gallbladder is more variable than suggested by most textbooks, some part of your thumb will now be resting over an area to which the patient's gallbladder can be brought by deep inspiration ("x" marks the spot in Fig. 20-7).

   2. Abduct your extended left thumb, rotating it in opposition down and into the patient's belly and hold it there.

   3. Instruct the patient to take a deep breath.

   4. Keep your thumb where it is. Do not lean on the patient's rib cage. If you are doing the test correctly, you should feel the rib cage move up toward you during the inspiration.

   5. When the inflamed gallbladder is driven down to a point at or near the indentation produced by your thumb, the patient will experience pain or tenderness sufficient to cause an abrupt halt in inspiration. This often occurs only toward the end of inspiration.

   6. Repeat with a placebo maneuver. Put your hand in the same position, but do not push in with your thumb. If the patient can now complete a full inspiration, whereas he could not do so before, Murphy's sign is positive for acute cholecystitis.

   Unfortunately, Murphy's sign has a sensitivity of only 27% (Gunn & Keddie, 1972).

Other

Signs of an acutely inflamed gallbladder are Boas' sign (p. 375) and the gallbladder rub (p. 379).

Courvoisier's Law

Courvoisier's "law" states that an enlarged gallbladder in the presence of (obstructive) jaundice is due to cancer rather than to cholecystitis with cholelithiasis. The underlying thesis is that the chronically scarred gallbladder cannot expand, but the one acutely obstructed by neoplasia can. But in fact, the gallbladder *was* enlarged in 20% of cases of jaundice due to cholelithiasis. In the same series, the gallbladder was *not* enlarged in 8% of cases of jaundice due to a cause other than a stone (e.g., cancer) (Courvoisier, 1890).

Caveats:

   1. The law is applicable only in jaundiced patients.

   2. The law is based upon a pathologic experience in 19th century Europe. We have no information about the operation of the law for a 20th century clinician trying to palpate, in vivo, the gallbladder of an obese American.

   3. Since neither the normal-sized gallbladder nor the enlarged gallbladder perfectly predicted the presence or absence of either stones or cancer, it is doubtful that Courvoisier's law is actually a law, except in the sense that a speed limit is a law.

The Kidneys

Falstaff: Sirrah, you giant, what says the doctor to my water?
Page: He said, sir, the water itself was good healthy water; but

for the party that owned it, he might have more diseases than he knew of.*

Shakespeare, *King Henry IV*, Part II, Act I, Scene II

Inspection

In modern times, kidneys are inspected by means of intravenous pyelography or ultrasound. Curiously, the sectional area of both kidneys as measured planimetrically in square centimeters is about the same as the individual's height in inches (Black, 1962).

As a rule, the kidneys will not differ in size by more than 1.5 cm. Irrespective of the adult patient's body size, a kidney less than 10 cm in length is suspicious, as is one greater than 15 cm.

Much can be learned about the kidney by inspection of the urine (see Ch. 28, p. 548).

Palpation

In thin subjects, it is possible to palpate one and often both kidneys bimanually.

A method. Attempt to palpate the right kidney in the following manner:

1. With the patient supine and the examiner standing comfortably at the patient's right, put the left examining hand behind the patient's right loin. Put your right hand in the right upper quadrant or below the lower edge of the liver (which you have already located) and gently push your right hand down and your left hand up.

2. Before you begin to push, and as you move your hands toward each other, say to the patient in a gentle, calm voice, "I want you to pretend that my hand is going to fall down through your belly; all the way through the back of your body; all the way through the bed; down to the floor," all the while increasing the pressure.

3. In the case of a palpable kidney, you are most likely to feel the rounded edge by moving your right hand down and medially. If you can palpate the kidney but are not hitting the lower edge, work your fingers inferiorly and medially to be sure that you are not feeling a horseshoe kidney.

4. Then work your right hand as high up as you can, and try to get some estimate of the size and texture of the kidney.

5. Repeat for the left kidney, mutatis mutandis.

Variations on the theme. Some workers palpate for the kidney with one hand, putting four fingers under the flank and pressing the thumb down from above. Others use the bimanual approach, but have the patient assume the lateral decubitus position, always examining the superior side.

Findings. As with other findings that have come down to us from the 19th century masters, kidney palpation was perfected in underfed middle European clinic patients. Except for a few ectomorphs, such persons are less frequently encountered these days. Inability to feel the kidneys through several centimeters of adipose tissue is of little use in the negative sense. (In fact, if you can feel the kidneys in a fat person, it might suggest an abnormality, the strength of the suggestion being in direct proportion to the patient's adiposity.)

To emphasize the fact that normal subjects (especially if large

and skinny) may have palpable kidneys, consider a recent study of members of a family that had some members with polycystic kidney diseases, wherein the examiners found at least one palpable kidney in 14% of those family members subsequently shown *not* to have polycystic kidneys (Gabow et al., 1984).

Palpably enlarged kidneys bilaterally should suggest the possibility that the patient has polycystic kidney disease or bilateral hydronephrosis.

If *one* kidney is palpably enlarged, think of hydronephrosis if it is tender and firm. If it is stony hard, the diagnosis is carcinoma until proven otherwise.

But we can rarely be certain that a hard mass in the right or left upper quadrant is carcinoma of the kidney.

A hard mass on the right is more likely to be colonic carcinoma than a kidney carcinoma. And the more caudally that one feels the hard mass, the more likely it is to be colonic rather than renal.

On the left, one is more likely to be feeling carcinoma of the kidney than carcinoma of the colon. Pancreatic carcinoma comes in a distant third followed by the spleen, the *bête noire* of the novice. (See p. 385 to review distinguishing features of the palpable spleen.) These discriminatory features are mentioned here in an archival sense as I expect them to be lost in the coming decades due to the technique of abdominal ultrasound, the Golem* of modern medicine.

The horseshoe kidney is the only type that will be palpable crossing the midline.

Percussion

A method. Simply punch with the ulnar surface of your fist over the right and left kidneys (with equal force). One wishes to strike hard enough to jar diseased bone or viscera, but not so hard as to produce pain in normal structures. For this purpose, start the blow no more than 6 inches (15 cm) from the back.

Significance. Acute pyelonephritis, perinephritis, and renal abscess may manifest as punch tenderness over the kidney. These tend to be unilateral as do the false positives due to the rare retrocecal appendix (on the right) or an inflamed Meckel's diverticulum. False positives due to musculoskeletal disease are usually, but not always, bilateral.

"Intrinsic renal disease," such as chronic interstitial fibrosis, arteriolar nephrosclerosis, and Kimmelstiel-Wilson disease, does *not* cause tenderness either to punch or thumb pressure (vide infra), despite statements to the contrary.

Thumb pressure test. Sometimes, the thumb pressure test may be helpful in making the distinction between tenderness due to kidney disease and that due to musculoskeletal disease. Applying pressure very slowly, push your thumbs as firmly as you can over the same costovertebral areas that elicited punch tenderness. If this procedure does *not* cause tenderness, it is presumed that the patient is more likely to have pyelonephritis than musculoskeletal disease of the back. However, a positive test (tenderness) is of no help.

Auscultation

Auscultation of the renal arteries is discussed in Chapter 18 (p. 348).

---

*Examination of the urine was a well-established practice in Elizabethan times.

---

*The Golem was a homunculus created out of inanimate matter by magic, as in the Frankenstein legend. Abdominal ultrasound reminds me of the Golem of Prague in that it is quite useful provided that it comes down from the attic only when its master calls for it. It is like the Golem of Chelm in that it can create terrible confusion when it is permitted to run amuck among the thoughtless. Remember, Frankenstein was the name of the doctor.

The Bladder

The urinary bladder may be palpable in thin persons if greatly distended, or fibrosed due to radiation therapy. Otherwise, bladder distention must be diagnosed by auscultatory percussion (Guarino, 1981) as follows:

With the patient supine, place the diaphragm (Guarino, 1985) of the stethoscope above the symphysis pubis in the midline, and hold it there with one hand (Fig. 20-15A). With the pulp of one finger of the other hand, percuss along the vertical midline, beginning above the umbilicus and proceeding caudad one finger width at a time until there is a sharp change: an increased volume of the percussion note. This is the upper edge of the bladder, as can be verified with phonoscopy (Fig. 20-15B).

The distance above the symphysis pubis at which the percussion note changed was shown to predict accurately the likelihood that the patient had a full bladder, defined as at least 250 ml of urine on subsequent catheterization (Table 20-4).

If you think you have detected a large bladder by this technique, try percussing the lateral borders in a similar manner. The distended, enlarged bladder assumes an ellipsoid outline in the frontal percussed representation.

The great Czech physician and professor of medicine at Vienna, Joseph Skoda, could diagnose bladder stone by ausculting at the symphysis pubis and listening to the friction of a catheter rubbing against the bladder stone (Sakula, 1981).

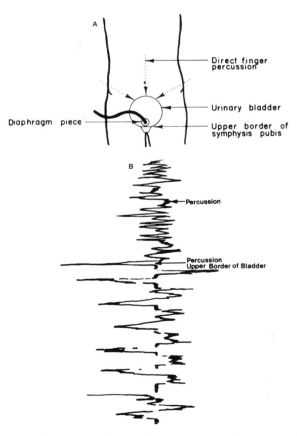

Figure 20-15. *A, Auscultatory percussion of the bladder. B, Phonoscopy tracing of a 33-year-old woman with a distended urinary bladder. A sharp, loud change in note with auscultatory percussion defines the upper border of the bladder.*

Table 20-4. Auscultatory Percussion for Determining Bladder Distention

Distance Above the Symphysis Pubis at Which the Percussion Note Changed	Likelihood of a Full Bladder
0–6.5 cm[a]	0%
6.5–7.5 cm	43%
7.5–9.5 cm	91%
Greater than 9.5 cm	100%

Source: *Guarino (1985).*

[a]*Measurements to the right of the decimal point not to be taken too seriously.*

The Pancreas

The pancreas is an organ that, in its normal condition, cannot be inspected, palpated, percussed, or ausculted. The diagnostic perfidiousness of the pancreas was remembered by medical students of my time when they were asked in anatomy class: "How is the pancreas like a faithless woman?" (Because all day long it lies in the arms of the duodenum, but at night gives its tail to the spleen.)

Nevertheless, in a diseased state, the pancreas can produce physical findings.

Inspection

A pancreatic pseudocyst or hemorrhagic pancreatitis may produce visible signs (see pp. 371 and 372).

Palpation

Between 45% and 65% of pancreatic pseudocysts are palpable (Shatney & Lillehei, 1979), and a diminishing abdominal mass might be a spontaneously draining pseudocyst. Patients with acute or chronic pancreatitis may have Mallet-Guy's sign. Have the patient assume the right lateral decubitus, knee-chest position, and press deeply in the area where splenomegaly might be (but isn't) present. The presence of tenderness, not otherwise elicited, is a positive sign. The explanation is that the overlying organs fall to the right in this position, exposing the body and tail of the pancreas to the direct pressure ("Bailey," Clain, 1973).

Auscultation

Pancreatitis often causes secondary ileus manifesting as absent bowel sounds. A murmur due to compression of the splenic artery occurs in 37% of cases of pancreatic carcinoma (Bauerlein & de la Vega, 1963).

Appendix 20-1. Differential Diagnosis of Patient in Figure 20-5

In the patient shown in Figure 20-5, pregnancy is doubtful from the apparent age. Ovarian cyst would not explain the tissue in the patient's hand. She might be coughing due to metastatic disease or tuberculous disease, which might also involve the liver and/or peritoneum. Therefore, I favor the diagnosis of ascites.

Appendix 20-2. Which Side Has the Perinephric Abscess?

If the patient in Figure 20-7 actually had a perinephric abscess, it would be on the right, because the patient is bent over toward that side. The pain could be aggravated by having the patient bend back toward the left.

Appendix 20-3. Answer to Self-Study on Page 386.

The diagnostic possibilities for the triad of hepatomegaly, massive splenomegaly, and a normal hematocrit are myeloid metaplasia, chronic granulocytic leukemia, and Gaucher's disease.

References

Aito H: The estimation of the size of the spleen by radiological methods. *Ann Clin Res* 15 (Suppl 6):5–54, 1974.

Ariel IM, Briceno M: The disparity of the size of the liver as determined by physical examination and by hepatic gammascanning in 504 patients. *Med Pediatr Oncol* 2:69–73, 1976.

Bauerlein TC, de la Vega F: A diagnostic sign of carcinoma of the body and tail of the pancreas. *Gastroenterology* 44:816, 1963.

Benner EJ, Labby DH: Hepatoma: Clinical experiences with a frequently bizarre tumor. *Ann Intern Med* 54:620–635, 1961.

Berris B: The incidence of palpable liver and spleen in the postpartum period. *Can Med Assoc J* 95:1318–1319, 1966.

Bjorkman SE: On the occurrence of a vascular murmur over greatly enlarged spleens. *Acta Med Scand* 145:79–83, 1953.

Black DAK: *Renal Disease*. FA Davis, Philadelphia, 1962.

Blendis LM, McNeilly, Sheppard L, Williams R, Laws JW: Observer variation in the clinical and radiological assessment of hepatosplenomegaly. *Br Med J* 1:727–730, 1970.

Bloom HJG: Venous hums in hepatic cirrhosis. *Br Heart J* 12:343–350, 1950.

Bremen JG: Spleen palpation aided by gravity. *Lancet* 1:1448–1449, 1973.

Cassel WG, Spittel JA, Ellis FH Jr, and Bruwer, AJ: Arteriovenous fistula of the splenic vessels producing ascites. *Circulation* 16:1077–1083, 1957.

Castell DO: The spleen percussion sign. *Ann Intern Med* 67:1265–1267, 1967.

Castell DO, Frank BB: Abdominal examination role of percussion and auscultation. *Postgrad Med* 62:131–134, 1977.

Castell DO, O'Brien KD, Muench H, Chalmers TC: Estimation of liver size by percussion in normal individuals. *Ann Intern Med* 70:1183–1189, 1969.

Cattau EL, Benjamin SB, Snuff TE, Castell DO: The accuracy of the physical examination in the diagnosis of suspected ascites. *JAMA* 247:1164–1166, 1982.

Celoria GM, Friedmann P, Rhee SW, Berman J: Fistulas between the aorta and the left renal vein. *J Vasc Surg* 6:191–193, 1987.

Cheng TO, Sutton GC, Sutton DC: Cruveilhier-Baumgarten syndrome: Review of the literature and report of a case. *Am J Med* 17:143–150, 1954.

Clain A, ed: *Hamilton Bailey's Demonstrations of Physical Signs in Clinical Surgery*, ed 15. Williams & Wilkins, Baltimore, 1973.

Clain D, Wartnaby K, Sherlock S: Abdominal arterial murmurs in liver disease. *Lancet* 2:516–519, 1966.

Courvoisier LG: *Casuistisch-Statistische Beiträge zur Pathologie und Chirurgie der Gallenwege*. Verlag von FCW Vogel, Leipzig, 1890.

Cullen TS: A new sign in ruptured ectopic pregnancy. *Am J Obstet Gynecol* 78:457, 1918.

Cummings S, Papadakis M, Melnick J, Gooding GAW, Tierney LM Jr: The predictive value of physical examinations for ascites. *West J Med* 142:633–636, 1985.

Dell JM, Klinefelter HF: Roentgen studies of the spleen. *Am J Med Sci* 211:437–442, 1946.

Delp MH, Manning RT: *Major's Physical Diagnosis*. WB Saunders, Philadelphia, 1975.

Dennis C: Current procedure in management of obstruction of the small intestine. *JAMA* 154:463–470, 1954.

Dickson AP, Imrie CW: The incidence and prognosis of body wall ecchymosis in acute pancreatitis. *Surg Gynecol Obstet* 159:343–347, 1984.

Edwards AJ, Hamilton JD, Nichol WD, Taylor GW, Dawson AM: Experience with coeliac axis compression syndrome. *Br Med J* 1:342–345, 1970.

Fenster LF, Klatskin G: Manifestations of metastatic tumors of the liver. *Am J Med* 31:238–248, 1961.

Fischer J: Hypersplenismus. *Internist* 12:176–186, 1971.

Fischer J, Wolf R: Die Milzszintigraphie [the spleen scan]. *Deutsche Artzeblatt* 7:401–408, 1973.

Gabow PA, Ikle DW, Holmes JH: Polycystic kidney disease: Prospective analysis of nonazotemic patients and family members. *Ann Intern Med* 101:238–247, 1984.

Ghosh PB, Rabbat AG, Trudel J, D'Amico P, Lecours R, Trudel J: Celiac compression syndrome. *Can J Surg* 25:377–379, 1982.

Goldstein LI: Enlarged tortuous arteries and hepatic bruit. *JAMA* 206:2518–2520, 1968.

Grim CE, Luft FC, Weinberger MH, Grim CM: Sensitivity and specificity of screening tests for renal vascular hypertension. *Ann Intern Med* 91:617–622, 1979.

Guarino JR: Auscultatory percussion of the bladder to detect urinary retention. *N Engl J Med* 305:70, 1981.

Guarino JR: Auscultatory percussion of the urinary bladder. *Arch Intern Med* 145:1823–1825, 1985.

Guarino JR: Auscultatory percussion to detect ascites. *N Engl J Med* 315:1555–1556, 1986.

Gunn A, Keddie N: Some clinical observations on patients with gallstones. *Lancet* 2:230–241, 1972.

Hackett LW: Spleen measurement in malaria: I. the importance of the spleen survey. *J Natl Malaria Soc* 3:121–133, 1944. [The National Malaria Society is the only American philanthropic society of which I am aware that achieved its goal and then voted itself out of existence.]

Halpern S, Coel M, Ashburn W, Alazraki N, Littenberg R, Hurwitz S, Green J: Correlation of liver and spleen size: Determination by nuclear medicine studies and physical examination. *Arch Intern Med* 134:123–124, 1974.

Harati Y, Niakan E: Diabetic thoracoabdominal neuropathy: A cause for chest and abdominal pain. *Arch Intern Med* 146:1493–1494, 1986.

Hardison JE: Venous hum of the Cruveilhier-Baumgarten syndrome. *Arch Intern Med* 137:1623–1624, 1977.

Hatano R, Iwai T, Goseki N, Kudo G, Hiranamu S, Kojima S, Murakami T, Suzuki S, Aoki N: Multiple aneurysms of the visceral arteries with migrating vascular bruit on postural change: A case report. *Jpn J Surg* 10:48–54, 1980.

Homeida M, Roberts CJC, Halliwell M, Jackson L, Read AE: Ultrasonic measurement of liver size. *Br Med J* 2:1561, 1976.

Jones IG, Lowenthal MN, O'Riordan EC: Hepatic bruit in Hodgkin's disease. *Med J Zambia* 12:80–81, 1978.

Julius S, Stewart BH: Diagnostic significance of abdominal murmurs. *N Engl J Med* 276:1175–1178, 1967.

Kelley ML Jr: Discolorations of flanks and abdominal wall. *Arch Intern Med* 108:132–135, 1961.

Kingston M, Ali MA, Lewall D: Hepatic tumors in Saudi Arabia: A practical approach to diagnosis. *Cancer* 55:1579–1585, 1985.

Kukowka A: Auskultorische Methode zur Bestimmung der Lebergrösse: ein einfaches, probates, Schnellverfahren. *Z Allg Med* 48:1645–1646, 1972.

LaFortune M, Constantin A, Breton G, Légaré AG, Lavoie P: The recanalized umbilical vein in portal hypertension: A myth. *AJR* 144:549–553, 1985.

Lawson JD, Weissbein MC: The puddle sign—an aid in the diagnosis of minimal ascites. *N Engl J Med* 260:652–654, 1959.

Lee RV: Abdominal bruits. *N Engl J Med* 277:313, 1967.

Lipp WF, Eckstein EH, Aaron AH: The clinical significance of the palpable spleen. *Gastroenterology* 3:287–291, 1944.

Mabin TA, Gelfand M: Cullen's sign, a feature in liver disease. *Br Med J* 1:493–494, 1974.

Macklem PT: Respiratory muscle dysfunction. *Hosp Pract* 21:83–96, 1986.

Magee HR, Mellick SA: Aortocaval fistula as a complication of leaking aortic aneurysm. *Br J Surg* 64:239–241, 1977.

Malchow-Moller A, Rasmussen SN, Jensen AM, Keiding N, Skovgaard LT, Juhl E: Clinical estimation of liver size. *Dan Med Bull* 31:63–67, 1984.

McBurney C: Experience with early operative interference in cases of disease of the vermiform appendix. *NY Med J* 50:676–684, 1889.

McFadzean AJS, Gray J: Hepatic venous hum in cirrhosis of liver. *Lancet* 2:1128–1130, 1953.

McIntyre RO, Ebaugh FG: Palpable spleens in college freshmen. *Ann Intern Med* 66:301–306, 1967.

McLaughlin MJ, Colapinto RF, Hobbs BB: Abdominal bruits. *JAMA* 232:1238–1242, 1975.

McLean AC: Diagnosis of ascites by auscultatory percussion and hand-held ultrasound unit. *Lancet* 2:1526–1527, 1987.

McSherry JA: The prevalence of epigastric bruit. *J R Coll Gen Pract* 29:170–172, 1979.

Meyhoff HH, Røder O, Andersen B: Palpatory estimation of liver size. *Acta Chir Scand* 145:479–481, 1979.

Missal ME, Robinson JA, Tatum RW: Inferior vena cava obstruction. *Ann Intern Med* 62:133–138, 1965.

Mitchell JS: Palpation of the spleen. *Lancet* 1:886–887, 1973.

Mohun GE: Abdominal bruits. *N Engl J Med* 277:313, 1976.

Naftalis J, Leevy CM: Clinical estimation of liver size. *Am J Dig Dis* 8:236–243, 1963.

Nixon RK: The detection of splenomegaly by percussion. *N Engl J Med* 250:166–167, 1954.

Odom NJ: Facial expression in acute appendicitis. *Ann R Coll Surg Engl* 64:260–261, 1982.

Peternel WW, Schaefer JW, Schiff L: Clinical evaluation of liver size and hepatic scintiscan. *Am J Dig Dis* 11:346–350, 1966.

Povzhitov NM, Mironets VI: [Methods of spleen palpation]. *Vrach Delo* 5:96–97, 1978.

Ramakrishnan T: Venous hum of the Cruveilhier-Baumgarten syndrome. *Arch Intern Med* 138:826, 1978.

Ratnoff OD, Patek AJ; The natural history of Laennec's cirrhosis of the liver. *Medicine* 21:207–268, 1942.

Riemenschneider PA, Whalen JP: The relative accuracy of estimation of enlargement of the liver and spleen by radiologic and clinical methods. *AJR* 94:462–468, 1965.

Rivin A: Abdominal vascular sounds. *JAMA* 221:688–690, 1972.

Rob C: Surgical diseases of the celiac and mesenteric arteries. *Arch Surg* 93:21–32, 1966.

Rosenfield AT, Laufer I, Schneider PB: The significance of a palpable liver. *Am J Roentgenol Radiat Therapy Nucl Med* 122:313–317, 1974.

Sakula A: Joseph Skoda 1805–1881: A centenary tribute to a pioneer of thoracic medicine. *Thorax* 36:404–411, 1981.

Sapira JD: . . . And how big is the spleen? *South Med J* 74:53–60, 1981.

Sapira JD, Williamson DL: How big is the normal liver? *Arch Intern Med* 139:971–973, 1979.

Sarr MG, Dickson ER, Newcomer AD: Diastolic bruit in chronic intestinal ischemia: Recognition by abdominal phonoangiography. *Dig Dis Sci* 25:761–762, 1980.

Serebro H: A diagnostic sign of carcinoma of the body of the pancreas. *Lancet* 1:85–86, 1965.

Shatney CH, Lillehei RC: Surgical treatment of pancreatic pseudocysts: Analysis of 119 cases. *Ann Surg* 189:386–394, 1979.

Sherman HI, Hardison JE: The importance of a coexistent hepatic rub and bruit: A clue to the diagnosis of cancer in the liver. *JAMA* 241:1495, 1979.

Shumacker HB, Waldhausen JA: Intrahepatic arteriovenous fistula of hepatic artery and portal vein. *Surg Gynecol Obstet* 112:497–501, 1961.

Silen W, ed: *Cope's Early Diagnosis of the Acute Abdomen*, ed 15. Oxford University Press, New York, 1979.

Smith GC, Lohr JA, Malcolm BS, Kesler RW: Hepatic hemangioendotheliomas and hyperbilirubinemia. *South Med J* 71:1439–1441, 1978.

Smith I, Wright FJ: Cullen's sign in ruptured ectopic gestation. *Lancet* 1:930–932, 1935.

Smythe CM, Gibson DB: Upper quadrant bruit due to tortuous splenic artery. *N Engl J Med* 269:1308–1309, 1963.

Snapper I, Kahn AI: *Bedside Medicine*, ed 2. Grune & Stratton, New York, 1967.

Strodel WE, Eckhauser FE, Lemmer JH, Whitehouse WM Jr, Williams DM: Presentation and perioperative management of arterioportal fistulas. *Arch Surg* 122:563–571, 1987.

Sullivan S, Krasner Williams R: The clinical estimation of liver size: A comparison of techniques and an analysis of the source of error. *Br Med J* 2:1042–1043, 1976.

Sullivan S, Williams R: Reliability of clinical techniques for detecting splenic enlargement. *Br Med J* 2:1043–1044, 1976.

Thompson H, Francis DMA: Abdominal-wall tenderness: a useful sign in the acute abdomen. *Lancet* 2:1053–1054, 1977.

Turner GG: Local discoloration of the abdominal wall as a sign of acute pancreatitis. *Br J Surg* 7:394–395, 1920.

Videbaek A, Christensen BE, Jonsson V: *The Spleen in Health and Disease*. Fadl's Forlag A.S., Copenhagen, 1982.

Watson WC, Williams PB, Duffy G: Epigastric bruits in patients with and without celiac axis compressiion. *Ann Intern Med* 79:211–215, 1973.

Westin J, Lanner L, Larsson A, Weinfeld A: Spleen size in polycythemia: A clinical and scintigraphic study. *Acta Med Scand* 191:263–271, 1972.

Wiener SL, Nathanson M: *Med Times*, 1976–1977. [See reference in Chapter 29.]

Williams DB, Payne AS, Foulk WT, Johnson CM: Splenic arteriovenous fistula. *Mayo Clin Proc* 55:383–386, 1980.

21
Male Genitalia

" . . . The husband had long been suffering from ulcers in the private parts, and his wife insisted on seeing them, promising that no one would give him a more candid opinion whether the disease was curable. She saw that there was no hope and urged him to take his life; she went with him, even led him to his death herself, and forced him to follow her example by roping herself to him and jumping into the lake."

The Letters of the Younger Pliny, Book 6

Penis

A Method

1. Put on a pair of gloves, remembering that some organisms such as *Treponema pallidum* can be infective through abraded skin* (Harrison et al., 1978).

2. Inspect the penis, remembering to retract the foreskin, if present, or to have the patient do so. (Be sure to return the foreskin to its usual state; unconscious patients have developed severe edema after the examiner failed to do this.)

3. Open the terminal urethra by compressing the glans anteroposteriorly between your thumb and forefinger, in order to inspect for ulcers and discharge.

4. Palpate the length of the shaft for induration and tenderness.

Ulcers

The distinguishing features of ulcers of various etiologies are given in Table 21-1 (see also Figs. 21-1 through 21-3).

The mucous membrane of the urethra may be involved in systemic diseases that cause mucosal ulcerations, such as Behçet's syndrome, pemphigus, and Stevens-Johnson syndrome.

Circumcision

The note in the case record as to whether or not the man is circumcised is of particular importance if he is suspected of having disseminated tuberculosis. Such patients often have urine cultures sent for mycobacteria as a way of demonstrating renal tuberculosis (evidence of extrapulmonary dissemination). If the receiving laboratory cannot distinguish species, the culture of *Mycobacterium smegmatis*, a contaminant present in the smegma of uncircumcised males, could be mistaken for *Mycobacterium tuberculosis*.

---

*The minimal infective dose of *Treponema pallidum* in rabbits has been determined to be one treponeme injected intratesticularly and four organisms inoculated intradermally (Public Health Service, 1968).

A circumcised man is less likely to have carcinoma of the penis, and his wife less likely to have carcinoma of the cervix.

Peyronie's Disease

This condition is also known as plastic induration of the penis. The patient may complain of curvature of the penis during erection. Nontender plaques may be felt in the corpora cavernosa laterally, or in the intercorporeal septum dorsally.

Priapism

Priapism is a prolonged, usually painful erection, initially unaccompanied by sexual desire. It may signify a neurologic lesion from the cerebrum to the nervi erigentes; a local mechanical cause, such as thrombosis, hemorrhage, neoplasm, or inflammation of the penis; or a thrombotic diathesis due to a hematologic condition such as leukemia or sickle cell anemia (hemoglobin S-S), or even sickle trait (hemoglobin S-A). (Hemoglobin S undergoes sickling when the pO_2 decreases. Persons with hemoglobin S-A usually have pO_2 levels sufficient to prevent sickling—except when they fly.)

Phimosis

This condition is the inability to retract the foreskin, either due to a congenital malformation or to adhesions from infection.

Paraphimosis

Paraphimosis is the inability to replace the foreskin, once retracted, due to edema of the glans.

Skin Lesions

Nonulcerating dermatologic diseases that characteristically involve the penis include psoriasis, scabies, and lichen planus. In secondary lues, a papulosquamous eruption typically involves the penis, palms, and soles (Fig. 21-4).

Table 21-1. Ulcers of the Penis

Etiology	Usual Number	Pain?	Lymphadenopathy?
Syphilis	One	No (unless superinfected)	Usually bilateral
Chancroid	Multiple	Tender	Bilateral, but usually more pronounced on one side
Granuloma inguinale	One (more likely to be inguinal)	No	No
Lymphogranuloma venereum	One (tiny, vesicular)	Not usually, but the lymphadenopathy is painful	Usually unilateral
Herpes simplex	Multiple (vesicular at first), occur in clusters	Yes	No
Cancer	Single	Not initially	Eventually

Reiter's syndrome is frequently accompanied by circinate balanitis, a painless eruption on the glans. This begins as small blebs, which coalesce into a large circular ring about the size of a dime.

Condylomata lata (Fig. 22-3, p. 402) are flat growths about the genitalia or anus seen during the secondary stage of syphilis. Condylomata acuminata (venereal warts), which also occur on the genitals or about the anus, have villous projections. Being caused by a virus, they are infectious.

Congenital Malformations

In hypospadius, the urethra opens on the ventral surface of the penis. This may occur as an isolated anomaly (in 1 of 700 newborn males). In about 15% of cases, there is some pathogenetic mechanism identified, such as Klinefelter's syndrome (karyotype XXY); other chromosomal abnormalities; maternal ingestion of estrogens or progestogens; or virilizing congenital adrenal hyperplasia in a genetic female (Williams, 1974). Hypospadius may accompany nondescent of the testicle.

In epispadius, the urethra opens dorsally.

Urethral Discharge

A thick, purulent-appearing discharge is likely to be due to gonorrhea. A slight, whitish discharge is more likely to be due to one of the causes of "nonspecific" (nongonococcal) urethritis such as chlamydia, ureaplasma, or even a presumably noninfectious condition such as Reiter's syndrome. Place a drop of the discharge on a slide, allow it to air dry, and prepare a Gram stain to look for leukocytes and gonococci (see Ch. 28, p. 553).

Impotence

The physical examination of the penis is seldom helpful in evaluating one of the major causes of morbidity in the male, sexual impotence, unless this is due to an end organ problem such as Peyronie's disease, phimosis, microphallus, or chordee (Nelson, 1987).

One special maneuver, the postage stamp test (see Ch. 3, p. 42) is useful for distinguishing impotence of a central origin from that due to a more peripheral cause (endocrine, vascular, peripheral neuropathy, etc.)

A 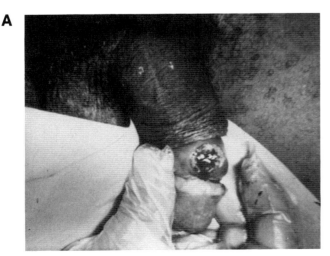   **B**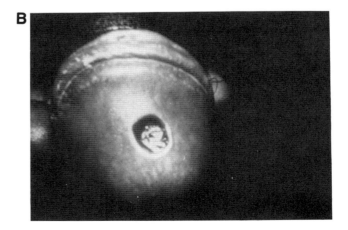

Figure 21-1. *Primary syphilis. A, Typical chancre at coronal sulcus; B, chancre of the glans. Photographs courtesy of Division of Sexually Transmitted Diseases, Center for Prevention Services, Centers for Disease Control, Atlanta, GA.*

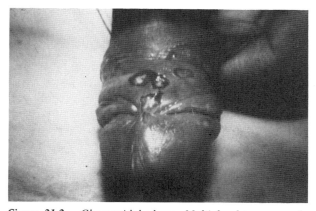

Figure 21-2. Chancroidal ulcers. Multiple chancres on the shaft. *Photograph courtesy of Division of Sexually Transmitted Diseases, Center for Prevention Services, Centers for Disease Control, Atlanta, GA.*

Vascular impotence may be evaluated by the penile-brachial blood pressure gradient (see Ch. 18, p. 347), but this requires Doppler equipment to make the penile artery pressure determination.

Neurologic impotence is usually accompanied by other neurologic signs (see bulbocavernosus reflex, Ch. 26, p. 504), but in some diabetics, no other neurologic sign is evident on routine examination.

Finally, the combination of hypogonadotrophic hypogonadism and hypoosmia occurs in Kallman's syndrome, and probably with zinc deficiency (Burch & Sullivan, 1976) (see Ch. 12, p. 218).

Scrotum

Skin Infections

In secondary syphilis, papulosquamous (Fig. 21-4) or annular squamous lesions (Fig. 21-5) may occur on the scrotum.

Mycoses commonly afflict the skin of the groin; *Tinea cruris* usually does not involve the scrotum, whereas *Candida albicans* frequently does. The diagnosis of candida is also suggested by scattered satellite lesions beyond the main area of dermatitis (Harrison et al., 1978).

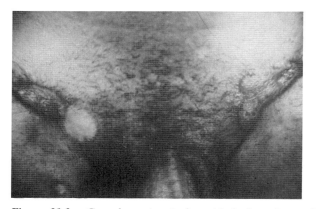

Figure 21-3. Granuloma inguinale, with both active and healed areas. *Photograph courtesy of Division of Sexually Transmitted Diseases, Center for Prevention Services, Centers for Disease Control, Atlanta, GA.*

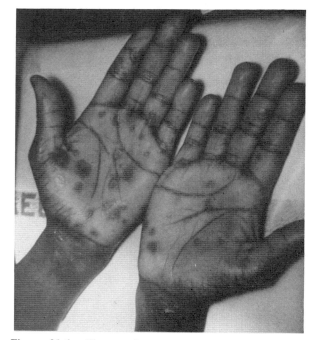

Figure 21-4. The papulosquamous eruption of secondary syphilis. *Photograph courtesy of Division of Sexually Transmitted Diseases, Center for Prevention Services, Centers for Disease Control, Atlanta, GA.*

The Fordyce Lesion

The Fordyce lesion (Fig. 21-6) consists of multiple minute (petechia-sized) dark nodules, hyperkeratotic over a vascular core, slightly raised, with a discrete border. They exactly resemble

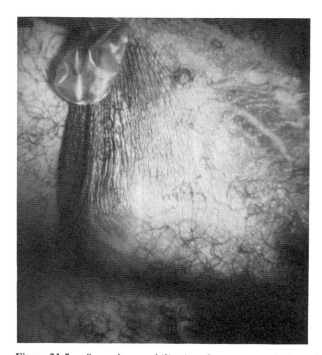

Figure 21-5. Secondary syphilis. Annular squamous lesions of the scrotum. *Photograph courtesy of Division of Sexually Transmitted Diseases, Center for Prevention Services, Centers for Disease Control, Atlanta, GA.*

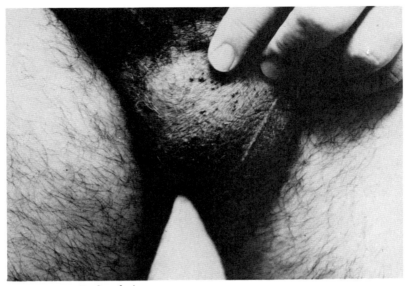

Figure 21-6.   Fordyce lesions.

caviar lesions of the tongue (black caviar, not red), with which they may coexist. They may be confused with the lesion of Fabry's disease (angiokeratoma corporis diffusum universale); however, the latter, as indicated in the Latin, are not confined to the scrotum. More recently, they have been confused with the early lesions of Kaposi's sarcoma (Fig. 7-9). But the Fordyce lesions are much smaller.

Fordyce lesions are seen in 15% of men over the age of 50 (Bean, 1958). They may be transmitted from father to son, but do not generally appear until after age 40 (although the patient shown in Fig. 21-6 was 39 years old.)

○   The lesion is benign and need not be biopsied. However, it may bleed, and thereby be associated with psychic morbidity. Accordingly, the patient should be reassured and advised to maintain a high order of hygiene to prevent itching and the need for abrasive scratching.

Gangrene of the Scrotum

In the universe of anaerobic and mixed (synergistic) gangrene (cellulitis and/or fasciitis), "Fournier's" (1883) refers to that of the scrotum, regardless of organism. "Meleney's" refers to that regardless of locus attributed to the pepto Streptococcus and Staphylococcus but indistinguishable at the perineum from cutaneous amebiasis (Davson et al., 1988). Fournier's gangrene is almost
○   always associated with an underlying urologic or colorectal problem, including postsurgical states. Rarely, it may be related to small vessel disease such as that of diabetes mellitus or polyarteritis nodosa (Downing & Black, 1985). Often, more than one of these factors is present (Lamb & Juler, 1983; Spirnak et al., 1984).

Varicocele

A varicocele looks like a bag of worms. Most varicoceles (98%) occur on the left, *supposedly* (vide infra) because of the greater hydrostatic pressure in the left testicular vein (compared with the right) due to the unique junction of the left testicular and left renal vein. A right varicocele should prompt a search for an anatomic irregularity or a testicular neoplasm.

1.   In a low-pressure venous system, the single most important factor affecting hydrostatic pressure is the height difference (Zerhouni et al., 1980). Therefore, if the patient is in the upright position, both testicles are subjected to the same amount of hydrostatic pressure when the valves are incompetent, regardless of the angle of junction of the testicular vein and the larger venous tributary.

In a study of patients with left varicocele, in whom a pressure difference was found between the left renal vein and the inferior vena cava, no such pressure difference was found between the right renal vein and the inferior vena cava. In a control group, the pressures in the right renal vein, left renal vein, and inferior vena cava closely approximated each other.

In conclusion, the left renal vein in subjects with varicocele seems to be anatomically obstructed. Such obstruction apparently is rare on the right (Zerhouni et al., 1980.)

2.   In a patient with nephrotic syndrome, the *appearance of any varicocele* justifies a search for renal vein thrombosis.

3.   A pulsating varicocele is seen in tricuspid insufficiency (Fred, 1988).

Edema

Edema of the scrotal wall can occur in any condition causing massive fluid retention (see Ch. 25, p. 446). Local causes include thrombosis of the pelvic veins, acute epididymitis, and torsion of the spermatic cord (DeGowin, 1965).

Lymphedema results from obstruction of the pelvic lymphatics. In filariasis, the condition may be so severe that it is called elephantiasis.

Transillumination of Scrotal Swelling

A Method

1.   Pull the blinds or take the patient to a darkened room.

2.   Make the swelling tense by grasping the neck of the scrotum between the fingers and thumb.

3.   Place a strong light behind the scrotum.

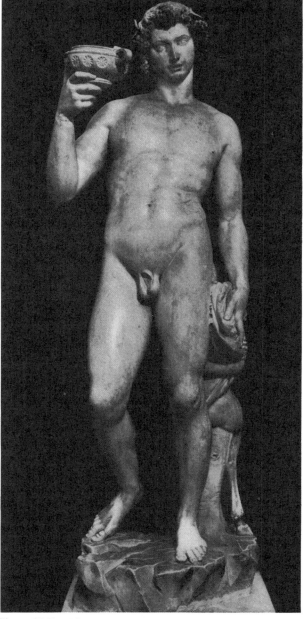

Figure 21-7. *The right testicle hangs lower than the left. Bacchus, by Michelangelo.*

Findings

A hydrocele or epididymal cyst should be translucent, and the opaque shadow of the testis may be visible. A hematocele will not transilluminate.

Testes and Epididymes

The testes (pronounced *tes-tease*)* are composed of a right testis and a left testis (pronounced *tes-tis*). *Testis* is the Latin word for testicle. The words "testament" and "testify" are derived from the same root. (In the ancient world there was no Bible to swear upon, and witnesses were required to take the oath of the court while holding onto their gonads, the implication being that if

they did not tell the truth, something would fall off. This also explains why women were not called to court.)

Inspection

For many years, I inspected the testicles to see whether the right or the left hung lower. I reasoned that if the hydrostatic pressure was, as supposed, greater on the left (thus causing varicoceles to be much more common on that side), the left testicle should normally hang lower, as in Figure 24-4. That being the case, one might not have to wait for the appearance of the right varicocele to get a clue to a right testicular tumor, but could simply observe for a right testicle that was lower than the left, as in Figure 21-7. However, I observed that the relative dependency of one testicle vis-à-vis the other had a great intersubject, and even intrasubject, variability. On searching the literature, I could find none on the relative position of the two testicles. Furthermore, none of the subjects who apparently had a lower right testicle had evidence of a testicular tumor on either side. Hence, I have abandoned this inspection.

Palpation

A Method

1. The testicles are exquisitely sensitive and should be handled by the physical diagnostician with great care. Not only should they be palpated *gently*, but physicians practicing in cool times or places should warm their hands by friction before beginning the examination. The most common cause of an undescended testicle is a physician with cold hands.

2. Feel the testis between your thumb and fingertips. Most important is to distinguish the testis from the epididymis. These are clearly two separate structures, the latter being superior to the former when the patient is erect (Fig. 21-8). The testis is the size, shape, and consistency of a hard-boiled pigeon's egg. The epididymis feels like a knotted strand of *al dente* spaghetti. (This elementary distinction apparently escapes many physicians; an oncologist from Massachusetts once told me that he had never seen a patient with a seminoma who had not first received a course of antibiotics for the treatment of "epididymitis"!)

3. While performing the examination, teach the technique to the patient (just as when examining the female breast).

Cancer of the testis is the most common solid tumor in men between the ages of 20 and 34 years, and there is some evidence that testicular self-examination will permit the early detection of stage I tumors (Garnick et al., 1980). Unfortunately, it is still possible for testicular germ cell tumors to metastasize to clinically detectable extragonadal sites at a time when the primary testicular tumor is still detectable only by ultrasound, not by palpation (Kirschling et al., 1983).

4. When a swelling is found, the examiner should be able to feel the *top* of the swelling within the scrotum if the swelling is of testicular origin. (If he is unable to do so, other possibilities such as a hernia should be considered.)

---

*Similarly, fomites is not pronounced *foam-heights*, but rather *foam-it-tease*. Fomites is the plural of the Latin word for kindling, sticks, or splinters, meaning inanimate objects other than food that transmit infectious particles. The singular is a fomes (pronounced *foams*), *not* a "fomite."

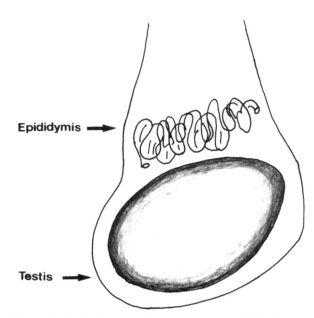

Figure 21-8.   *Relative positions of testis and epididymis.*

Findings

Testicular size.   The scientific literature on testicular size uses volumetric measurements and devices not available from the usual supply houses (Takihara et al., 1983).

As a rule of thumb, I have noticed that the average testicle of androgenically normal men is always at least the same length as the distal two phalanges on the patient's little finger (except in patients with a Marfanoid habitus). Using calipers (see Ch. 7, p. 121) one can accurately measure the long axis of the testicle for which normal values are available (Tishler, 1971). The lower limits of normal (mean minus two standard deviations)* are 31 mm for whites and 34 mm for blacks. Japanese testicles are normally smaller than white testicles (Takihara et al., 1983).

Bilaterally small testes occur in Klinefelter's syndrome, myotonic dystrophy, and secondary hypogonadism. A small testicle (usually unilaterally but sometimes bilaterally) may result from atrophy after involvement with mumps, syphilis, trauma, filariasis, maldescent, or repair of an inguinal hernia.

Testicular lesions.   Pain and swelling of the testis occur in orchitis, which may be due to mumps, syphilis, gonorrhea, or other infections. A nontender swelling or mass in the testis may occur with neoplasm, tuberculosis, or tertiary syphilis (with the formation of a gumma). A hard nodular mass in the testicle is usually neoplastic.

A swelling due to the accumulation of fluid or blood within the tunica vaginalis will feel smooth and resilient. It may be due to a hydrocele (which transilluminates, see p. 395) or a hematocele (which does not).

🖗 In testicular torsion, a twisting of the spermatic cord results in occlusion of the arterial supply and venous drainage. The condition

---

*I abandon here the use of 95% confidence limits because the raw data were not corrected for body size, and the lower 95% confidence limits (41 mm for whites, 44 mm for blacks) would falsely diagnose many small, but androgenically normal, men.

is an acute emergency; failure to make the diagnosis may result in loss of the testis due to gangrene. The patient, usually a young man in severe distress, has a tender, edematous mass in the scrotum. The differential diagnosis includes acute epididymo-orchitis and strangulated scrotal hernia. It is stated that the following signs favor testicular torsion ("Bailey," Clain, 1973):

1.   The affected testis lies higher than its fellow.

2.   Because the developmental anomaly permitting the torsion, namely the presence of a mesentery between the testis and epididymis, is almost always bilateral, the unaffected testis will be seen to lie perfectly horizontally (not slightly inclined), if the patient is examined erect. (The sign is obscured on the affected side.)

3.   In testicular torsion, it is unusual to be able to distinguish the epididymis from the testis.

4.   Elevation and support of the testis for 1 hour will diminish the pain of epididymo-orchitis, but not of a torsion.

Epididymal lesions.   Polyarteritis tends to confine itself to the epididymes as does *C. trachomatis* and postprostatectomy Gramnegative epididymitis.

Enlarged and/or cystic epididymes in the region of the caput are frequently seen in Young's syndrome, which is associated with obstructive azoospermia (but motile sperm), chronic sinopulmonary infections, and a normal sweat test (Handelsman et al., 1984).

Tuberculosis and gonococcal infections may begin in the epididymis and secondarily spread to the testes. An examination of the epididymis is especially important in patients suspected of having disseminated tuberculosis.

Hernias

Ordinarily, a hernia is diagnosed by seeing or palpating a bulge. Occasionally, bowel sounds can be heard over a mass in the scrotum, confirming the presence of intestine.

A Method

1.   The patient stands, stripped below the waist, while the examiner sits in front of him.

2.   Carefully look for a bulge. Keep your eyes glued on the external inguinal ring, and ask the patient to cough; observe whether there is an impulse or a bulge. Ask the patient to cough again, and compare the two sides.

3.   If you do not see a swelling, but the patient has reported a pain or swelling, ask him to point to the spot where he felt it. Then look again as he coughs.

4.   Using the right hand for the right side, and the left hand for the left side, invaginate the scrotum upon the little finger. Rotate the finger so that the nail lies against the spermatic cord.

5.   Introduce the finger into the superficial inguinal ring; the normal size ring will just admit the tip of the little finger. (A larger ring does not necessarily imply the presence of a hernia.)

6.   Ask the patient to cough. A palpable impulse confirms the presence of an inguinal direct hernia.

Zieman's Method ("Bailey," Clain, 1973)

1.   Follow steps 1 to 3 above.

2.   Adjust the patient's position. Have him turn his head to the side, and hold it erect, instead of looking down to see what you are doing.

3. With the patient still standing, the examiner rises. For examining the right, he stands behind and somewhat to the right, and for examining the left, behind and somewhat to the left. Using the hand corresponding to the side to be examined, spread the fingers as if catching a ball, and place the third finger over Hesselbach's triangle (the site of a direct hernia). The second finger will then be over the site of an indirect hernia, and the fourth finger over the site of a femoral hernia. Instruct the patient to hold his nose and blow. Feel for the gliding motion of the walls of an empty sac or the pushing sensation caused by the protrusion of a viscus into the sac.

Prostate and Seminal Vesicles

These structures are palpated in the course of the digital rectal examination (see Ch. 23), which is an indispensable part of the examination of the male genitalia.

References

Bean WB: *Vascular Spiders and Related Lesions of the Skin*. Charles C Thomas, Springfield, IL, 1958.

Burch RE, Sullivan JF: Clinical and nutritional aspects of zinc deficiency and zinc excess. *Med Clin North Am* 60(4):675–685, 1976.

Clain A, ed: *Hamilton Bailey's Demonstrations of Physical Signs in Clinical Surgery*, ed 15. Williams & Wilkins, Baltimore, 1973.

Davson J, Jones DM, Turner L: Diagnosis of Meleney's synergistic gangrene. *Br J Surg* 75:267–271, 1988.

DeGowin EL: *Bedside Diagnostic Examination*. Macmillan, New York, 1965.

Downing R, Black J: Polyarteritis nodosa: An unrecognized cause of Fournier's gangrene. *Br J Urol* 57:355–356, 1985.

Fournier AJ: Gangrene soubroyante de la verg. *Med Pract* 4:589–597, 1883.

Fred HL: *Elephant Medicine—and More*. Mercer University Press, Macon, 1988.

Garnick MB, Mayer RJ, Richie JP: Testicular self-examination. *N Engl J Med* 302:297, 1980.

Handelsman DJ, Conway AJ, Boylan LM, Turtle JR: Young's syndrome: Obstructive azoospermia and chronic sinopulmonary infections. *N Engl J Med* 310:3–9, 1984.

Harrison JH, Gittes RF, Perlmutter AD, Stamey TA, Walsh PC: *Campbell's Urology*, ed 4. WB Saunders, Philadelphia, 1978.

Kirschling RJ, Kvols LK, Charvoneau JW, Grantham JG, Zincke H: High-resolution ultrasonographic and pathologic abnormalities of germ cell tumors in patients with clinically normal testes. *Mayo Clin Proc* 58:648–653, 1983.

Lamb RC, Juler GL: Fournier's gangrene of the scrotum. *Arch Surg* 118:38–40, 1984.

Nelson RP: Male sexual dysfunction: Evaluation and treatment. *South Med J* 80:69–74, 1987.

Public Health Service, U.S. Department of Health, Education, and Welfare: *Syphilis: A Synopsis*. U.S. Government Printing Office, Washington, DC, 1968 (Public Health Service Publication No. 1660).

Spirnak JP, Resnick MI, Hampel N, Persky L: Fournier's gangrene: Report of 20 patients. *J Urol* 131:289–291, 1984.

Takihara H, Saktoku J, Fuji M, Nasu T, Cosentino MJ, Cockett ATK: Significance of testicular size measurement in andrology: I. A new orchiometer and its clinical application. *Fertil Steril* 39:836–839, 1983.

Tishler PV: Diameter of testicles. *N Engl J Med* 285:1489, 1971.

Williams RH: *Textbook of Endocrinology*, ed 5. WB Saunders, Philadelphia, 1974.

Zerhouni EA, Siegelman SS, Walsh PC, White RI: Elevated pressure in the left renal vein in patients with varicocele: Preliminary observations. *J Urol* 123:512–513, 1980.

22
Female Genitalia

"Members of generation are common to both sexes, or peculiar to one; which, because they are impertinent to my purpose, I do voluntarily omit."

Robert Burton, *Anatomy of Melancholy,* Part 1, Section 1, Member 2, Subsection 4

Overview

Importance of the Pelvic Examination in General Medicine

For many women, a pelvic examination is a traumatic event, sometimes because of past experience with insensitive examiners (Magee, 1975). Apparently, many physicians find it bothersome also, judging from the frequency with which the examination is "deferred" (i.e., not done). This omission can cause an important diagnosis to be missed (e.g., pregnancy). (A surprising number of women in their first trimester have had major surgical procedures that would have been postponed had the surgeon known they were pregnant.) The pelvic examination is particularly crucial in patients with abdominal signs or symptoms, fever of unknown origin, or urinary complaints. Many a pelvic abscess has remained undiagnosed for days, and many a case of vaginitis has been inappropriately treated as "cystitis." While hidden, the female organs are seldom impertinent to the physician's medical purpose.

•

A Case History

An immensely obese, alcoholic patient was admitted late at night to the medical service of a well-known county hospital. The chief complaint was abdominal pain. The intern diagnosed pancreatitis, passed a nasogastric tube, ordered intravenous fluids, and went to bed.

The next morning, the nurse called frantically to inform him of the presence of a newborn infant in the patient's bed.

•

The Environment

Every effort should be made to protect the patient's privacy. When equipping a room for performing pelvic examinations, be sure that the table does not have its foot facing the door. The patient will be worried about someone opening the door, and will not be able to relax. The room should be provided with a curtained off area where the patient can undress and leave her clothing. This area should be supplied with tissues, individually packaged sanitary pads, and a wastebasket, for the patient's use after the examination.

It goes without saying that the room should be kept warm, with an extra space heater if necessary.

$$ *Equipment*

The physician will need the following for the routine pelvic examination:

1. A good light source. A gooseneck lamp is best. A flashlight, with someone to hold it, is second best.

2. An examining table with stirrups, and a low stool with wheels. If it is absolutely necessary to examine a hospitalized patient in bed, an upside-down bedpan may be used to elevate her hips. This should give adequate elevation for performing the speculum examination (vide infra).

Remember that the stirrups are always both cold and hard. Oven mittens of the type with the thumb in the middle (Fig. 22-1) make perfect coverings. Alternately, the patient may wish to leave her shoes on.

3. *Three* disposable gloves. You may want to begin with two gloves on the hand that will eventually be used for the rectovaginal examination (see p. 407).

4. Lubricant, such as KY jelly (for the bimanual examination, not for the speculum).

5. Two slides for the Papanicolaou smear and fixative. (For the latter, one pathology laboratory simply pastes a different label on a can of commercial hair spray).

6. Several other slides and cover slips for examining cervical mucous and/or vaginal discharge.

7. Transport medium that the laboratory supplies for gonococcal cultures, warmed to room temperature. (Warming can be speeded by carrying the plate around in your armpit.)

8. Supplies for other microbiologic tests, if indicated (tubes for viral cultures, slides for *Chlamydia*, etc., obtained from the laboratory that is to perform the tests). The viral medium may need to be kept frozen, and thawed just before it is inoculated.

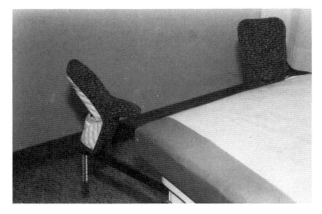

Figure 22-1. Oven mitts can serve as coverings for the stirrups.

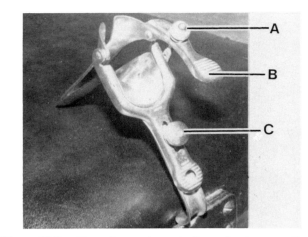

Figure 22-2. Graves' speculum. A, Lateral set screw; B, thumbpiece; C, central set screw.

9. Nitrazine paper, available through various mail order catalogues offering medical or chemistry supplies, for checking the pH of vaginal secretions (see p. 403).

10. Sterile swabs and wooden scrapers.

11. A selection of vaginal speculums. The Graves (duckbill) speculum comes in various widths and lengths. The Pederson speculum, which is narrower and flatter, can be used in virginal patients and those with a narrow introitus due to senescence, scars, or radiation. Disposable plastic speculums have the advantage that the vaginal wall can be seen through the speculum. However, the ratchets do not permit as fine an adjustment as the screw on the metal speculums.

12. Guaiac card for testing the stool for occult blood.

13. A microscope and a Gram stain kit (see Ch. 28, p. 553). The microscopic examination of any abnormal vaginal discharge should be considered an intrinsic part of the physical examination.

A Self-Study

Before attempting to examine a patient, the neophyte physician needs to examine the speculum and to practice manipulating it. Move the distal ends of the blades apart (like a duckbill) by pushing on the thumbpiece (which elevates the anterior blade) and pulling on the handle with your fingers (to lower the posterior blade). The blades are then held in position by tightening the screw located laterally. The center set screw allows for adjustment of the distance between the proximal ends of the blades (Fig. 22-2).

Preparing for the Examination

A few simple courtesies can make the examination less distressing to the patient, and easier for the doctor. Besides the obvious humanitarian considerations, it is not possible to do a good examination of a patient who is uncomfortable and tense.

Whenever possible, interview the patient while she is fully dressed, preferably in a consultation room. Never introduce yourself to the patient for the first time while she is in the stirrups, unless forced by circumstances such as precipitous delivery or other emergency. Even if you are simply being asked to confirm a finding on the pelvic examination, the patient should at least be allowed to sit up for the introduction (Magee, 1975).

Provide for adequate draping. The double draping technique described in Chapter 15, with the gown opening in the back, permits the upper body to be well covered during the pelvic examination. The sheet is draped over the patient's abdomen and knees.

It is best to have a female attendant present during the examination, even if the physician is a woman, to reassure the patient and to help with the procedure. (For male physicians, this is absolutely necessary. If a patient accuses a physician of sexual abuse, however unjustly, the testimony of the attendant may be his best defense.)

Before you begin the examination, the patient should be given the opportunity to go to the bathroom. A full bladder can obscure or be confused with pelvic pathology. Similarly, a full rectum can make the examination inconclusive. (If there is any difficulty in distinguishing hard stool from an area of nodularity, the patient would have to be reexamined after emptying the rectum anyway.)

The "dorsal lithotomy" position is preferred (i.e., feet in the stirrups, hips abducted as widely as possible, buttocks at the very edge of the table). In patients who are unable to abduct the hips, the Sims position may be used (the patient on her side, with the lower arm behind the back and the thighs flexed, the upper more than the lower.)

Order of Examination

The examination begins with inspection and palpation of the external genitalia. Next, the vagina and cervix are gently palpated with one gloved finger, lubricated with warm water only (vide infra), enabling the examiner to determine the direction in which to point the speculum. Also, clues to vaginal pathology may be felt. (In some instances, the need for gynecologic consultation will become obvious at this point, and the patient can be spared a second speculum examination.) The vagina and cervix are inspected with the aid of the speculum (see p. 403), and specimens for pathologic and microbiologic examination are obtained. Then the internal genitalia are palpated bimanually, between the abdominal wall and the fingers within the vagina. In most instances, the rectal examination concludes the examination. Sometimes, it may be desirable also to examine the standing patient to reveal a prolapse or hernia that was not apparent in the dorsal lithotomy position. While the patient is dressing, the physician carries out the microscopic examination of the cervical and vaginal secretions, if indicated.

External Genitalia

Pubic Hair

The appearance of a male-type escutcheon (see Ch. 7, p. 124) can be a virilizing sign. However, there is normally a continuum. Terminal* hair was found on the abdomen (above the pubic triangle) of 35% of 400 English and Welsh university women (McKnight, 1964).

In patients afflicted with pubic lice, nits may be seen at the base of the hairs, along with signs of excoriation of the skin.

The Vulva

Labia Majora

The skin covering the labia majora may be afflicted with the same lesions as the skin of the rest of the body, including malignant melanomas, psoriasis, and seborrheic dermatitis. The labia are particularly rich in sebaceous glands, hence subject to sebaceous retention cysts and hair follicle infections. The apocrine glands may be afflicted with hidradenitis suppurativa (Fox-Fordyce disease).

Since the labia majora are the analog of the scrotum, the occurrence of labioinguinal hernias, while rare, should not be surprising. In certain hermaphrodites, testicles are found in the labia majora.

An abscess of Bartholin's† gland, when fully formed, is an obvious tender red mass in the posterior labium. However, considerable enlargement of the gland (due to a retention cyst or rarely adenocarcinoma) can be missed unless it is searched for. Palpate the posterior part of the labia majora between the finger and thumb, searching for a swelling. In patients with a Bartholin's abscess, there is a high incidence of sexually transmitted disease; Gram stain and cultures for gonorrhea and chlamydia should be performed, and diagnostic tests for syphilis should be considered.

The Clitoris

Enlargement of the clitoris is an unmistakable sign of virilization. The adult clitoral index, defined as the vertical times the horizontal dimensions, is normally from 9 to 35 mm (Rittmaster & Loriaux, 1987). Borderline values, often seen in idiopathic hirsutism, are from 36 to 99 mm. If the index is 100 mm or more, it is a sign of severe hyperandrogenicity (Tagatz et al.,

1979), and demands an explanation. In the infant, clitoral enlargement may signal an adrenogenital syndrome or a maternal ovarian tumor.

The Urethra

A purulent discharge from the urethra can result from gonorrhea, a urethral diverticulum, or another cause of urethritis. Sometimes the discharge is apparent only after stroking the anterior vaginal wall in the direction of the meatus.

A urethral caruncle, a tender, inflamed red mass at the meatus, may be a complication of urethritis.

A prolapsed urethra may form a hemorrhagic, painful mass, superficially resembling a cancer because of its friability. The condition may occur in children or elderly women, especially after straining.

In gonorrhea, pus may be expressed from the ducts of Skene's glands, located just lateral and somewhat posterior to the urethral orifice.

The Hymen

Inspection of the genitalia should be a part of the examination of all infant girls in order to check for the presence of a vagina, and for imperforate hymen. In the event of the latter, the examiner should perform a rectal examination with his little finger to determine whether there is a bulging in the vagina (i.e., an accumulation of endocervical mucus [hydrocolpos] due to maternal hormone secretion). (This can become very large and could lead to laparotomy for an "abdominal mass" [Green, 1971].)

Imperforate hymen should be ruled out in adolescent girls with abdominal pain. Painful hematocolpos and hematosalpinx, sometimes with rupture into the abdomen, have resulted from failure to recognize this condition before several menstrual periods have occurred. Even before menarche, mucus accumulation behind an imperforate hymen has occasionally caused obstruction of the ureters and bilateral hydronephrosis.

An excessive amount of tough, fibrous tissue can be the cause of dyspareunia.

Labia Minora

Simple adherence of the labia minora (labial agglutination or labial adhesions) in young girls is to be distinguished from imperforate hymen and congenital absence of the vagina. In one study, the incidence was fivefold higher (2.9%) in children who were proven victims of sexual abuse (Muram, 1988).

Trauma

A very large hematoma may result from trauma, such as falling astride a hard object. If there is evidence of trauma without a persuasive history, the possibility of rape or sexual abuse must be considered.

○   In examining any patient in whom rape or sexual abuse is a possibility, a medicolegal protocol must be strictly followed in order to collect evidence required by the court (such as the presence of semen, and signs of the use of force). Consultation with a specialist is strongly advised.

The adverse consequences of misdiagnosing sexual abuse when it has not occurred can be devastating. The differential diagnosis includes scurvy, bleeding disorders, mongolian blue spots, osteogenesis imperfecta, and lichen sclerosus et atrophicus (see p. 402), with or without superimposed infection (Handfield-Jones et al., 1987).

---

*Terminal hairs are coarse, dark, and long. Normally, they develop only in certain areas such as the axilla, scalp, pubic triangle or diamond, and beard.

†Casper Bartholin, the third in a line of famous Danish physicians, also described Bartholin's duct from the sublingual gland. His father Thomas was the re-discoverer of the lymph nodes (see p. 139). Thomas's father, who was also named Casper, was a polymath from Malmo who accepted the Chair in Medicine at Copenhagen (and later the one in Theology) after refusing chairs in Philosophy, Anatomy, and Greek! There is no record of any of them having served on a committee.

Sexually Transmitted Diseases

Lesions that can occur on the penis (see Ch. 21, p. 391) can also occur on the vulva or inside the vagina. These include the primary chancre of syphilis, the lesion of lymphogranuloma venereum, granuloma inguinale, chancroid, the ulcerating vesicles of herpes, condylomata lata (due to secondary syphilis, see Fig. 22-3), and condylomata acuminata (venereal warts). The last are caused by the human papilloma virus, some serotypes of which have been implicated in the recent increased incidence of cervical carcinoma in young women (Raymond, 1987a, 1987b).

A diffuse reddening and edema of the vulva may result from the presence of certain types of vaginal discharge (Table 22-1).

Gonorrheal vaginitis may be distinguished by its tendency to involve the urethra, the vulvovaginal glands, and Bartholin's and Skene's glands.

Other Infectious Diseases Affecting the Vulva

The vulva may be involved by parasites such as pinworms (especially in children) or scabies. Impetigo, a staphylococcal and/or streptococcal lesion characterized by yellow-crusted erosions, is a common accompaniment of scabies (Whiting, 1983).

Numerous fungi are saprophytes in the vulvar area and may become pathogens under conditions of lowered resistance or increased heat or friction. Predisposing conditions include pregnancy, diabetes, oral contraceptives, and the use of broad-spectrum antibiotics. The most common fungi are *Tinea cruris* and *Candida* (monilia). The rash of *Tinea cruris* tends to have a butterfly appearance, with clearly defined, raised, scaly borders, also affecting the upper, inner thighs. Usually, monilial vulvitis is accompanied by a curdy, white vaginal discharge. There may be red maculopapular lesions, "satellite lesions," lying beyond the border of the inflamed area.

Ulcerations of the vulva and vagina can be caused by *Entamoeba histolytica* (generally after a bout of uncontrolled diarrhea).

Other Systemic Diseases

Draining sinuses, abscesses, and deep ulcerations may result from Crohn's disease. Other conditions causing vulvar ulcers include Beçhet's syndrome, pemphigus vulgaris, dermatitis herpetiformis, and erythema multiforme.

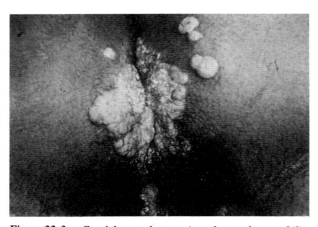

Figure 22-3. *Condylomata lata, a sign of secondary syphilis. Photograph courtesy of Division of Sexually Transmitted Diseases, Center for Prevention Services, Centers for Disease Control, Atlanta, GA. (See p. 392.)*

Atrophic Vulvitis

After the menopause, the labia shrink and flatten due to the loss of subcutaneous fat. The skin becomes thin and shiny, and elasticity diminishes. The vaginal orifice may become stenotic. Changes of a similar nature generally coexist in the vagina. (vide infra).

Vulvar Dystrophies

Vulvar skin is more sensitive to irritants than peripheral skin, and additionally is exposed to a wide variety of potential sensitizers and irritants, such as laundry powders, douches, contraceptive creams, and deodorants (Friedrich, 1985). A long-standing itch-scratch cycle can cause a hyperplastic dystrophy, which is a variant of lichen simplex chronicus (neurodermatitis). This may produce a diffuse erythema, or localized, elevated lesions, often with a white appearance due to hyperkeratosis. Chronic irritation is also thought to cause malignant changes.

Lichen sclerosus (also called lichen sclerosus et atrophicus) typically produces white to pale pink flat macules, which may coalesce into plaques, involving the vulva, medial thigh, and/or perianal region. The skin may come to resemble parchment or cigarette paper. Agglutination and fusion of the interlabial folds, and a concentric stenosis of the introitus may occur. Half to two thirds of the patients are postmenopausal, but the disease does occur in children (of whom only 35% have genital lesions). Extragenital sites such as the axilla may be involved. A 34% incidence of clinically manifest autoimmune diseases has been reported in patients with this condition (Soper & Creasman, 1986).

Carcinoma develops in about 3% of patients with lichen sclerosus (Soper & Creasman, 1986). Conversely, lichen sclerosus was an associated lesion in 16 of 30 (53%) of patients with invasive vulvar carcinoma (Punnonen et al., 1985).

At the time of presentation, 2% to 5% of women with a vulvar dystrophy have an invasive carcinoma of the vulva, and an additional 4% to 8% have some cellular atypia (Soper and Creasman, 1986).

Carcinoma-in-Situ of the Vulva

The lesions of squamous cell carcinoma in situ (sometimes referred to by the ambiguous terms Bowen's disease or erythroplasia of Queyrat) can be unifocal or multifocal, discrete or coalescent. About 20% are pigmented; the remainder are white or red. The relationship to invasive carcinoma is not as strong as with cervical carcinoma-in-situ. There is an increasing incidence in younger women, with 42% being under the age of 25 years, compared with 14% in an earlier era (Kistner, 1986).

Paget's Disease

Although formerly considered synonymous with carcinoma-in-situ, Paget's disease of the vulva is a separate entity (Nichols & Evrard, 1985), an adenocarcinoma that has an occasional tendency to invade and metastasize to lymph nodes (Kistner, 1986). It presents as a sharply demarcated, florid, red, pruritic, moist area, with occasional crusting. Islands of whitened skin appear between the reddened areas. The lesion may spread to the perineum and thighs. Adenocarcinoma of the vulvar apocrine glands or of the breast (also an apocrine gland) are sometimes associated with this condition (Kistner, 1986).

Invasive Carcinoma of the Vulva

Vulvar cancer is extremely variable in appearance. In its early form it may be an elevated papule or a small ulcer, and may be easily confused with condyloma acuminatum, papilloma, ulcerated chancroid, gumma, or tuberculosis. (Thus, biopsy is very important.) A typical later lesion is an ulcerating mass. Although young women

Table 22-1. Differential Diagnosis of Vaginal Discharge

Etiology	Odor	Appearance of Discharge	Appearance of Vulva/Vagina	pH	Microscopic	Symptoms
Normal	—	Thick	Pink, white	3.8–4.2	Lactobacilli	—
Candida	—	Curdy, white	Erythema, edema	4.0–4.7	Pseudohyphae on KOH prep	90%; itching
Trichomonas	Fishy	Green, yellow, gray; frothy in 10%	Diffuse erythema or "strawberry vagina" or gray pseudomembrane	5.0–7.0	Organisms; many WBCs	Itching; dysuria
Gardnerella vaginalis	Fishy	Thin, "flour paste"	Usually no gross vulvo-vaginitis. Frothy in 7%	5.0–5.5	Clue cells; lactobacilli eliminated; few WBCs unless another infection present	Few have irritation
Gonococcus	—	Purulent	Bartholinitis, skenitis may be present		Gram-negative intracellular Diplococci	May have dysuria; acute abdominal pain if PID develops
Senescent vaginitis	—	Mucoid	Smooth, shiny, lacking rugae; pale; telangietasia	5.5–7.0	Parabasal cells, WBCs, various bacteria; "dirty" background	Burning; itching; dyspareunia

WBC, white blood cells; PID, pelvic inflammatory disease.

may develop this disease, about 70% of patients are postmenopausal (Kistner, 1986).

Vaginal Examination

External Inspection

Several types of hernias may present as a bulge covered with vaginal mucosa at the introitus. A colpocele consists simply of redundant vaginal mucosa. A cystocele contains part of the bladder, and a rectocele part of the rectum. An enterocele is a herniation of the peritoneal lining of the posterior cul-de-sac into the posterior vaginal fornix, which can also protrude beyond the introitus in severe cases. Asking the patient to strain, cough, or bear down may make any of these hernias more apparent, as will an examination in the standing position. In extreme cases, the cervix will prolapse through the introitus. All of these abnormalities result from relaxation of the endopelvic fascia, usually due to childbirth.

Occasionally an obturator hernia will form a bulge in the vaginal wall; this is more likely to be felt than seen (vide infra).

Palpation

As noted above, a digital examination of the vagina precedes the insertion of the speculum to determine the approximate location of the cervix. Avoid pressure on the sensitive anterior structures (urethral meatus and clitoris) when inserting your finger. Although jelly lubrication would make the examination easier, it will also interfere with interpretation of the Pap smear, so nothing except water lubrication should be used on the glove at this point, unless you are definitely not planning to take a Pap smear.

It is important to talk to the patient and explain to her what you are going to do before you do it. For example, "I'm going to touch the outside of your vagina and spread it apart. Now, I'm

going to put my finger in" (Magee, 1975). It is generally not very helpful to command the patient to relax. If you push down and out from just inside the introitus, and ask her to relax the muscle you are pushing on (the levator ani), she will probably understand what you mean. Or ask her to do the opposite of what she does when she has to go and can't get to the bathroom (Magee, 1975).

Feel all the vaginal walls, particularly the anterior fornix, which is the usual site of vaginal carcinoma. Clear-cell adenocarcinoma may present as a nodule about the size of a green pea under the vaginal vault.

The mouth of a rectovaginal fistula may be palpable as an area of induration in the posterior vaginal wall.

A tender swelling on vaginal examination, in the region of the obturator foramen (the large rounded opening between the pubis and the ischium, palpable through the lateral wall of the vagina) can be an important clue to the diagnosis of an obturator hernia ("Bailey", Clain, 1973). This rare condition, which occurs almost exclusively in thin women over the age of 60, can be an obscure cause of strangulation of the bowel, frequently of the Richter* type. The swelling in the groin is likely to be overlooked because it is covered by the pectineus muscle. Pain may be referred along the obturator nerve and its geniculate branch to the knee (the Howship-Romberg sign), and may limit movement of the hip joint, which tends to be held in a semiflexed position (also see Ch. 26, p. 500).

Speculum Examination

A Method

1. Choose a speculum of the appropriate size, based on your previous digital examination. Use the largest speculum that will

---

*In a Richter's hernia, only a portion of the circumference of the intestine is strangulated.

fit comfortably. In 90% of cases, the medium Graves' speculum is best.

2. Before inserting a metal speculum, be sure to warm it up with some hot water, which also helps to lubricate it a little. If you think it might be a little too warm, touch it to the inner thigh and ask the patient if the temperature is comfortable for her.

3. Seat yourself on a low stool at the foot of the examining table.

4. It is best to insert the instrument with the blades horizontal, *very slowly*. (Many textbooks recommend inserting the speculum with the blades vertical and rotating it once it is inside. The sensation has been compared with that of scraping a steel beam across the urethra [Magee, 1975].)

Some insert the instrument right over the index and third fingers of the left hand, which are pushing down on the posterior vaginal wall. (Others just use the fingers of the left hand to keep the labia apart and the pubic hair out of the way.) Aim posteriorly (the object being to get the posterior blade behind the cervix), and try to avoid putting pressure on the roof of the vagina. (Any pressure should be applied posteriorly.)

5. After the speculum is in place, open it so that you can visualize the cervix. If you are using a plastic speculum, forewarn the patient about the click that it makes when locking into place. If a greater anteroposterior exposure is needed, the central set screw may be released and the blades separated further. Be sure that this screw is again tightened securely; if the blades suddenly move closer together, they may pinch the vaginal mucosa or labia.

6. The cervix will seem to be much more conveniently located in the second thousand patients that you examine than in the first thousand. If you can't at first see it, and you are using the right size speculum, it may be hiding behind either the anterior or the posterior blade of the speculum. The longer posterior blade is supposed to act as a scoop to slide the cervix between the two blades as the speculum is opened. You may have to withdraw the speculum a little to look behind the anterior blade, then possibly to insert it deeper and more posteriorly. In cases of redundant vaginal mucosa or a retroverted uterus, a "pusher" (which might be made of a cotton pledget held in a curved uterine dressing forceps) may help to expose the cervix (Green, 1971).

7. Look at the cervix for signs of disease (vide infra).

8. Obtain a Pap* smear from the posterior vaginal pool of secretions, and another from the cervix: Wipe off any heavy mucus from the cervix, then insert a cotton swab or a wooden scraper into the endocervical canal and rotate it a full 360 degrees. Some state that you should see punctate bleeding as evidence that an adequate specimen has been obtained (Demarest, 1985). Others note that the bleeding may be a sign of chlamydia infection (F. Abbas, personal communication, 1987). Check your Pap smear reports; if they do not specifically state that endocervical cells are seen, reevaluate your technique.

The frequency with which Pap smears should be taken for routine screening is the subject of controversy. The American Cancer Society now recommends routine smears only every 3 years, once consecutive annual smears are negative. However, because the Pap smear is only about 86% sensitive (Kistner, 1986), and because the progression from mild dysplasia to frank carcinoma may be much more rapid than previously thought (Raymond,

1987a), the American College of Obstetrics and Gynecology continues to recommend annual screening (Gunby, 1980).

9. Spread the specimen onto a glass slide and *immediately* spray it with fixative. Deterioration of the cells occurs rather rapidly. Label the slides with the patient's name.

10. Obtain a specimen for gonococcal culture if indicated by the history. (In a patient population with a high incidence of sexually transmitted disease, this may be done routinely in all patients.) Place a sterile swab in the endocervical canal and rotate it. Count slowly to 30, then remove the swab and roll it across the surface of the transport medium (which you have previously warmed to room temperature.) Obtain other specimens as indicated by the history or epidemiologic setting, for example, slides for chlamydia, according to the directions supplied by the laboratory.

11. Where clinically indicated, make two slides of vaginal secretions to examine yourself as quickly as possible: a wet mount and a thin smear for Gram stain. Some place a drop of normal saline on the slide for a wet mount; but a small drop of secretions under a cover slip may be just as satisfactory. Place a drop of secretions on some nitrazine paper for determining the pH (Table 22-1). If more than a few minutes will elapse before you can get to a microscope, place the wet mount under an incandescent lamp to keep it warm, so that trichomonads, if present, do not lose their motility.

12. Look at the vaginal mucosa carefully, especially as you begin to withdraw the speculum. As before, be certain that any pressure is exerted posteriorly rather than anteriorly. Release only the lateral set screw, to allow the tips of the blades to come together as the speculum is withdrawn, *not* the central set screw (because releasing the latter might cause the blades to pinch the vaginal mucosa.)

13. Perform the bimanual examination (vide infra).

The Cervix

The ectocervix is covered by pink squamous epithelium, and the endocervix by a red columnar epithelium. The location of the boundary between these two types of epithelium varies. During childhood and after the menopause, the boundary is located out of view within the cervical canal. With estrogenic stimulation, the boundary may migrate so that the columnar epithelium is visible. This cervical eversion or ectropion may be confused with cervical erosion, a term that implies denudation of the epithelium.

Endocervical glands may become plugged, forming

---

*"Pap" was the nickname of the method's inventor, George Nicholas Papanicolaou, M.D. (Athens), Ph.D. (Munich). After the Balkan war, he emigrated to the United States, where he was working as a rug salesman in a department store, when he finally secured a position as instructor in anatomy at Cornell. While using exfoliative cytology to study female endocrinology, he noticed that cancer cells stained differently. He presented and published in the *Proceedings of the Third Race Betterment Conference*, Battle Creek, Michigan, January 2–6, 1928, noting that, "It is not an exaggeration to say that certain cases of carcinoma of the cervix may be diagnosed by the presence of only one of these cells." This was ignored, and he resumed endocrinology research for a dozen years. When the Cornell dean happened to read the old paper, he encouraged Papanicolaou (then 57) to return to cancer diagnosis, with salubrious results for all. The "Pap" smear is the only eponymous nickname that I know of in medicine.

mucinous retention (nabothian) cysts. These are visible as spherical elevations or small cysts 2 to 10 mm in diameter. They are of no pathologic significance.

The cervical os is round in a nulliparous woman. After childbirth, the os may appear slitlike, or may be distorted in shape due to scarring if lacerations occurred. A patulous (Latin for "distended, spread apart") cervix may be a sign of recent abortion (spontaneous or induced).

Polyps may be seen protruding from the cervix.

Chronic cervicitis, a term defined as epithelial necrosis and neutrophils, has been found in about 98% of cervices (Kistner, 1986), and is not necessarily of clinical importance. Clinically significant cervicitis may show a beefy, friable cervix with a mucopurulent discharge (Levin et al., 1987). (This will appear yellow on a white cotton swab.)

Several infectious diseases may produce cervical lesions, including syphilis (Fig. 22-4), tuberculosis, and chancroid. Herpes simplex may produce cervical inflammation, vesicles, ulcers, or occasionally a fungating mass indistinguishable from carcinoma. Condylomata are sometimes found on the cervix.

Although hyperkeratosis is not itself premalignant, it is frequently found in association with cervical neoplasia. Thus all patients with white lesions of the cervix should be biopsied (Kistner, 1986).

A bluish appearance of the vagina and introitus, Chadwick's sign of pregnancy, usually appears near the end of the second month. This sign was first described by Jacquemier, and so is also known by his name. A bluish appearance of the cervix is called Goodell's sign, an eponym that is also attached to softening of the cervix. The physical signs of pregnancy are summarized in Table 22-2. (See p. 102 for the rollover test of pregnancy-induced hypertension.)

In patients who have had a hysterectomy, the cervix is usually absent. (However, in former times abdominal hysterectomy was performed leaving the cervix in place.) If the cervix is absent, a Pap smear from the vaginal vault is still recommended by some, although carcinoma of the vagina is rare (1% of all genital malignancies).

Vaginal Discharge

Vaginal discharge (or leukorrhea) is one of the most common reasons for visits to gynecologists. The major causes are listed in Table 22-1.

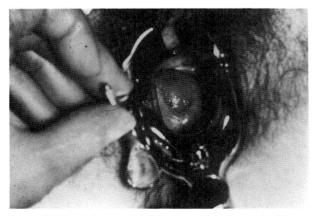

Figure 22-4. *Primary syphilitic chancre on the cervix. Photograph courtesy of Division of Sexually Transmitted Diseases, Center for Prevention Services, Centers for Disease Control, Atlanta, GA.*

As many as one in five women may harbor *Trichomonas vaginalis*, and it has been found in 37% of men with nonspecific urethritis (Kistner, 1986). Many infested persons of either sex are completely asymptomatic, but women may have a profuse, irritating discharge with a fetid odor. Multiple small round red papules may cover the vaginal mucosa ("strawberry vagina"). Prompt microscopic examination of the wet mount may reveal this motile, flagellated, pear-shaped protozoan, often in the company of many leukocytes. Trichomonads may resemble leukocytes, particularly if they have rounded up and lost their motility due to a chilling delay in the examination. In 600 patients, the sensitivity of the wet mount for this diagnosis was 60%; the specificity was 100% (Krieger et al., 1988).

Candida is the second most common cause of vaginal discharge. The symptoms of vulvar burning and itching may seem to be much more severe than might be expected from the amount of discharge. Predisposing conditions include diabetes, pregnancy, corticosteroids, obesity, systemic antibiotics, and possibly oral contraceptive use. Severe, recurrent vaginal candidiasis

Table 22-2. Pelvic and Extra-Pelvic Signs of Pregnancy

Name or Eponym	Description
Chloasma	"Mask of pregnancy": irregular brownish patches on the face and neck
Linea nigra	Brownish black color in midline of abdominal wall
Palmar erythema	Occurs in two thirds of white and one third of nonwhite women
Spiders telangiectasia	Occur in about two thirds of white and 10% of black women
Epulis	A focal, highly vascular swelling of the gums
Montgomery's glands	Small elevations (hypertrophic sebaceous glands) scattered through the areola
Other breast change	Increased size and nodularity; colostrum secretion; delicate veins become visible beneath the skin; nipples become pigmented and more erectile;
Ladin's sign	An area of elasticity on the anterior face of the uterus just above the cervix; felt on palpation through the vagina as early as the 5th or 6th week
Hegar's sign	Softening of the isthmus between cervix and uterine corpus
Goodell's sign	Bluish appearance and softening of the cervix
Chadwick's sign	Bluish vaginal mucosa
McDonald's sign	Uterine corpus and cervix can be easily flexed on each other (because of the softening responsible for Hegar's sign)
Piskacek's sign (von Braun-Fernwald's sign)[a]	Asymmetry of the uterus with a well-defined soft prominence of the cornu, due to implantation near one of the cornua

Source: *Hellman and Pritchard (1971) and Danforth and Scott (1986).*

[a] *Actually, the sign should be attributed to Robert Latou Dickinson (Munsick, 1985).*

has preceded development of clinically apparent immune deficiency syndrome (AIDS) (Rhoads et al., 1987). Budding yeast or pseudohyphae may be seen on the wet mount, and may become more visible if 10% KOH is added. The Gram-positive organism also is easily seen on the Gram stain, being much larger than bacteria.

"Nonspecific" vaginitis (or bacterial vaginosis) is due to *Gardnerella vaginalis* (previously called *Hemophilus vaginalis*). Its discharge has a fetid odor like that of trichomoniasis, so that the physician could suspect the diagnosis during the examination or by sniffing the speculum. An amine produced by the bacteria can be volatilized by adding a drop of KOH to the discharge. Smell the slide quickly—the fishy odor may be apparent only in the first whiff. On the wet mount, the vaginal epithelial cells look speckled (because of the adherent bacteria), and may appear to lose their borders. These are called clue cells. The Gram stain shows sheets of pleiomorphic Gram-negative coccobacilli, and a notable absence of the normal lactobacilli, which are plump Gram-positive rods.

Patients with gonorrhea often do *not* complain of a vaginal discharge. But of course the physician will look for kidney-bean-shaped, intracellular Gram negative diplococci in all Gram stains. In prepubescent girls, the gonococcus is the most common cause of a vaginal discharge. The physician who discovers it is obligated to investigate the possibility of sexual abuse, although in children this organism may also be inoculated by fingers or towels, because of the greater susceptibility of the thin immature mucosa and the alkaline pH of the vagina (Monif, 1982).

The discharge in atrophic or senescent vaginitis is seldom profuse. Although this condition may cause a blood-tinged discharge, such patients need to be referred for evaluation of a co-existing endometrial carcinoma.

Vaginal Carcinoma

A blood-tinged discharge may be the presenting symptom of vaginal carcinoma.

A polypoid mass or a fungating grapelike mass may be a sarcoma. Any polyp in the vagina of a child must be biopsied without delay because of the possibility of the extremely aggressive tumor, sarcoma botryoides.

Other Findings in the Vagina

Look for the opening of a rectovaginal fistula.

Vaginal ulcers may occur from the same etiologies as ulcers of the vulva (see p. 401).

Transverse ridges in the vagina (or on the cervix), abnormal vaginal mucosa, and vaginal adenosis (the presence of glandular epithelium capable of secreting copious quantities of mucus) are often seen in patients with in utero exposure to DES (Kistner, 1986).

Bimanual Examination

A Method

1.   Stand either at the foot of the table or at the patient's left side, outside the abducted leg.

2.   Explain to the patient that you are going to feel her womb and ovaries. Ask her to "take slow, deep breaths, and try to make your abdomen very soft."

3.   Use whichever hand you wish for the next step. In fact, some physicians switch intrapelvic hands halfway through so as to optimize their palpation of each adnexa.

4.   Insert your index and third fingers (well lubricated with jelly) into the vagina, again taking care to avoid pressure on the anterior structures. Fold the fourth and fifth fingers into the palm, which is supine (i.e., facing upward). If the introitus is very small, you may be able to insert only the index finger.

5.   Locate the cervix. You may wish to take this opportunity to tell the patient, "Your cervix is right here. It feels like the end of your nose." (Make sure that it does feel that way, vide infra.) Remind her that if she uses a diaphragm for contraception, she needs to check that it covers the cervix. Or if she has an intrauterine device, she needs to check periodically to be sure its string is in place in the cervical os.

6.   Place the vaginal fingers under the cervix and push it (and the uterine corpus) toward the abdominal wall. Watch the patient's face; tenderness is an important sign of pelvic inflammatory disease. Place the external hand gently on the abdominal wall and feel for the fundus of the uterus, starting just under the umbilicus and proceeding toward the symphysis pubis. By palpating the uterus between the two hands, you can ascertain its size, shape, consistency, and mobility.

If you are not able to feel the fundus of the uterus in this way, it may be retroflexed, in which case it is felt in the cul-de-sac, posterior to the cervix. Another clue to a retroflexed uterus is that the cervix tends to be almost parallel to the axis of the vagina, instead of perpendicular to it.

7.   To palpate the left adnexal area, move your fingers to the left of the cervix. Move the external hand just medial to the anterior superior iliac spine, and bring it over the ovary by a series of inferior displacements. Feel for the size, shape, and mobility of the ovary. Remember that ovaries, like testicles, are tender, so gentleness is very important.

Examine the right adnexal region, mutatis mutandis.

(Don't be discouraged. Palpating the ovaries is not like feeling for a coin in your pocket. It has been compared with trying to determine which grocery bag has the oranges or the hot dog buns in the middle, by feeling through the sides of the bag.)

8.   The examination concludes with a rectovaginal examination. First, change your glove or remove the outer (soiled) glove from the hand to be used for the rectovaginal examination. While gynecologists have always been careful to avoid introducing rectal organisms into the vagina, it may be equally important to keep infectious agents (e.g., lymphogranuloma venereum; human papillomavirus, the cause of venereal warts; and the human immunodeficiency virus, the cause of AIDS) out of the rectum (Wilbanks, 1986).

Inspect the anal area for hemorrhoids, fistulae, and other signs of pathology (see Ch. 23, p. 412).

Making sure that the fingers are well lubricated, insert the index finger into the vagina, and the third finger into the rectum.

Feel the rectovaginal septum between your two fingers for thickening and nodularity. If the uterus is retroverted, outline the fundus. Finally, move the rectal finger through 360 degrees to check for masses in the rectum (see Ch. 23, p. 412). (You may remove the finger from the vagina before doing this.)

Check the stool on the glove for occult blood.

Some Pedagogic Notes

1. Gynecologists disagree on whether the abdominal hand is pushing structures toward the vaginal fingers to be examined by them, or the vaginal fingers are lifting structures to be examined by the external hand.

Since the external hand is closer to the ventral side of the structures, and the internal hand to the dorsal side, both hands should be used to obtain information. It may be helpful to think of first one, and then of the other, as the "examining" hand.

2. It may be quite difficult to distinguish an adnexal mass from a uterine mass. If you apply downward pressure to a uterine mass, or move it from side to side, you should feel pressure and movement of the cervix against your fingers. If you do not, the mass may be ovarian, or a leiomyoma suspended on a long pedicle.

3. Students should never pass up an opportunity to examine a patient under anesthesia. The use of mannikins would also be very helpful in improving skill in this examination.

The Cervix

In either pelvic inflammatory disease or in ruptured ectopic pregnancy (p. 408), the cervix will be exquisitely tender, especially with motion. This is sometimes called the "chandelier sign" because the patient seems to jump for the chandelier.

A stony hard consistency of the cervix is a sign of carcinoma. Softening is a sign of early pregnancy (Table 22-2), but also may occur with leiomyoma.

The Uterine Corpus

The normal uterus feels like a small ripe pear. It should be firm, smooth, and freely movable.

Retrodisplacement

Although once treated with enthusiastic surgical intervention, retrodisplacement of the uterus is itself of no pathologic significance, being found in about 20% of women who presented at a large gynecologic clinic (Kistner, 1986).

Infections

◗ On examination, the uterus may be boggy and tender. A purulent exudate may be seen coming from the cervical os. This may signal endometritis, which following a septic abortion can rapidly lead to shock and death.

Tumors

The most common type of tumor of the uterine corpus is the benign leiomyoma, commonly but incorrectly termed a "fibroid." These tumors can grow to be extremely large and may cause symptoms due to impingement on other pelvic structures. The differential diagnosis includes: 1) pregnancy, 2) ovarian tumor, 3) a redundant or distended cecum filled with feces, 4) a redundant sigmoid, 5) an appendiceal abscess, 6) diverticulitis, 7) carcinoma of the sigmoid colon (Kistner, 1986), and 8) endometrial carcinoma.

Endometrial cancer may not cause any abnormalities detectable on pelvic examination. Vaginal cytologies occasionally pick up a case, but have a high incidence of false negatives.

Pregnancy

The physical signs of pregnancy are summarized in Table 22-2. With laboratory testing, pregnancy is usually diagnosed before the uterus is significantly enlarged on the physical examination.

The presence of Piskacek's sign reliably shows the placental site, and its unequivocal presence nearly precludes the existence of a tubal pregnancy (Munsick, 1985).

The Adnexae

The mature ovaries are almond-shaped structures, almost the size of the distal half of your little finger. Normal ovaries are impalpable in 13% of premenopausal women and 70% of postmenopausal women (Granberg & Wikland, 1988).

Cysts of the Ovary

A cyst of 6 cm or less could be a follicle cyst or a corpus luteum cyst. The former often disappears after the next menstrual period. The corpus luteum cyst, if it ruptures, can result in all the signs and symptoms of intraperitoneal bleeding.

Ovarian cysts of large size may be associated with hydatidiform mole, chorioadenoma destruens, or choriocarcinoma (Kistner, 1986). In the Stein-Leventhal syndrome, the polycystic ovaries may each be larger than the uterus.

False positives. Midline "tumors" that have occasionally simulated an ovarian cyst include a distended urinary bladder and the pregnant uterus.

If an ovarian cyst becomes very large, it must be distinguished from ascites. 1) The differentiation might be made by percussion. Ascites displaces the small intestine centrally, producing a tympanitic percussion note in midabdomen and dullness in the flanks. With an ovarian cyst, the intestine is pushed laterally so that there is midabdominal dullness and lateral tympany. (Be sure that the bladder is empty before performing this test.) 2) An ovarian cyst never produces a fluid wave. 3) With extremely large cysts, Blaxland's method may be used: Place a flat ruler on the abdomen just above the anterior superior iliac spines, and press firmly backwards. If the swelling is due to a cyst, the pulsations of the aorta are transmitted to the fingers and can be demonstrated by the ruler ("Bailey", Clain, 1973). Ascites will not produce this effect.

Tumors of the Ovary

Most ovarian neoplasms are lateral or posterior to the uterus, and so must be sought both bimanually and on rectovaginal examination. Unfortunately, about 72% have disseminated before the diagnosis is made.

The differential diagnosis of an ovarian mass includes: a low-lying distended cecum, a redundant sigmoid colon, appendiceal abscess, impacted feces in the rectosigmoid, diverticulitis, carcinoma of the sigmoid, pedunculated leiomyoma, desmoid tumor, urachal cyst, or retroperitoneal neoplasm or abscess. A hematoma of the rectus muscle, which may occur without history of trauma in anticoagulated patients, can be distinguished by its superficial location, demonstrated by voluntarily tensing the abdominal muscles. An ectopic pelvic kidney deserves special note.

About 25% of ovarian malignancies are accompanied by ascites at the time of discovery. Rarely, benign ovarian tumors are associated with nonmalignant ascites and right pleural effusions (Meig's syndrome) (Kistner, 1986).

The Oviducts (Fallopian Tubes)

The oviducts are generally not palpable. However, when involved with pelvic inflammatory disease, they may be felt as rubbery, cordlike structures, which may eventually become fixed in the posterior cul-de-sac.

🠾 The mass due to tubo-ovarian abscess may be felt either anterior or posterior to the uterus. If a previously palpable mass suddenly disappears in the setting of a hard, tender abdomen, one may be dealing with a ruptured tubo-ovarian abscess, a potential cause of death.

Pelvic tuberculosis, usually of the oviduct, is found in about 10% of women with the pulmonary disease (Kistner, 1986). At first, the pelvic examination is completely normal. Later, slight thickening of the tubes and tubo-ovarian masses may occur. Finally, ascites may develop because of peritoneal involvement.

Synthesis

Ruptured Tubal Pregnancy

In the event of an acute abdomen occurring in a woman who *could* be pregnant, one must consider this diagnosis, which is responsible for 2% to 3% of all obstetric deaths. This diagnosis is treacherous because the pregnancy test is often negative, and the physical findings are highly variable.

🠾 If there has been a leakage of blood, manipulation of the cervix may cause a chandelier sign. The cul-de-sac may have a feeling of fullness due to liquid blood, or there might even be a mass if the blood has clotted. Cullen's sign (Turner's sign) (see Ch. 20, p. 372) is quite rare (Smith & Wright, 1935).

Endometriosis

Endometriosis is defined as the presence of functioning endometrium outside of its normal situation. On physical examination, check for fixed ovarian masses, nodularity in the rectovaginal septum, and induration in the cul-de-sac. Among other areas affected are the lower genital tract (cervix, vulva, and vagina), pelvic peritoneum, umbilicus, and laparotomy scars (Kistner, 1986).

Pedagogic Inspiration

In the following story, one of the central figures was a very fine observer, who told the story on herself at a time when our paths were about to part.

•

A patient was admitted to the woman's medical floor at a very prestigious hospital located in a very cosmopolitan city on the West Coast. The admitting diagnosis was fever of unknown origin, which remained the diagnosis for 48 hours. At that time, the resident reviewed the chart with the intern and asked what the pelvic examination showed. The intern replied that she had not done a pelvic. My informant, who was then the resident, told

the intern to do it immediately, because it was part of the workup for fever of unknown origin.

Two days later, while reviewing the chart, the intern was again asked about the results of the pelvic, and again responded that she had not done the pelvic examination. The resident pointed out the various diagnoses that could cause the fever in this patient, which would be manifested in the pelvic examination, and again instructed her intern to do the pelvic.

The next day, the pelvic still had not been done, so the resident instructed her intern to do it instantly. The intern returned a few minutes later announcing that the patient refused the examination.

At this point, the resident did what she should have done at the beginning. She went to the patient herself and announced that she, the resident, was going to perform the long-overdue pelvic examination.

"But you *can't* perform an internal pelvic examination on me," the patient retorted.

"And why not?" asked the resident.

"Because," said the patient, "I'm a man."

•

References

Bloom HJG: Venous hums in hepatic cirrhosis. *Br Med J* 12:343–350, 1950.
Clain A, ed: *Hamilton Bailey's Demonstrations of Physical Signs in Clinical Surgery*, ed. 15. Williams & Wilkens, Baltimore, 1973.
Danforth DN & Scott JR, eds: *Obstetrics and Gynecology*, ed 5. JB Lippincott, Philadelphia, 1986.
Demarest CB: Getting the most from the Pap smear. *Patient Care* 19(Feb 28):63–86, 1985.
Friedrich EG Jr: Vulvar dystrophy. *Clin Obstet Gynecol* 28:178–187, 1985.
Granberg S, Wikland M: A comparison between ultrasound and gynecologic examination for detection of enlarged ovaries in a group of women at risk for ovarian carcinoma. *J Ultrasound Med* 7:59–64, 1988.
Green TH Jr: *Gynecology: Essentials of Clinical Practice*, ed 2. Little, Brown, Boston, 1971.
Gunby P: Aftermath of the ACS bombshell. *JAMA* 243:2372–2374, 1980.
Handfield-Jones SE, Hinde FRJ, Kennedy CTC. Lichen sclerosus et atrophicus in children misdiagnosed as sexual abuse. *Br Med J* 294:1404–1405, 1987.
Hellman LM, Pritchard JA: *Williams Obstetrics*, ed 14. Appleton-Century-Crofts, New York, 1971.
Kistner RW: *Gynecology: Principles and Practice*, ed 4. Year Book Medical Publishers, Chicago, 1986.
Krieger JN, Tam MR, Stevens CE, Nielsen IO, Hale J, Kiviat NB, Holmes KK: Diagnosis of trichomoniasis: Comparison of conventional wet-mount examination with cytologic studies, cultures, and monoclonal antibody staining of direct specimens. *JAMA* 259:1223–1227, 1988.
Levin S, Benson CA, Goodman LJ, Pottage JC Jr, Kessler HA, Trenholme GM: The office approach to the sexually transmitted diseases: Part I. *DM* 33(3):1–179, 1987.
Magee J: The pelvic examination: A view from the other end of the table. *Ann Intern Med* 83:563–564, 1975.
McKnight E: The prevalence of "hirsutism" in young women. *Lancet* 1:410–413, 1964.
Monif GRG: *Infectious Diseases in Obstetrics and Gynecology*. Harper & Row, New York, 1982.

Muram D: Labial adhesions in sexually abused children. *JAMA* 259:352–353, 1988.

Munsick RA: Dickinson's sign: Focal uterine softening in early pregnancy and its correlation with the placental site. *Am J Obstet Gynecol* 152:799–802, 1985.

Nichols DH, Evrard JR: *Ambulatory Gynecology.* Harper & Row, New York, 1985.

Punnonen R, Soidinmaki H, Kauppila O, Pystynen P: Relationship of vulvar lichen sclerosus et atrophicus to carcinoma. *Ann Chir Gynaecol* 197 (Suppl):23–25, 1985.

Raymond CA: Cervical dysplasia upturn worries gynecologists, health officials. *JAMA* 257:2397–2398, 1987a.

Raymond CA: For women infected with papillomavirus, close watch counseled. *JAMA* 257:2398–2399, 1987b.

Rhoads JL, Wright C, Redfield RR, Burke DS: Chronic vaginal can-

didiasis in women with human immunodeficiency virus infection. *JAMA* 257:3105–3107, 1987.

Rittmaster RS, Loriaux DL: Hirsuitism. *Ann Intern Med* 106:95–107, 1987.

Smith I, Wright FJ: Cullen's sign in ruptured ectopic gestation. *Lancet* 1:930–932, 1935.

Soper JT, Creasman WT: Vulvar dystrophies. *Clin Obstet Gynecol* 29:431–439, 1986.

Tagatz GE, Kopher RA, Nagel TC, Okagaki T: The clitoral index: A bioassay of androgenic stimulation. *Obstet Gynecol* 54:562–564, 1979.

Whiting D: Puzzling genital lesions: How to make the Dx. *Mod Med* 55(4):58–77, 1983.

Wilbanks GD: Changing gloves between vaginal and rectal examination: Reinstitution of old practices for new diseases. *JAMA* 256:1893, 1986.

23
The Rectum

"They say man has succeeded where the animals fail because of the clever use of his hands, yet when compared to the hands, the *sphincter ani* is far superior. If you place into your cupped hands a mixture of fluid, solid and gas and then through an opening at the bottom, try to let only the gas escape, you will fail. Yet the sphincter ani can do it. The sphincter apparently can differentiate between solid, fluid and gas. It apparently can tell whether its owner is alone or with someone, whether standing up or sitting down, whether its owner has his pants on or off. No other muscle in the body is such a protector of the dignity of man, yet so ready to come to his relief. A muscle like this is worth protecting."

Walter C. Bornemeier, 1960

Preparation

Before performing a rectal examination on the patient, you should have acquired some minimum physical skills that will permit you to make your examination at least as discomforting as possible and certainly painless. In bygone days, it was expected that all of the medical students would have performed rectal examinations upon each other before being set loose upon patients. The type of diligent preceptorship requisite to such an activity is now as rare as a xebec.

Similarly, medical schools previously had a required proctology rotation. Among other educational opportunities, this included the chance to perform (with the patient's prior permission) a rectal examination on an anesthetized patient under the direct supervision of the patient's personal proctologist, who was about to perform surgery.

There are excellent mannikins that will permit the student to gain some initial experience in inserting a lubricated gloved finger through a sphincter and palpating a variety of prostatic prostheses. If your school does not have such a mannikin, volunteers should be solicited from your Curriculum Committee.

A Method

In the woman, the rectal examination is generally performed as part of the pelvic examination (see Ch. 22, p. 406). However, in cases in which the pelvic examination has been deferred, the rectal examination can still be done by the method used for the man.

Positioning the Patient

Usually, the examination is best performed with the patient standing with his legs spread a few feet apart, leaning forward, his chest resting on the examining table.

The bed-bound patient can be examined in one of two modi-

fied Sims' positions, the two differing as to whether the dependent leg is extended or flexed: The patient may be placed in the left lateral decubitus position, as for a lumbar puncture, with the knees and hips flexed, the trunk flexed forward, and the arms holding the hips and knees in maximum flexion. The second position would be obtained by having the lower (left) leg fully extended at the knee and, more importantly, at the hip. This actually rolls the patient another 45 degrees toward the prone position. Which position is optimum depends on the given patient's skeletal mobility and/or the obscuring quality of his buttocks.

If the patient is in an immovable supine position, the hips can be flexed, the knees flexed (passively, if need be, and held by an assistant), the anus thus exposed to the examiner. While one can do a rectal examination and even obtain stool samples from a patient held in this position, one may not always be completely confident about what one is palpating.

Protecting the Patient's Dignity

The patient should be handed some toilet paper or tissue at this time to hold for later use at the end of the examination. Say to the patient, "I am going to use some lubricant to make the examination more comfortable for you. I will tell you when I'm done." (This last statement is made as a part of physicianhood. The patient will know very well when you are done.)

You can also hand the patient the tissue at the end of the examination, but some doctors become so busy with the guaiac test that they forget. Besides, handing the patient the tissue in the beginning shows the patient that you are sensitive to and anticipate his feelings. Having him hold the tissue makes him a more active participant and less acted upon, a matter that could become exquisitely important in light of the psychodynamics of some male patients.

Alternatively, Dr. Douglas Lindsey of Arizona instructs the students to do the wiping, because they are wearing gloves. If you do this, tell the patient that you are cleaning off the lubricant. Then ask him to get dressed while you run a test for occult blood. Leave the room, being sure that a box of tissue and a covered wastebasket are conveniently within his reach. Before returning, allow the patient sufficient time to restore his dignity, and wash his hands if he likes.

The Actual Examination

1. Put your gloves on, spread the patient's cheeks, and examine for hemorrhoids, tumors, condylomata, ulcers, fissures, excoriations, prolapsing internal hemorrhoids, or anything that you have never seen before. You will probably fail to see a fissure if you do not spread the cheeks and put a little bit of stretch on the anus.

Dr. Frank Iber of Illinois adds:

> You can gain a great deal of information from inspection prior to the rectal examination. If the person, with a little straining, can show you the margin between the skin and the mucosa, this will reveal external hemorrhoids and skin irritation. If he is unable to relax sufficiently to show you this margin it may indicate pathology to be encountered with the finger or proctoscope.

While performing this part of the examination, you might also want to check the patient for the anal wink (see Ch. 26, p. 504).

2. Put a generous amount of lubricant on your gloved index finger and say, "I am going to put some lubricant on you now. It might feel cold."

3. Place the lubricant at the anal orifice. If the patient has asked whether this is going to hurt, you have said, "No, it will be uncomfortable but it shouldn't produce a pain in the sense of being a sharp sensation. If I do anything during the examination that makes you feel a sharpness, or a pain, be sure to tell me."

If the patient has not raised this issue, at this point you should say, "This might feel a little uncomfortable," or "You'll feel a pressure." (Don't call it a "pain.") Depending on the individual patient, you might add, "But it shouldn't be painful." You want to encourage him to report any such sharp painful sensation, because it is a clue to the presence of a mucosal tear, a prostatic inflammation, or a rectal abscess.

4. At this point, it is assumed that you have practiced the rectal examination upon a mannikin or an anesthetized patient. Accordingly, you may have become inappropriately cavalier about the rectal sphincter.

Gently press the tip of your index finger through the center of the sphincter, so that the entire circumference of your finger is coated with lubricant. Note the anal sphincter tone.

5. Insert the examining finger as far as possible and prepare to sweep the four quadrants searching for abnormalities (vide infra).

6. Finally, ask the patient to perform a Valsalva maneuver ("bear down") so that you can make a final check of the lumen, feeling for polyps and other masses, and the farthermost rectal mucosa. Say "we're almost done" or words to that effect.

7. Withdraw the examining finger and inspect it for stool. Note its appearance, and place a smear on a slide for occult blood testing, or sometimes for other tests such as stool fat stains (see Ch. 28, p. 554). If you wipe off the lubricant, dispose of the tissue paper inside the glove, which you turn inside out on removing it.

Findings on Rectal Examination

Inspection

Fissures or Fistulae

The presence of perianal fistula and/or fissure suggests that a patient with inflammatory bowel disease has Crohn's regional enteritis rather than chronic ulcerative colitis.

Pilonidal Sinus

Although often misdiagnosed as a "fistula-in-ano," a pilonidal sinus is actually located some distance away from the anus, in the midline near the base of the coccyx. Purulent fluid may be expressed by pressure over the sacrum ("Bailey," Clain, 1973).

Skin Lesions

Pruritis ani, with erythema and lichenification of the perianal skin, may result from a variety of causes, such as sensitivity to various foods, condiments, coffee, drugs, irritants in toilet tissue and undergarments, and topical preparations used to treat itching. A symmetrical pink discoloration is said to be characteristic for sensitivity to dairy proteins (Friend, 1987). Parasitic infestations (most commonly pinworms) and fungal infections (such as monilia) are also a possibility. Be attentive for evidence of sexually transmitted diseases (see Table 21-1), which may present in the perianal region rather than on the genitalia, especially in homosexual men.

Perianal Ecchymosis

A ringlike perianal ecchymosis (Bryant's sign) may occur with intraperitoneal bleeding.

Palpation

Sphincter Tone

One of two abnormalities may be found. A pathologic tenderness and resistance to a properly performed insertion indicates a local abnormality. Insufficient resistance of the sphincter indicates a neurologic abnormality, frequent practice of receptive anal intercourse, or the residuum of a mechanical problem (e.g., a laceration occurring during childbirth). (The ability of the patient to squeeze the clinician's finger with the rectal sphincter is an excellent alternate test of spinal cord integrity—also see the bulbocavernosus reflex, Chapter 26 (p. 504).

Internal Findings

Anteriorly, everyone should be able to palpate the prostate (vide infra). With a little more experience, one can also detect a distended bladder as well as seminal vesicles that have enlarged secondary to disease. Cowper's bulbourethral glands, situated inferior to the prostate, are usually palpable only if inflamed.

In women, note enlargement and displacement of the uterus, and—in the pouch of Douglas—swellings, carcinomatosis, or the bulging of a pelvic abscess.

Laterally to the patient's right, one can elicit tenderness from an inflamed and swollen appendix. This is especially important if the patient has a retrocecal appendix, which may *not* produce the expected findings on abdominal examination. Laterally to the patient's left, one might find tenderness due to diverticulitis or abscess.

Posteriorly, one can palpate the pyriformis muscle and an occasional tumor in the presacral area. One may demonstrate tenderness in the sacrococcygeal joint. An aneurysm of the internal iliac artery may be felt as a pulsating mass.

Higher in the canal, one can find stricture of the rectum due to cancer or fibrosis, rarely postobstructive dilation of the canal, and very rarely the apex of an intussusception. The feeling that there are multiple small adenomas in the rectal mucosa should suggest that one is palpating the pseudopolyps of chronic ulcerative colitis.

Tumors may be found in *any* of the above locations.

The presence of impacted stool may explain diarrhea (which occurs around the obstructing feces), abdominal discomfort, and even difficulty with voiding.

The Prostate

Size of the prostate. The size of the prostate in the normal young man and in the senior citizen with benign prostatic hypertrophy is best learned from the mannikin in the teaching lab. For those without such a tool, the young man's prostate is roughly the size of a walnut, and the older man's enlarged prostate is the size of a lemon. Given the difficulties in assessing the size of a globular object from palpation of a restricted area of its surface, one should probably just say "normal" or "enlarged," after achieving sufficient experience.

A teaching trick. One can teach students to describe the consistency of the palpated prostate gland by using one's own flexed thumb as a model. "Hard" means like any bony prominence. "Indurated" is like the extensor pollices as they are stretched taut over diaphyseal bone. "Normal" is like the tensed thenar eminence. "Boggy" is like the relaxed thenar eminence (in imitation of acute prostatitis).

It is important to keep checking your descriptions against your own thumb because with fatigue and distraction, you may be changing your usage of the last two terms.

1. "Boggy" is a word that should probably be eliminated from the terminology of clinical examination, as it is now used only as a shibboleth with prostatitis. It is true that peat bog is soft and some *acutely* inflamed glands do seem soft like peat bog. This is partly due to cysts or abscesses and partly due to the fact that the gland is so tender that one cannot get a good feel of it without causing the patient to move away. However, in some books, "boggy" refers to *chronic* prostatitis, incorrectly I believe, since the chronic form of prostatitis is more likely to be "indurated," sometimes with sufficient fibrosis that it is "hard" enough to raise a suspicion of neoplasia.

2. *False positives*: Wiener and Nathanson (see Ch. 29) warn that elderly men with atrophic prostate glands may have their bony symphysis pubis palpated and a "stony hard" gland misidentified.

Prostatic nodules. Prostatic nodules are a sign of neoplasm and are an indication for biopsy. Oddly enough, in some series only about 50% of prostate nodules actually turn out to be neoplasm, the rest being nodular hyperplasia. If the nodular induration is due to tuberculosis, one or both seminal vesicles and the vas deferens are also involved in most cases ("Bailey," Clain, 1973).

While we were formerly taught to feel for a bony hard spot in the prostate, more recent thinking points out that a bony hard spot in the prostate is a relatively late finding. Even a spot of induration should be noted and biopsied (Chodak & Shoenberg, 1985).

Rectal examination has the highest sensitivity for prostate cancer of all screening tests, including both cytologies and chemical tests, such as random acid phosphatase measurements (random means those not drawn immediately after the rectal examination—see "pearl" (O)). However, the sensitivity is still only 69%,

the specificity 89%, the predictive value of a positive test 67%, the predictive value of a negative test 91%, and the efficiency of the test 85% (Guinan et al., 1980).

A self-study: *Considering that a lymphoma metastatic to the prostate can also produce a hard prostate, what would happen to the specificity of the test (hard prostate as a test for prostatic carcinoma) in an oncology clinic? To the predictive value of a positive test? (See Appendix 23-1.)*

Three-Glass Test. This special test is described in Chapter 28 (p. 551).

Alleged Adverse Effects of the Rectal Examination

1. The rectal examination does not cause false-positive elevations of the serum acid phosphatase or of prostatic-specific antigen (Brawer et al., 1988) in patients with benign prostatic enlargement. It is therefore not necessary to draw the enzyme levels prior to rectal examination. The examination can, however, cause a rise in the acid phosphatase level in patients with malignant prostatic enlargement or in those whose malignancy has become refractory to hormonal therapy (Osegbe & Magoha, 1982).

O   Thus, to improve the sensitivity of the serum acid phosphatase for detecting prostatic malignancy, it should specifically be drawn *after* the rectal examination, the exact opposite of the usual teaching.

2. Students are often admonished not to perform a rectal examination in a patient suffering a myocardial infarction because of the possibility of precipitating a fatal arrhythmia by stimulating a reflex. This is an old wives' tale.

In a series of 86 patients with documented acute myocardial infarction, a *gentle* rectal examination was performed within 24 hours of admission and not found to produce a single example of death, arrhythmia, or even angina. The unsuspected findings of occult blood, prostatic enlargement, and voluminous hard stool were encountered rather frequently. Thus, the value of rectal examination in planning anticoagulant therapy and bowel and bladder care outweighs the hypothetical risk (Earnest & Fletcher, 1969). As the pre-1968 medical school aphorism goes: "If you don't put your finger in it, you'll put your foot in it."

Appendix 23-1. Answer to Self-Study

The false positives for prostatic cancer would increase, because of the increasing proportion of cases of lymphoma. Since the specificity is equal to the true negatives divided by the sum of the true negatives and false positives, the specificity in this instance would decrease.

Also the predictive value of a positive test (true positives over the sum of the true positives and false positives) would decrease.

References

Brawer MK, Schifman RB, Ahmann FR, Ahmann ME, Coulis KM: The effect of digital rectal examination on serum levels of prostatic-specific antigen. *Arch Pathol Lab Med* 112:1110–1112, 1988.

Chodak GW, Shoenberg HW: Early detection of prostate cancer by routine screening. *JAMA* 252:3261–3264, 1985.

Clain A, ed: *Hamilton Bailey's Demonstrations of Physical Signs in Clinical Surgery*, ed 15. Williams & Wilkins, Baltimore, 1973.

Earnest DL, Fletcher GF: Danger of rectal examination in patients with acute myocardial infarction—fact or fiction? *N Engl J Med* 281:238–241, 1969.

Friend WG: Pruritis ani. *Med Times* 115(11):89–94, 1987.

Guinan P, Bush I, Ray V, Vieth R, Rao R, Bhatti R: The accuracy of the rectal examination in the diagnosis of prostatic carcinoma. *N Engl J Med* 303:499–583, 1980.

Osegbe DN, Magoha G: The effect of rectal examination on serum acid phosphatase levels in benign and malignant prostatic disease. *Postgrad Med J* 58:763–766, 1982.

24
The Musculoskeletal System

About Domitius Tully:

Crippled and deformed in every limb, he could only enjoy his vast wealth by contemplating it and could not even turn in bed without assistance. He also had to have his teeth cleaned and brushed for him—a squalid and pitiful detail—and when complaining about the humiliations of his infirmity was often heard to say that every day he licked the fingers of his slaves.

The Younger Pliny, *Letters*, Book Eight:18

Muscles

Inspection

Myopathy

The sculpture sketched in Figure 24-1 has what appears to be a myopathy. Notice that the subject is unable to arise unassisted from the tailor position. This indicates disease of the pelvic girdle; when severe, the subject will also be unable to arise unassisted from a squatting position.

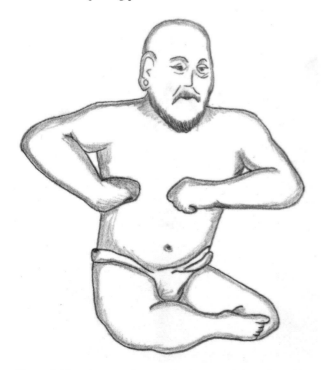

Figure 24-1. *A case of myopathy (see text.) Drawing of late Olmec period sculpture, on display in the Mexico City Museum of Anthropology.*

The position of the hands gives rise to speculation about a myopathy afflicting the shoulder girdle. In some such diseases, the patient first notices weakness during acts requiring vigorous repeated motion with the hands held at or above the shoulder level, such as brushing the teeth, combing the hair, or shaving. This man has indeed grown a beard, but direct inspection of the shoulder girdle reveals no apparent atrophy; in fact there might even be some hypertrophy. Accordingly, I believe that his upper extremities are simply postured in the synkinesia of a man with pelvic girdle weakness trying to arise. (For more on synkinesia, see Ch. 26, p. 487).

Given the above, what is your diagnosis? Write it down. (Answer is in Appendix 24-1, p. 431.)

Atrophy

Using nature's own control, compare the development of muscles on both sides, or measure the circumference at comparable points along the two limbs (see Ch. 19, p. 367.)

Muscle atrophy can result from neuropathy as well as from myopathy (Fig. 26-36.)

A Bulge in the Muscle

A ruptured biceps or other muscle will have a bulge that occurs only and always during contraction. In a reversal of the usual order for the clinical examination, the history should confirm the diagnosis. The patient can usually recall the exact time of onset. The appearance of the bulge immediately follows a violent effort and a popping sound. Associated symptoms are some discomfort on contraction and some weakness. In the absence of such a history, consider the alternate diagnosis of a muscle herniation through a defect in the covering aponeurosis.

In part A of Fig. 24-2, the arm is extended at the elbow. All the muscle seen is of normal consistency. There is nothing hard to palpation. The photograph in B, with the elbow flexed, was taken just seconds after the first. The bulge is about halfway between the acromion and the contracted biceps. It is the consistency of contracted muscle. What is your diagnosis? Write down your answer, then see Appendix 24-2 (p. 432).

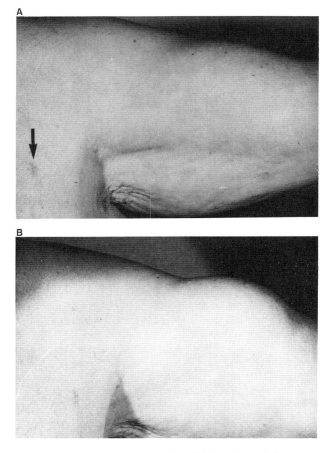

Figure 24-2. *A, The biceps relaxed. The pointer indicates a spider telangiectasis. (It is poorly seen, but demonstrates the usual size.) B, The biceps contracted. What is your diagnosis?*

Rhabdomyosarcomas usually feel hard both during and between contractions, but may rarely *appear* to be a localized bulge, occurring only and always during contraction. In such cases, the contraction probably just throws the rhabdomyosarcoma into relief. Similarly, myositis ossificans should not be confused with muscle herniation or muscle rupture since it will also be hard during muscle relaxation.

Fibrillation and Fasciculation

These phenomena are discussed in Chapter 26 (p. 493).

Tetanus

A sustained tonic spasm of the muscles, most notably in the jaw, where it is called trismus or lockjaw, results inter alia from the toxin produced by *Clostridium tetanus*. Such spasm can be precipitated by almost any type of stimulus.

Tetanic equivalents are discussed in Chapter 26 (p. 488).

Torticollis

Torticollis is an abnormal sustained posture of the head and neck involving lateral deviation and rotation (Fig. 24-3). The patient may complain of stiffness and spasm in the neck muscles before the postural abnormality is apparent. The muscles of the neck, including the sternocleidomastoid, trapezius, levator scapulae, and posterior cervical muscles may become visibly hypertrophied.

Torticollis is a dramatic presentation in patients who have

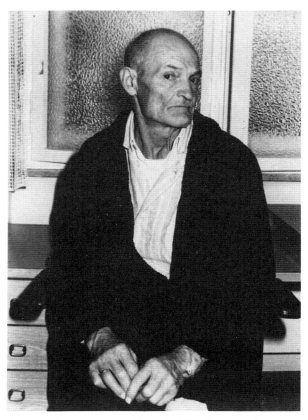

Figure 24-3. *A patient with torticollis. Photograph courtesy of Dr. W.H. Poewe, reprinted with permission (Poewe, 1987).*

been treated with high-dose phenothiazines or butyrophenones. The differential diagnosis is listed in Table 24-1.

A classic finding in spasmodic torticollis is that the abnormal head posture can be easily corrected by a light touch with one hand to the side of the chin (*geste antagonistique*) or counterpressure to other parts of the head, perhaps by enhancing proprioceptive input (Poewe, 1987). This might lead some to conclude (erroneously) that the problem is "psychogenic."

Palpation

Localized Tenderness

Fibrositis, a form of nonarticular rheumatism, may be diagnosed more conveniently by palpation of the muscles than by demonstrating the sleep-laboratory abnormalities that also accompany it (Smythe & Moldofsky, 1977–1978). There are 14 points whose normal tenderness becomes exaggerated. The first 12 of these are paired (Figs. 24-4 and 24-5). The points are these:

1. The midpoint of the upper border of the trapezius
2. The tennis elbow site, the origin of the third (long) extensor muscle from the lateral epicondyle
3. The second costochondral junction
4. The fat pad overlying the medial collateral ligament of the knee
5. The origin of the supraspinatus muscle near the medial border of the scapula
6. The upper outer quadrant of the buttock
7. The unpaired structures
    a. The intervertebral ligaments between C-4 and C-6;
    b. The interspinus ligaments between L-4 and S-1.

Table 24-1. Causes of Torticollis

Mechanical

Osteogenic
Osseous malformations (e.g., Klippel-Feil)
Traumatic bone lesions
Cervical spondylitis/osteomyelitis
Cervical spondylosis/osteoporosis

Arthrogenic
Rheumatoid arthritis (involvement of lateral atlantoaxial joint)

Myogenic
Traumatic lesions of neck muscles
Ruptures, hematomas
Shortening of neck muscles
Developmental, scarring
Myositis (e.g., polymyalgia rheumatica)
Acute stiff neck

Compensatory
Ocular palsies (e.g., fourth-nerve palsies)
Cervical syringomyelia
Posterior fossa tumors
Cervical disc disease

Dystonic
Spasmodic torticollis
Drug-induced
Acute neuroleptic-induced dystonia
Tardive dyskinesia
Levo-dopa-treated Parkinson's disease

Source: *Poewe (1987).*

Generalized Tenderness

Generalized muscle tenderness may be found *acutely* in polymyositis, infectious diseases (malaria, rubella, influenza, rheumatic fever, dengue, rat-bite fever, and trichinosis); in hyponatremia, and myopathies, such as McArdle's disease and march myoglobinuria. *Chronically,* the muscles may be tender in hypoparathyroidism, polymyalgia rheumatica, and other collagen vascular disorders.

Percussion

See Chvostek's sign (Ch. 26, p. 490).

Special Maneuvers

Myotonia and Myoedema

A patient with myotonia is unable to relax his hand after a handshake and so continues to grip your hand. (Of course, this must be distinguished from the intentionally held handshake of the disturbed patient who wishes to hold your attention as he speaks.) (See Ch. 13, p. 221 for a method of diagnosing myotonia of the tongue, and Ch. 25, p. 438 for other diagnoses that can be made by shaking a patient's hand.)

The most interesting of the myotonias is Thomsen's disease or myotonia congenita. If you strike the muscles of the thenar eminence with a reflex hammer, they immediately undergo a prolonged tonic contraction.

The most common myotonia is myotonia dystrophica or Steinert's disease. These patients have what is known as a hatchet face due to atrophy of the temporalis, masseter, and sternocleidomastoid muscles (the latter becoming pencil-like). The patients may also develop premature temporal baldness, testicular atrophy, and cataracts. Myotonia dystrophica (Steinert's disease) should never be translated into English, as it might be confused with muscular dystrophy, to which it is not related.

Thomsen's disease (myotonia congenita) has lifelong myotonia but no other abnormalities and is quite benign.

Eulenburg's paramyotonia congenita is a very rare disease in which sudden spastic muscle contractions occur during or immediately after cold exposure.

Myotonia can also be seen in adynamia episodica (hyperkalemic periodic paralysis) and chondrodystrophical myotonia, among the naturally occurring diseases (Furman & Barchi, 1986). Vincristine and propranolol may unmask latent myotonia dystrophica, but other chemical substances may actually produce myotonia de novo (e.g., aromatic carboxylic acids, sulfhydryl-inhibiting para-substituted mercuribenzones, and inhibitors of sterol synthesis including clofibrate). The roles of iodine and hypochloremia in some myotonic syndromes is even more obscure.

Myotonia must be distinguished from a different sign known by the misnomer myoedema, which is also elicited by direct mechanical stimulation of muscle. In myoedema, the muscle contracts slowly and relaxes at the same rate (about $1^1/_2$ seconds). This finding can be produced in almost anyone, given a sufficiently vigorous pinch on the biceps. However, it is easily produced in abnormal states by light percussion with a hammer. Myoedema is not specific for neurologic or muscle disease, and is seen with hypoalbuminemia and/or catabolism (Conn & Smith, 1965); myotonia, on the other hand, is due to primary muscle disease. Myoedema normally requires a much harder striking force than myotonia, which can be elicited with a very light tap in some circumstances. Myoedema is not usually elicited on the thenar eminence; myotonia is. Finally, the after-contraction of myoedema (actually the failure of relaxation) is much briefer in duration than that of myotonia.

Other Maneuvers

Methods for testing muscle strength are given in Chapter 26 (for resistance testing and for the timed stands test, p. 482).

Muscle tone (the tension in resting muscle) is affected in various neurologic conditions (see Ch. 26: spastic and flaccid paralysis; p. 483, the Babinski tonus test, p. 488; and tests for Parkinson's disease, p. 475.)

Joints and Extra-Articular Structures

Inspection and Palpation

In general, joints are checked for erythema (rubor), swelling (tumor), heat (calor), tenderness (dolor), crepitus, and deformity (see Ch. 25). Details pertinent to individual joints are discussed below in the sections on the regional examination.

Special Maneuvers: Range of Motion

A Method

The joints should be put through their range of motion both actively and passively.

If the patient has less than a full range of motion, the angle through which the joint moves should be measured. A simple device (a jointed plastic stick attached to a protractor) is avail-

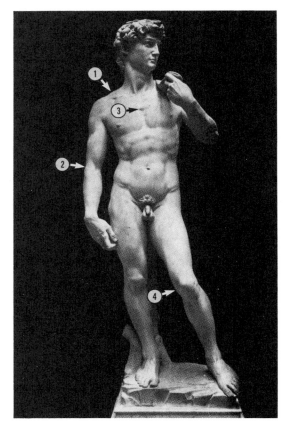

Figure 24-4. *Points of exaggerated tenderness in the fibrositis syndrome. See text for anatomic description. David, by Michelangelo.*

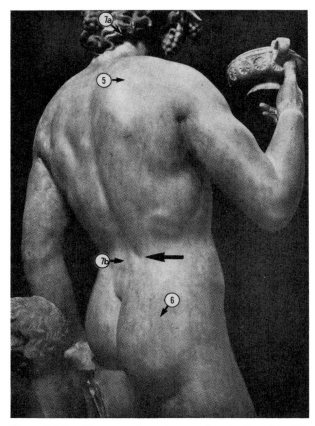

Figure 24-5. *The posterior trigger points in fibrositis. The large arrow indicates the dimple of Venus, which is not a trigger point. See "Modified Schober flexion test" on p. 422. Bacchus, by Michelangelo.*

able for this purpose, or can be improvised. The normal range of motion for various joints is given in Table 24-2. Special features important in the range-of-motion examination of particular joints are discussed when that joint is separately considered below.

A self-study.   Perform each of the maneuvers listed in the table on your partner or on yourself.

○ If the patient has much more pain and resistance to motion when it is performed actively rather than passively, the source of the pain is likely to be the extra-articular structures, such as muscles or tendons. When the pain is just as great when the joint is supported and passively moved by the examiner, intra-articular inflammation is likely.

Increased Range of Motion

Ehlers-Danlos syndrome (cutis laxa) is the affliction of cutaneous hyperelasticity and joint hypermobility (Figs. 24-7, A and B), which are only the dramatic external heralds of important internal cardiovascular, mesenchymal, clotting, and gastrointestinal abnormalities.

Thorax

The examination of the musculoskeletal structures of the chest wall is discussed in Chapter 16 (pp. 245–249).

Shoulder

Range of Motion

Simple maneuvers that can serve as a screening test for range of motion about the shoulder are these: 1) Have the patient extend both arms fully at the elbow, then swing the arms upward in the frontal (coronal) plane, attempting to touch the palms together above the head (abduction); 2) Have the patient perform a similar motion except with the arms in a sagittal plane (flexion); 3) Have the patient place the back of each hand as high as possible between the shoulder blades (internal rotation).

Neer and Welsh Impingement Sign

This sign, along with point tenderness of the greater tuberosity and anterior acromion, and pain on shoulder abduction, forms the diagnostic trinity of supraspinatus tendinitis seen in competitive swimmers (Johnson et al., 1987).

A method.   With one hand, hold the sitting patient's arm straight up, pointing at the ceiling, the patient's palm facing medially. With the other hand, push the tuberosity of the humerus against the anterior inferior surface of the acromion.

Interpretation.   The test is positive if the resultant facial expression shows pain and the patient reports that this reproduces his experience of the original pain. The positive test is confirmed if it is subsequently negated by the injection of 10 ml of 1% lidocaine into the subacromial bursa.

Table 24-2. Normal Range of Motion for Various Joints

Joint	Motion	Range
Shoulder	Abduction (in frontal plane)	0° to 180°
	Forward flexion (Fig. 24-6)	0° to 180°
	Internal, external rotation (humerus, held laterally so that it is parallel to floor and perpendicular to body; forearm moved in sagittal plane)	0° to 90°
Elbow	Flexion-extension	0° to 160°[a]
	Pronation	0° to 90°
	Supination	0° to 90°
Wrist	Flexion-extension	90° to 70°
	Ulnar-radial deviation	50° to 20°
Metacarpo-phalangeal	Flexion-extension	90° to 30°
Spine	Extension	0° to 30°
	Lateral motion	0° to 50°
	Rotation (trunk)	90°
	Rotation (lower thoracic, lumbar)	30°
Cervical spine[b]	Flexion	45°
	Extension	60°
	Rotation	60° to 80°
	Lateral bending	40°
Hip	Extension	0° to 15°
	Flexion (knee flexed)	0° to 120°
	Flexion (knee extended)	0° to 90°
	Abduction	0° to 40°
	Internal rotation (see p. 425)	0° to 40°
	External rotation	0° to 45°
Knee	Hyperextension-flexion	−15° to 130°
Ankle	Plantar flexion-dorsiflexion	−45° to 20°
	Inversion-eversion	−30° to 20°

Source: *Polley and Hunder (1978).*

[a]*Some normal individuals lack 5 to 10 degrees of full extension at the elbow, and some have an additional 5 to 10 degrees of hyperextension.*

[b]*Manipulation of the neck must always be undertaken with caution, and avoided altogether in patients with suspected instability (e.g., subluxation of the atlanto-axial joint) due to trauma, rheumatoid arthritis, ankylosing spondylitis, or other condition.*

Tests for Bicipital Tenosynovitis

In this condition, there is direct tenderness over the biceps tendon in its groove. In many cases, this can be demonstrated by flipping the tendon back and forth above its junction with the muscle belly.

Speed's test. This test is performed by having the patient flex his shoulder (elevate it anteriorly) against resistance, while the elbow is extended and the forearm is supinated. The test is positive when pain is localized to the bicipital groove (Crenshaw & Kilgore, 1966).

Yergason's test. This test is also based upon the remote production of pain at the bicipital groove or insertion.

1. Have the patient sit with his palms on his thighs.

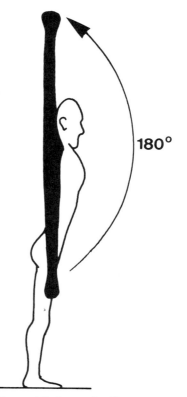

Figure 24-6. *Forward flexion at shoulder.*

2. Starting with the good side, grasp his wrist firmly, and ask him to turn his palm up, against the resistance you are supplying. This causes the biceps to contract.

3. Repeat on the painful side.

Pain localized to the anteromedial aspect of the shoulder is a positive sign ("Bailey," Clain, 1973).

Drop-Arm Test for Rotator Cuff Tear

Tears of the rotator cuff impair active abduction of the arm.

A method:

1. Passively abduct the patient's arm to a horizontal position. Test his ability to maintain that position against resistance.

2. Ask the patient to raise his arm over his head, then lower it to the horizontal position.

3. Have the patient lower his arm below the horizontal position, and observe whether it falls suddenly to his side.

Interpretation. The patient with a rotator cuff tear will have difficulty maintaining the horizontal position against resistance, or holding the arm in abduction if it falls below the horizontal (i.e., a 90-degree angle to the body). Such a patient usually does not have difficulty in raising the affected arm over his head, once it is brought to a 90-degree angle, because of the action of the deltoid muscle (Polley & Hunder, 1978).

Elbow

Tests for Epicondylitis

1. Lateral epicondylitis may be confidently diagnosed in tennis players (or others who stress the radioulnar and radiohumeral joints) by reproducing pain at the lateral epicondyle in any of three ways.

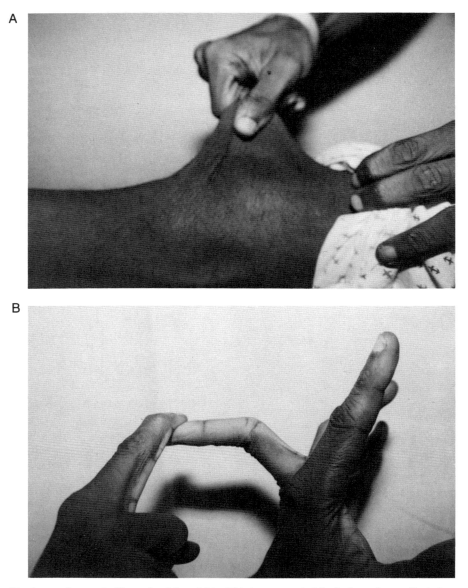

Figure 24-7. *Ehlers-Danlos syndrome. A, Hyperelasticity of skin. This is not seen in Marfan's syndrome. B, A demonstration of increased joint mobility (which is not, in itself, diagnostic of the syndrome). Photographs courtesy of Dr. Renee Ridzon of Massachusetts.*

a. With the patient's elbow fully extended, passively pronate his forearm. This stretches the common extensors (Mills's maneuver).

b. With the patient's arm fully extended in supination and flexed at the wrist, have him attempt to extend his wrist against resistance.

c. Have the patient make a fist, knuckles facing the floor. Holding his forearm in a pronated position by grasping his wrist with one hand, place your other hand on the top of his fist and provide resistance to his extending the wrist. Ask him to push your hand up toward the ceiling (Cozen's test).

2. Medial epicondylitis, common in golfers, may be confidently diagnosed by reproducing the pain at the medial epicondyle in the following manner: With the patient's arm in the position for test b above, place your resisting hand on the palmar side of his fist and challenge the patient to keep you from extending his wrist.

Wrist and Hand

Finkelstein's Test

To diagnose chronic stenosing tenosynovitis of the extensor pollicis brevis and abductor pollicis longus, ask the patient to grasp his own thumb, then push the patient's hand in the direction of his ulna (Fig. 24-8). This will produce remote pain in the region of the tenosynovitis, at the radial styloid process.

Temporomandibular Joint

On ausculting over an inflamed temporomandibular joint, one may be able to hear crepitus or a click. The sensitivity and specificity of this test are unknown.

Cervical Spine

Neck Compression Test

Simply tilt the head and neck toward the symptomatic side and see if pressure on the top of the head intensifies the (radicular and

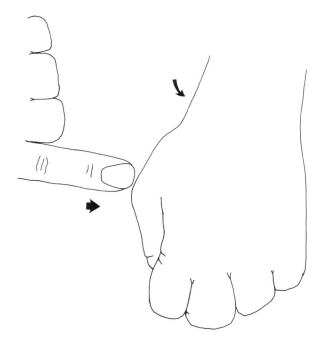

Figure 24-8. *Finkelstein's test for chronic stenosing teno-synovitis. Arrowhead indicates area at which physician exerts pressure. Curved arrow indicates site of remote pain in positive test.*

chronic) neck, shoulder, arm, and hand pain. The neck compression test is 100% sensitive for the diagnosis of lateral rupture of a cervical intervertebral disc and is "almost pathognomonic" (Spurling & Scoville, 1944). In half the cases of this entity, the scalenus anticus syndrome (see Ch. 18, p. 344) develops.

Shoulder Abduction Test

Relief of radicular pain in the shoulder, arm, and/or hand by placing the ipsilateral palm on the top of the head is diagnostic of cervical extradural compressive monoradiculoneuropathy, especially that due to disc herniation or spondylosis (Davidson et al., 1981). The sensitivity of this test is 68%.

Thoracic and Lumbosacral Spine

Inspection

The curvature of the spine is normally concave forward (kyphotic) in the thoracic and sacral regions, and convex forward (lordotic) in the lumbar region.

Kyphosis. In adolescents, an exaggeration of the normal thoracic kyphosis can result from Scheuermann's disease, vertebral osteochondritis, lateral malcurvature (scoliosis, vide infra), or just bad posture. Pathologic kyphosis may also accompany rickets. In older women, the so-called dowager's hump may result from osteoporosis. A more angular deformity (in contrast to a gentle curve), called a gibbus, should suggest tuberculosis of the spine (Pott's disease) or metastatic carcinoma (Fig. 24-9).

Lordosis. An exaggerated lordosis can be primary (as in rickets, cretinism, or spondylolisthesis), but is usually compensatory for other deformity of the spine or diseases in the lower limbs (e.g., flexion contracture of the hip, congenital dislocation of the hip, progressive muscular dystrophy, paralysis from poliomyelitis, obesity of the abdomen, dorsal kyphosis, and short-

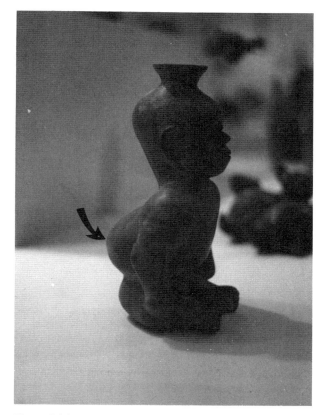

Figure 24-9. *A gibbus. This deformity is most likely due to tuberculosis. However, a case could be made for "gargoylism" (i.e., Hurler's or Morquio-Brailsford types of mucopolysaccharidosis). The ornamental figure, from a 2nd or 3rd century pre-Columbian vessel from Colima, Mexico, is displayed in the Baltimore Museum of Art.*

ening of the Achilles tendons [Raney & Brashear, 1971]). Most commonly, an increase in lordosis results from poor posture, pregnancy, or wearing high heels.

Flattening of the lumbar lordosis may occur in painful conditions of the lower back such as sacroiliitis or a herniated intervertebral disk.

Scoliosis. Scoliosis is a lateral curvature of the spine that usually becomes apparent during the years of growth. If neglected, it can progress to cause severe deformity and impairment in respiratory mechanics. Therefore, a check for this condition is part of the screening physical examination of children and adolescents.

The curve may either be S shaped or C shaped. The former is more likely to be structural, and the latter to result from a paralytic condition.

Look for a high shoulder, a prominent hip, or a projecting shoulder blade. Have the patient lean forward as you observe from behind, with his shoulder blades at eye level. Look for asymmetry in the scapulae and the erector spini muscle masses.

Structural scoliosis may be congenital, resulting from developmental errors such as a hemivertebra or asymmetric fusion of two or more vertebrae. Cryptogenic scoliosis might result from a slight unilateral weakness of the trunk musculature, or asymmetric growth at the epiphyseal plates of the vertebral bodies. Known causes of structural scoliosis include neurofibromatosis, osteogenesis imperfecta, osteomalacia, or unilateral thoracic conditions such as chronic empyema. Paralytic scoliosis may be a sequela of poliomyelitis, progressive muscular dystrophy, Friedrich's ataxia, or syringomyelia. Compensatory scoliosis is due to muscle spasm and/or pain in the spine or its associated soft tissues.

Pointing test.   Patients with pain from herniated discs or the posterior apophyseal joints tend to point to the back, the buttocks, or the posterior thighs as the site of maximal pain. Pain due to nerve root irritation tends to radiate distally to the leg. A pain drawing may also be used. Open-ended questions about the anatomical pattern of pain showed a high degree of reproducibility (90%) over time (Waddell et al., 1982).

Palpation

Paravertebral muscle spasms may be detected by palpation, especially if unilateral. To check for localized points of tenderness along the spine, first palpate the spinous processes.

▆ Consider the possibility of a fracture dislocation of the spine in all accidents that could produce a violent hyperflexion of the spine. (If it is necessary to turn the patient, he must be turned without twisting the vertebral column. Three or four persons are needed.) Palpate along the spinous processes for a gap or step-off. Tenderness of a spinous process is another cardinal sign of fracture.

Percussion

If there is no tenderness on palpation, try percussion of the spinous processes.

Provocative maneuvers for eliciting localized pain:

▆   1.   With lesions that involve compression of the spinal cord or nerve roots, pain may be increased by anything that raises the cerebrospinal fluid pressure. Ask the patient to cough or strain, then point to the painful site.

    2.   Have the patient jump and land on his heels or raise up on his toes and land on his heels (the heel drop) and point to any areas that are painful. (Of course, one would not want to do this in a patient with a history of trauma.)

    3.   Place one hand flat on the patient's head and punch it with your other hand's fist. Is remote pain produced in the suspect area?

Interpretation.   Localized or referred pain over a vertebral body should suggest a compression fracture or involvement in an infectious or neoplastic process. Radicular pain (pain radiating peripherally) indicates nerve root compression.

Range of Motion

Forward flexion.   Forward flexion of the lumbar spine may be measured by having the patient stand barefoot, heels at shoulder width, knees straight. He then attempts to touch his toes by maximally flexing the trunk and holding the position for 15 seconds. The dependent variable is the distance from the middle fingertip to the floor, after one trial run. The mean in normal subjects is 4.0 cm, with a standard deviation of 6.9 (Merritt et al., 1986).

This test assumes that patients with "organic" back problems can get within 20 cm of the floor because most such flexion occurs at the hips, not the back. But some control patients with tight hamstrings and tall stature cannot get within 20 cm (Merritt et al., 1986), so failure on this test alone should *not* be considered evidence of compensation neurosis, malingering, or other "uncooperativeness" (Nehemkis et al., 1979).

Another disadvantage of the forward flexion test is the substantial interrater and intra-rater variability, studied in 50 normal subjects (Merritt et al., 1986). (Presumably, variability would be even greater in diseased subjects.) For this reason, the test, although standard in most textbooks, is inferior to the Schober flexion test.

Original Schober test.   Mark the skin where the spine is crossed by an imaginary line between the posterior iliac spines. With the patient still standing, a second mark is made 10 cm above the first. Have the patient bend forward maximally as in the above test, attempting to touch the floor with his hands, and remeasure the distance between the two marks. In normal men, the distance increases an average of 4 to 6 cm (Schober, 1937). Normally, it is greater than 15 cm (14 cm in shorter subjects). False positives (lesser increases not due to disease) occur in joggers, persons over 50, and persons with prior back surgery (Fries, 1985).

Modified Schober flexion test.   With the patient erect, the examiner estimates the top of the sacrum by drawing a line between the dimples of Venus (Fig. 24-5). Mark spots 10 cm above and 5 cm below this, in the midline. Then have the subject bend forward maximally. The dependent variable is the distance between the two spots, minus 15 (all measured in centimeters.) In normals, the range was from 4.3 to 10.3 cm (Merritt et al., 1986). Only 2% of the normal population had less than 5 cm of flexion in a study that showed this test to have a statistically significant 91% interobserver agreement (Waddell et al., 1982). There is an increase in mobility from the 15 to 24 decade to the 25 to 34 decade, followed by a progressive decrease with advanced age. Mobility may decrease by as much as 50% between youth and old age (Moll & Wright, 1971).

Forestier's sign.   Observe the patient from the rear, while he alternately flexes his trunk to the right and to the left. Normally, if the patient flexes to one side, the paraspinal muscles on that side relax, and those on the opposite side contract. However, if the back is stiff enough, the muscles contract to the side to which the patient is laterally flexing, and the contralateral muscles relax. The contracting muscles purse up as a bowstring (the curved spine is the bow), so this is also called the bowstring sign. This sign is stated to be of low sensitivity but high positive predictive value for ankylosing spondylitis (Fries, 1985).

Straight-Leg Raising Tests

Lasegue's sign.   The history of Lasegue's sign is discussed in Ch. 26 (p. 469).
    A method (after Bailey):

    1.   With the patient supine, place your hand beneath the lumbar spine to be sure there is no compensatory lordosis. Also, observe it during the test because a change in the lumbar curve invalidates the test result.

    2.   Grasp the ankle of the leg to be tested, and place your other hand on the front of the thigh to keep the knee extended. Slowly raise the leg until the patient experiences pain or until the leg has been flexed to 90 degrees at the hip (less in the elderly). If the test produces pain (a positive test), note the angle at which pain was experienced.

    3.   Put the leg back on the table, then repeat the above maneuver, moving very slowly toward the maximum painless angle. At that point, take your hand off the thigh and dorsiflex the foot, producing additional traction on the sciatic nerve. Note whether the patient experiences pain.

    4.   Repeat the maneuver on the other side.
    Interpretation: A positive straight-leg raising test, especially when confirmed by the maneuver in step 3, suggests im-

pingement on the sciatic nerve somewhere along its course. Pain evoked before 40 degrees suggests pressure on the nerve root from a protruding intervertebral disc. Pain after that point suggests nerve root tension from another cause. (This test is also positive in meningitis, in which case it is usually called Kernig-Lasegue sign [see Ch. 26, p. 469].)

A false positive (pain at about 60 degrees) in persons with no abnormality of the sciatic nerve, as in Scheuermann's disease, may result simply from tight hamstring muscles.

The interobserver reliability of the straight-leg raising test is 100% within 10 degrees (Nelson et al., 1979.)

Alternate criteria: If 75 degrees of flexion is used as the cutoff, only 2% of normal subjects had a positive test in a study that showed a highly significant 77% agreement between examiners (Waddell et al., 1982).

The straight-leg raising test is one key to the diagnosis of sciatica; weakness of extension of the great toe (see Ch. 26, p. 485) is another. A third trick is to press right over the sciatic notch to see if one can perfectly reproduce a pain thought to be sciatica.

Crossed Straight-Leg Raising Sign.

As Fajerstajn originally pointed out in 1901, straight-leg raising of the nonpainful leg may worsen the pain on the other side (a positive crossed straight-leg raising test.) This sign is almost pathognomonic of disc herniation (Hudgins, 1977). *Mechanism*: stretching the nonpainful, ipsilateral root exerts a lateral pull on the dural sac, thus stretching the opposite (affected) root to some degree.

The predictive value of a positive test is 97% for the crossed straight-leg raising test, compared with 64% for a positive straight-leg raising test on the painful side only. If the patient has a positive crossed straight-leg raising test, Hudgins suggests that myelography is unnecessary for the diagnosis of disc herniation, and that a negative myelogram should in fact be disregarded in such patients since up to 20% of lumbar myelograms fail to detect a disc herniation when it is present. Finally, a positive crossed straight-leg raising test predicts a good surgical result in 91% of the patients, compared with only 70% of the patients with the sign on the painful side only (Hudgins, 1977).

Crossover pain: In one more variant to this test, raising the painful side causes the appearance of pain radiating down the nonpainful leg (Hall, 1983). This indicates a central disc rupture.

Femoral Nerve Traction Test

In the straight-leg raising maneuver, most of the tension is placed upon the fifth lumbar and first sacral nerve roots, and very little upon the third and fourth lumbar roots (Dyck, 1976). To remedy this problem, Dyck invented the following test:

A method:

1. Have the patient lie on his asymptomatic side, so that the symptomatic side is superior.

2. Holding the patient's knee in full extension, the examiner gently hyperextends the superior hip to about fifteen degrees. Pain in the anterior thigh is a positive test for lumbar disc protrusion. A false positive may occur in the case of radiculitis of the fourth lumbar root, and in all conditions that directly or indirectly afflict the superior psoas muscle (since maximal tension is produced on this muscle.)

3. Next, while the hip is kept in 15 degrees of hyperextension, gently start to flex the knee. This intensifies the traction on the femoral nerve. If this maneuver intensifies or produces the anterior thigh pain, the test is positive.

4. Repeat with the afflicted side down. This is called the contralateral femoral test and is analogous to the crossed straight-leg

raising test. In this instance, the asymptomatic superior side is manipulated, and the symptomatic side (which is "down") experiences symptoms.

There are two additional points to interpreting the test:

1. Sensory examination changes can also be used as the dependent variable.

2. Pain radiating beneath the knee is seen in fourth, but not in third, lumbar root disease.

Herron-Pheasant Test

This is a new bird (Herron & Pheasant, 1980). After testing the patient's ankle jerks, knee jerks, and motor function (see Ch. 26, p. 481), have him lie prone on the examining table, with his knees hyperflexed so that the heels are close to the buttocks. After maintaining this posture for 45 to 60 seconds, the knees are allowed to return to only 90 degrees of flexion (with the patient still prone), in which position the reflexes and motor function are retested.

If the hyperflexion produces any suppression or abolition of a reflex, or any weakness, it is attributed to lumbar disc protrusion.

Additionally, traction on the femoral nerve during hyperflexion may provoke anterior or groin pain, suggesting further study of the femoral nerve by the femoral nerve traction test (vide supra). Or, depending upon the distribution of the anterior thigh pain, it may signify an iliofemoral or other entrapment neuropathy.

In all of these tests, there is an issue of interpretation.

Evaluation for Impaired Patient Cooperation

One general class of tests is based on the method of inducing the patient to perform a specialized movement with his body in a given position, which he was unable to perform in another position.

Aird's test. This test is positive when a patient who could not touch his toes in a standing position is able to do so while sitting on an examining table with his legs extended in front of him. Similarly, persons who, when supine, cannot flex their hips and knees because of back pain, will be able to achieve a superior degree of flexion when you are concentrating on their ankle jerks.

In the converse of Aird's test, I have found male patients who cannot touch their toes while sitting on the examining table (even with hip and knee flexion allowed), but who can quickly pick up their underwear and pants after the rectal examination, especially if a knock at the door signals that an intrusion may be imminent.

Similarly, the straight-leg raising test can be performed with the patient sitting, simply by extending the knee; the hip is already flexed at 90 degrees by the sitting posture. There should be less than 15 degrees of difference between the results of the test in the sitting and the recumbent posture. In one version, the two tests are performed under different circumstances. For example, when the maneuver is repeated with the patient in the supine position, it is done as part of the neurologic exam under the guise of striking the patella with a large, impressive Queen's Square hammer (that I display prominently as a memento from Dr. Chuck Herlihy *fils.* of Alabama, but which is used for no other purpose.) Or, the second testing may be done with the patient sitting, in the guise of positioning the foot for a Babinski test (see Ch. 26, p. 501).

Burns' bench test. Ask the patient to kneel (with his hips and knees flexed) on a bench and to place his fingers on the floor. The patient with low back pain can "pass" this test because the kneeling position relieves strain, stress, and tension upon and within the low back. Inability to perform this maneuver probably results from a cause other than back pain.

Magnuson's test. This a low-back gambit from Bailey (Clain, 1973). Mark the site that the patient indicates as the site of his pain. (I like to use chalk dust. A felt-tipped marker can cool the skin and so be a reminder for the patient as well as the examiner.) After the rectal examination, or checking the reflexes, or some other activity, the patient is asked to indicate the site of pain again, as if the examiner were confused and wished to double-check himself.*

Double leg raising.   When unilateral nerve root impingement is present, both legs can often be elevated together without pain to a higher level than the affected leg alone. This is because of flexion of the lumbar spine and the lack of the contralateral tethering of the nerve roots. In patients whose disease is not located in the spine, double leg raising is frequently painful at a lower elevation than the single leg lift. These patients apparently believe that if one is bad, two should be worse (Hall, 1983).

There are so many possibilities that the reader is invited to invent a test and name it for himself.

Sacroiliac Joint

A comparison of the Schober test and six pressure maneuvers used to examine the sacroiliac joints revealed none of them to be either sensitive or specific for sacroiliac disease (Russell et al., 1981).

Gaenslen's Sign

With the patient supine, hold the hip and knee of the nontested side in flexion, and allow the other lower extremity from the hip down to hang over the edge of the examining table. Then press down on the (tested) leg so as to produce hyperextension at the hip. The test is positive when this maneuver produces pain in the ipsilateral back. Originally offered as an operating room test for lumbosacral disease, it is now used to diagnose sacroiliitis (Winchester et al., 1987). Sensitivity, specificity, and predictive value are unknown for either diagnosis.

Patrick's Test

Ask the patient, who is lying supine, to place the lateral malleolus of the tested leg on the opposite knee. Then push the patient's flexed knee toward the examining table. Check for pain, muscle spasm, or limitation of motion of the hip.

This test was first described by Dr. Hugh Talbot Patrick, a neurologist, who called this the fabere sign† (Polley & Hunder, 1978) for the motions that were tested: *f*lexion, *ab*duction, *e*xternal *r*otation, and finally *e*xtension. The test is positive if it produces hip pain. Patrick thought this was a sign of arthritis of the hip, but lately the test has been used to diagnose sacroiliitis (Winchester et al., 1987). Sensitivity, specificity, and predictive value are unknown for either diagnosis.

A Pedagogic Note

Elsewhere in this text I have suggested that one can always find someone who *cannot* do something. However, with regard to the tests for sacroiliitis I have accepted the negative conclusions of others because they fit so well with my own clinical experience.

Beware. Dr. Tinsley Harrison of Alabama used to say that "clinical experience" was like "military experience," and he

then would cite Napoleon on the general's own pack mule: "My mule has more military experience than any general I have faced, yet still is unfit to lead an army."

Accordingly, my clinical experience, as remembered, could be in error in this situation. If so, will I have made a type I (alpha) error or a type II (beta) error? (*A reminder*: Alpha is the error of accepting a chance difference as a true one; beta is the error of rejecting a true difference as a chance one.)

Hip

Inspection

Pointing test.   When asked to point to the site of pain, the patient with hip joint disease will usually point to the groin. Less frequently, pain is felt deep in the buttock or posterior to the greater trochanter. In some instances, pain may be referred to the knee.

Trendelenburg's sign.   Have the patient stand, unassisted, on each leg in turn. Normally, the buttock on the weight-bearing leg is lower because the contralateral hip is lifted up so as to move inward toward the center of gravity. The patient with hip dislocation is unable to lift the abnormal buttock into this elevated position. Thus, a positive Trendelenburg sign is a lower buttock on the *non*-weight-bearing side. Figure 24-10A shows a true negative Trendelenburg sign.

Trendelenburg's sign is positive with hip dislocation or with a completely fractured femoral head. False positives may occur if the test is done incorrectly, for example, if the patient is permitted to lean against an assistant or wall or piece of furniture. False positives may also occur (after an initally negative test) with weak hip abductors, as in models who become fatigued (Fig. 24-10B). They adduct the nonsupporting leg and rotate it downward towards the center of gravity. Both of these false positives can be prevented by having the patient perform the test unassisted in the middle of the room away from furniture, and by requiring the legs to be kept separate.

A self-study: The next time you are nude, you can check this sign on yourself in the mirror. After seeing a true negative, you can also produce the false positive by adducting the nonsupporting leg, flexing your knee, and putting your toe on the ground like the model in Figure 24-10B.

Palpation

In greater trochanteric bursitis (also see p. 426), the pain is reproduced by palpation over the greater trochanter.

The pain due to meralgia paresthetica (an entrapment neuropathy of the lateral femoral cutaneous nerve as it exits from the lateral aspect of the inguinal ligament) may be reproduced by compressing the inguinal ligament against the nerve and bone at the medial aspect of the anterior superior iliac spine (McBeath, 1985). (An area of hyperesthesia is also present on the anterior lateral aspect of the thigh.) The sensitivity and specificity of this test is not known; it does not always work, partly because the entrapment tends to come and go.

Auscultation

A snapping sound may emanate from the hip due either to intraarticular disease (during motion of the femoral head on the acetabulum) or extraarticular disease (because of a sudden jump of the fascia lata of the gluteus maximus over the greater trochanter, or from a snapping of the iliopsoas tendon over the iliopectineal prominence during extension from flexion) (Lyons & Peterson, 1984).

---

*This demonstrates the truth of the old saying, "Liars ought to have good memories," attributed to Algernon Sidney in 1698. This worthy apparently got it from Corneille (*La Menteur*, Act IV, Scene 5, 1642), who must have been familiar with Montaigne's reference in his chapter on liars. The latter in turn was supposedly familiar with Quintilian's *"mendacem memorem esse oportere."* A Greek reference would convince me that they were all plagiarists, while a Sumerian one would suggest the existence of a universal truth.

†I have already seen this sign capitalized and spelled without the "e," so that Drs. Fabere and Faber should soon take their places in the pantheon of nonexistent physicians next to Drs. Jod, Austin, Grey, Graham, Seabright, and Bantam.

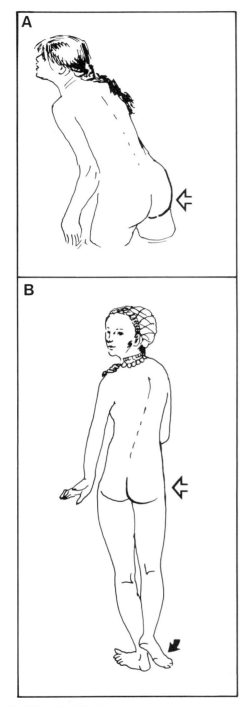

Figure 24-10. *Trendelenburg's sign. A, A true negative. The walking bather is supporting her weight on her left leg. Note that Renoir has properly shown the right buttock to be higher than the left. This rules out a congenital dislocation of the right hip only. To rule out a left congenital dislocation, the bather would now have to stand on her right leg. Redrawn from* The Bathers *by Renoir.*

B, A false positive. The model is tired, and although supposedly standing on her unassisted left foot has actually put her right foot back on the ground. Thus, although her right buttock is lower than the left, this results from the adduction of the legs. Note the slight flexion of the right knee. Redrawn from The Judgment of Paris *by Lucas Cranach.*

Special Maneuvers

Range of motion. When checking range of motion at the hip, it is important to fix the pelvis and spine, or pelvic and lumbar compensatory movements may be confused with hip mobility. One way to accomplish this is to sit on the other femur. Another way is have the patient lie supine and use his hands to hold the leg not being tested in a position of 90 degress of flexion at the hip and maximal flexion at the knee.

To test internal and external rotation, one can have the patient lie supine or prone with the knee flexed to 90 degrees. If the patient is prone, swing the foot across the midline to test external rotation, and away from the midline to test internal rotation. If the patient is supine, flex both the knee and the hip to 90 degrees, and push the knee laterally to test external rotation, medially to test internal rotation.

Hip dislocation and subluxation. When the hip is completely dislocated, Trendelenburg's sign (p. 424) will be positive as will auscultatory percussion (p. 430). A special problem is congenital dysplasia or subluxation of the hip. These children usually do not have a complete dislocation initially, and the diagnostic goal is to detect the subluxation before it progresses to complete dislocation. There are three tests, presented in order of efficiency.

1. *Limitation of external rotation*: With the infant supine, flex the knees and the hips to right angles. Then externally rotate the hips by attempting to push the knees laterally to the examining table. Normally both knees will go to the table, or almost to the table, and the angles formed with the table will be symmetric. But in congenital subluxation, the knee on the affected side will not either reach the table or come as close to the table as the other side.

2. *Ortolani's "click and jerk"*: With the child supine, each hip is tested in turn. First, flex the hip to a right angle and then internally rotate it very slowly, with gentle downward pressure on the knee. A click may be heard, and/or a jerk felt, as the femoral head moves out of the acetabulum. Next, externally rotate the hip slowly as far as it will go. Again, a click and/or a jerk may occur as the femoral head reenters the acetabulum.

3. Asymmetric internal rotation can sometimes be detected by maneuvers akin to the above, sometimes without the "click and jerk" (Barness, 1972).

Psoas spasm sign. We have previously discussed the psoas sign to inspection (Ch. 5, p. 80) and the reverse psoas maneuver for appendicitis (Ch. 20, p. 379). A second psoas maneuver can be used to separate psoas spasm from pain in the hip joint.

1. Place the patient on his abdomen.

2. With the knee flexed, pull upon the ankle so as to hyperextend the hip, while your other hand presses down lightly on the ipsilateral lumbosacral area.

3. Repeat for the other side.

Pain and limitation of motion with the above maneuver is a sign of psoas spasm.

or

Test each leg for abduction, adduction, and flexion at the hip joint, with the patient supine. Generalized disease of the hip (in contrast to psoas spasm) will cause pain and limitation in all of these directions.

Psoas spasm is seen in psoas hematoma, psoas abscess (both the old kind from tuberculosis and the new pyogenic forms), hypertrophic arthritis of the spine, perinephric abscess, and (on the right) appendiceal abscess (Cabot, 1937).

Resistance Testing

Having the patient resist attempts to abduct his hip, starting from the adducted position, will reproduce the pain due to *greater trochanteric bursitis*.

The Knee

Inspection

Pointing test. Ask the patient to point to the part of the knee that hurts. There are two areas that should suggest the need for some of the advanced tests to be given below. In recurrent displacement of the medial meniscus, the sore spot, as viewed from the medial side of the knee, will be about one fourth of the way posterior from the anterior edge, just a bit above where the tibia ends. From the same view, a sore spot halfway posterior (that is, equidistant from the front and back) is just over the medial (tibial) collateral ligament. (See Fig. 24-11.)

Asymmetry. In senile rupture of the quadriceps near its insertion at the superior border of the patella, the usual suprapatellar meat is missing. Use your own suprapatellar space or the patient's good side as a control.

The ligament holding the lower edge of the patella to the tibial tuberosity (the ligament of the patella) can also rupture. At first it is swollen, and later the infrapatellar meat is missing, but at all stages the best sign is that the patella on the afflicted side is higher than the normal patella due to the unopposed effect of the quadriceps.

Swelling. Look for swellings with the knee in both flexion and extension. An effusion within the knee joint itself may obliterate the hollows lateral to the patella.

The most common swellings not due to effusion in the joint are: infrapatellar bursitis ("clergyman's knee"); anserine bursitis (which produces a fluctuant swelling on the medial aspect of the knee, just below the medial femoral epicondyle); cystic swellings of the menisci (localized to the anteromedial or lateral side of the joint space); and prepatellar bursitis ("housemaid's knee" or "genu remoris" [vide infra].)

Very advanced: Prepatellar bursitis resulting from vigorous prayer (with genuflexion and kneeling) was reported in a woman who suffered severe remorse after violating instructions from a health clinic not to have sexual relations for an unspecified time. (She had been treated 4 weeks earlier for a positive syphilis serology.) (This genu remorsi was renamed genu remoris to pun with genu amoris (see p. 427) (Rutstein & McCutchen, 1977).

A Baker's cyst is an abnormal communication between the knee joint space and one of the bursa, usually the gastrocnemius-semi-membranosus bursa (Schmidt et al., 1974). Such potential communications are found in over half the population (Good, 1964) but do not usually attract attention until and unless there is an intraarticular chronic effusion that expands the Baker's cyst (producing "dissection"). Look for swelling distal to the transverse popliteal crease. This may only be seen with the patient erect and the knee fully extended. Prominent popliteal fat pads may obscure, or be mistaken for a Baker's cyst. (The crescent sign of a ruptured Baker's cyst is shown in Fig. 25-11.)

Varus and valgus. Varus was a Roman general, famous for being knock-kneed. In fact, he became eponymic in the Latin language for his affliction. Valgus, on the other hand, is the Latin word for bow-legged. The ignorant have perverted these words by exporting them in adjectival form to other portions of the body. The confusion may have started from the fact that when the varus knees point in, the valgus hips point out, compensatorily. In distant climes, the words were so abused and tortured that when they were finally returned to the knees, they were assigned a meaning exactly opposite to that which they possessed prior to their diaspora. At the present time, the English medical dictionaries and Latin-English dictionaries define these words oppositely. So, it is now impossible to use either of them in an intelligent manner. I suggest a moratorium on the use of words by persons who know not the language. Knock-kneed and bowlegged have the inestimable advantages of being precise and unambiguous. Those wishing to retain the Latin so as to sound impressive should remember, *"Qui stultis videri eruditi volunt stulti eruditis videntur"* (Quintilian, IX, 7, 22).*

Palpation

1. If the patient complains of pain, try to reproduce it by palpating the knee. Tenderness in the area of the medial (tibial) collateral ligament may be due to a problem with that ligament or with the medial meniscus. Maximal tenderness over the femoral attachment suggests a tear of the ligament (Fig. 24-11,B), but maximal tenderness directly over the joint line in front of the ligament suggests a bucket-handle tear of the medial meniscus (Fig. 24-11,A). Be sure to check this spot with the knee flexed before reporting the test to be negative, as medial meniscus problems may show palpation tenderness during knee flexion, but not extension.

If the tenderness is posterior to the collateral ligament, think of a torn posterior horn of the medial meniscus.

A false positive for medial collateral ligament damage may be obtained in saphenous nerve entrapment neuropathy. The latter diagnosis can be made when pressure high above the point of ligamentous attachment also causes pain, which radiates all the way down the medial surface of the leg (Koppel & Thompson, 1960).

2. If you suspect a transverse fracture of the patella, scrape the anterior surface of the patella in a cephalad-caudad dimension, with a long fingernail held transversely. The nail will get stuck in a groove made by the fracture. (This is one type of fracture that can be diagnosed before the X rays are developed; see also "Auscultatory Percussion," p. 430.)

3. Bilateral tenderness of the tibial tuberosities (Fig. 24-11,C) in a youngster is probably pathognomonic of Osgood-Schlatter disease (Fairbank, 1937). In this condition, there is partial separation of the epiphysis of the tibial tuberosity, usually resulting from a sudden pull by the ligament of the patella during exercise.

Special Maneuvers

Effusion in the knee joint. Relatively large amounts of fluid in the joint may be detected by ballottement.

1. Have the patient lie supine with knees extended.

2. Encircle the suprapatellar region with one hand, compressing the suprapatellar pouch.

3. Tap on the patella sharply with the other hand. If there is a sufficient quantity of fluid, you will feel the patella click against the femur.

Relatively small amounts of fluid may be demonstrated by the bulge sign:

1. Have the patient lie supine with the knee fully extended and the muscles relaxed.

2. Stroke the medial aspect of the knee to express the synovial fluid from this area.

3. Tap the lateral aspect of the knee and watch for the appearance of a bulge on the medial side. It may be necessary to repeat several times to find the optimal percussion area; usually, the area just above the midportion of the patella.

---

*Whosoever wishes to appear learned among the stupid will appear stupid among the learned.

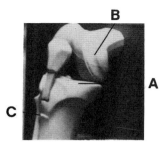

Figure 24-11. *Areas of tenderness in various afflictions of the right knee. A, Tenderness over the joint line suggests a tear of the medial meniscus; B, maximal tenderness over its femoral attachment suggests a tear of the medial collateral ligament; C, a tender, bony lump over the tuberosity of tibia occurs in Osgood-Schlatter disease. Model courtesy of Syntex Laboratories.*

A reversal of this method (i.e., stroking the lateral side and tapping on the medial side) may give the same result, but is usually not as effective (Polley & Hunder, 1978).

Knee creaking:
A method:

1. With the patient supine, passively move the patella in a cephalad-caudad dimension several times to see whether creaking can be produced.

2. Then swing the patella from left to right.

3. Wiggle the femur and the tibia, then flex the knee.

Interpretation: Creaking elicited by the first two maneuvers indicates chondromalacia of the patella. Creaking elicited by all three suggests chondromalacia of the femur. Creaking elicited only by the third maneuver suggests arthritis of the knee (Lewin, 1952).

Brittain's test:
A method:

1. Place your index finger above the upper edge of the patella when the patient has that knee flexed at a right angle.

2. As the patient extends his knee, gently exert pressure on the patella with your finger. A grinding or grating sensation—not just creaking—may be produced in the event of patellar chondromalacia or osteochondral fracture of any contiguous bone (patella, distal femur, or proximal tibia).

Interpretation: Even if you cannot feel the grating, the test is still positive if the finger pressure produces pain. *A caveat:* the patient should *not* be told what to expect.

•

Genu amoris: A case. A 31-year-old woman presented with intractable pain in her knee, such that she had had to give up bicycling and skiing. The examination was unrevealing except for creaking in the knees and a positive Brittain's test. A diagnosis of chondromalacia was made. Due to the unusual severity and persistence of symptoms, her daily activities were reviewed in detail, revealing nothing of an injurious nature. At the end of the interview she confided a previously unmentioned practice: "I always have sex on my knees." A hard surface was frequently utilized. Although the patient experienced no pain during the activity, it apparently did involve repetitive patellar concussion, which has been recognized as an aggravating factor in some cases of chondromalacia. Upon abandoning this position for intercourse, the patient's symptoms improved remarkably (Pinals, 1976).

•

There are numerous special maneuvers designed to diagnose what have been called "internal derangements of the knee (IDK)." It has been noted by Smillie ("Bailey," Clain, 1973) that the abbreviation "IDK" also stands for "I don't know."

McMurray's test. This test provides information on the posterior horns of both the lateral and medial menisci.
A method:

1. Have the patient lie supine, and flex the hip and knee until the heel touches the buttock.

2. Steady the knee with one hand, and grasp the patient's heel with the other. Rotate the patient's foot laterally as far as possible, and then bring the knee back to a 90-degree angle.

The test is positive for a torn medial meniscus if, during the extension of the leg thus held in external rotation, the patient's symptoms are reproduced, especially if you hear or feel a click. The patient should be able to state that the sensation is the same as he experienced when his knee previously gave way (McMurray, 1942).

3. Now relax the rotation and return the heel back toward the buttock. Rotate the foot medially, thus placing the knee in internal rotation, and slowly extend the knee. Results analogous to those in step 2 are a positive test for disease of the lateral meniscus.

There is a version of the McMurray test (Apley, 1977) in which the knee is moved through varying degrees of flexion while being subjected to an abduction force. This seems to constitute a more precise test. (It is *not* called Apley's test; he has his name on several others.)

False positives: In children and some adults with abnormally lax cartilaginous attachments, clicks can be produced during this maneuver, even in the absence of any cartilaginous lesion. Such clicks are not accompanied by pain (McMurray, 1942).

Childress' test:
A method: Have the patient squat, raise his heels, then waddle across the room toward you as you observe. A patient with a rupture of the posterior horn of the middle meniscus will be unable to flex completely the knee on the affected side. Additionally, such a patient will usually experience pain on the affected side, and sometimes a clicking sound can be heard.

This test cannot be done by patients with proximal girdle myopathy because they cannot waddle; nor by patients with posterior column disease because they cannot maintain their position when they waddle; nor by patients with peroneal neuropathy or muscular dystrophy because they cannot raise up on their toes.

Please note that none of the conditions affecting the patient's ability to perform this test normally can be detected by the routine X-ray examination.

Apley's test. This test sounds rather gruesome, and is the one test I was afraid to perform during my required junior orthopedic rotation at Pitt. The test was called the "grinding test," and I was afraid of hurting the patient. But, to paraphrase Shakespeare, desperate diseases are diagnosed by desperate remedies, or not at all.

A method (after Apley, 1977; Helfet, 1982):
Part I: Testing the medial collateral ligament.

1. Have the patient lie prone.

2. Holding his foot with one hand, flex his knee to a right angle.

3. Rotate his foot laterally (i.e., so that the toes point away from the midline).

4. Sit on his hamstrings, to hold his femur against the examining table or floor.

5. Try to flex the knee further. This will produce pain when there is disease of the medial collateral ligament.

Part II: Testing for disease of the medial meniscus.

6. Grind the tibial condyles against the femoral condyles with a rotating motion, placing your upper body weight on the plantar surface of the foot. This will produce pain in cases of disease of the medial meniscus.

In order to do this test correctly, something has to be holding the femur against the table or floor. As noted above, this can be your lower body weight. But when you push down on the foot with your upper body weight, be careful not to lift your weight off the hamstrings. If you are large enough, you can do this test from the side, using one knee to hold the hamstrings in position.

Apley's distraction test:

A method: Hold the femur immobile as in the above test and repeat the rotation, but instead of grinding the tibia down (step 6), exert traction on the leg and pull the foot up toward the ceiling.

Interpretation: This maneuver will not increase the pain due to disease of the medial meniscus, but will increase the pain due to ligament disease (Helfet, 1982).

General Varus test for the medial meniscus:

A method:

1. Have the patient stand like a Roman general (i.e., with the knee to be tested slightly flexed and the foot slightly forward and applied flat to the floor).

2. Forcefully try to push the knee medially to make the patient knock-kneed like General Varus (see p. 426).

Interpretation: Pain is produced in diseases of the medial meniscus.

Fairbank's apprehension test.

Recurrent subluxation of the patella in young women may masquerade as meniscus injury. Fairbank's apprehension test (Fairbank, 1937) is positive in the former but not the latter. With the patient sitting so that the knee is flexed, grab the patella and slowly begin to push it laterally. The patient with patellar subluxation will immediately begin to become apprehensive. She may even grab your wrists because she "knows" that "it" is going to happen again if you keep pushing in that direction.

Cruciate ligaments, customary test:

A method:

1. With the patient sitting on the edge of the bed or examining table, let him dangle his legs.

2. Have the patient hold his own femur, while you wiggle the tibia under the femoral head.

Interpretation: Usually there is no excursion of the tibia. If there is, the anterior and/or posterior cruciate ligaments are abnormal.

Ghormley's test for the cruciate ligaments:

A method:

1. If the patient is sitting on a bed or examining stool and his feet reach the floor, place your own feet in front of and behind the patient's foot to keep it from slipping forward and backward on the floor.

2. Now grasp the proximal tibia and see how far it moves in an anterior-posterior direction.

Interpretation: Normally, there is almost no displacement achievable. Anterior displacement of $1/2$ inch or more indicates a tear of the anterior cruciate ligament. Posterior displacement indicates a tear of the posterior cruciate ligament (Lewin, 1952).

Drawer sign:

1. Have the patient lie supine on the bed or examining table with his knee flexed from 30 to 90 degrees.

2. Fix the patient's foot to the bed by sitting on it.

3. Pull the superior tibia (just under the femur) forward and backward. If it slides like a drawer, the test is considered positive.

The interpretation is probably the same as for Ghormley's test, although Bailey notes that in extreme cases of anterior displacement, the medial collateral ligament is probably also torn in addition to the anterior cruciate ligament.

Quadriceps active test to diagnose posterior cruciate ligament disruption:

1. Have the supine patient flex the knee to be tested to 90 degrees.

2. Support the patient's thigh with one hand, and check that the thigh muscles are relaxed.

3. Use your other hand to stabilize the patient's foot, resting your elbow on the table.

4. Keeping your eyes on the patient's flexed knee, ask him to slide his foot gently down the table.

If the posterior cruciate ligament is disrupted, contraction of the quadriceps (induced by step 4) will cause about 2 mm of anterior displacement of the tibia with the knee in this position.

The sensitivity of the test is 98%. No false positives were found in normal knees or knees with known *anterior* cruciate ligament disruption (Daniel et al., 1988).

Yushiva-Bücher's* tibial and fibular collateral ligaments test:

1. Have the patient sit on the examining table with his legs dangling.

2. Passively extend the knee to be examined to within 10 or 15 degrees of full extension.

3. Put your hand on the distal femur and wiggle it from side to side. Normally, there should be a little bit of movement. This is your control value for the test.

4. Now fully extend the knee and see if you can still wiggle the femur.

Interpretation: Normally, the femur will not move when the knee is locked in full extension. If the femur does so move even as much as the control maneuver in step 3, there is presumably disease of the collateral ligaments.

Fouché's ausculted internal rotation of the tibia:

This maneuver was first demonstrated to the authors by Fouché, who has taught it to several generations of surgeons. It has been a source of interest to visiting military orthopedic surgeons from abroad, and we have come to regard it as an invaluable contribution to the diagnosis of internal derangement of the knee. The test is carried out on the right knee, with the patient flat on his back on a couch, with his hip and knee fully flexed. The left fingers of the examining surgeon are held on the anteromedial joint line, the right hand firmly grasping the patient's right foot, which is used as a lever in internally rotating the tibia on the femur. The motion is carried through as a complete circumduction movement, starting with the knee fully flexed, and ending with it slightly flexed. The menisci move with the tibia, and the posterior end of the medial meniscus is nipped between the femoral and tibial condyles, the tendency being for the femoral condyle to force the meniscus toward the center of the joint. It may move a small distance, and then slip back, producing an audible and palpable thud. With practice, one is able to

---

*Since no orthopedic knee test should go without an eponym, I claim this test for Dr. Feldsher Yushiva-Bücher, the fabulous Galician clinician.

recognize this normal thud, and to distinguish it from other sounds. The sound which a torn meniscus may produce varies with the type of tear. From a grossly torn and frayed meniscus may be elicited a crunch or squelch; from a narrow bucket-handle strip of cartilage, a high-pitched click; or from multiple splits in the posterior part of the meniscus, a succession of clicks. A broad rim of meniscus which is partly loose may cause only exaggeration of the normal thud; while the reduction or the dislocation of a wide bucket-handle portion causes a loud crack and a jolt. This test should be distinguished from the McMurray sign, in which the knee is held in full flexion, with the tibia in external rotation, and then gradually extended until a click occurs as the medial femoral condyle crosses the lesion in the meniscus. The maneuver we describe is just the reverse, in that it does not reduplicate the strain which produces the original lesion, as the McMurray test is supposed to do. (DuToit & Enslin, 1945)

Ankle

Inspection

An effusion into the ankle joint produces bulging beneath the extensor tendons and a fullness just anterior to the lateral and medial collateral ligaments. The foot tends to be held in slight dorsiflexion and inversion. The best way to detect an early effusion is to view the joint from behind and look for fullness in the normal fossae behind the malleoli, comparing them with the normal side ("Bailey," Clain, 1973).

Palpation

In a rupture ("sprain") of the calcaneofibular (lateral malleolar) ligament, due to forced inversion of the foot, the tenderness is located anterior and possibly inferior to the lateral malleolus, rather than over the malleolus itself. This finding helps to differentiate a sprain from a fracture (see p. 430 for fractures).

Tenderness and swelling are found along the course of the tendons below and behind the lateral malleolus in chronic stenosing tenosynovitis of the peroneal tendon sheath (vide infra).

Special Maneuvers

1. To distinguish a partial from a complete avulsion of the lateral malleolar ligament, invert the ankle slowly and check for an obvious gap between the tip of the malleolus and the talus.

2. In recurrent dislocation of the peroneal tendons, the tendons of the peroneus longus and brevis slip from behind and under the lateral malleolus, due to laxity in the superior peroneal retinaculum. Check for pain and a clicking sensation during dorsiflexion with eversion. If the patient or examiner is unable to demonstrate these findings, one may have to rely on their historical occurrence.

3. Chronic stenosing tenosynovitis of the peroneal tendon sheath causes pain on inversion of the foot.

4. To perform Helfet's test of the tibiofibular joint, have the patient stand on the afflicted leg only, then flex that leg at the knee. The patient with instability of the tibiofibular joint cannot complete this test. The patient with arthritis or sprain of that joint will be able to support his weight briefly without putting his other foot down, but will refuse to do so because of pain. Such a patient will be able to perform the test successfully after the joint is injected with 25 mg of hydrocortisone and 1% topical anesthetic.

The differential diagnosis includes trauma, especially to the ankle (not the knee); rheumatoid arthritis; and exostosis of the head of the fibula (Helfet, 1982).

Synthesis

In the pride of victory Bajazet threatened that he would besiege Buda; that he would subdue the adjacent countries of Germany and Italy; and that he would feed his horse with a bushel of oats on the altar of St. Peter at Rome. His progress was checked not by the miraculous interposition of the apostle, not by a crusade of the Christian powers, but by a long and painful fit of the gout. The disorders of the moral are sometimes corrected by those of the physical world; and an acrimonious humor* falling on a single fiber of one man may prevent or suspend the misery of nations. (Edward Gibbon, *The Decline and Fall of the Roman Empire*, Ch. 64, J.M. Dent, Everyman's Library)

Diagnostic Criteria for Major Arthritides

Some criteria for entities to be considered in the differential diagnosis of arthritis are listed in Tables 24-3 to 24-7. Hand findings are described in detail in Chapter 25 (pp. 435–442).

Reiter's Syndrome

The sensitivity for the criteria in Table 24-9 is 84%, and the specificity 98% (Willkens et al., 1981).

Keratoderma blenorrhagica (see Ch. 7, p. 115) and circinate balanitis (see Ch. 21, p. 392) are considered pathognomonic of Reiter's syndrome by some.

Caveat: Late keratoderma blenorrhagica is identical to pustular psoriasis.

Osteoarthritis

Osteoarthritis is thought to result from the excessive wear and tear of repetitive trauma or from other predisposing factors, such as: acquired or developmental structural abnormalities; metabolic disturbances affecting articular cartilage (alkaptonuria and acromegaly); repeated joint hemorrhage; disordered proprioception (leading to the Charcot joint, vide infra); and a genetic predisposition (especially for certain forms of the disease such as Heberden's nodes).

Tenderness to palpation may be observed, but signs of inflammation, except for effusion, are relatively uncommon (Rodnan et al., 1973).

The joints most commonly involved are: the distal interphalangeal joints (see Ch. 25, p. 435), the proximal interphalangeal joints, the first carpometacarpal joint (radial side), the hips, the knees, the apophyseal and the intervertebral articulations, and the joints of the foot.

Charcot Joint

Usually a knee or ankle, this joint is anesthetic due to neuropathy, predominantly diabetic or luetic. Unable to sense position or pain, it grinds itself into deformity, frequently with pieces of loose bone and cartilage floating within the joint ("joint mice").

Bone

Question: *Roentgen (also spelled Rontgen) won the Nobel prize in physiology or medicine for discovering X rays. True or false? (See Appendix 24-2 for the answer.)*

Inspection

Inspect for obvious bony deformities. (Abnormal overall proportions are discussed in Ch. 5, p. 83.) Note any asymmetry; one

---

*Gibbon was at least partly right. *Gout* comes from the Latin *gutta* or "drop." This reflected the belief that gout was caused by an acrimonious humor falling, one drop at a time, into the fibers of the joint.

Table 24-3.   Diagnostic Criteria for Rheumatoid Arthritis

1.   Morning stiffness
2.   Pain with motion or tenderness (apparent at the time of examination)
3.   Swelling (seen)
4.   A second swollen joint (seen) not more than 3 months after criterion 3.
5.   Symmetric joint swelling (not including distal interphalangeal joints)
6.   Subcutaneous nodules (see Ch. 25, p. 435)
7.   Characteristic radiographic changes
8.   Positive rheumatoid factor
9.   Poor synovial fluid mucin
10.   Characteristic synovial histology
11.   Characteristic nodule histology

Source: *Rodnan et al. (1973).*

In classic rheumatoid arthritis, 7 of the 11 findings are present. Items 1 through 5 must be continuous for 6 weeks to be counted. The diagnosis is definite if five features present; probable if three are present; possible if two are present. Excluders: increased concentration of LE cells; SLE rash; dermatomyositis, sclerodactyly; rheumatic fever; tophi; erythema nodosum, multiple myeloma, and so forth.

special method of determining asymmetry is to measure the length of the limbs.

A Method for Measuring the Legs (Length)

1.   Have the patient lie supine on an examining table, with his pelvis level, his hips and knees fully extended, and both hips equally abducted or adducted.

2.   Locate the anterior superior iliac spines, and mark their lower margins.

3.   Measure from the point marked in step 2 to the medial malleolus on the same side.

(Measurement of leg circumference is in Ch. 19, p. 367.)

A Method for Measuring the Arms

1.   Have the patient extend his arm with the shoulder adducted.

2.   Measure the distance from the tip of the acromion to the tip of the middle finger (Raney & Brashear, 1971).

Diagnostic Measurements

1.   In a Pott's fracture* of the ankle, usually resulting from forced eversion, the distance between the malleoli may be increased.

2.   In a Dupuytren's fracture, which usually results from falling from a height onto the feet, the talus is driven upwards, greatly increasing the width of the ankle between the malleoli and shortening the distance from the malleoli to the sole.

Palpation

I. Snapper once made a diagnosis of Paget's disease by palpating the patient's shins and finding warm spots over the hyperperfused bone. (See also Ch. 9, p. 149.)

Tenderness at the neck of the fibula is a sign of a spiral fracture.

---

*A Pott's fracture is a fracture of the lower end of the fibula, often associated with a fracture of the tip of the medial malleolus. Often there is also displacement of the talus laterally or medially (second-degree fracture) and backward (third-degree fracture).

Table 24-4   Diagnostic Criteria for Systemic Lupus Erythematosus

1.   Malar rash
2.   Discoid rash
3.   Dermal photosensitivity
4.   Oral (or nasal) ulcers (seen)
5.   Nonerosive arthritis of at least two joints
6.   Pleuritis or pericarditis
7.   Persistent proteinuria (3+ or 500 mg/day) or cellular casts (white or red blood cells)
8.   Seizures or psychosis
9.   Hemolysis or white count less than 4,000 on two occasions or lymphocytes less than 1,500 on two occasions or platelets less than 100,000
10.   LE cells or anti-native DNA or anti-Smith or biologic false positive serologic test for syphilis more than 6 months
11.   Antinuclear antibody

The diagnosis is made by the presence of 4 of the 11 criteria (Tan et al., 1982).

Percussion

Tenderness to light finger percussion may be a sign of osteomyelitis. (Rolling a pencil along a long bone, exerting pressure, is another way to elicit tenderness.)

Special Maneuvers

Induced Crepitation

A very crude test, that can be used by anyone with a sufficient knowledge of peripheral nervous anatomy to avoid avulsing a nerve, is to grasp the ends of a long bone and twist so as to produce a diaphyseal torque. The test is positive for fracture if crepitation is heard.

The test may produce pain without crepitation in hematomas, sprains, or other injuries that have not resulted in a fracture.

This test is not as sensitive as auscultatory percussion.

Findings Associated with Fractures

Remote findings that may be associated with fractures include fat embolization (Ch. 28, p. 551; Ch. 7, p. 108), Battle's sign (see Ch. 9, p. 145), Purtscher's retinopathy (Ch. 10, p. 199), palpation of the ribs, and observation for heightened inspiratory retraction of an area of the chest wall (see Ch. 16, pp. 246 and 249).

Auscultatory Percussion

We find, for example, that among tissues of the body, bone is the best conductor of sound. (Cammann & Clark, 1840)

A method.   To detect fractures of the femur or of the pubic rami, place your stethoscope at the symphysis pubis, and with the earpieces in your ears, percuss each patella in turn, taking

Table 24-5.   Diagnostic Criteria for Ankylosing Spondylitis

A.   Moderate to advanced or ankylosed bilateral sacroiliitis plus at least one of the following:

1.   Limitation of motion of the lumbar spine
2.   Pain at the dorsal lumbar junction or in the lumbar spine
3.   Chest expansion of 2.5 cm or less (see Ch. 16, p. 246)

B.   Minimal bilateral sacroiliitis *or* moderate, advanced, or ankylosed unilateral sacroiliitis *plus* clinical criterion 1 above or both criteria 2 and 3.

Source: *Fries (1985).*

Table 24-6. Diagnostic Criteria
for Progressive Systemic Sclerosis (Scleroderma)

Proximal scleroderma, or any two of the following criteria:

1. Sclerodactyly
2. Digital pitting scars
3. Bibasilar pulmonary fibrosis

Source: *Subcommittee for Scleroderma Criteria (1980).*

care to strike the patella with exactly the same force on both sides (Carter, 1981).

On the side of the fracture (Fig. 24-12), the percussion note will be softer, and missing some high-frequency components. Sound transmission gradually returns to normal as the fracture heals. (The same principle has also been applied to diagnose fractures of the humerus (Berger, 1982).

Caveats:

1. This test assumes the presence of patellae, the absence of knee effusions, and the existence of a fracture on one side only (Peltier, 1958).

2. To avoid inducing false positives and false negatives, the patient's legs should be unencumbered by blankets or heavy dressings (Peltier, 1958). Both legs must be in the same position (i.e., symmetric—not with one hip or knee in flexion and the other in extension).

3. The test may also be positive in pseudoarthrosis (Berger, 1982), hip dislocation without fracture, unilateral bone cysts, and bone tumors (Sotos, 1982). But it may miss hip effusion (Peltier, 1958), aseptic necrosis of the femoral head, and impacted fractures of the femoral head.

False positives. Impaired transmission on the right in a patient whose right hip fracture was years remote was found to be due to a prosthesis, which must have dampened the cortical bone vibrations.

False negatives. Dr. John Guarino finds that some fractures may be missed if the diaphragm is placed upon the symphysis pubis; he places the stethoscope head on the iliac crests (J. Guarino, personal communication, 1988).

A schizophrenic patient who was reputed to have a fracture on

Table 24-7. Diagnostic Criteria for Gout

Pathognomonic: urate crystals in the joint fluid. (See Ch. 28, p. 552)

The presence of six or more of the following is considered diagnostic; but 11% are false positives due to pseudogout (Wallace et al., 1977).

1. More than one attack
2. Peak inflammation within 1 day
3. Monoarticular
4. Rubor
5. First metatarsophalangeal (MTP) dolor or tumor (podagra—see Table 24-8)[a]
6. Unilateral first MTP involvement
7. Unilateral tarsal involvement
8. Tophus (33% sensitive, 93% specific, see Fig. 25-3)
9. Increased serum uric acid
10. Asymmetric swelling
11. Subcortical cysts with erosions
12. Negative cultures

[a]*Podagra is Greek for "pain in the foot." In current usage, it means pain in the big toe, or more specifically the first metatarsophalangeal joint.*

Table 24-8. Etiologies of Podagra

Gout
Pseudogout (calcium pyrophosphate dihydrate deposition)
Calcium hydroxyapatite

Less frequent causes
    Rheumatoid arthritis
    Osteoarthritis
    Mechanical

One-upsmanship causes
    Sarcoidosis
    Ankylosing spondylitis
    Reiter's syndrome
    Psoriatic arthritis
    Arthritis reactive to inflammatory bowel disease
    Charcot joint of syphilis, diabetes mellitus, etc.
    Infectious
    Paget's disease
    Hemochromatosis

Striped unicorns[a]
    Sesamoiditis
    Pancreatic disease
    Thyroid acropachy
    Palindromic rheumatism
    "Psychogenic" rheumatism

Source: *Bomalaski and Schumacher (1984).*

[a]*A striped unicorn is an imaginary zebra (see Ch. 27, p. 530).*

the right was shown to have impaired transmission on the left. On reviewing the radiographs, it was found that the patient had a congenitally dislocated hip on the left with a false acetabulum, in addition to the recent fracture on the right! The fractured side actually transmitted sound better than the dislocated side because the fractured femoral head was still in the normal acetabulum.

Appendix 24-1. Myopathy: Answer to Question on Page 415

Given the fact that the myopathy is not generalized, and that there is no atrophy at a time when the pelvic girdle is afflicted, most of the myopathies have already been ruled out. His baldness should not suggest myotonia dystrophica, since that typically causes temporal baldness, not alopecia totalis. Further, his masseter muscle seems well preserved, as does the temporalis. Alcoholic myopathy should not be localized to the pelvic girdle, nor should that of hypothyroidism. Chronic thyrotoxic myopathy should also show more atrophy of the shoulder girdle, and so perhaps should polymyositis. Thyrotoxic periodic paralysis, and for that matter the other periodic paralyses, including myasthenia gravis, should not so selectively affect the pelvic girdle. The patient does not look Cushingoid, and there is no evidence that corticosteroids were known to the Olmecs. I will discount sarcoid myopathy, central core myopathy, and nemeline myopathy on the basis of rarity.

Do you see how much easier this analysis would be if we could just elicit a history?

In summary, we have an adult male with pelvic girdle disease,

Table 24-9. Diagnostic Criteria for Reiter's Syndrome

1. Peripheral arthritis of more than 1 month's duration, and
2. Associated urethritis and/or cervicitis

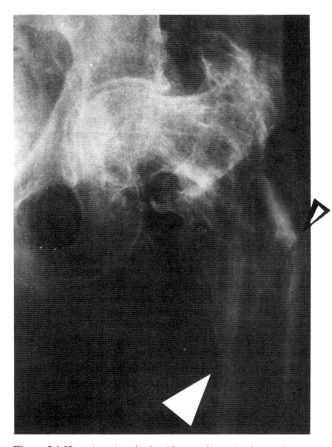

Figure 24-12. *A patient had evidence of impaired auscultatory percussion in a hip fractured many years previously (with no recent trauma). Admission hip films now revealed no evidence of nonunion to at least two observers. On the insistence of the examiner who had noted the physical findings, another film was obtained. Note the new fracture line running about halfway from the upper arrow toward the lower arrow.*

no diffuse atrophy, perhaps even some hypertrophy. I would diagnose this as a case of Duchenne's pseudohypertrophic muscular dystrophy, mild sex-linked variant. (It would have to be the mild variant for the patient to reach this age without yet showing atrophy of the biceps and brachioradialis muscles.)

If you diagnosed myositis ossificans, give yourself a raspberry.

Appendix 24-2. Answer to Question Concerning Figure 24-2

The resident said that the bulge shown in Figure 24-2 was a bicipital head whose tendon insertion had ruptured. The attending said it was a herniation through an aponeurotic defect, noting that the patient could not recall the onset. The resident rebutted that the patient often could not remember things and seemed to have a chronic organic brain syndrome, either directly due to alcohol or indirectly through the effects on the liver (remember the spider?). If you diagnosed either one of these, your answer is as good as anyone else's. Although one aims for diagnostic closure, sometimes the information that is sought does not justify the risk required to obtain it, and we go without a final answer.

Appendix 24-3. Roentgen: Answer to Question on Page 429

The answer to the question is: False. Roentgen won the Nobel prize in physics for that discovery. In fact, it was in the first set of Nobel prizes awarded, in 1901. But Roentgen never won the prize in physiology or medicine despite the fact that his invention changed medicine probably more than any other. It is clearly the gold standard for diagnosing fractures and other bone diseases.

References

Apley AG: *System of Orthopaedics and Fractures*, ed 5. Butterworths, London, 1977.

Barness LA: *Manual of Pediatric Physical Diagnosis*, ed 4. Yearbook Medical Publishers, Chicago, 1972.

Berger EY: More on diagnosing fractures of the hip or pelvis. *N Engl J Med* 308:971, 1982.

Bomalaski JS, Schumacher HR: Podagra is more than gout. *Bull Rheum Dis* 34(6):1–8, 1984.

Cabot RC: *Physical Diagnosis*, ed 11. William Wood and Co, Baltimore, 1937.

Cammann P, Clark A: Cammann and Clark on percussion. *NY J Med Surg* 3(July):62–96, 1840.

Carter MC: A reliable sign of fractures of the hip or pelvis. *N Engl J Med* 305:1220, 1981.

Clain A, ed: *Hamilton Bailey's Demonstration of Physical Signs in Clinical Surgery*, ed 15. Williams & Wilkins, Baltimore, 1973.

Conn RD, Smith RH: Malnutrition, myoedema, and Muehrcke's lines. *Arch Intern Med* 116:875–878, 1965.

Crenshaw AH, Kilgore WE: Surgical treatment of bicipital tenosynovitis. *J Bone Joint Surg [Am]*, 48:1496–1502, 1966.

Daniel DM, Stone ML, Barnett P, Sachs R: Use of the quadriceps active test to diagnose posterior cruciate-ligament disruption and measure posterior laxity of the knee. *J Bone Joint Surg [Am]* 70-A:386–391, 1988.

Davidson RI, Dunn EJ, Metzmaker JN: The shoulder abduction test in the diagnosis of radicular pain in cervical extradural compressive monoradiculopathies. *Spine* 6:441–446, 1981.

DuToit GT, Enslin TB: Analysis of one hundred consecutive arthrotomies for traumatic internal derangement of the knee joint. *J Bone Joint Surg* 27:412–425, 1945.

Dyck P: The femoral nerve traction test with lumbar disc protrusions. *Surg Neurol* 6:163–166, 1976.

Fairbank HAT: Internal derangement of the knee in children and adolescents. *Proc R Soc Med* 30:427–432, 1937.

Fries JF: The reactive enthesiopathies. *DM* 31(1):24–26, 1985.

Furman RE, Barchi RL: Pathophysiology of myotonia and periodic paralysis. In: Asbury AK, McKhann GM, McDonald WI (eds), *Diseases of the Nervous System*, vol 1. Ardmore Medical Books, WB Saunders, Philadelphia, 1986.

Good AE: Rheumatoid arthritis, Baker's cyst, and "thrombophlebitis." *Arthritis Rheum* 7:56–64, 1964.

Hall H: Examination of the patient with low back pain. *Bull Rheum Dis* 33(4):1–8, 1983.

Helfet AJ: *Disorders of the Knee*, ed 2. JP Lippincott, Philadelphia, 1982.

Herron LD, Pheasant HC: Prone knee-flexion provocative testing for lumbar disc protrusion. *Spine* 5:65–67, 1980.

Hudgins WR: The crossed-straight-leg-raising test. *N Engl J Med* 297:1127, 1977.

Johnson JE, Sim FH, Scott SG: Musculoskeletal injuries in competitive swimmers. *Mayo Clin Proc* 62:289–304, 1987.

Koppel HP, Thompson WAL: Knee pain due to saphenous nerve entrapment. *N Engl J Med* 263:351–353, 1960.

Lewin P: *The Knee and Related Structures*. Lea & Febiger, Philadelphia, 1952.

Lyons JC, Peterson LFA: The snapping iliopsoas tendon. *Mayo Clin Proc* 59:327–329, 1984.

McBeath AA: Some common causes of hip pain: Physical diagnosis is the key. *Postgrad Med* 77(8):189–195, 198, 1985.

McMurray TP: The semilunar cartilages. *Br J Surg* 29:407–414, 1942.

Merritt JL, McLean TJ, Erickson RP, Offord KP: Measurement of trunk flexibility in normal subjects: Reproducibility of three clinical methods. *Mayo Clinic Proc* 61:192–197, 1986.

Moll JMH, Wright V: Normal range of spinal mobility. *Ann Rheum Dis* 30:381–386, 1971.

Nehemkis AM, Carver DW, Evanski PM: The predictive value of the orthopedic examination in identifying the low back pain patient with hysterical personality features. *Clin Orthop* 145:158–162, 1979.

Nelson MA, Allen P, Clamp SE, de Dombal FT: Reliability and reproducibility of clinical findings in low-back pain. *Spine* 4:97–101, 1979.

Peltier LF: The transmission of sound by the femur. *Gen Pract* 17(1):109, 1958.

Pinals RS: Genu amoris. *Arthritis Rheum* 19:637–638, 1976.

Poewe WH: Torticollis: Causes, clinical presentation, and management in the elderly. *Geriatric Med Today* 6(1):54–63, 1987.

Polley HF, Hunder GG: *Rheumatologic Interviewing and Physical Examination of the Joints*, ed 2. WB Saunders, Philadelphia, 1978. [This book was distributed by the Medical Information Service of Merck Sharp & Dohme.]

Raney RB, Brashear HR: *Shands' Handbook of Orthopaedic Surgery* ed 8. CV Mosby, St Louis, 1971.

Rodnan GP, McEwen C, Wallace SL, eds: *Primer on the Rheumatic Diseases*, ed 7. The Arthritis Foundation, New York, 1973. [Reprinted as a Supplement to *JAMA* 224(5), 1973.]

Russell AS, Maksymowych W, LeClercq S: Clinical examination of the sacroiliac joints: A prospective study. *Arthritis Rheum* 24:1575–1577, 1981.

Rutstein JE, McCutchen JW: An unusual complication of genu amoris. *Arthritis Rheum* 20:906, 1977.

Schmidt MC, Workman JB, Barth WF: Dissection or rupture of a popliteal cyst: A syndrome mimicking thrombophlebitis in rheumatic diseases. *Arch Intern Med* 134:694–698, 1974.

Schober P: Lendenwirbelsule und Kreuzschmerzen. *Münchener Med Wochenschr* 84:336–338, 1937.

Smythe HA, Moldofsky H: Two contributions to understanding of the "fibrositis" syndrome. *Bull Rheum Dis* 28(1):928–931, 1977–1978.

Sotos JG: Diagnosis of fractures of the hip or pelvis. *N Engl J Med* 306:366, 1982.

Spurling RG, Scoville WB: Lateral rupture of the cervical intervertebral discs: A common cause of shoulder and arm pain. *Surg Gynecol Obstet* 78:350–358, 1944.

Subcommittee for Scleroderma Criteria of the American Rheumatism Association Diagnostic and Therapeutic Criteria Committee: Preliminary criteria for the classification of systemic sclerosis (scleroderma). *Arthritis Rheum* 23:581–590, 1980.

Tan EM, Cohen AS, Fries JF, Masi AT, McShane DJ, Rothfield NF, Schaller JG, Talal N, Winchester RJ: The 1982 revised criteria for the classification of systemic lupus erythematosus. *Arthritis Rheum* 25:1271–1277, 1982.

Waddell G, Main CJ, Morris EW, Venner RM, Rae PS, Sharmy SH, Galloway H: Normality and reliability in the clinical assessment of backache. *Br Med J* 284:1519–1523, 1982.

Wallace SL, Robinson H, Masi AT, Decker JL, McCarty DJ, Yu, T-F: Preliminary criteria for the classification of the acute arthritis of primary gout. *Arthritis Rheum* 20:895–900, 1977.

Willkens RF, Arnett FC, Better T, Calin A, Fisher L, Ford DK, Good AE, Masi AT: Reiter's syndrome: evaluation of preliminary criteria for definite disease. *Arthritis Rheum* 24:844–849, 1981.

Winchester R, Bernstein DH, Fischer HD, Enlow R, Solomon G: The co-occurrence of Reiter's syndrome and acquired immunodeficiency. *Ann Intern Med* 106:19–26, 1987.

25
The Extremities

"A man's reach must exceed his grasp, or what's a heaven for?"

Robert Browning

Upper Extremities

Nodules

The extensor surfaces of the upper extremities are the best places to find rheumatoid nodules. However, they can also occur in a number of other subcutaneous locations (Table 25-1).

Rheumatoid nodules are not diagnostic for rheumatoid arthritis, but in patients with rheumatoid arthritis, the presence of nodules predicts a 90% chance of having rheumatoid factor (Kaye et al., 1984).

Table 25-2 shows diseases associated with subcutaneous nodules similar to those found in rheumatoid arthritis. Those in boldface letters have the best track record for fooling the clinician. Fortunately, most of these diseases have either decreased somewhat in prevalence (rheumatic fever, tophaceous gout, gummatous syphilis) or the diagnoses can be made on other grounds.

Self-Study Question: *In your practice, you see 95 patients with rheumatoid arthritis for every five with rheumatic fever. What then is the likelihood (irrespective of the clinical setting) that a patient with an occipital nodule has one versus the other disease? (Use Table 25-1. Answer is in Appendix 25-1.)*

Elbows

In hypothyroidism, the elbows are said to look unwashed. That is, they are grey and keratotic and surrounded by normal skin.

Plummer's sign is named for the Mayo Clinic endocrinologist who noticed that some hyperthyroid patients were so agitated that they inflamed their elbows by repeated movement against the starched white bedsheets. (Dr. Jack D. Myers of Pennsylvania taught me this sign.)

Hands

Acromegaly

Acral enlargement, the literal translation of "acromegaly," involving the hand, foot, and head, occurs in 98% of cases of this disease. Actually, the hand develops a characteristic appearance that is easy to recognize once seen. This is called the "spade hand" because the hand vaguely resembles the garden implement (Fig. 25-1). (However, the diagnosis of acral enlargement may also be based on the history of an increase in glove, ring, shoe, and/or hat size [Braunstein, 1986].)

Findings in Rheumatic Diseases

Rheumatoid arthritis (see Ch. 24, p. 430) can be diagnosed in some cases simply by inspecting the hand, even when no nodules are present. First, there may be interosseus atrophy, best noted by inspecting the dorsum of the hand in oblique lighting, but with practice discernible in direct light. Second, there is ulnar deviation of the hand and the fingers. The best fingers to check for ulnar deviation are the third and index fingers since many normal older persons will appear to have mild ulnar deviation of the other fingers. However, in severe carpal rheumatoid arthritis, all the fingers show a clear ulnar deviation.

It is worth remembering that rheumatoid arthritis of the wrist tends to spare the radial side of the joint. In fact, a severe arthritis of the wrist that spares the ulnar side and vigorously attacks the radial side is likely to be osteoarthritis (degenerative joint disease or DJD). Also remember that classic rheumatoid arthritis never attacks the distal interphalangeal joints.

Psoriatic arthritis, a seronegative rheumatoid variant, does attack the distal interphalangeal joints. The diagnosis is suggested by the associated skin and nail changes (see Ch. 7, p. 131). Psoriatic arthritis may be severely deforming, whereas osteoarthritis is not.

Other manifestations of rheumatoid arthritis include: 1) loss of grip strength; 2) limited flexion in one or more fingers due to nodular tenosynovitis (felt as a small movable nodule in the flexor tendon as you passively flex and extend the joint); 3) vasculitic lesions, which may herald serious systemic vasculitis (Weiss, 1984); and 4) Haygart's nodes (actually not nodes but fusiform synovial swellings of the proximal interphalangeal joints [PIPs]).

Patients with hemochromatosis are prone to a degenerative type of arthritis that can affect the hands and fingers as well as the joints of the lower extremities. The PIPs of the middle and ring fingers may be affected, mimicking Haygart's fusiform swelling of rheumatoid arthritis confined to those joints.

Table 25-1. Principal Sites of Subcutaneous Nodules

Site	RA (%)	RF (%)
Elbows	91	80
Fingers	14	19
Knees	13	48
Ankles	7	20
Occiput	5	20

Source: *Benedek (1984).*

(Figures refer to percentage of patients with the disease and nodules whose nodules occur in the given location. The prevalence of nodules in rheumatic fever (RF) averages about 9%, varying with the stage of the disease. The prevalence of rheumatoid nodules in rheumatoid arthritis (RA) is similarly variable, averaging around 28% (Benedek, 1984).

Self-Test: *See Figure 25-2.*

Osteoarthritis produces characteristic nodules of the distal interphalangeal joints (DIPs) called Heberden's nodes. These feel like two little dried split peas placed subcutaneously on the lateral and medial dorsal surface of the finger at the DIP. When they are present on the proximal interphalangeal joint, they are called Bouchard's nodes. Osteoarthritis tends to spare the metacarpophalangeal joints.

Progressive systemic sclerosis (see Ch. 24, p. 431) is characterized by sclerodactyly, which is discussed further on page 441.

Finally, a tophus on the hand is diagnostic of gout (see Table 24-7), although these occur more frequently on the ears and feet, and when present on the hand (Fig. 25-3) could be initially confused with a rheumatoid nodule.

Bony Anomalies

Short fourth metacarpal.
One can diagnose a short fourth metacarpophalangeal bone without taking a radiograph by having the patient make a fist and noticing that the fourth knuckle is dimpled inward. Shortening of the fourth metacarpal bone is seen in pseudo-hypoparathyroidism, pseudo-pseudohypoparathyroidism, gonadal dysgenesis (Turner's syndrome), and 10% of normals (Levin & Kupperman, 1964; Slater, 1970).

The hypothesis that pseudohypoparathyroidism resulted from end-organ resistance to a circulating hormone was first proposed by the Boston endocrinologist Fuller Albright. This possibility, previously unknown as a mechanism for human disease but subsequently confirmed, was suggested to him by analogy with the Sebright bantam rooster, which fails to develop secondary sex characteristics owing to end-organ resistance to circulating male sex hormones. A careless typesetter changed the Sebright bantam syndrome to the "Seabright-Bantam" syndrome, allowing Drs. Seabright and Bantam to join Dr. Jod (see p. 234) in the pantheon of eponymously immortalized, albeit nonexistent, endocrinologists.

Metacarpal index.
By palpation, one can estimate the metacarpal length-to-width ratio (metacarpal index) as a method of quantitating the elongation of the metacarpal bones in Marfan's syndrome. The independent covariable is PA hand films taken with the hands flat against the plate, which are used for measurement of the second through fifth metacarpals. The ratio of the length of the bone divided by the width (at the midpoint of the length) is used to generate an average, whose upper limit of normal is 8.8 for men and 9.4 for women (Eldridge, 1964). This ratio distinguished the patients with Marfan's syndrome from those without it, something

Table 25-2. Diseases Associated with Subcutaneous Nodules Similar to Those Found in Rheumatoid Arthritis

Rheumatic and immunologic diseases
Rheumatic fever
Systemic lupus erythematosus
Tophaceous gout
Discoid lupus erythematosus
Anarthritic rheumatoid syndrome
Degenerative joint disease (Heberden's nodes)
Sarcoidosis
Weber-Christian disease
Agammaglobulinemia with polyarthritis

Dermatologic disease
Granuloma annulare
Erythema elevatum diutinum
Acrodermatitis chronic atrophicans
Discoid lupus erythematosus
Basal cell carcinoma
Sebaceous cysts

Metabolic diseases
Tuberous xanthomatosis (see Ch. 7, p. 116)

Neoplastic diseases
Multicentric reticulohistiocytosis
Basal cell carcinoma

Infectious diseases
Syphilis
Synovial tuberculosis
Candidiasis
Bejel
Yaws
Pinta
Leprosy (Hansen's disease)

Miscellaneous conditions
Para-amyloid
Ganglions of the hand or wrist
Foreign body reactions
Chemical irritations
Delayed local reaction to tuberculin

Source: *Kaye et al. (1984).*

not achieved by the upper segment/lower segment or height/span ratios (see Ch. 5, p. 83).

Hand-Foot Syndrome in Sickle-Cell Disease
The earliest manifestation of sickle-cell disease in infants may be a painful, symmetrical swelling of the dorsa of the hands, or feet, or both. This sign of sickle-cell crisis occurs exclusively in children less than 8 years of age (Watson et al., 1963).

Bulimia
Calluses and abrasions on the dorsal surface of the hands may be acquired by a patient with bulimia, in the course of inducing emesis. These are produced by the patient's teeth (Wynn & Martin, 1984).

The Palms

Skin. Lesions of the palmar skin may be divided into: 1) dermatologic conditions and 2) those that reflect and are part of a systemic medial illness.

1. The former include ichthyosis vulgaris, X-linked ichthyosis, recalcitrant pustules, hand-foot-and-mouth disease, lichen planus, pompholyx, some psoriasis, the dermatophytoses (including tinea), and a variety of contact dermatitides.

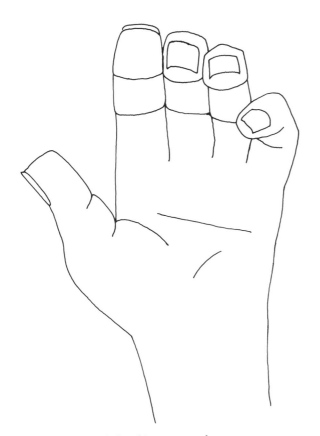

Figure 25-1. *Spade hand in acromegaly.*

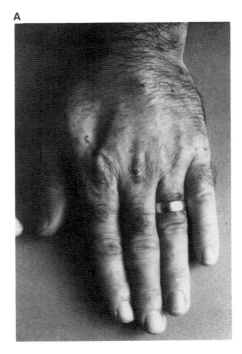

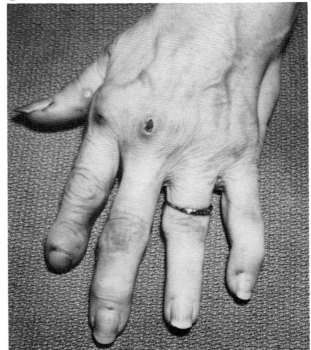

Figure 25-2, A and B. *Self-test: One hand belongs to a patient with rheumatoid arthritis, and one to a patient with porphyria cutanea tarda. Identify the diagnosis, and then the skin lesions.*

You should be having difficulty because skin lesions must always be considered in the context in which they occur. Neither of these diagnoses could easily be made from the skin lesions alone. Therefore, look for interosseus muscle atrophy and slight ulnar deviation, the signs of rheumatoid arthritis, but not porphyria. (See Appendix 25-2 for the answer.)

2. The latter include those that are part of a generalized eruption —secondary syphilis (Fig. 21-4, p. 393), Reiter's syndrome, rare cases of disseminated gonococcemia, erythema multiforme (from any of its causes), and roseola—and arsenical and other hyperkeratoses, which are confined to the palms and soles.

Palmar keratoses, especially when multiple, may be associated with arsenic toxicity. Skin bladder and lung cancer may also be associated with palmar keratoses (Cuzick et al. 1984), but here the keratoses may be few or single (see also Ch. 7, p. 113).

Palmar and finger crease xanthomas are discussed in Chapter 7 (p. 117).

Hyperpigmented macules and patches of the palms were present in 35% of black adults and in over 60% of those over the age of 65 (McDonald & Kelly, 1987).

Palmar dermatoglyphs. In patient's with Down's syndrome, one may see a bilateral simian crease (Fig. 25-4), in which the normal (two) transverse palmar lines are replaced by a single line that completely crosses the palm. However, the diagnosis of Down's syndrome should never be based on this finding in isolation. (See Ch. 10, p. 164 for more on Down's syndrome.)

If both transverse lines are maintained, but the proximal one completely crosses the palm, it is referred to as a Sydney crease (see Fig. 25-5). It indicates an increased propensity to develop granulocytic leukemia. It is also seen in Down's syndrome and congenital rubella (Wertelecki, 1979). It was first described by Purvis-Simith of Australia and shown to me by Dr. W. Wertelecki of Alabama.

In ichthyosis vulgaris, there are extra vertical palm creases between the thenar and hypothenar eminences (Fig. 25-6).

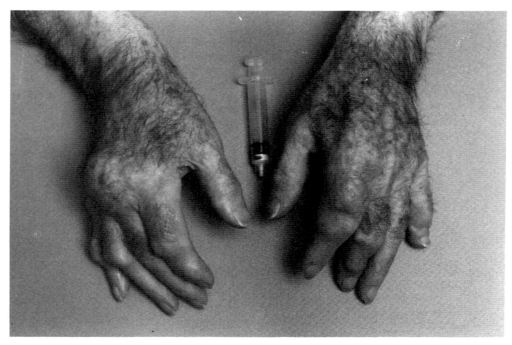

Figure 25-3. *This phlegmatic patient accepted the diagnosis of "arthritis" for many years. No one seemed to realize that the development of these tophi was not an inevitable consequence of "arthritis." Aspiration of the joint by Dr. Renee Ridzon of Massachusetts revealed the milk of urate shown in the syringe. Examination of the fluid by means of the improvized polarizing microscope and first-order compensator (see Ch. 28, p. 552) revealed the pathognomonic urate crystals. Photograph courtesy of Dr. Ridzon.*

Dupuytren's* contracture. This condition may affect only one finger or two fingers (as in Fig. 25-7). However, the thumb is always spared. It is caused by a stenosing tenosynovitis or fibrosis of the palmar tendons, producing the respective trigger finger(s). During maximum attempted extension of the fingers, the afflicted fingers are held in flexion. Sometimes the tendons can be felt better than seen.

Dupuytren's contracture especially occurs in older, white male patients who smoke cigarettes and have a family history of Dupuytren's contracture. (See Tables 25-3 and 25-4 for associations.)

Diagnoses Made by Shaking the Patient's Hand

I have observed three physicians make a diagnosis simply by shaking the patient's hand:

1. Dr. Gerry Rodnan of Pennsylvania diagnosed rheumatoid arthritis by squeezing the metacarpal heads during a handshake. This is a good sign, but painful. Some do not shake hands with patients suspected to have rheumatoid arthritis, but simply ask what would happen if one were to squeeze their hand.

*Dupuytren, being of humble origin, would probably never have become a physician were it not for the educational reforms that followed the French Revolution. These reforms consisted of lowering the barriers to, not the standards of, a medical education. Their success may be judged from the fact that Dupuytren went on to become a full professor, much feared but much respected by the students. At Dupuytren's funeral, when the hearse reached the medical school, the students stopped it, unhitched the horses, and pulled the hearse the remaining distance to the cemetery themselves.

2. Dr. Eugene Robin of California correctly diagnosed apathetic thyrotoxicosis in an elderly man who had orthopnea and warm moist palms.
3. Dr. Gunther Haase of Pennsylvania diagnosed myotonia on handshake (and so can you, see Ch. 24, p. 416).

Osler's Nodes and Janeway Lesions

In trying to determine whether a given case is more probably due to endocarditis or to another malignant process, I have found that attention to the position of the hemorrhages is at times very helpful. Several times I have noted numerous small hemorrhages with slight nodular character in the palms of the hand and the soles of the feet, when possibly the arms and legs had but a scanty crop in malignant endocarditis, whereas this has not been my experience with processes likely to be mistaken for it. (E. Janeway, 1899; cited in Farrior & and Silverman, 1976).

Ephemeral spots of a painful nodular erythema chiefly in the skin of the hands and feet . . . . The spots came out at intervals as swollen areas, some the size of a pea, others a centimeter and a half in diameter, raised, red, with a whitish point in the center. I have known them to pass away in a few hours but more commonly they last for a day or even longer. The commonest situation is near the tip of the finger which may be slightly swollen. (W. Osler, 1885–1909; (cited in Farrior & Silverman, 1976)

Red spots, some erythematous and some hemorrhagic, of a macular or papular nature, with or without a nodular and/or white center, may appear on the hands, feet, digits, toes, and extremities of patients with acute, subacute, or chronic bacterial endocarditis or endarteritis.

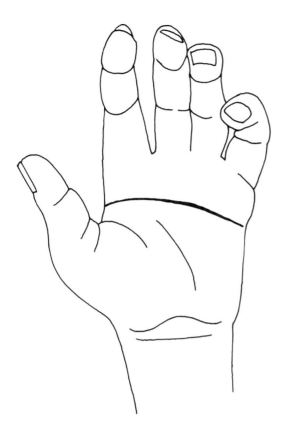

Figure 25-4.   *A simian crease.*

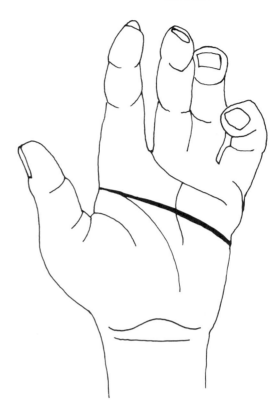

Figure 25-5.   *A Sydney crease.*

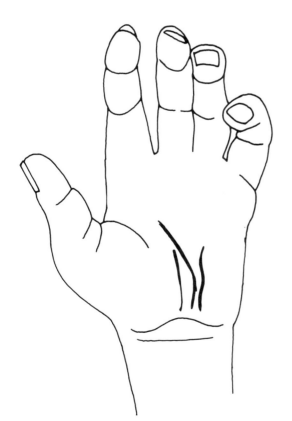

Figure 25-6.   *Palmar creases in ichythosis vulgaris.*

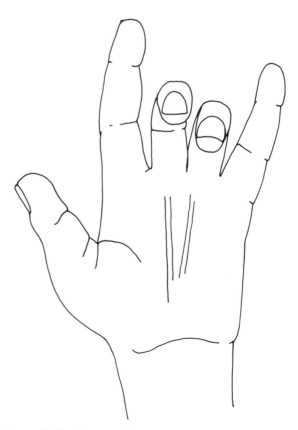

Figure 25-7.   *Dupuytren's contracture.*

Table 25-3.   Prevalence of
Dupuytren's Contracture in Various Diseases

Liver disease (Attali et al., 1987; Early, 1962; Pojer et al., 1972;
    Su & Patek, 1970; Wolfe et al., 1956)
    Alcoholic cirrhosis (18%–66%)
    Noncirrhotic alcoholic liver disease (19%–22%)
    Nonalcoholic chronic liver disease (19%–28%)
    (Chronic alcoholism without liver disease (6%–45%)
        (Hueston, 1960);
        (Control groups had a prevalence of 1%–12%)

Tuberculosis (chronic pulmonary) (13%–42%) (Hueston, 1960)

Epilepsy, treated (8%–56%) (Critchley et al., 1976; Pojer et al.,
    1972)

Men over 60 years of age (>35%) (Hueston, 1960)

Possible, but not proven:
    Systemic lupus erythematosus
    Fibrosing diseases other than Peyronie's (Dalinka & McGee,
        1970; Lund, 1947)
    Coronary artery disease (Hueston, 1960; Kehl, 1943)

Disproven:
    Manual labor (Hueston, 1960)
    Brewery workers (Hueston, 1960)

J.A. Mullin, M.D., of Canada first showed these lesions to Osler in 1893 (Farrior & Silverman, 1976), although they had already been described by Lancereaux (Yee & McAllister, 1987). During Osler's writings, Janeway described "his" lesion. The only remaining distinction between them (Farrior & Silverman, 1976) devolves upon the arbitrary statement that Janeway lesions are never painful or tender. Yet there is no basis for this distinction in Janeway's own description (vide supra), and no less an authority than Kerr has given us the clinicopathologic correlation of a tender Janeway spot (Kerr, 1955; Kerr & Tan, 1979). Probably tenderness depends upon whether neural structures are involved (Kerr & Tan, 1979; von Gemmingen & Winkelman, 1967).

I cannot tell the difference between the two. For those wishing to maintain a distinction, I will simply note that on occasion "both" have been shown to be due to septic emboli based upon Gram stain or culture of the lesion or the nearby tissue (Alpert et al., 1976; Cross & Ellis, 1966; Fanning & Aronson, 1977; Kerr, 1955; Lin et al., 1980; Puklin et al., 1971) and at other times "both" have been sterile and shown to be due to an immune vasculitis (Farrior & Silverman, 1976; von Gemmingen & Winkelman, 1967).

In the preantibiotic era, the lesions were found in 40% to 90% of cases of endocarditis, but now are reported in only 10% to 23% of cases (Thapar et al, 1978; Yee & McAllister, 1987). The pronouncement that they are now rarely *seen* should be amended to read that they are now rarely *recognized* . . . in some quarters.

Table 25-4.   Prevalence of Other
Diseases in the Dupuytren's Contracture Population

Alcoholism	31%–48%	
Peptic ulcer	18%–31%	
Cholecystitis	10%–34%	
Diabetes mellitus	6%–25%	(especially correlates with retinopathy) (Larkin & Frier, 1986)
Glucose intolerance	93%	(Nardoni et al., 1981)
Cirrhosis	7%–9%	
Peyronie's disease	2.4%	
Chronic hepatitis	2.4%	

Source: *Pojer & Jedličková (1970).*

False positives.   These lesions have also been seen in lupus erythematosus (Farrior & Silverman, 1976), infected intraarterial lines (Michaelson & Walsh, 1970), bacteremia without endocarditis, gonococcal sepsis, typhoid fever, hemolytic anemia (Fanning & Aronson, 1977; Yee & McAllister, 1987), and nonbacterial thrombotic (marantic) endocarditis (Yee & McAllister, 1987).

Fingers

Digital Gangrene

Digital gangrene (Figs. 25-8 and 25-9) can occur in a variety of embolic and immune complex diseases such as subacute bacterial endocarditis, polyarteritis nodosa, systemic lupus erythematosus, and atheromatous embolization, as well as in frostbite, cryofibrinogenemia, cryoglobulinemia, and progressive systemic sclerosis. However, if the lesions do not have a sharply demarcated border, or are *not* in the distribution of the terminal artery (i.e., at the fingertips), or if the lesion is single, one may well be dealing with posttraumatic ecchymoses, an especially frequent red herring in the foot. (See the legend to Fig. 25-8 for some points to consider in making the distinction.)

Some experts expect cryoglobulinemias to produce lesions on the toes more frequently than on the fingers, because the toes should get colder.

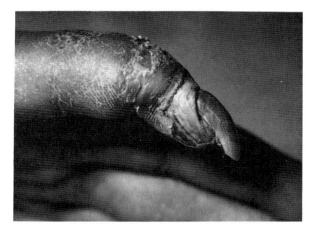

Figure 25-8.   *This patient with mixed cryoglobulinemia has digital gangrene. How can you distinguish his thumb lesion from a simple posttraumatic ecchymosis? (See Appendix 25-3 for the answer.)*

It may be objected that the above legend is incorrect in referring to "this patient" because it describes a photograph of just the thumb. In point of fact, most pictures are not pictures of an entire person, but only of the face, head, bust, and so forth. The thumb is no less noble than any other portion of a person.

More importantly, the advanced reader should form the habit of referring to all parts of Smith as being Smith himself, because of an unfortunate occurrence during the physician's maturation: As he becomes technically confident, the physician begins to see the individual parts as being somehow greater than, and also different from, the whole.

You can see this occur in others more easily than in yourself. At bedside rounds, senior students will often touch another person's patient in order to examine a finding but will not even say to the patient as much as "May I?" or "Excuse me, please." This happens with otherwise polite persons who suddenly become so interested in a part that they forget that it is a part of *a person.*

Thus, this figure is truly a picture of Smith, not just of his thumb.

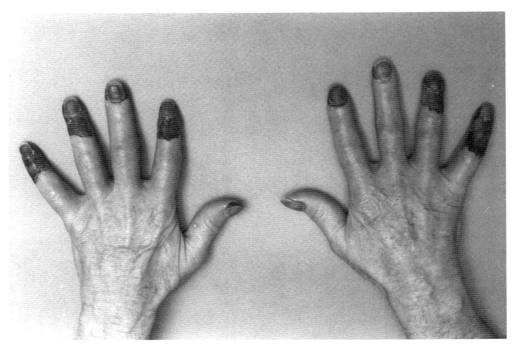

Figure 25-9. *Diagnosis? Write your answer down, then see Appendix 25-4. Photograph courtesy of Dr. Renee Ridzon of Massachusetts.*

Other Finger Markings

Distal purpleness of the fingers, resembling the cyanotic phase of Raynaud's phenomenon (see also Ch. 18, p. 345), may be seen in dermatomyositis, less commonly in the other collagen vascular diseases such as systemic lupus erythematosus or progressive systemic sclerosis. The most specific finger sign for dermatomyositis is scaling knuckle patches known as Gottron's knuckle patches (not the same as Gottron's sign, described in Ch. 7, p. 107).

Stains. Black stains appear under gold rings during exacerbations of diabetes mellitus, in psychotic depression, and during the first few days of the menstrual period. The substance responsible for this may be the same as the one that appears on the skin of menstruating women, which hastens the death of flowers touched by their hands (Reid, 1974).

Brachydactyly

Brachydactyly may be seen as part of the trichorhinophalangeal syndrome, type I (Giedion's syndrome), which is further characterized by sparse and slowly growing hair, a long pear-shaped nose, clinodactyly (a permanent lateral or medial deviation of one or more fingers), and sometimes multiple exostoses and Perthes' disease of the hip. Type II may have mental retardation, microcephaly, and skin and joint laxity (Howell & Wynne-Davies, 1986).

Brachydactyly or a unilaterally small hand may be seen in association with Poland's syndrome (see Ch. 15, p. 240).

Arachnodactyly

This word literally means "spider fingers." In 1896, Marfan described only the skeletal aspects of what is now called Marfan's syndrome in a 5-year-old whose long thin delicate fingers were flexed by fibrous contractures so as to make them resemble the bent legs of a spider (Eldridge, 1964). Six years later, Achard suggested the term arachnodactyly. The term is now used incorrectly to refer to the thin long fingers, without the contracting

fibrous bands. The latter, as it turns out, are rather unusual, even in a syndrome known for its peculiar associations.

Oddly enough, arachnodactyly is no longer part of the criteria for diagnosis of Marfan's syndrome, which are an upper segment-to-lower-segment (crown-to-pubis/pubis-to-floor) ratio of 0.85 or less, dislocated lenses, a substantiated family history of the disorder, and aortic root disease. But in one recent series, these individual criteria were present in only 42%, 61%, 42%, and 70% to 76% (depending upon criteria for inclusion), respectively (Chan et al., 1987).

Marfan's thumb sign.

A method: Have the patient open his hand and cross his thumb across the palm as far as possible (Fig. 25-10A). Next, have him fold the fingers down across the thumb (Fig. 25-10B).

Interpretation: The test is positive if any part of the tip of the thumb can be seen sticking out beyond the ulnar surface of the fist. (Compare with yourself.) This sign, not described by Marfan, occurs in Marfan's syndrome, its various forme frustes, Ehlers-Danlos syndrome, and other conditions of joint hypermobility (Fig. 25-10C).

Sclerodactyly

○ In sclerodactyly, the distal interphalangeal folds are lost. To make this more clear, have the patient maximally flex all interphalangeal joints. (Many patients with severe scleroderma are unable to do this.) If one examines one's own distal interphalangeal skin lines, one will see that they are retained during flexion, whereas with sclerodactyly they are lost. (Dr. Margaret MacLachlan of Pennsylvania taught me this trick.)

Sclerodactyly is so frequent in the disease progressive systemic sclerosis (scleroderma) that the clinical neophyte should probably not diagnose it in the absence of the finding. Criteria for the diagnosis are given in Table 24-6.

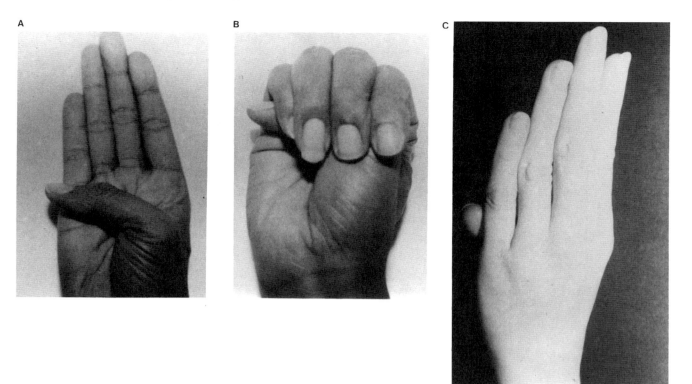

Figure 25-10. *Marfan's thumb sign. A, A patient with Marfan's syndrome showing the thumb sign with his fingers still extended; B, the same patient after making a fist; C, a rare positive test (dorsal view) in a person who does not meet the criteria for Marfan's. Photographs courtesy of Dr. Renee Ridzon of Massachusetts.*

Note that rare persons over the age of 40 will have sclerodactyly diagnosed by the test described above without having scleroderma. I have also seen it several times in patients with carcinoma of the esophagus. The reason for such an association is unknown.

Other Findings

Fingernails (including the nail beds and clubbing of the fingers) are discussed in Chapter 7 (p. 127).

Hand and finger signs of cardiology have been catalogued by Silverman and Hurst (1968).

Lower Extremities

Some lesions affecting both the upper and the lower extremities have already been discussed (e.g., see Osler's nodes p. 438, digital gangrene, p. 440, and hand-foot syndrome, p. 436).

Inspection

Lipoatrophy

Lipoatrophy can be seen and (usually) palpated as the abrupt absence of fat under the skin. Lipoatrophy may be seen on any part of the body as in systemic lupus erythematosus and insulin injection sites, but if found on the lower extremities of a febrile patient it suggests the diagnosis of Weber-Christian disease (relapsing febrile nodular panniculitis).

Lipoatrophia semicircularis, a form of pseudolipoatrophy that occurs most commonly in young women, consists of symmetric bilateral bandlike depressions on the anterolateral aspect of the midthighs. The asymptomatic lesions develop over a period of weeks, persist for a variable period, and may have spontaneous, total, or partial remissions as well as recurrences. They may result from repetitive external mechanical trauma. One young woman who had no history of trauma or familial metabolic diseases had a remission of lesions when she stopped wearing tight blue jeans (Mascaro & Ferrando, 1982). However, her sister developed similar lesions after wearing the same pair of jeans for 2 weeks (Mascaro & Ferrando, 1983).

These cases show the importance of taking a broad view of the patient's problem. They also provide an example of a disease that is familial without being either congenital or inherited, and transmissible without being infectious.

Anterior Tibial Compartment Syndrome

🖝 The anterior tibial compartment syndrome develops following vigorous exercise, trauma, or vascular occlusion. It may also be due to one of the other etiologies listed in Table 25-5. It presents as anterior lower leg pain, erythema, and tenderness. Entrapment of the deep peroneal nerve by the swollen muscles causes inability to evert the foot or dorsiflex the foot or toes (see Table 26-7). There is also sensory loss in the interdigital space between the big and second toes. This is an important syndrome to recognize because without immediate surgical decompression, there can be extensive myonecrosis of the anterior tibial compartment and permanent loss of deep peroneal nerve function (Rorabeck et al., 1972).

Changes Found in Diabetics

Necrobiosis lipoidica diabeticorum. This pretibial lesion, the color of dried blood, begins as a plaque with sharp borders.

Then it becomes shiny and atrophic and may ulcerate. It is almost pathognomonic for diabetes mellitus, but it is very rare.

Xanthoma diabeticorum. Any eruptive xanthoma (described in Ch. 7, p. 116) occurring in a diabetic can be called xanthoma diabeticorum. These are round papules, not plaques.

Diabetic shin spots. Also called "diabetic dermopathy," these are sharply circumscribed depressed atrophic shin patches that look as if the patient had bumped his shins on a coffee table (with poor healing and scarring), although most patients with the lesion recall no such events. Their prevalence is 49% in juvenile-onset diabetics, 46% in adult-onset diabetics, 20% in nondiabetic endocrine patients, and 1.5% in nondiabetic medical students (Danowski et al., 1966).

Shin spots are different from the papules of perforating collagenosis, another skin sign of diabetes mellitus (discussed in Ch. 7, p. 119, which also has a predilection for the extensor extremities.

Pretibial Myxedema

This violaceous induration of the skin, first described by Osler (Graner, 1985), is observed over the shins and sometimes over the dorsum of the feet. Despite its name, it is associated with hyp*er*thyroidism, *not* hyp*o*thyroidism. (Mnemonic: myxedema doesn't cause myxedema.)

The word *myxedema* just means "slimy edema." Thus, any liquid swelling accompanied by a noncellular proteinaceous component is myxedema, be it the generalized subcutaneous form of hypothyroidism (from which that disease takes its other name) or this peculiar localized cutaneous form of hyperthyroidism.

Erythema Nodosum*

This literally means "knotty redness" or red nodes, which can occur anywhere but are most characteristic pretibially. At one time thought to be a dermatologic equivalent of rheumatic fever, it is now recognized to be a nonspecific although highly enlightening skin sign of a wide variety of diseases whose only common denominator seems to be an allergic component in the acute stages. Thus, it is seen during acute activations or onset of tuberculosis, coccidioidomycosis, lymphoma, ulcerative colitis, leprosy (if it can be said to have an acute phase), and in a wide variety of drug reactions. It is most useful in: 1) excluding the diagnosis of rheumatoid arthritis and most seronegative spondyloarthropathies, and 2) making the diagnosis of sarcoidosis since the combination of bilateral hilar lymphadenopathy with erythema nodosum is so certain to be sarcoid that biopsy is not required (Winterbauer et al., 1973).

Ecchymoses

The crescent sign of *pseudothrombophlebitis* (Good & Pozderac, 1977; Kraag et al., 1976) is shown in Fig. 25-11. Common causes of nontender ecchymoses of the leg are trauma, venous stasis, sclerosis of superficial vessels, and coagulopathy.

---

*Why do we say, correctly, erythema nodos*um*, when we say polyarteritis nodos*a*? Although it would seem that erythema is a first declension feminine noun (so that the modifying adjectives would also end in *a*), it is actually a Greek noun (meaning redness, as in erythrocyte). Thus, it is in group IV of the third declension, whose nominative singulars end in *a* but whose gender is neuter.

Table 25-5. Etiologies of the Anterior Tibial Compartment Syndrome

"Idiopathic"
Onset some hours after exertion (e.g., marching ["march gangrene"] or horseback riding)
Posttraumatic
Fracture of the tibia (Gershuni et al., 1987)
Soft-tissue trauma
Burns (Justis et al., 1976)
Vascular compromise
Postembolic
Sickle-cell trait (Hieb & Alexander, 1988)
Use of the MAST suit (Johnson, 1981)
Other
Following embolectomy with restoration of normal arterial flow
Ergotamine ingestion (Elliott & Glass, 1976)
Systemic capillary leak syndrome (Madrenas et al., 1987)
After Caesarian section in a diabetic (Lecky, 1980).

Source: *Rorabeck et al. (1972).*

Most of the latter are painless when seen, not associated with swelling of the calf, and hence not likely to be confused with thrombophlebitis. (The ecchymoses of scurvy are discussed in Ch. 7, p. 110.)

Chronic Venous Insufficiency

A swollen brawny hyperpigmented pair of lower extremities with an ulcer near the medial (internal) malleolus permits the diagnosis of chronic venous insufficiency simply by inspection.

Pes Cavus

This term means "arched (or cavernous) foot." In fact, it appears as if the foot has been prepared by nature for the wearing of high heels, as the plane surface of the heel is several inches above the plane surface of the metatarsal heads and the toes. It may be unilateral or bilateral, depending on the etiology, and is often accompanied by "hammer" toes (so called because they are "cocked back" like a gun hammer). Pes cavus can be seen only with the shoes and socks removed.

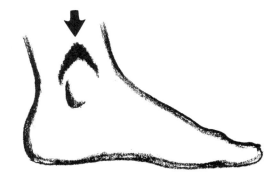

Figure 25-11. *Following the rupture of a Baker's cyst (or other cause of a calf hematoma), the blood dissects down the fascial planes and emerges as a crescent either above the malleolus (as shown) or sometimes below it. Since the Baker's cyst was often missed prior to rupture, the early signs of leg tenderness and swelling point to the erroneous diagnosis of thrombophlebitis. But the delayed emergence of the crescent sign permits the confident diagnosis of "pseudothrombophlebitis," which of course requires no anticoagulation.*

Pes cavus is sometimes called "horse foot" (pes equinus) because the toes and the metatarsal heads resemble the hoof and the heel resembles the higher portion of the horse's foot. However, this is a misnomer because patients with pes cavus do bear weight on their heels, albeit the more posterior portions.

The etiology is usually neurologic (e.g., Friedrich's ataxia, Charcot-Marie-Tooth peroneal atrophy, old poliomyelitis, spastic hemiplegia or diplegia) or muscular (e.g., muscular dystrophy). I have also seen it in Sipple's syndrome and neurofibromatosis.

Toe Amputations

Amputation of the toes may occur on the little toe (as in the disease ainhum, which only affects those of African descent). Or it may affect any of the other toes due to accidental strangulation by a hair or a thread from a piece of clothing. The latter is more likely to occur in an infant and may also involve the finger. The archetypal case was reported by Morganstern in 1898 when a human hair wrapped around a penis causing strangulation of the latter and urinary retention (Manfredi, 1981).

Palpation

Toe Temperature

The temperature of the toes is a highly reliable and highly reproducible estimate that correlates with cardiac output and prognosis in shock (Fagan, 1988; Joly & Weil, 1969).

Acromegaly

The feet enlarge in acromegaly, and the heel pad thickens. Although originally a radiographic finding, the latter can be adapted to the physical examination.

A method.   Put your fingers on your heel. Indent the heel pad 2 cm. Can you feel the calcaneus? If so, you are most likely normal.

In point of fact, there have been some acromegalics of recent onset or arrested disease in whom the heel pad is within normal bounds (Kho et al., 1970; Steinbach & Russell, 1964). There are also many normals whose heel pads exceeded the initial cutoff values of 21 mm (Puckette & Seymour, 1967; Steinbach & Russell, 1964), even though 21 mm supposedly was 80% sensitive for the diagnosis, with no false positives. However, we now know that the heel pad normally increases as a function of maleness, age, body weight, and black race.

The sensitivity and specificity of various criteria are given in Table 25-6.

Since most of the patients examined for acromegaly will not have the disease (due to the prevalence factor again), one really

wants to minimize the false positives. Accordingly, figures of 23 mm for women and 25 mm for men could be used, or the graph showing correction for weight (Kho et al., 1970) could be consulted. Since the examiner must make this metric estimation from indentation, the reader is cautioned not to go beyond the bounds of the method.

Edema

The Starling Equation*:

$$J_v = k \left[(P_i - P_o) - \sigma (\pi_i - \pi_o) \right]$$

Dependent edema is usually demonstrated pretibially. However, there are some cases of very slight dependent edema that appear first in the more dependent foot, and bed-bound supine patients accumulate their extra interstitial fluid at the sacrum. Wherever the edema, its extent has been traditionally graded from 1+ to 4+. This may now be abandoned since loop diuretics will quickly convert the latter to the former, and one is more interested in the simpler question whether the edema is present or absent. If present, one wants to know how far up the body it goes, since 1+ pitting edema reaching the chest wall may be more significant than 3+ pretibial edema.

The pit recovery time (i.e., not how deep is the pit one's finger can make, but how long it takes for the pit to refill) is a very valuable diagnostic sign.

○ *A method for pit recovery time.*   Although the original method used a constant pressure device, I have attempted to modify the test so that it can be done with the fingers. The neophyte is advised to start with a few patients of known serum albumin and try to find the amount of pressure that reproduces the results (Fig. 25-12) described by the original authors (Henry & Altmann, 1978).

1. Press down firmly all the way to the bone. Start the stopwatch.
2. Shine a light at a tangent across the pit and do not call the pit recovery time until there is no shadow remaining anywhere in the area of the pit.

The test is very crude. After 10 years, one still makes mistakes in the 35- to 40-second range. Notice the scatter around the regression line given in the original paper (Fig. 25-12).

---

*J_v is the rate of fluid formation, k is the filtration coefficient (which is related to permeability), P is hydrostatic pressure, and π is oncotic pressure. σ is the permeability coefficient whose change is probably most important for postanoxic states (vide infra). The subscript o refers to pressures outside the vessel (membrane), and the subscript i to the pressure inside.

Table 25-6.   Sensitivity and Specificity of Heel Pad Thickness for Diagnosis of Acromegaly

Reference	Population	Cutoff	Sens	Spec
Steinbach & Russell, 1964	Combined	21 mm	79%	100%
Fields et al., 1967	White male	24 mm	75%	98%
	Black male	27 mm		
Kho et al., 1970[a]	Female	21.5 mm	95%	88%
	Male	23 mm		
Langfeldt, 1968	European	23 mm	94%	100%
Gonticas et al., 1969	Acromegaly & eruthyroid controls	17.83 + .0863 BW	100%	98%
	Myxedematous patients		100%	81%

Sens = sensitivity; Spec = specificity; BW = body weight in kg.

[a]All controls were white.

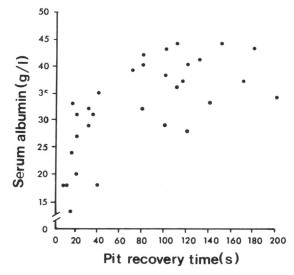

Figure 25-12. *Relation between serum albumin concentration and pit recovery time in 31 patients (from Henry & Altmann, 1978, reprinted with permission of the* British Medical Journal*).*

Interpretation. In *acute* edema (i.e., of less than 3 months' duration), there is a direct relation between the serum albumin concentration and the pit recovery time (Henry & Altmann, 1978). Thus, in hypoalbuminemic edema, the pit recovery time is very short (i.e., 40 seconds or less). (See Fig. 25-13 for an example of a short pit recovery time.)

In the edema due to congestive failure, or other causes of increased venous pressure in the lower extremities, the pit recovery time will regularly be over 40 seconds, provided there is not also hypoalbuminemia (see p. 446 for a more complete differential diagnosis).

In capillary edema (as opposed to lymphedema, vide infra), the pit recovery time is greater than 40 seconds if the serum (and tissue) albumin are normal. (Capillary edema is due to increased permeability of the capillaries, as in vasculitis, idiopathic edema of women, and post total-body anoxia.)

I have seen at least one patient with an unrelated *low* serum albumin and post anoxic edema in whom the pit recovery time was still greatly prolonged. Perhaps in post anoxic edema the reflectance coefficient of the Starling equation is changed and the pressures and protein concentration become less important.

It is stated that some cases of glomerulonephritis have a high protein content and a long pit recovery time; these are obviously nonhypoalbuminemic nonnephrotic cases (Henry & Altmann, 1978).

During hot weather, aldosterone concentration increases in normal persons, and the serum albumin stays normal, but pedal edema (especially observable at the top of elastic socks) may be seen at evening, especially if the individual is in an occupation requiring him to stand all day. This normal edema also has a long pit recovery time, presumably because the edema has a normal (high) protein concentration.

I have additionally observed a peculiar inexplicable two-component pit recovery time in which the edema begins to recover very quickly and then turns out to have a delayed pit recovery time. This is seen in the *combination* of increased venous pressure and hypoalbuminemia, most commonly in cirrhotic patients with severe ascites compressing the inferior vena cava and concomitant hypoalbuminemia due to impaired hepatic synthesis.

I had one patient with congestive heart failure and nephrotic

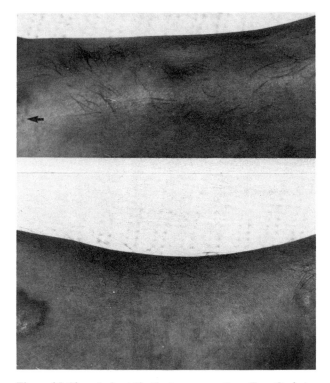

Figure 25-13. *A short (fast) pit recovery time. Top, On being told of a patient with pitting edema and a normal albumin, I went to take a picture of his pit recovery time, which I expected to be prolonged (see text). In the top view, you can see two pits made with my thumb, one in the center and one made just before it, to the right. (Ignore the arrow for now.) Bottom, After taking the top picture, I quickly advanced the film in the camera, reset the flash, and brought it back to my eye for focusing. But already the pit had disappeared! (In fact, the lower picture shows a completely different distribution of hairs and a different focal plane, as I had to hunt for the pit that had so quickly disappeared. However, it is the same region of the same foot. The lesion to the left was cropped out of the upper photograph; the edge is marked by an arrow.) Do not attempt the following questions until you have finished reading the chapter:*

1. *This is surely a quick pit recovery time, but what could have caused it? If it is true that the pit recovery time is proportional to the interstitial protein concentration (and it is), then how could a patient with a normal serum albumin have a fluid with such a short pit recovery time?*

2. *And what will the pit recovery time be in 4 months? (Write your answer down before consulting Appendix 25-6.)*

syndrome due to Kimmelstiel-Wilson disease, in whom there was a two-component pit recovery,. However, a measured serum albumin was normal! It later developed that he had experienced a precipitous fall in his glomerular filtration rate just prior to admission, which was associated with a precipitous fall in his (measured) proteinuria. This apparently permitted his liver to "catch up" and his comparatively low serum albumin to rise to a normal level at the time I saw him. This case confirms the original authors' contention that the quick pit recovery time (component) is a reflection of the albumin level in the interstitium, not just in the serum.

Finally, it must be reemphasized that in all the above cases we are talking about acute (less than 3 months' duration) edema. If the edema is chronic, the scarring and fibrosis in the interstitium will make *all* types of edema have a prolonged pit recovery time because the fibrous and collagen strands will demarcate the pit and produce a slow pit recovery even in the presence of pure hypoalbuminemia (Henry & Altmann, 1978).

Differential diagnosis of pitting edema. Pitting edema is a leading sign and symptom whose pathophysiology has been understood for half a century. Furthermore, there is a discrete number of items in the differential diagnosis (Table 25-7). Each of these items has specific and characteristic physical findings apart from the edema itself. The first branch point (hypoalbuminemia versus increased venous pressure) can even be achieved without a laboratory by utilization of the pit recovery time.

Very advanced. It has been forgotten that an increase in venous pressure, comparable to that seen in congestive heart failure, reduces the flow of lymph in the thoracic duct, and that this decrease in lymphatic clearance is part and parcel of fluid accumulation in the interstitial spaces (Wegria et al., 1963). Thus, the edema found in the leg in congestive heart failure, which we call pedal edema, might be called, correctly, "lymph" or "lymphedema" by some. Accordingly, in this text note that we call it simply edema.

Table 25-7. Differential Diagnosis of Pitting Edema

I. Hypoalbuminemia
  A. Impaired synthesis
    1. Decreased intake of the amino acid precursors as in starvation or protein-calorie malnutrition (kwashiorkor)
    2. Decreased absorption of amino acid precursors as in malabsorption syndrome
    3. Impaired synthesis due to hepatic insufficiency
  B. Increased loss
    1. Skin loss—from burns, pemphigus, or other such "weeping" skin diseases including some drug reactions
    2. Urinary loss—nephrotic syndrome
    3. Fecal loss—for example, everything from Menetrier's disease to inflammatory bowel disease with azorrhea. (In some inflammatory bowel diseases both malabsorption and azorrhea occur at the same time.)
II. Increased venous pressure—This may be visualized by working backward from the heart down to the foot veins, as follows:
  A. Systemic venous hypertension
    1. Congestive heart failure
    2. Restrictive cardiac disease
    3. Tricuspid valve disease
    4. Constrictive pericarditis
    5. Pericardial tamponade
  B. Regional venous disease
    1. Inferior vena caval syndrome
    2. Venous thrombosis
    3. Lower extremity venous insufficiency
    4. Using round circumferential elastic thigh garters to hold up stockings (This disease has been made obsolete by the pantyhose industry, but formerly one saw a case a year. Since fashions tend to cycle it is included for prospective completeness.)
III. Capillary edema due to increased permeability (rare and diagnostically obvious)
  A. Vasculitis (rare)
  B. Post anoxic syndrome (a futile, but not diagnostically difficult situation)
  C. Idiopathic edema of women (this also affects the hands and is cyclic)

Lymphedema is a term we reserve for the interstitial fluid that accumulates in cases of pure lymphatic disease (vide infra).

Lymphedema

Lymphedema may be classified by age of onset or by etiology (Stone & Hugo, 1972).

Lymphedema at birth. Lymphedema at birth may be due to prematurity, from amniotic bands, from congenital lymphangiectasia (Goodman, 1962), or from Milroy's form of congenital familial lymphedema (Milroy, 1928).

Lymphedema in childhood. Lymphedema appearing after birth but before age 10 could be due to a familial form such as Meige's; to Turner's, Bonnevie-Ulrich (Goodman, 1962), or Noonan's syndrome (Mendez & Opitz, 1985), or even from a congenital defect (Goldrick & Ahrens 1964).

Lymphedema after age 10. Between the ages of 10 and 29, most cases are primary (Meige's), never malignant, and rarely infectious (Smith et al., 1963).

From 30 to 49 years of age, the idiopathic primary cases continue to appear and should probably carry the name "Kinmonth" (Schirger et al., 1962). These occur with a 10:1 female preponderance. In this same epoch, malignancy appears as an etiology and infectious causes become more prevalent, although both of these together make up only half the cases, the idiopathic still forming the other half (Smith et al., 1963).

Of new cases appearing after age 50, malignancy persists, the infectious causes begin to wane, and the idiopathic cases have disappeared.

More about etiologies:

For the resident: The infectious causes can be secondary to lymphedema (Schirger et al., 1962), the lymphedema secondary to the recurrent infection (Young & DeWolfe, 1960), or the lymphedema simply transient due to the lymph node enlargement and obstruction of the infectious disease, as in cat-scratch fever (Filler et al., 1964). Tumorigenic lymphedema is usually seen in men and is most likely to be due to prostatic carcinoma, which infiltrates the lymphatics. When it occurs in women, it is usually due to lymphoma, except for the peculiar situation of the Stewart-Treves syndrome: upper extremity lymphedema associated with (fatal) aggressive lymphangiosarcoma in asymptomatic female subjects who have previously had an ipsilateral mastectomy for breast carcinoma (Goodman, 1962).

As a rule, infectious causes have a 2:1 ratio in favor of women, and for the malignant causes, the sex preference is the exact reverse.

Bilaterality of lymphedema is seen in many of the congenital cases, in many of the infectious cases including sarcoidosis (Silver et al., 1966), but not in cases due to neoplasia (Smith et al., 1963).

Lymphedema may be part of the yellow-nail syndrome (see Ch. 7, p. 133).

The history of the description of familial lymphedema is given in Appendix 25-5.

Pit recovery time. Initially, the pit recovery time should be quite short since the edema fluid has a low protein content (Goodman, 1962) and the venous pressure and circulation time would be normal. However, with the passage of time, the tissues become brawny and fibrotic, and as with hemic edema, the pit recovery time becomes prolonged strictly due to the chronicity of the process. Thus, in Milroy's (adult) index case, "Deep pressure with the finger over the crest of the tibia, at a point near its middle, produced a depression which was distinctly apparent to both touch and sight ten minutes after the pressure was removed" (Milroy, 1892).

Consider the question posed in the legend to Figure 25-13.

Appendix 25-1. Answer to Self-Study Question on Nodules in Rheumatoid Arthritis and Rheumatic Fever (see p. 435).

A diagnostic ratio may be computed as follows: 28% of the 95 rheumatoid arthritis patients (26.6) would have nodules. Of these, 5% or 1.33 would appear on the occiput. Of the rheumatic fever patients, 9% would have nodules (0.45), and 20% of these would be on the occiput (0.09). Thus the ratio of rheumatoid to rheumatic fever patients with this finding would be 14.8:1.

This question reemphasizes the importance of prevalence. Although occipital nodules are rare among patients with rheumatoid nodules, and are four times more common among all rheumatic fever patients with nodules, the relative prevalence of the disease would actually make an occipital nodule favor the diagnosis of rheumatoid arthritis in that physician's practice, all other things being equal.

Appendix 25-2. Answer to Question in Figure 25-2 (Porphyria Cutanea Tarda Versus Rheumatoid Vasculitis)

A.   Porphyria cutanea tarda causes hypermelanotic pigmentation and atrophic scars, especially on the exposed surfaces of the hands and face. Photograph courtesy of Dr. Renee Ridzon of Massachusetts.

B.   Rheumatoid vasculitis may also cause pinhead-sized hemorrhagic spots and necrotic areas. Photograph courtesy of *Consultant* (Cliggott Publishing Company) and Thomas E. Weiss, MD, Alton Ochsner Medical Foundation.

Appendix 25-3. Answer to Question in Figure 25-8

First, a posttraumatic ecchymosis would never cause loss of tissue, such as digital pulp, muscle, and subcutaneous tissue. This thumb has obviously undergone considerable loss of volume distally. Second, the lesion is chronic, as evidenced by the scale; however, it is still dark. A posttraumatic ecchymosis might be dark acutely, but would have faded by the time it became chronic.

Appendix 25-4. Answer to Question in Figure 25-9

After celebrating the kalends of February at a symposium, this gentleman walked home in a snowstorm. Losing his house keys in a snowbank, he searched for them with ungloved hands. The unsuccessful search leaving him weary, he decided there and then to retire for the night, and awakened with this classic case of frostbite, not distinguishable from the other causes of digital gangrene without the history.

Appendix 25-5. Historical Note on Familial Lymphedema

Familial lymphedema was first described by Letesier in 1865 (Goodman, 1962).

Milroy's disease was first described by Nonne in 1890. The next year Milroy saw his cases in Omaha, a city that was then new. He noted that the "consequent dearth of medical libraries in Omaha is a serious obstacle in the way of the study of pathological and other questions here." Milroy wrote to Delafield in New York and Welch in Baltimore. The latter showed the case report to Osler, who agreed that it was not angioneurotic edema, the subject of a paper by Osler that he sent to Milroy. The latter was appreciative of the reprint about a disease they both knew Milroy's patients not to have, since that disease too "is not so much mentioned in any textbook or encyclopedia that I have been able to find in Omaha" (Milroy, 1892). Finally, Osler, still oblivious to Nonne's priority, named the disease after Milroy (Milroy, 1928).

Appendix 25-6. A Note on the Pit Recovery Time: Answer to Question in Legend to Figure 25-13

If the pit recovery time is as short as indicated in Figure 25-13, then the fluid *must* be hypoproteinemic. If the serum albumin is normal, the edema fluid cannot be coming from the blood vascular compartment. (Vasculitis and venous hypertension both produce edema fluids of high protein content [Henry & Altmann, 1978].) The only remaining conclusion is that the edema is actually *lymph*edema (see p. 446).

The answer to the second question in the legend is that the pit recovery time would eventually become prolonged, assuming that the lymphedema had not resolved.

This particular patient had lymphedema secondary to Kaposi's sarcoma, a spot of which can be seen on the left.

References

Alpert JS, Krous HF, Dalen JE, O'Rourke RA, Bloor CM: Pathogenesis of Osler's nodes. *Ann Intern Med* 85:471–473, 1976.

Attali P, Ink O, Pelletier G, Vernier C, Jean F, Moulton L, Etienne J-P: Dupuytren's contracture, alcohol consumption, and chronic liver disease. *Arch Intern Med* 147:1065–1067, 1987.

Benedek TG: Subcutaneous nodules and the differentiation of rheumatoid arthritis from rheumatic fever. *Semin Arthritis Rheum* 13:305–321, 1984.

Braunstein GD: Diagnosis. In: Melmed S (moderator), Pituitary tumors secreting growth hormone and prolactin. *Ann Intern Med* 108:238–253, 1986.

Chan K-L, Callahan JA, Seward JB, Tajik AJ, Gordo H: Marfan syndrome diagnosed in patients 32 years of age or older. *Mayo Clin Proc* 62:589–594, 1987.

Critchley EMR, Vakil SD, Hayward HW, Owen VMH: Dupuytren's disease in epilepsy: Result of prolonged administration of anticonvulsants. *J Neurol Neurosurg Psychiatry* 39:498–503, 1976.

Cross DF, Ellis JG: Occurrence of the Janeway lesion in mycotic aneurysm. *Arch Intern Med* 118:588–591, 1966.

Cuzick J, Harris R, Mortimer PS: Palmar keratoses and cancers of the bladder and lung. *Lancet* 1:530–533, 1984.

Dalinka MK, McGee JW: The variable manifestations of sclerosing fibrosis. *J Assoc Can Radiol* 21:280–286, 1970.

Danowski TS, Sabeh G, Sarver ME, Shelkrot J, Fisher ER: Shin spots and diabetes mellitus. *Am J Med Sci* 251:570–575, 1966.

Early PF: Population studies in Dupuytren's contracture. *J Bone Joint Surg [Br]* 44B:602–613, 1962.

Eldridge R: The metacarpal index: A useful aid in the diagnosis of the Marfan syndrome. *Arch Intern Med* 113:248–254, 1964.

Elliott MJ, Glass KD: Anterior tibial compartment syndrome associated with ergotamine ingestion. *Clin Orthop* 118:44–46, 1976.

Fagan MJ: Relationship between nurses' assessments of perfusion and toe temperature in pediatric patients with cardiovascular disease. *Heart Lung* 17:157–165, 1988.

Fanning WL, Aronson M: Osler node, Janeway lesions, and splinter hemorrhages. *Arch Dermatol* 113:648–649, 1977.

Farrior JB, and Silverman ME: A consideration of the differences between a Janeway's lesion and an Osler's node in infectious endocarditis. *Chest* 70:239–243, 1976.

Fields ML, Greenberg BH, Burkett LL: Roentgenographic measurement of skin and heel-pad thickness in the diagnosis of acromegaly. *Am J Med Sci* 254:528–533, 1967.

Filler RM, Schwachman H, Edwards EA: Lymphedema after cat-scratch fever. *N Engl J Med* 270:244–245, 1964.

Gershuni DH, Mubarak SJ, Yaru NC, Lee YF: Fracture of the tibia complicated by acute compartment syndrome. *Clin Orthop* 217:221–227, 1987.

Goldrick RB, Ahrens EJ Jr: Unilateral chylous lymphedema and xanthomatosis. *Am J Med* 37:610–622, 1964.

Gonticas SK, Ikkos DG, Stergiou LH: Evaluation of the diagnostic value of heel-pad thickness in acromegaly. *Radiology* 92:304–307, 1969.

Good AE, Pozderac RV: Ecchymosis of the lower leg: A sign of hemarthrosis with synovial rupture. *Arthritis Rheum* 20:1009–1013, 1977.

Goodman RM: Familial lymphedema of the Meige's type. *Am J Med* 32:651–656, 1962.

Graner JL: "Osler's sign": Pretibial myxedema of Graves' disease. *Can Med Assoc J* 132·745–746, 1985.

Henry JA, Altmann P: Assessment of hypoproteinaemic oedema: A simple physical sign. *Br Med J* i:890–891, 1978.

Hieb LD, Alexander AH: Bilateral anterior and lateral compartment syndromes in a patient with sickle cell trait: Case report and review of the literature. *Clin Orthop* 228:190–193, 1988.

Howell CJ, Wynne-Davies R: The tricho-rhino-phalangeal syndrome: a report of 14 cases in 7 kindreds. *J Bone Joint Surg [Br]* 68:311–314, 1986.

Hueston JT: The incidence of Dupuytren's contracture. *Med J Aust* 47:999–1001, 1960.

Johnson BE: Anterior compartment syndrome following use of MAST suit. *Ann Emerg Med* 10:209–210, 1981.

Joly HR, Weil MH: Temperature of the great toe as an indicator of the severity of shock. *Circulation* 39:131–138, 1969.

Justis DL, Law EJ, MacMillan BG: Tibial compartment syndromes in burn patients: a report of four cases. *Arch Surg* 111:1004–1008, 1976.

Kaye BR, Kaye RL, Bobrove A: Rheumatoid nodules: Review of the spectrum of associated conditions and proposal of a new classification, with a report of four seronegative cases. *Am J Med* 76:279–292, 1984.

Kehl KC: Dupuytren's contracture as a sequel to coronary artery disease and myocardial infarction. *Ann Intern Med* 19:212–223, 1943.

Kerr AJ Jr: *Subacute Bacterial Endocarditis.* Charles C Thomas, Springfield, IL, 1955.

Kerr A Jr, Tan JS: Biopsies of the Janeway lesion of infective endocarditis. *J Cutan Pathol* 6:124–129, 1979.

Kho KM, Wright AD, Doyle FH: Heel pad thickness in acromegaly. *Br J Radiol* 43:112–125, 1970.

Kraag G, Thevathasan EM, Gordon DA, Walker IH: The hemorrhagic crescent sign of acute synovial rupture. *Ann Intern Med* 85:477–478, 1976.

Langfeldt B: Heel-pad measurement as an aid to diagnosis of acromegaly. *Dan Med Bull* 15:40–43, 1968.

Larkin JG, Frier BM: Limited joint mobility and Dupuytren's contracture in diabetic, hypertensive, and normal populations. *Br Med J* 292:1494, 1986.

Lecky B: Acute bilateral anterior tibial compartment syndrome after Caesarian section in a diabetic. *J Neurol Neurosurg Psychiatry* 43:88–90, 1980.

Levin J, Kupperman HS: Skeletal abnormalities in gonadal dysgenesis. *Arch Intern Med* 113:730–736, 1964.

Lin CS, Lee RL, Kuo CM, Lee LC: Positive culture of the Janeway lesion in acute bacterial endocarditis. *Taiwan I Hsueh Hui Tsa Chi* 79:99–102, 1980.

Lund M: Dupuytren's contracture and epilepsy. *Acta Psychiatr Neurol* 16:465–492, 1947.

Madrenas J, Garcia-Bragado F, Fernandez JM: Anterior tibial compartment syndrome secondary to systemic capillary leak syndrome. *J Neurol Neurosurg Psychiatry* 50:943–944, 1987.

Manfredi SJ: Accidental appendage strangulation. *Plast Reconstr Surg* 67:60–61, 1981.

Mascaro JM, Ferrando J: Lipoatrophia semicircularis: The perils of wearing jeans? *Int J Dermatol* 21:138–139, 1982.

Mascaro JM, Ferrando J: The perils of wearing jeans: lipoatrophia semicircularis. *Int J Dermatol* 22:333, 1983.

McDonald CJ, Kelly AP: Diseases of black skin. In: Demis A (ed), *Clinical Dermatology*, ed 4. Harper & Row, New York, 1987.

Mendez HMM, Opitz JM: Noonan syndrome: A review. *Am J Med Genet* 21:493–506, 1985.

Michaelson ED, Walsh RE: Osler's node—a complication of prolonged arterial cannulation. *N Engl J Med* 27:472–743, 1970.

Milroy WF: An undescribed variety of hereditary edema. *NY Med J* 56:505–508, 1892.

Milroy WF: Chronic hereditary edema: Milroy's disease. *JAMA* 182:14–22, 1928.

Nardoni A, Baldissera A, Iacono M, Copetti R, Cella R: Malattia di Dupuytren: Prospettive etiopatogenetiche attuali. *Minerva Med* 72:859–864, 1981.

Nonne*: Elephantiasis congenita. *Dtsch Med Wochenschr* 16:1124, 1890.

Pojer J, Jedličková J: Enzymatic pattern of liver injury in Dupuytren's contracture. *Acta Med Scand* 187:101–104, 1970.

Pojer J, Radivojevic M, Williams TF: Dupuytren's disease: Its association with abnormal liver functions in alcoholism and epilepsy. *Arch Intern Med* 129:561–566, 1972.

Puckette SE Jr, Seymour EQ: Fallibility of heel-pad thickness. *Radiology* 88:982–983, 1967.

Puklin JE, Ballis GA, Bentley DW: Culture of an Osler's node: A diagnostic tool. *Arch Intern Med* 127:296–298, 1971.

Reid HR: The brass-ring sign. *Lancet* 1:988, 1974.

Rorabeck CR, MacNab I, Waddell JP: Anterior tibial compartment syndrome: A clinical and experimental review. *Can J Surg* 15:249–259, 1972.

Schirger A, Harrison EG Jr, Janes JM: Idiopathic lymphedema: Review of 131 cases. *JAMA* 182:124–132, 1962.

Silver HM, Tsangaris NT, Eaton OM: Lymphedema and lymphography in sarcoidosis. *Arch Intern Med* 117:712–714, 1966.

Silverman ME, Hurst JW: The hand and the heart. *Am J Cardiol* 22:718–728, 1968.

Slater S: An evaluation of the metacarpal sign (short fourth metacarpal). *Pediatrics* 46:468–471, 1970.

Smith RD, Spittell JA Jr, Schirger A: Secondary lymphedema of the leg: Its characteristics and diagnostic implications. *JAMA* 185:80–82, 1963.

Steinbach HL, Russell W: Measurement of the heel-pad as an aid to diagnosis of acromegaly. *Radiology* 82:418–423, 1964.

Stone EJ, Hugo NE: Lymphedema. *Surg Gynecol Obstet* 135:625–630, 1972.

Su C-K, Patek AJ Jr, Dupuytren's contracture: Its association with alcoholism and cirrhosis. *Arch Intern Med* 126:278–281, 1970.

Thapar MK, Rao S, Feldman D, Linde LM: Infective endocarditis: A review I. Incidence, etiology, pathology and clinical features. *Paediatrician* 7:65–84, 1978.

von Gemmingen GR, Winkelman RK: Osler's node of subacute bacterial endocarditis: Focal necrotizing vasculitis of the glomus body. *Arch Dermatol* 95:91–94, 1967.

---

*His initials are unknown. Sometimes Nonne is listed as "MH," but those initials actually refer to the greeting "Meine Herren" (gentlemen) at the start of his presentation.

Watson RJ, Burko H, Megas H, Robinson M: The hand-foot syndrome in sickle-cell disease in children. *Am J Dis Child* 102:215, 1963.

Wegria R, Zekert H, Walter KE, Entrup RW, De Schryver C, Kennedy W, Paiewonsky D: Effect of systemic venous pressure on drainage of lymph from thoracic duct. *Am J Physiol* 204:384–288, 1963.

Weiss TE: Painful hands: Differential diagnosis by physical examination only. *Consultant* 24(12):51–65, 1984.

Wertelecki W: The simian and Sydney crease. In: Wertelecki W, Plato CC, Paul NW (eds), *Dermatoglyphs—Fifty Years Later*. Alan R. Liss, New York, 1979.

Winterbauer RH, Belic N, Moores KD: A clinical interpretation of bilateral hilar adenopathy. *Ann Intern Med* 78:65–71, 1973.

Wolfe SJ, Summerskill WHJ, Davidson CS: Thickening and contraction of the palmar fascia (Dupuytren's contracture) associated with alcoholism and hepatic cirrhosis. *N Engl J Med* 255:559–563, 1956.

Wynn DR, Martin MJ: A physical sign of bulimia. *Mayo Clin Proc* 59:722, 1984.

Yee J, McAllister CK: Osler's nodes and the recognition of infective endocarditis: A lesion of diagnostic importance. *South Med J* 80: 753–757, 1987.

Young JR, DeWolfe VG: Recurrent lymphangitis of the leg associated with dermatophytosis: Report of 25 consecutive cases. *Cleve Clin Q* 27:19–24, 1960.

26
The Neurologic Examination

"The chief features of interest in the case, to which the attention of the Society is directed, are, that during life the existence of a tumour was diagnosed in the brain, and its situation localized, entirely by the signs and symptoms exhibited without any external manifestations on the surface of the skull."

Medico-Chirurgical Transactions,
published by the Royal Medical and Chirurgical Society of London,
vol. 68, J.E. Adlard, London, 1885

Cranial Nerves

A Caveat for the Sophomore

By now you have probably noted some discrepancies between the sequence of examination taught in your school and the one offered here. In a little while, you will realize that there are some potential conflicts even between the latter and the outline presented in Chapter 4 (e.g., many of the cranial nerves were already examined earlier *en passant*). Even within this chapter there are inevitably arbitrary divisions. For instance, the vestibular and cerebellar systems really should go together. The cerebellum and the dorsal columns might be considered together. But in fact, signs of disease in these three systems are actually in three different sections of the work. Similarly, some of the tests of gaze are not considered with the skilled movements but rather with the cranial nerves whose testing might first reveal such gaze abnormalities. The principle of medicine is clear in all these situations: if you have already learned one order of examination, stick with it. Consistency is more important than the specific virtues of any necessarily arbitrary linear system of organization.

Cranial Nerve I

The testing of the first cranial nerve is discussed under the regional examination of the nose, in Chapter 12 (p. 218). Although performed regionally, the results are recorded under the neurologic examination in the case record.

Cranial Nerve II

The testing of vision is presented in detail in Chapter 10 (pp. 155–157).

Cranial Nerves III, IV, and VI

Pupil (Cranial Nerve III)

Horner's syndrome, or the sympathetic-ocular syndrome, consists of anisocoria (with the homolateral pupil smaller), en-ophthalmos, ptosis, and anhidrosis with decreased pilomotor response. It is frequently seen in the Pancoast syndrome (see Ch. 10, p. 170).

The anisocoria of Horner's syndrome results from a failure of dilatation (which normally acts as an opposing force to miosis). This can be demonstrated by looking through the ophthalmoscope at the iris. First shine the light into the pupil, and then move it away from the pupil to the iris. In the normal eye, you can observe the iris to relax when the light is not shining into the pupil; this does not occur in the affected eye (S. Horenstein, personal communication, 1988).

Anisocoria is also discussed in detail in Chapter 10 (p. 170).

Extraocular Muscles (Cranial Nerves III, IV, and VI)

A difficult self-test. The extraocular muscles are discussed in Chapter 10 (p. 158), but it is time for a review. The next few cases are difficult but very revealing. Go slowly through the questions that follow. Make good clinical observations, and reason carefully from your data.

The answers to the questions will be found at the end of the section (p. 452) so that you will not inadvertently glance at them.

1. Look at Gregory (Fig. 26-1). His eyes are in the primary position. (We refer to the eyes as being in the primary position when the patient is following instructions to look directly at the examiner.) What's wrong with Gregory? Write down your full answer.

2. Moses (Fig. 26-2A) is apparently being seen in the dermatology clinic for a keratotic problem. For the time being, ignore that. a) If the photograph was taken with Moses looking at you in the primary position, what is the most likely diagnosis? b) Before turning to page 453 for the answer, what diagnosis would you make if the picture was taken while Moses was watching your finger move from the midline to his left (your right)?

3. What's wrong with the virgin in Fig. 26-3A? She is not exactly in the primary position, but rather is gazing down toward your right hand. However, if you ask her to look at you, she will

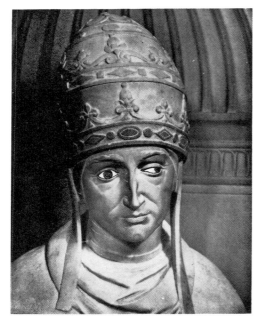

Figure 26-1. Self-test (see text). Saint Gregory, by Michel-angelo, from the Piccolomini altar.

do so, but without moving her head. (If you have gotten the correct answer by now, you have either studied Ch. 10, pp. 158–160, or you should be writing books like this instead of reading them.)

4. Look at the eyes in Fig. 26-4. a) If this is the primary position, what are the *two* most likely diagnoses? b) If you were checking the extraocular motions, and the patient was supposed to be looking to his right (to your left), what would be the two most likely diagnoses?

Answers:

1. If you said oxycephaly, you are 100% wrong; that's just his hat. Go back and look at the eyes.

Gregory has a left third cranial nerve oculomotor palsy. Any other answer is wrong. This cannot be a coincidental palsy of the individual muscles innervated by cranial nerve III on the left side. Why not? (The answer to that question explains why all other explanations are incorrect). Go back and look at the picture again.

Did you notice the ptosis on the left but not the right? This clearly implicates cranial nerve III. If Gregory were suffering only from disease of the individual oculomotor muscles (as unlikely as William of Occam* would consider that), there would be no ptosis.

The left eye looks laterally because the lateral rectus, which is innervated by cranial nerve VI, is unopposed by the medial rectus, which is innervated by cranial nerve III.

The superior oblique muscle, which is innervated by the trochlear nerve, is unaffected. Although it is used for turning the eye down and in, it is not much use without the superior rectus,

---

*William of Occam was a philosopher whose "razor" was a logical device used to cut through intellectual problems that have multiple solutions. Basically, it said that the most likely solution is the simplest. Or, a single explanation that explains all findings is more likely to be true than multiple explanations for the same things. In medicine, this means that the least complex diagnosis is most likely to be correct. Stated another way, it tells us never to make two diagnoses, when one would explain all the findings.

Now that our technology has developed to the point that we are able to keep patients alive with their diseases (and the attendant signs and symptoms) for prolonged periods, the rule must be modified. It should state that signs and symptoms not yet explained by previous known diagnoses are best explained by a single additional diagnosis, as opposed to two or more additional diagnoses. Most good clinicians understand this intuitively.

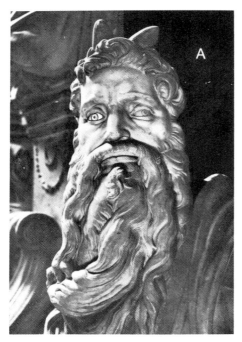

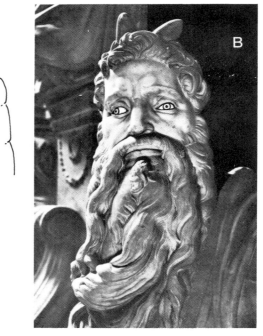

Figure 26-2. Self-test (see text). Monument of Pope Julius II. Moses, by Michelangelo.

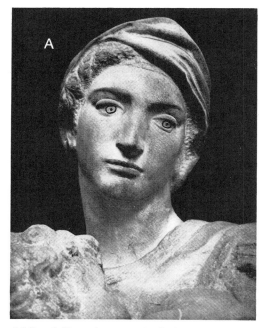 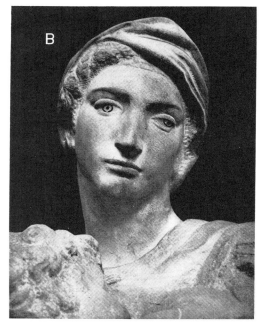

Figure 26-3. *Self-test (see text). Bielschowsky's sign. The Medici Virgin, by Michelangelo.*

inferior rectus, and inferior oblique muscles, all of which are lost here, being innervated by cranial nerve III.

2. a) In the primary position, Moses has a left medial rectus muscle paralysis. It is probably not an oculomotor nerve paralysis since there is no ptosis. Again, the unopposed lateral rectus can pull the eyeball laterally when it is not opposed by the medial rectus. (If you got that wrong, go back and do both questions over before reading on, because you probably got the second one wrong also.)

b) If Moses was following your finger to his left, the single lesion most likely to explain the finding is a right medial rectus palsy, since he is unable to pull the right eyeball around so that it will point toward your finger, although the left has moved normally.

This case illustrates why one must always describe the examination carefully: the same appearance can indicate disease in

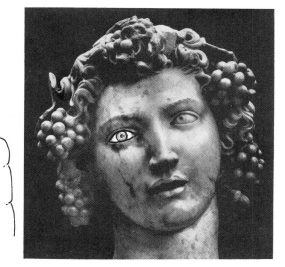

Figure 26-4. *Self-test (see text). Bacchus, by Michelangelo.*

three different places, depending upon what instructions the patient is following when the appearance is observed.

Yes, *three* different places. There is one other lesion that could produce this appearance while gazing to the left (your right). But you could only detect it by testing the cardinal directions of gaze. What if you saw the appearance in Figure 26-2B when Moses gazed to his right (your left)?

It now appears that each lateral rectus can work. A patient with these findings would look normal when asked to look directly at the examiner, because each medial rectus also works. This, then, is a disturbance of conjugate gaze called *bilateral internuclear ophthalmoplegia*. (This is to be distinguished from *internal* ophthalmoplegia, which refers to paralysis of the pupil, and is usually used in distinction to *external* ophthalmoplegia or impaired mobility of the eye.) *Unilateral* internuclear ophthalmoplegia occurs with gaze palsy only to one side.

Internuclear ophthalmoplegia is important to know about for two reasons: 1) If you are not aware of it, you can miss it. 2) It is, like other disorders of conjugate gaze, not a peripheral muscle or nerve sign but a central nervous system sign. Bilateral internuclear ophthalmoplegia (Moses, Fig. 26-2,A and B) is often seen in multiple sclerosis; unilateral internuclear ophthalmoplegia often occurs after vascular accidents to the medial longitudinal fasciculus.

3. This patient has a right trochlear nerve palsy or a paresis of the muscle it innervates, the right superior oblique. The patient's head is tilted away from the lesion. This is the natural position of about half the patients with this exceedingly rare problem (Younge & Sutula, 1977). Even if you did notice the head position, you would have to make the definitive diagnosis by going through the six cardinal motions of gaze.

The cardinal positions of gaze (Fig. 26-5) would reveal the lesion as follows: In the primary position, the right globe would show some slight but definite hyperdeviation. This would implicate either the right superior oblique or right inferior rectus (the only two muscles that pull the right globe down). When the patient looked up and to the left, the right globe would still be hyperdeviated. This

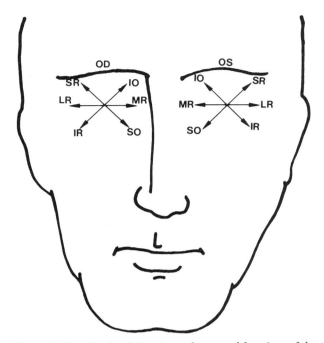

Figure 26-5. *Cardinal directions of gaze and functions of the extraocular muscles (after Younge & Sutula, 1977).*

maneuver would exclude the right inferior rectus and would implicate the right superior oblique. (If the patient had a right inferior rectus palsy, the right eye would show hyperdeviation on looking up and to the right, since that maneuver requires right inferior rectus contraction and takes the strain off the right superior oblique.)

The girl in Figure 26-3B is the virgin's twin sister. She also has a cranial nerve IV (or superior oblique muscle) paralysis, but on the left side. When she came in, her head was tilted toward her right. The present figure shows what happens when you tilt her head (examiner's hands not shown) out of its natural position, toward the side of the lesion. The sign is very subtle, but definite. Look carefully at the illustration and describe what has happened.

The left pupil and iris have floated up. Notice that you can now see a little bit of sclera and all of the limbus on the left, but not on the right.

4. a) In the primary position, this would be a left lateral rectus muscle paralysis or a left cranial nerve VI lesion. The left eye is turned inward because the sixth cranial nerve innervates only the lateral rectus, and all of the other unopposed muscles, especially the medial rectus, are pulling the eyeball in.

b) If, on the other hand, you were testing the extraocular motions (with your finger positioned as shown), this would probably be a right lateral rectus paralysis (or a right cranial nerve VI lesion) because the patient is unable to bring his right eyeball laterally.

○   Cranial nerve VI is the most common cranial nerve to be afflicted, presumably because it travels the longest course.

Red Glass Test

When an ocular palsy is slight, the examiner may not be able to see a defect in the ocular movement, although the patient is expe-

riencing diplopia. The red glass test may help to confirm the presence of a defect and to identify the muscle involved.

A method:

$$ 1.   Place a *red glass* (or cellophane) over the patient's right eye.

2.   Hold a flashlight at a distance of 1 meter in each of the cardinal directions of gaze. Ask the patient to state the position of the red and the white images.

A caveat: Be sure to keep the flashlight beyond the point of convergence. (Testing within the point of convergence is the most common cause of diplopia, with or without the red glass [S. Horenstein, personal communication, 1988], because neither eye can aim at the target, and a physiologic diplopia is thus induced. Try it on yourself: hold your forefinger in front of your nose. As it is moved from say 12 inches away to 2 inches away, attend to how many images you see.)

Interpretation:

1.   The direction in which the separation between the images is maximum is the direction of action of the paretic muscle. For example, if the greatest separation occurs on looking to the left, either the left lateral rectus or the right medial rectus is weak.

2.   The image formed by the paretic eye is the one projected most peripherally. Why is this true? (Hint: draw a picture. Consider the distance of the retinal image to the macula of each eye.) In the previous example, if the red image is farther to the left as the patient looks to the left, it is the right medial rectus that is weak (Victor & Adams, 1970).

Case report.   A physician, on noting that "things just didn't look right," ascertained that she had transient diplopia on gaze to the right. Performing the red glass test on herself, she observed that there were two images when the flashlight was held to the right, but only one image when it was held to the left. Having thereby persuaded herself that she was not imagining things, she consulted a neurologist, who was not able to detect any defect in testing the cardinal directions of gaze. The diagnosis of multiple sclerosis was made on the basis of a nuclear magnetic resonance scan.

The patient noted that the distance between the two images was a semiquantitative measure that correlated with subjective severity of symptoms. Over the next couple of weeks, while on prednisone therapy, she performed the red glass test daily. The white image was to the right. Gradually, the distance between the images diminished, until only one image was present.

Paralysis of Gaze

Horizontal Gaze Palsy

When the patient is unable to shift his gaze to a particular direction, or when the eyes do not move together (conjugately) in the expected manner, the cause is inevitably central in origin. For instance, in acute cerebral cortical disease, especially involving a frontal lobe, the eyes conjugately gaze toward the side of the lesion, and cannot, on command, move to the opposite side, although they will move together to the extent that they can move. On the other hand, with destructive lesions below the cerebral cortex, as in the pons, the eyes tend to look away from the side of the lesion. The patient is unable to look in the other direction on command, though the motions that can occur are conjugate. With irritative lesions, the rules are reversed.

Gaze preference refers to conjugate deviation of a spontaneous nature that is inconstant. That is, the eyes can be made to cross the midline, as during caloric stimulation (see p. 480), thus ruling out brain stem disease, but the eyes customarily look at one and only one side, usually the side of a cortical lesion and usually in the parietal lobe.

In frontal lobe lesions, conjugate gaze deviation is very short-lived. By the time the patient gets upstairs from the ER, it has generally resolved. If it persists, think of parietal lobe disease (S. Horenstein, personal communication, 1988).

If there were bilateral cortical infarcts involving the frontal areas controlling the initiation of horizontal gaze, a patient could lose the ability to track on command, but would retain the ability to track by reflex. That is, the patient would be unable to follow the instruction "look to the right," but would be able to look to the right in the course of following the examiner's finger, or sometimes the examiner's head were the latter to be used as a tracking target.

Of course, metabolic disturbances can do this, and probably other lesions could interrupt the cortical projections to the midbrain centers controlling the eye movements. But the most common cause of this phenomenon on a general medical ward is simply a patient who is too fatigued or confused to cooperate with the tracking or looking command, but who will reflexly follow the physician's head (as a tracking target) while staring into the physician's eyes.

Parinaud's Syndrome

Parinaud's syndrome is paralysis of conjugate vertical gaze due to damage near the posterior commissure. In some cases downward conjugate gaze is preserved, but upward conjugate gaze seems almost always to be lost. If this syndrome is found in a sexually precocious prepubertal boy, make a diagnosis of pinealoma.

For the intermediate student.   This Parinaud's syndrome is not to be confused with Parinaud's conjunctivitis, which is the same as Parinaud's oculoglandular syndrome. The latter refers to a preauricular lymph node in combination with an ipsilateral (but unilateral) conjunctivitis (see Ch. 8, p. 141). This is mentioned to point out the peculiar principle that a majority of clinical syndromes have been described by a small minority of physicians.

For the advanced student.   Some authorities consider the neurologic Parinaud's syndrome to be a triad including, in addition to supranuclear paralysis of upward conjugate gaze, defective convergence and (nonconstricted) pupils that react more briskly to accommodation than to light (Maciewicz, 1983). These latter two signs point to the same midline structures as the first, so the distinction between the two definitions is not always important.

For the intern.   Does the patient have some sort of myopathy or peripheral neuropathy that prevents the eyeballs from moving upward, or is he unable to look up *on command*? One trick is to have the patient track upward (e.g., ask him to follow your finger with his eyes.) Many patients can track but cannot voluntarily look up. A second trick is to use the vertical version of the oculocephalic (doll's eye) reflex (sign, test) discussed later on page 479. If passive head tilting downward causes the globes to rotate superiorly (in relation to the skull), one has demonstrated: 1) absence of a mysterious myopathy or combination of peripheral neuropathies inhibiting upward gaze, and 2) that the projections from the midbrain loci controlling eye movements have become severed from their higher (frontal) projections.

For the resident.   Although Parinaud's syndrome is most famous as a sign of pinealoma, hydrocephalus is probably its most common cause (Chattha & DeLong, 1975).

For the guru.   What Parinaud actually described is a triad of disturbances of the three components of normal convergence. These signs taken together he referred to as "essential." Additionally, he recognized a second form called "combined," in which the "essential" form was combined with paralysis of elevation and/or depression (Parinaud, 1886). Thus, it is quite possible for someone to have Parinaud's syndrome according to Parinaud's definition, and not have a paralysis of upward conjugate gaze! The es-

sential Parinaud's syndrome is a peculiar triad, the individual features of which are quite inconstant:

1. Paralysis of convergence, indicated either by the examiner's recognition that convergence does not occur and/or by a peculiar subjective diplopia of variable salience.
2. Paralysis of accommodation in one eye, both eyes, or neither eye (Maciewicz, 1983). (See Table 10-7.)
3. Pupillary reflexes exactly reverse to those of the Argyll Robertson pupil (Parinaud, 1886). Note that this can also occur in Wernicke's encephalopathy (see Ch. 10, p. 173).

In the same paper, Parinaud described a number of other gaze palsies. Most intriguing to the medical historian is the fact that not a single one of the patients reported in Parinaud's original paper (Parinaud, 1886) had a pinealoma.

For the scholar.   By reading the paragraphs in this section in reverse sequence, much as an archeologist examines the superimposed levels of civilization in a slit trench, from the oldest at the bottom to the newest at the top, one can observe the transmogrification of an original syndrome (Parinaud, 1883). Such distortions are euphemistically referred to as "the advance of modern science."

For the clinician.   Parinaud's syndrome due to trauma may be distinguished from Parinaud's syndrome due to pinealoma in that the former, but not the latter, has a segmental palsy of the iris in response to light stimulation (Thompson, 1978).

Parinaud's syndrome remains important in the age of modern imagery because it is an early sign of midbrain dysfunction, occurring before the CT scan becomes abnormal.

Cerebellar Hemorrhage

The diagnosis of cerebellar hemorrhage is discussed here because of the historical importance attributed to its eye signs, especially the conjugate gaze palsies (Table 26-1). Note that the cerebellar hemorrhage has a wide variety of neurologic signs and symptoms by which it may be distinguished from other intracranial hemorrhages.

The sign of "ocular bobbing" (referred to in Table 26-1) is abrupt spontaneous downward jerks of the eye with a slow return to the midposition, *plus* paralysis of spontaneous and reflex horizontal eye movements (Bosch et al., 1975).

In the mid-1960s, it was believed that one could, and must, make the emergent diagnosis of cerebellar hemorrhage based upon the eye findings. However, the eye signs are not as necessary to the diagnosis as once thought (Heiman & Satya-Murti, 1978).

Newer eye signs are not included in the table (e.g., spontaneous unilateral eye closure [Messert et al., 1976], which occurs because the patient develops an ipsilateral VII nerve palsy due to displacement of the brain stem by the hematoma, and attempts to avoid diplopia by closing the only eyelid still under his control, the contralateral one. The eye on the side of the hematoma is the one that remains open).

Very advanced.   The maximal predictive value of a positive test is about 0.85 for decreased corneal reflex (see p. 457),* about 0.67 for facial paresis, and about 0.71 for the presence of hypertension. The minimal predictive value of a negative test was less than 0.40 for any of the signs in the table. Even the old historical pearl, "Don't diagnose cerebellar hemorrhage in a nonhypertensive patient," breaks down. The minimal predictive value of a negative test for normotension was only 0.40 (Rosenberg & Kaufman, 1976).

A note on terminology.   We have invented two new statistical terms, the *maximal* predictive value of a positive test and the *mini-*

---

*The corneal reflex will be impaired in all conditions wherein the facial muscles are paralyzed.

Table 26-1. Differential Diagnoses of Intracranial Hemorrhages

Finding	Cerebellar Hemorrhage	Thalamic-subthalamic Hemorrhage	Putaminal Hemorrhage	Pontine Hemorrhage	Ruptured Aneurysm Without Intracerebral Clot
Hemiplegia	No	Yes	Yes	Quadriplegia or bilateral motor signs	No
Size of pupils	Small, often	Small, often	May be normal	Small	Variable
Pupillary reaction	Yes	No	Yes	Maybe	Yes
Facial weakness	Ipsilateral peripheral mild	Contralateral central	Contralateral central	Contralateral [??]	No
Sensory deficit	No	Yes	Yes	Yes	No
Conjugate gaze palsy	Common	Uncommon	Yes	Yes	No
Side	Ipsilateral	Contralateral	Contralateral	Ipsilateral	—
Reversed by ice water?	No	Usually	Yes	No	—
6th nerve palsy	Yes	Yes	No	Yes	Maybe
Hemianopia	No	Yes, clears early	Maybe	Maybe	Maybe
Early inability to walk	Yes	No	No	Yes	No
Vomiting	Severe and repeated	Occasional	Occasional	Yes	Yes
Convulsion	No	No	Yes	No	Yes
Unconscious at presentation	Maybe	No	No	Yes	Often
Eyes deviate downward	No	Yes	No	No	No
Ocular bobbing	Yes	No	No	Yes	No
Preretinal hemorrhage	No	No	Occasional	No	Yes
Abrupt evolution	No	No	Occasional	No	Yes
Decerebrate posture	Bilateral, usually late	Unilateral	Unilateral	Unilateral	Late

Sources: *Brennan and Bergland (1977), Fisher et al. (1965), and Vincent (1976).*

mal predictive value of a negative test. These are defined as the predictive value of tests calculated from series in which there were control subjects free of the disease being studied, but which control subjects were probably not present in the same proportion as in real life. With the prevalence of the diseased subjects inflated, the apparent predictive value of a positive test can be considered the maximal predictive value of a positive test, since it would decrease were the subjects without the disease entered into the study in proportion appropriate to their prevalence. Conversely, the predictive value of the negative test defined in the artificial test population is the minimal predictive value of a negative test.

Cranial Nerve V: Motor

A Method for the Beginner

1. Place your hands over both of the patient's temporalis muscles and instruct the patient, "Grind your teeth." Normally, you should feel both of the temporalis muscles contracting. (Try it on your partner.)

2. Next slip your hands down to the masseter muscles at the lower posterior angle of the mandible. Again, instruct the patient to perform bruxism (teeth grinding) or simply ask him to chew. Again you should feel both masseters contract under your hands. (Try it on your partner.)

A Rounding Ploy

The most common cause of reported bilateral temporalis muscle failure is examination of an edentulous patient (not realized to be such) by a senior medical student on a neurology elective. (A senior medical student who is already specializing in neurology apparently no longer needs to examine the mouth. Since the cranial nerves do not show up on a CT scan, there is nothing that can be missed by not looking inside the mouth, that will be detected by anyone else.)

Rather, the edentulous patient should be instructed to gum his lips or lower jaw. (Skip the temporalis muscle examination and go directly to the masseter examination, since without real teeth, even this maneuver will not generate as good a contraction of the temporalis as of the masseter.)

Additionally, when examining the mouth, perform the following maneuvers:

1. Rotate the tongue blade within the mouth to a vertical position.
2. Instruct the patient to grasp the tongue blade between his teeth.
3. Then ask him to wiggle the grasped tongue blade.

I prefer this to the usual method of having the patient simply grasp the horizontal tongue blade between his clamped teeth and "hold it in place." By requiring the patient to hold a vertical tongue blade and wiggle it, we also check the internal and external pterygoid muscles. The former method tests only the masseter and temporalis.

○ Do not check the pterygoids in a patient with a weak masseter because the jaw may dislocate (S. Horenstein, personal communication, 1988).

For the advanced resident. The Landry-Guillain-Barré-Strohl* syndrome tends to spare the masseter muscle, which is frequently involved in myasthenia gravis. This distinction is empiric but not scientific since we have no underlying basis for explaining it (see Ch. 1, p. 4).

Cranial Nerve V: Sensory

Skin Sensation

Because the detailed examination takes the same amount of time as the screening examination, one might as well do the detailed examination. The technique is called double simultaneous stimulation (DSS).

A method:

1. Ask the patient to report which side(s) is (are) touched.

2. Standing in front of him, have him stare at your nose. Moving both your index fingers constantly so as to eliminate visual cuing, occasionally bring one or both fingers close enough to the face to tap the skin lightly.

3. Start at the top and work down, being careful to perform testing within each of the three divisions of the trigeminal nerve. Within each division, tap on both sides at once as well as on one side only.

If you wish to be very fancy, you can perform the same test with cotton wisps, instead of your fingers.

Interpretation. If the afflicted side does not perceive touch with DSS, while it may perceive touch when stimulated by itself, there is generally a cortical lesion. With peripheral disease, the subject will not perceive either a single or double stimulus.

You may wonder why one is sure to tap on one side only in each of the three divisions, if DSS is superior to single stimulation. First, the subject may have peripheral disease. But even with cortical disease, the single stimulation in each division must be randomly performed so as to break up the "halo" effect. That is, if the subject with the cortical disease always sees the fingers wiggling, even when they are not tapping him, and he is always tapped doubly, he may learn to report the sensation of DSS each time even when he is not experiencing it, thus defeating the purpose of the test.

Despite the verbosity of the description, DSS with control single-sided stimulation of all three divisions of the trigeminal nerve can be performed in 8 seconds.

Corneal Reflex

The sensory nerve V also supplies the corneal surface.

A method:

1. Moisten a soft piece of cotton or other material that will not scratch the cornea. This should of course be clean. It should not have been used on another patient, especially one with Jakob-Creutzfeldt disease, AIDS, or herpetic keratitis.

2. Touch the cornea. This sounds simple, but one must steer between the Scylla of the sclera and the Charybdis of the visual

*Strohl was actually the medical student who found the patients and presented them at neurology conference (Guillain et al., 1916).

startle reflex. You may have the patient look up (so that you do not touch the eyelids), or to the side, or at the top of your forehead. In any event, approach the patient from the side, so that the eyes cannot see the wisp of cotton. When the wisp is over a portion of the cornea not covering the pupillary aperture, go straight in, observing both eyes for the blink.

3. Repeat on the other side.

What might be wrong with the technique of the examiner shown in Figure 26-6? Assuming the technique to be adequate, what do you think is the diagnosis for each of the patients illustrated in Figure 26-6? (Write your answers down before looking in Appendix 26-1.)

$$ *An alternate method.* The French method, which avoids the potential for contagion as well as the problems listed in step 2, is to take a straw or syringe and squirt air at the cornea (S. Horenstein, personal communication, 1988).

Interpretation. The corneal reflex involves two different cranial nerves, V for the afferent limb and VII for the efferent limb. Not knowing this can get you into a pickle. This should remind you of the advertisement for the 57 varieties of Heinz pickles. That pickle ($5 \rightarrow 7$) can remind you of the afferent limb (V) and the efferent limb (VII). Accordingly, we can progress to the study of the VIIth cranial nerve, with relish.

Corneal reflexes may be lost in coma of any etiology if the corneas are allowed to dry out and so become hyposensitive. Thus,

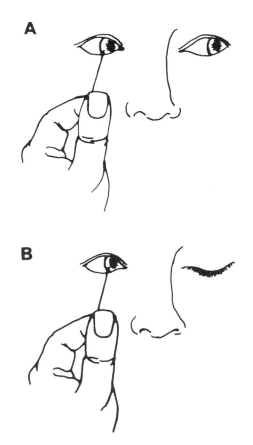

Figure 26-6. *The corneal reflex: two self-tests. See text and Appendix 26-1.*

about 12% of absent corneal reflexes in comatose patients occur in those who regain consciousness, and with corneal lubrication, their corneal reflexes as well (S. Horenstein, personal communication, 1988).

Corneomandibular reflex. If corneal stimulation also produces a lateral deviation of the mandible, it is called the corneomandibular reflex. This is probably an associated movement more than a true reflex. It indicates supranuclear interruption of the corticotrigeminal tract on the side of the stimulated cornea.

While the corneomandibular reflex is abnormal in the awake patient, its presence in a comatose patient indicates that the brain stem is intact. It is one of the "brain stem release" signs rarely used today.

Perioral Reflex

A method:

1. Place a finger in the angle of the mouth and strike it to see the reflex closure.
(Alternately, stroke the nasolabial fold.)

Interpretation:

1. This reflex tests V as the afferent, and VII as the efferent.

2. Except in infants, there is normally no response. In an adult, the infantile response of contraction of the nearby facial muscles is a cortical release sign, signifying severe damage.

Cranial Nerve VII: Somatomotor Portion

Routinely, we test only that somatomotor portion of cranial nerve VII, which supplies the muscles of facial expression.

Peripheral Versus Central Palsy

A method:

1. Observe the patient for greater than normal facial asymmetry, including inspection of the lateral palpebral commissures. Also look for flattening of a nasolabial fold.

2. Ask the patient to raise his eyebrows, and look for symmetrical wrinkling of the forehead.

3. Ask the patient to close his eyes tightly. Try to force the lids open with your thumb, rolling the skin against the supraorbital rim, *not* against the globe, in order to detect weakness of one eyelid.

4. Ask the patient to show his teeth (or gums) and to puff out his cheeks.

Interpretation. Central facial palsies are due to cortical (upper motor neuron) lesions, and peripheral palsies are due to lesions of the facial nerve or its brain stem nucleus (lower motor neurons). Note that "peripheral" as used here includes a portion of the central nervous system, the nucleus in the brain stem.

The upper third of the face, including the muscles of the forehead and the orbicularis oculi, is supplied by nucleus that receives fibers from both sides of the cerebrum. The lower part of the face is supplied by nucleus that receives fibers from only one side of the cerebral cortex. Therefore, if the patient experiences a supranuclear lesion (e.g., a lesion of the motor cortex or of its fibers descending to the nucleus) that produces a facial palsy, the forehead will be spared. Such a patient would be able to perform step 2 normally, but not step 4. On the other hand, if the facial palsy is due to a lesion of the peripheral nerve or of the brain stem nucleus, the forehead and eyelids will also be paretic. (See the Bells of Scotland, which follow.)

In the case record, be sure to describe the findings (e.g., "upper face [not] spared"); "peripheral" and "central" palsy are conclusions, not findings.

When localization of a lesion based upon loss of the upper third of the facial muscle is not completely compatible with the rest of the examination, the former should be abandoned, as about 5% of the population does *not* have crossed innervation of the motor supply to the upper third of the facial nerve. In such patients, total facial hemiparesis cannot be used as evidence of nuclear (brain stem) disease. Of course, if the upper third is preserved, that is still evidence of supranuclear disease.

Emotional Versus Volitional Pathways

Some patients with facial palsy are wrongly suspected of malingering because they cannot seem to move the facial muscles on the examiner's command, but are capable of moving them if the examiner can make the patient laugh involuntarily. This retention of motor function in response to strong emotion is called *volitional palsy.* It may be seen when the frontal lobes are spared, and the lesion occurs somewhere between the motor cortex and the pons, just above the nucleus (DeJong, 1979). *Emotional* (or mimetic) *palsy* is seen when the above pathways are spared, and the lesion is in the frontal lobes or its projections into the reticular pons just above the nucleus. Such patients can move their facial muscles on command, but not during the spontaneous expression of strong emotion. They may be misdiagnosed as Parkinsonian or schizophrenic. It is for the latter reason that the instructions on judging affect (see p. 522) require the examiner to measure more than just facial appearance.

A person who can smile but not whistle might also be accused of malingering. But this is exactly what is seen as an early manifestation of progressive muscular dystrophy of the fascioscapulohumeral type (Landovzy-Dejerine) where the seventh cranial nerve is intact, but the oribicularis oris is asymmetrically involved (Perkoff & Tyler, 1953).

Bell's Palsy

Bell's palsy is a subset of the peripheral variety of facial palsies, referring to lesions distal to the geniculate ganglion (DeJong, 1979).

Hunt's syndrome, which is herpes of the geniculate ganglion, produces a peripheral facial palsy and herpetic vesicles on the eardrum. This situation is the only one in which it is useful to know that the eardrum, parts of the ear canal, and parts of the tragus are supplied by the somatosensory branch of cranial nerve VII. The actual distribution is quite variable from person to person.

A method. The best test* for Bell's palsy is to ask the patient to close each eye, individually, in turn. In very mild cases, the patient will not be able to close the eye on the afflicted side without also closing the contralateral (normal) eye.

Two caveats. If you don't know the history, merely observing the patient's facial appearance, especially around the eyes, can be misleading. With recovery, partial contractures may set in on the paralyzed size, making it appear to be the more contracted side. Hence the normal side may appear comparatively paretic.

Similarly, a third nerve lesion can produce upper lid ptosis (mim-

---

*Because of the extremely large number of talented people who have worked in the field of neurology over the past century, we are blessed with a surfeit of neurologic tests for each lesion. Accordingly, we will often try to pick one simple test, and ask the reader to consult DeJong for a fuller catalog.

icking the contractures mentioned above), but not the lower lid droop seen in cranial nerve VII lesions.

During an eye blink, the lower lid normally moves 2 to 5 mm horizontally and nasally, thereby producing a partial vacuum in the lacrimal system that helps to clear it and to wipe the tears away from the globe. However, in facial palsy, the lateral motion is lost, and in fact the lower lid does not move up much at all. This is best demonstrated with a camera, but the effects can be seen without it (Arrigg & Miller, 1985). The tears build up on the affected side. Since they form a stagnant pool, they can permit bacterial overgrowth and infection.

Bell's Phenomenon

Ordinarily, when one attempts to close the eye against a resistance by contraction of the orbicularis muscle of the eyelids, the globe rotates upward. This is not pathologic, but rather is a normal synkinesia (i.e., associated movement). Hence, we speak of "Bell's phenomenon," not "Bell's sign." Usually, it is not noticed because the closing eye obscures the globe.

A method. Ask a naive medical student to try to keep his eyes closed while you try to open them by opposing them with your thumbs. Press extra hard on one side only to keep that eye from closing, and you will see Bell's phenomenon. On the other side, you must let the eyelid win over your thumb, or your subject may visually fix on a spot as he concentrates on his task. Such visual fixation can eliminate Bell's phenomenon bilaterally.

Interpretation. Bell's phenomenon may be significant only when it is absent. (Such phenomena are often likened to Sherlock Holmes's barking dog*.)

Bilateral absence occurs in: 1) visual fixation by a neurologically intact person; 2) brain stem or lower motor neuron oculomotor disease, but not supranuclear oculomotor disease; 3) bilateral disease of the third cranial nerves (unlikely by Occam's Razor); 4) 15% of normal persons (Adams & Victor, 1985).

The phenomenon is absent unilaterally in ipsilateral third cranial nerve disease (not seventh).

In Bell's palsy, whenever the orbicularis muscle closes it must do so against an effective "resistance." Because of this, it is particularly easy to observe the unmasked (normal) Bell's phenomenon on the afflicted side (DeGowin, 1965; "Major," Delp & Manning, 1975). This has led to the unfortunate conclusion that Bell's phenomenon is a "sign" of Bell's palsy. This convoluted reasoning is reinforced by the similarity in names and the unhappy practice of describing both palsy and phenomenon in the same physical diagnosis textbook passage. This emphasis on one situation in which the phenomenon is present has unfortunately detracted from its more salient use in those situations—outlined above—in which it is absent.

---

*Just as Willie ("the Actor") Sutton never actually authored the words of Sutton's Law (p. 531), so Holmes never referred to the dog as the "barking dog." In the adventure called *Silver Blaze*, Watson asks Holmes:

"Is there any point to which you would draw my attention?"
"To the curious incident of the dog in the night-time."
"The dog did nothing in the night-time."
"That is the curious incident," remarked Sherlock Holmes.

Later, Holmes explains,

" . . . I had grasped the significance of the silence of the dog, for one true inference invariably suggests others. The Simpson incident had shown me that a dog was kept in the stables, and yet, though someone had been in and had fetched out a horse, he had not barked enough to arouse the two lads in the loft. Obviously the midnight visitor was someone whom the dog knew well."

Thus, this should be called the silent dog, not the barking dog (as Sutton's Law should be named after William Dock, who actually described it).

Because it is a normal synkinesia, Bell's phenomenon has been used by others to distinguish an oculomotor conversion reaction from "organic" pathology. (If the synkinesia occurs, the innervation of the eye muscles must be intact; therefore, the patient is "malingering" if unable to move his eyes on command.) However, there are problems with relying on this phenomenon alone, since if the phenomenon persists, the patient might actually have supranuclear disease.

Bell's phenomenon has also been confused in some texts with Negro's sign, the movement of the globe up and out when the patient looks up at the ceiling. Negro's sign is present in both central and peripheral facial palsies. Negro's sign, like Bell's phenomenon, is more pronounced on the side of the lesion.

Historical Note: The Bells of Scotland

Both Bell's palsy and Bell's phenomenon were named for Sir Charles Bell (1774–1842). However, this was not the Bell whose clinical acumen so impressed the medical student Arthur Conan Doyle that he became the model for Sherlock Holmes (Doyle, 1958). The latter, Joseph Bell, was a scion of the other Scottish family of eminent surgeons, also named Bell.

Other

Unilateral hyperacusis may be due to palsy of the stapedius muscle, which normally functions to dampen the oscillations of the ear **\$\$** ossicles. For detecting this finding, one may use the tape recorder and earpiece described for interviewing patients who are hard-of-hearing (see Ch. 2, p. 25). The two sides may be compared by noting the volume setting that elicits the acoustic reflex (a startle, wince, grimace, or blink in response to a sound sufficiently loud to be unpleasant). Pure tones and white noise appear to be the best discriminators, not music (Johns, 1986).

Cranial Nerve VII: Visceral Sensory

Taste is more complicated than smell, because the anterior two thirds of the tongue is innervated by cranial nerve VII, the back of the tongue by cranial nerve IX, and the epiglottal taste buds by cranial nerve X.

A Method

The following technique may be adapted for use in lieu of a formal taste sensation laboratory:

\$\$ **1.** Make up 1/4% aqueous solutions of table salt, table sugar, quinine (about 1/2 tsp/l) and about 1tsp/cup kitchen vinegar. These solutions should be strong enough for an older person (who will have fewer taste buds) to taste. Remember, you are not testing for threshold but for total absence of taste.*

2. Write on a piece of paper the words "sweet," "salty," "sour," "bitter," and "plain water." (If the patient is unable to indicate his choice by pointing to one of the words, you may have trouble with the test. a) If the patient is allowed to open his mouth to speak his answer, the solutions will run from one side to the other and from front to back, so the loss of taste on one side or the other, or in the area supplied by a specific cranial nerve, may be missed. b) If the patient is allowed simply to signal "yes," the vinegar may stimulate cranial nerve V in the mouth and nose, and this sensation may be reported as a "positive" response, even though the patient is not experiencing taste.)

3. Have the patient protrude his tongue, and paint on the solutions one at a time, in one place at a time, and on only one side at a time.

---

*The median detection threshold/median recognition threshold, in mmol/l, for normal subjects, is as follows: sodium chloride 12/30; sucrose 12/30; hydrochloric acid 3/6; urea 120/150 (Henkin et al., 1971).

Rules of thumb. To test cranial nerve VII, use the salt and sugar solutions on the anterior tongue. To test cranial nerves VII and IX, paint the sour solution (the vinegar) on the lateral surface, anteriorly for VII, and posteriorly for IX. To test cranial nerve IX, paint the bitter quinine solution posteriorly, but do not let the patient swallow. (He will not be able to as long as his tongue is sticking out.) The quinine solution should be used last.

4. With the tongue still out, ask the patient to make a response.

5. After each response, let the patient rinse with some water, which should be expectorated, not swallowed.

Very advanced. The patient should not be allowed to eat artichokes before the test, as they will make many substances subsequently seem sweet.

Testing with sugar solutions is very difficult because it tends to roll across the midline. Some examiners only use salt on the side of the tongue (S. Horenstein, personal communication, 1988).

An Alternate Technique

$$ Wire two 9-volt hearing aid batteries in series to make an 18-volt battery. Then place the end leads on the tongue 3 mm apart. No matter what type of taste bud is touched, the patient with intact taste sensation will report a metallic taste (S. Horenstein, personal communication, 1988).

Interpretation

Unilateral impairment of taste on the anterior two thirds of the tongue is due to a lesion of cranial nerve VII, located above its exit from the stylomastoid foramen, either in the portion that passes through the auditory canal (the chorda tympani) or in the portion that proceeds to the geniculate ganglion. Contrariwise, supranuclear lesions are not accompanied by alteration in taste (Fig. 26-7).

Causes of bilateral decrease or loss of taste are listed in Table 26-2.

○ Complaints of dysgeusia (as in gold therapy) or hypogeusia may actually have normal taste tests but abnormal olfactory nerve testing.

Cranial Nerve VII: Visceral Motor

The visceral motor branches of cranial nerve VII supply the salivary (Ch. 13, p. 222) and lacrimal glands (see the Schirmer test, Ch. 10, p. 157). Unilateral dryness of the eyes and mouth could be due to a lesion of this nerve. If bilateral, the problem is probably end organ damage as in Sjögren's syndrome.

Cranial Nerve VIII

The auditory portion of cranial nerve VIII has already been tested with the Rinne, Weber, and Schwabach tests during the examination of the ear (see Ch. 11, p. 211).

One aspect of the vestibular portion of cranial nerve VIII was tested during the examination of the extraocular movements, when the presence or absence of nystagmus was noted.

The findings from these two examinations might have been recorded under the respective regional examinations.

Additionally, screening tests for vestibular function, the Barany test, and the caloric response are discussed on page 479, since the vestibular system is mostly easily tested as a system.

Arbit's Hearing Test

$$ A device constructed of a stethoscope, a tuning fork (512 Hz), and a suction cup or feeding nipple (designed to attach the tuning fork

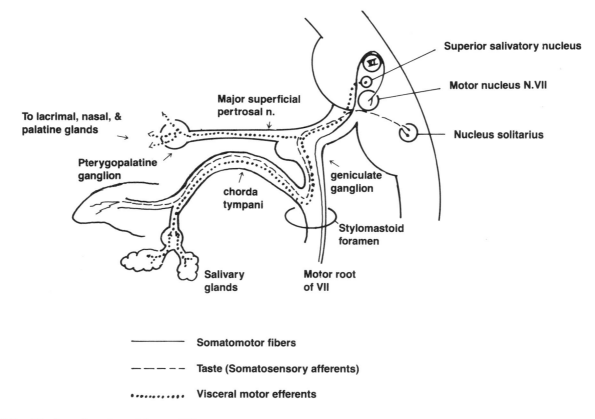

Somatomotor fibers

– – – – Taste (Somatosensory afferents)

•••••••••• Visceral motor efferents

Figure 26-7.   The branches of cranial nerve VII.

Table 26-2.   Causes of Bilateral Loss of Taste or Hypogeusia (Decreased Taste)

Neurologic Disease
    Familial dysautonomia

Local Afflictions
    Facial hypoplasia
    Sjögren's syndrome
    After radiation therapy
    Laryngectomy

Drug Therapy
    Steroids
    Diuretics
    Aspirin

Nutritional Deficiencies
    Niacin deficiency
    Zinc deficiency

Endocrine Conditions
    Cushing's syndrome
    Hypothyroidism
    Diabetes mellitus (abnormal taste of glucose only)
    Pseudohypoparathyroidism

Infectious Diseases
    Dengue fever
    Influenza-like infections

Other Systemic Conditions
    Sarcoidosis
    Cancer
    Chronic renal failure
    Cirrhosis of the liver
    Burns
    Hypertension (abnormal taste of salt only)

Sources: *Clee et al. (1983), Schiffman (1983), and Wechsler (1963).*

to the stethoscope diaphragm) has been described for improved bedside testing of hearing (Arbit, 1977). One also needs a device such as a hemostat for clamping (occluding) the stethoscope tubing.

A method:

1.   Preinstruct the patient that he is to indicate when he is no longer able to hear the sound of the tuning fork.

2.   Place the earpieces of the stethoscope in the patient's ears.

3.   Strike the tuning fork, which is attached to the stethoscope diaphragm by the feeding nipple.

4.   Listen to the tuning fork while watching the patient for the preestablished signal.

Hearing is said to be normal if the patient hears the sound at least 15 seconds longer than the examiner.

Comment.   While this test seems to work as well or better than the contemporary "customary" examination, it has not been compared with the Rinne and Weber tests.

A unilateral method.   Test each ear individually by clamping the tubing leading to one ear. The patient again signals when he no longer hears the sound (in the ear served by the unoccluded tubing). At that instant, unclamp the tubing and ask the patient if he now hears the sound. If he does, you have identified a definite hearing difference between the two ears.

Loudness Recruitment

The device described above can also be used to detect loudness recruitment, by comparing the two ears at different tuning fork intensities (for details, vide infra).

If you could carry around an audiometer in your pocket, and use it as an independent variable for testing your diagnosed patients with unilateral deafness, you would soon make an interesting discovery: Patients with unilateral sensorineural deafness due to the involvement of the hair cells of the organ of Corti would show very strange audiograms (Fig. 26-8).

The schematic audiogram demonstrating recruitment (*solid circles*) would not be seen in non-end-organ deafness (*squares*). Looking at the circles, we see that the infirm ear has a very high threshold. The difference between the good ear and the infirm ear decreases at higher decibels (louder sound). In fact, at very high amplitudes (sound intensities), the good ear and the bad ear hear equally well! The bad ear is thus said to have "recruited" something which permits it to be equal to the good ear at very suprathreshold intensities.

For the attending.   Recruitment is almost never found in sensorineural deafness due to involvement of the cochlear nerve (VIII) (i.e., its presence implies disease of the end organ rather than of the communicating neural tissue). The exception has been the report of this phenomenon in a few cases of acoustic neurinoma (cerebellopontine angle tumor) (Alpers & Manchall, 1971). In a general medical practice, recruitment most often is due to Meniere's syndrome.

A bedside test for unilateral recruitment:

A method: Hit the tuning fork very lightly, and rapidly present it to each ear in sequence. Repeat several times, each time with a lighter touch on the tuning fork, varying the ear that is stimulated first. The purpose is to search for evidence that threshold or near-threshold sound is significantly different between the two ears. This point is operationally defined as the softest touch on the tuning fork that will permit an ear to perceive the sound as softer (than the opposite ear) regardless of the sequence of presentation.

Next, hit the tuning fork as hard as you can and quickly present it to each ear. If the subject now reports that the infirm ear hears just as well as—or sometimes better than—the good ear, recruitment is said to be present (Chandler, 1958).

This test was developed by Chandler, who noticed that the patient who has recruitment will often give visual signals of discomfort when the maximally activated tuning fork is presented to the infirm ear.

Of course, the patient with nonrecruiting sensorineural deafness, or one with a conductive deafness, will continue to report that the sound is much louder in the "good" ear, no matter how hard you hit the fork.

Obviously, Chandler's test for recruitment can be modified as by Arbit in that the clamped and unclamped tubing permits the same tuning fork to be presented to each ear in sequence without actually moving the fork around the patient's head.

For the guru.   We need to acknowledge that the distinction between sensorineural and conduction deafness derives from 19th century concepts. They were based upon tuning fork tests and therefore are still convenient. However, with increasing information about the cochlear portion of the ear, exceptions to the old concepts have arisen (Goodhill, 1979).

Low-Frequency Hearing Loss in Meniere's Syndrome

Meniere's syndrome should not be diagnosed without vestibular signs and low-frequency hearing loss. One way to detect the latter is to see if the patient can hear the dial tone on the telephone. This test works all over the world, except in Vienna, where the dial tone is the 440-Hz A to which the Vienna Philharmonic tunes up (S. Horenstein, personal communication, 1988). Additionally, the diagnosis should not be made in the absence of vestibular signs (see p. 479).

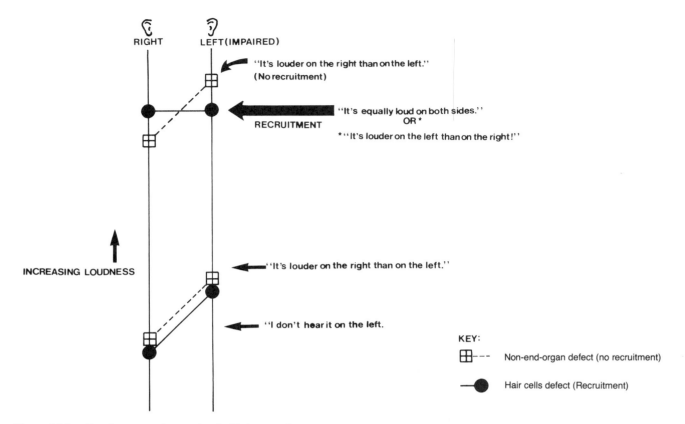

RIGHT   LEFT(IMPAIRED)

"It's louder on the right than on the left."
(No recruitment)

"It's equally loud on both sides."
OR *

RECRUITMENT

*"It's louder on the left than on the right!"

INCREASING LOUDNESS

"It's louder on the right than on the left."

"I don't hear it on the left.

KEY:

⊞--- Non-end-organ defect (no recruitment)

●— Hair cells defect (Recruitment)

Figure 26-8. *Loudness recruitment thresholds (see text).*

Syndrome of Acoustic Neurinoma (Cerebellopontine Angle Tumor)

The major neurologic abnormality is, of course, disease of cranial nerve VIII. Hearing loss is found in 98% of these patients, tinnitus in 70%, disequilibrium in 67%, and nystagmus in 26% (Harner & Laws, 1983).

On vestibular testing (see p. 479), over 80% of patients will have at least some decrease on one side.

Cranial nerves V and VII may also be involved: 26% to 29% of the patients have facial numbness, and 10% to 12% have facial weakness. Either dysgeusia or lingual numbness from involvement of chorda tympani fibers is found in 6%. An abnormal corneal reflex is found in 33%.

Only about 10% have diplopia, and abnormal eye movements are found in but 11% (due to involvement of cranial nerves III, IV, and VI).

Cranial nerves I, II, IX, X, XI, or XII are collectively and individually involved but rarely. (Rarely means less than 1% of the time.) Abnormalities of these cranial nerves, especially in a discontinuous fashion (i.e., not in numerical sequence), should suggest an alternate diagnosis.

As with other retrocochlear diseases, there is a disproportionate impairment in speech discrimination, as opposed to pure-tone audiometry.

With present imaging techniques, acoustic neurinoma is diagnosed so early that the classical picture is no longer seen, just as brain tumors no longer present with papilledema (S. Horenstein, personal communication, 1988).

Cranial Nerves IX and X

Where accessible to the physical diagnostician, cranial nerves IX and X overlap so much that they can be considered together.

A Method for the Beginner

Examine the palate to see whether the uvula is in the midline position. In asymptomatic patients, it usually is.

Also perform a gag reflex, at the conclusion of the examination of the throat. Simply let your tongue depressor slide back toward the posterior third of the tongue. In all likelihood, you will have already produced many gag reflexes inadvertently by the time you are polished enough to produce one intentionally. Accordingly, by the time you do it, you will know what it looks like.

The Uvula in Pathologic Conditions

A great deal can be learned from the position of the uvula in pathologic conditions. In Figure 26-9, each row refers to a pathologic condition, except for the top row, which illustrates the normal. Each column represents a condition of examination. The figures in the left hand column are the palate and uvula as observed at rest. The second column is the result of following the command to say "ahh."

If the individual has a palsy, the uvula will be deviated toward the good (healthy) side. Please note that the uvula may not exactly point to the good side (as shown in the figure) but rather may seem to be hanging straight down on the good side of the midline.

In some cases of partial palsy, the uvula will hang in the middle, but on induced phonation ("ahhh") will move toward the good side. Again, in actual practice the whole area moves. The uvula again does not really point at the good side as shown in the figure, which is intended as a mnemonic.

Sometimes the uvula is in the midline but does not move on phonation. Here we must be dealing with a bilateral paralysis. But does it result from upper or lower motor neuron disease? To find out, simply touch a cotton applicator to the uvula. If it does not move, one is obviously dealing with a bilateral lower motor neuron

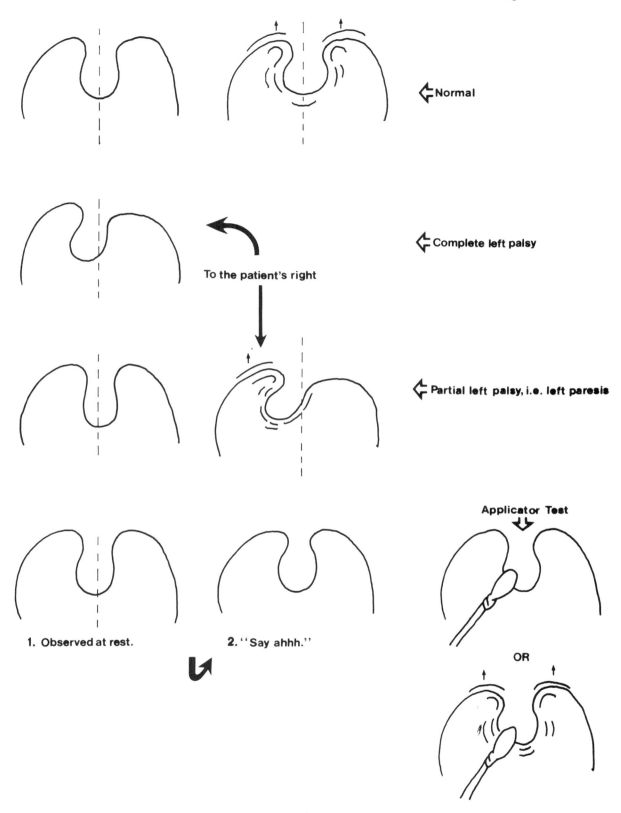

Figure 26-9.   *The uvula in various pathologic conditions. Left column: at rest. Middle column: on phonation ("ahhh"). Right column: applicator test. First row: normal. Second row: complete left palsy. Third row: partial left palsy (i.e., left paresis). Fourth row: lower motor neuron disease of IX and X. Fifth row: upper motor neuron disease of IX and X.*

palsy. If, as in the bottom panel, it does respond (bilaterally) to direct stimulation, one is dealing with a bilateral upper motor neuron palsy.

Notice that we have not said whether IX, X, or both cranial nerves were involved in this palsy. That is because they usually go together. The most common causes seen in practice are involvement of the IX and X cranial nerves in brain stem disease. Sometimes, there is unilateral involvement due to the syndrome of the jugular foramen. In that instance, one also sees homolateral involvement of XI in addition to IX and X (syndrome of Vernet, vide infra).

Distinguishing Lesions of IX and X

If one wishes to separate lesions of IX and X, one is obliged to find a testable function served by one but not the other.

While IX does supply taste to the posterior third of the tongue, it should be noted that X supplies the taste buds even further back. Given the vagaries of testing for taste in general, and without touching the anterior two thirds of the tongue in particular, the distinction can probably not be made on these grounds.

However, X does have some accessible and testable functions. Old-time neurologists used to perform the *oculocardiac reflex*. This was done by pressing on the eyeball and observing the slowing of the heart. If the visceral motor branches of X were interrupted, no such slowing would take place. (However, interruption of the afferent fibers of V also leads to loss of the reflex.)

X also has somatosensory branches that supply the anterior aspect of the tragus, sometimes the posterior aspect of the tragus, sometimes a little spot of skin on the back of the ear, and sometimes the external auditory canal. Unfortunately, IX also supplies these areas in some persons. The best place to search for an anesthetic spot is on the tragus. If you find it, you have fair evidence of involvement of cranial nerve X.

Finally, X supplies somatomotor branches to the vocal cords.

Vocal Cord Paralysis

For the attending. The following discussion presumes that you have performed indirect laryngoscopy or have consulted a laryngoscopist.

Total bilateral loss of X is usually associated with a fatal outcome, although the loss of X itself is not fatal, because both sides of the medulla oblongata must be damaged for a long distance in order to destroy all of the nucleus of X. A person can live with bilateral paralysis of the recurrent laryngeal branches of X, although he will have dyspnea and impaired phonation. If there is bilateral disease of the adductor branches, there will be impaired phonation, but no respiratory difficulties. If there is bilateral paralysis of the abductor branches, there will be no difficulties with phonation to speak of, but there will be severe dyspnea. The last is known as Gerhardt's syndrome.

Unilateral laryngeal nerve palsies are a little more common. Unilateral recurrent laryngeal nerve palsy is associated with a raspy voice that easily fatigues. Its differential diagnosis is to some degree dependent on the laterality. If the left recurrent laryngeal nerve is affected, one should think of aortic aneurysm, trauma (e.g., thyroidectomy), mitral stenosis, or other causes of left pulmonary artery enlargement. If the right recurrent laryngeal nerve is involved, one should look for disease of the right pulmonary apex. Recurrent laryngeal nerve palsy of either side may be caused by pericarditis, goiter (Hamburger, 1986), tumors, and (rarely) tabes dorsalis. Unilateral superior laryngeal nerve palsy is usually the result of trauma.

Cranial Nerve X in Combination with Other Cranial Nerve Lesions

All of these are homolateral syndromes. When IX, X, and XI are involved together, that is the syndrome of Vernet and indicates disease at the jugular foramen, if unilateral. The syndrome of Vernet plus involvement of the XII cranial nerve and the sympathetics is known as the syndrome of Villaret and Collet, and indicates that the lesion is in the retroparotid space, if unilateral. However, if only X and XI are involved, that is the syndrome of Schmidt, and should be attributed to disease of the central nervous system (rather than the peripheral nerves) until proved otherwise.

Cranial Nerve XI

The trapezius muscles may be tested by having the patient shrug his shoulders. The sternocleidomastoid muscles may be tested by having the patient rotate his head *away* from the side being tested (when facing you) against the resistance of the examiner's hand placed on the lateral aspect of the mandible opposite the side being tested (Fig. 26-10).

1. If the sternocleidomastoid muscles are intact, and the trapezius muscle is paretic on one side, this suggests that the weakness is due to a lesion above the brain stem, because 95% of the population has bilateral cortical representation in the cranial nerve XI nucleus which controls the sternocleidomastoid (but not in that part that controls the trapezius). (It does not *prove* supranuclear palsy because the problem might also be in the paretic muscle or its nerve branch.)

However, if both the sternocleidomastoid and the trapezius are weak, one cannot always be sure that this is due to a brain stem lesion. It could also be a supranuclear problem occurring in a patient from the 5% of the population lacking the bilateral cortical representation in the motor nuclei of the sternocleidomastoid.

2. The function of the spinal accessory nerve may also be impaired by neck lesions that cause entrapment.

3. Weakness of neck forward flexion is found in 100% of myopathies of any cause. Do not test the side-to-side or rotational strength. Instead, tell the patient to put the chin on the chest and keep it there while you try to extend the neck (forcing the head up and back). The absence of sternocleidomastoid weakness as demonstrated by this maneuver calls into question the diagnosis of myopathy (S. Horenstein, personal communication, 1988).

Cranial Nerve XII

A Method

Instruct the patient to stick his tongue out at you and then, as you lightly hold his mandible, ask him to point the tongue first to the right and then to the left.

In the *acute* stage of lower motor neuron (peripheral or nuclear) hypoglossal paralysis, the tongue points toward the paralyzed side *and* the paralyzed side may *appear* higher and more voluminous (Dinkler's sign, see Fig. 26-11). This *may* also be seen in *acute* supranuclear hypoglossal palsies.

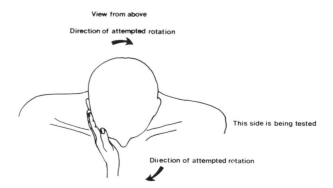

View from above

Direction of attempted rotation

This side is being tested

Direction of attempted rotation

Figure 26-10. *Testing the sternocleidomastoid. (See text.)*

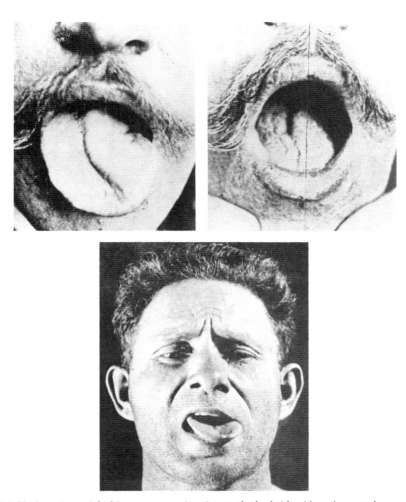

Figure 26-11.   Top, *When Dinkler's patient sticks his tongue out, it points to the bad side. Also, the acutely paralyzed left side seems to be bunched up (Dinkler's sign), while the normal right side is relatively flat. When the patient puts his tongue back in his mouth, both sides are flat. Notice also that the tongue goes in on the right side—that is, it is pulled back to the good side by the good muscle. Bottom, This patient is faking an acute hypoglossal nerve palsy. Notice that his tongue is quite flat, in contrast to the photographs on top. Reproduced with permission from Alexander L: The neurologic examination. In:* Pullen's Medical Diagnosis. *WB Saunders, Philadelphia, 1950.*

A true-negative Dinkler's sign is not seen in acute malingering or acute conversion reactions.

A false-positive Dinkler's sign may be seen in facial nerve palsy. The tongue appears to be pointing to the side of the facial nerve lesion on casual inspection, but closer examination will reveal that the tongue is pointing straight out but the patient is unable to open his mouth completely on the affected side.

Dinkler's sign associated with pain is now usually due to carcinomatous involvement of the peripheral nerve XII. It may also be due to basilar meningeal carcinomatosis, usually from breast cancer in women and prostate or lung cancer in men.

An uncomplicated *chronic* unilateral cranial nerve XII palsy will not usually "point to the bad side" when the patient first protrudes his tongue. The tongue will usually come straight out of the mouth, at which time you should inspect and palpate it for atrophy of the diseased side. (The bulging deformity of Dinkler's sign will not be seen if atrophy has supervened.)

But the patient with chronic hypoglossal nerve palsy (just like the patient with acute hypoglossal nerve palsy) will not be able to move his protruded tongue to the normal side of his mouth. Be aware that if commanded to point the tongue to the good side, some such patients will move their mandible and facial muscles so as to bring the normal angle of the mouth over to the midline tongue. (If the tongue cannot come to the angle of the mouth, the mouth will come to the tongue. That is why you *lightly* hold the mandible.)

If there is ipsilateral basal occipital bone tenderness in the region of the hypoglossal canal (through which nerve XII exits the skull), one is most likely dealing with neoplasia (especially prostatic in the male), even if the patient has already survived long enough to have chronic hypoglossal nerve palsy with hemiatrophy.

The (relaxed) tongue can be examined for fasciculations at rest as well as for myotonia (see Ch. 13, p. 221). The tongue is the *only* muscle in which one can see fibrillations (see p. 493) at the bedside. A fibrillating tongue usually resembles a bag of worms. But at other times, there may just be slight "revolutions" of the tongue near the molars. These findings, of course, have no specific significance related to cranial nerve XII.

For tongue signs of chorea, see page 474.

Skilled Acts

Aphasia and Other Disorders of Speech

How could we arrest scientific and industrial progress? By closing down, or by controlling, laboratories for research, by suppressing and controlling scientific periodicals and other means of discussion, by suppressing scientific congresses and other conferences, by suppressing Universities and other schools, by suppressing books, the printing press, writing, and, in the end, speaking. All these things which indeed might be suppressed (or controlled) are social institutions. Language is a social institution without which scientific progress is unthinkable, since without it there can be neither science nor a growing and progressive tradition. (Popper, 1964, p. 154)

Aphasia is a word coined by Trousseau, meaning loss of speech. Horenstein of Missouri defines aphasia as the inability to initiate or sustain conversation. Technically, most patients categorized as aphasic have some speech and so are actually dysphasic, but the question of the extent of the abnormality is much less important than two other questions: 1) Does the patient actually have an abnormality of speech itself, or of something else (e.g., the mechanism for articulation) that is revealed in the process of speaking? 2) For those patients who truly do have aphasia, what is the specific type?

What Aphasia Is Not

Aphasia is not mutism. Patients with mutism are unable to make sounds, but language function is retained, as may be demonstrated (in literate patients) by reading and writing, two functions that are almost always impaired in the true aphasia.

$$ One method of testing is to show the mute patient the following message, printed in large block letters: "Put your left thumb on your right cheek." Some aphasic patients will not be able to follow this written instruction, but all literate mute patients can. Some patients with mutism can hear, and thus can follow spoken instructions or respond appropriately to "yes-or-no" questions and questions permitting small number responses to be given by holding up fingers. Usually, if one understands the distinction between aphasia and mutism, the diagnosis of mutism will have been made long before reaching the formal neurologic examination.

Aphasia is also not dysarthria. Dysarthria is the inability to articulate clearly. A dysarthric patient does get the approximate sounds in the correct order in the correct words in the correct arrangement. Dysarthria may be due to a neurologic deficit involving the control of the apparatus of sound making (e.g., cranial nerve palsies of VII, IX, X, and XII), or it may simply be due to intrinsic disease of one of the end organs of sound making such as the nasopharynx or tongue. If one remembers the distinction between dysarthria and aphasia, one will usually have made the diagnosis early in the interview. If there is a question, remember that language function is intact in dysarthria, so the patient will be able to respond to written instructions, make nonverbal responses, and write linguistically coherent material, as described above in mutism.

Good repeat-after-me test phrases for dysarthria (but not always for aphasia, vide infra) are, "Methodist Episcopalian," "around the rock the ragged rascal ran," and "Peter Piper picked a peck of pickled peppers."

Persons who distort the vowel /r/ or who substitute /w/ for /r/, tend to engage in destructive behavior toward self or others (Mehrhof & Rousey, 1971).

Aphasia is also not cerebellar speech (see p. 479).

Some apparent abnormalities of speech that are actually abnormalities of mental status may also be detected during the interview. These could conceivably be confusing to the sophomore who did not know the correct definitions of these types of speech. *Word salad* refers to a verbal output characteristic of some (but not all) schizophrenic patients. It sounds jumbled up, like a salad, in the sense that a salad is a mixture of small amounts of many things with no predominant theme. Such patients are quite fluent, but the content of their speech makes no sense. However, this is not aphasia, because the language function is not disturbed. With the schizophrenic patient, it is the thought content that is abnormal, as reflected perfectly in the language that is produced. Fortunately for the sophomore, the schizophrenic patients who produce word salad usually do so in the context of so many other peculiar actions and mannerisms so that the diagnosis is not long in doubt (see p. 520 for diagnostic criteria).

Manic patients may also demonstrate their disease through language. *Push of speech* refers to an accelerated rate of speech and a relative inability to be quiet; it is therefore almost never confused with aphasia. *Flight of ideas* is just that. The main content of the speech is difficult to follow, not because of language problems but because the main subject of the monologue changes so rapidly. *Tangentiality* and *circumstantiality* (see Ch. 2, p. 19, footnote) could also be confused with aphasia by the jejune. However, within the context of the other abnormalities of mania (see p. 525), the distinction should be obvious.

Depressed patients may produce a small quantity of speech, slowly and sometimes softly, but the grammar, syntax, and word choice are all normal.

Caveats

The student must realize three critical facts: 1) The perfect correlation between anatomic localization and abnormality of function that is seen in other areas, say with valvular heart disease or spinal cord disease, does not always exist for aphasia. 2) Most patients will not present with one of the "pure culture" clinical pictures about to be described. 3) The clinical picture resulting from etiologies as diverse as metabolic encephalopathies or brain tumors or Alzheimer's disease may vary from day to day in the same patient, even though the anatomical substrate is presumably unchanged. Nevertheless, there are still useful concepts and methods of examination.

A Method

The examination for aphasia and other disorders of speech (broadly conceived) is carried out in two parts. The first consists of observations of the usual doctor-patient conversation. Look for fluency (the rate of speech) and the latency to beginning speech (S. Horenstein, personal communication, 1988). The second, which is used to classify aphasias, is based upon the patient's response to specific instructions. The specific abstractions from conversations and the specific maneuvers including test phrases are presented throughout this section *ad seriatim*.

The first part of the examination is not in itself sufficient to rule out an aphasia; active testing is necessary.

Table 26-3. Some Common Kinds of Aphasia

Aphasia Type	Spontaneous Speech	Comprehension	Repetition	Associated Findings
Broca's aphasia	Nonfluent	Intact		Paresis of right face and arm
Conduction aphasia	Fluent	Intact	Impaired	
Isolation aphasia	Fluent	Impaired	Intact	
Wernicke's aphasia	Fluent	Impaired	Impaired	Right superior quadrantanopsia
Nominal aphasia	Fluent	Intact	Intact	

Source: *Geschwind (1971).*

Fluent Versus Nonfluent Aphasias

Having determined that the patient does truly have an aphasia, one next wishes to determine whether it is fluent or nonfluent. (Some characteristics of various aphasias are summarized in Table 26-3.)

1. The nonfluent aphasia is characterized by spontaneous speech that is slow, labored, increased in latency, often mumbled, and lacking grammatical niceties such as definite articles or appropriate suffixes. It resembles what one composed in the days of 10-words-per-telegram. For younger readers, it sounds as if the patient is imitating Hollywood's idea of an American Indian speaking English in 1880.

The nonfluent aphasia signifies a lesion in Broca's area (Fig. 26-12).

The patient with bilateral frontal lobe isolation (see p. 515) may at first appear to have a nonfluent aphasia.

2. Fluent aphasias are characterized by speech of normal grammar and at least normal speed, but failure to use the correct words. If asked what class of objects comprises a Plymouth, a Cadillac, and a Toyota, the patient may use an indefinite ("you know,

the thing"), an operational definition ("what you come to work in"), a paraphrasia ("a horse"), or a paranymy ("a bar"). (Paraphrasia has a better prognosis than paranymy. For example, if someone means to say "my sister," but says "my niece," he is at least within the correct class of objects; whereas the paranym "my blister" is not even close.)

Fluent aphasia indicates temporal or parietal lobe lesions.

All of the phenomena of fluent aphasia described above were once called alexia. (There was even thought to be a specific "alexia" center.) Worse, some use the word "alexia" to mean the inability to read words, but that malfunction is usually due to ocular, visual pathway, or occipital disease, not temporal or parietal lesions.)

a. *Conduction aphasia.* To test for conduction aphasia, ask the patient to say, "No ifs, ands, or buts, please." Patients with conduction aphasia understand the directions to repeat the test phrase because their comprehension is intact. But their attempted repetition is impaired, and they will stumble over this particular test phrase. Oddly enough, some of those who cannot do this test phrase can easily repeat some of the longer, seemingly more diffi-

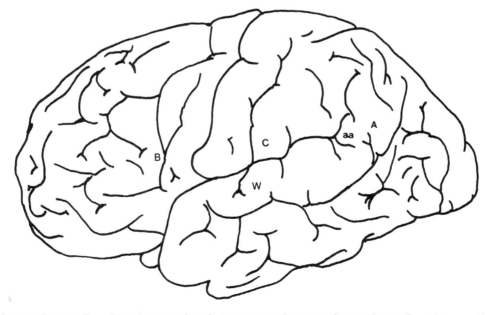

Figure 26-12. *The speech areas. B = Broca's area, where lesions can produce a nonfluent aphasia. C = the general area where lesions produce a conduction aphasia, a fluent aphasia in which the patient will attempt to follow the examiner's instructions, which he does understand. But he will not be able to repeat the test phrase "No if, ands, or buts, please." W = Wernicke's area, where lesions may produce a fluent aphasia, in which the patient can neither understand nor respond to verbal repetition or other tasks.*

In the unhappy circumstance that both Wernicke's and Broca's area are afflicted, the patient will have global (total) aphasia. A = the old "alexic" area where a lesion may leave competence in the spoken language but incompetence in selecting specific words or in writing a letter. Region aa = one area associated with what was formerly called amnestic aphasia, or anomic aphasia in the old classification. Younger neurologists restrict the designation anomia to fluent aphasias in which there is no difficulty with repetition tasks. Younger neurologists would also consider the areas A and aa as overlapping, or perhaps as more appropriate to a phrenology text. Also see Figure 26-13.

cult phrases that have been used. In fact, I have had patients with large cerebral metastases in the area C in Figure 26-12, who could initiate and maintain long goal-oriented discussions (such as those concerned with obtaining cigarette privileges) without any evidence of apparent error in their spontaneous speech, but who could not repeat this phrase with any amount of practice. (Southerners are not penalized for dropping the terminal "s's.")

b. *Isolation aphasia.* These patients are like parrots in that they can repeat any test phrase, but do not understand what they are repeating. They may sometimes fool the examiner, but they can be detected by using a test phrase with a command in it, such as, "put your left thumb on your right ear."

These patients have lesions that surround but do not involve either Broca's area or Wernicke's area. They are very rare.

c. *Wernicke's aphasia.* These patients are unable to comprehend the instructions and are also unable to repeat the instructions. Thus, they fail to produce any test sentence on command.

Additionally, if given spoken instructions and asked to nod yes or no as to whether they understand the instructions, patients with impaired comprehension (as well as those with isolation aphasia) do *not* nod affirmatively. They just stare at the examiner. It is easy to see why this was formerly called receptive aphasia or "word-deafness," although such patients are not deaf. (This can be demonstrated by continuing to speak as you walk in a circle around the patient and observe his head movements.)

(Another way of testing for comprehension is to give spoken instructions or instructions printed on a piece of paper, e.g., "Tear this piece of paper in four parts; give me one, put one on the table, and keep two for yourself, one in each hand." Such instructions require no use of speech in the response. If the patient cannot comprehend, he will not be able to follow the written instructions.)

These patients have lesions in the classical Wernicke's area as shown in Figure 26-12.

d. *Nominal aphasia.* This type of aphasia is most often missed because the patient has intact comprehension and repetition and so passes all the tests above. But, like all aphasic patients, the patient with nominal aphasia has trouble naming objects. Sometimes, a rather long list of objects must be presented. Some neurologists use objects of increasing rarity, such as: 1) a wristwatch, 2) the strap, 3) the buckle, and finally 4) the part of the buckle that fits into the leather hole. Hardly anyone knows the name of the latter (the tongue of the buckle). Thus, it permits testing for neologism: "Make up a word to describe this." (Aphasic patients cannot make up words.) "Pin" would be a good neologism. "Din" would be paranymy.

These patients may have lesions located at the angular gyrus or the adjacent portion of the temporal lobe or sometimes at other places (Fig. 26-12). Sometimes there is no focal lesion but rather a metabolic encephalopathy. Sometimes, this type of aphasia occurs during recovery from one of the other types of aphasia.

You can see why the classification of aphasias has occupied the best minds of neurology for a long time, with a perfect solution not yet in sight.

Determining Cerebral Dominance

Handedness is sometimes a useful piece of information in the aphasic patient who has suffered a stroke, since more than 99% of right-handed persons have their language function in the left cerebral cortex (Baker & Joynt, 1986; DeJong, 1979). Unfortunately, about half of practicing left-handers also have their language function in the left cortex, and a small percentage of these sinistrals may even have bilateral representation.

Still more confusing is the situation with persons who have learned two alphabetic languages and often lose only the newer one after a stroke; yet others will retain the newer language and

instead lose their mother tongue (sometimes through simple disuse, perhaps especially if there is a psychologic reason why the patient wishes to forget the mother tongue). The rule of Ribot states that the oldest language learned is most likely to be kept, and if lost, will be the first to return during recovery. This rule does not always work. Pitres' Law states that the most practiced language, regardless of when it was learned, is the language most resistant to loss and quickest to return. This law too is often repealed. Still worse, there is some evidence that with nonalphabetic languages like Chinese, language function may reside in the right cortex of a right-handed person, although if such persons learn English or another alphabetic language, the language function for the latter resides in the left cortex of a right-handed person. Finally, to show the severe limitation of all the "rules," we have the situation of the Japanese language, which includes both alphabetic and morphogrammatic letters (the latter called kanji). These are learned in school at the same time and are used together in many kinds of printed matter. Yet, when a 32-year-old dextral Japanese woman suffered a proved hemorrhage of the left posterior inferior temporal gyrus, she lost her ability to read the kanji, but retained her ability to read the alphabetic letters and words (Kawamura et al., 1987).

All the above notwithstanding, how does one ascertain handedness in a stuporous, comatose, aphasic, or otherwise uncommunicative patient? One can measure the size of the biceps or attempt to assess venous drainage. These signs, while often indeterminate, have the virtue of being reliable when asymmetric. Sometimes, it is possible to determine the dominant hand of workmen who use specialized tools by searching for calluses that are exclusively or predominantly on the working hand. Beer drinkers who remove the twist-off caps can develop a callus on the inner (opposing) surface of the dominant thumb. Guitar players develop calluses on the fingertips of the nondominant (fret-board) hand; fortunately, sinistrals (like Paul McCartney) usually play their guitars "backward." Tar stains (misnomered "nicotine stains") from burning cigarettes are usually on the fingers of the dominant hand, except in those who smoke while using their dominant hand constantly, such as crossword puzzle enthusiasts or beer drinkers (whose dominant hand is kept busy moving the beer to the mouth), who therefore may have their tar stains on the other hand.

It has been stated recently that the proximal part of the thumbnail on the dominant hand is more square, but in a prospective study this was wrong so often that I have abandoned it. Fraying of the cuff is said to be more exaggerated on the dominant side, but except for some rare occupations not yet encountered among my patients, this has also not been useful.

Agnosias

The agnosias are disorders in which the patient cannot recognize common objects, nor tell their meaning. The patient is not able to answer questions such as, "Is it yours?" "Whose is it?" "Is it bigger or smaller than (something else)?" "What does it mean if it is bigger?"

$$ Usually, only tactile stereoagnosia is tested for. Common objects are placed in the patient's hand without allowing him to see them, and he is asked to identify them. Examples include pens, keys, and coins. It is not necessary for the patient to be able to tell the exact denomination of the coin.

A remarkable case of visual agnosia is described in a classic collection of clinical essays (Sacks, 1985).

Apraxias

Apraxia is the inability to perform a task, and by tradition refers to nonverbal tasks, for example, getting dressed (Fig. 26-13).

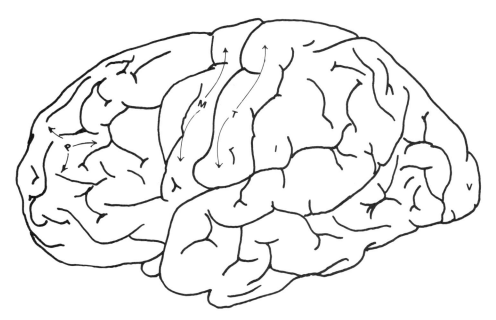

Figure 26-13. *Major areas of the brain. P = the general area where lesions can produce changes in personality. (Such changes can also result from lesions in other areas.) M = the motor area, located just in front of the central gyrus (which is indicated by the hollow arrow). Compare this with Figure 26-12, and you can see why afflications of Broco's area are likely to be accompanied by hemiplegia. T = the sensory area, which includes tactile sensation. It is not surprising that lesions in this area may lead to asterognosis.*

V = vision areas of the occipital lobe where lesions may cause blindness. I = the old ideomotor apraxia area. In ideomotor apraxia, the patient cannot carry out instructions to perform complex motor behavior, although he can understand the instructions and attempt to perform them (e.g., "show me how to blow up a balloon"). However, the patient may be able to perform the same acts spontaneously or in an appropriate emotional imitative context, since the motor area itself is intact. Note the similarity to conduction aphasia in the current aphasia classification, and the fact that the areas are about the same.

$$\$\$$ There are two kinds of apraxia: ideational (due to posterior hemispheric lesions) and kinetic (due to frontal lesions). To distinguish them, take out a wooden match box and ask the patient to strike a light. Patients with ideational apraxia will not be able to slide the box open. (They cannot dial a telephone either.) They may rip it open to get the matches inside. Patients with kinetic apraxia will go to strike the match but will hold it wrong so that it doesn't light or so that it breaks (S. Horenstein, personal communication, 1988).

Meningitis

Stiff Neck

The first physical sign of meningitis is a stiff neck that is resistant to passive motion. However, this sign can also be present in rheumatoid arthritis, cervical osteoarthritis, polymyalgia rheumatica, and a wide variety of other cervical afflictions of the bones, joints, ligaments, and muscles of the cervical area. Thus, if the neck is supple, one can (usually) be reassured of the absence of meningitis. But if the neck is stiff, the problem has still not been localized to the meninges.

In this text, the word "meningismus" is not used to mean stiff neck because it has three other current meanings, all different: 1) signs of inflammation of the brain cortex and its coverings in or near the cervical area (*Dorland's Medical Dictionary*); 2) hysterical mimicry of same (*Dorland's*); 3) (in pediatrics) the same signs occurring in children with infectious diseases or febrile processes as a reaction additionally characterized by an increased cerebrospinal fluid pressure but normal fluid composition (DeJong, 1979). Therefore, *meningismus delende esse.*

Amoss' Sign (also called Hoyne's Sign)

Sometimes the patient with meningitis will sit on the bed with his hips and knees flexed and the neck extended, the spinal column arched lordotically and the extended arms supporting the thorax from behind. This is also called the "tripod sign" because the two arms and the spinal column form a tripod holding up the head extended maximally at the neck. (Actually, the flexion of the hip and the knees is an equally important feature of this sign, although this was not appreciated originally.) The position can be understood as the best way to relieve stretch on the spinal cord and the nerve roots, as will become apparent in the discussion of semiopathophysiology on page 470. A false positive may be seen in ruptured intervertebral disc.

Since not all patients with meningitis are conscious at initial presentation (or for other reasons cannot attain this tripod position), the physician is obligated to perform maneuvers that will evoke the patient's attempt to relieve induced stretch on the nervous system and its coverings. These are the signs to be discussed next.

Kernig-Lasegue and Brudzinski Signs

History

The Kernig-Lasegue sign was first described in 1880 by a Yugoslav physician, Lazarevic ("Bailey," Clain, 1973). He has never received credit for it. His sign is known by two other names to two different groups of specialists, who use it for different purposes. (Having encouraged the student to describe something original in the hope of eponymous immortality, it must now be recalled how many times the original innovator's name is lost to posterity. As Shaw noted, virtue is its own punishment.)

The next year, 1881, the sign was published by Forst, in French, in his M.D. dissertation. Forst credited his teacher Lasegue with having taught him the sign, but Lasegue had not previously published this sign under his own name (Wartenberg, 1950).

In 1882, Kernig published the same test in a Russian journal, and again in German in 1884. Up until this point, it is not clear that any of the authors knew of each other's work, or that they realized they were all describing essentially the same sign.

In 1909, Brudzinski, a Polish physician, described his "neck phenomenon" sign in French, and 2 years later in German. Brudzinski also described a number of other signs (also see DeJong, 1979), but this is the only one that has survived in popular usage, and is the one referred to by physicians as "the" Brudzinski sign.

Methods of Eliciting the Nerve Stretch Signs

The Kernig version had many forms. Sometimes the legs were passively lifted from the bed in an extended position until there was resistance and flexion at the knee. Sometimes they were lifted with the knees in a flexed position until maximal hip flexion was obtained, at which point the knees were extended to check for resistance. And sometimes just one leg was manipulated. Kernig himself usually performed the maneuver with the patient sitting, as described in his own words:

In the majority of cases of meningitis, contractures are not present in the extremities while the patient is lying down, whereas if one tries to extend the knee while the patient remains sitting, one succeeds only to an angle of about 135 degrees. In cases in which the phenomenon is pronounced, a right angle is maintained. The phenomenon is so striking that the difference between the entire absence of this contracture in the reclining position and its presence in the sitting position is so readily seen that it is worthwhile to pay particular attention to this symptom and to look for it in every case (Verghese & Gallemore, 1987).

The Lasegue version has been described in Chapter 24 (p. 422).

In the Brudzinski ("nape-of-the-neck") sign, the legs were not manipulated. Rather, the meninges and nerves were stretched by flexing the neck, while the examiner looked for a flexion response in the lower extremities.

Other signs described by Brudzinski prior to the nape-of-the-neck sign were the identical contralateral reflex sign and the reciprocal contralateral reflex sign. The former is a flexion of the contralateral leg when the hip and knee on one side are passively flexed by the examiner. The reciprocal contralateral reflex occurs when the leg that has flexed responsively begins to extend spontaneously (a motion that resembles a little kick). (Verghese & Gallemore, 1987).

All of these nerve stretch signs are essentially the same (Wartenberg, 1950).

Semiopathophysiology

With vigorous flexion of the neck, the spinal cord moves upward about 1 cm in the lumbar region, and the medulla oblongata may elevate as much as 4 mm. In fact, all maneuvers that put a stretch upon the nervous tissue and its coverings can elicit a limited number of responses. The pain (which will be in the correct distribution of one of the nerve roots) causes resistance to further movement, as in the "tight hamstrings" of the Kernig-Lasegue sign. The stretch can also be mechanically relieved by flexion at the hips and knees. Conversely, when the knee is extended (or flexed), the sciatic nerve root moves down (or up), tightening (or relaxing) in turn the stretch on the spinal cord, mutatis mutandis.

O   In meningitis, the stiff neck is a problem of *forward flexion only*, since that is the motion that puts strain on the meninges. Resistance to lateral flexion, rotation, or extension must be due to some other etiology.

Significance

The sensitivity of Kernig's version was 87% in the hands of Kernig (Kernig, 1907) and 57% in the hands of Brudzinski (Verghese & Gallemore, 1987), who found his own version to be 96% sensitive. More recent series are in the same range although one can no longer be certain that the authors personally examined the patients. The contralateral reflex was present in 66% of the cases of meningitis observed by Brudzinski (Verghese & Gallemore, 1987).

False negatives. With localized inflammation of the meninges, as with the localized meningitis that follows bacterial contamination of a neurosurgical wound, the stretch signs will be negative, since almost all of the meninges that are stretched are not inflamed. Cryptococcal "meningitis" (actually, predominantly an encephalitis) is an especially common cause of false negatives.

False positives. These include the musculoskeletal conditions named in Chapter 24 (p. 423), spinal cord tumor, myelitis, tetanus, cauda equina tumor, "high sciatica," radiculitis, cerebrospinal syphilis, cervical cord trauma, multiple sclerosis, poliomyelitis, subarachnoid hemorrhage, "cystic serofibrinous arachnoiditis," spina bifida (Wartenberg, 1950), sphenoid sinusitis, and other diseases of the spinal cord and its nerve roots, such as carcinomatous meningitis, sarcoid meningitis, and Mollaret's meningitis. Thus, the stretch signs are not as diagnostic for infectious meningitis as many seem to think.

Pediatric Cranial Bruits

In children less than 5 years of age, cranial bruits may be heard in 82% of the patients with purulent meningitis, lasting only 1 to 4 days after the initiation of therapy. Such bruits are not heard in adults with meningitis, and are heard in only 16% of children without fever and only 18% of children with fever but without meningitis (Mace et al., 1968).

Posture

Rigidity

Disease processes that effectively cause transection of the brain at a low mesencephalic level remove the cerebrum from control over the rest of the body. This results in *decerebrate rigidity,* which is characterized by full extension of the head and four limbs.

Decorticate rigidity is due to lesions at a higher level, or even just functional removal of the frontal lobes. This type of rigidity is characterized by flexion of the upper limbs and extension of the lower limbs. If the head is passively rotated to face one side, the arm (as well as the leg) on that side will be extended, but the upper and lower limb on the other side will be flexed. If the head is then rotated to face the opposite direction, the formerly flexed side will now extend and vice versa. If the head is replaced straight forward, the original position is resumed.

Asterixis

Asterixis* is the inability to sustain posture. It is commonly sought in the upper extremities especially as a diagnostic for impending hepatic encephalopathy. It consists of an intermittent, relatively unrhythmic loss of posture, followed by a regaining of posture.

A Caveat for the Sophomore

Asterixis is sometimes referred to as the "liver flap." This is a bad term for several reasons. First, there are many etiologies other than hepatic disease. Second, "flap" implies that the phenomenon occurs only in the hands. While the hands are most frequently examined for this finding, asterixis also may be shown by the fingers, eyelids, tongue, toes, or, for that matter, any part of the voluntary musculature that is required to maintain posture. Finally, the word "flap" implies something rhythmic, while asterixis is really not rhythmic compared with tremors.

A Method

1. Have the subject extend his raised arms at the elbows and wrists, with the fingers extended and spread. Ask him simply to maintain this posture. Do *not* consider any *rhythmic* shaking of the fingers to be asterixis; such movements are tremors.

2. Concentrate on lapses in posture, which is quickly regained, then lost again. These may be rapid, like a tremor, but will be *intermittent* and *nonrhythmic*. Or, there may be a slow flapping of the hands that may seem appear to be rhythmic, but only for a few beats. This can appear like the motion of a child episodically waving an irregular "bye-bye."

Other Methods

Dr. Gert Muelheims of Missouri became frustrated with trying to teach encephalopathic patients to keep their hands maximally extended at the wrist for the purpose of demonstrating asterixis, and so produced an original modification: He requests the patient to squeeze the doctor's hand or the doctor's extended fingers. Patients who are unable to maintain a posture are unable to maintain a steady squeeze.

Dr. J. Posner of New York has the patient squeeze a semi-inflated blood pressure cuff with instructions to maintain the reading. The readings bounce around dramatically in patients with asterixis.

Significance

Although asterixis was discovered in 1949 by Foley and Adams in patients with hepatic encephalopathy, it quickly became obvious that other abnormalities could produce the same lesion.

---

*Asterixis was a made-up word composed in a Greek bar (the Taverna) across from Boston City Hospital. Foley, a well-known wit, used it in a paper, never expecting it to be taken seriously (S. Horenstein, personal communication, 1988).

Perhaps the current importance of asterixis is not the length of the differential diagnosis it suggests, but rather its implication that, whatever the diagnosis, the condition is at a serious point. For instance, in one study of alcoholic liver disease, asterixis was the *only* admitting physical finding that had a statistically significant predictive value for mortality, the rate being 56% in those with asterixis, as opposed to 26% in those without it (Hardison & Lee, 1966).

A list of etiologies, no doubt incomplete, is given in Table 26-4.

Gait

If there is any portion of the physical examination even more difficult to teach didactically than the general appearance, it must be gait. The best way to learn it is to have a more experienced person point out to you the various abnormalities in actual patients. Accordingly, what follows is mostly in the nature of attempting to alert you to the kinds of abnormal gaits that you might see. Since gait is also dependent upon normal bones, joints, and all portions of the nervous system, there will inevitably be some cross-references between this section and others.

Spontaneous Manifestations

The spontaneous manifestations of a gait abnormality consist of what can be seen and heard as the patient attempts to ambulate normally. There are many apocryphal stories of diagnosticians whose consulting rooms were at the end of a long hall so that, watching the patient walk down the hall from the waiting room, the clinician might be able to make the diagnosis even before shaking hands with the patient. This is how they did it.

Table 26-4. Causes of Asterixis

Liver Disease
    Laennec's or other severe cirrhosis
    Drug-induced or other deterioration of prior liver disease

Pulmonary failure, usually due to CO_2 retention, but sometimes from hypoxia (Kilburn, 1965) or bronchogenic carcinoma with bronchial obstruction

Renal failure

Other metabolic encephalopathies (after Conn, 1960)
    Hypokalemia
    Hypomagnesemia
    Bromide intoxication
    Phenytoin intoxication (DeJong, 1979)
    Glutethimide intoxication
    Prochlorperazine intoxication
    Chloral hydrate intoxication
    Intravenous ammonium chloride

Gastrointestinal disease
    Whipple's disease
    Malabsorption syndrome
    Idiopathic steatorrhea
    Toxic megacolon of ulcerative colitis

Miscellaneous
    Congestive heart failure
    Leukemia with sepsis
    Focal brain lesions (Degos et al., 1979)

Inspection

1.   Patients with painful skin lesions on the bottom of the feet or with hyperesthesia (increased sensitivity) due to neurologic disease or dysesthesia (unpleasant, painful sensations) walk with a peculiar light-footed step, carefully putting the foot down and quickly lifting it. They seem to be walking on a bed of hot coals.

2.   Patients with girdle muscular dystrophy, hip dislocation, or weakness of the glutei walk with a waddle like a duck, due to extensor overpull. (Some of these patients also have increased lordosis, but this is usually not possible to see from the front as they walk toward you.)

3.   Patients with ankylosing spondylitis have a normal pace although their stooped position might at first suggest parkinsonism. They tend to take small steps, and to keep their head forward and their hands in front of their body.

4.   The hallmark of the parkinsonian gait (also see p. 475) is that the patient takes very small steps. This is called the *marche a petit pas* (*pas* as in *pas-de-deux*), roughly translatable as "walk of little steps." However, *marche a petit pas* by itself can also be seen in cerebral and spinal conditions. The full demonstration of the specifically parkinsonian gait involves the addition of slowness and the absence of normally associated movements, such as swinging the arms as one walks. Further, the parkinsonian may exhibit difficulty in getting started (first step retardation), festination (a speeding up of the rate of movement after walking is begun), and propulsion (the tendency to fall forward as if the body's center of gravity was always just a little bit ahead of the patient.) Finally, the "peacock phenomenon" may be demonstrated as the patient is about to change directions or speed. As the hip reaches its maximum flexion (as part of the normal gait), it suddenly hitches up like a peacock step. This is actually due to dystonia superimposed upon normal flexion. It is best seen with the patient walking around the room nude, although many patients of either sex are initially reluctant to do this (S. Horenstein, personal communication, 1988).

5.   Patients with spastic paraplegia take short steps, but in contrast to parkinsonism, the toes never seem to leave the floor. Additionally, the knees cross in front of each other as the patient walks, and it is this latter peculiarity that has christened this the "scissors gait."

6.   The circumduction gait is similar to the scissors gait, and is seen in spastic hemiplegia. The afflicted foot seems to be dragged through a convex semicircle as it steps forward in turn, due to inability to flex the hip. If the hall is long enough, the patient will eventually turn toward the wall on the afflicted leg's side.

7.   The "steppage" gait is characterized by a foot drop so that with each step the foot is lifted very high as if the subject were going up steps, but the toe of the lifted foot points down toward the ground in midstep. The foot seems to be walking through invisible tar or bubble gum. This gait is caused by any muscular or neurologic disease that afflicts the tibialis anterior and the long extensors of the toes.

8.   The gait may be very *wide based* in dorsal column disease and other afflictions of light touch and proprioception. The patient with such sensory ataxia may also slap his feet down so as to get increased input from the sensory endings in the feet.

These patients have more difficulty walking with their eyes closed, in contrast to patients with wide-based gait due to cerebellar disease.

9.   Weakness causes "pseudosensory ataxia" and possibly the inability to walk at all. This occurs in any patient who has been bed-bound for a long time, or who has become weakened for other reasons. Such patients ask for help even before they stand up because they think they are going to fall (and they are often right.) They are sometimes erroneously labeled as having a conversion reaction, but their facial expression is not that of *la belle indifference* (the beautiful lack of concern), but of true apprehension (also see gait 10).

10.   Patients with cerebellar disease lurch from the knees, looking exactly like someone who is intoxicated with alcohol and is about to fall to the knees (hence the folk description of "knee-crawling drunk"). The gait is also likened to atrial fibrillation, in that it is an irregular irregularity of rate, range (how far each step is), and direction (S. Horenstein, personal communication, 1988). Sometimes such patients are labeled as malingerers if their doctor does not make accurate observations or does not complete his neurologic examination.

The cerebellar gait is also wide pedestaled, so inspect the intermalleolar distance of patients as they walk. Also ask them to stand with the feet as close together "as is comfortable" and so that they do not fall. The distance between the internal malleoli should normally be 4 cm or less (S. Horenstein, personal communication, 1988).

11.   The malingerer feigning a gait disorder actually lurches from the hips, not the knees. Additionally, the malingerer may intermittently be so uncooperative as to exhibit astasia-abasia ("can't stand, can't move). The latter is also seen in pseudosensory ataxia, but the manner of falling in the two entities is different. The patient with gait 9 or 10 will go down all at once, and so will fall in a sprawl, as if the ankles had been knocked out from under him. The malingerer will instead exhibit a biphasic fall: first, some prefall upper extremity movement from a very stable hips-down pedestal, and then a moment later a "fall" or a crumple in a relatively narrow space on the floor. Such a patient will not sprawl widely, if at all, until the upper torso and arms are quite near the floor. As a rule, he will not hurt himself, although patients with gaits 9 and 10 often will. Accordingly, all these patients should be tested by a strong examiner who stands with his arms surrounding, but not touching, the patient, so as to catch the patient in case of loss of balance.

12.   A very bizarre gait may be seen in Huntington's chorea (see p. 474), although technically it is not truly a gait abnormality, since it is often *not* the same on every step. It is dancelike, unpatterned, and unpredictable. The chorea ("dance") movement disorder may sometimes be complicated by the patient's trying to minimize it or cover it or make it "more natural" by adding purposeful movements on top of the abnormality. Since the latter are truly and obviously volitional, and since the total effect is quite bizarre, these patients are also sometimes misunderstood as uncooperative or malingering.

13.   Patients who walk with their toes turned out simply have fallen arches. This is of little systemic significance outside of countries that have unusual health requirements for military conscription.

Auscultation

At one time, it was possible to make diagnoses by listening to the patient walk down the hall while he was still around the corner and out of sight. Recently, I have not often been with house staff in such quiet places, but will give the tricks of the erstwhile trade for the fans of Sherlock Holmes.

Patients who slap their feet when they walk either have fallen arches or sensory ataxia. Some of the latter, but none of the former, may actually slap with two beats on each step, first putting their weight on the heel and then striking the forefoot separately in an apparent attempt to increase sensory input. You can study this yourself after your foot "falls asleep." Notice the first steps you take with the afflicted foot before "the circulation comes back." (Actually, it is not the circulation, but the nerve transmission.)

A scraping sound alternating with a normal step will sound like a syncopated "slide-thump, slide-thump." This is heard in spastic hemiplegia as well as in unilateral musculoskeletal conditions.

"Slide-slide," without the syncopation, is heard in bilateral musculoskeletal disease, spastic paraplegia, or Parkinson's disease.

A soft plopping step is heard in the steppage gait.

Induced Abnormalities of Gait

1. Have the patient walk once with his eyes open and then again with his eyes closed. If the patient does noticeably worse with the eyes closed, it is a strong clue to a sensory ataxia. If the patient does equally poorly with eyes open or closed, the problem could be in the cerebral motor cortex (motor ataxia) or in the vestibular system or cerebellum.

2. Have the patient walk a straight line in tandem, that is, heel to toe. This exacerbates all gait problems, especially vestibular ones, and is often used for distinguishing the subtypes of cerebellar disease. Patients with lesions of the vermis will have truncal ataxia, and so will fall toward either side, in random distribution. But patients with disease of a cerebellar hemisphere will tend to fall preferentially to the side of the lesion. Be sure to stay close enough to the patient to catch one who falls.

3. Have the patient walk eight steps forward and eight back (the "compass test"). It is best to remove all visual clues: walk with the patient and say, "Keep your eyes closed; I won't let you bump into anything" (S. Horenstein, personal communication, 1988). Those with vestibular or cerebellar disease will stray away from the original path, moving toward the side of the lesion. (With cerebellar disease, the turning may occur only on walking backward.) Eventually, the patient will touch all points of the compass.

4. Have the patient start from a sitting position in a chair. Patients with limb girdle dystrophy and patients with Parkinson's disease have great trouble getting started, as may some patients with motor ataxia.

5. Ask the patient to walk on his heels. This cannot be done in motor ataxia, or with spastic paraplegia or foot drop (steppage gait).

6. Ask the patient to walk on his toes. This cannot be done by patients with Parkinson's disease, sensory ataxia, pseudosensory ataxia, cerebellar disease, spastic hemiplegia, or paresis of the soleus or gastrocnemius muscles.

Movement Disorders

Tremors

Rate

One can make a diagnosis with 90% certainty simply by *watching* the tremor (Jankovic & Fahn, 1980).

If the tremor is slow (3 to 5 Hz*), it is either a cerebellar tremor, which becomes worse with intention, or a parkinsonian tremor, which is worse (i.e., of greater amplitude) at rest. (This last point may be confusing to some in that the parkinsonian tremor may speed up with intention, and this increase in rate is sometimes wrongly described as a "worsening.")

If the tremor is rapid (6 to 12 Hz), it is either primary, chemical, or, if observed with intention, parkinsonian.

State

Try to find a situation in which there is no tremor (usually at rest). If the tremor is persistent only at rest, this almost guarantees the diagnosis of Parkinson's disease. Then try to determine what brings on the tremor. If it appears with the initiation or cessation of a movement, it is probably cerebellar or other "movement-related" tremor. If it appears when holding a posture (e.g., holding the limb out against gravity), it is probably essential, or senile, or chemical (e.g., coffee) or catecholamine induced.

Things are not always as simple as indicated in the last paragraphs. However, there are other clues (e.g., see the "pill-rolling tremor," p. 475).

Etiology

The various etiologies of tremor are summarized in Table 26-5.

Chorea

Chorea means dance, and the term is quite descriptive of this disorder of coordinated movement. As a rule, chorea begins in just one limb and may be interpreted as fidgeting. Later, there may be involuntary facial grimaces, and finally the chorea spreads to the whole body. The chorea may become so violent that the patient throws himself off the bed (*folie musculaire*) in a manner that appears to be the volitional act of an insane person.

Chorea is aggravated by strong emotion. That is worth keeping in mind because of the current tendency to be suspicious of the patient who is worse with strong emotion and a diagnosis that cannot be made by the laboratory. Chorea is a clinical diagnosis; there is no laboratory or imaging procedure.

Chorea may be superimposed upon athetosis (see p. 474).

Types of Chorea

1. Sydenham's chorea (St. Vitus' dance) occurs in acute rheumatic fever. Nowadays, it may be more common in systemic lupus erythematosus (Greenhouse, 1966). It is a state (i.e., it is self-limited).

The disease commonly begins by slight twitchings in the muscles of the face, which gradually increase in violence and variety. The eyelids are kept winking, the brows are corrugated,

---

*One hertz = 1 cycle/second. A cycle is one to-and-fro movement.

Table 26-5. Etiologic Classification of Tremors

Cerebellar
  Cerebellar degenerations and atrophies
  Multiple sclerosis
  Wilson's disease
  Drugs, toxins: phenytoin, barbiturates, lithium, alcohol, mercury, 5-fluorouracil
  Hereditary sensory neuropathy (Dejerine-Sottas)
  Midbrain ("rubral") tremor
  Miscellaneous cerebellar lesions
Parkinsonian tremor
  Idiopathic
  Other: postencephalitic, basal ganglia toxicity (carbon monoxide, manganese, carbon disulfide), striatal toxicity (reserpine, phenothiazines, "designer drugs," etc.), tumor, trauma, vascular, chronic hepatocerebral degeneration, striatonigral degeneration, olivopontocerebellar atrophy, progressive supranuclear palsy, Shy-Drager disease, Wilson's disease, Huntington's chorea, normal pressure hydrocephalus
Chemical and metabolic
  Thyrotoxicosis, hypoglycemia, pheochromocytoma, epinephrine, isoproterenol, caffeine, theophylline and other catecholamine-like agents, levodopa, amphetamines, lithium, tricyclic antidepressants, butyrophenones, thyroid hormone, adrenocorticosteroids, alcohol withdrawal, mercury, lead, arsenic, bismuth, carbon monoxide, methyl bromide, monosodium glutamate, sodium valproate
Primary
  Autosomal dominant
  Senile
  Sporadic
  With peripheral neuropathy: Charcot-Marie-Tooth disease
  With other movement disorders: torsion dystonia, spasmodic torticollis

Source: *Jankovic and Fahn (1980).*

and then elevated, the nose is screwed first to the one side and then to the other, and the mouth is drawn in various directions, giving the patient the most ludicrous appearance imaginable.

If the patient attempts to protrude the tongue it is accomplished with a great deal of difficulty and uncertainty. The hands are kept rolling—first the palms upward, and then the backs. The shoulders are shrugged, and the feet and legs kept in perpetual motion; the toes are turned in, and then everted; one foot is thrown across the other, and then suddenly withdrawn, and, in short, every conceivable attitude and expression is assumed, and so varied and irregular are the motions gone through with, that a complete description of them would be impossible. (Huntington, 1872)

Chorea mollis is a form of Sydenham's chorea in which the patient appears as if weakened on one side of the body because only the other side is contorting. He comes limping down the hallway with only half of the body twisting, grimacing, and gesticulating.

Young persons may also have Dubini's chorea or the electrical chorea of Bergeron and Henoch, which resemble Sydenham's chorea in that they are states (i.e., self-limited).

   2. Huntington's chorea is a trait, not a state (i.e., it does not get better). It comes on gradually, often taking years to develop fully, "until the hapless sufferer is but a quivering wreck of his

former self" (Huntington, 1872). It may begin in any decade; those cases inherited from the paternal side tend to have an earlier onset (S. Horenstein, personal communication, 1988).

The first description of Huntington's chorea was actually given by Elliotson, not Huntington:

> When it [chorea] occurs in adults, it is frequently connected with paralysis or idiotism, and will perhaps never be cured. It is very rare for you to remove the affection if it occurs in an adult, or if it occurs in a local form. It will sometimes take place in one arm only, or in the head, or some of the muscles of the face, so that the person makes faces continually. In cases of this description I have never seen the affection cured. It then appears to arise for the most part from something in the original constitution of the body, for I have often seen it hereditary. (Elliotson, 1832)

A Method

○ **1.**   A simple trick for diagnosing chorea is to ask the patient to stick his tongue out and keep it there.

   2.   The patient with manifest chorea cannot maintain the tongue in a protruded position. (The patient with advanced Parkinson's disease or Wilson's disease cannot keep the tongue *in* the mouth.)

Athetosis

Athetosis* literally means "without posture" or "not capable of being fixed in a position." It differs from chorea in that the athetoid movements are more confined to the head, neck, and distal extremities, especially the upper. Athetoid movements are slower but larger in amplitude (excursion) than normal movements. They differ from asterixis by being continuous between two extremes (e.g., between flexion and extension, or perhaps between internal and external rotation). They frequently contain a pause, in what is called the "habitual attitude." When athetosis ends in dystonia, the habitual attitude is the position in which the patient "gets stuck."

Sometimes it is difficult to decide whether the patient has chorea or athetosis. In such cases, the patient is said to have "choreoathetosis" by analogy with "fib-flutter."

Pseudoathetosis is seen in diseases of sensory input such as tabes dorsalis. The patient seems to be making wide, deliberate, slow excursions of the limbs for the purpose of increasing sensory input. Pseudoathetosis of the hands has been called "the piano-playing tremor."

Hemiballismus

Hemiballismus may be initially confused with chorea, but it is characterized not so much by a dancing motion as by a throwing out of one side of the body in an uncontrolled, episodic, and sometimes violent manner. The patient resembles a hemiparetic playing the net in a volleyball game, hence the Greek name *hemi* (a lateral half of the body) plus *ballismus* (jumping or throwing.) Unlike the other movement disorders, hemiballismus is due to a subthalamic lesion (the nucleus of Luys contralateral to the movement.) Also unlike the movement disorders above, the primary movement occurs at the shoulder (rather than the hand). Physiologically, it is a

---

*The word "athetosis" was invented by Dr. Hammond, who was remarkable for writing the first North American neurology textbook, for being the only neurologist who ever became Surgeon General of the United States, and finally for being the only Surgeon General of the United States who was court-martialed (S. Horenstein, personal communication, 1988).

rebound of the arm (above the head) from a decerebrate posture. Thus, it is actually the limb that is "thrown."

Rubral Tremor

A peculiar kind of tremor is seen in lesions of the superior cerebellar peduncle. The arm is held in extension at the elbow in what is essentially a decerebrate position (see p. 470). It then relaxes, but returns to the decerebrate position. The alternation of the two positions gives the appearance of a tremor. In fact, it more resembles someone with an extended elbow screwing the top on a marmalade jar. Here, all the screwing action is at the wrist, so the Germans call this "Bindearm," an untranslatable word that means something at "wrist-arm" in the sense of "arm motion done by the wrist." Since the tremor is believed to be due to the inhibition of impulses coming from the cerebrum to the red nucleus (nucleus ruber), it is also called the "rubral tremor."

Dystonia

In dystonia, the distortions of movement are due to abnormal tonus in certain muscle groups. Sometimes the dystonia is a minor complication of a neurologic disease *sui generis*. Thus, the extraocular muscles of the globe are actually experiencing dystonia in oculogyric crises of postencephalitic parkinsonism. But in other diseases, the dystonia is the main clinical feature of the disease (e.g., Brueghel's syndrome—isolated blepharospasm and oromandibular dystonia) (Fig. 9-5).

Parkinsonism

These feelings of inward blame and depression became greatly exacerbated and almost unbearable during the oculogyric crises from which Miss H. suffered. These crises, which started in 1928, would come with great regularity, every Wednesday; so much so that I could always arrange for my students to come on Wednesdays if they wished to witness such a crisis. Nevertheless, the times of these crises were modifiable to some extent: on one occasion, I informed Miss H. that my students could not come on Wednesday, but would be coming on Thursday. "OK," said Miss H., "I will put off the crisis to Thursday," and she did. (*Awakenings*, Oliver Sacks)

Disease of the basal ganglia-striatal dopaminergic system can take many forms. The archetype of these is Parkinson's disease*, once misnomered paralysis agitans (shaking palsy). (There is no paralysis, which is a loss of motor function as opposed to a paresis or weakness.) In most cases, the cause is unknown. Cases following viral encephalitis are increasingly rare and carbon monoxide poisoning always was a rare cause. Currently, many cases seem to be pharmacogenic (Table 26-5).

Signs

Gait and tremor. The characteristic gait (p. 472) and tremor (p. 473) have already been discussed. An additional aspect of the parkinsonian tremor is the so-called "pill-rolling" movement of the fingers, in which the thumb moves in opposition to the four fingers, especially the first two. Since pharmacists no longer roll pills, perhaps the term should be changed to the "stem-winding" movement of a watch owner. As such watches

---

*Parkinson's disease was first described by James Parkinson in 1817, 5 years before he described appendicitis and its fatal complication of perforation.

become rare, perhaps we should change to a "jeweler's screwdriver" movement.

Cogwheel rigidity. The best test of the extrapyramidal system (now generally understood to be inclusive of the basal ganglia, the striatum, the substantia nigra, and the descending connections) in terms of diagnosticity is *cogwheel rigidity*. It was once almost pathognomonic of Parkinson's disease, but as both L-dopa and phenothiazines became widely prescribed, drug-induced parkinsonism became a more common cause. However, the latter has recently become less common, due to the popularity of haloperidol as a substitute for phenothiazines.

A method:

1. With the patient relaxed, passively extend the upper extremity at the elbow over a period of about 4 seconds. Then flex the elbow back to the original position over about 3 seconds. Repeat a few times.

2. If the patient has cogwheeling, you will feel alternate periods of resistance and relaxation, occurring about three or four times per 90 degrees of flexion or extension.

3. The sensation is as if you were pulling against a very soft ratchet or cogwheel, each spoke representing an area of resistance, regularly placed. The spaces between the spokes of resistance are the areas of normal easy passive movement. Once you have elicited the finding, it is unforgettable.

An alternate method: Dr. Simon Horenstein of Missouri does not flex at the elbow but rather rotates the arm at the radioulnar joint.

Other signs. Patient's with Parkinson's disease have difficulty performing two tasks simultaneously, as may be demonstrated by asking the patient to "tap the top of your head and stick your tongue out at me" (after you have determined that each task can be performed separately). Although this will exacerbate many movement disorders, it was specifically used in the pre-dopa era as a way of bringing out the movement disorder of Parkinson's disease.

Another useful test, which is based upon the paucity of associated movements in parkinsonism, is *Souques' leg sign*. This may be demonstrated by suddenly thrusting the seated patient backward in his chair. Normally, the legs would kick out as a synkinesia (see p. 487), but in parkinsonism there is no such movement.

As the Parkinson's disease advances, the face becomes very stiff. This can cause interpersonal difficulties because someone interacting with the parkinsonian patient may get no visual facial feedback to what he is saying, and such absence of visual cues is often misinterpreted as sullenness, hostility, or indifference on the part of the patient.

Other features of parkinsonism are a tendency to protrude the tongue (just like Wilson's disease), increased salivation, a monotonous tone to the speech, a general stiffness of all movements, and micrographia (small handwriting). The latter can best be seen by collecting signatures (sometimes from medicolegal release forms) made over a long period of time.

The most eloquent description of the disease and its progression is that of Parkinson himself, who defined the disease as:

involuntary tremulous motion, with lessened muscle power, in parts not in action and even when supported; with a propensity to bend the trunk forwards, and to pass from a walking to a running pace: the senses and intellects being uninjured . . .

The first symptoms perceived are, a slight sense of weakness [not paralysis], with a proneness to trembling in some particular part; sometimes in the head but most commonly in one of the hands and arms [especially the nondominant hand, i.e., the left in most persons]. The symptoms gradually increase in the part first affected; and at an uncertain period, but seldom in less than twelve months or more, the morbid influence is felt in some other part. . . . After a few more months the patient is found to be less strict than usual in preserving an upright posture: this being most observable whilst walking, but sometimes whilst sitting or standing. Sometime after the appearance of this symptom, and during its slow increase, one of the legs is discovered slightly to tremble, and is also found to suffer fatigue sooner than the leg of the other side: and in a few months this limb becomes agitated by similar tremblings, and suffers a similar loss of power.

Hitherto the patient will have experienced but little inconvenience; and befriended by the strong influence of habitual endurance, would perhaps seldom think of his being the subject of disease, except when reminded of it by the unsteadiness of his hand, whilst writing or employing himself in any nicer kind of manipulation. But as the disease proceeds, similar employments are accomplished with considerable difficulty, the hand failing to answer with exactness to the dictates of the will. Walking becomes a task which cannot be performed without considerable attention. The legs are not raised to that height, or with that promptitude which the will directs, so that the utmost care is necessary to prevent frequent falls. . . .

The propensity to lean forward becomes invincible, and the patient is thereby forced to step on the toes and the fore part of the feet, whilst the upper part of the body is thrown so far forward as to render it difficult to avoid falling on the face. In some cases, when this state of the malady is attained, the patient can no longer exercise himself by walking in his usual manner, but is thrown on the toes and forepart of the feet; being, at the same time, irresistibly impelled to take much quicker and shorter steps, and thereby to adopt unwillingly a running pace. In some cases it is found necessary entirely to substitute running for walking; since otherwise the patient, on proceeding only a very few paces, would inevitably fall, . . . as first noticed by Gaubius, who says, "I have seen one, who was able to run, but not to walk."

His words are now scarcely intelligible; and he is not only no longer able to feed himself, but when the food is conveyed to the mouth, so much are the actions of the muscles of the tongue, pharynx, and &c. impeded by impaired action and perpetual agitation, that the food is with difficulty retained in the mouth until masticated; and then as difficultly swallowed. Now also, from the same cause, another very unpleasant circumstance occurs: the saliva fails of being directed to the back part of the fauces, and hence is continually draining from the mouth, mixed with the particles of food, which he is no longer able to clear from the inside of the mouth. (Parkinson, 1817)

Question: *Why does this elegant description omit the cogwheel rigidity that was later described by Duchenne? Write down your answer before consulting Appendix 26-2.*

One must be very cautious not to misdiagnose early Parkinson's as some form of psychiatric illness. For instance, the shaking and the pill-rolling may get worse under emotional duress, but improve when the patient is removed from the actual or threatened noxious situation. In fact, they often disappear completely when the patient is observed during sleep. Even the oculogyric crisis of postencephalitic parkinsonism (basically a spasm of upward gaze) can be delayed by the patient for a considerable period of time (see the

epigram on p. 475). And finally, there is the kinesic paradox of Souques in which the patient can perform under noxious circumstances activities that had been lost in the course of the disease. For example, one immobilized patient in the pre-dopa era suddenly ran into his burning home to successfully rescue a valued object of great weight; following this, he again became immobile. It is easy to see why the neurologically inexperienced could misinterpret some or all of these facts.

Phenothiazine-Induced Movement Disorders

Obviously, any drug that can block striatal dopaminergic receptors can result in an imbalance between the dopaminergic and cholinergic systems in such a way that the dopaminergic system is relatively defective. Thus, dopaminergic blockers, including but not limited to the phenothiazines, can acutely produce a picture that mimics parkinsonism. The cure is obviously to inhibit the cholinergic system by the administration of an anticholinergic drug.

Technically, the above movement disorder could be called a dyskinesia, which simply means an abnormality of movement. However, dyskinesia has been adopted for another movement disorder, *tardive dyskinesia*, which is biochemically the opposite of drug-induced parkinsonism. It tends to come on in patients who have been on chronic dopaminergic blockade, which is being withdrawn or diminished. (Sometimes, the dose has not been changed, but the dopaminergic system just seems to age and to exhibit tachyphylaxis. Often, these patients are also receiving chronic anticholinergic medication.) At this point, tics and dyskinesias of various types suddenly emerge. In this case, the treatment is to increase dopaminergic blockade (the "hair-of-the dog-that-bit-you" approach) and/or to increase cholinergic activity— the exact opposite of the approach to the drug-induced parkinsonism discussed above.

Because these two movement disorders have exactly opposite biochemical causes and treatments, a word about nomenclature is in order. "Tardive" means late or after a long period of treatment. It is used to highlight the fact that tardive dyskinesia (which can almost be thought of as dopaminergic-blocker withdrawal) comes on after a long period of time.

Similarly, "dyskinesia" can and should be modified by indicating the muscle groups involved. The classic fly-catcher dyskinesia, wherein the tongue darts in and out of the mouth like that of a frog catching flies should be called a buccolingual dyskinesia, and if it is a *tardive* dyskinesia, that word should be added to the description.

"Dyskinesia" by itself does not imply a specific etiology, and it should not imply only a facial or lingual dyskinesia. For instance, some patients with tardive dyskinesia can present with chest muscle spasms mimicking cardiopulmonary disorders; others have abdominal wall spasms; and some with diaphragmatic tardive dyskinesia can be quite confusing to the unwary.

Coordination

Dorsal Column Signs
(or Signs Potentially Related to the Dorsal Columns)

The dorsal columns carry the tracts conducting vibratory and position sense up to the higher centers. Therefore, examination of the dorsal columns' integrity really begins with the peripheral examination of vibratory and position (proprioception) sensations (see p. 507ff).

○   Other tests of the dorsal columns, especially of proprioception, may also test cerebellar and vestibular functions. A general principle is that if the patient can perform the task with his eyes open (visual cues available) but not with his eyes closed, it is a sign of impaired proprioception (dorsal column disease); but if the individual cannot perform the test even with his eyes open, it is a sign of vestibular-cerebellar dysfunction.

Romberg Test*

A method:

1. Have the patient stand with his feet together, and his arms at his sides.

2. Stand nearby, not touching the patient but ready to catch him if he falls.

3. Observe the patient for about 20 seconds.

4. Tell the patient to close his eyes. Continue the test for another 30 seconds.

Interpretation. If the patient is able to maintain posture with his eyes open, and then loses it when his eyes are closed, this is evidence of impaired proprioception. But if the patient falls even with his eyes open, the test is positive for cerebellar and vestibular disease. (It is stated that if the patient falls repeatedly to one side, that is a sign of ipsilateral cerebellar disease; however, in the course of the required repeated testing many patients learn that they will fall to that side and so sometimes overcompensate by going to the other side in a lurch. Accordingly, it is suggested that if cerebellar disease is suspected on the basis of the Romberg test, the examiner should immediately proceed to some of the more specific and sensitive cerebellar signs described below.)

False positives: Malingerers will also fall, but they will first flex their knees and engage in other activities to lower the center of gravity and decrease the painful impact. When they learn that they will be caught and protected, they may bend into the protecting examiner from the waist, keeping the legs straight. However, if they are not certain that they will be caught, they may simply collapse in a heap, straight down and not to one side or the other.

False negative: This test was previously known to Morgagni. Romberg reinvented it because his practice as a neurologist was greatly concerned with tabes dorsalis. Nowadays we do not see much tabes, but we see a lot of diabetic neuropathy. This leads to an important false negative: the modern diabetic may have lost position sense in his toes but still have position sense at the ankles, and so be able to perform the Romberg test perfectly.

Cerebellar Signs or Predominantly Cerebellar Signs or Potentially Cerebellar Signs

Also see page 169 for nystagmus, page 456 for the eye signs of acute cerebellar hemorrhage, page 471 for gait, and "Freebies" at the end of this section (p. 479).

Dysdiadokokinesia

Dysdiadokokinesia is clumsiness in performing rapid alternating movements, such as alternating pronation and supination of the hands, or difficulty with the tongue movements required to pronounce "k," "t," or "cu."

---

*Romberg wrote the first neurology textbook. Prior to his work, there was only Morgagni's notebook.

A method:

1. Tell the patient to imitate you and begin by rapidly (150 times/minute) patting your own chest with both hands, using, say, the radial side of each hand.

2. While watching the patient's imitation, increase the speed, looking for differences in rate, range, amplitude, and direction between the patient's two sides (a very sensitive test of unilateral cerebellar disease in itself).

3. Next, begin alternating the side of the hand striking the chest, going to, say the ulnar side for 10 beats and then back to the radial side for 5 beats and finally alternating sides on each blow. Watch the patient to see if one side "lags behind" or falls out of rhythm. Of course, any limb or set of alternating movements may be used (though forearm rotation is generally best), but the test should always be done bilaterally.

Another method. Ask the patient to repeat "Topeka" or "Katy, K-Katy" as fast as possible.

Interpretation. Abnormalities of rate, range, amplitude, and direction occur only in cerebellar disease, so the predictive value of a properly performed positive test is quite high.

Sometimes it is easier to make a determination by listening, not just to "Topeka," but also to the hand-patting test (steps 1 and 2 above). Are rhythm and amplitude maintained, or do you hear a ritardo and diminuendo?

False negatives: Wiener and Nathanson (1976–77) note that many physicians miss unilateral cerebellar disease through not having the patient perform with both hands at the same time. Such a failure obviously deprives the physician of his control side. On the other hand, Dr. Horenstein of Missouri feels that the hands should be done separately because the "good" cerebellum sometimes compensates for the "bad," another type of false negative.

False positives: A false-positive test should be considered a possibility any time the test for dysdiadokokinesia is positive and other cerebellar tests are negative. This can occur in the nondominant hand, which is often less skilled at fine motor performance than the dominant side. It can also occur with frontal lesions that which produce apraxia, due to the fact that the cerebellum, whose posterior lobe receives its major projections from the frontal lobe, is thus rendered "deaf" (i.e., suffers sensory deprivation).

Heel, Knee, Shin Test

A method:

1. Tell the supine patient to place one of his heels on the opposite knee and then to slide the heel all the way down the shin to the great toe.

2. Repeat with the other heel, mutatis mutandis.

Interpretation. Patients with cerebellar disease cannot do this test. If the cerebellar disease is unilateral, the impairment will only be seen with the ipsilateral heel.

As with many of the vestibulo-cerebellar tests, this test may be converted to a proprioception-dorsal columns test by having the patient also perform it with his eyes closed. Patients with cerebellar disease will have an abnormal test with the eyes closed or open;

but patients with proprioception-dorsal columns disease will be markedly improved with the eyes open.

Norman Bass' razor. Repeat the above test on both sides, insisting that the heel be *exactly* 1 inch above the shin. The induced "locking" of the hip joint actually improves the performance of this step in patients with cerebellar ataxia, but does not improve the performance of the test in persons with other causes of poor performance such as malingering.

Finger-to-Nose Test

A method:

1. Hold your finger about 2 feet in front of the patient's face and instruct him, "Touch my finger with your right forefinger."

2. After he does this, say, "Now touch your nose."

3. While he is moving his finger back to his nose, relocate your own target finger in a different quadrant.

4. After he touches his nose, say, "Now touch my finger again."

5. Repeat steps 3 and 4. Increase the speed slightly and do about five trials.

6. Repeat the whole procedure with the patient's other hand.

Interpretation. Look for cerebellar ataxia, which will be manifested by a jerky, asynergic pointing at the target finger of the examiner. Also look for dysmetria (abnormal movement/judgment of distance), which will be manifested by missing the target through lateral displacement at termination of the movement.

Dysmetria is found not only in cerebellar disease, but also in upper extremity proprioceptive disease (which is somewhat rare, occurring in tabes dorsalis and untreated pernicious anemia), as well as in vestibular disease.

But if upper extremity position sense is intact and there are no vestibular signs elicitable, then this is an excellent test for cerebellar disease. In that case, if the abnormalities noted above are found only on one side, then the patient has ipsilateral hemispheric cerebellar disease. (If the signs are abnormal *bilaterally*, the patient either has bilateral cerebellar hemispheric disease or disease of the midline cerebellar structures.)

In unilateral disease, if the test is done rapidly with alternate hands, the "bad" hand will drift or drop toward the floor during the "good" hand's turn (while the "bad" hand is waiting its turn).

A different response. Overpointing can be a sign of loss of depth perception (e.g., in parietal lobe dysfunction, see p. 514).

Because the subject must be allowed to look at the target finger, the test in its present form does not lend itself to repetition without visual clues; therefore, an alternate method is described to permit the differentiation of cerebellar and vestibular disease.

An alternate method:

1. Have the patient extend his arm laterally. The movements here are initiated with the patient looking straight ahead and therefore lacking visual cues.

2. With flexion permitted only at the elbow joint, ask him to place his forefinger on the tip of his nose.

This test could be modified to permit visual clues by having the patient rotate his head toward the side of the tested forefinger.

Truncal Ataxia

While limb ataxia is a sign of unilateral cerebellar hemisphere disease, truncal ataxia is a sign of disease of the posterior vermis and archecerebellum. It is not necessary to get the patient to stand up for this, an important point since many of the patients so afflicted are unable to get out of bed. Even if the patient can simply be made to sit up in bed, patient observation will often be rewarded within 30 seconds by a torso that sways like a palm tree in a gusting Beaufort-scale-six wind.

Alternately, if the patient can sit on the side of the bed, sit down next to him. Normal patients will adjust their position; patients with truncal ataxia will not. This may be the first or only sign to occur in children with posterior midline tumors (S. Horenstein, personal communication, 1988).

Rebound Phenomenon of Stewart and Holmes

A method:

1. Have the patient flex his arm at the elbow, and attempt to extend it against the examiner's resistance, as during the testing of triceps strength.

2. Suddenly release the resistance.

Interpretation. If the arm goes into *complete* extension, with a force jerking the patient upward and forward, the test is positive. This is, of course, just one more test of the impaired reciprocal inhibition seen in cerebellar disease, since normally one can stop the contraction of the extensors and initiate the contraction of the antagonistic flexors prior to reaching full extension.

Other authors' instructions to the contrary, this test should not be done in the opposite direction (as during testing of the biceps' motor strength) as the patient with cerebellar disease may strike himself in the face. Although this has been used as a test for malingering (since the malingerer has normal reciprocal inhibition and so will not strike his own face), it is a test for *cerebellar* malingering only. Contrary to some opinion, the absence of flexion rebound in a patient with simple asthenia of that upper extremity does *not* prove malingering. It simply proves that the patient has no detectable cerebellar disease.

Cerebellar Drift

Because of the inability to maintain posture in vestibulo-cerebellar disease, there are a number of signs based upon "cerebellar drift," the inability of the patient to maintain a limb in a given posture without its "drifting away" from its original position. The Romberg test (see p. 477) is one of these. The test given here is done without the patient seeing the limb and so should be used when vestibular and proprioceptive disease have been otherwise excluded, or else modified by repeating the test with and without visual clues. This test is optimal for unilateral disease since the limb ipsilateral to the cerebellar lesion is the one that drifts and the other is the control.

A method:

1. Ask the patient to hold his arms in front of him, extended at the wrists and elbows, palms down.

2. Have him close his eyes, and instruct him to keep his arms "there."

3. Watch the patient for 2 minutes to see if one limb begins to drift away from its position.

False positives. Patients with noncerebellar disease may fail this test, but in ways different from the patient with cerebellar disease. In the latter, the drift may occur in any direction from the shoulder, whereas the paretic arm will never drift superiorly or laterally. Further, the paretic arm may begin to "drift" inferiorly, but then instead of continuing a steady drift as with cerebellar disease, it will simply collapse downward. More frequently, the paretic arm will roll into the pronator drift sign (see p. 483), as may also occur with Sydenham's or Huntington's chorea. Also see Barre's sign (p. 483).

Freebies

There are other cerebellar signs that may be casually noticed during the examination of the patient but that are not usually specifically sought.

1. *Cerebellar speech* is irregular, jerky, and briefly monotonous and slow, with sudden punctuations by exposive increases in rate and volume, as if a poorly tuned motorcycle were speaking.

2. After the patellar jerk has been elicited, the leg will continue to swing back and forth several times before it comes to rest. (*Before* eliciting the knee jerk, make sure there is room for the leg to swing back, should this sign be present.) This is called the *pendular knee jerk.* (The test also works with the triceps jerk.) It is the best test for hypotonia, which may also be noted by the experienced examiner during muscle testing.

3. Eye signs of cerebellar hemorrhage have been listed in Table 26-1 (p. 456). But there is a special type of eye sign seen in unilateral cerebellar disease, called *skew deviation.* Both eyes deviate away from the side of the cerebellar disease, the eye ipsilateral to the lesion also turning downward, while the contralateral eye turns upward. This sign results from a lesion of the cerebellar peduncle as it enters the brain stem.

The cerebellar signs are intellectually appealing for two reasons. First, they are easy to learn to perform; and second, when one of them is present, others usually will be found. (This is true for clinicians beginning with the patient and progressing toward the diagnosis. If one begins with the CT scan and then tries to reason back to the physical, one can occasionally find a cerebellar metastasis that has not yet caused any physical findings.)

Vestibular Signs and Predominantly Vestibular Signs

Doll's Eye Reflex

Also called Bielschowsky's doll's-head eye reflex (the original term), the doll's head, or the doll's eye sign or maneuver, or the oculocephalic reflex, sign, or maneuver, this is a useful test in comatose patients in whom there is a question as to whether the midbrain and its reflexes have been preserved.

In a comatose patient over 6 months of age with an intact midbrain and vestibular reflexes, the eyes will maintain the original direction of gaze as the patient's head is passively turned. This means that the eyes are fixed on the same point in the room as the patient's head is moved, which means that the globes move within the head proportionally to the movement of the head but in a direction opposite to the passive motion of the head. If you stare at the right edge of this page as you rotate your head to the left, you are maintaining the *"original* direction of gaze."

Interpretation. The slow rotation activates the vestibular apparatus, which provides input to the midbrain, which instructs the extraocular muscles to move the globes so as to maintain the original direction of gaze, as if the patient were still focusing on an object. But if there is midbrain damage or dysfunction, these reflexes are lost, and passive rotation of the head will not result in movement of the globes to maintain the original direction of gaze. Rather, the eyes will continue to stare in whatever direction the head is pointed. It is as if they were the eyes of a doll, which are painted onto the skull.

Caveat. Since the doll's eye test involves the passive rotation of the skull in a patient who is unconscious, we must remember to assure ourselves of the integrity of the cervical vertebrae before performing this test. If one cannot be assured of this, one should proceed directly to caloric testing.

Very advanced. If the patient is awake and has intact cerebral function, he will probably continue to look wherever you point his head. This is clearly not evidence of midbrain disease. Thus, the test has been used by some to test for bilateral cerebral disease. That is, if the original direction of gaze is maintained on rotation of the head of a noncomatose patient, it becomes evidence for bilateral cerebral hemisphere disease (with the unmasking of the "normal" midbrain reflex). I personally don't use this test for this purpose since some normal patients will maintain their original direction of gaze as you turn their head because they assume you want them to do so.

Amanuensis. The doll's eye test should *never* be reported as positive or negative. Rather, the reporter should state whether or not the eyes maintained their original direction of gaze on lateral rotation of the head.

First, if the examiner is testing a comatose patient for midbrain disease, the test will be "positive" for disease if the eyes *do not* maintain their original direction of gaze. But if the examiner is testing for bilateral cerebral disease, the test is "positive" if an awake patient *does* maintain his original direction of gaze.

Second, the doll's eyes reflex also operates in the vertical direction ("setting sun sign"), and has been so used in the study of paralysis of upward voluntary gaze (see p. 455). Unfortunately, dolls have been manufactured in which the lid-globe apparatus is so counterbalanced against gravity that when the doll is moved from an erect to a supine position, the globes move and the eyes close (the doll "goes to sleep"), unlike the usual doll's eyes that are painted on. Thus, the use of "positive" and "negative" (or doll's eyes "present" or "absent") guarantees almost endless confusion.

Vestibular Finger-to-Nose Test

This is a test of upper extremity proprioception, of the cerebellum, and of the vestibular apparatus. Because upper extremity proprioception is usually normal (as can be independently determined, see position sense testing on p. 508), this is used as a test for the cerebellum and the vestibular apparatus. For the latter, the test is used in conjunction with one of the vestibular stimulation tests (calorics and the various motion tests, vide infra).

A method:

1. Have the patient touch your fingertip, as in the original version of this test on page 478.

2. After he touches your finger, have the patient touch his nose as before.

3. Tell him to close his eyes.

4. Immediately ask him to touch your (*unmoved*) finger again.

Interpretation:

1. With cerebellar disease, the patient will probably show a cerebellar intention tremor.
2. If the lesion is not unilateral, the patient will "past point" on either side (randomly) an equal number of times. With unilateral vestibular or cerebellar disease, the patient will past point only to one side.

Spontaneous Nystagmus

Before performing the tests for induced nystagmus (vide infra), check for baseline nystagmus (see Ch. 10, p. 161, for a description of various types of nystagmus).* In the awake patient, nystagmus has two components: the fast (jerk) cerebral component and the slow vestibular component. If there is a destructive lesion of one vestibular nerve or labyrinthine apparatus, there may be a spontaneous nystagmus in which the *slow component looks at the diseased side*. This simple observation has saved a lot of people a lot of time.

If the fast component is always in the same direction (regardless of whether the eyes are looking to the left or the right), the lesion is labyrinthine. If the fast component labyrinthine (vestibular-ear unit) changes direction with changing direction of gaze, always showing the fast component in the direction of gaze, then the problem is not labyrinthine but in the brain stem (including drug intoxications).

If the nystagmus is *always* rotatory, regardless of position or stimulus, then the lesion is in the brain stem and not vestibular.

Vertical nystagmus is always due to a lesion in the brain.

If nystagmus is present only and always together with vertigo, then the patient has vestibular disease, and thus may have Meniere's disease (see p. 461). However, if the nystagmus and vertigo are dissociated, Meniere's is excluded because the lesion must be in the brain stem (S. Horenstein, personal communication, 1988). With Meniere's syndrome, there is no nystagmus between spells with eyes open, but it may be present with eyes closed (Alford, 1972).

Nystagmus on rapid rising results from disease in the posterior semicircular canals, not the brain stem. Thus, it is important to make the physical examination appropriate to the history. If the patient complains of vertigo (not lightheadedness) on rapid rising, have him stand up quickly and check whether nystagmus occurs at the same time (S. Horenstein, personal communication, 1988).

Additional comments on nystagmus are found in Chapter 10 (p. 161).

Caloric Testing

To test the integrity of the labyrinthine apparatus, the midbrain, and the oculomotor efferents, heat and cold are used to induce thermal currents in the vestibular endolymph. These in turn produce nystagmus, provided that the neural tissue specified above is intact.

A method:

1. If the patient is supine, tip his head up about 30 degrees. This ensures that you get maximal stimulation of the horizontal canals and so produce horizontal nystagmus.

For the conscious patient: If the patient is sitting, tip his head back about 60 degrees. If you leave his head upright, you will get maximal stimulation of the vertical canals, which produces rotatory nystagmus. Having the conscious patient wear a pair of strong convex lenses prevents him from accommodating to the stimulus by visual fixation, yet still permits the examiner to see the nystagmus. Alternately, Dr. Broadwater of Missouri simply has the patient close his eyes; nystagmus can be detected from the corneal bulges in the lightly closed lids.

This test may cause the conscious patient to vomit. Be sure to have a bucket close by.

---

*Also see Chapter 4 (p. 68) for instructions about the *naming* of nystagmus. In this chapter the convention of neurology tests will be followed when possible: the nystagmus is named for the *fast* component.

O   Cerebellar nystagmus, unlike caloric nystagmus, is not position dependent.

2. Pour 100 ml of very cold water in one of the external canals after you have assured yourself that there is no perforation of the tympanic membrane.

Comment: The purpose of the ice water is not to give the patient frostbite of the tragus, but to set up a thermal current in the endolymph. If you use cool water (20°C), you can eventually get the same effect, but it will require about a quart of water. With ice water, you can get a nice effect with only 5 to 30 ml, starting in about 20 to 30 seconds and lasting about 1 minute.

The same thing goes for warm water, should you care to use it. You can use a quart of 50°C water, or smaller volumes of hotter water. The fact that this test is usually performed on unconscious patients should not encourage you to scald the tympanic membrane; test the temperature against the back of your hand.

3. Look for nystagmus in the conscious patient, or deviation of the eyes in the unconscious patient. In the conscious patient, the cold-induced slow component comes toward the stimulated ear, and the fast jerky compensatory cerebral component, for which the nystagmus is named, moves opposite. With warm water, the directions are reversed. (Thus, the mnemonic COWS = cold opposite, warm same.)

Interpretation:

1. In unconscious patients, there can be no nystagmus because there is no fast cerebral component. The unopposed slow cerebellar/vestibular component appears as tonic deviation toward the cold side. If both sides are stimulated with cold, the eyes look downward (Plum & Posner, 1972).

2. In conscious patients, the absence of thermally induced nystagmus on just one side means that a destructive lesion (labyrinth or vestibular nerve) is ipsilateral. The absence of an inducible response bilaterally means there is bilateral disease, which by Occam's Razor is probably in the brain stem.

3. In conscious patients, a trick for amplifying the nystagmus so that it is more easily seen is to have the patient look to the side away from the cold-stimulated ear rather than straight ahead.

Lateral past-pointing and falling, which can be checked for at the same time, are, however, still *toward* the side of the cold irrigation.

4. Some lesions such as expanding tumors, abscesses, vascular aneurysms, and so forth initially go through an irritative phase before they become destructive. At this point, there is simply an exaggeration of all normal responses. For instance, cold stimulation of the diseased side will produce nystagmus (fast component to the healthy side), which can be accentuated on lateral gaze to the healthy side. There is also falling and past-pointing to the afflicted side. This phase of the disease does not usually last long, but can occasionally be confusing if one does not know about it.

Barany Chair Test

If you can find an old-fashioned barbershop chair with a headrest and a spinning base, you can try this one. (Remember that most Veterans Administration hospitals have a barbershop with such a chair.) A desk swivel chair could also be used.

A method:

1. Instruct the patient to close his eyes and place his head against the headrest, which is tilted 60 degrees backward (from vertical) or 30 degrees forward (from horizontal).

2. Spin the chair to the patient's right 10 times as fast as you can and abruptly stop it with the patient facing you.

3. Tell the patient to open his eyes.

4. Normally, the patient will have nystagmus with the slow component going to the right (the direction in which the patient was spun).

5. If the patient attempts to stand, he will fall, or more commonly will lean to his right while seated.

6. Hold a finger up directly in front of the patient and ask him to touch it with his forefinger. Normally, he will past point to his right.

7. Repeat, spinning the chair to the patient's left (mutatis mutandis).

Interpretation:

1. Destructive lesions cause the absence of the normally elicited responses (Steps 4 to 6 above).

2. If only some of the responses are lost, the patient may have an intramedullary lesion.

3. Various other interpretations of these tests have been offered without any good data from large series. But the availability of the CT scan increases the opportunity for definitive analysis of all patterns of response. Unfortunately, it has also made these tests less urgent for cerebellar and midbrain lesions, which can now be imaged in vivo.

Drop Test (Nylen, Barany, Hallpike Maneuver)

This is a unilateral vestibular stimulation test for positional vertigo.

A method:

1. Rehearse the patient once before doing the test.

2. Have the patient, sitting on his bed, maximally extend his head (to 45 degrees) and turn it 45 degrees to one side.

3. Hold his upper body.

4. Let the patient suddenly drop backwards, his head over the edge of the bed.

5. Repeat, with the head rotated to the opposite direction. (The "down" ear is the one being tested.)

Interpretation. Whichever down side produces nystagmus is the side causing the positional vertigo.

With labyrinthine disease, there is a 4- to 5-second latent period between the movement and the onset of nystagmus. In brain stem disease, there is no latent period.

Other Tests

Nystagmograms and formal Barany chairs permit quantitation and extension of these principles but are usually not available to the generalist. Similarly, alteration in the position of the head permits stimulation of different semicircular canals in both the caloric and the Barany chair tests (see DeJong, 1979).

The Politzer maneuver is discussed in Chapter 11 (p. 213).

Motor Examination

I had to report on papers along with everyone else, and the first one I was assigned was on the effect of pressure on cells —Harvey chose that topic for me because it had something that had to do with physics. Although I understood what I was doing, I mispronounced everything when I read my paper, and the class was always laughing hysterically when I'd talk about "blastospheres" instead of "blastomeres," or some other such thing.

The next paper selected for me was by Adrian and Bronk. They demonstrated that nerve impulses were sharp, single-pulse phenomena. They had done experiments with cats in which they had measured voltages on nerves.

I began to read the paper. It kept talking about extensors and flexors, the gastrocnemius muscle, and so on. This and that muscle were named, but I hadn't the foggiest idea of where they were located in relation to the nerves or to the cat. So I went to the librarian in the biology section and asked her if she could find me a map of the cat.

"A *map* of the *cat* sir?" she asked, horrified. "You mean a *zoological chart!*" From then on there were rumors about some dumb biology graduate student who was looking for a "map of the cat."

When it came time for me to give my talk on the subject, I started off by drawing an outline of the cat and began to name the various muscles.

The other students in the class interrupted me: "We *know* all that!"

"Oh," I say, "you *do*? Then no *wonder* I can catch up with you so fast after you've had four years of biology." They had wasted all their time memorizing stuff like that, when it could be looked up in fifteen minutes.

(Reprinted from "*Surely You're Joking, Mr. Feynman!*," *Adventures of a Curious Character*, Richard P. Feynman, as told to Ralph Leighton. Edited by Edward Hutchins. By permission of W.W. Norton & Company, Inc. Copyright ©1985 by Richard P. Feynman and Ralph Leighton.)

Muscle Strength

Resistance Testing

Initially, one should test muscle strength in classmates and patients with no known muscle or neurologic disease, using the time-honored method of opposition (vide infra). Because all of these folks are presumably normal, one is testing to become familiar with the routine and to learn of the range of biologic variability. Also, one can become familiar with the sensation of uniform resistance that occurs when a muscle is overpowered.

Muscles that are truly weak give way smoothly when resistance is overcome. This is to be distinguished from voluntary release, which occurs in one of two ways: some will actively and successfully resist for a few moments, then suddenly let go, while others will attempt to simulate the gradual release of true weakness. Deliberate relaxation always produces a series of small "cogwheel" steps (Hall, 1983).

Although establishing the patient's cooperativeness during the examination is important, the discovery of voluntary release does not necessarily guarantee that the disease is of the higher centers. Patients may feign gross weakness to ensure that the doctor will not overlook a minor degree of real muscle power loss (Hall, 1983). Also, voluntary release may occur because of pain.

1. *Biceps*: Have the patient make a fist, with his elbow partly flexed and the distal knuckles pointing toward himself. Place your hand on his knuckles or wrist and offer a resistance to further flexion. Say, "Pull my hand against your shoulder."

2. *Triceps*: With the forearm positioned to move in a plane parallel to the floor, offer resistance to the dorsum of the hand, instructing the patient, "Push me away from you." Be sure to start resistance at 130 degrees of extension, since before that point the muscle is disadvantaged mechanically. It is easier to detect weakness if much resistance is expected.

3. *Deltoids and shoulder girdle*: Exert pressure on the lateral aspect of the resting upper arm, and ask the patient to, "Push my hand up in the air as far as you can."

○ Inside 15 degrees of abduction, the supraspinatus (predominantly C4) acts, but the deltoid (C5) does not. When tested within that 15-degree arc, the shoulder will elevate if the supraspinatus is weak, as the trapezius is recruited to substitute.

4. *Palmar interossei*: Instruct the patient to spread his fingers. Insert your own fingers into the interspaces and urge the patient to "Cut my fingers off, like with scissors." Do not allow the patient to flex his fingers during this maneuver.

5. Flexion and extension of the wrist may be tested next, and any individual muscle groups of special interest (see advanced section, Table 26-6).

6. *Lower extremity*: Check flexion and extension of the knee and flexion, extension, abduction, and adduction of the hip. As with the upper body, it is important to test girdle strength (hip flexion), because some myopathies preferentially afflict the proximal muscles and pelvic girdle while sparing the more easily tested distal muscle groups. In addition to resistance testing, a good test of the pelvic girdle is to have the patient arise from the squatting position without the use of the hands. Another is the "timed stands" test (vide infra).

○ The importance of checking abduction at the hip is that this motion is affected in L5 root disease, but not in disease of the peroneal nerve below the knee (S. Horenstein, personal communication, 1988).

7. In testing the power of plantar flexion, it may be helpful to have the patient perform 10 toe raises on both feet and 10 more on each foot separately. This fatigues the calf muscles and accentuates minimal differences in strength (Hall, 1983).

○ To test the soleus (always S1), one must put the gastrocnemius muscle out of action by flexing the knee to 90 degrees, then having the patient perform plantar flexion against your hand's resistance.

8. Testing extension (dorsiflexion) of the big toe alone (exclusively or almost exclusively L5) is one of the keys to diagnosing sciatica. A subtle weakness in the extensor hallucis longus is much more easily detectable than slight weakness in a much larger muscle.

"Timed Stands" Test

To evaluate and follow patients with polymyositis, the following standardized test has been described (Csuka & McCarty, 1985):

Using a stopwatch, measure to the nearest tenth of a second the time required for a subject to complete ten full stands from a sitting position in a plastic molded straight-back chair 44.5 cm high and 38 cm deep. Subjects are permitted one practice stand to learn the task, and are then encouraged to perform it as quickly as possible. Use of the arms is not allowed. Subjects with symptomatic arthritis, morbid obesity, or incapacitating lung or heart disease cannot perform the task. Normal times in women varied from 10.9 seconds at age 20 to 21.8 seconds at age 85, and for men ranged from 8.8 seconds at age 20 to 21.5 seconds at age 85. The prediction equations were: for women, time (seconds) = 7.6 + 0.17 × age, and for men, time = 4.9 + 0.19 × age.

Of course, this test which evaluates endurance, rather than just momentary force, can be used to follow patients with any cause of muscle weakness.

Testing Gentle Motor Exertions

A test that detects patients who are uncooperative or suffering from conversion, suggestion, or autohypnosis relies on the fact that persons with motor weakness (e.g., from a stroke) also lose the ability to perform slight, gentle motor exertions. Hold up something that will bend on the application of slight force, such as a calling card, an index card, a plastic ruler, or a wound piano string. Ask the patient to touch the top of it "as lightly as possible." Patients with motor weakness from stroke, for example, press down so hard that they visibly bend the object. Patients with the other types of diagnosis *are* able to touch it lightly.

Detailed Testing of Individual Muscles

In testing patients with neuromuscular disease, each pair of muscles should be scored individually, according to Table 26-6 (the muscle examination sheet of the National Foundation for Infantile Paralysis). This may seem unnecessarily finicky, as a provident nature has given us paired muscles, allowing right-left comparisons. However, in cases of symmetric impairment, these operational definitions are very useful.

The interrater agreement on precise grade of muscle strength is between 48% and 75%; intrarater agreement is 54% to 65%. Allowing a difference of one grade, interrater agreement was 90% to 95% and intrarater agreement 96% to 98% (Iddings et al., 1961).

Table 26-6. Muscle Examination

				Key
100%	5	N	Normal	Complete range of motion against gravity with full resistance.
75%	4	G	Good*	Complete range of motion against gravity with some resistance.
50%	3	F	Fair*	Complete range of motion against gravity.
25%	2	P	Poor*	Complete range of motion with gravity eliminated.
10%	1	T	Trace	Evidence of slight contractility. No joint motion.
0%	0	O	Zero	No evidence of contractility.
	S or SS			Spasm or severe spasm.
	C or CC			Contracture or severe contracture.

*Muscle spasm or contracture may limit range of motion. Place a question mark after grading a movement that is incomplete from this cause.

	LEFT		RIGHT
NECK		Flexors	
		Extensors	
TRUNK		Flexor	
		Extensors—thoracic	
		Extensors—lumbar	
		Rotators—External oblique	
		Internal oblique	
HIP		Flexors	
		Extensors	
		Abductors	
		Adductors	
		External rotators	
		Internal rotators	
KNEE		Flexors—hamstrings	
		Extensors	

continued

Table 26-6—*continued*

	LEFT	RIGHT
ANKLE	Plantar-flexors—gastroc. & soleus	
	Dorsiflexor (tibialis anterior)	
FOOT	Invertors—anterior and posterior	
	tibial	
	Evertors—peroneus longus and	
	brevis	
TOES	Flexors	
	Extensors	
SCAPULA	Abductor—serratus anterior	
	Adductor—rhomboids	
	Elevators—levator scapulae,	
	trapezius	
SHOULDERS	Abductor—deltoids	
	Abductor—supraspinatus	
	Adductor—pectoralis major	
	Extensors—latissimus dorsi, teres	
	major	
	Flexors—coracobrachialis,	
	ant. deltoid	
	External rotators	
	Internal rotators	
ELBOW	Flexors	
	Extensors	
FOREARM	Supinators	
	Pronators	
WRIST	Flexors—radial deviation	
	Flexors—ulnar deviation	
	Extensors—radial deviation	
	Extensors—ulnar deviation	
THUMB	Abductors—abductor pollicis	
	longus	
	Abductors—abductor pollicis	
	brevis	
	Adductors	
	Flexors	
	Extensors	
	Opponens	
FINGERS	Opponens—5th finger	
	Flexors—metacarpophalangeal	
	Flexors—proximal interphalangeal	
	Flexors—distal interphalangeal	
	Extensors	
	Abductors	
	Adductors	

Source: *Leopold (1952).*

More detailed methods of testing each function are given in Table 26-7.

○ In using Table 26-7, remember that *innervation is written in protoplasm, not stone.* No two authorities agree on all the branches of the nerves because there is a wide range of biologic variability.

A Note on Muscle Tone

A spastic paralysis, associated with muscle hypertonicity and exaggerated deep tendon reflexes, results from lesions of the brain or from interruption of the descending tracts. In contrast, lower motor neuron or peripheral nerve lesions produce a flaccid paralysis. (Also see Ch. 24.)

A Note on Hemiparesis

Localizing Cortical Lesions

The areas of the motor cortex controlling various parts of the body have been determined experimentally (Fig. 26-14).

Signs of Fatigue

Pronator drift. Rather subtle weakness may be detected by having the patient close his eyes and hold both arms, palm up, extended at the wrist and elbow. The hand of the hemiparetic arm will tend to pronate (also see cerebellar drift, p. 478).

Barré's sign. Have the patient lie prone with his knees flexed at a 90-degree angle. The weak leg will tend to flex or extend further. False positives occur in cerebellar disease.

Costal Excursion

In hemiparesis of cerebral origin or in regional disease of the spinal cord, the vigor of costal excursion is lessened as well as the vigor of movement of the skeletal muscles. It is not detected when only the extent of costal movement is observed and the vigor of movement is neglected. The intercostals have a bihemispherical supply quite like the frontalis.

The familiar method of differentiating a supranuclear from a nuclear or infranuclear facial palsy is to determine the share of the frontalis in the paresis. We find, however, that, although the forehead may be symmetrically wrinkled in cases of cerebral facial paresis, the wrinkles are not so firmly held against a smoothing pressure on the affected side. It is exactly the same with the intercostal muscles.

In some cases of cerebral palsy, the thorax of the affected side can be seen to have a diminished extent of excursion; in other cases, the two sides are seen to move symmetrically. But in all cases of complete cerebral hemiparesis or when the upper and lower extremities of one side are involved, the vigor of costal excursion is diminished on the affected side. The neurologists have differed in their opinions on this subject because they have observed only the extent of costal movement. It is true that in many cases the extent of excursion is symmetrical on the two sides, but if the patient makes forced inspirations and the vigor of costal movement on the two sides alternately is compared, the ribs on the paretic side will always be found to move with less vigor. (Hoover, 1926)

Differentiation from Disorders of Higher Cortical Centers

Dr. Bill Domm of Virginia was wont to examine the shoes of patients claiming hemiparesis. If the patient was truly hemiparetic around the clock and not just in front of the doctor, the shoes would be worn asymmetrically in a manner congruent with the patient's observed gait.

Of course, some patients with disorders of the higher centers, such as a conversion reaction, may well be hemiparetic all of the time regardless of the doctor's presence. These are also the patients who may eventually develop a disuse atrophy of the concerned muscles, which atrophy is misinterpreted as evidence that the patient does not have a disorder of the higher centers but rather a peripheral neuropathy. Accordingly, we will now discuss

Table 26-7.   Testing Motor Function

Maneuver	Muscles Tested	Peripheral Nerve	Spinal Cord Segments
Neck flexion. Have supine patient raise head from the bed. Place your hand on his forehead and instruct him to push against it.	Sternocleidomastoids Profundi colli	Spinal accessory Cervicales	(Cranial nerve XI) C1-C4
Neck extension. Place patient prone, with head extending beyond the top of the table. Place your hand on his occiput and ask him to push against it.	Longissimus capitis and cervicis Trapezius	Cervicales Spinal accessory	C1-C4 (Cranial nerve XI)
Trunk flexion. Have patient lie on a firm surface with knees flexed. Hold his knees and have him do a sit-up.	Rectus abdominus	7th–12th intercostals	T5-T12
Flexion of hip. Have the seated patient lift his thigh from the table and resist your effort to push it down.	Iliopsoas	Branches from the lumbar plexus & the femoral nerve	T12-L4
Extension of hip. Have patient lie prone. With his knee extended, have him extend the thigh (i.e., lift it up from the table) and resist your effort to push it down.	Gluteus maximus "Hamstrings" (semi-membranosus, semitendinosus, biceps femoris)	Inferior gluteal Sciatic branches	L5-S2 L4-S3
Abduction of hip. Have patient lie on his side, raise the upper leg to about 45 degrees and resist your effort to push it down.	Gluteus medius and minimus	Superior gluteal	L4-S1
Adduction of hip. Have patient lie on his side with both legs straight. Have him raise both legs off the table, and resist your effort to push down on the *lower* leg.	Adductors, gracilis, and pectineus	Obturator	L2-L4
External rotation of hip. Have patient lie supine with one foot resting on the table and the leg to be tested dangling beyond the edge of the table, with the knee at a 90-degree angle. Have him rotate the leg so that the foot moves medially, until the lower leg makes an angle of about 30 degrees with the vertical. Place your hand above the medial malleolus and have him resist your effort to push the leg down to a vertical position.	Obturator, quadratus femoris, pyriformis, gemelli	Obturator	L2-L4
Internal rotation of hip. Similar to the above, except that patient rotates leg so that the foot moves laterally. Place your hand above the lateral malleolus, and have him resist your effort to push the leg toward the vertical.	Gluteus medius and minimus	Superior gluteal	L4-S1
Flexion of knee. Have patient lie prone, flexing the leg at right angles. Place one hand on his thigh, and one on the Achilles tendon. Have the patient resist your effort to pull the foot down to the table.	"Hamstrings"	Sciatic branches	L4-S3
Extension of knee. Have patient lie supine, with his knee extended and at the edge of the table. Place one hand on his thigh and one at the ankle. Have him resist your effort to push the foot toward the floor.	Quadriceps femoris	Femoral	L2-L4
Plantar flexion of ankle. Have the patient stand on the leg to be tested and raise his heel a couple of inches from the floor. (If strength is not a grade 5, repeat against examiner's resistance with patient supine.)	Gastrocnemius, soleus, plantaris (triceps surae)	Tibial	L5-S2
Dorsiflexion of ankle. With the patient supine, place your hand on the dorsum of his foot, and have him pull the foot up (toward his face) against your resistance.	Tibialis anterior	Deep peroneal	L4-S1
Inversion (supination) of foot. Have the patient invert the foot (if he is sitting, the big toe will be farther from the floor). Place your hand under the foot from the lateral side, and have the patient resist as you try to pull the foot down into neutral position.	Tibialis anterior, tibialis posterior	Deep peroneal, tibial	L4-S1

continued

Table 26-7—*continued*.

Maneuver	Muscles Tested	Peripheral Nerve	Spinal Cord Segment
Eversion (pronation) of foot. Have the patient evert the foot and hold that posture as you try to pull the foot back into neutral position.	Extensor digitorum longus, peroneus longus and brevis	Deep peroneal; superficial peroneal	L4-S1
Flexion of toes. Place one hand under the tips of the patient's toes, and the other hand on top of the toes. Push upward on the tips of the toes as the patient pushes down.	Flexor hallucis longus and brevis, flexor digitorum longus	Tibial	L5-S2
Extension of toes. Place one hand on the dorsum of the foot and the fingertips of the other on the dorsal side of the toes. Have the patient push his toes against your fingertips as you resist.	Extensor hallucis longus, extensor digitorum longus	Deep peroneal	L4-S1
Abduction and upward rotation of scapula. With his arms in front of him, have the patient push hard against some immovable object. Observe the medial borders of the scapulae, which should remain close to the thoracic wall.	Serratus anterior	Long thoracic	C5-C7
Adduction and downward rotation of scapulae. Have the patient brace his shoulders backward against resistance. The muscle bellies can be felt and sometimes seen.	Rhomboids	Dorsal scapular	C4-C5
Elevation of the shoulders. Have the patient shrug his shoulders against resistance.	Levator scapulae Trapezius (upper)	Dorsal scapular Spinal accessory	C3-C5 (cranial nerve XI)
Abduction of shoulder. Have patient maintain abduction against resistance. To test the deltoid muscle, the angle between the arm and the patient's chest must be more than 15 degrees but less than 90 degrees.	Deltoid	Axillary	C5-C6
Abduction of shoulder. With his arm at his side, have patient try to abduct the arm against resistance.	Supraspinatus	Suprascapular	C4-C6
Adduction of shoulder. Have the patient adduct the arm against resistance. (If the arm is above the horizontal, the clavicular part is tested; if the arm is below the horizontal, the sternocostal part of the muscle is tested.)	Pectoralis major	Medial and lateral pectoral	C5-T1
Extension of shoulder. Have the patient lie prone with arms at his side, and lift the arm off the table as you resist.	Latissimus dorsi, teres major	Subscapular	C5-C8
Flexion of shoulder. With patient seated on the examining table, have him lift the upper arm against resistance (with elbow extended), so as to parallel the thighs.	Coracobrachialis Anterior deltoid	Musculocutaneous Axillary	C6-C7 C5-C6
External (lateral) rotation of shoulder. Keeping his elbow at his side, have the patient try to carry the flexed forearm backward against resistance. The muscle belly can be felt over the scapula. Alternately, have the patient lie prone, with shoulder abducted to 90 degrees and elbow flexed 90 degrees, with his hand pointed toward his head. Place one hand at his wrist, and have him resist your effort to push his forearm toward the floor.	Infraspinatus	Suprascapular	C5-C6
Internal (medial) rotation of shoulder. Have the patient lie prone as in testing external rotation, except that his hand points toward his feet. Have him resist your effort to push his wrist toward the floor.	Subscapularis, teres major, latissimus dorsi	Subscapular	C5-C8
Flexion of elbow. Have the patient flex his elbow and resist your attempt to straighten his arm. (Put one hand on the patient's humerus, and the other at the wrist.)	Biceps, brachialis	Musculocutaneous	C5-C6

continued

Table 26-7—*continued.*

Maneuver	Muscles Tested	Peripheral Nerve	Spinal Cord Segment
Extention of elbow. Position the patient's arm so that it is parallel to the ground, to eliminate the effect of gravity on the forearm. Have him extend the forearm against resistance, starting from an angle of about 130 degrees.	Triceps	Radial	C6-T1
Supination of forearm. Have the patient extend his arm by his side, with the hand in supination (palm forward), and resist your attempt to pronate the hand.	Biceps, supinator	Radial	C5-C7
Pronation of forearm. Have the patient extend his arm by his side, with the hand in pronation, and resist your attempt to supinate the hand.	Pronator teres	Median	C6-C7
Flexion of wrist. (a) Have the patient try to flex the wrist toward the radial side against resistance.	Flexor carpi radialis	Median	C6-C8
Flexion of wrist. (b) Place the patient's hand, palm upwards, on the table, with the fingers extended. Have the patient try to abduct the little finger strongly against resistance. If the flexor carpi ulnaris is intact, the tendon can be seen and felt as it fixes the point of origin of abductor digiti minimi, even when the abductor digiti minimi is paralyzed.	Flexor carpi ulnaris	Ulnar	C7-T1
Extension of wrist. (a) With the fingers extended, have the patient try to extend the wrist to the radial side against resistance.	Extensor carpi radialis longus	Radial	C5-C8
Extension of wrist. (b) With the fingers extended, have the patient try to extend the wrist to the ulnar side against resistance.	Extensor carpi ulnaris	Radial	C6-C8
Abduction of thumb. (a) With the thumb in the plane of the palm, have the patient try to abduct it at right angles against resistance.	Abductor pollicis longus	Radial	C6-C8
Abduction of thumb. (b) Place the patient's thumb so that the nail is in a plane at right angles to the palm, with a fountain pen or similar object between thumb and palm. Have the patient try against resistance to bring the edge of his thumb to a point vertically above its original position, maintaining the nail in the original plane.	Abductor pollicis brevis	Median	C6-T1
Adduction of thumb. Have the patient resist your attempt to abduct the thumb. (Alternately, have the patient try against resistance to hold a strip of paper between the thumb and the palm, with the thumb lying along the palmar aspect of the index finger, its nail in a plane at right angles to the palm.)	Adductor pollicis	Ulnar	C8-T1
Flexion of thumb. Fix the proximal phalanx of the thumb between your thumb and index finger. Have the patient flex the terminal phalanx and resist your effort to extend it by pulling with your index finger.	Flexor pollicis longus and brevis	Median Ulnar	C6-C7 C8-T1
Extension of thumb. Have the patient resist attempts to flex the thumb at (a) the MCP joint, and (b) the IP joint.	Extensor pollicis (a) brevis and (b) longus, respectively	Radial	C6-C8
Opposition of thumb and fifth finger. Have the patient touch his thumb and little finger together, while you try to pull them apart, using the thumbs of both hands.	Opponens pollicis and opponens digiti quinti	Median (former) and ulnar (latter)	C6-T1, C8-T1 respectively
Flexion of fingers at metacarpophalangeal joints (MCPs). Keeping the fingers extended at the proximal and distal interphalangeal joints, have the patient flex at the MCPs, and maintain flexion while you attempt to extend the fingers by exerting pressure with your thumb.	Lumbricales	Median (two lateral lumbricals); ulnar (others)	C6-T1; C8-T1

continued

Table 26-7—*continued.*

Maneuver	Muscles Tested	Peripheral Nerve	Spinal Cord Segment
Extension of fingers at MCPs (while flexed at the interphalangeal joints). Fix the metacarpals, and have the patient try to keep his fingers extended at the MCPs while you exert pressure on the proximal phalanges.	Extensor digitorum communis, extensor indicis proprius, extensor digiti quinti proprius	Radial	C6-C8
Flexion of fingers. Using your index finger, fix the proximal phalanx in extension at the MCP joint, and have the patient flex at the PIP joint and resist your attempts to straighten the finger, using your other index finger.	Flexor digitorum sublimis	Median	C7-T1
Flexion of fingers. Fix the second phalanx in extension, using your index finger, and have the patient flex the distal phalanx and resist attempts to straighten it.	Flexor digitorum profundus	Median (index and middle); ulnar (ring and little finger)	C7-T1; C8-T1, respectively
Extension of fingers. With wrist and fingers extended at all joints, have the patient resist attempts to flex the fingers by pressing on the middle phalanges.	Extensor digitorum communis and interossei	Radial	C6-C8
Abduction of fingers. With the fingers in extension, have the patient try to abduct the index finger and then the little finger against resistance.	First dorsal interosseus and abductor digiti quinti	Ulnar	C8-T1
Adduction of fingers. With the fingers in extension, and close together, have the patient try to spread the fingers, while you exert resistance.	Palmar interossei	Ulnar	C8-T1

Sources: *Gray (1966), Leopold (1952), Medical Research Council (1943), and Vick (1976).*

the diagnosis of motor disease due to problems with no known anatomic correspondence.

Synkinesias in Diagnosis of Paresis

A common trick for revealing the diagnosis of malingering is to get the patient to use a muscle group in one position after having claimed inability to use it in another. At the crudest level, this involves such maneuvers as telling the patient, who had claimed the inability to flex at the knee, "You can pick up your pants now," following a rectal examination performed with the patient leaning over the examining table. But a more sophisticated and reliable method of making the same assessment is to check for the absence of the associated motor movements (synkinesias) that normally occur with certain activities (Table 26-8).

The simplest sort of synkinesia is swinging the arms during rapid walking. The absence of same is a clue to Parkinson's disease. But the synkinesias shown in Figures 26-15 through 26-24 are more concerned with distinguishing the various etiologies of paresis. The illustrations by Dr. R.S. Lyman are from Dr. Leo Alexander's superb chapter on the neurologic examination in Pullen's *Clinical Diagnosis* (see Ch. 29). These should be studied now.

A Self-Study

To see what some of the synkinesias look like in a malingerer, ask a naive colleague to "fake" a lesion. Then try the maneuvers. The synkinesias that are normally present with effort (such as Souques' and Hoover's) will usually "drop out" of the examination. To imitate the synkinesias in patients with paralysis due to a gross brain lesion, offer an external resistance to your colleague's "paralyzed" limb. For example, overcome his effort to lift his arm by pressing down with all your weight on his humerus; Souques' synkinesia (see legend to Fig. 26-20B)

should appear. Similarly, pressing down on his thigh will permit the opposite heel to dig in as in Hoover's synkinesia (see legend to Fig. 26-24).

Hoover's Sign as a Guide to Prognosis

The Hoover sign can also be used to help predict recovery of a paralyzed leg following a stroke, because the synkinesia is a bilateral motor event originating in only one hemicortex (the good one). In fact, this is the way that Hoover initially used his test

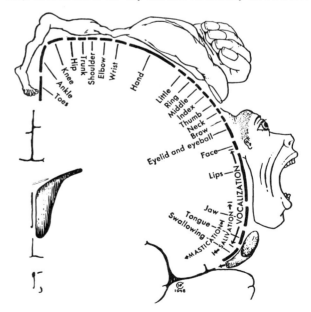

Figure 26-14. *The motor homunculus. Reproduced from Penfield W, Rasmussen T:* The Cerebral Cortex of Man. *Macmillan, New York, 1950.*

Table 26-8.   Synkinesias

Name	Motion
Babinski's rising synkinesia	Flexion of the paretic thigh associated with flexion of the trunk (Figs. 26-15 and 26-19A)
Leaning backward synkinesia	Triple extension of paretic legs associated with extension of trunk (Figs. 26-16 and 26-19C)
Néri's sign	Knee flexion of paretic leg associated with flexion of trunk in standing position (Figs. 26-17 and 26-19B)
Triple flexion	Dorsiflexion of the foot in association with flexion of knee and hip of paretic limb (Figs. 26-18 and 26-19E)
Climbing asynergia	Extreme plantar flexion with inner rotation of the foot associated with flexion of hip and knee in certain frontal lesions (Fig. 26-18C)
Babinski's tonus test	Tonus judged by degree of passive flexion of elbow when upper arm elevated (Figs. 26-20A, 26-21A, and 26-22A)
Sougue's test (interossei phenomenon)	Overextension and spreading of fingers associated with elevation of paretic arm (Figs. 26-20B, 26-21B, and 26-22C)
Babinski's pronation sign	Pronation of hand occurs when supinated, abducted paretic arm is dropped toward body (Figs. 26-20C, 26-21C, and 26-22B)
Strümpell's pronation sign	Pronation of hand associated with flexion of the elbow (Figs. 26-20D, 26-21D, 26-22D)
Raimistes' hand sign	Flexion of paretic wrist (Figs. 26-20E, 26-21E, and 26-22F)
Bechterew's arm sign	Exaggeration of normal "hang" when arms (flexed at the elbow) are elevated (Figs. 26-20F, 26-21G, and 26-22E)
Contralateral triceps contraction	Associated with forceful biceps action in normal individuals (Figs. 26-20G, 26-20H, 26-21F, 26-22G)
Triceps or biceps contraction	Associated with coughing in normal persons (Figs. 26-20I, 26-20J, 26-21H, and 26-22I)
Klippel-Weil test	Flexion of the thumb in association with passive extension of the other fingers in paretic arm (Figs. 26-20K, 26-21I, and 26-22H)
Raimistes' leg sign	Paretic limb carries out motion (adduction or abduction) that is forcibly prevented in the normal limb (Fig. 26-23)
Hoover test	Normal heel presses down on table as patient attempts to lift paretic leg (Fig. 26-24)

(while Barré used his test to check for conversion). (See Barre's sign, p. 483.)

Ask the patient to raise the healthy leg, and keep your hand behind the heel of the weak leg to see if it presses down. If it does, the patient has a good prognosis for regaining the ability to walk. If it does not, no statement can be made about prognosis (S. Horenstein, personal communication, 1988).

Tetanic Equivalents

Of the many tetanic equivalent tests, I use only three: Trousseau's; a test whose name I do not know; and the Chvostek. Many more tests are described in DeJong (1979). Additionally, Erb's test is frequently alluded to in textbooks, but it is rarely performed now because it requires a device for electrically stimulating the patient.*

Trousseau's Sign

A method:

1.   Place the blood pressure cuff around the biceps, and inflate the cuff well over systolic blood pressure. Observe the hand for an arbitrary minimum of 3 minutes, unless the test has already become positive.

DeJong leaves the tourniquet on for up to 4 minutes; other authors leave the cuff on for 5 minutes. In the von Bonsdorff test, the tourniquet is left on for 10 minutes. Then it is removed and the patient is made to hyperventilate before the test is considered negative. One Chvostek-positive hypoparathyroid patient required 20 minutes of the tourniquet before the Trousseau test became positive (Simpson, 1952). In the original Trousseau test, there is no mention of how long the band must be left on the patient's arm before the test is considered negative. Similarly, the extent of blood pressure cuff inflation was never specified, since in the original version of the test Trousseau simply gripped the arm and squeezed it with his hands (Trousseau, 1861).† Later Trousseau learned to use a constricting band when he observed a blood-letting at the Necker Hospital performed upon a woman with this sign. When the tourniquet (constricting band) was applied to her arm, the spasm appeared quickly. Only much later, after Trousseau's death, was the blood pressure cuff employed as the constricting band.

Historical note. Trousseau was one of those encyclopedic clinicians produced in 19th century France. Once Trousseau made an incorrect diagnosis in a case in which a local dolt made the correct diagnosis. Recognizing that all diagnostic medicine is merely a clever playing of the odds, Trousseau is reputed to have said, "Even a broken clock gives the correct answer twice a day." In addition to his test for tetany, he also described Trousseau's syndrome: migratory thrombophlebitis as a sign of internal malignancy, which he later found in himself (see Ch. 19, p. 368). Nowadays, when I ask, "Who was Trousseau?", I am variously told that he was an oncologist, an endocrinologist, a neurologist, or a phlebologist, according to the situation in which his name has arisen. It was all the same Trousseau.

2.   A positive test is shown when the tested hand voluntarily demonstrates the tetanic equivalent of flexing at the wrist and extending all the fingers. Trousseau referred to this as the *main d'accoucheur* (hand of the obstetrician). I personally avoid this

---

*Erb wrote the book on electrical stimulation that Freud first used when he entered the private practice of neurology. Today, Erb is best known for Erb's palsy, a birth injury of the C5 and C6 nerve roots, which leaves the arm lying limply by the side, the hand internally rotated posteriorly and flexed in the position used by New York headwaiters when receiving bonuses for placing one at ringside.

†Oddly enough, this original Trousseau maneuver later reappeared as the Hochsinger phenomenon. (Hochsinger was an Austrian pediatrician who was not born until 1860.) One suspects that this may be another epiphenomenon of the Franco-Prussian War, akin to Traube's sign (see p. 312).

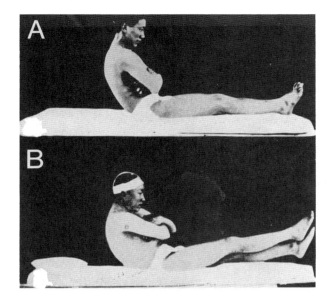

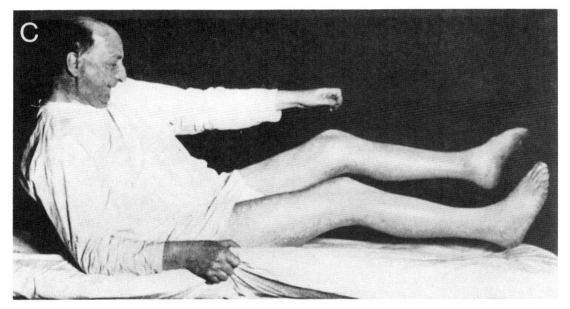

Figure 26-15. *Babinski's rising synkinesia. A, Normal individual. B, Patient with spastic paraparesis of both legs, presumably due to a lesion of the leg area of the motor cortex caused by a gunshot wound at the vertex. C, Patient with a right frontostriatocallosal lesion, presumably due to occlusion of the right anterior cerebral artery. Reproduced with permission from Alexander L: The neurologic examination. In: Pullen's Medical Diagnosis, WB Saunders, Philadelphia, 1950.*

name because it might be confused with the hand of the gynecologist, a term applied to the benediction hand (papal hand) of median nerve palsy (see p. 506).

Significance. The Trousseau test has a sensitivity of 66% in hypocalcemia and a false-positive rate of 4% (Simpson, 1952).

Other false positives. The Trousseau test has also been reported as positive in a case of hysteria (Thomson et al., 1977), and the muscle contractions seen in some cases of Addison's disease may appear to produce a positive Trousseau sign (Archambeaud-Mouveroux et al., 1987; Bornstein et al., 1962). However, the case for a positive Trousseau in experimental hyponatremia is confounded (McCance, 1936), and the case for a positive Trousseau sign in nonalkalotic hypokalemia is unconvincing (Jacob et al., 1986).

General significance. These tests all have the same basic significance, although the Chvostek test has some special considerations that will additionally be discussed (see p. 490). In summary, all these tests may be positive in hypocalcemia, less frequently in situations where the measured amounts of calcium and magnesium are normal but their ionized (physiologically active) fractions are decreased due to alkalosis (0.16 mg/dl of ionized calcium adjustment for every 0.1 pH unit), and *rarely* in hypomagnesemia uncomplicated by concurrent hypocalcemia (Kingston et al., 1986). (Also see the case report on p. 492).

Usually, the magnesium and pH are normal and the tetanic equivalent is due to one of the classic causes of hypocalcemia,

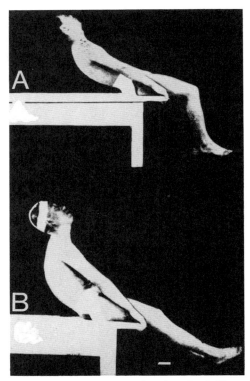

Figure 26-16. *Learning backward synkinesia. A, Normal individual. B, Patient with spastic paraparesis (same as in Fig. 26-15B). Reproduced with permission from Alexander L: The neurologic examination. In: Pullen's Medical Diagnosis, WB Saunders, Philadelphia, 1950.*

hypoparathyroidism, vitamin D deficiency, steatorrhea, or renal insufficiency. At other times, there are mixed etiologies, as when hypomagnesemia inhibits the normal release of parathormone from the parathyroid glands, causing a secondary hypocalcemia.

A Second Sign

A method. An extremely valuable test for tetany is to tap *lightly* the broad portion of the triangular-headed reflex hammer above the lateral malleolus. A tetanic equivalent is adduction, extension, and eversion.

(This is the same response as is evoked in Lust's peroneal phenomenon. However, in Lust's phenomenon or sign, the stimulus is a tap at the lateral surface of the proximal fibula just below the knee, where the common peroneal nerve wraps around the lateral aspect of the fibula.)

Significance. In my limited experience, this is one of the most sensitive of the tetanic equivalents. It is often the first to appear, and following treatment, the last to correct. However, nowadays it is impossible to gather good data on this test because of the rapidity with which house staff correct the various chemical etiologies of the tetanic equivalents.

Chvostek Test

The Chvostek test is named in honor of the 19th century Viennese clinician who described it.

A method. To perform the Chvostek test, tap the cranial nerve VII as it emerges *and* in the area of its first branches. Areas to be tapped are shown in Fig. 26-25. Use the reflex hammer for the

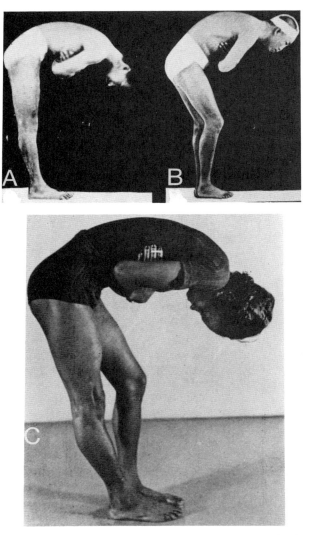

Figure 26-17. *Néri's bending over synkinesia. A, Normal individual. B, Same patient as in Figure 26-15B with spastic paraparesis. C, Flexion of the paretic left leg in a patient with a right front lesion. Reproduced with permission from Alexander L: The neurologic examination. In: Pullen's Medical Diagnosis, WB Saunders, Philadelphia, 1950.*

points labeled "C" and "S." Percuss lightly with the tips of your fingers held together over the "sideburn" area.

A positive Chvostek test is obtained if tapping over this nerve causes a "reflex" contraction of some or all of the muscles it serves (muscles of facial expression.)

Significance. The Chvostek test has a sensitivity of 27% (Simpson, 1952) in latent tetany.

In addition to the tetanic conditions of hypocalcemia, hypomagnesemia, and alkalosis, the test can also be positive in disease of the pyramidal tract supplying the facial muscles. This is in essence a clonic reflex, whereas the true Chvostek sign of tetany is not a reflex but simply a sign of motor irritability.

Other false positive. The Chvostek test is also positive in diphtheria, measles, smallpox, scarlet fever, pertussis, typhoid fever, tonsillar disease, tuberculosis, myxedema, "joint neu-

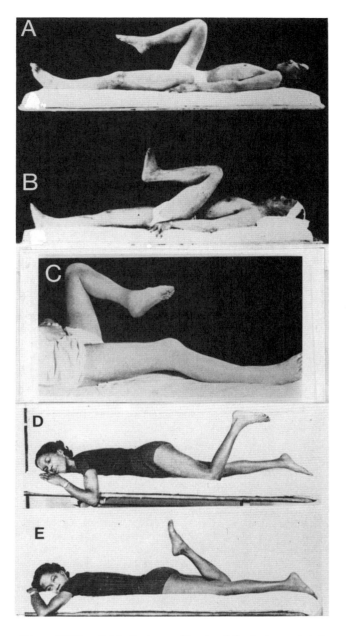

Figure 26-18. Triple flexion synkinesia of the foot associated with active voluntary flexion of the hip and knee joints. A, The normal foot shows plantar flexion. B, The pyramidally hemiparetic limb shows dorsiflexion of the foot. C, In certain frontal lesions, extreme plantar flexion with inner rotation (supination) of the foot (climbing asynergia) may become associated with hip and knee flexion. D, Same phenomenon of "triple flexion" in a prone patient asked to flex only the knee of the paretic left leg. (Note hip flexion.) E, Active voluntary flexion of the normal right leg, without hip movement and with plantar flexion (i.e., extension) of the foot. Reproduced with permission from Alexander L: The neurologic examination. In: Pullen's Medical Diagnosis, WB Saunders, Philadelphia, 1950.

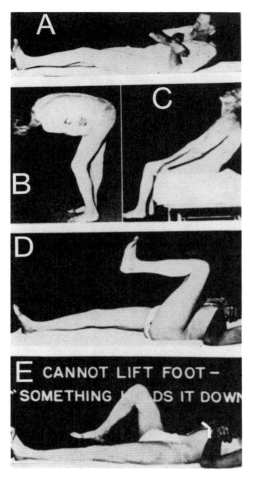

Figure 26-19. Synkinesias associated with active trunk and leg movements missing in a patient with a right-sided conversion hemiparesis. A, Babinski's rising synkinesia. Note that the heels remain on the bed. B, Néri's bending over synkinesia. Note that he bends the normal leg, rather than the "paretic" one. C, The bending backward synkinesia. The legs do not extend. D, The synkinesia of the foot associated with active voluntary hip and knee flexion on the left. Note that the normal foot (paradoxically) shows dorsiflexion. E, Note the absence of the expected dorsiflexion in the "paretic" foot. Compare with Figures 26-18, A and B. Reproduced with permission from Alexander L: The neurologic examination. In: Pullen's Medical Diagnosis, WB Saunders, Philadelphia, 1950.

ralgia," and "enteroptosis"* (Hoffman, 1958). Some of these may actually represent a fortuitous coincidence, because of the high false-positive rates in normals (vide infra.)

The Chvostek yields false positives in 19%, 20%, 30%, 40%, 45%, and 74% of variously reported series of normal children (Hoffman, 1958; Simpson, 1952). In adults, the comparable false positive rates are 4% (Dodelson, 1963); 5%, 16%, and 25% (Hoffman, 1958), and 29% (Simpson, 1952).

---

*Enteroptosis (or visceroptosis) means "fallen viscera." It was a non-disease of medical progress. Doctors learned anatomy on recumbent cadavers and surgical patients, and so later saw the same organs "fallen" (through the effects of gravity) when viewed fluoroscopically on erect patients. This non-disease has been eradicated by eliminating both fluoroscopy and the vigorous teaching of gross anatomy.

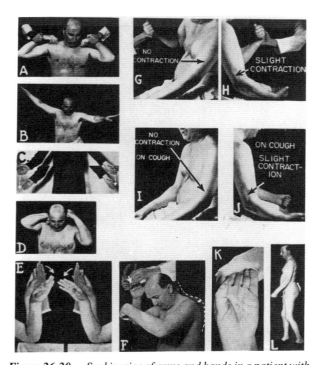

Figure 26-20. *Synkinesias of arms and hands in a patient with neurologic left-sided hemiparesis with asynergia and athetoid phenomena, presumably due to right-sided frontostriato-callosal lesion caused by occlusion of the right anterior cerebral artery. A, Babinski's tonus test. (This is not, strictly speaking, a synkinesia, but a phenomenon indicative of the state of tonus.) Note that the paretic, hypertonic left arm cannot be bent to quite as acute an angle as the right arm. B, Souques' test (interossei phenomenon). When a patient with a disturbance of the frontal or pyramidal system carries out a request to elevate his extended arms, the fingers of the paretic hand show overextension and spread. C, Babinski's pronation sign. If the arms are passively abducted with the hands in supination, and then suddenly released, the hemiparetic arm usually shows pronation of the hand when falling back toward the body, while the normal extremity remains in a supinated posture. If the sign is only suggestively positive, it must be interpreted in the light of the general condition of tonus of the arm. If it is negative, it does not exclude involvement of the frontal or pyramidal system. D, Strümpell's pronation sign. When asked to bring his hand to his shoulder by flexion of the elbow, the normal individual will bring the palm of the hand to the shoulder with the hand in supination. In neurologic hemiparesis, this movement will be accompanied by pronation, so that the dorsum of the hand will approach the shoulder with the palm facing forward. This phenomenon is not present in the photograph, though the movements do show some apraxic clumsiness. E, Raimistes' hand sign (Raimistes' arm sign). If the elbow of the patient is placed on a table, with the forearm and hand held vertical by the examiner's hand, then the examiner's hand is suddenly removed, the hand that is paretic due to pyramidal involvement will drop to form an angle of 130 to 140 degrees with the forearm. F, Bechterew's arm sign. If both arms, flexed at the elbow, are passively elevated at the shoulder and then suddenly released, normal arms will not drop immediately, but for a moment or longer will "hang" in midair. This "hang" may be exagerated in case of neurologic hemiparesis even if not associated with an appreciable increase in tonus.*

A number of suggestions have been made for reducing the number of false positives:

1. Require the test to be positive bilaterally. (But the false positives were bilateral in 40%, 50%, and 80% of various series. Also, it is not known how many true positives are bilateral. A similar limitation in knowledge applies to many of the following techniques, any or all of which might also decrease the sensitivity of the test while trying to eliminate the false positives.)

2. Especially attend to percussion within the "sideburn area." In a series of false positives (Hoffman, 1958), the test was falsely positive at *both* Chvostek's and Schultze's points (Fig. 26-24) in 71%, only at Schultze's point in 24%, and only at Chvostek's point in about 5%. Very few false positives seem to be produced by percussing lightly in the "sideburn" area.

3. Require that the corner of the eyes be involved in the contraction of the facial muscles.

4. Ignore the slight motions of the angle of the mouth (and sometimes the corner of the nostrils) that result from the tap itself rather than from an actual contraction.

5. Keep the masseter muscle tense. The other muscles can still respond to the tetanic stimulus. This would also help eliminate the problem of the appearance of motion due to the impetus of the blow.

6. Require both of two taps, administered within seconds of each other, to be positive. In the case of false positives, the first response may be positive and the second negative (Hoffman, 1958).

Case report. A patient was admitted with a serum calcium of 5.5 mg/dl, an albumin of 2.5 g/dl, a serum magnesium of 0.7 mEq/l (normal greater than 1.5), and an arterial pH of 7.60. Yet he had no Chvostek, Trousseau, or lateral malleolus sign, on repeated testing by many. The significance of a serum potassium of 2.3 mEq/l as a modifying factor was discounted because it was not sufficiently low to cause paralysis. Dr. Gert Muehlheims was consulted and pointed out that the hypokalemia was a "well-known" modifying factor in the production of tetanic equivalents, operating at the membrane, without the requirement that it be severe enough to paralyze independently the muscle.

The membrane equation states that the excitability of the neuromuscular unit is proportional to the ratio:

$$[potassium][hydroxide]/[calcium][magnesium]$$

Some patients with conversion paralysis will show no "hang" (see Fig. 26-21G). G and H, The test of triceps contraction on contralateral forceful biceps innervation. In the patient with neurologic hemiparesis, this contraction occurs in the normal arm when the paretic arm performs the forceful biceps flexion (H), but may be absent (as in G) in the paretic arm when the normal arm performs the forceful biceps flexion. I and J, The arm muscle reaction to coughing. This is present in the normal arm (J). It may be either absent or exaggerated in the paretic arm (I). K, The Klippel-Weil test. Flexion of the thumb associated with passive extension of the other fingers occurs in neurologic hemiparesis (but not in normal individuals). L, The arm in walking. The normal arm swing is absent or reduced, and the paretic arm tends to be held in flexion. Reproduced with permission from Alexander L: The neurologic examination. In: Pullen's Medical Diagnosis, WB Saunders, Philadelphia, 1950.

A high ratio leads to tetany; a low one to weakness or paralysis.

(This analysis is inadequate in a number of ways. First, the intracellular/extracellular ratios are not shown. Second, the extracellular concentrations have no precise mathematical relationship to each other. Third, the actions are misrepresented. For example, alkalosis acts through decreasing the ionized fraction of calcium, not through a direct effect on the resting membrane.)

Nevertheless, the utility of the above may be considered in the light of subsequent events. The house staff, unimpressed by two antediluvian professors ranting about fluxes of ions across membranes, proceeded to do that which they do best—repletion therapies. The patient had difficulty elevating his magnesium, in part because the house staff was careful to go slow and low and avoid magnesium intoxication, and in part because his intracellular depletion was even greater than his serum depletion. The continued hypomagnesemia also inhibited his response to calcium repletion, probably through inhibiting the release of parathyroid hormone. His potassium repletion alone was briskly achieved. Then the nurses called the house staff to report the occurrence of a grand mal seizure, surely one of the more dramatic of the tetanic equivalents.

Fibrillation and Fasciculation

Though involving the muscles, these phenomena are signs of neurologic disease. Basically, they both tell us that the observed muscle units are undergoing a slow denervation. In *fibrillation,* small muscle units appear to undergo slow contraction and relaxation as if something wormlike were turning over in the muscle mass. Actually, the individual fibers are contracting quite quickly, just like the "f" waves in the EKG of atrial fibrillation. It is the wavelets of the battalions of individual contracting fibers that produce the slow motion of the "turning worm," just as in Schrödinger's example, in which a glass of freshly poured water loses its turbidity by the slow motion of a wave front, which on closer inspection is the (mathematically determined) change in the boundary of a zone of very fast activity (Brownian motion, the collision of high-speed atoms).

The tongue (see p. 465) is the only muscle in which one can see fibrillation at the bedside. It may resemble a bag of worms.

Fasciculations are simply twitches of larger muscle units and exactly resemble the kind of muscle twitch that many normals have from time to time in the absence of denervation. Accordingly, fasciculations alone should never be considered significant.

Pernicious fasciculations have the following four characteristics:

1. They are stereotyped, that is, they always affect the same muscle fibers.
2. They are present at rest.
3. They may even be present at sleep.
4. They are perfectly rhythmic or periodic.

The patient may also have atrophy and/or weakness in the same muscles.

Pernicious fasciculations may be seen in amyotrophic lateral sclerosis, syringomyelia, bulbar palsy, and progressive spinal muscle atrophy of whatever eponym. Most importantly, they are *not* seen in *acute* denervation. In order for fasciculations to appear,

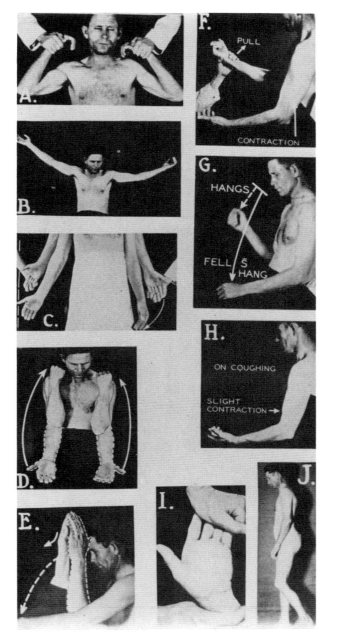

Figure 26-21. *Synkinesias of arms and hands in malingered left-sided "hemiparesis." A, Babinski's tonus test. The "paretic" arm shows exaggerated flexibility, not hypertonus. B, Souques' test. The test is negative (i.e., there is no overextension and spread of the fingers, as there should be with neurologic hemiparesis). C, Babinski's pronation sign: suggestively, but not completely positive. D, Strümpell's pronation sign is negative (i.e., the "paretic" side is not "palm forward" as in neurologic hemiparesis (see Fig. 26-20D).) E, Raimistes' hand sign. The malingerer allows his whole arm to drop. The hand does not form an angle with the forearm as in Fig. 26-20E). F, The test of triceps contraction on contralateral forceful biceps innervation. The normal contraction is present. G, Bechterew's arm sign. The "paretic" arm drops without a "hang." H, Arm muscle reaction to coughing is normal. I, On the Klippel-Weil test, the synkinesia expected in central hemiparesis is absent. J, The arm in walking is allowed to hang down limply, such as it does in*

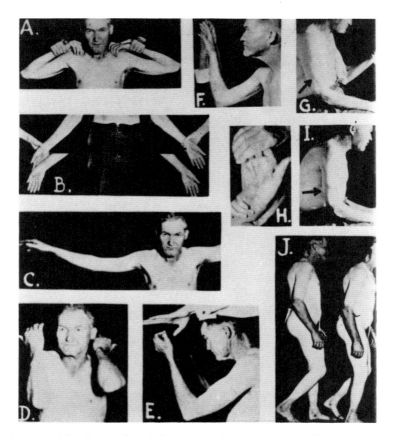

Figure 26-22. *Synkinesias of arms and hands in right-sided conversion hemiparesis. A, Babinski's tonus test. The "paretic" right arm shows exaggerated flexibility. B, Babinski's pronation sign is negative. C, Souques' test is negative (i.e., the synkinesia is absent when it should be present if he had neurologic paralysis). D, Strümpell's pronation sign is negative (i.e., the "palm forward" synkinesia is absent when it should be present due to neurologic paralysis). E, Bechterew's arm sign. The normal "hang" is observed. F, Raimistes' hand sign. The hand does not make the expected angle with the forearm (as it does in Fig. 26-20E). G, Triceps contraction of the "paralyzed" side is present on contralateral forceful biceps innervation. H, Klippel-Weil test is negative (i.e., the flexion synkinesia is missing). I, The "paralyzed" arm muscle reaction to coughing is present. J, The arms swings normally with walking. Reproduced with permission from Alexander L: The neurologic examination. In: Pullen's Medical Diagnosis, WB Saunders, Philadelphia, 1950.*

the neuromuscular unit must have had time to die (i.e., both fibrillations and pernicious fasciculations may be rhapsodized as the dying agitations of neurally abandoned muscle units).

Reflexes

Question: *Who invented the word "reflex"? (See Appendix 26-3.)*

Deep Tendon Reflexes

A Digression on Reflex Hammers

$$ The first reflex hammers that were used were winemakers' hammers. These had already been adopted for percussion of the chest and in fact the use of the pleximeter for mediate percussion derived directly from the way that winemakers percussed barrels. Later it was realized that immediate percussion (see Ch. 16) was just as good, and only the little hammer was kept (for a while) for percussion. Later it was adapted for deep tendon reflexes.

The first hammer made specifically for the neurologic examination was the Taylor hammer, the rubber triangular-headed hammer shown in Figure 26-26.

The Queen's Square hammer pictured in Figure 26-27 was first made as a gift by the head nurse in radiology for her beau, a neurologist, by sticking a radiator handle on a piece of Malaccan cane. Soon everyone wanted one. Since the Empire no longer provides Malaccan cane, they are now made of wood.

The cabinet maker's "deadfall hammer" is said to be the best, although difficult to obtain (S. Horenstein, personal communication, 1988). This hammer has a hollow head filled with petroleum sludge and buckshot such that every blow is struck with exactly the same impact.

General Observations on Reflexes

Note the strength and symmetry of the reflexes. A grading system is given in Table 26-9.

Alternately, if you tap *lightly* initally, gradually increasing the strength of your blow to the gentlest rap that will elicit a reflex, you can grade the reflex according to the degree of your own effort.

The only reflex that is always abnormal is clonus.

In children, the upper extremity reflexes are normally stronger than the lower extremity reflexes. In senescence, this is reversed (S. Horenstein, personal communication, 1988).

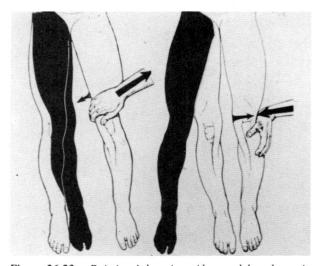

Figure 26-23. Raimistes' leg sign. Abnormal leg shown in black, normal in white. If the examiner opposes active adduction of the normal leg, the abnormal leg adducts. If the examiner opposes abduction of the normal leg, the abnormal leg abducts. In other words, the pyramidally paralyzed or paretic leg will carry out a movement identical with that which was forcefully prevented in the other, normal leg. This maneuver brings out a latent tendency to symmetric homologous associated movements, following the same general rules as those of the arms. Reproduced with permission from Alexander L: The neurologic examination. In: Pullen's Medical Diagnosis, WB Saunders, Philadelphia, 1950.

Jaw Reflex (Masseter or Mandibular Reflex)

Standard method:

1. Place your finger over the top of the patient's chin, opening his jaw sufficiently to enable you to detect a reflex closing.

2. Hit your finger sufficiently hard to put a stretch on the masseter muscles. The masseters will contract.

Interpretation. The presence of the reflex implies that the trigeminal nerve's sensory and motor portions are intact on at least one side, as is the reflex center in the pons. This is the only deep tendon reflex innervated from above the foramen magnum.

This reflex is sometimes absent in normal people.

The jaw jerk provides the "normal" control for the patient with spinal cord disease, when you are trying to find the level of disease and want to know if a lower reflex is hypo- or hyperactive. As a general rule, the jaw jerk is the same strength as the biceps and the knee jerks, while the triceps seem to equal the ankle jerks (S. Horenstein, personal communication, 1988).

A better method. It is more useful to test one side at a time by placing a tongue blade over the mandibular molars and lightly tapping the portion of the tongue-blade lever that protrudes from the mouth. This permits a comparison of the two sides. The reflex will be lost or diminished ipsilateral to a trigeminal (pontine) nucleus lesion, but will be hyperactive with supranuclear palsies or pyramidal tract disease.

Biceps Reflex

A method (Fig. 26-26):

1. Have the patient's arm flexed at the elbow in the range of 90 to 130 degrees. This can be done by grasping his elbow in your hand, supporting both the elbow and the forearm by resting

them on your own forearm. In this way, the patient can be perfectly relaxed while the proper angle is maintained. Or, if the patient is sitting, you could have him place the arm palm-up in his lap or on the physician's desk as if to prepare for the blood pressure measurement.

2. Place your thumb on the patient's bicipital tendon in the antecubital fossa. This is easy to find because it is the only tendon crossing this space. If you have trouble finding the first one (when you are practicing on your partner), ask your partner to rotate his hand externally just a few centimeters (i.e., to move the thumb laterally and then inferiorly and the ulnar surface of the hand superiorly). As soon as the motion is initiated, you will feel the bicipital tendon jump up against your thumb.

3. Push your thumb against the tendon, but leave some "slack" in it. (With all these stretch/tendon reflexes, there must be some slack. If the tendon is pressed too hard, the reflex may not be obtained even from a normal person.)

4. Hit your thumb with the reflex hammer. The arm should flex at the elbow.

Interpretation. The afferent limb of this reflex is the musculocutaneous nerve; the efferent limb comes from segments C5 and C6.

A caveat: Of course, the afferent and efferent for all reflexes meet in the same segment at the internuncial neuron, and travel in the same peripheral nerve trunk. *As a teaching convention, we will name the segment as the efferent and the peripheral nerve as the afferent.*

○ Remember the biologic variability observed in freshman anatomy class. All of these listings of neuroanatomic segments are written in protoplasm, not stone. They are probably only 99% accurate in actual practice.

Triceps Reflex

A method (Fig. 26-27):

1. Lift the *upper* arm (the brachium) so that the humerus is approximately parallel to the floor. The radius and ulna (the antebrachium), being unsupported, will hang down at approximately a 90-degree angle.

2. Hit the triceps tendon as it runs along the humerus, 2 or 3 inches proximal to the olecranon process of the ulna. (Do not hit the ulna itself, as there will be no reflex unless the patient is a physician, in which case he will simply shake his head in wonderment at the new curriculum. But that is not the reflex you are trying to elicit.)

3. A positive reflex consists in extension of the arm at the elbow.

A caveat: With an overly cooperative patient, who postures the arm (thereby abolishing the reflex) out of a wish to help you, it may be necessary to say, "Let me do all the work, now" and to wiggle the elbow joint through about 30 degrees of extension and flexion.

Another trick to help the patient relax is to have him place his hand upon his hip.

Interpretation. The afferent limb is the radial nerve and the efferent limb comes from spinal cord segments C6 through T1.

Teeth clenching is a proven Jendrassik maneuver (vide infra) for the triceps reflex (Tarkka & Hayes, 1983) as is contraction of a

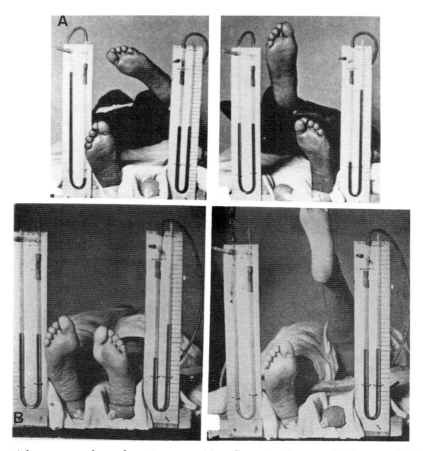

Figure 26-24.   *Hoover test (phenomenon of complementary opposition, Grasset and Gaussel). If a normal individual in the recumbent position raises one leg up high, the other will press down on the examining table, with a pressure that can be quantitated by means of a manometer, with the rubber bulb placed under the heel. A, When a patient suffering from a neurologic hemiparalysis or weakness (in this case on the left) lifts the paretic leg or attempts to lift the paralyzed leg, the other leg will press down with great force. However, when he lifts the normal leg, the pressing down movement of the paralyzed or paretic leg will be absent or reduced respectively. B, The opposite is the case in malingered or conversion paralysis or weakness. When lifting the normal left leg, the hysterically paralyzed right leg will press down like a normal leg. However, when attempting to lift the "paralyzed" leg, the down-pressing movement of the normal leg will be absent or trifling, commensurate to the absence or paucity of the effort made. Reproduced with permission from Alexander L: The neurologic examination. In:* Pullen's Medical Diagnosis, *WB Saunders, Philadelphia, 1950.*

lower extremity muscle (Delwaide & Toulouse, 1981). The amplitude of the reflex may also be increased by having the patient turn his head toward the side being tested; this maneuver will also shorten the latency time. Turning the head away from the side being examined has the opposite effect (Tarkka & Hayes, 1983).

Brachioradialis Reflex

A method (Fig. 26-28):

1.   Place the forearm so that the radial surface is superior. If the patient is sitting, he may rest the forearm across his thigh or place his arm on the physician's desk. In other circumstances (as with the bed-bound, frail patient), the physician may simply lift the arm into position by holding the patient's hand or by holding the forearm from beneath.

2.   Strike the radial surface about midway between the ends of the radius.

3.   A positive response is extension at the wrist and inversion (medial rotation of the radial hand).

Interpretation.   The afferent limb is in the radial nerve, and the efferent limb comes out of spinal cord segments C5 to C8.

If the brachioradialis reflex gives finger flexion as a response, without the other motor activities, and the finger flexion is spastic, this indicates a segmental transverse spinal cord lesion at the level of the missing muscle response. *Explanation:* The descending intraspinal sublesional fibers cause the fingers to respond, but they are disconnected from the inhibitory pathways of the higher centers by the segmental lesion and hence their response is spastic. This is a general rule of reflexes that is less often noted at the biceps and triceps jerks.

Finger Flexion Reflex

A method (Fig. 26-29):

1.   Place your fingers over the volar surface of the patient's fingers, which are held together and slightly curved.

2.   Strike your own fingers, which extends the patient's fingers somewhat and activates the stretch reflex.

3.   A normal response is flexion of the fingers.

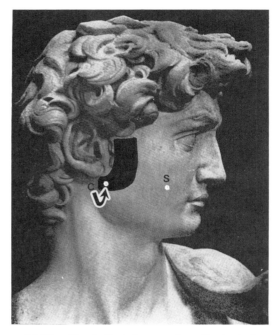

Figure 26-25. *The indicated areas show the best places to search for the Chvostek "reflex," which is really not a reflex but rather a tetanic equivalent. Chvostek percussed the area marked "C," where the facial nerve is accessible in front of and below the external auditory meatus. Schultze preferred to percuss the region between the zygomatic arch and the corner of the mouth (marked "S"). One can also percuss at the "sideburn" area, marked in black (see text). Detail from David, by Michelangelo.*

Interpretation. This reflex gives information about segment C8.

Thumb Reflex (after Rask, 1979)

A method (Fig. 26-30):

1. After assuring yourself that the brachioradialis reflex is intact, grasp the patient's hand with your non-hammer-wielding hand and supinate the patient's hand. Then extend (dorsiflex) it at the wrist to about 45 degrees by exerting pressure on the palm with your grasping hand. But do not touch the patient's thumb (since thumb flexion is the anticipated response.)

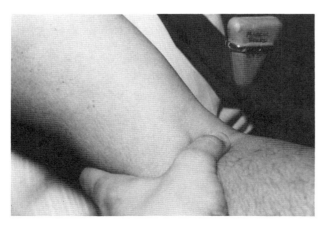

Figure 26-26. *The biceps reflex (see text).*

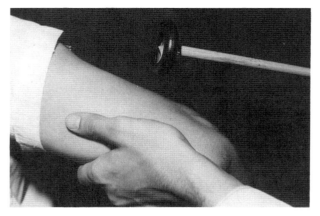

Figure 26-27. *The triceps reflex. The Queen's Square hammer is not really going to strike the side of the arm as it seems, but rather the triceps tendon, obscured in this view by the examiner's thenar eminence. Why has the examiner intruded his hand into the picture? Because he is supporting the patient's arm. Why is the patient being examined wearing clothing? Because he is not a patient, and this is a posed picture.*

2. Find the tendon of the flexor pollicis longus (Fig. 26-30). One way is to have the patient alternately flex and extend his thumb while you press down with the free fingers of your hammer-wielding hand above the radius on the volar surface, trying to feel the wiggling. (If the patient's thumb is paralyzed, you may have to do the same maneuver on yourself and transpose the information to the patient.) A good place to start your search is a thumb-length proximal to the navicular tuberosity on the volar aspect of the patient's wrist. (Try it on yourself, now.)

3. Hit the tendon and watch the thumb flex at the distal interphalangeal joint.

Hint: Sometimes you have to reinforce the reflex. This can be done by asking the patient to clench and unclench his teeth or to push his feet together. (See the Jendrassik maneuver at the end of this section, p. 499.)

Interpretation. This reflex is altered in disease of C7 or in five of seven cases of entrapment neuropathy of the anterior interosseus nerve (the Kiloh-Nevin syndrome) (Rask, 1979).

Pronator Reflex

A method:

1. Lift the patient's forearm straight up by holding onto the patient's fingertips, with the patient's elbow resting on the bed, examining table, or other stationary object. Do *not* hold the fingers too tightly since the normal reflex response will be pronation of the forearm.

Table 26-9. Grading System for Deep Tendon Reflexes

Grade	Reflex
0	No contraction perceptible
1+	Contraction barely but definitely perceptible
2+	Contraction obviously perceptible; barely perceptible relaxation phase
3+	Vigorous contraction apparent from across the room
4+	Hyperactive contraction; most neurologists equate this with the presence of clonus, though some use "5+" to designate clonus

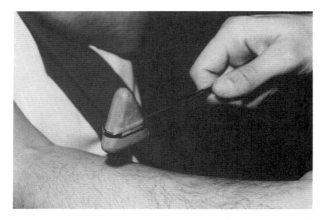

Figure 26-28. *The examiner is testing for the brachioradialis reflex. Although the text calls for striking the antebrachium about halfway, this particular examiner is striking more proximally than that; others will go more distally. This is a good reflex for beginners because the reflexogenic zone is so large.*

2. Hit the ulnar surface and watch for hand pronation.

Significance. The afferent fibers are carried in the median nerve and the efferent fibers come from spinal cord segments C6 through T1.

Modifications. DeJong elicits the response with the patient's forearm in semiflexion and the wrist in semipronation, but I favor the starting position of DeGowin, given above. One may also hit the radial surface and get the same pronation response. (Try it on your partner or yourself.)

Pectoral Reflex

A method:

1. Rest the patient's arm and forearm so that the humerus is abducted about 30 degrees out from vertical zero.

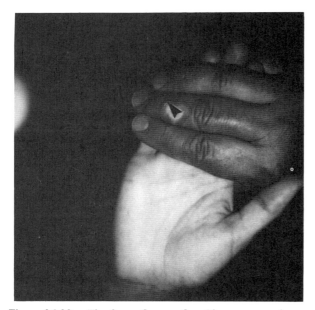

Figure 26-29. *The finger flexor reflex. The arrow marks one place where the hammer could strike. Actually, a blow to any of the examiner's fingers would stretch the patient's fingers and thus elicit the reflex.*

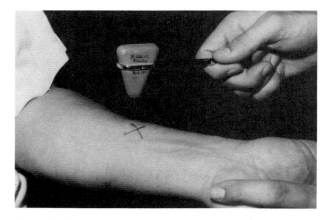

Figure 26-30. *The thumb reflex. In this subject, the tendon of the flexor pollicis longus, shown as an "x," is more proximal than indicated by the text, reemphasizing the importance of searching in the individual patient.*

2. As with the biceps reflex, you will not strike the tendon directly, but rather through the intermediary of your thumb or forefinger. So, place your mediate thumb or forefinger in the front of the axilla where it joins the anterior body wall. That little "curtain" that separates the axilla from the anterior chest is the insertion of the pectoralis major muscle on the greater tubercle of the humerus.

3. Strike your digit (with the hammer coming from below), and you will feel rather than see the contraction of the muscle, accompanied by internal rotation and adduction of the humerus.

Significance. This tests spinal cord segments C5 through T1. Can you see why a clinician might go a lifetime and never check this reflex? The reason is that it basically checks the same spinal cord segments as the triceps reflex plus the biceps reflex or the brachioradialis reflex. In fact, its only use is to check those segments in someone in whom these reflexes cannot be checked (i.e., someone with an above-the-elbow amputation). Its other reputed use—detecting a lesion of the anterior thoracic nerve—is more simply and specifically achieved by having the patient push down with his hands on his own anterior iliac spines. The little "curtain" representing the insertion of the pectoralis major will be missing on the side of the lesion.

Knee Jerks (Patellar Tendon Reflexes)

A method:

1. Have the patient sit so that the leg to be examined is flexed but hanging in a free-swinging condition. This can be done by having the patient sit on the edge of the bed, which is raised to a sufficient height that the patient's feet do not rest on the floor.

   If the patient is sitting in a chair, the legs can be crossed (with first one and then the other on top) and the upper one examined.

2. Find the patella, and just below it the inferior patellar tendon, which inserts on the anterior superior surface of the tibia (Fig. 26-31).

3. Give the tendon a sharp tap.

Some neurologists check this reflex with the feet flat on the floor. However, it should not be done with just a *part* of the foot touching the floor, as the patient may tense the limb.

A method for the bed-bound patient. One method is to strike the superior edge of the patella. This can be done with the legs extended; the patella moves superiorly.

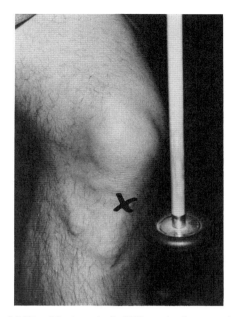

Figure 26-31. *The knee jerk. "X" marks the spot. Any lower and you will be beating upon the tibia. Much higher, and you will hit the patella.*

For the attending. The following technique, which involves the customary infrapatellar tendon as the object of the hammer blow, is preferred for purposes of group demonstration:

If you are right-handed, stand at the supine patient's right. Slip your left hand under the patient's right knee and lift it from the bed to produce sufficient passive flexion to elicit the reflex. Tell the patient to let you support the entire weight of his leg. Tap the tendon with the hammer in your right hand. Elicit the left knee jerk in the same manner *mutatis mutandis.*

Significance. The knee jerk tests spinal cord segments L2 to L4.

In the 19th century, several large series demonstrated an absence of knee jerks in 0.04% to 4.8% of healthy subjects. Jendrassik (1885) studied 1,000 controls "of various ages" and found the knee jerks missing in 1.6% of these. Of these 16 subjects, one had diabetes mellitus, which was already known as a cause of missing knee jerks, and in the other 15, the "missing" knee jerks could be "restored" by using Jendrassik's maneuver (vide infra).

○ No reflexes should ever be described as "absent" unless Jendrassik's maneuver has been done.

Jendrassik's Maneuver

Jendrassik first described voluntary contraction of the upper extremities so as to facilitate remote deep tendon reflexes, specifically the knee jerks (Jendrassik, 1883, 1885). This method may be applied to any recalcitrant reflex, including the ankle jerks.

Jendrassik's maneuver is sometimes called "reinforcement" or "distraction," but after a century of study we still do not know the exact mechanism or mechanisms (Hayes, 1972).

A method:

1. Say to the patient, "Grab your wrists tightly and when I say 'pull,' try to pull them apart." Demonstrate this for the patient yourself.

2. When you are positioned to elicit the reflex, say "Ready, . . . 1 . . . 2 . . . 3 . . . pull!" At the last word, rap the patellar tendon.

Some observations. A few empiric observations that have been scientifically studied are worth noting:

1. Having the patient turn his head toward the side being tested will facilitate the facilitation (Tarkka & Hayes, 1983).

2. The louder the signal ("pull"), the greater the facilitation (Scheirs & Brunia, 1982).

3. The amount of facilitation is directly proportional to the intensity of the maneuver. If at first unsuccessful, be sure that the patient is exerting maximal effort on the voluntary contraction of the remote muscles (Hayes, 1972).

4. The facilitation only lasts from 1 to 6 seconds after initiation of the voluntary contraction (Hayes, 1972), and is maximum for only 300 milliseconds (Kawamura & Watanabe, 1975), so be expeditious.

False positives. There are three kinds of neurologically intact patients in whom an unmodified Jendrassik's maneuver does not work (i.e., the finding of "absent reflex despite Jendrassik maneuver" is a false positive). The first of these is the tense patient who responds to the instruction "pull" by tensing all the voluntary muscles, not just the ones remote from the area where you are trying to elicit the reflex. This effectively suppresses the deep tendon reflexes.

A remedy: Neurophysiologic studies of facilitation (Kawamura & Watanabe, 1975) reveal that the facilitation begins after the instruction "pull" but 100 milliseconds *before* muscle contraction begins. Accordingly, to elicit the reflex in such total-body contractors you need to catch them in the 100 milliseconds before they respond to your instruction "pull." To do this, advance the timing of your blow, so that you are starting your swing as you begin to pronounce "pull," thus catching the patient before he can begin the muscle contraction. (As with most of medicine, one learned this empirically before there was a scientific explanation available.) It may take a little practice to perfect your timing, because different examiners have different speeds of striking and different response times of their own, but as is usually the case, once mastered, this invaluable skill will not be lost.

The second group of patients in whom an unmodified Jendrassik's maneuver does not work includes the tense people I call "anticipators." They are like linemen in football who go offside by anticipating the quarterback's cadence and so are moving before the signal. Similarly, the anticipators contract before being asked to "pull." Thus, the anticipator's maximum facilitatory period may have passed even before you have started your hammer motion.

A remedy: Again, the solution is to advance the timing of the hammer blow still further. After the patient has gotten used to the "Ready . . . 1 . . . 2 . . . 3 . . . pull" cadence, just say "Ready . . . 1 . . . 2 . . . 3 . . . " and begin tapping for the reflex before "pull." You may start tapping on "3" or in some patients even on "2.75." (It may take some time to "catch" the individual patient.)

The third and final normal group in whom Jendrassik's maneuver will not elicit the knee jerks (or the ankle jerks) are the 20% of classical ballet dancers (especially women who have been going "on point" for 8 to 10 years) who do not have knee jerks or ankle jerks (Goode & Van Hoven, 1982). Whether or not these are truly "false positives" is left to the wise discretion of the thoughtful reader. The reflexes are as truly absent in these patients as they are in those with neuropathy, myelopathy, radiculopathy, and so forth. On the other hand, these are neurologically healthy persons whose missing reflexes are discovered by a thorough clinician who has usually been consulted for some other reason.

Other Methods of Aiding Relaxation

Simply having the patient change position may help to bring out a reluctant reflex. A general method of helping patients relax that is also applicable to other parts of the physical examination is to ask the patient to *tense* briefly the part in question. Relaxation must follow the tensing, and sometimes will go beyond the baseline state.

Inverted Knee Jerks

If you strike the patellar tendon and the knee flexes (instead of extending), the patient has an "inverted" knee jerk. This is evidence of a spinal cord lesion at L2, L3 and/or L4 (Boyle et al., 1979), almost always a transverse spinal cord lesion.

Adductor Reflex

A method.   Place your finger transversely about 5 cm above the medial femoral epicondyle, with the patient's thigh in slight abduction. A blow to your finger will cause thigh adduction. (Other stimulus points are given by DeJong, 1979)

Interpretation.   This reflex is not customarily tested because it is often absent, and also because it tests L2 to L4, segments that are more easily evaluated with the patellar reflex. However, the motor nerve for the patellar reflex is the femoral nerve, whereas the motor nerve for the adductor reflex is the obturator nerve, the latter being the one that is trapped in an obturator hernia (Young et al., 1988). This leads to an excellent test for strangulated obturator hernia—*the Hannington-Kiff sign* (Hannington-Kiff, 1980). It consists of an ipsilateral loss of the adductor reflex with intact patellar reflexes. In the presence of acute abdominal obstruction, the Hannington-Kiff sign makes the diagnosis of a strangulated obturator hernia. The patient may also have referred pain just above the knee in the skin area served by the obturator nerve, in which case the Howship-Romberg sign is also said to be present (see Ch. 22, p. 403).

Ankle Jerks (Achilles Reflex)

A method:

   1.   Have the patient sit comfortably with his feet dangling down and not touching the floor. After you gently dorsiflex the foot, rap the Achilles tendon (Fig. 26-32).

Recalcitrant ankle jerks.   First, remember to wiggle the foot passively in the extension–flexion dimension (prior to placing it in dorsiflexion (extension) and striking the tendon with the hammer) so as to determine that the patient is not posturing his foot. Next, try Jendrassik's maneuver (see p. 499), which can also be used with the special positions and manipulations described below.

   If all else fails, and the patient is not bed bound, have him kneel on a chair, with the upper extremities and thorax supported by the back of the chair, the abdomen and pelvic girdle being supported on the knees, and the ankles hanging from the front edge of the chair. With the patient's weight so distributed, it is nearly impossible for him to posture the feet; thus, the ankle jerks can usually be elicited if present.

   If the patient is bed bound, the physician should place the ankle

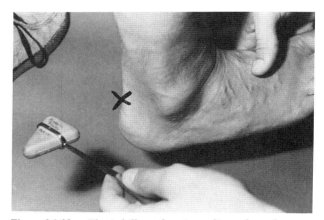

Figure 26-32.   *The Achilles reflex. According to legend, young Achilles was made almost impervious to harm when he was dipped in the magic river. However, since he was held by the heels, he remained vulnerable at that point, hence, the Achilles heel and tendon. The Achilles tendon reflex is vulnerable to disc herniations and other causes of S1 nerve root impingement or damage. The examiner is using the broad edge of the rubber hammer (plexor) and will strike the spot marked "x."*

to be tested lateral to the opposite shin by flexing the patient's knee and slightly rotating the hip externally. Here, the legs resemble a figure four: the vertical stroke is represented by the nontested leg, which supports the lateral surface of the leg being tested, permitting the ankle to be clear of the bed (Fig. 26-33).

   Alternately, one can use *mediate percussion* in the bed-bound patient as follows: Place your own finger over the plantar surface of the patient's passively dorsiflexed foot, as the patient lies supine, both legs comfortably resting side by side. Strike your own finger, thereby dorsiflexing the foot further and activating the tendon reflex.

   A third method for the bed-bound patient is to have the patient "sit in a chair" while lying supine. Flex his hip to 90 degrees, his knee to 90 degrees, and hold your hand against his sole in place of the "floor." Then strike either the "floor" or the Achilles tendon.

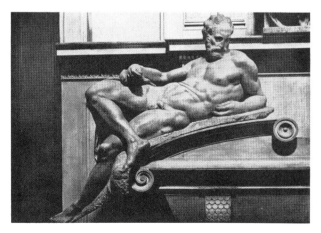

Figure 26-33.   *This illustrates the figure-four position for examining the Achilles tendon reflex in the bed-bound patient. If the patient has difficulty getting his foot above the knee, it is permissible to have the foot recline instead on the shin, or to use a mediate blow as described in the text. The Twilight by Michelangelo, from the tomb of Lorenzo de Medici.*

Significance. The afferent limb of the reflex is the posterior tibial nerve; the efferent limb comes from segments L5 to S2.

In practice, absence of the ankle jerk is not very good for picking up root compression syndromes involving L5. It is useful for root compression syndromes involving S1, in which it is 85% sensitive with a "false-positive" rate of 10%. The latter figure refers to patients who have no myelographic evidence of disease such as a herniated disc, but many of these could actually be true positives for other diseases (Rico & Jonkman, 1982).

Ankle jerks are absent in 15% of all patients (Reinfrank et al., 1967). Most of these (78%) have diabetes mellitus (although only 32% of all diabetics are without ankle jerks (Abraham et al., 1966). The remainder will almost inevitably have a disease such as the ones listed in Table 26-10. Only 0.2% of patients under the age of 60 will have absent ankle jerks without such a cause.

This leaves the issue of how often the ankle jerks are missing in persons over the age of 60 for no reason other than age (or an unskilled examiner). A review of the reported literature figures for absent ankle jerks in the elderly gives a range of 27% to 50% of persons over age 65, 40% of those over age 75, and 38% to 80% of those over age 80 (Impallomeni et al., 1984), but these figures are undoubtedly due to improper technique. For instance, in a prospective study (Impallomeni et al., 1984), reflexes were elicited as follows: Patients were not examined until the day after admission (when they were more calm), and both mediate percussion (p. 500) and the Jendrassik maneuvers were used. Using this method, only 6% of all elderly patients (mean age 82 years) had missing ankle jerks, and most of these had a known explanation. *Only 1.5% of the patients studied had missing ankle jerks that had to be attributed to age.*

Speed of contraction and relaxation. The rapidity of contraction may be increased in some neurologic disorders as well as in hyperthyroidism.

The relaxation phase of the ankle jerk has been well studied. It is discernibly briefer than normal in 14% to 93% of patients with hyperthyroidism (Abraham et al., 1966: Rives et al., 1965) and immediately following exercise (Martin et al., 1970). It is diagnostically prolonged in 62% to 100% of patients with hypothyroidism (Abraham et al., 1966; Reinfrank et al., 1967; Rives et al., 1965) as well as in some other disorders (see Table 26-11). (Of course, if the patient is known to have a neuropathy of the lower extremities only, there is no reason why one could not estimate the deep tendon reflex relaxation time from a biceps tendon reflex.)

Table 26-10. A Few Causes of Missing Ankle Jerks, Not Due to Poor Technique

Diabetes mellitus
Tabes dorsalis
Eadie's syndrome
Myotonic dystrophy
Ankle joint disease
Pernicious anemia
Systemic lupus erythematosus or other rheumatic diseases including rheumatoid arthritis
Severe myxedema
Alcoholic polyneuropathy
Amyloidosis
Spondylolisthesis with compression of nerve roots
Neuropathy of unknown etiology

Table 26-11. Causes of Prolonged Achilles Tendon Reflex Relaxation Time (Other Than Hypothyroidism)

Neuropathic disorders
  Neurosyphilis (common)
  Syringomyelia
  Pernicious anemia
  Diabetes mellitus
  Sarcoid
Muscle disorders
  Myotonia congenita
  Other myotonic disorders
Local edema
Hypothermia
Drug therapy
  Beta blockers
  Reserpine
  Glucose infusion
  Potassium infusion
  Quinidine
Female sex (including pregnancy, ballet dancers, and anorexia nervosa)
Aging

Sources: *Abraham et al. (1966), Carel et al. (1979), Ingbar and Woeber (1974), Martin et al. (1970), Simpson et al. (1963), and Zachmann (1967).*

Using a recording device, the positive predictive value of fast reflexes (i.e., a shortened half-relaxation time) was found to be 92% for hyperthyroidism. The positive predictive value for prolonged relaxation time was 72% for hypothyroidism. The predictive value of normal reflexes was 99.3% for the euthyroid state (Reinfrank et al., 1967).

In a study that stratified patients by age, an Achilles reflex time (from tapping the tendon to muscle half-relaxation) less than 240 milliseconds had a true-positive rate of 37% and a false-positive rate of 0% for hyperthyroidism in patients aged 30 to 59 years. The true-positive rate was 48% and false-positive rate 0% in patients aged 60 to 83 (Nordyke et al., 1988).

Other tricks

1. The prolonged ankle jerk of diabetic neuropathy (Roberts' sign) can sometimes be elicited after repetitive tapping of the ankle jerk, every 1 or 2 seconds, for at least six taps (Roberts, 1982). Sometimes the reflex could even be extinguished. These phenomena are not seen in myasthenia gravis or thyroid disease.

2. The absence of deep tendon reflexes has received adequate emphasis as a sign of Eaton-Lambert syndrome (Doi's sign). However, in the individual patient it is sometimes difficult to decide whether the absent reflexes are due to the Eaton-Lambert syndrome or to a peripheral neuropathy.

In Eaton-Lambert syndrome the reflexes may be made to reappear following a brief (10-second) period of maximal voluntary contraction (Doi et al., 1978). This will easily distinguish Eaton-Lambert syndrome from neuropathy, or for that matter from myasthenia gravis.

The Babinski Reflex

Actually, there are several Babinski "reflexes," the first four of which are synkinesias (see p. 487).

First, the platysma muscle contracts on maximal opening of the mouth. Second, there is Babinski's rising reflex (Fig. 26-15) in patients with a lower limb paresis. Third is the Babinski tonus test Figs. 26-20A, 26-21A, and 26-22A). Fourth is the Babinski pronation sign (Figs. 26-20C, 26-21C, and 26-22B).

However, when most people speak of "the" Babinski reflex, they are referring to one of the many eponymic tests based upon dorsiflexion of the great toe with fanning of the other toes in response to a noxious stimulus applied to the lower extremity, which occurs in pyramidal (corticospinal) tract disease.

This reflex is not a proprioceptive reflex, but a nociceptive one, and the response is hierarchical, not "all-or-none" like the proprioceptive stretch reflexes.

A Method

1.   Grasp the patient's ankle with one hand.

2.   Using either the sharp handle of a percussion hammer or a splinterless broken jagged edge from a tongue depressor (in your other hand), stroke the sole of the foot, beginning at the calcaneus and proceeding up the *lateral* aspect and then across the metatarsal heads toward the great toe.

(Much nonsense has been written about what sort of objects can and cannot be used to stroke the sole. While the patient should not be injured, the whole point of the procedure is to produce a noxious stimulus.)

3.   Observe the toes throughout the procedure, because by the time one reaches the great toe, the reflex or sign has already occurred if it is present.

Interpretation

The normal response is brisk plantar flexion.

However, one may *rarely* see a slow, *tonic* plantar flexion, which is a pathologic sign. It resembles the foot's equivalent of a frontal grasp reflex (see p. 504).

Two criteria are required for a positive response: 1) the big toe must move up (dorsiflex) and 2) the other toes fan in a beautiful sequential toe ballet fashion. (In older patients, the toes do not always fan, but do undergo sequential or lateral independent movement.)

Although often occurring in tandem with clonus, the Babinski sign is not always diagnostic of pyramidal tract disease, in contrast to clonus, which is pathognomonic. Because the Babinski sign results from the release of a spinal extensor reflex, interruption of ascending sensory pathways may be the explanation for the rare Babinski seen with a normal pyramidal tract.

True positives (*with* fanning of the toes) must be distinguished from false positives, in which there is rapid withdrawal flexion at the hip and knee, dorsiflexion of the foot, and sometimes dorsiflexion of all the toes, but no toe fanning. This false-positive toe dorsiflexion of withdrawal is abrupt, and looks like a hand or foot being pulled back from a hot stove. In the true Babinski reflex, the movement is much slower. It may take half a second or more for the toe dorsiflexion and fanning to be completed.

Of course, the false-positive abrupt toe withdrawal from a noxious stimulus may also be produced by an adverse, but not completely unpleasant sensation—the tickle. Accordingly, one should never stroke too lightly nor confine one's stroking to ticklish areas of the foot. In fact, the particular path recommended avoids going over the ticklish part of the soles, as this powerful stimulus (tickling) may produce the confounding withdrawal reflex (which might either be misinterpreted as a positive Babinski, or conceivably could disguise a true-positive Babinski and

make it appear to be a withdrawal response). Unfortunately, there is a photograph of Babinski himself performing the Babinski reflex, and he appears to be stroking the ticklish part of the sole (Schoenberg & Schoenberg, 1977)!

It is believed that some false positives, especially those due to withdrawal, may be abolished by moving the hand at the ankle to exert pressure on the ball of the foot at the great toe.

In perfectly alert patients, false positives may be seen following physical exhaustion, during the apneic phase of Cheyne-Stokes respiration, and when the short toe flexors are paralyzed. Some patients with athetosis and chorea are erroneously thought to have Babinski signs simply because their hyperactivity results in a coincidental extension following the stimulus.

Other false positives are seen in a variety of unconscious states. After the patient is aroused, the Babinski reflex can no longer be found. Scopolamine and barbiturates probably produce their false positives (when they occur) in a similar way.

False negatives occur from time to time in patients with other long tract signs such as clonus (see p. 503) and hyperreflexia. The reason for this is not known, although concurrent disease of the spinal cord from L4 to S2 will of course obliterate any response including a positive one. Sometimes the Babinski can be made to disappear with an injection of physostigmine (DeJong, 1979).

Equivalents

A large number of other stimuli have produced eponymic reflexes, but all of them should require the same *two* toe movement response criteria to be considered positive. (Similarly, the normal response to these maneuvers is the same plantar flexion of the toes.)

Oppenheim's test requires a noxious stimulus to be applied to the anterior tibial periosteum, beginning near the knee and moving caudally. Scrape with two knuckles. This test is recommended when there is distal sensory impairment.

In Gordon's test, one simply squeezes the calves (more vigorously than when checking for thrombophlebitis) and observes for toe changes.

Stransky's test is performed by slowly and vigorously abducting the little toe, maintaining it in maximal abduction for 1 to 2 seconds, and then suddenly letting go. Dorsiflexion of the big toe occurs either while the little toe is abducted or immediately after it is released.

Chaddock's test is closest to Babinski's in that the noxious stimulus is applied to the foot, slowly stroking, but this time going around the back of the lateral malleolus and then across the lateral dorsum of the foot.

An historical note.   In his time it was said that the best neurologist in St. Louis was C.G. Chaddock; and the second best was C.G. Chaddock, drunk. The number of observations which prompted this encomium may be deduced from the following story:

•

One day a St. Louis University medical student stopped in Frank John's bar (known as Frank's) for a tipple and found himself standing next to Chaddock. The student became flustered, saying, "Gosh, I'm sorry, Professor Chaddock. I'm not supposed to be here. I'm actually supposed to be attending a neurology lecture."

"Don't worry, son," said Chaddock, "I'm supposed to be giving it."

•

In addition to the foot extensor response, persons with a positive Babinski also have motor activity at the hip and ankle that can usually be palpated better than seen. This becomes important in patients who have had their toes amputated but who may thus still be examined for a long tract sign. Thus, Brissaud's reflex is a contraction of the tensor fascia lata upon stimulation of the sole of the foot.

It may be asked what one is to do if the entire foot has been amputated. As with Gordon's and Oppenheim's reflexes, the afferent arc may sometimes involve an area beyond the sole; thus one is encouraged to apply a noxious stimulus over a wide area.

In summary, the Babinski, Oppenheim, and Gordon reflexes have served well. Probably any three of this cornucopia would be sufficient.

Plantar Flexion Equivalents

There are several tests named after Rossolimo that produce plantar flexion in cases of pyramidal system lesions. One involves hitting the ball of the foot at the point of articulation with the metatarsal bones, and another a quick snapping with the examiner's fingers applied to the tips of the small toes. Yet another plantar equivalent is Mendel-Bechterew's sign, which involves hitting the cuboid bone with reflex hammer.

These plantar flexion signs are tonic foot responses, which include plantar flexion, toe flexion, and inversion. Thus, they are pedal equivalents of the grasp reflex (see p. 504).

Because of the tendency to confuse students, I perform none of these plantar flexion signs. Wartenberg (cited by Alexander in Pullen's Medical Diagnosis, see Ch. 29) points out that other plantar flexion stretch reflexes include those by Yoshimura, Boveri, Villaret, Faure-Beaulieu, Kempner, Foerster, Weingrow, Zhukowski, Kornilow, Sicard and Cantaloube, Markow, and the alternate reflexes of Bechterew, Yoshimura, and Rossolimo. There was even a Guillain-Barré reflex described in 1916 by authors better known for another entity.

(If one wished to catalogue in a similar fashion all the dorsiflexion reflexes, one could undoubtedly produce a longer list. For that matter, given the large number of sensory end organs located in the lower extremity, there is no reason why an enterprising young physician could not invent his own reflex and name it after himself. In fact, I encourage the reader to do this.)

Fortuitous Variants

1. When the Babinski reflex is due to interruption of the pyramidal tract within the spinal column, it is possible for the afferent arc to involve the area all the way up to the level of the lesion. This is called "an increased reflexogenic zone." In fact, there are even several situations in which the afferent arc is on the opposite side from the upgoing toe. For example, one might stimulate the right foot and observe the classic Babinski response on the left. This is called a crossed Babinski reflex, and like the crossed extensor reflex (vide infra) is seen in bilateral (albeit incomplete) spinal cord lesions, as well as bilateral intraspinal pyramidal tract disease, and bilateral cortical lesions.

2. Sometimes plantar flexion responses are followed by extension. Such reflexes are known as " biphasic pyramidal tract signs." They too indicate involvement at the spinal cord level, especially in the thoracic cord.

3. The *direct extensor thrust* is an extension of the entire limb in response to the physician pressing up against the sole. It is sometimes followed by plantar flexion or stepping movements. It is supposedly not seen in complete lesions of the spinal cord.

4. The *crossed extensor reflex* occurs when any kind of stimulation of the lower extremity causes ipsilateral withdrawal and contralateral extension. It is seen in severe spinal cord diseases other than unilateral pyramidal tract disease. This is also known as Phillipson's reflex, and given the opportunity for confusion, this is one place in which the eponym might be more useful than the operational description.

Clonus

Ankle Clonus

A method:

1. Grasp the patient's foot and rapidly put it through its entire range of extension and flexion three times in a row. On the last "wiggle," thrust it in full extension and vigorously maintain it so. (This whole step should take only about 2 seconds.)

2. Clonus is present when there is rhythmic resistance to your maintained extension. (Rhythmic means that there must be at least three "beats" of clonus. Sometimes the clonus is sustained, and the foot will beat against the resistance for as long as you maintain it; sometimes, there are only three or four beats of clonus, each successively weaker than the last. Either of these is a positive sign. Feigned clonus is either not rhythmic, or continues during plantar flexion when the tendon is no longer stretched.)

Teaching hint.   Don't search for clonus until you have seen a patient with pyramidal tract disease. Elicit the sign in that patient. Once obtained, it is impossible to forget.

Significance.   Ankle clonus, usually occurring in tandem with a positive Babinski reflex, *always* means pyramidal tract disease (or adrenergic hyperstimulation as from drugs). It may be relied upon to the exclusion of all else including the plantar responses above.

Clonus in Other Locations

Clonus can also be obtained from the quadriceps longus by grasping the patella, sharply pulling it downward, and maintaining the downward stretch. Alternately, one can strike the superior edge of the patella with a rubber reflex hammer, aiming the blow downward (so as to stretch the tendon of the quadriceps longus); however, it is difficult to maintain stretch on the tendon with this maneuver, a problem some have solved by placing their finger over the patella, striking their finger with the hammer, and then maintaining pressure with the finger.

Jaw clonus is obtained by placing the examiner's finger on the patient's symphysis mentis (as for the jaw reflex, p.) stretching the tendons either manually or with a hammer blow, and again maintaining the stretch pressure.

It is also possible to elicit clonus from the fingers and wrist by passively extending them and maintaining tension.

Other Reflexes

Grasp Reflex

In adults, this is not a stretch or tendon reflex, but rather a contactual automatism, of which there are two types: positive, in which the patient attempts to maintain stimulus contact, and negative, in which he avoids the stimulus contact. The grasp reflex is of the first type. It is never present in normal adults. (In babies, the "grasp" reflex is actually performed as a tendon-stretching reflex.)

There are a variety of methods of testing, all of which have in common the stimulation of the palm of the hand and the response of finger flexion. One way to do this is to stroke with your fingers starting at the palm then out to the fingers and the distal (volar surface) of the fingers, just touching them. The positive response is the patient's fingers curling up to maintain contact. To avoid false positives, do *not* stretch tendons, and do *not* pull on the fingers. (The latter may elicit the thalamic traction response, another false positive.)

Sometimes, this is such a strong reflex that the flexed fingers of a comatose patient will hold the examiner's fingers (which had stroked the patient's palm in a distal direction) and permit the examiner to lift the patient's arm up from the bed as if the patient were cooperating. (This one version is mentioned to explain why families sometimes believe that comatose patients are responding to them by squeezing their hands.)

○   This pathologic reflex is based upon parietal lobe release, and so it can be found in any disease of the nervous system *except* parietal lobe disease. Although the grasp reflex has been championed as a frontal lobe sign, and it is true that frontal lobe is a common source of lesions that produce the sign, it is *not* diagnostic of lesions in this area.

The tonic foot response, the pedal equivalent of the grasp reflex, is discussed on pages 502 and 503.

An Avoidance Contactual Automatism

Gently stroke the ulnar side of the hand, going distally. In a positive response, the fingers or the whole hand may move away, and in some cases the whole arm may elevate.

This finding occurs only in parietal lobe disease; in fact, it is the only pure parietal lobe sign (S. Horenstein, personal communication, 1988). (Other parietal lobe signs are discussed on p. 514.)

Ciliospinal Reflex

This reflex is elicited by scratching the skin over the maxilla or by pinching the skin on the side of the neck, depending upon whether one wishes to check the afferent limb in cranial nerve V or in the cervical nerves. The efferent limb is pupillary dilatation mediated through the sympathetics.

The extent and time course of a positive (normal) response may be learned by going to the mirror and staring at the pupil ipsilateral to the cheek you scratch.

Cutaneous Abdominal Reflexes

The stimulus for the upper abdominal cutaneous reflexes (right and left) consists of stroking with a noxious stimulus from above to below in a line about 2 inches beneath the costal border. The noxious stimulus can be either the wooden edge of a Queen's Square reflex hammer, or the rough end of a fractured wooden tongue depressor.

The response is a contraction of the abdominal musculature, which pulls the umbilicus up and laterally toward the site you are stroking. This tests T7 to T9.

The middle abdominal cutaneous reflex consists of stroking from the side toward the umbilicus, exactly at the level of the umbilicus. Again, a normal response consists of abdominal muscular contraction moving the umbilicus toward the site of the stimulus. This tests T9 to T11.

The inferior abdominal reflex is elicited by stroking from below to above on a line parallel with the inguinal ligament but about 2 inches higher. Again the umbilicus moves toward the stimulus. This is a test of T11 to L1.

Caveats:

1. The test should be considered abnormal only if a) asymmetric results are obtained (either right versus left, or above versus below the umbilicus), or b) the response is missing bilaterally in one or two segments only. In other words, if all the responses are missing, the test is inconclusive.

2. If all the responses are missing, there may be an error in your technique. Optimally, the patient should be examined in a relaxed, supine position, with the stimulus applied at the end of expiration. Attend to the amount of pressure applied. Pressing too hard causes a defensive reaction, with voluntary contraction of all the muscles, thus eliminating the chance to see the segmental pulling of the umbilicus which constitutes a positive response. Pressing too lightly will fail to elicit a response. The ideal stimulus is a wiping motion like that of a man shaving.

Cremasteric Reflex

Any noxious stimulus (such as stroking, light pinprick, or light pinching) is applied to the medial thigh. The normal response is homolateral contraction of the cremasteric muscle, with a gradual elevation of the testicle. This tests segments L1 and L2. It is seldom used today.

Scrotal Reflex

Contraction of the dartos, but not the cremasteric, can be elicited by stroking the perineum or applying an ice cube to the scrotum.

Bulbocavernosus Reflex

If the dorsum and/or sides of the glans penis are subjected to a noxious stimulus such as a squeeze, the bulbocavernosus muscle contracts. This response may be palpated by placing a finger on the perineum right behind the scrotum. Additionally, there is contraction of the urethral constrictor (midline in the same area) and of the external anal sphincter (the "anal wink"). The latter is best detected by placing a gloved finger in the patient's anal canal. (However, the anal wink is also the less specific efferent limb of other reflexes involving the application of a noxious stimulus [vide infra].)

This reflex checks S3 and S4 and is especially useful in evaluating some of the neurologic causes of male impotence (see Ch. 3, p. 42).

The bulbocavernosus reflex may be checked in women by parting the labia and squeezing the clitoris. The efferent limb is sensed by feeling the bulbocavernosus muscle through the perineum.

Anal Reflex (Anal Wink)

The external anal sphincter contracts in response to a variety of noxious stimuli (such as a pin scratch) nearby. I do not check it routinely, although it is popular among neurologists for checking the terminal spinal cord, among anesthesiologists for checking epidural anesthesia and other blocks, and among pediatricians since it is one of the normal newborn reflexes. It checks S2 to S5.

A Note

This list of reflexes is incomplete. As with the rest of the neurologic examination, a more detailed listing can be found in De-Jong (1979).

Selected Peripheral Nerves

A Quick Test of the Nerves to the Hand

Horenstein's "Handy Guide" to the hand nerves:

The entire hand innervation (motor) can be tested by examining the forefinger, which is chosen because the innervation is most constant. The radial nerve is tested by finger extension at the metacarpol phalangeal joint. The median nerve is tested by extension at the distal interphalangeal joint (DIP). Brace the finger straight with the DIP flexed and then ask for the DIP to be extended so that "the whole finger is straight." (This is the action of the lumbricales.) The ulnar nerve is tested by having the extended forefinger perform abduction or adduction, the former being easier for the patient. (This is the action of the interossei.)

Radial Nerve

One test for acute radial nerve damage is a motor test: see if the patient can extend his hand at the wrist against the resistance of gravity or of your own hand.

In chronic disease of the radial nerve, look for a spontaneous wrist drop.

There are two branches of the radial nerve. If the deep branch is the only one involved, the patient can have the finger drop but *not* the wrist drop. This is important because one cannot refute the hypothesis of radial nerve damage based upon the absence of the wrist drop (hence the reason for using the forefinger in the Handy Guide). Physicians involved in worker's compensation should be especially chary about diagnosing such patients as conversion reactions.

If motor evidence of a radial nerve injury is found, clinch the diagnosis by demonstrating the specific sensory involvement. The best place to test the sensory branches of the radial nerve is on the dorsum of the thumb and adjoining dorsum of the hand proper (see area indicated on Fig. 26-34).

Ulnar Nerve

Froment's Newspaper Sign

A good test for acute ulnar nerve damage.

A method:

1.   Have the patient grasp a piece of newspaper (or writing paper, or a tape) with each hand between the tips of the thumb and index finger.

2.   Instruct him to pull laterally with each hand to tauten the test object. In cases of acute ulnar neuropathy, the paper will slip from the thumb on the affected side. *A caveat:* Please note that this test requires that the median nerve be intact, so that the index finger can flex.

Prescription Paper Test

This is the best test for chronic ulnar nerve damage, or for acute ulnar nerve damage with coexisting median nerve damage. (See also Table 26-7.)

A method:

1.   Ask the patient to spread his extended fingers and hold a piece of prescription paper between two of them.

2.   Instruct the patient to clamp the paper with the sides of his fingers (closing them like a scissors.)

3.   Ask the patient to hold onto the paper while you try to pull it out.

Claw Hand Deformity

Patients with a chronic ulnar palsy will be unable to extend the little finger at its interphalangeal joints. Sometimes the ring finger shares this posture. The fingers are hyperextended at the metacarpophalangeal joints, the hypothenar eminence is flattened, and the palm is hollowed. Together these produce the characteristic *main en griffe*, which has been translated as "claw" hand, but should probably be translated as "talon" because some think of "claw" in connection with "hammer," whereas the hand more closely resembles a bird's talon, rather than the claw of a hammer.

1.   The same posture also occurs in median nerve palsy when the patient is asked to *flex* his fingers (vide infra).

2.   In combined median and ulnar nerve damage, all four fingers will be clawed.

3.   When the patient with an ulnar palsy is asked to extend his fingers, the resulting posture resembles that of some gynecolo-

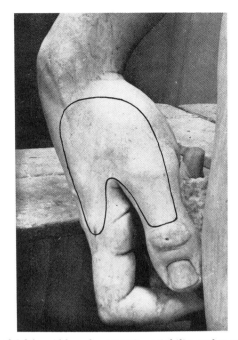

Figure 26-34.   *Although anatomic variability makes most universal statements suspect, sensation within the marked area is carried by the radial nerve in almost everyone. Detail from David, by Michelangelo.*

gists at the introitus, with one or two of the ulnar-most fingers tucked in flexion, and the index and third fingers straight. (This should *not* be referred to as the *main d'accoucher* because that phrase literally means the hand of the obstetrician, not the gynecologist. The obstetrician extends all fingers at the interphalangeal joints and flexes at the metacarpophalangeal joints, and Trousseau has already taken that name for the posture of carpal spasm.)

Sensory Abnormalities

Once you have detected motor evidence of ulnar nerve disease, clinch the diagnosis by checking sensation on the little finger.

Palpation

The ulnar nerve is probably the only nerve in the body that is readily palpable in vivo. It lies in the groove between the olecranon process and the medial epicondyle of the humerus. This groove is posterior and distal to the place where you palpated for epitrochlear nodes. (Mail carrier's ulnar neuropathy has a dimple distal to this point [Massey, 1989].)

Try finding your own. It has the size and shape of the thin plastic refill of some ballpoint pens and the consistency of spaghetti cooked al dente. When it is pressed lightly, you may experience a noxious sensation. If the nerve is touched too vigorously, the result is paresthesias or the sensation known as "hitting the funny bone"—probably thus named because it lies near the humorous humerus.

If an ulnar nerve feels enlarged and stiffened, you can diagnose interstitial hypertrophic neuritis.

Median Nerve

Motor Signs

A good motor test for acute median nerve disease is Ochsner's clasp sign. Have the patient clasp his hands together as if in prayer, but more tightly. If the motor branch of the median nerve is diseased, it will not be possible for the patient to flex the index finger on that side and it will stick up from the clasped hands.

The best chronic motor sign is also based on the inability to flex the index finger, and sometimes the middle finger. When the other two fingers are flexed, the result is the benediction sign or the papal hand.

The patient with a chronic median nerve palsy will also have loss of wrist flexion, thenar atrophy, and inability to flex the distal phalanx of the thumb, index finger, and usually the third finger. Taken together, this results in the appearance of a "monkey paw." If asked to flex all of his fingers, the patient will assume the posture of a gynecologist at the introitus (benediction hand).

Sensory Abnormalities

To confirm your diagnosis of a median nerve lesion, you must demonstrate a sensory component. The best place (in terms of consistency of innervation by the median nerve) is the tip of the index finger. It will be easy to remember this after studying Figure 26-35.

Carpal Tunnel Syndrome

This neuropathy is due to entrapment of the median nerve in the carpal tunnel. The volar carpal ligament looks and feels thickened and somewhat nodular. If the palmaris longus tendon can be seen all the way past the volar carpal ligament, the patient does not have carpal tunnel syndrome.

Tinel's sign is the reproduction of tingling paresthesias over the volar radial aspect of the hand by percussing the volar wrist over the carpal tunnel. Begin over the area of the wristwatch band, moving up toward the "life line"* on the palm back to the wristband, and then a bit radially to the palmaris longus tendon, if you can feel it. Tinel's sign is 65–66% sensitive (Phalen, 1970; Spinner et al., 1989).

Phalen's sign is the reproduction of tingling and paresthesia in the median nerve region by holding the patient's wrist in acute passive flexion for a minute. The significance is the same as Tinel's sign, but the sensitivity is 70–77% (Phalen, 1970; Spinner et al., 1989).

Median nerve hypesthesia is 43–73% sensitive for the diagnosis, and thenar atrophy (Fig. 26-36) is 37–40% sensitive (Phalen, 1970; Spinner et al., 1989).

Both the signs and the nerve conduction studies correlate exactly with the symptoms. If the patient is asymptomatic when seen, the signs may not be present.

---

*The palm reader's "life line" is the palmar crease separating the thenar eminence from the rest of the palm.

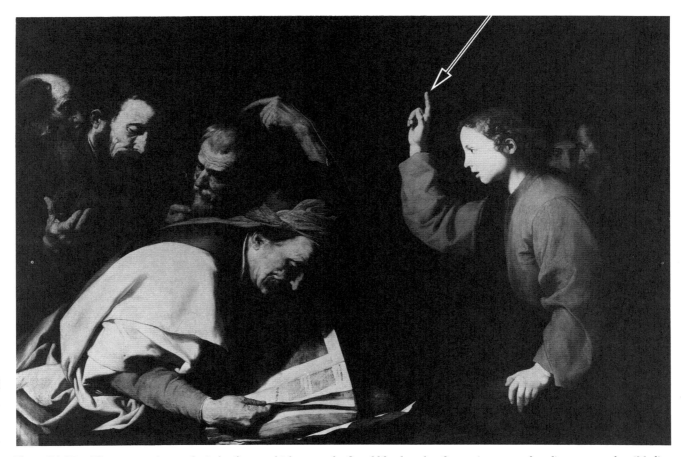

Figure 26-35.   *The arrow points to the index finger, which cannot be flexed like the other fingers in a case of median nerve palsy. (Median nerve palsy can also cause the benediction hand—not illustrated here—in which the index and middle finger are extended at the MCP joint, as if to give a papal benediction.) One of the doctors is trying to find the anatomic basis for the test in his textbook, while the one immediately behind him is apparently testing the sensory division of his own median nerve by thumping his forefinger on his head.* Christ Among the Doctors *by Ribera, courtesy of the Kunsthistorisches Museum, Vienna.*

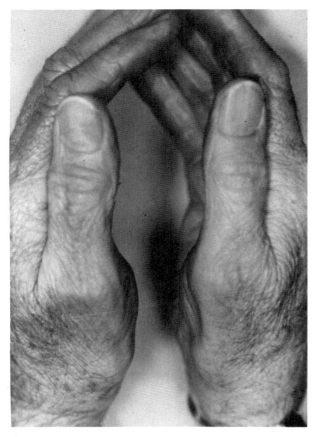

Table 26-12. Tuning Forks for Vibratory Sensation

Frequency	Advantages	Disadvantages
64 Hz	Meissner's fibers lose this first (S. Horenstein, personal communication, 1988)	
128 Hz	Higher threshold than 256 Hz	
256 Hz	1. Lowest vibratory threshold 2. More sensitive than 128 Hz in pernicious anemia (Herbert, 1988) 3. Paccinian fibers lose this first	
512 Hz	Higher threshold than 256 Hz	Many normal old persons give false positives (S. Horenstein, personal communication, 1988)

Sources: *Threshold data from Plumb and Meigs (1961) and Lofvenberg and Johansson (1984).*

Figure 26-36. *Thenar atrophy due to carpal tunnel syndrome. Photograph courtesy of* Consultant *and Thomas E. Weiss, M.D., Alton Ochsner Medical Foundation.*

Other Peripheral Nerves

The anterior interosseous branch of the median nerve is involved in some unusual lesions of the forearm ("Bailey," Clain, 1973). This nerve innervates the flexor pollicis longus and is tested by the method in Table 26-7, and by the thumb reflex (see p. 497).

Other upper extremity entrapment syndromes have been reviewed (Esposito, 1972).

Other lower extremity entrapment neuropathies (e.g., femoral nerve entrapment [Ch.24, p. 423], and anterior compartment syndrome [Ch.25, p. 442]) have been reviewed (Kopell & Thompson, 1960). Most of the latter are still diagnosed by history, but there is no reason that manipulations to reproduce symptoms or produce signs could not be developed for some of them as for the carpal tunnel syndrome (see p. 506).

The bible for peripheral neuropathy is Dyck et al. (1984).

Sensory Testing

Vibratory Sensation

Vibratory sensation does not really exist as a separate sensory modality. It is rather an interpretation of deep pressure sensation, the bone acting as a resonator. However, it is still a clinically useful modality, if not a neuroanatomic one, and when tested in concordance with position sensation is a helpful assay of the human dorsal columns.

$$ There has been a great deal of discussion about which frequency tuning fork is truly the best. Based upon the data sum-

marized in Table 26-12, the 256-Hz fork is recommended for testing vibratory sensation. But the others have their champions. Dr. Simon Horenstein of Missouri carries an *additional* 64-Hz fork because that is the frequency first lost by the Meissner's fibers. Some prefer the 128-Hz fork because the threshold is higher for this frequency than for 256 Hz; thus, a more difficult task is created. There are even those who like the 512-Hz fork on the grounds that one can save money by using the same tuning fork for testing both hearing and vibratory sensation.

(The last remind me of the surgeon who showed the patient his X-ray films and advised an operation. The patient asked how much it would cost. "Ten thousand dollars," said the surgeon. The patient said, "Well, I am in debt, I have no insurance and no prospects. All I have in the world is the 10 dollars in my pocket. What can you do for 10 dollars?" "Well," said the surgeon, "for 10 dollars I could touch up the X rays." Moral: the practice of medicine is full of false economies.)

More important even than the frequency are the strength of the blow to the fork and the duration between the blow and the application of the tuning fork to the patient. Young persons probably get more variable results than older examiners because the older examiners are more constant in their motions. (Also, as Jack Myers once said to a medical student, "The most important aspect of the neurologic examination is knowing which findings to ignore.")

A Method

1. If you have not already done so during the performance of the Weber test (Ch. 11, p. 211), give the patient a reference sensation for vibration by placing the base of the vibrating tuning fork on his forehead or sternum. Ask the patient, "What do you feel?" He should say "buzzing," "tingling," "humming," or some other word that indicates that he feels vibrations, not simply the pressure of the base of the fork. If you must help the patient by asking, "Is it vibrating?," you should place the *non*vibrating fork over the same area and ask if the patient can feel the difference. Then say, "It's just the first sensation that we're looking for. Pressure alone, like now, doesn't count. Okay?"

Then wait to see if the patient indicates that he understands. In this manner, almost all patients can be taught to report vibration specifically and not just pressure.

Another reference sensation can be elicited by placing by vibrating fork on the edge of the great toenail.

2. When the patient has indicated that he understands the instructions, say, "Now close your eyes. I will touch you, and you tell me if you feel the (vibration equivalent) or if you don't. I won't hurt you. Keep your eyes closed." Then strike the fork and place the base firmly against the bony prominence to be tested. (Vibration is always and only tested over bone!)

Say, "What do you feel?" (Don't say: "Is it vibrating?" or "Do you feel anything?")

The patient should respond with one of the chosen words. If you are uncertain as to whether he is feeling the vibrations, ask, "Or are you just feeling the pressure?" You may have to hit the fork again since the intensity of the vibrations is constantly decreasing, and an overly cooperative patient may wait until he can no longer feel vibration in order to give an affirmative response to the last question!

3. Additionally, if the patient can truly feel the vibrations, he should also be able to detect their sudden cessation. Accordingly, say to the patient, who has already said that he can feel the vibrations, "Keep your eyes closed and tell me the moment it stops." With your free hand, suddenly damp the tines. This sharp cutoff can easily be identified and is thus preferable to the more common practice of letting the tuning fork "run down on its own." When the latter happens, some overly cooperative patients spend a lot of time silently trying to decide if "it is all gone," while the frustrated examiner can clearly see that the tines are no longer moving.

Alternately, one can begin the testing with a very soft or even a damped blow so that the patient initially feels nothing, and increase the intensity on successive tests until getting above the threshold of perception (S. Horenstein, personal communication, 1988).

4. Some overly cooperative patients also learn to pair the sound of the examiner striking the fork with the subsequent vibratory sensation. Control for this at least once by hitting the fork, silently damping it, and then applying it to an area previously determined to be normal. The patient should report pressure, but no vibration.

5. Routinely, one should test both index toes. ("Routinely" means there is nothing in the history and nothing on the neurologic examination [including the position sense testing] to suggest neurologic disease.) Spending time on the thumbs routinely is less profitable.

Herbert noted that the index toe lost vibratory sensation before the big toe in pernicious anemia (Herbert, 1988).

6. When testing the toes on a cold day, allow time for the patient's feet to warm up, as cold increases the vibratory threshold and so may give a false positive for impaired vibratory sensation (Keighley, 1946).

7. If vibratory sense is impaired in the toes, sequentially test at the malleoli, the shins, the patellae, and so forth.

If diabetic neuropathy is suspected, one should also check vibratory sensation over the sacrum. Although the longest nerves in the body go to the toes, some diabetics actually have a myelopathy in addition to or without the peripheral neuropathy. Since the sacrum is the most convenient place to check the longest passage through the spinal cord, this examination improves the sensitivity of the neurologic examination as a screening test for complications of diabetes mellitus.

Validity

Each time the patient correctly identifies vibration versus pressure, or identifies the cessation of vibration on damping, it is considered a correct response. Seven correct responses with no incorrect responses is a valid test for normal vibratory sensation. One incorrect response and eight or nine correct identifications is also a valid test for normal vibratory sensation. But two or more incorrect responses out of seven, eight, or nine suggests either impaired vibratory sensation or lack of cooperation.

The statistical basis for the validity testing is called the sign test (Edwards, 1954), which is based on the binomial distribution. The question we are asking is whether or not the patient's responses are random. The probability of seven out of seven correct responses by chance alone is 0.0078. The probability of six or more correct out of seven (by chance alone) is 0.0625, which is greater than the 0.05 cutoff customarily used as a criterion for statistical significance.

Questionable Results

If the test results are questionable because of the manner of the patient's response, what should the examiner do? According to Susann's Law, he should repeat the testing later. This law, named for its author Jacqueline Susann, states that "Once Is Not Enough." It was taught to me by Dr. Bruce McClain of Virginia.

Discordance of Vibratory and Proprioceptive Sensation

Vibratory sensation is carried along fibers that are predominantly located in a different portion of the dorsal column than the proprioceptive fibers, according to some experts. Also, some believe that the two sets of fibers diverge in the higher portions of the spinal cord. Nevertheless, in a large teaching experience, reported dissociation of vibratory and position sense usually turns out to be not an unusual lesion, but a young doctor and an old patient. This still happens even though the "free" tuning forks once given to sophomore medical students by drug hucksters are not so ubiquitous now. These forks were so poorly made that they could not possibly be used for their stated purpose. Entire classes, unable to elicit vibratory sensation in anyone, abandoned such testing.

Proprioception (Position)

Proprioception is customarily tested in the lower extremities on a routine basis. Some physicians test the little toes in the belief that the longest nerve tracts in the body are best suited to a screening test. Others find the little toes clumsy to work with, and so test the big toe. Although the method is given for the big toe, the same principles apply to other toes as well as to the thumbs and fingers. The latter should be tested if one suspects a diagnosis affecting the upper extremities, such as syringomyelia, some diabetic Charcot joints, or myelopathy (in which a level must be determined).

A Method

1. The first trick is to position yourself so as to eliminate visual cues to the patient, or instruct the patient to close his eyes and glance up from time to time to see that he has done so. If the patient is bed bound, and you are wearing a white coat, you can drape it over the patient's feet. (Alternately, use the bed sheet or a blanket.) It must be emphasized that many patients, especially those with decreased proprioception, will open their eyes in the middle of testing to see the position of their toes, no matter how clearly and pleasantly the examiner gives his instructions. This is not a reflection of the perverse nature of humankind, but an example of how anxious patients are to please. If unable to succeed at the task with his eyes closed, the patient may wish to help the doctor in his work by opening his eyes, thus being able to give the correct answer to the questions.

Validity

If the patient gets seven out of seven, or eight out of nine correct, proprioception is intact (see p. 508, "Validity"). If fewer than this, either proprioception or reporting is impaired.

Pinprick (Superficial Pain) Sensation

A Method

1. Ask the patient to close his eyes, touch him with a sharp pin on a normal part of his skin, and tell him that, "This is sharp." Then touch him with the dull end of the pin and tell him that, "This is dull." Have the patient identify the sharp sensation to be sure he has understood the instructions, before proceeding to the areas where abnormal results may be obtained.

2. Apply the sharp and dull parts of the pin in a random sequence, and ask the patient to identify them. Seven correct responses in a row is statistically significant, and evidence for intact sensation.

What kind of pin? The use of a single pin for all patients, as was standard practice in the past, is no longer advisable. Viruses, slow viruses, virions, and prions could be transmitted from patient to patient, especially by an examiner who stabbed vigorously to be sure of hypesthesia. While it is not necessary to puncture the skin in order to test superficial pain sensation, this does happen from time to time. Accordingly, each patient gets his own safety pin (the head can be used for "dull"). A disposable syringe needle (the hub can be used for dull) is sometimes used, but these are very sharp and often cause the patient to bleed. Alternately, break a wooden applicator stick or tongue blade in half so as to obtain a sharp point, or use a Japanese or Korean chopstick. (Chinese chopsticks are not so pointed, but a hand-held pencil sharpener will make a point that is perfect for testing, as well as a clean new point for each patient.)

\$\$

Another Method

With very intelligent patients, one can use the Wartenberg wheel, a series of sharp arms radiating out from a roller hub, which can be lightly passed over a large area, producing a relatively uniform "sharp" stimulus at regular intervals. Ask the patient to tell you if there is a change in the sensation.

With this method, there is no control "dull." Also, there may be bizarre responses due to the stimulus-response summation from many points within a segment.

If one does use this method, one must take care not to puncture the skin. Since the question of whether or not there has been a slight puncturing of the skin is in the domain of metaphysics (it being impossible to prove a negative proposition), some would advise soaking the wheel in a disinfectant such as chlorine bleach, or autoclaving it, before using it on another patient.

\$\$ A chrome-plated Wartenberg wheel is not necessary. The original device was a tailor's tracing wheel, available at any fabric shop.

Localization of Lesion from Distribution of Sensory Loss

Sensory loss due to a lesion in a peripheral nerve or a nerve root should be located in the appropriate region of the skin (Fig. 26-37). A lesion that interrupts the ascending fibers in the lateral spinothalamic tracts will cause sensory loss in the dermatomes below that level (a "sensory level," a key finding in spinal cord compression). Acute central disc herniation causes saddle anesthesia (Hall, 1983). Peripheral neuropathy often causes sensory loss in the distal extremities, the "stocking-glove" distribution. For localizing lesions in the cerebral cortex, there is a sensory homunculus (Fig. 26-38), comparable to the motor homunculus (Fig. 26-14). (The homunculi were constructed from data gathered by direct intraoperative stimulation of the brain of a conscious patient. You might want to compare it with results obtained in your own patients in the era of the CT scan.) Finally, findings that do not correspond to the neurologic anatomy may be attributed to problems in the higher cortical centers (see p. 510).

Do not attempt to memorize the figures; you can always look them up. Your time is better spent examining patients.

When testing for sensory deficits, a good maneuver is to have the patient draw out the perceived deficit on his skin. Begin your testing in the center of the region so indicated and work out to the periphery (S. Horenstein, personal communication, 1988).

Deep Pain

Deep pain, or noxious deep pressure, is different from other proprioceptive sensation in that the fibers ascend in the lateral spinothalamic tracts. These have already been tested by superficial pain. Thus, deep pain is seldom tested for these days. Formerly, its absence was sought as an early sign of tabes dorsalis.

The absence of deep pain is eponymized according to the part of the body that the examiner squeezes. The Achilles tendon is Abadie's, the testicle is Pitres', the ulnar nerve (see p. 505) is Biernacki's. The eyeball and the ovary have not yet been claimed.

Piesthesia Versus Light Touch Sensation

Piesthesia is the sensation of pressure. This is based upon the stimulation of subcutaneous corpuscles whose messages are carried in the dorsal columns. It is also important because it is distinct from superficial light touch (tactile) sensation, which is carried in \$\$ the fibers of the ventral spinothalamic tract. Light touch is tested for with a camel's hair brush.

Temperature Sensation

Temperature sensation is not usually checked routinely, because it is carried in the lateral spinothalamic tracts, which have already been tested with pinprick. However, in cervical syringomyelia, the syrinx may occur at the site of fiber decussation and produce the puzzling result that pain sensation is decreased while light touch is intact. In this setting, temperature testing is used as the "tie-breaker" and usually reveals that pain and temperature sensation in the area served by the involved segment are clearly decreased or missing, while light touch (carried in the ventral spinothalamic tract) is intact.

A Method

While considerable blarney has been spoken about the importance of using warm or cold water of specific temperatures, the point to remember is that the water should be neither so hot nor so cold that it produces pain in addition to temperature sensation.

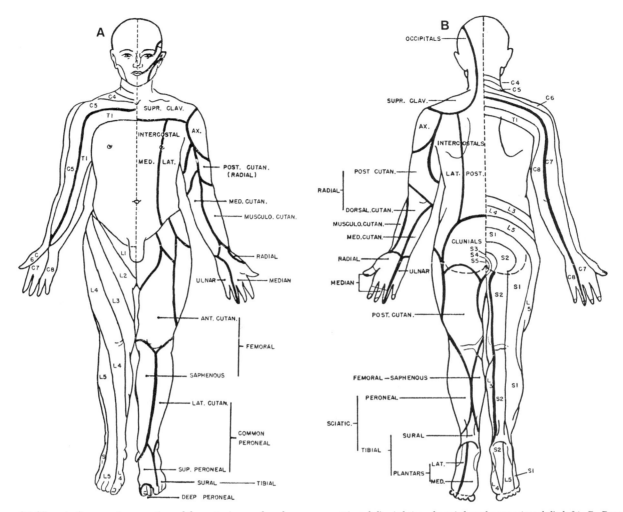

Figure 26-37. *A, Sensory innervation of the anterior surface by nerve root (model's right) and peripheral nerve (model's left). B, Posterior view of same.*

Similarly, the two temperatures must be far enough apart for the difference to be detectable. This is most important when using thick-walled glass test tubes. (Although metal containers are more difficult to find, they are preferable because they conduct heat much better than glass does.)

1. Have the patient close his eyes, place one of the test tubes against his skin and ask, "Hot, cold, or neither?" (It is important to include the "neither" because tactile sensation may be intact, and the overly cooperative patient may guess even without temperature sensation. By reducing the odds of success at guessing from 50% to 33%, one can more quickly and confidently complete the testing.)

2. Keep changing the areas of the test tubes that are applied to the patient's skin because the skin itself may warm the wall of a glass tube, causing false positives.

3. Similarly, it is a good idea to check occasionally the temperature by touching the tubes to your own skin.

Alternate Methods

One could use a cold object (such as a cold tuning fork) or solid objects that may be cooled in the office refrigerator to avoid the inconvenience of tubes and water.

To eliminate the confounding tactile sensation that leads the overly cooperative patient to make guess responses, one could use radiant heat (e.g., an incandescent light source pointed or

focused on the skin) and thus test heat sensation only. (Although different receptors sense heat and cold, the fibers for both ascend in the lateral spinothalamic tract.)

Sensory Signs of Abnormal Activity in Higher Nervous Centers

As in all types of sensory testing, there must be internal consistency. That is, pinprick, thermal, and "tickle" sensation (a type of pain) are lost together. (When comparing the cotton on the left side to that on the right, the patient may say, "I could feel it, but it didn't tickle me" [S. Horenstein, personal communication, 1988].)

Patients with malingering, conversion reactions, "compensation neurosis," and hysteria may sometimes present with complaints referable to the peripheral nervous system, when the basic problem is actually higher in the nervous system. The various motor manifestations of this diagnostic problem have already been covered (see p. 487). Four sensory manifestations are especially useful.

1. Lateral Anesthesia to Pinprick Ending Sharply at Midline

Also known as "sharp midline cutoff," this finding signifies that there is no peripheral neurologic explanation for the patient's problems.

This is logical because the peripheral nerves from each side

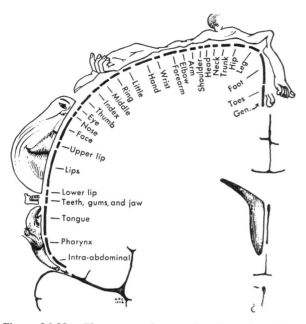

Figure 26-38.   The sensory homunculus. Reproduced from Penfield W, Rasmussen T: The Cerebral Cortex of Man. *Macmillan, New York, 1950.*

jointly supply the midline, where they overlap. Thus, midline stimuli can be sensed even if one side is completely anesthetic. (You will note that when you have a nerve block for your dental work, the numbness is not midline and the cutoff or demarcation area for the anesthesia is gradual rather than sharp.)

2. Sharp Cutoffs for Vibratory Sensation

Often used over the sternum, this method can also be used to find sharp cutoffs (either midline or peripheral) over other bones.

A method.   Place your vibrating tuning fork against the bone. For each trial, reposition it no more than the diameter of the base of the tuning fork, especially as you approach the area where there was a sharp border for other sensations. Patients whose "lesion" is in the higher information-processing centers may report the sharp cutoff of vibratory sensation at the same skin area as it occurred with other sensory modalities. This does not occur in patients with peripheral nerve lesions because the vibrations are amplified by the bone, and the bone vibrates for some radius around the base of the tuning fork. Patients who have not had a course in neurophysiology do not know this, and believe that the fork is testing some purely localized skin sensation.

Some doctors feel that the hallmark of patients with the "lesion" in the higher centers is their unreliability, causing the lines of sensory cutoff to shift when the patient was examined repeatedly with the same modality. Thinking that the malingerer would "forget" between trials where the sensory cutoff was supposed to be, these doctors marked the cutoff in plain view of the patient. This maneuver assumes that malingering patients would not notice the line! To get around this new problem, other doctors marked the line in a different location from the finding, believing that if the patient, on second testing, indicated a cutoff at the marked line, the examiner had demonstrated a shifting cutoff. This practice is also to be eschewed since some overly cooperative patients will follow the implied suggestion even though they are not malingerers.

An alternate method.   Place a quarter or other coin in the midline or over the sharp cutoff, and then place the base of the vibrating tuning fork against it so that the entire coin vibrates. Patients who are composing a neurologic examination, for whatever rea-

son, may report that they feel the vibrations only under one half of the coin (e.g., 12½ cents of vibration.)

Another method.   In the case in which you mark the sharp cutoff line of the skin, try sliding the "insensitive" skin over the sensitive bone and repeating the test. Also try sliding the "sensitive" skin up over the insensitive bone and repeating the test. The patient who is "composing a neurologic examination" may "regain" vibratory sensation over previously insensitive bone (and lose it over the previously sensitive bone) because he believes the sensation to be carried by the skin.

3. Topographic Confusion

This third gambit (after Bowlus & Currier, 1963) is actually a variation of a traditional children's game.

A method.   Stand in front of the patient and tell him to mimic your actions exactly.

a.   Hold your arms forward, extended at the elbows, with the palms facing each other.

b.   When the patient has copied you exactly, quickly (as if testing him for his reaction time) rotate your wrists 180 degrees so that the thumbs are now pointing down, with the palms facing laterally. (If you did not play this game as a child, practice now so that the motions will be second nature when you do it on a patient.)

c..   Flexing your arms at the elbows, let your hands cross over and under each other in the midline, so that the palms now face each other again with the thumbs still pointing toward the floor (Fig. 26-39A).

d.   Now clasp your hands together with the fingers from each hand alternately placed. Your arms, hands, and body should form a sort of crude figure "8" (Fig. 26-39B).

e.   Bring your clasped hands under your chin. (To do this, move both elbows first out then down.) The thumbs will now be farthest from you (Fig. 26-39C).

f.   Looking down your fingers, you will be confused as to which side the fingers are coming from. The patient would also be confused if he looked, but he is looking at you for the next instruction because he believes that you are testing some motor function.

g.   Say, "Keep your hands clasped just like that for a minute," as you release your own clasped hands and pick up the examining pin.

Note that the distal phalanges are on the same side of the clasped fingers as the side of the body they are from. But the middle digits resemble so many sausages squeezed together. There is an uncanny ignorance of the viewed parts of one's own anatomy. (This explains why this was a popular children's game in the pretelevision era, when children were more easily amused than today.) The test is based on this ignorance.

h.   Say to the patient, "I am going to stick two fingers. Tell me which you can*not* feel—the first or the second."

i.   Jab any two adjacent fingers.

The neurologically impaired patient will not be able to feel the fingers whose distal phalanges are on the side of the hemianesthesia. They will make an immediate response. (However, these genuine peripheral neuropathy patients often ignore your instructions and tell you which finger they *can* feel.)

The person whose symptoms are not due to a peripheral lesion has a completely different response. He will be stumped and often unable to answer quickly without thinking, although he will usually say something while trying to figure out which finger he is not supposed to be able to feel. Sometimes, he will release his hands and "quit." Sometimes, he can be hurried into making an answer before he has figured out the topography of his clasped fingers. He might say that he felt no pin with either finger or that he felt it with

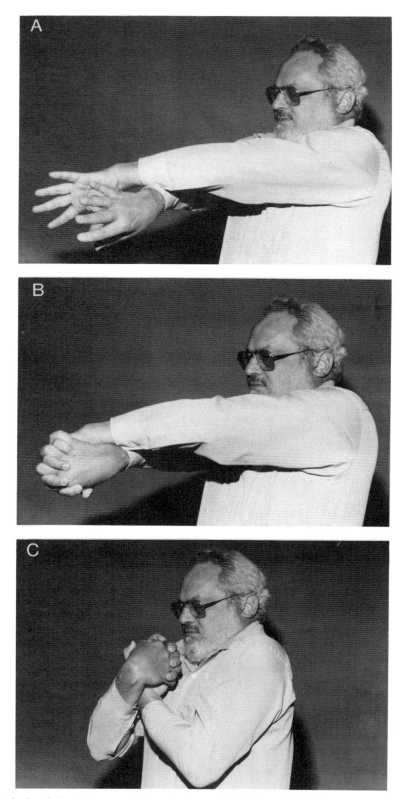

Figure 26-39.   *Positioning the hands for the topographic confusion test for hemianesthesia. The patient, who unlike the model will not be anticipating a flashbulb, should keep his eyes open throughout the test.*

both. These are equally bogus, since any two adjacent fingers must come from opposite sides of the body.

A caveat: Definition of "higher centers." Be not too quick to judge. While the detection of the entity "malingering" makes assumptions about the higher center's representation of motivation, parietal lobe lesions can also produce some interesting examination results (see p. 514). For instance, some patients with parietal lobe lesions will also be unable to do this particular test.

A variation. This test may be converted to a test of motor function by pointing to—not touching—any two adjacent digits, beginning with the "healthy one," and asking the patient to wiggle the fingers.

4. Another Confusion Technique
This final test works only with very simple people.

a. Ask the patient to close his eyes.

b. Beginning on the healthy side of the cutoff line, begin rhythmically sticking the patient with the pin.

c. As you continue to move toward the cutoff line, ask the patient, "Can you feel that?"

d. When the patient answers in the affirmative, say, "Good. Now say 'yes' each time I stick you and you can feel it, and say 'no' when you cannot feel it."

e. At a place on the healthy side of the cutoff line, continue rhythmically sticking the patient so that he gets in a few "yeses." Then quickly move the pin-sticking at the same rhythm so that you reach the cutoff line in about two beats. Continue sticking as you move across the line.

The person with a peripheral neuropathy will simply stop responding when you cross the line.

Some persons with disease of the higher centers will say "no" each time you touch them, once you have crossed the line. (Of course, if they had no sensation, they would not be able to tell when you were touching them.)

A positive test is so amazing the first time you observe it that I suggest resting your pin in one "anesthetic" place and slightly varying the rhythm so as to convince yourself that you are not getting automatic "noes."

To the attending. Don't do this test with a Wartenberg wheel.

A caveat. To get results on these tests, you should be quick, professional, brusque, and almost bored in manner. You should remember that although these tests are tricks in a sense, you are still working for the patient. You are using these tricks not to hurt or fool him, but rather to solve problems for him. The purpose of the tests is not to abuse or humiliate patients.

If the test is positive, I sometimes say to the patient, "This will go away in a few days." In others, I might refer the patient for evaluation for long-term psychotherapy. In some cases, I might confront the patient, pointing out that his nervous system is working better than he thinks, taking care to do so in a positive and encouraging way. At other times, I have encouraged an insurance company to go to trial or at least to take my deposition, because in patients with "compensation neurosis," the findings do not get better until the trial is over or the case dropped. There is no pat rule for all patients in whom these tests are positive except one: you are still working for the patient, albeit in a somewhat paternal fashion.

Intracranial Lesions
Evidence of space-occupying lesions (such as tumors, hemorrhages, or arteriovenous malformations) or vascular problems may be sought by auscultatory percussion (see Ch. 9, p. 152) or auscultation for bruits (see Ch. 18, p. 343).

Further Reflections on the Neurologic Examination (or, The Patient as an Active Participant)

In olden days, a patient would say to the doctor, "Give me a *good* physical," as if one might get a *bad* physical. This statement derived, on inquiry, from several sources: A personal service involving touching of an excellent quality was desired. The physician was seen as superior to the machine. Touching was in itself therapeutic. Finally, the patient was passive, acted upon. The last concerns us here.

In the neurologic portion of the physical examination, the patient is sometimes required to make responses that are correct or incorrect. Their correctness is communicated (nonverbally) to the patient by the physician, and so in this portion of the examination the patient is no longer passive. This has two practical interpersonal implications. First, the patient who does not give correct answers should not be made to feel a failure. The best way to prevent this is to indicate in the instructions that some incorrect answers are to be expected. Second, a cluster of incorrect answers will often indicate to the patient that something is wrong. Many times the problem is a peripheral neuropathy, appearing as a complication of another problem that is of greater concern to the physician. The problem needs to be explained to the patient so that he will not worry. This could be done as soon as one finds the neuropathy, although in general one wishes to avoid premature reassurance (Sapira, 1972). Alternately, the physician may wait until the examination is complete and the patient dressed to explain the conclusions of the consultation, (e.g., "You have a little nerve damage in your legs, but that is from your diabetes and doesn't explain why you have been getting short of breath. I am more concerned about the shortness of breath, which seems to be due to . . . ")

Autonomic Nervous System

Examination of the Skin
The normal vasodilation that follows a scratch is a simple test of the intact autonomic nervous system. This may be formalized and exaggerated as the triple response to the intradermal injection of 0.1 ml of 1:1,000 histamine phosphate (DeJong, 1979).

Sweat Test
$$ A simple sweat test consists of placing the patient in an uncomfortably warm room and observing the skin with a magnifying lens.

Alternate Stimuli
If a hot room is not available, heating blankets or a rack of heat lamps may be used. Pilocarpine injections should be avoided as they are unreliable.

Alternate Detectors
$$ Drag the bowl of a spoon across the skin. If there is no sweating, it drags, but if there is sweating, it slides. Or, apply a piece of tissue or paper towel, say to the forehead, and observe whether only one side is wet.

The various indicator dusts that turn color when wet are useful for formal presentations, but are not needed for close work by the individual physician. They should specifically be avoided in the hospital as they stain the bed linens, in some cases permanently.

Finger Wrinkling

Normally, when the hands are immersed in water at 40°C for 30 minutes, the volar surfaces (which are devoid of sebaceous glands) wrinkle or pucker or "prune." This sign is lost in diabetic autonomic neuropathy, in Guillain-Barré syndrome, in the distribution of the median nerve in median nerve neuropathy, in postsympathectomy states, and in an anesthetized finger (ring block) (Bull & Henry, 1977). The fingers may also fail to wrinkle in cases of severe edema.

Cardiovascular Examination

Postural hypotension (see Ch. 6, p. 89) is a useful autonomic sign, assuming that one has eliminated volume depletion as its etiology. (The absence of a pulse rise is not seen in volume depletion.) The presence of a pressor and/or pulse response to mental arithmetic localizes the lesion to the central afferent limb. Unfortunately, these maneuvers, the pharmacologic tests, the cold pressor test, and the chemical determination of autonomic neurohumor levels all have little therapeutic implication. See also "Oculocardiac Reflex" (p. 464).

Selected Syndromes

Parietal Lobe Syndrome

Classical Approach

1. Parietal lobe lesions may interfere with the visual pathways and produce a lower homonymous quadrantanopsia (in the ipsilateral nasal field and contralateral temporal field).

2. A gaze preference (see p. 454) may result from a parietal lobe lesion.

3. The only pure parietal lobe sign is an avoidance contactual automatism (see p. 504).

4. Parietal lobe lesions may produce loss of sensory modalities or, more likely, loss of all sensory representation of the affected surface. These lesions may be very difficult to detect unless one uses Bender's technique of double simultaneous stimulation. If the clinician taps simultaneously on both sides of the body (e.g., the face, see also p. 457), at exact mirror image points, patients with a parietal lesion will not feel the stimulus on the side opposite the lesion (that is, the part of the body served by the afflicted cortex). However, the stimulus will be perceived if the same spot is touched singly! This interesting phenomenon is also known as parietal cortical extinction.

5. More posteriorly placed parietal lobe lesions may produce peculiar sensory syndromes characterized more by loss of awareness of the part than by loss of a discrete modality. With *implicit neglect,* the patient verbally admits that there is a problem, but operationally and behaviorally ignores the problem in his contemporary behavior and his plans for the future. With *explicit neglect,* the syndrome itself is denied, as in the final worst stages of cortical blindness (vide infra).

One example of the latter is *contralateral* (to the lesion) *neglect,* in which the patient pays no attention to the limb or other body part whose parietal lobe representation has been afflicted. The patient may not wash it, or in some cases move it, even though motor function is perfectly intact. However, contralateral neglect is not of itself diagnostic for parietal lobe lesions and may be seen with temporal lobe lesions, occipital lobe lesions, frontal lobe lesions, or lesions of the connections between them.

In other versions of contralateral neglect, there are various forms of agnosia in which the patient may variously deny that there is anything wrong with the body part or even that it belongs to him. Or there may be preservation of sensation with an alteration in the dimensions of identity, depth of sensation, and general stereognosis (not simply position sensation).

These forms of agnosia may also be part of other peculiar syndromes, which may tempt the superficial physician to believe that he is dealing with some sort of malingering. One such syndrome, long a snare to the gullible, is Gerstmann's syndrome. (While some authorities believe that Gerstmann's syndrome is simply a concatenation of events with no specific localizing significance, it is peculiar enough to be noted.)

Gerstmann's syndrome may be seen in middle cerebral artery strokes, especially on the left. It comprises acalculia, alexia, finger agnosia, and right-left confusion. The latter is not simply the inability to name right and left parts, but an unawareness of their distinction. This was best illustrated by a patient of Dr. Andy Lonigro of Missouri.

After completing the examination of one leg, which the patient had extended out to him, Dr. Lonigro released his grasp on that leg and said to the patient, "Now, give me your other leg."

The patient did not move, but merely glanced at Dr. Lonigro quizzically and said, "But Doctor, that *is* my other leg."

For some other clinical histories, see Sacks (1985).

Finger agnosia may be detected in severe cases by grasping the patient's fingers in such a way as to intertwine alternately the examiner's own fingers with those of the patient. When the digital braids are presented to the patient, he is unable to say which of the fingers belong to him.

Density Approach

It is more useful and clinically clearer to note the density of the parietal lobe syndromes than it is to attempt a treacherous topologic diagnosis, as discussed under classical approach. Thus, there is a hierarchy of disease starting with mild disease and progressing to more severe, dense disease.

Tactile sensation. For this modality, the mildest disease is that which is only detected using the technique of double simultaneous stimulation. Next, there is impaired localization of the singly presented stimulus. At the next level, there is inability to perform the tests for two-point discrimination (vide infra), inability to identify numbers drawn on the tip of the finger (where there are abundant nerve endings, as opposed to the palm on which there are few), and inability to recognize (not name) objects placed in the patient's palm (out of sight). Then, there is inability to dress that side of the body. If the patient wears spectacles, he may put them on so that they fit only the good side. At the very worst level of function, the patient will deny the limb on the affected side.

$$ A method for two-point discrimination: Using a compass or EKG calipers or a bent paper clip, determine the minimum separation between the points at which the patient can determine whether he is being touched with one or two points. Always compare the two sides, using the healthy side as nature's own control. Where this is not possible, be aware that the normal distance varies greatly from person to person and on different parts of the body. The normal ranges are: fingertips, 3 to 8 mm; palm, 8 to 12 mm; back of the hand, 25 to 30 mm; chest, forearm, and shin, 40 mm; back, 40 to 70 mm; thigh and arm, 60 to 70 mm (Wechsler, 1963).

Vision. A similar hierarchy exists for visual events. At the first level, the only way to detect a defect is by double simultaneous stimulation (e.g., hold up two pens, one in each lower temporal quadrant at the same relative position, and determine whether the patient sees both or only one). At the next level, the patient loses his capacity for linear bisection.

$$ A method for linear bisection: Hold your tape measure horizontally in front of the patient, so that any numbers facing him are upside down. Instruct him not to look at the numbers and to point to the "middle" of the segment. Normal persons will come close to the middle (say about 50 cm on a 100-cm tape). Patients with parietal lobe disease will deviate to the good side in proportion to their defect.

With more severe disease, depth perception is lost. The patient will overpoint at the target (say your finger), but only when it is held on the side served by the damaged parietal lobe. At the next level of dysfunction, the patient will lose the ability to construct overlap-
$$ ping polygons, either with matches or toothpicks or when drawing card #8 of the Bender Gestalt test. Finally, with the most severe lesions, the patient is cortically blind and not aware of the fact.

Cerebral Hemorrhage

Hypertensive patients tend to have gray matter cerebral hemorrhages in an isohexahedron bound by the corpus callosum anteriorly, posteriorly, and superiorly; the thalamus-hypothalamic border inferiorly; and the claustrum laterally. These are often related to Bouchard aneurysms. Outside this isohexahedron, the gray matter hemorrhages are predominantly due to other causes such as trauma or the cerebral bleeding that frequently ends the life of patients with severe liver disease.

Wallenberg's Syndrome

This syndrome is also known as the lateral medullary syndrome, or the lateral plate syndrome, from the anatomic area affected. It is also called the syndrome of the posterior inferior cerebellar artery (PICA), after the vessel whose insufficiency most commonly causes it, but actually this waterfall area can become ischemic due to disease in other vessels, including the vertebral artery, and the superior, middle, and inferior lateral medullary arteries.

Significance

This syndrome is important for the generalist for a number of reasons: First, it is the most frequent of the medullary syndromes. Second, it is a syndrome of crossed sensory (pain and temperature) deficit, and therefore likely to be misinterpreted by some psychologically suspicious but anatomically lax physicians. Finally, it has an excellent prognosis for at least partial recovery of function, which can be gratifying for the practitioner, albeit a pitfall for the unsophisticated designer of therapeutic trials.

Appearance

Because it is a syndrome, not all of the findings will "run together" (syndrome) in the individual case. All the findings are ipsilateral to the lesion, except one: the loss of pain and temperature sense on the limbs and trunk, which is contralateral to the loss of pain and temperature on the face. This harlequin sensory defect is the clue to the diagnosis, which in the individual patient can be associated with a large variety of additional defects and their historical counterparts. These include palsies of cranial nerves VI, VII, and VIII; and paralysis of the soft palate, larynx, and pharynx, with their presenting symptoms of dysphagia and dysphonia. The corneal reflex may be lost, and there may even be a Horner's syndrome. Occasionally, cerebellar involvement may produce asynergy and hypotonia. (Again, all of these defects are ipsilateral to the lesion.) Cerebellar involvement may also be responsible for the "midline symptoms" of vertigo, nausea, and vomiting.

It should be specifically noted that there may be ataxia with falling toward the side of the lesion, but true motor weakness of the limbs is not seen and should suggest another diagnosis.

Lesions of the Reticular Activating System

Basilar artery thrombosis, encephalitis, Wernicke's encephalopathy, trauma, neoplasm, and other entities capable of producing a bilateral lesion in the upper brain stem can damage the reticular activating system and the corticospinal and corticobulbar pathways, producing a syndrome of almost total paralysis and impaired consciousness.

Coma Vigil

Patients in coma vigil can apparently be awakened by stimuli. The eyes can open and at times sweep the room from side to side or follow moving objects and persons. Because they seem to respond to loud noises, they are said to be "standing vigil." This state is also called akinetic mutism to emphasize the absence of movement (except of the eyes) and the patient's silence, but this term does not highlight the peculiar retention of eye movement. There are two other inconstant paradoxes: although there are no deep tendon reflexes, there sometimes is withdrawal from noxious stimuli, and although such patients cannot chew, they can sometimes swallow.

Unfortunately, when the family first sees the reflex withdrawal or the eye tracking, they become convinced that the patient is recovering. They must then be disabused by the doctor, who does them the same cruel favor as the friends of the Athenian maniac, who had believed that all the ships arriving in the harbor were his own.

This syndrome must be distinguished from bilateral frontal lobe isolation.

Locked-in Syndrome

Although caused by the same etiologies as the entities above, the locked-in syndrome is not accompanied by impairment of consciousness, possibly because the reticular formation on one side is spared. The patient can communicate with the examiner by blinking his eyes (once for "yes" and twice for "no"; or by counting with eye blinks). Trousseau had such a patient, whom he described to his friend Alexander Dumas *fils*, who portrayed the syndrome in his short story "The Notary." In this story, a young girl recites the alphabet while the patient selects the correct letter by blinking, thus spelling out whole words and sentences.

Bilateral Frontal Lobe Isolation

This entity presents as transcortical motor aphasia. Afflicted patients do not speak spontaneously (although they may grunt from time to time). It requires a great deal of input to get them aroused sufficiently to speak, but when they do, they are quite fluent. Repetition of the test phrases is clear and accurate, and they can read instructions, even aloud, but their writing is poor. Because of their usual silence and their general lack of motor spontaneity, they are often erroneously believed to have coma vigil. Dr. Simon Horenstein of Missouri points out that if you throw a damp (soft) washcloth at such a patient, he will leap into action and catch it. (The cloth should be soft so that the patient will not be injured in the event that your diagnosis is incorrect.)

(Landry-)Guillain-Barré(-Stohl) Syndrome

This syndrome is predominantly an ascending paralysis accompanied by "albuminocytologic dissociation" (i.e., the cerebrospinal fluid shows an elevated protein but relatively few, if any, cells). It often follows viral infections, inoculations, mycoplasma infections, or surgery, and is more frequent in the setting of lymphoma or lupus erythematosus. None of these is essential to the diagnosis (Committee, 1978).

The diagnosis requires progressive weakness of more than one limb, with areflexia. The diagnosis is in doubt if there is marked persistent asymmetry of weakness, bladder or bowel dysfunction at onset, or a sharp sensory level.

"Funny Spells"

Many persons, especially over the age of 40, have lightheadedness for which no etiology can be found. Many of these patients may have impaired vasomotor reflexes due to aging, caffeine, cigarettes, alcohol, sleep deprivation, and an exciting life-style in which catecholamines are continuously being released with or without the aid of drugs. Try reproducing the lightheadedness by having the patient rapidly flex and extend his neck (back and forth and from side to side), and/or rotate it at a rate of about three times per second for a few seconds.

This syndrome has been seen in patients with several negative workups including angiography and CT scan.

Other Syndromes

Also see Meniere's syndrome (p. 461), acoustic neuroma (p. 462), the syndromes of Vernet, Villaret-Collet, and Schmidt (p. 464), the Klippel-Feil syndrome (Ch. 14, p. 231), and carotid sinus syncope (see Ch. 18, p. 340).

Mental Status Examination

While I say my thoughts are in my head, everything's all right; it becomes harmful when we say thoughts aren't in my head,

they're in my mind. (Wittgenstein, *Philosophical Remarks* #230)

If one finds that a patient seems peculiar or uncanny in some poorly defined way, one is required to make further investigation. At the very least, one should do a complete and thorough mental status examination. One should never find one's self describing a patient as "weird" or having "a funny kind of personality," without subsequently making sufficient detailed examination as to be able to elucidate the ultimate nature of such a puzzle. Noting that the patient is odd should be the beginning of a diagnostic move, not its termination.

Self-test: *See Figure 26-40.*

Cognition and Consciousness

I think that both mind and matter are merely convenient ways of grouping events. (Lord Russell, *A History of Western Philosophy,* Ch. 31)

The cognitive portion of the mental status examination must be performed before the history is completed in that one third of all patients who are suspected of having one of the organic brain syndromes (Table 26-14) or any other cause of disorientation. Accordingly, this material has already been covered in Ch. 2 (p. 18) even though it is recorded under "neurologic exam." (Of course, if the patient is not a reliable reporter, that fact should be recorded on the first page of the case report under "reliability," see Ch. 4, p. 64.)

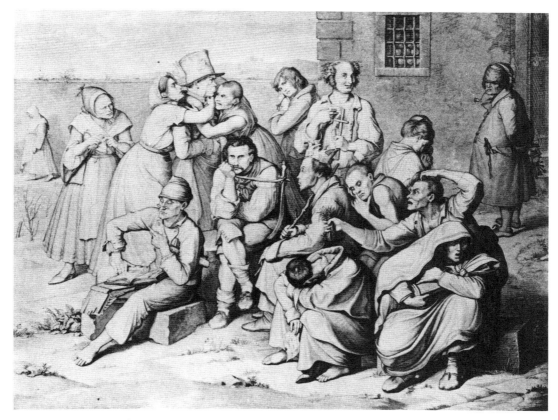

Figure 26-40.   *Self-test: What diagnoses can you make from observing these patients? Some suggestions are in Appendix 26-4.* The Madhouse, *engraving by Casper Heinrich Merz, after the drawing by Wilhelm von Kaulbach. The artist called the work* ein Rettungsmittel aus einer geistigen Erkrankung *(a means of rescue from a mental illness.) Reproduced from* Medicine and the Artist (Ars Medica) *by permission of the Philadelphia Museum of Art.*

Table 26-13. Definitions of Altered Levels of Consciousness

Acute organic brain syndrome (delirium) or chronic organic brain syndrome (dementia): The patient is in contact with his surroundings and will respond to questions, but is disoriented at least in the sphere of time. This is the mildest form of impaired consciousness.

Stupor: This state may be defined as anything between delirium and coma. A stuporous patient is arousable and so is usually in partial or intermittent touch with his environment. Auditory contact is the last to be lost. (Note: It is often impossible to prove that a stuporous patient is disoriented since such patients may not be able to maintain appropriate contact with the interviewer for a sufficient period of time to permit the determination to be made.)

Coma: The patient is out of touch with his surroundings. He appears to be sleeping but cannot be aroused. This is the most severe state of altered consciousness.

An Illustrative Case

The actual transcription of an interview with a dementia patient follows. Its purpose is to illustrate some points already covered: the importance of specific testing for orientation; the importance of testing as soon as the confused patient becomes confusing; and the recognition that although this portion of the mental status examination is done while speaking with the patient, it is still part of the physical examination.

This particular patient was seen at a time when the author was in charge of a psychosomatic service. This was the fifth medical patient in a row who had an organic brain syndrome discovered in a consultation for a "functional" disorder. We were once again falsely assured that the patient was oriented.

In all fairness, and to illuminate the pedagogic difficulty in convincing the very best of young minds that one must specifically test for orientation and not assume that it is present, note the following: The tape recording of this interview has been played for many generations of medical students, who could be taught to enjoy the macabre humor of the senior medical resident struggling to get the correct diagnostic information. In later years, one could see these very same medical students have the same experiences in their turn. This may mean that the best way to teach medicine is at the bedside with real patients, rather than by "show and tell."

●

Doctor: Can I talk with you for a while?
Patient: . . . .
Doctor: How are you doing?
Patient: All right . . . .
Doctor: Having any problems?
Patient (quickly): No . . . .
Doctor: You been feeling all right?
Patient: Yeh . . . .
Doctor: Any complaints?
Patient: No . . .
Doctor: Anything bothering you at *all*?
Patient (quickly): No . . . .
Doctor: (20-second pause): . . . Do you know where you are?
Patient: Yeh (mumbled statement)
Doctor: Where are you?
Patient: In, uh, Birmingham Hospital.
Doctor: Which hospital?
Patient: The VA? (the correct answer)

Doctor: The VA, yuh . . . And, uh, do you know what day it is?
Patient: No.
Doctor: Do you have any idea what day it is?
Patient: No, I don't.
Doctor: Do you know what month it is?
Patient: (mumbles) . . . Is it Christmas month?
Doctor: What month is that?
Patient: December.
Doctor: That's correct. . . . What year is it?
Patient: Forty . . . three . . . I believe. (It is 1971.)
Doctor: Forty-three?
Patient: Yeh? . . .
Doctor: Is that what you think it is? Forty-three?
Patient: Yeh, that's about what I think it is. Nineteen forty-three.
Doctor: I see. . . . How old are you?
Patient: February 12, 1912.
Doctor: How *old* are you?
Patient: Sixty years old.
Doctor: Huh?
Patient: Sixty years old.
Doctor: Sixty years old. . . . And you were born when?
Patient: February 12, 1912.
Doctor: . . . . 1912 . . . Where do you live?
Patient: Russelville.
Doctor: Russelville, huh?
Patient: Yeh.
Doctor: What's your address?
Patient: . . . . Russelville, General delivery . . .
Doctor: General delivery . . .
Patient: Yeh.
Doctor: Are you living in a house down there somewhere?
Patient: No, I stay with my sister.
Doctor: Who's that?
Patient: Fannie Mae. Fannie Mitchell.
Doctor: Fannie Mitchell.
Patient: Yuh.
Doctor: Where does *she* live?
Patient: In Leeton, Alabama.
Doctor: In Meeton, Alabama.
Patient: In *Leeton*, Alabama.
Doctor: Leeton?
Patient: Yeh.
Doctor: And you live with her?
Patient: Yeh.
Doctor (perplexed): How come they send your mail to Russelville?
Patient: Well, uh, that's my route. That's my route . . . having been changed on me.
Doctor: You mean . . . what *do* you mean?
Patient: Well, it had changed down in Alabama.
Doctor: What did you have changed?
Patient: My mail.
Doctor: Your, mail, huh?
Patient: Yeh.
Doctor: And your sister's name is what again? (The sister's stated name does not match the patient's last name.)

Patient:	Fannie Mitchell.
Doctor:	Fannie Mitchell, huh?
Patient:	Yeh.
Doctor:	How old is she? (A question that could be skipped.)
Patient:	Seventy-something years old.
Doctor:	Seventy *something* years old. . . . What brought you to the hospital?
Patient:	. . . (mumbles) . . . I was brought by the railroad agent. . . . I had no power . . . The railroad agent. I was pretty broken down.
Doctor:	You were paralyzed?
Patient:	(mumbles)
Doctor:	*Almost* paralyzed.
Patient:	And the railroad agent brought you here?
Doctor:	. . . . When did you become paralyzed?
Patient:	Just that night. The night before I came.
Doctor:	Um hm . . . What else happened?
Patient:	. . . Well, he come and got me . . .

●

It may be argued that this patient was so severely disoriented in the dimension of time that he must have had chronic organic brain syndrome (i.e., dementia). It might be argued further that there was very little likelihood of finding a reversible dementia, and thus no point in making the diagnosis. I am unwilling to accept this latter position for three reasons. First, even if the dementia were irreversible, knowing that the patient has impaired cognition helps the doctor understand some of the patient's behavior; it will also help the doctor avoid inappropriate behavior of his own, such as expecting the patient to remember appointments or adhere to medical regimens involving several medications of different schedules. Second, many of the dementias are in fact reversible. And third, the assumption that the problem is irreversible initiates a vicious cycle wherein doctors cease testing for impaired cognition, stop finding most cases, and so never find reversible dementia even when it is present.

Reversible Dementia

Pedagogic inspiration. While the workup for reversible dementia in a patient with no focal signs is partly an essay in laboratory medicine (Table 26-14), it might be worthwhile to review the outcome of such evaluations.

A review of 890 dementia evaluations in the modern era revealed that only 80% were clearly irreversible (Delaney, 1982; Fox et al., 1975; Freemon, 1976; Garcia et al., 1981; Harrison & Marsden, 1977; Heilman & Wilder, 1971; Larson et al., 1984; Marsden & Harrison, 1972; Rabins, 1981; Smith et al., 1976; Smith & Kiloh, 1981).

Of 790 cases with etiologies assigned (all of the above except the series of Heilman and Wilder), 7% had depressive pseudodementia. Additional psychiatric diagnoses encountered were mania and schizophrenia.

Normal pressure hydrocephalus was encountered in 3%, although it is not clear how many of these were still reversible. Drug intoxication was correctly diagnosed and reversed in 2%. In 2%, a resectable brain mass was detected, although some of these were metastatic. Hypothyroidism was found in only 1%, although a surprising number of cases of hyperthyroidism were found. Subdural hematomas were found in 1%. Other entities that individually contributed less than 1% of cases were: portosystemic encephalopathy, neurosyphilis, fungal meningitis, and pernicious anemia.

Table 26-14.   Clinical Evaluation of the Patient with a Chronic Organic Brain Syndrome

A *real* history and physical examination by a physician

Lumbar puncture:
 Opening pressure
 Cells
 Sugar, protein, and gamma globulin
 AFB, fungal, and bacterial cultures
 Serology and counterimmunoelectrophoresis (CIE) for antigens (India ink if cryptococcal antigen not available)
BSP[a] or other liver function test to rule out portosystemic encephalopathy
Thyroxine and T3-resin uptake
Glucose, BUN, sodium, potassium, bicarbonate, calcium, phosphate, magnesium, with calculated and/or measured osmolality
Folate and vitamin B_{12} levels
CT head scan
Human immunodeficiency virus (HIV) antibodies

The "full court press"[b]
 Skull films in absence of basal skull fracture
 Arteriography in the absence of focal signs
 RISA cisternography without hydrocephalus (high yield with hydrocephalus and normal CSF pressure)
 Ceruloplasmin without Kayser-Fleischner rings
 Drug and heavy metal screen
No longer done: closing pressure and volume, serum or CSF chloride, serum bromide, or CSF alcohol

 [a]*The Bromsulphalein (BSP) test is no longer widely available, nor is indocyanine green or rose bengal. Portosystemic encephalopathy is extremely unlikely in the presence of a normal serum bilirubin, serum albumin, prothrombin time, and blood ammonia level. Again, this should be a clinical diagnosis.*

 [b]*A phrase coined by Dr. Gaeton Lorino of Alabama, a basketball fan, to describe that part of the evaluation done in desperation with little expectation of success.*

Hallucinations and Delusions

"Hallucinations are quite possible in your present condition," the doctor decided, "although we should really check on them . . . " (Dostoevsky, *The Brothers Karamazov*, Part 4, Book 11, Ch. 9)

Definitions

Terms for this section are defined in Table 26-15.

Table 26-15.   Definitions

Illusion: a false perception occurring in response to a sensory stimulus

Hallucination: A false perception occurring in the absence of a sensory stimulus

Delusion: A firmly held belief not in keeping with the individual's culture or level of education

Examples: If you hear a car backfire, and you believe that it may be a pistol shot, that is an illusion. If you hear a pistol shot when there has been no sound (either of a pistol or of a car backfiring), that is a hallucination. If you hear a pistol shot and believe that it is God firing a pistol at you because you have ordered inappropriate laboratory tests, that is a delusion. (If someone decides he is ordering too many laboratory tests in the absence of an external sensory stimulus, that is called enlightenment.)

Eliciting the History of Hallucinations

It can be very difficult to evoke evidence of a hallucination from the person who has hallucinated. This is especially true when the person does not recognize that he has hallucinated, or if he is embarrassed by it.

One way to elicit the information is to ask, "Have you ever had an experience like dreaming, when you were not asleep?" Let the patient attempt an answer without much more structuring of the question. In this way, there is an excellent chance that you will quickly learn about the hallucinations.

Some doctors ask, "Have you ever seen something (or heard something) that other people couldn't see (or hear)?" This question is a little more specific and a bit less sensitive. Of course, the question must be changed for haptic (touch) and olfactory hallucinations.

A less sensitive question is, "Do you have special powers that other people don't have?" Notice that this question has little to do with hallucinations but rather is one test for eliciting paranoid delusional systems. Thus, while it may lead into a delusional system and from there into a hallucinatory system (should one exist in the same patient), the overlap is not perfect.

Some interviewers ask, "Have you ever had an experience like taking LSD or PCP when in fact you have not taken those chemicals?" This question presumes that the individual has in fact had past psychotomimetic experiences. In that event, the occurrence of such an experience remote from drug use raises a cause-and-effect problem: Could the current experience be a flashback? Hence, this question is neither sensitive nor diagnostic and is included here only for the sake of completeness.

In conclusion, I prefer the questions at the beginning of this section as the most powerful in a screening interview.

A caveat for the beginner. Scotomata, illusions, "floaters," and figures of speech have all been misrepresented as "visual hallucinations." The use of the suggested questions will increase your batting average in obtaining the history of hallucinations, but you should also beware of the false positives.

The most difficult false positive is the auditory illusion. We have all heard noises in the middle of the night that could be misinterpreted as an intruder. The best distinguishing feature is that the illusion is accompanied by perplexity, and the hallucination is not. (The pseudoperplexity of a patient who reports seeing a dead relative who speaks a puzzling message is perplexity about the content of the hallucination, not its existence. But the perplexity of a sound in the night is this: If it is an intruder, how could he have gotten in through a locked door?)

Orientation has been suggested as a requirement for hallucinations, but should not be used as such. Hallucinating patients with affective disorder or schizophrenia may or may not be disoriented at the time they hallucinate, and patients with organic brain syndrome who hallucinate will definitely be disoriented. This raises the question of the differential diagnosis of hallucinations, which includes: primary affective disorder (depression and mania) (p. 524); schizophrenia (p. 520); alcoholism (p. 522); hysteria (p. 522); and organic brain syndromes (p. 516). No type of hallucination is diagnostic for any disease (Goodwin et al., 1971).

Delusions

As implied by the definition (Table 26-15), a belief that is delusional for one person might not be so for another.

For example, believing that departed relatives inhabit environmental flora would be appropriate for adherents to an animist religion, but inappropriate for a Catholic bishop whose culture and education advise him that the souls of the departed are somewhere else.

A delusion must also meet the criterion of being firmly held, which means that the person adheres to it in the face of reasonable contradictory information or when adherence to the belief poses a real threat to the believer.

Note that both criteria must be satisfied. Religious beliefs that are in keeping with the group religious belief are not classified as delusions, even when so firmly held as to lead to martyrdom, because there is no available evidence that can be used as "reasonable contradictory information." Martyrdom per se would be considered evidence of delusional behavior only if it occurred because of a religion to which the martyr was the sole adherent. Nevertheless, it is possible to diagnose delusional behavior in a religious setting. For example, three charwomen were members of a fundamentalist church that held all-day Sunday services. At these services, the women regularly wore special robes and as part of the religious event engaged in a musical activity during which they had an ecstatic spiritual experience. For this group, this experience represented transport to the presence of the deity. One particular Sunday, one of these women refused to remove her robes at the end of the service. She continued singing and communing with the deity throughout the night, until the next day, when the other two women correctly brought her to the emergency room. Thus, what is "in keeping with the individual's culture" on one day, might not be on the next day.

Similarly, a belief about health matters that would not be delusional for an uneducated person might be delusional if held by a physician. The second criterion ("firmly held") is decisive here.

Scientific hypotheses are beliefs to which there may be tenacious adherence. But until contradictory evidence appears, adherence to a hypothesis (no matter how bizarre) is not delusional. Even adherence to disproved hypotheses may, on further inquiry, turn out to represent narcissism rather than delusion.

Self-Test: *Which, if any, of the following are evidence of delusional thinking?*

a. *A man caring for a demented wife came to believe that the electricity and telephone lines coming into his home were poisoning him, so he cut them down. He also believed that the water lines and gas lines were sucking his money out of the house, so he had those services disconnected. In this state, he and his wife perished during inclement weather.*

b. *A patient reported that on awakening from sleep, he believed he saw an elephant in his bedroom. When he gasped aloud, the startled elephant turned into a lion and vanished upwards through the ceiling.*

c. *Regardless of weather, a woman stands in front of a television store window for hours because the television sets are showing her private messages (concerning her role in an earlier life), which are being sent to her by the head of the Central Intelligence Agency.*

d. *A man believed that his country's legal system existed for the purpose of providing social stability for an economic system that the man believed to be unfair and inefficient. In order to bring his beliefs to a wider audience, he engaged in public protests against the economic system, which led to his incarceration.*

Write your answers down. Now go back and look at the definitions at the top of this section. Reread your answers. Do you want to change any of them? The correct answers are found in Appendix 26-5 (p. 523).

While these examples refer to persons who brought themselves to the attention of others, there are many persons who have delusions but who do not present them so openly. Sometimes this is because the delusion, while firmly held, does not in any way intrude into their social intercourse. Some delusional patients have learned to conceal the delusion from examiners until assured of a hospitable reception. The following sequence of questions may be useful for eliciting delusions in such cases (and for performing this part of the mental status examination in all patients in whom it is to be done).

1. "Do you have some opinions that are not held by other people?" (Most people believe they do.) "Could you tell me about them?" Or, "Could you tell me about some of them?" Or, "Could you tell me about some of the more interesting ones?"

2. "Do you have any special abilities?" (Most people believe they do.) Or, "Do you have any special skills?" Or, "Can you discern things other people cannot?" Or, "Can you pick up on messages that other people might not?" Or, "Do you ever get special messages in public?" Or, "Do you ever get special messages from loudspeakers?" Or, "Are there ever special messages for you on the radio (on television, in the newspaper, in musical songs, crossword puzzles, etc.)?"

3. "Do other people ever try to influence how you think?" (Politicians always do.) Or, "How do they do this?" Or, "Who are they?" Or, "What do they want?" Or, "Do they ever try to influence your behavior?" (Advertisers do.) Or, "How do they go about it?"

Each of the above sets is arranged in order from open-ended, vague, nonthreatening questions (which will elicit a lot of false positives) descending to more diagnostic ones. With much practice, careful attention to the patient during the interview will permit the examiner to move quickly through this portion of the examination.

However, the most important aspect of this examination is the physician's unspoken thoughts about the meaning of delusions, as these will color his demeanor and influence his nonverbal and verbal signals to the patient. Thus the doctor's thoughts may influence the patient's answers to the doctor's questions.

This is known as the "experimenter effect" in experimental psychology. That is, the experimenter, without realizing it, gives a subtle cue to the subject and gets a predetermined response. This chapter of epistemology began with the performing horse Clever Hans, which could answer, by tapping on the stage, very complicated arithmetic and geographical questions. Collusion was suspected because Clever Hans could answer correctly only those questions to which the owner knew the answer. But the owner cooperated for years in all studies of the phenomenon, and was as surprised as anyone when finally shown photographs revealing that he slightly changed the inclination of his head when Clever Hans had tapped a sufficient number of times. Clever Hans was reading a subtle nonverbal signal (Rosenthal, 1966).

Differential Diagnosis of Delusions

Delusional thinking is often found in schizophrenia and the schizophreniform disorders, the latter including, but not being limited to, paranoia, amphetamine psychosis, and hallucinogenic psychosis. Delusional thinking may also be seen in the patient with mania, severe depression, and a severe organic brain syndrome. Of these, it is most common in the latter, when it is acute. It can also be acute in the affective disorders, but this is rarely a diagnostic challenge since mania is easily diagnosed on other grounds and depression so severe as to be accompanied by a delusion will have probably already brought the patient to the attention of the medical community.

Paranoid Ideation

Technically, paranoid ideation is characterized by persecutory thoughts and feelings that are strongly held (i.e., not subject to modification by logic or experience). The most frequent type of paranoid ideation seen on a general medical ward is ideas of reference. These are the continual impression that the conversation, facial expressions, and behavior of other persons have reference to one's self. (These "other persons" need not be present in fact but may be viewed on a television set. They may be true historical persons such as the Director of the FBI or the President.)

Paranoid ideation may be part of several different syndromes:

1. *Paranoid schizophrenia*: If so, that patient may fulfill the research diagnostic criteria for schizophrenia (Table 26-16). It should be noted that "paranoid schizophrenia" as a *label* is one of the most common incorrect working diagnoses extant (vide infra, "suspiciousness").

2. *Acute organic brain syndrome, or even dementia, with a paranoid component*: This is probably the most frequent etiology of paranoid ideation on a general medical service, especially in patients with partial sensory deprivation such as those who are deaf, blind, immobilized, or in isolation.

3. *Paranoid states*: These are very, very rare. Some such patients may be developing paranoid schizophrenia, or they may have misdiagnosed delirium. However, most of them have a pure paranoid state, called paraphrenia by the British. It can be diagnosed from the fact that the delusional and/or hallucinatory system is confined to one area, and there is no other affective, cognitive, or thought disorder.

Table 26-16.   Research Diagnostic Criteria for the Diagnosis of Schizophrenia

A through C are all required:

A.   Both of the following are necessary:
1. A chronic illness with at least 6 months of symptoms prior to the index evaluation without return to the premorbid level of psychosocial adjustment
2. Absence of a period of depressive or manic symptoms sufficient to qualify for affective disorder or possible affective disorder

B.   The patient must have at least one of the following:
1. Delusions or hallucinations without significant perplexity or disorientation associated with them
2. Verbal production that makes communication difficult because of a lack of logical or understandable organization (This must be distinguished from aphasia, see p. 466.)

   Many patients with schizophrenia have a detached affect; however, when it occurs in mild form, interrater agreement is difficult to achieve. On the basis of presently available information, blunted affect probably occurs rarely or not at all in the absence of B-1 or B-2.)

C.   At least three of the following manifestations must be present for a diagnosis of "definite" schizophrenia, and two for a diagnosis of "probably" schizophrenia:
1. Single
2. Poor premorbid social adjustment or work history
3. Family history of schizophrenia
4. Absence of alcoholism or drug abuse within 1 year of onset of psychosis
5. Onset of illness prior to age 40.

Source: *Feighner et al.* (1972).

4. Finally, some patients who are labeled "paranoid" are in fact merely frightened and suspicious, and do not have true paranoid ideation. (These are the ones commonly mislabeled as "paranoid schizophrenia.")

On a university psychiatric unit, 40% of all patients admitted during a 10-month period had some sort of paranoid symptoms, ranging from true paranoid delusions down to ideas of reference or simple suspiciousness (Freedman & Schwab, 1978).

Of the patients with paranoid symptoms, 42% had only suspiciousness or ideas of reference. Of the others with true paranoid delusions, only one half had paranoid schizophrenia. The rest had organic brain disorders or the affective disorders (depression or mania). Three of the latter patients were inadequately treated for their affective disorders because the presence of paranoid symptoms had led to an incorrect diagnosis of schizophrenia.

Diagnosing Schizophrenia

Criteria for the diagnosis of schizophrenia are given in Table 26-16.

For the attending. In this section, the Research Diagnostic Criteria for psychiatric disorders is used, not those in the DSM-III. Although the criteria are similar, there are a number of differences. My preference for the former is based upon long familiarity with them. Later, as psychopharmacology research shifted to the use of these criteria in defining study populations, that additional rationale was added.

There are two drawbacks to the use of these criteria. First, whether it is the DSM-III or the Research Diagnostic Criteria, there is a deemphasis on the individual patient's developmental history, without which it becomes impossible for the physician to understand such issues as noncompliance, the patient's responses to hospitalization or disease, modification of the illness by the patient's social situation, and other items that are impossible to teach from a book but are of overwhelming importance in the actual practice of medicine. (As Hippocrates said, "It is more important to know what kind of patient has the disease, than what kind of disease the patient has." Of course, there is no reason why a modern physician should have to choose only one of the two.)

Second, with the rigid Research Diagnostic Criteria, one finds that the most common psychiatric diagnosis made is that of an undefined psychiatric disorder, and the originators of the system are very proud of this fact as a demonstration that their system is really pulling out "pure cultures" of disease, as it were. This is not true with the DSM-III, which has a diagnosis (or diagnoses) for almost everyone who comes to the psychiatric department, of which diagnoses not all have been subjected to the same rigorous scientific evaluation as the Research Diagnostic Criteria. That said, the individual attending can select his own criteria, or even no criteria.

Other Troubling Thoughts and Behavior

Delusions are to be distinguished from obsessions. The latter are troubling thoughts (not actions) that may dominate thinking and that cannot be excluded upon the wish of the patient. A phobia is a morbid fear of some object or situation; the patient usually recognizes an irrational aspect to the fear but still cannot overcome it volitionally. A compulsion is an irresistible urge to perform some act (not a thought) despite the patient's realization that the performance of the act cannot be rationally understood.

For example: If one had a morbid fear of open places, one would have the phobia called agoraphobia. If one could not stop thinking of the word "agoraphobia," one would have an obsession. And if one could not eat breakfast without first writing the word "agoraphobia" 100 times, one would have a compulsion.

Asking About Phobias

Open-ended questions that are useful for eliciting clues to phobias are: "What kind of situations do you dislike?" and "What kinds of things do *you* like to avoid?" The answers are not always about phobias, and sometimes even the patient with phobias will need a little encouragement to talk, not yet believing that any of his doctors really want to hear about *that*. But if these questions are asked with a warm genuine interest (and not monotonously as items on a printed questionnaire), one will get leads to phobias if they exist.

To determine whether one is hearing about a phobia, and not simply a nonneurotic fear, the trick is to get the patient talking and to *let* the patient keep talking. The patient's fearful affect and the web of detail and inhibition revealed will let the sensitive listener know that he is hearing about things that are truly disturbing to the patient.

The phobia entire is ego-alien. A normal fearful response is neither ego-alien nor ego-syntonic (see Ch. 2, p. 23), but always a response to a circumstance (e.g., fear of surgery). If a patient fearful of surgery is given a nonsurgical alternative treatment, the fearful response disappears. But a phobic patient is keenly aware of his phobia even when not in the presence of the feared situation or object. Merely looking at a picture of a phobic object, or thinking of the phobic circumstance, may be noxious.

Affect: Some Definitions

I have reigned over fifty years in victory and peace, beloved by my subjects, dreaded by my enemies, respected by my allies. Riches and honors, powers and pleasures have waited on my call. Nor does any earthly blessing appear to have been wanting in my years. During this life of wonder I have kept count of the days of happiness which have been given to me. They number fourteen. O, man, place not thy confidence in this world. (Caliph Abd-ar-Rahman III, found postmortem in his private prayer room)

Depressed Affect

A depressed affect is a predominant and persistent mood tone of sadness, despondency, and/or despair (see epigram). It is a major diagnostic clue to depression and to the *normal* process of grief-and-mourning when it occurs coincidental with and/or following the real or perceived or expected loss of a significant other or significant personal function. Thus, the loss can be wife, mother, arm, motor function of the arm, expectation of continued life, independence of life-style, sexual ability, or a combination of these or similar functions or ego objects.

Besides in grief-and-mourning and endogenous depression (see Appendix 26-8), a depressed affect can also occur in characterologic (neurotic) depression, in drug-induced depression, and in the depression associated with occult neoplasms, especially of the abdominal viscera.

Even grief reactions can be pathologic, as in anticipatory pathologic grief. Here, a characterologic (personal) neurotic conflict is activated during the grief reaction toward the imminent death of some significant other. The significant other is usually a person with whom the patient's relationship solved a preexisting neurotic conflict, a conflict that then reemerges with the death of the significant other (Viederman, 1987).

Elevated Affect

A predominant and persistent mood tone of euphoria, characterized by an optimistic mental set and feeling of well-being and confidence, inappropriate to the subject and/or circumstances, is a major diagnostic clue to mania. (See Appendix 26-9.)

Inappropriate Affect

An inappropriate affect is an apparent mood tone that is discordant with what would be expected in the company of the patient's verbal productions. For example, the patient might appear happy when discussing sad things, or sad when discussing joyous things. This may be a diagnostic clue to schizophrenia.

Detached Affect

This type of affect is also called flat, blunted, or inadequate. The patient is emotionally dull and detached and appears insensitive to stimuli in an environment that normally causes pleasure, pain, or some other emotion that has observable accompanying manifestations. This is seen in some cases of schizophrenia and depression, inter alia.

Assessment of Affect

A Method

1. Listen to the patient's speech. Does he sound depressed, joyful, frightened, detached, or none of the above?

2. Watch the patient's face. Does he appear depressed, joyful, frightened, detached, or none of the above?

3. Pay attention to the way that *you* feel. Does speaking with the patient make you feel depressed, happy, or frightened?

4. Is any of the above discordant with the subject or content of the patient's speech? Why?

Interpretation

As a rule, concordance between the estimated affect of any two of the above dimensions suggests that a significant affective diagnosis is possible. For instance, depressed patients tend to look and sound depressed; they may also make the physician feel depressed "for no special reason." Manic patients in their euphoric phase tend to be joyous or excited in their speech and joyous in their appearance, and to make the physician feel happy in the sense of being amused (see Appendix 26-9).

Discordance between the verbal output and the simultaneous affect may suggest either an inappropriate affect or an inadequate affect. A special maneuver is useful for the latter. Ask the patient to describe both the happiest and saddest memories of his life. If he consistently maintains an unchanged affect while recalling these experiences vividly, he is likely to have a detached affect.

Affect may not always permit a specific diagnosis. If a patient looks or sounds frightened, this is rather a diagnostic cue to evaluate the cause of the fear, which may be rationally related to the experience of hospitalization or illness. Similarly, a patient may episodically appear detached either because of depression, organic brain syndrome, or simply momentary exhaustion from his illness.

Self-Assessment Test: *Describe the affect of the following two patients, and write your answer down before consulting Appendix 26-6.*

1. *A woman tells her doctor that she fears her husband is going to kill their children. While telling him this, she giggles with barely contained glee.*

2. *A young woman was elected president of her sorority. Two days later, both of her parents were killed in an automobile accident. While describing these events to the physician, she neither smiles, frowns, nor shows any other facial expression of emotion, speaking in a monotonous way without accenting any words.*

Hysteria

There are at least six major uses of the word hysteria (Ford, 1983) (Fig. 26-41):

1. Conversion reaction
2. Somatization disorder (Briquet's syndrome)
3. Description of a histrionic personality
4. A contagious group process (e.g., an epidemic of hysterical fainting, or the reaction of the crowd when the Beatles appeared)
5. As a pejorative term: "another male hysteric"
6. As a specific term within psychoanalytic theory

In the present work, we will confine ourselves mostly to the first three definitions.

A conversion reaction implies the existence of an unconscious conflict that is converted into a bodily symptom or neurologic sign of symbolic meaning to the patient. Supposedly, the conflict would be noxious to the conscious mind so its expression in body language is adaptive.

A less psychoanalytically derived definition would emphasize the appearance of neurologic signs and symptoms of no known anatomic explanation and so would also include some examples of malingering and "compensation neurosis."

Somatization disorder is diagnosed by the criteria in Table 26-17.

Histrionic personality may be diagnosed by the DSM-III, or in some clinics, by the Minnesota Multiphasic Personality Inventory (MMPI).

Note that a conversion reaction or conversion symptom can be part of the criteria for somatization disorder, but each can occur without the other. Similarly, the concurrence of a conversion reaction and hysterical personality was 9%, less than 50%, and more than 50%, in three different studies (Ford, 1983).

Drug Abuse (Including Alcohol)

Any one of the following is diagnostic for drug abuse (Feighner et al., 1972), which is discussed in detail in Chapters 2 and 3 (pp. 23 and 45):

1. History of withdrawal symptoms
2. Hospitalization for drug abuse or its complications
3. Indiscriminate prolonged use of central nervous system active drugs

For alcoholism specifically, two questions are useful: "Have you ever had a drinking problem?" and "When was your last drink?". If the answers are "yes" and "within the last 24 hours" the sensitivity for the diagnosis of alcoholism (using the MAST, Michigan Alcoholism Screening Test, as a gold standard) is 92% (Cyr & Wartman, 1988). (A brief version of the MAST is presented as Appendix 26-10).

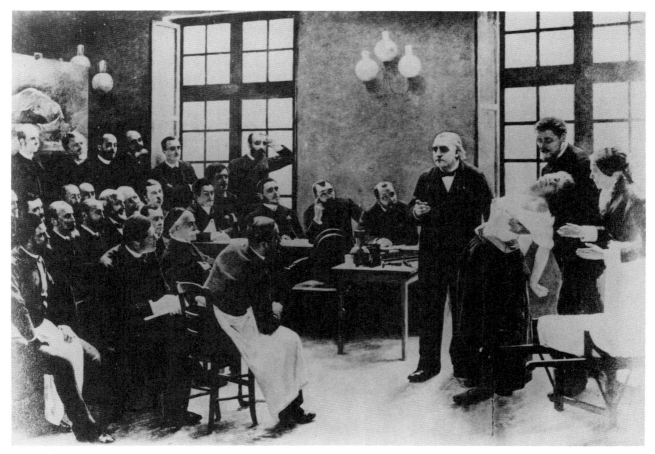

Figure 26-41. *Grand rounds with Charcot, who is demonstrating the hysterical* arc de cercle. *Note the large painting of the* arc de cercle *at the rear of the auditorium in full view of the patient. Could this have been used to help the suggestible discern what was expected? (Self-test: in which sense is the word "hysterical" being used? Write your answer down before consulting Appendix 26-7.) Photograph courtesy of the National Library of Medicine.*

Appendix 26-1. Self-Test on the Corneal Reflex

In Figure 26-6, the examiner seems to be approaching the patient from below and not the side, and *might* well touch the lower lid before getting to the cornea. Assuming that the examiner does touch only the cornea, the patient in Figure 26-6A has a lesion of the ophthalmic branch of the right cranial nerve V (or conceivably a lesion of only the nasociliary branch).

In the patient in Figure 26-6B, the afferent (sensory) limb of the reflex arc seems to be intact because a left blink reflex has been evoked. So, the efferent (motor) limb of the reflex arc is intact on the left but impaired on the right (because the orbicularis oculis is innervated by VII). This must be a lesion of the right nerve VII.

Appendix 26-2. Why Parkinson Could Not Detect Cogwheeling

Answer to the question on page 476: Parkinson practiced in the era of the gold-headed cane. At this time, doctors were so elevated above patients that they did not actually touch them except with the cane. Thus, there was no way that even an astute observer like Parkinson could detect cogwheeling.

Appendix 26-3. The Origin of the Word "Reflex"

Thomas Willis, who is today remembered only for his circle, invented the word "reflex" in his 1664 text on the brain, illustrated by Sir Christopher Wren (Chassis & Goldring, 1965). (Willis also invented the word "voluntary" for striated muscle movement, adopting it from scholastic philosophy, thus explaining his unusual definition that such movements occurred by the will of the person, who therefore took full moral responsibility for them.)

Appendix 26-4. Mental Status Suggested by General Appearance

Some diagnoses suggested by the general appearance of patients pictured in Figure 26-40 include: postpartum depression, schizophrenia (with intact cognition), normal control, *folie a trois*, melancholy, depression, paranoia, hallucination. (Actually, the last two are signs, not diagnoses.)

Appendix 26-5. Delusions

Answers to questions on delusions (p. 519):

Table 26-17.   Perley-Guze Criteria for the Diagnosis of Hysteria (Somatration Disorder)

1.   Complicated or dramatic history with onset prior to the age of 35 years
2.   Minimum of 25 symptoms in at least 9 of the 10 symptom groups with no known medical explanation

Group 1
  Headaches
  Sickly most of life
Group 2
  Blindness
  Paralysis
  Anesthesia
  Aphonia
  Fits or convulsions
  Unconsciousness
  Amnesia
  Deafness
  Hallucinations
  Urinary retention
  Ataxia
  Other conversion
    symptoms
Group 3
  Fatigue
  Lump in throat
  Fainting spells
  Visual blurring
  Weakness
  Dysuria
Group 5
  Anorexia
  Weight loss
  Marked fluctuations in
    weight
  Nausea
  Abdominal bloating
  Food intolerances
  Diarrhea
  Constipation
Group 6
  Abdominal pain
  Vomiting

Group 7
  Dysmenorrhea
  Menstrual irregularity
  Amenorrhea
  Excessive bleeding
Group 8
  Sexual indifference
  Frigidity
  Dyspareunia
  Other sexual difficulties
  Vomiting during 9 months of
    pregnancy or hospitalized for
    hyperemesis gravidarum
Group 9
  Back pain
  Joint pain
  Extremity pain
  Burning pains of the sexual
    organs, mouth, or rectum
  Other bodily pains
Group 10
  Nervousness
  Fears
  Depressed feelings
  Need to quit working or inability
    to carry on regular duties
    due to feeling sick
  Crying easily
  Feeling life is hopeless
  Thinking a good deal about
    dying
  Wanting to die
  Thinking of suicide
  Suicide attempts

Source: *Perley and Guze (1962).*

a.   The man was delusional. The culture's belief about the function of utility lines is rather unambiguous. Furthermore, physical inspection of the behavior of water pipes provides compelling contradictory evidence against their being used to suck money out of houses. The criterion of "firmly held" belief appears to be met because of the extreme state of privation and even death that resulted from adherence to this belief system.

It is not possible to state whether his wife was delusional because we know nothing about her belief system. Even if they both had the same belief system, it would still be delusional and not exceptable on the grounds of religion because of the compelling contradictory evidence. Instead, we would refer to this as a *folie a deux* (the madness of two).

b.   This probably represents a hallucination, not a delusion. If he simply reported his visual experiences without the qualification of the phrase "he believed," we could make a definite diagnosis of hallucination. The patient's statement that he "be-

lieved" he had the reported sensory experiences is not sufficient to qualify as a delusional belief system.

c.   Our culture does not teach this use for television programs. Assuming that standing in front of a public store window for hours qualifies the belief as "firmly held," this is a delusion.

d.   The behavior may be fanaticism, and it may be dangerous, but it probably does not constitute a delusion based on the material presented. The judgments "unfair" and "inefficient" are value judgments that do not admit of an external comparison. Thus, although the belief does meet the criterion of "firmly held," it is not out of keeping with his culture. It could only be so if he lived in a culture that prohibited the judgments "unfair" and "inefficient" (in which case he could be considered delusional!)

Appendix 26-6. Assessment of Affect

Answers to questions on page 522:

1.   This is not an elevated or manic affect, but rather an inappropriate one. There is no expressed optimism or feeling of well-being concordant in verbal production and observed affect. Rather there is a discordancy.
2.   This is a detached or flat affect.

Appendix 26-7. Hysteria

Answer to question in legend to Figure 26-41, Grand Rounds with Charcot:

It is hard to know for certain which are the correct answers, since none could be proved from the photograph alone. It is more important that the student attempt an answer from his observation and reasoning. Such answers might include the following considerations:
a.   The patient could have a conversion reaction.
b.   A somatization disorder is an alternate or additional possibility (conversion and somatization disorder can coexist).
c.   The patient could have a histrionic personality, or simply be a suggestible person.
d.   Although there is no group process demonstrable in the photograph, if one *believed* that the painting at the rear of the hall was being used to inform a contagious "group" process (by serial presentation), this too could be an acceptable answer. (There is some historical precedent for this belief.)
e.   Diagnoses should not be pejorative. (Specifically, the example of male hysteria would require the additional diagnosis of transvestism, as both the figure in the painting and the patient are dressed as women.)
f.   No evidence can be adduced from the figure for the doctrinaire psychoanalytic response, partly begun with Charcot's offhand comment to Freud, *"Toujours meme chose. Toujours la genitale."* (Always the same thing. Always the genitals.) (Note that hysteria is derived from the Greek *hystera* [uterus].)

Appendix 26-8. Criteria for Depression

For a diagnosis of [endogenous] depression, A and B are required.
   A. Dysphoric mood characterized by symptoms such as the

following: depressed, sad, blue, despondent, hopeless, "down in the dumps," irritable, fearful, worried, or discouraged.

B. At least five of the following criteria are required for "definite" depression; four are required for "probable" depression. (1) Poor appetite or weight loss *(positive if 2 lb a week or 10 lb or more a year when not dieting)*. (2) Sleep difficulty (include insomnia or hypersomnia). (3) Loss of energy, e.g., fatigability, tiredness. (4) Agitation or retardation. (5) Loss of interest in usual activitiess, or decrease in sexual drive. (6) Feelings of self-reproach or guilt (either may be delusional). (7) Complains of or actually diminished ability to think or concentrate, such as slow thinking or mixed-up thoughts. (8) Recurrent thoughts of death or suicide, including thoughts of wishing to be dead. (Feighner et al., 1972)

Appendix 26-9. Criteria for Mania

For a diagnosis of mania (Woodruff et al., 1971), symptoms 1 through 3 are required (numbers in parentheses indicate the percentage of untreated manic patients who have this symptom or sign at some time during their illness).

1. Euphoria (90%) or irritability (100%)
2. At leat three of the following categories: a) hyperactivity (100%) or increased sexual activity (80%); b) push of speech (pressure to keep talking) (100%); c) flight of ideas (racing thoughts) (70%); d) grandiosity, which may be delusional (100%); e) decreased sleep (100%); f) distractability (70%)
3. A psychiatric illness lasting at least 2 weeks with no preexisting psychiatric conditions such as schizophrenia, anxiety neurosis, phobic neurosis, obsessive compulsive neurosis, hysteria, alcoholism, drug dependency, antisocial personality, ego-alien homosexuality or other sexual deviations, mental retardation, or organic brain syndrome (Feighner et al., 1972).

Appendix 26-10. The Brief MAST (Pokorny et al., 1972)

1. Do you feel you are a normal drinker? (No = 2)
2. Do friends or relatives think you are a normal drinker? (No = 2)
3. Have you ever attended a meeting of Alcoholics Anonymous? (Yes = 5)
4. Have you ever lost friends or girlfriends/boyfriends because of drinking? (Yes = 2)
5. Have you ever gotten into trouble at work because of drinking? (Yes = 2)
6. Have you ever neglected your obligations, your family, or your work for two or more days in a row because you were drinking? (Yes = 2)
7. Have you ever had delirium tremens (DTs), severe shaking, heard voices or seen things that weren't there after heavy drinking? (Yes = 2)
8. Have you ever gone to anyone for help about your drinking? (Yes = 5)
9. Have you ever been in a hospital because of drinking? (Yes = 5)
10. Have you ever been arrested for drunk driving or driving after drinking? (Yes = 2)

Scoring: 0–5 = nonalcoholic; 26 or more = alcoholic. Intermediary scores are predominantly alcoholic.

References

Abraham AS, Atkinson M, Roscoe B: Value of ankle-jerk timing in the assessment of thyroid function. *Br Med J* 1:830–833, 1966.

Adams RD, Victor M: *Principles of Neurology*, ed 3. McGraw-Hill, New York, 1985.

Alford BR: Meniere's disease: Criteria for diagnosis and evaluation of therapy for reporting. *Trans Am Acad Ophthalmol Otolaryngol* 76:1462–1464, 1972.

Alpers BJ, Manchall EL: *Clinical Neurology*, ed 6. F.A. Davis, Philadelphia, 1971.

Arbit E: A sensitive bedside hearing test. *Ann Neurol* 2:250–251, 1977.

Archambeaud-Mouveroux F, Treves R, Fressinaud C: Acute adrenal failure with diffuse paroxysmal contracture. *South Med J* 80:1202, 1987.

Arrigg P, Miller D: A new lid sign in seventh nerve palsy. *Ann Ophthalmol* 17:43–45, 1985.

Baker AB, Joynt RJ: *Clinical Neurology*, revised ed. Harper & Row, New York, 1986.

Bornstein B, Kott E, Tamir M: The syndrome of muscle contraction in Addison's disease. *Presse Medicale* 70:2448–2450, 1962.

Bosch EP, Kennedy SS, Aschenbrener CA: Ocular bobbing: The myth of its localizing value. *Neurology* 25:949–953, 1975.

Bowlus WE, Currier RD: A test for hysterical hemianalgesia. *N Engl J Med* 269:1253–1254, 1963.

Boyle RS, Shakir RA, Weir AI, McInnes A: Inverted knee jerk: A neglected localising sign in spinal cord disease. *J Neurol Neurosurg Psychiatry* 42:1005–1007, 1979.

Brennan R, Bergland R: Acute cerebellar hemorrhage. *Neurology* 27:527–532, 1977.

Bull C, Henry JA: Finger wrinkling as a test of autonomic function. *Br Med J* 1:551–552, 1977.

Carel RS, Korczyn AD, Hochberg Y: Age and sex dependency of the Achilles tendon reflex. *Am J Med Sci* 278:57–63, 1979.

Chandler JR: A simple and reliable tuning fork test for recruitment. *Arch Otolaryngol* 67:67–68, 1958.

Chassis H, Goldring W (eds.): *Homer William Smith Sc.D.: His Scientific and Literary Achievements*. New York University Press, New York, 1965.

Chattha AS, DeLong GR: Sylvian aqueduct syndrome as a sign of acute hydrocephalus in children. *J Neurol Neurosurg Psychiatry* 38:288–296, 1975.

Clain A (ed): *Hamilton Bailey's Demonstration of Physical Signs in Clinical Surgery*, ed 15. Williams & Wilkins, Baltimore, 1973.

Clee MD, Burrow L, Delaney P, Garcia-Pont PH, Schiffman SS: Taste and smell in disease. *N Engl J Med* 309:1062–1063, 1983.

Committee: Criteria for diagnosis of Guillain Barré syndrome. *Ann Neurol* 3:565–566, 1978.

Conn HO: Asterixis in non-hepatic disorders. *Am J Med* 29:647–661, 1960.

Csuka M, McCarty DJ: Simple method for measurement of lower extremity muscle strength. *Am J Med* 78:77–81, 1985.

Cyr MG, Wartman SA: The effectiveness of routine screening questions in the detection of alcoholism. *JAMA* 259:51–54, 1988.

Degos J, Verroust J, Bouchareine A, Serdaru M, Barbizet J: Asterixis in focal brain lesions. *Arch Neurol* 36:705–707, 1979.

DeGowin EL: *Bedside Diagnostic Examination*. Macmillan, New York, 1965.

DeJong RN: *The Neurologic Examination*, ed 4. Harper & Row, New York, 1979.

Delaney P: Dementia: The search for treatable causes. *South Med J* 75:708–709, 1982.

Delp MH, Manning RT: *Major's Physical Diagnosis*. WB Saunders, Philadelphia, 1975.

Delwaide PJ, Toulouse P: Facilitation of monosynaptic reflexes by voluntary contraction of muscles in remote parts of the body. *Brain* 104:701–719, 1981.

Dodelson R: Checkup on Chvostek. *N Engl J Med* 268:1199, 1963.

Doi H, Murai Y, Kuroiwa Y: Deep tendon reflex in Eaton-Lambert syndrome. *Folià Psychiatr Neurol Jpn* 32:109–113, 1978.

Doyle AC: *Famous Tales of Sherlock Holmes*. Dodd, Mead, and Co, New York, 1958.

Dyck PJ, Thomas PK, Lambeert EH, Bunge R: *Peripheral Neuropathy*, ed 2. WB Saunders, Philadelphia, 1984. [There are 2, 323 pages in two volumes.]

Edwards AL: *Statistical Methods for the Behavioral Sciences*. Rinehart & Co, New York, 1954.

Elliotson J: St. Vitus's dance. *Lancet* 1:162–164, 1832.

Esposito GM: Peripheral entrapment syndromes of the upper extremity. *NY State J Med* 72:717–724, 1972.

Feighner JP, Robins E, Guze SB, Woodruff RA Jr., Windkur G, Munoz R: Diagnostic criteria for use in psychiatric research. *Arch Gen Psychiatry* 26:57–63, 1972.

Fisher CM, Picard EH, Polak A, Dalal P, Ojemann RG: Acute hypertensive cerebellar hemorrhage diagnosis and surgical treatment. *J Nerv Ment Dis* 140:38–57, 1965.

Ford CV: *The Somatizing Disorders: Illness as a Way of Life*. Elsevier, New York, 1983.

Fox JH, Topel JL, Huckman MS: Dementia in the elderly—a search for treatable illnesses. *J Gerontol* 30:557–564, 1975.

Freedman R, Schwab PJ: Paranoid symptoms in patients in a general hospital psychiatric unit: Implications for diagnosis and treatment. *Arch Gen Psychiatry* 35:387–390, 1978.

Freemon F: Evaluation of patients with progressive intellectual deterioration. *Arch Neurol* 33:658–659, 1976.

Garcia CA, Reding MJ, Blass JP: Overdiagnosis of dementia. *J Am Geriatr Soc* 29:407–410, 1981.

Geschwind N: Current concepts: Aphasia. *N Engl J Med* 284:654–656, 1971.

Goode DJ, Van Hoven J: Loss of patellar and Achilles tendon reflexes in classical ballet dancers. *Arch Neurol* 39:323, 1982.

Goodhill V: *Ear Diseases and Dizziness*. Harper & Row, New York, 1979.

Goodwin DW, Alderson P, Rosenthal R: Clinical significance of hallucination in psychiatric disorders: A study of 116 hallucinatory patients. *Arch Gen Psychiatry* 24:76–80, 1971.

Gray H: *Anatomy of the Human Body*, ed 28 (Goss CM, ed). Lea & Febiger, Philadelphia, 1966.

Greenhouse A: On chorea, lupus erythematosus, and cerebral arteritis. *Arch Intern Med* 117:389–393, 1966.

Guillain G, Barré JA, Strohl A: [On a syndrome of radiculoneuritis with hyperalbuminosis of the cerebrospinal fluid but no cellular reaction: Remarks on the clinical characteristics and deep tendon reflex graphs.] *Bull Soc Med Hop Paris* 40:1462–1470, 1916.

Hall H: Examination of the patient with low back pain. *Bull Rheum Dis* 33(4):1–8, 1983.

Hamburger JL: The various presentations of thyroiditis: Diagnostic considerations. *Ann Intern Med* 104:219–224, 1986.

Hannington-Kiff JG: Absent thigh adductor reflex in obturator hernia. *Lancet* 1:180, 1980.

Hardison WG, Lee FI: Prognosis in acute liver disease of the alcoholic patient. *N Engl J Med* 275:61–66, 1966.

Harner SG, Laws ER Jr: Clinical findings in patients with acoustic neurinoma. *Mayo Clin Proc* 58:721–728, 1983.

Harrison MJG, Marsden CD: Progressive intellectual deterioration. *Arch Neurol* 34:199, 1977.

Hayes KC: Jendrassik maneuver facilitation and fractionated patellar reflex times. *J Appl Physiol* 32:290–295, 1972.

Heilman KM, Wilder BJ: Evaluation and treatment of simple dementias. *Mod Treat* 8:219–230, 1971.

Heiman TD, Satya-Murti S: Benign cerebellar hemorrhages. *Ann Neurol* 3:366–368, 1978.

Henkin RI, Schechter PJ, Hoye R, Mattern CFT: Idiopathic hypogeusia with dysgeusia, hyposmia, and dysosmia: A new syndrome. *JAMA* 217:434–440, 1971.

Herbert H: Don't ignore low serum cobalamin (vitamin B12) levels. *Arch Intern Med* 148:1705–1707, 1988.

Hoffman E: The Chvostek sign. *Am J Surg* 96:33–37, 1958.

Hoover CF: The diagnostic aid in evaluating the vigor of inspiratory costal excursion. *Arch Intern Med* 37:773–779, 1926.

Huntington G: On chorea. *Med Surg Reporter* 26:317–321, 1872.

Iddings DM, Smith LK, Spencer WA: Muscle testing: Part 2. Reliability in clinical use. *Phys Ther Rev* 41:249–256, 1961.

Impallomeni M, Kenny RA, Flynn MD, Kraenzlin M, Pallis CA: The elderly and their ankle jerks. *Lancet* 1:670–672, 1984.

Ingbar SH, Woeber KA: The thyroid gland. In: Williams RH (ed), *Textbook of Endocrinology*, ed 5. WB Saunders, Philadelphia, 1974.

Jacob J, De Buono B, Buchbinder E, Rolla AR: Case report: Tetany induced by hypokalemia in the absence of alkalosis. *Am J Med Sci* 291:284–285, 1986.

Jankovic J, Fahn S: Physiologic and pathologic tremors: Diagnosis, mechanism and management. *Ann Intern Med* 93:460–465, 1980.

Jendrassik E: Beitrage zur Lehre von den Sehnen-reflexen. *Deutsch Arch Klin Med* 33:177–199, 1883. [This paper also has a good discussion of clonus.]

Jendrassik E: Zur Untersuchung des Kniephanomens. *Neurol Zentralbl* 4:412–415, 1885.

Johns DR: Assessment of hyperacusis in Bell's palsy. *Ann Intern Med* 105:973, 1986.

Kawamura M, Hirayama K, Hasegawa K, Takahashi O, Yamura A: Alexia with agraphia of kanji (Japanese morphograms). *J Neurol Neurosurg Psychiatry* 50:1125–1129, 1987.

Kawamura T, Watanabe S: Timing as a prominent factor of the Jendrassik manouevre on the H reflex. *J Neurol Neurosurg Psychiatry* 38:508–516, 1975.

Keighley G: An instrument for measurement of vibration sensation in man. *Milbank Mem Fund Q* 24:36–48, 1946.

Kernig W: Ueber die Beugekontraktur im Kniegelenk bei Meningitis. *Z Klin Med* 64:19–69, 1907.

Kilburn KH: Neurologic manifestations of respiratory failure. *Arch Intern Med* 116:409–415, 1965.

Kingston ME, Al-Sibai MB, Skooge WC: Clinical manifestations of hypomagnesemia. *Crit Care Med* 14:950–954, 1986.

Kopell HP, Thompson WAL: Peripheral entrapment neuropathies of the lower extremity. *N Engl J Med* 262:56–60, 1960.

Larson EB, Reifler BV, Featherstone JH, English DR: Dementia in elderly outpatients: A prospective study. *Ann Intern Med* 100:417–423, 1984.

Leopold SS: *The Principles and Methods of Physical Diagnosis*. WB Saunders, Philadelphia, 1952.

Lofvenberg J, Johansson RS: Regional differences and interindividual variability in sensitivity to vibration in the glabrous skin of the human hand. *Brain Res* 301:65–72, 1984.

Mace JW, Peters ER, Mathies AW: Cranial bruits in purulent meningitis in childhood. *N Engl J Med* 278:1420–1422, 1968.

Maciewicz RJ: Case records of the Massachusetts General Hospital. *N Engl J Med* 309:542–549, 1983.

Marsden CP, Harrison MJG: Outcome of investigation of patients with presenile dementia. *Br Med J* 2:249–252, 1972.

Martin FIR, Chow E, Alford FP: Age and sex dependency of the Achilles tendon reflex. *Am J Med Sci* 1:759–763, 1970.

Massey EW: Dimple sign in mail carrier's ulnar neuropathy. *Neurology* 39:1132, 1989.

McCance RA: Experimental sodium chloride deficiency in man. *Proceed R Soc Med* 119:245–268, 1936.

Medical Research Council: *Aids to the investigation of peripheral nerve injuries: War Memorandum No. 7*. Her Majesty's Stationery Office, London, 1943.

Mehrhof EG, Rousey CL: Speech difficulties symptomatic of destructive behavior toward self or others. *J Nerv Ment Dis* 152:63–67, 1971.

Messert B, Leppik IE, Sato S: Diplopia and involuntary eye closure in spontaneous cerebellar hemorrhage. *Stroke* 7:305–307, 1976.

Nordyke RA, Gilbert FI Jr, Harada ASM: Graves' disease: Influence of age on clinical findings. *Arch Intern Med* 148:626–631, 1988.

Parinaud H: Paralysie des movements associes des yeux. *Arch Neurol* 5:145–172, 1883.

Parinaud H: Paralysis of the movement of convergence of the eyes. *Brain* 9:330–341, 1886.

Parkinson J: *An Essay on the Shaking Palsy*. Whittingham and Rowland, London, 1817. Reprinted in: *Medical Classics* 2:964–997, 1938.

Perkoff GT, Tyler FH: The differential diagnosis of progressive muscular dystrophy. *Med Clin North Am* 37:545–563, 1953.

Perley MJ, Guze SB: Hysteria—the stability and usefulness of clinical criteria: A quantitative study based on a follow-up period of 6–8 years in 39 patients. *N Engl J Med* 266:421–426, 1962.

Phalen GS: Reflections on 21 years' experience with the carpal tunnel syndrome. *JAMA* 212:1365–1367, 1970.

Plum P, Posner JB: *The Diagnosis of Stupor and Coma*, ed 2. FA Davis, Philadelphia, 1972.

Plumb CS, Meigs JW: Human vibration perception. *Arch Gen Psychiatry* 4:611–614, 1961.

Pokorny AD, Miller, BA, Kaplan HB: The Brief MAST: A shortened version of the Michigan Alcoholism Screening Test. *Am J Psychol* 129:342–345, 1972.

Popper KR: *The Poverty of Historicism,* Harper Torchbook Edition. Harper & Row, New York, 1964.

Rabins PV: The prevalence of reversible dementia in a psychiatric hospital. *Hosp Community Psychiatry* 32:490–492, 1981.

Rask MR: The flexor pollicis longus deep tendon reflex (FPL–DTR). *Muscle Nerve* 2:503–504, 1979.

Reinfrank RF, Kauman RP, Wetstone JH, Glennon JA: Observations of the Achilles reflex test. *JAMA* 199:670–672, 1967.

Rico RE, Jonkman EJ: Measurement of the Achilles tendon reflex for the diagnosis of lumbosacral root compression syndromes. *J Neurol Neurosurg Psychiatry* 45:791–795, 1982.

Rives KL, Furth ED, Becker DV: Limitations of the ankle jerk test: Intercomparison with other tests of thyroid function. *Ann Intern Med* 62:1139–1146, 1965.

Roberts HJ: Timed repetitive ankle jerk responses in early diabetic neuropathy. *South Med J* 75:411–416, 1982.

Rosenberg GA, Kaufman DM: Cerebellar hemorrhage: Reliability of clinical evaluation. *Stroke* 7:332–336, 1976.

Rosenthal R: *Experimenter Effects in Behavioral Research*. Appleton-Century-Crofts, New York, 1966.

Sacks O: *The Man Who Mistook His Wife for a Hat and Other Clinical Tales*. Summit Books, New York, 1985. [A compendium of life stories (not mere case histories) of patients afflicted with extraordinary neurologic illnesses.]

Sapira JD: Reassurance therapy. *Ann Intern Med* 77:603–604, 1972.

Scheirs JGM, Brunia CHM: Effects of stimulus and task factors on Achilles tendon reflexes evoked early during a preparatory period. *Physiol Behav* 28:681–685, 1982.

Schiffman SS: Taste and smell in disease. *N Engl J Med* 308:1275–1279, 1983.

Schoenberg DG, Schoenberg BS: Eponym: The upgoing toe. *South Med J* 70:1237–1238, 1977.

Simpson GM, Blair JH, Nartowicz GR: Prolonged Achilles reflex in neurosyphilis simulating "myxedema reflex." *N Engl J Med* 268:89–91, 1963.

Simpson JA: The neurological manifestations of idiopathic hypoparathyroidism. *Brain* 75:76–90, 1952.

Smith JS, Kiloh LG: The investigation of dementia: Results in 200 consecutive admissions. *Lancet* 1:824–827, 1981.

Smith JS, Kiloh LG, Ratnavale GS, Grant DA: The investigation of dementias: The results in 100 consecutive admissions. *Med J Aust* 2:403–405, 1976.

Spinner RJ, Bachman JW, Amadio PC: The many faces of carpal tunnel syndrome. *Mayo Clin Proc* 64:829–836, 1989.

Tarkka IM, Hayes KC: Characteristics of the triceps brachii tendon reflex in man. *Am J Phys Med* 62:1–11, 1983.

Thompson HS: Segmental palsy of the iris sphincter in Adie's syndrome. *Arch Ophthalmol* 96:1615–1620, 1978.

Thomson JE, Allam BF, Boyle IT: A case of misleading Trousseau's sign. *Scot Med J* 22:286, 1977.

Trousseau A: *Clinique Medicale de l'Hotel Dieu de Paris*, vol 2. JB Balliere, Paris, 1861.

Verghese A, Gallemore G: Kernig's and Brudzinski's signs revisited. *Rev Infect Dis* 9:1187–1192, 1987.

Vick NA: *Grinker's Neurology*, ed 7. Charles C Thomas, Springfield, IL, 1976.

Victor M, Adams RD: Common disturbances of vision, ocular movement, and hearing. In: Wintrobe MM, Thorn GW, Adams RD, Bennet IL Jr, Braunwald E, Isselbacher KJ, Petersdorf RG (eds), *Harrison's Principles of Internal Medicine*, ed. 6. McGraw-Hill, New York, 1970.

Viederman M: Presented at the annual meeting of the American Psychosomatic Society, Philadelphia, March 28, 1987.

Vincent F: Cerebellar hemorrhage. *Minn Med* 59:453–458, 1976.

Wartenberg R: The signs of Brudzinski and Kernig. *J Pediatr* 37:679–684, 1950. [He also discusses the Lasegue sign as being identical with the Kernig sign.]

Wechsler IS: *Clinical Neurology*, ed 9. WB Saunders, Philadelphia, 1963.

Wiener SL, Nathanson M: *Med Times*, 1976–1977. [See reference in Chapter 29.]

Woodruff RA, Guze SB, Clayton PJ: Unipolar and bipolar primary affective disorder. *Br J Psychiatry* 119:33–37, 1971.

Young A, Hudson DA, Krige JEJ: Strangulated obturator hernia: Can mortality be reduced? *South Med J* 81:1117–1120, 1988.

Younge BR, Sutula F: Analysis of trochlear nerve palsies: Diagnosis, etiology, and treatment. *Mayo Clin Proc* 52:11–18, 1977.

Zachmann M: Influence of glucose and insulin administration on the Achilles tendon reflex time. *Br Med J* 4:528–529, 1967.

27
Clinical Reasoning

"If the fresh facts which come to our knowledge all fit themselves into the scheme, then our hypothesis may gradually become a solution."

Sherlock Holmes in *The Adventures of Wisteria Lodge*

Principles of Clinical Reasoning

Falsifiable Hypotheses (See Ch. 1, p. 4)

A falsifiable hypothesis is not a fraudulent or inappropriate hypothesis, but rather one that is susceptible to being disproved. An example of a falsifiable hypothesis is: "The patient has consolidation in the left lower lobe." This is falsifiable because it is possible to demonstrate that there is *no* consolidation in the left lower lobe.

In contrast, Galen's hypothesis about his cure for the plague was not falsifiable: "This cure is efficacious in all cases in which it has been tried; except in those that were so sick that they were going to die anyway." One cannot prove that the survivors would have died if they had not received his cure (or that those who did die would not have lived without it).

A differential diagnosis (vide infra), as discussed in Chapter 3, should be a list of falsifiable hypotheses.

Negative Propositions

Negative propositions are frequent in medicine. Here are some clinical examples:

1. It is not possible to percuss the heart borders.
2. Persons who have one kidney removed never get compensatory hypertrophy of the remaining kidney.

Although negative propositions such as these are difficult to prove, they can be easily *disproved* (as by counterexample). In other words, they are falsifiable.

As a general rule, negative propositions, if universal, cannot be proven. For instance, if I say, "There are no unicorns," this implies that neither you nor I have yet seen a unicorn; furthermore neither of us will find a unicorn in the future; and finally there are no unicorns hiding in the basement (or perhaps on Mars) that we have overlooked. Such a universal proposition could not be proved. However, a sufficiently restricted negative proposition can be proved; for example, "There are no visible unicorns in this room right now." Further, the latter can be disproved (if you open your eyes and see one), so it is falsifiable.

Every positive proposition in a differential diagnosis list implies negative propositions regarding the other entries on the list, as-

suming that Occam's Razor (see Ch. 26, p. 452) holds. That fact, plus the general difficulty of proving negative propositions, may be the ultimate basis for the rule that "one should never say never in medicine."

Null Hypothesis

A restricted kind of negative proposition that is commonly used in science is called the *null hypothesis*. This is the hypothesis that states there are no differences between two groups.

Let us say that we have randomly allocated some patients suffering from a given disease into two groups. One group (the experimental group) is given a new medicine and the other (the control group) is treated identically except that it does not receive the new medicine. Differences in outcome between the two groups can legitimately be attributed to the new medicine; we avoid the *post hoc ergo propter hoc* fallacy (vide infra) by including a prospective control group.

Although we are seeking positive information by doing the experiment—about whether the new medicine does (or does not) work—we proceed by attempting to *disprove* the null hypothesis (i.e., by trying to refute the proposition that the two groups are as alike as two random samples drawn from the same population or universe). Customarily, we usually consider the null hypothesis to be disproved if the probability of the differences arising randomly is shown to be less than 5% ($p < .05$).

In clinical medicine, we examine one patient at a time. In this setting, the null hypothesis is that he falls within the normal distribution of the rest of the population of healthy people (or of people who do not have the disease that is under consideration.)

The student who is philosophically inclined will ask: Does this mean that medical research, and worse, clinical medicine, is basically probabilistic? The answer is yes. The conclusions are arrived at in medical research by probabilistically refuting the restricted negative proposition known as the null hypothesis. (The restrictions are generally hidden in the case record or in the "Materials and Methods" section of a journal article.)

Indeed, all "proofs" related to real phenomena (that is, phenomena outside the abstract worlds of mathematics and symbolic logic) involve just this type of probabilistic thinking. This tends to be frustrating to the medical student, who is not trying to do something negative, but rather to arrive at a positive diagnosis. In a fundamental sense, all positive diagnostic statements are umbilically related to the act of rejecting other possibilities (such as "normality"). In conditions like "essential hypertension," which are generally recognized to be "diagnoses of exclusion," the process is simply more obvious.

In summary, science cannot prove anything. The scientist is engaged in the activity of trying to *disprove* things.

•

To illustrate this point, there is an apocryphal story about Galileo. While he and a friend watched ice float down the river one winter, they fell into a dispute as to whether the ice floated because of surface tension and the flat shape of the ice floe, or because the specific gravity of the ice was less than that of the water. The sun was shining, and they reasoned that *if* the sun melted the ice floe from the sides and changed its shape and *if* it then sank while they were watching it, those events would support the surface tension theory. But the ice floated around a bend in the river and disappeared.

They then proposed to go to the laboratory and carve a small piece of ice in the shape of the ice floe they were observing. This model could be placed in a vessel containing hot water. Again, *if* it melted from the side and *if* it then sank, those events in tandem would support the surface tension theory.

As they were proceeding to place the ice model into the water, Galileo suddenly had an idea and changed the experiment. "Instead," he exclaimed, "let's place the ice at the *bottom* of the water and see what happens."

•

Some historians of science consider this a pivotal point in the history of ideas. The advantage of Galileo's modification of the experiment was that whether the ice floated to the top or stayed on the bottom, the result would admit of one and only one of the two available hypotheses, having effectively refuted the other. This is the same type of reasoning that an effective clinician employs in his handling of signs, symptoms, and laboratory tests. He seeks tests whose results exclude one of the possibilities.

To return to the ice floe experiment, if the piece of ice failed to float to the top, then it could not be of less specific gravity than the water, and the surface tension theory must be correct. If it did float, it refuted the idea of surface tension as the explanation, since surface tension did not operate at the bottom of the container, and so the specific gravity theory would stand. Of course, if there were a third explanation that neither Galileo nor his friend had considered, they could well draw an incorrect inference from the result of the experiment. Similarly, diagnosis by exclusion is treacherous if the differential diagnosis is incomplete.

Levels of Probability

To avoid error, it is important to keep the probabilistic nature of medicine constantly in mind whenever you listen to case presentations and read about clinical medicine. The probabilistic nature of your conclusions should be made as explicit as possible.

When negative propositions are presented, there are several possible levels of certainty. If someone makes a statement such as example 1 or 2 on page 529, it might mean a number of different things.

First, the speaker may simply be stating a belief. Second, he may be recounting a remembered experience. Without documentation, this level is approximately as reliable as a statement of belief. (I have done a number of clinical projects in which I collected data prospectively by writing the clinical experience on a card and filing it out of sight. On a regular basis, I have found, on reviewing the written records, one or more situations I

would otherwise have sworn I had never seen. Most clinical scientists have had similar experiences.) Third, the speaker or author may have documented personal experience. In this case, the proposition might be proved, if sufficiently restricted. (Proposition 1 is a good example. If the speaker cannot determine the heart borders by percussion, then the limited negative proposition might be true . . . for him. But a problem is born when he assumes that all others are equally lacking in this skill, i.e., when he extrapolates from a limited negative proposition to a universal one.) Fourth, the speaker may intend to a make much stronger, more general statement: "It never was and we don't expect it to." The expectation may be based upon a scientific body of work that predicts (but does not prove) that something will not happen in the future. But expectation, however reasonable, is still not a proof.

The scientific physician will strive to achieve the highest level of certainty that is possible, and not to overstate the level of certainty that exists.

Very advanced. The odd relationship between positive and negative propositions was illustrated by Wittgenstein's statement: "It appears to me that negation in arithmetic is interesting only in conjunction with a certain generality . . . . I don't write ~ (5 × 5 = 30), I write 5 × 5 ≠ 30, since I'm not negating anything but want to establish a relation between 5 × 5 and 30 (and hence something positive" (Wittgenstein, 1975).

A different example would be better for those not familiar with symbolic logic: we do not say "5 × 5 is roughly 26," we say "5 × 5 is definitely not 30." Although the former might appear "closer," the latter, as a technique, would eventually allow us to exclude all the incorrect answers and so arrive at the correct one. But the former eternally remains no more correct than the equivalent, but different, "5 × 5 is roughly 24."

Aphorisms

A Bestiary of Clinical Reasoning

A well-known aphorism says, "When you hear hoofbeats, they're probably coming from a horse, not a zebra" (Fig. 27-1).

Sometimes the hoofbeats are not coming either from a zebra or a horse (Fig. 27-2), thus the need for differential diagnosis, arranged in order of probability. For hoofbeats, we would list: 1) horse, 2) bull, 3) zebra and other unlikely possibilities. (One

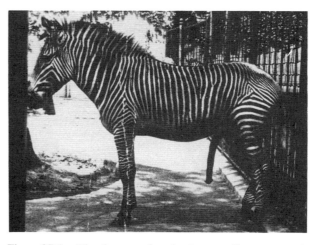

Figure 27-1. *That famous zebra that is generally not responsible for the hoofbeats.*

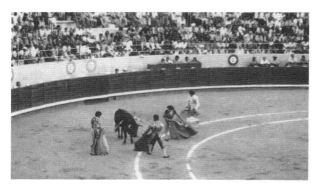

Figure 27-2. A nonzebra, nonhorse, which can produce hoofbeats.

always likes to put a zebra at the *end* of the differential: "If you don't think about it, you'll never diagnose it.")

Then there is always the confounding possibility that it is a horse, but you *don't* hear any hoofbeats (Fig. 27-3).

Sutton's Law

Ordering the differential diagnosis according to decreasing probability is a strategy in accordance with Sutton's Law, which mandates "go where the money is."

Historical note. The apocrypha states that Dr. George Dock was a visiting professor at Yale, long ago when visiting professors were presented interesting patients to be discussed *viva voce* with no specific forewarning or preparation. Dock was presented a patient whom he thought was an easy puzzle; namely, the obvious test to perform was a liver biopsy, which would completely resolve the problem. Instead, he was given the results of every other available laboratory test, none of which were capable of resolving the issue. "Why don't you follow Sutton's Law?" he finally asked.

No one had ever heard of Sutton's Law, so Dock told a story about the bank robber Willie "the Actor" Sutton. Sutton was famous for robbing banks, getting caught, and then escaping from prison by the use of subterfuge and costume (hence the nickname "the Actor.") Each time he escaped, he resumed robbing banks, and was eventually returned to prison. Dock said that a newspaper reporter, wondering why the recidivist did not desist from the ac-

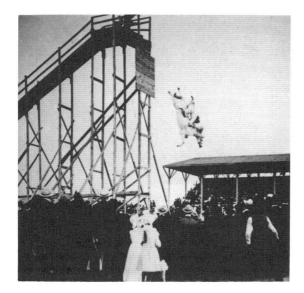

Figure 27-3. A horse that did not produce hoofbeats.

tivity that regularly landed him in prison, asked him, "Why do you keep robbing banks, Willie?"

Sutton allegedly replied, "Because that's where the money is."

Dock explained that in the case under discussion, the money was in the liver, and hence Sutton's Law dictated that one should biopsy the liver.

Years later, Sutton was asked if he had actually made that statement, and laughingly responded in the negative. But he allowed that it was a good answer, and he would have said it if he had thought of it. By that time, however, his name was already firmly ensconced in clinical lore.

The Law of Sigma

Sigma is the standard deviation of individuals around a group mean. If an individual is somewhat different from the group, consider first the possibility that he is simply located near one of the tails of the distribution, rather than a member of a different population altogether. (This rule might actually be considered a corollary of Occam's Razor [see Ch. 26, p. 452].) For example, if a patient with an organic brain syndrome enters the hospital with a problem that could be explained either by: 1) a new problem, or 2) too much or too little of a medication prescribed for an old problem, bet on the latter.

Case report. A patient had been discharged from the hospital with a prescription for phenytoin. Because most of his old records were lost, and the patient had Wernicke-Korsakoff syndrome, it was not certain whether he had taken his phenytoin.

The patient was readmitted with orthostatic hypotension, nystagmus, truncal ataxia, and macrocytic anemia. The resident wisely stopped the phenytoin while waiting for the drug level to return from the laboratory.

The patient had lost his truncal ataxia by the time he was examined by the attending, who wrongly attributed its absence to an incorrect prior examination by the house officer. Worse, the attending violated the rule above and diagnosed several new entities instead of phenytoin intoxication.

The admission phenytoin level came back markedly elevated.

Comment. Although this was not an easy case, following the rule would have enabled the attending to interpret better the loss of truncal ataxia. By the following day, the patient had also lost his nystagmus.

Other Aphorisms

For the Barking Dog and for Susann's Law, see Chapter 26 (pp. 458 and 508).

Inference

You will recognize inferential reasoning as illustrated in this anecdote:

●

Medical student: I saw Smith get on the bus this morning. He had been drinking and gambling.

Scientist: Did you see him drinking?

Medical student: No.

Scientist: Did you see him gambling?

Medical student: No.

Scientist: Then how can you scientifically make the statement that he had been drinking and gambling?

Medical student: When he got on the bus, he gave the driver a blue chip and told him to keep the change.

•

Still, inferential reasoning is full of potential for error (vide infra).

Frequently Violated Rules for the Logical Handling of Clinical Data

The logical handling of clinical data has been discussed in extended form (Bernard, 1957; Feinstein, 1967), but a few principles are listed here, in addition to those discussed above. I take them to be self-evident, and they were generally accepted by house staff, faculty, and students when presented in the form of an opinion questionnaire (Sapira, 1980). Nevertheless, they are frequently violated in practice.

Rule 1. If some of the findings supporting a new diagnosis can be reasonably rejected as either artifactual or related to a preexistent or coexistent diagnosis, such rejection of those findings does not, per se, refute either the new diagnosis or the verity of the other findings.

Rule 2. The fact that a finding is elicited by only a minority of observers does not mean that the finding can reasonably be rejected as artifactual.

Comment: If a finding is elicited, it is a finding, assuming that clinicians are not hallucinatory or tending toward intentional obfuscation. The finding could have been transient, or perhaps only a minority of the observers might have the skills to elicit it.

Dr. Claude Bernard was frequently asked how one could determine which of two identical experiments yielding contrary results should be considered the correct one. Dr. Bernard answered that both should be considered correct, since two identical experiments could not yield different results. He then pointed out that to yield opposite results, there must have been unrecognized and differing conditions between the two experiments, and these would ultimately be shown to be the cause of the differing results. I believe Bernard's rule is the antecedent of this second principle.

Rule 3. If there are findings whose validity is not contested, supporting a diagnosis with which a consultant does not agree, the consultant is obligated to offer an alternative diagnosis that will also explain the findings.

Rule 4. Positive findings are more important than negative findings, except for those negative findings that are known as "excluders." (For example, the absence of an increase in the serum bromide concentration would be an "excluder" for the diagnosis of bromism.)

Comment: The antecedent of this principle was apparently formulated by Dr. Jack Myers and popularized by Dr. Eugene Stead:

Jack Myers frequently said that much clinical learning could be summarized by the statement: any positive observation has greater weight than any negative observation. If a marble is found in a room, that is a positive observation and, in general, means that the room did contain a marble. If the doctor finds no marble on searching the room, it may mean that there is no marble there, but many times it will mean that the doctor is not good at finding marbles. (Stead, 1978)

Rule 5. If a patient has *n* findings, the patient's diagnosis (or diagnoses) should explain all *n* findings.

Comment: This principle is most frequently violated by sophomore medical students. Because of their praiseworthy intent to "get *the* diagnosis" (which they correctly assume to be a precondition for the patient's selection for examination by medical students), students emphasize those positive findings that support their first diagnosis, but fail to consider other findings that would suggest an alternative diagnosis.

Logical Fallacies

Post Hoc Ergo Propter Hoc

The Latin expression in this section heading means: "After this, therefore, because of this." It refers to one of the most common errors of logic committed in the daily clinical practice of medicine: assuming that if A follows B, A was caused by B. The fallacy's very ubiquity breeds a malignant tolerance: some persons are unable to accept the fact that an error is being committed even when it is pointed out. Enlightened clinicians may not like to believe themselves capable of making such an unreasonable assumption, but in fact, the inference that sequence is evidence of causality seems so eminently reasonable that the fallacy is easily perpetrated in our very best hospitals, books, journals, and offices. (In fact, sometimes the sequence *is* reasonable; so far, no one has suggested that Saint Sebastian [see Fig. 5-2] was secreting those arrows!)

Post hoc ergo propter hoc is a special case of an associative fallacy. For example, while it is true that there is a strong statistical association between height and weight, it would be erroneous to conclude that one could become taller simply by overeating. Otherwise the complaint of the fat man, "I'm not overweight; I'm just too short" would be true.

Go to the chart rack and pick up any chart. You might see in bold red letters on the outside: "Allergic to codeine." What is the scientific basis for such a statement?

To be sure that the patient had an allergic reaction, it should have been replicated on challenge, preferably blind, and must be the sort of reaction recognized as allergic, not simply the pharmacologic (e.g., a histamine-releasing effect) of codeine. However, upon interviewing the patient, one finds that the patient noticed some event that followed the administration of what was believed to have been codeine, and assumed a causal relationship. Sometimes the effect attributed to the drug, and the time interval described, are so unlikely that the chance of causal association is slight. But at other times, the effect (e.g., nausea) and the time interval are quite good for assuming a causal (if not necessarily allergic) association.

Of course, nothing is wrong with making an assumption as long as one recognizes what one is doing. However, with *post hoc ergo propter hoc* such an assumption is often accepted as if it had been proved.

The importance of establishing the likelihood of causality becomes apparent when the patient has a serious infection that is preferably treated by an antibiotic to which the patient is thought (by *post hoc ergo propter hoc* reasoning) to be allergic.

Open a chart, and you may find a statement like this in the progress notes: "The fever has responded well to antibiotics. Cultures still negative."

First of all, antibiotics are not hypothermic. *Infections* may respond to antibiotics, but fevers don't. At this point, we aren't sure that the antibiotics chosen are appropriate for the organism or even that the patient has an infection. In fact, the patient might have a collagen-vascular disease.

It would be much better to enter the note: "Patient afebrile. Cultures still negative." This contains the same information in fewer words, without the error in logic.

Although the argument may seem trivial, consider the patient who has unbeknownst to his doctors developed a febrile drug reaction due to one of the "covering" antibiotics. The logical fallacy may lead to treatment inadvertently based upon the hair of the dog, that is, more antibiotics are added to "cover" the fallaciously assumed microbial cause of the fever. (Perhaps a dog chasing its tail might be a more suitable image.)

Thus, the *post hoc ergo propter hoc* fallacy has a great potential for harm, especially in those situations in which it may seem the most reasonable.

Discounting of One Etiology by Eliminating Only One of Multiple Subcomponents

Consider a situation in which syndrome X can be caused by etiology 1 or etiology 2. Etiology 2 is usually due to condition a, although it is sometimes due to condition b. (You may wish to diagram this.) Suppose that a patient with syndrome X has been proven not to have a. It would then be erroneous to conclude that his syndrome must have been caused by etiology 1.

A specific case might be hypokalemia with hyperkaliuria, which can be caused by renal tubular acidosis type 1 or type 2. It can also be caused by mineralocorticoid excess. For the sake of discussion, assume that all other "nonrenal" causes of hypokalemia with hyperkaliuria (diuretics, other drugs, etc.) have been eliminated. Since the patient has a urinary pH of 5.2, it is accepted that he cannot have renal tubular acidosis type 1. However, it would be a fallacy to conclude that he must have mineralocorticoid excess. Why? Write your analysis down before consulting Appendix 27-1.

Differential Diagnosis

Use of Differential Diagnosis as a Guide to Reading

A Personal Perspective

When I was a depressed and anxious freshman in medical school, I approached one of the sophomores, Howie Reidbord, whom I had known in college. I asked what distinguished the students at the top of the class from the students at the bottom of the class, a question of more than casual interest since the bottom 20% didn't graduate. "Reading," said the future Dr. Reidbord. "The ones at the top read more than the ones at the bottom."

It is impossible to communicate what that time and place were like to those who were not there. But let me give one example.

When I was a medical resident, I was reading in the hospital library one evening. As I finished one article and lifted my head to the next article in the stack, I saw an orderly sitting across from me, reading a cardiology textbook. Each time I got another article from the stack, I noticed that he was still there, reading intently. Finally, I asked him what he was doing. "Reading about my patients," he answered, as if to say, why else would somebody be in the library reading medical texts.

I thought I might have misidentified his white uniform, but he truly was an orderly, who was serving a 2-year sentence to public service because of moral objections to the then-nascent Vietnam war. He too stayed after his duty hours to read about his patients. It would be misleading to say that everybody always read about all of his patients, but the story illustrates the intellectual environment of the times.*

---

*Readers who take exception to the author's comments about the deterioration in American medical education in the past 20 years (under the aegis of experts who say they are "in favor of education") are invited to consider how many of the more than 100 medical schools in the United States require demonstrated proof of competence in differential diagnosis for promotion (none that I have been able to determine.) Yet this keystone of the diagnostic process is pertinent even for those who rely on herbal teas for therapy, being utilized in parts of *A Barefoot Doctor's Manual!*

How Much Reading Is Necessary?

Once you have compiled a differential diagnosis, it becomes obvious that you must learn something about each entity in the list in order to find out how close the match is between the abstraction of the disease and the reality of the findings in each patient. Accordingly, if you have a differential of 10 diseases for one patient, then you must read about 10 diseases. If there are two differential diagnoses being developed for a patient, and each of them contains 10 different entities, then you must read about 20 diseases, unless some diseases appear on both lists. In the last case, by Occam's Razor, the patient should have one of the diseases that is on both lists (vide infra).

This investment of time will pay handsome dividends not only in learning specific facts about a disease, but in the inestimably valuable skill of learning how to teach yourself. The most effective self teaching occurs if you read about the patient before you go to sleep that night.

How Should One Begin the Differential Diagnosis?

If a patient presents with only one symptom, such as headache, or only one sign, such as a systolic murmur, it is obvious that the differential diagnosis must concern that symptom or sign. However, patients often present with many signs and symptoms. The beginning student needs a strategy for deciding which of the symptoms and signs on which to concentrate.

One good rule is to select the sign or symptom that has the fewest possible explanations. For example, if a patient complained only of headache, you would have to do the differential diagnosis of headache. However, if the patient also had fever, chest pain, nausea, vomiting, malaise, and leukocytosis, it would be unreasonable to start with the differential diagnosis of headache, since that symptom is a feature of so many different diseases. Chest pain would be a better symptom on which to focus.

As a case in point, two sophomore students saw a patient whose chief complaint was pauciarticular arthralgia of several days' duration. The patient was an intravenous drug abuser, who on physical examination had a grade 5 out of 6 holosystolic murmur radiating to the axilla. Starting with the arthralgias, and reading the usual rheumatology textbooks, one would have great difficulty arriving at the diagnosis of infectious endocarditis, and in fact might be led to the incorrect diagnosis of lupus erythematosus. On the other hand, starting with the description of the murmur, one could quickly eliminate all possibilities except disease of the mitral valve. The differential diagnosis of acute mitral insufficiency in a febrile drug abuser quickly leads to consideration of infective endocarditis. Reading about this entity in any good textbook would soon yield the explanation for the arthralgias.

For the attending. This method of teaching is highly structured. I refer to it as "iterative" (vide infra, p. 534) because it requires making a list and proceeding in an orderly fashion. Good diagnosticians, of course, do not actually make diagnoses that way, but rather by "model building," which requires processing vast amounts of information, mostly out of consciousness. (Actually, the example given above uses model building, to select the *combination* of findings from which to begin the differential diagnosis.) I cannot teach "model building" explicitly, but good students will acquire it. In the past, those who could not think this way did not get through medical school.

Preparing a Differential Diagnosis from a Case Record

A Method

The following method is presented for the beginner who has the task of analyzing a case record prepared by someone else (as for the traditional clinical pathologic conference).

Assumptions:

1. There is one major, "unknown," correct diagnosis.
2. The abstracter has included in the case record all the information required to arrive at the correct diagnosis.
3. The person analyzing the case record has access to a medical library.

Sequence of the analysis (Fig. 27-4):

1. Read the case history once.
2. Read it a second time, underlining all symptoms, signs, and abnormal laboratory results (collectively referred to as the "findings.")
3. Pick a single leading finding. (At first try, you might choose one with which you are familiar from prior reading.
4. Write down the differential diagnosis of this leading symp-

tom or sign. Until you are adept at composing your own differential, you should copy one from an expert. In addition to a medical textbook, you might wish to use Mac-Bryde's *Signs and Symptoms* (Blacklow, 1983) or a similar source.

5. List the findings that are "always" and "frequently" associated with the disease at the top of the differential diagnosis. You may need to read more about that particular disease.
6. Review the case history. Are there any findings "always" associated with the disease under consideration, which are specifically missing from the case record? If "yes," cross that disease from the list and repeat step 5 with the next disease in the differential. If "no," proceed to step 7.
7. Is there any outstanding finding in the case record that is not explained by the disease under consideration? If "yes," cross the disease off the list and go back to step 5 (but remember that in real life patients can have more than one disease). If "no," proceed to step 8.
8. Examine the list of "frequent" findings prepared in step 5. Do they match poorly with the findings in the case record? If so, cross the disease off the list and repeat step 5 for the next disease in the differential. If not, proceed to step 9.
9. Are there a number of findings in the case record that are

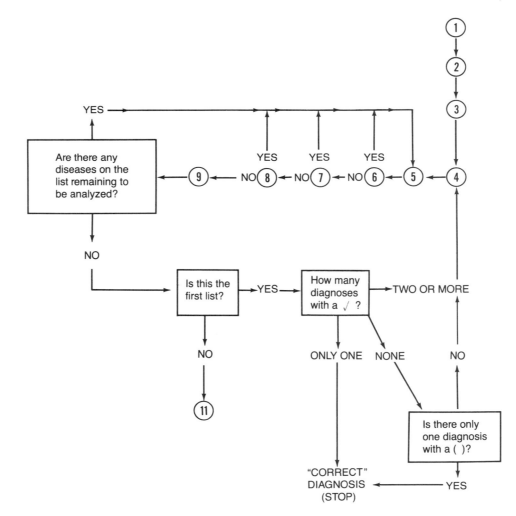

Figure 27-4. *Steps in preparing a differential diagnosis (see text).*

not explained by the diagnosis under consideration? If "yes," place parentheses around the diagnosis, and go back to step 5. If no, place a check next to the diagnosis and return to step 5.

10. When you have performed steps 5 through 9 for all the diseases on the list, you may have arrived at a diagnosis. If there is only one disease with a check, that is the most likely diagnosis. If there is more than one disease checked, or if no diseases are checked, but two or more are in (exclusionary) parentheses, you have identified the set that probably contains the correct diagnosis, and will need to proceed to step 11.

11. Repeat the procedure, starting with the second leading finding, and see what diagnosis appears most likely on *both* lists. You may need to use still more findings, until only one diagnosis emerges as the most likely.

An Example

The lists described in the method above are called iterative, from the Latin *iter* meaning "to plow again." To be more specific, let us give an example of the use of iteration.

Consider the situation of a patient whose hematocrit is rapidly dropping, and who has a negative stool guaiac, and no evidence of intravascular hemolysis. Such a case could be analyzed either by consulting a series of differential diagnostic lists, or by having access to a single differential list called, perhaps, "occult bleeding with a negative stool guaiac and no hemolysis":

1. Bleeding into the lung
2. Bleeding into the pericardium
3. Bleeding into the peritoneum
4. Bleeding into muscles, including the retroperitoneum
    a. Bleeding into muscles
    b. Bleeding retroperitoneally without muscle hematoma
    c. Bleeding both into muscles and the retroperitoneum
5. Bleeding into the central nervous system (presumably this would cause neurologic signs and symptoms)
6. Bleeding into the kidneys
7. Bleeding into the liver
8. Bleeding into the gastrointestinal tract (presumably outdated guaiac was used for the test)
9. Bleeding into joints

This differential diagnosis is not necessarily listed in order of decreasing probability for every patient (e.g., the presence or absence of neurologic signs would, as noted, move item 5 higher or lower).

Formulating Lists of Differential Diagnoses

A number of books that discuss leading signs and symptoms are still available. These vary from those with an extensive pathophysiologic emphasis to those that are nothing more than collections of lists. In an earlier era, students would compile and collect their own lists.

Formulating a list for differential diagnosis obviously requires some familiarity with medicine, but a student who has completed a course in sophomore pathology should be able to do so. A grid system may be composed, listing body organ (or physiologic system) on the horizontal axis and pathophysiologic process on the vertical axis. These processes traditionally include:

1. Inflammation
2. Neoplasia
3. Disturbance of flow
4. Metabolic

5. Congenital
6. Vascular

and sometimes others such as "iatrogenic."

Sometimes, one of these rows will be blank; for example, the thymus, being a solid organ, would not experience disturbance of flow. At other times, the entire system might collapse to only one column; for example, splenomegaly would only involve analyzing one organ, the spleen. Similarly, the category of diseases involving one organ or system might be subdivided into primary (e.g., diseases directly affecting the spleen) or secondary (e.g., secondary splenomegaly due to portal hypertension due to primary liver disease).

Sometimes, the pathophysiologic entry needs to be expanded. For example, inflammation could be split into primary inflammatory (e.g., sarcoidosis) versus infectious, and the latter in turn could be subdivided into classes of infectious agents (protozoal, bacterial, viral, fungal, etc.) Each of these could be divided still further. "Bacterial," for instance, could be classed by staining property, morphology, and so forth.

Separating clusters of findings in the dimension of time (acute versus chronic) and grouping them selectively in a meaningful manner is also useful, especially in the increasing number of chronic prediagnosed conditions. For instance: "The sudden appearance or worsening of dyspnea in a patient known to have chronic pulmonary insufficiency suggests the supervention of either pneumonia, pulmonary embolus, or left heart failure." Here, the prediagnosed condition is "*chronic* pulmonary insufficiency," and the "sudden appearance" or "worsening" of the dyspnea is the *acute* modifier.

Examples of some differential diagnoses are given in Chapter 20 (p. 386, Splenomegaly), Chapter 16 (p. 280, auscultatory findings in the chest), and Chapter 25 (p. 446, pitting edema).

A Self-Test

The following exercise tests whether a medical student can understand and apply these *concepts*. It is "information-free" (i.e., not dependent upon specific instructional experiences of the student):

•

Two astronauts are sent by spaceship to the distant planet Grlth, which is inhabited by a tribe of five-legged creatures known as Chmendricks. For 2 weeks the astronauts live among the Chmendricks, exchanging earth food and Grlth food, with no apparent adverse effects to either group. The astronauts learn that they can remove their spacesuits, since the planet's atmosphere is identical to that of the earth (i.e., astronauts and Chmendricks respire in a similar way). It is of interest that none of the astronauts or the Chmendricks that come in contact with them develop illness.

As the astronauts lift off for their return trip home, the King of the Chmendricks waves his right talon in a gesture of farewell. At this moment, one of the astronauts notices a discoloration of the third phalanx of the talon.

Give a 20-item differential diagnosis of this discoloration. The items do *not* have to be listed in order of probability. You have up to 1 week to conceptualize how you will perform the differential diagnosis. Once you start writing, you have 20 minutes.

•

Diagnostic Strategies

Introduction

Implicit assumptions about highly complex systems can often be made more salient and tested by means of oversimplified models that reflect basic characteristics of the system in a comprehensive manner. Here is such a model of diagnostic medicine.

Premises

A very simple model of a finite universe of diseases, each disease designated by a letter, is shown in Table 27-1. The diseases manifest varying symptoms, which are numbered. The table shows that symptom 1 can occur in diseases A through F. Symptom 2 is similarly nonspecific, occurring in diseases B through G, while symptom 3 may be seen in diseases E through J. Thus, not a single one of the symptoms is pathognomonic.

Similarly, the signs of this universe of diseases may be indicated by numbers. Again, the signs are not specific for any given disease. Furthermore, there are some diseases that have symptoms but no physical signs (diseases A, H, I, and J), which are in this respect like the real syndromes of acute hypercalcemia, hyponatremia, or some other metabolic disorders. Note that the sensitivity and specificity of the signs and symptoms are imperfect and unknown. We assume only that the patient has to have had at least one symptom in order to initiate contact with the diagnostician.

For each disease, let us assume that there is a laboratory test that is positive only and always in the presence of the corresponding disease (i.e., sensitivity and specificity are 100%). Each of these tests is indicated by a letter, corresponding to the respective disease. Let us further assume that the laboratory test always becomes positive early in the course of the disease, simultaneously with or preceding the appearance of the very first symptom of the disease. Of course, these assumptions would rarely, if ever, be true in real life. Nevertheless, a situation like this is the implicit goal of reductionistic medicine, and one is willing to accept the premise that it is a theoretically feasible one. So, these tests will be the "gold standards" of diagnosis for the purpose of this discussion (in mimicry of everyday beliefs in the value of the laboratory.)

The number of laboratory tests required to reach a diagnosis will be the dependent variable in the calculations to follow.

When shown this model, and asked to develop a diagnostic method, clinicians offer a variety of strategies, strikingly reminiscent of those utilized in daily practice.

"Shotgunning"

One could simply order every available laboratory test, the real-world technique known as "shotgunning." In this model, it is a more rational strategy than in the real world because here we are not concerned with the morbidity or the cost of the tests; also these

Table 27-1.   A Hypothetical Universe of
Diseases, with Their Signs, Symptoms, and Laboratory Tests

Disease	Symptoms			Signs			Laboratory Tests									
	1	2	3	1	2	3	A	B	C	D	E	F	G	H	I	J
A	X						X									
B	X	X		X				X								
C	X	X		X	X				X							
D	X	X		X	X					X						
E	X	X	X		X	X					X					
F	X	X	X			X						X				
G		X	X		X								X			
H			X											X		
I			X												X	
J			X													X

Source: *Sapira (1981)*.

idealized tests have perfect sensitivities. This would require an average of 10 tests for correct diagnosis.

Diagnosis by Exclusion

If one further assumes all the patients have one of the 10 diseases, it would be necessary to perform only nine tests to be certain of diagnosing every case. One test can be omitted; it doesn't matter which one. If all nine are normal, the patient obviously has the disease corresponding to the 10th (omitted) test. "Diagnosis by exclusion" may not work if the differential diagnosis is incomplete, but if it is complete there is an advantage over "shotgunning" in that only nine laboratory tests are required for correct diagnosis.

An example of "diagnosis by exclusion."   Given a two-pan balance, and 13 externally identical billiard balls, of which 12 weigh exactly the same, the 13th being lighter, how many trials on the balance would be required to identify that one lighter ball?

Amazingly, it can be done in no more than three trials. (Stop and figure it out before reading Appendix 27-2.)

Sequential Searching

Laboratory tests include more possibilities than blood chemistries and the like, which are performed on specimens removed from the patient's body. There are also testing modalities that require the presence of the patient, such as electrocardiograms, radiographs, echocardiograms, radionuclide scans, and so forth. Thus, it may not be possible to obtain all laboratory tests simultaneously.

Clinicians familiar with this reality tend to modify the "diagnosis by exclusion" strategy into that of "sequential searching," halting the process as soon as a positive result is obtained. Diagnosing disease A would require only one test, B would require two, C would require three, and so on down to I and J, each of which would require nine. If we let the diseases be equiprevalent, the average number of tests required to diagnose the patient by this strategy would be:

$$\frac{1 + 2 + 3 + 4 + 5 + 6 + 7 + 8 + 9 + 9}{10} = 5.4$$

which is a significant improvement over the previous two strategies.

A corollary to the "sequential searching" method is that there is no point in performing a test if it is not going to alter your diagnosis, prognosis, or treatment in some way.

A specific example is the case of a patient with an enlarged liver. The resident suspected the diagnosis of acute alcoholic hepatitis, although on questioning he acknowledged that it might actually be due to viral hepatitis, both diagnoses being reasonable given the patient's history and physical findings.

When asked what he could do to eliminate acute alcoholic hepatitis from the differential, he named a liver enzyme test. However, he could not say how the results of the test would refute the hypothesis (i.e., he could not name a level of the enzyme at which he would drop either diagnosis). Therefore, he was advised not to order the test.

Utilizing Data from History and Physical Examination

Up to this point, all the strategies have involved manipulation of the "perfect" data (i.e., the laboratory tests). Would a strategy that utilizes the "imperfect" data obtained from the clinical examination be useful?

To answer this question we first need to express the given information in the form of a matrix, as shown in Table 27-2. Each cell contains the diseases that could cause the concurrence of the symptoms indicated in the row, and the signs (if any) indicated in the columns. That is, each cell represents the differential diagnosis of the combination of symptom(s) and sign(s). In all the examples, the diseases are assumed to have equal prevalence.

(Only a few cells have been filled in; you may fill in the rest.)

For a patient presenting only with symptom 3 and none of the physical signs, the differential diagnosis would comprise diseases E, F, G, H, I, and J (assuming their other symptoms and signs had not yet appeared). The average number of laboratory tests required to reach the diagnosis would be:

$$(1 + 2 + 3 + 4 + 5 + 5)/6 = 3.3$$

For a patient with both symptoms 1 and 2, but no signs, the patient could have diseases B, C, D, E, or F (albeit in an early form). Here the average number of laboratory tests required to diagnose a patient with this clinical presentation would be:

$$(1 + 2 + 3 + 4 + 4)/5 = 2.8$$

For symptoms 1 and 3 together, but no signs, there are only two possibilities: diseases E and F. For this cell, only one laboratory test is required.

For symptom 3 and sign 1, Table 27-2 shows a dash. There is no disease which presents in this manner.

For the concurrence of symptom 3 and sign 2, there is only one possibility, disease E. Accordingly, zero laboratory tests would be required to find the single disease causing this particular presentation.

If one similarly calculates the average number of laboratory tests for each cell, the matrix shown in Table 27-3 is obtained. If one then assumes the various clinical presentations to be equiprevalent, one could calculate, for the 34 cells representing possible clinical presentations, the average number of laboratory tests that would be required to diagnose a patient within this universe of possibilities. It comes out to an astonishingly low 1.13 laboratory tests.

In other words, a strategy involving combinations of imperfectly sensitive and imperfectly specific findings obtained from the clinical examination is a more powerful strategy than any of those exclusively involving direct manipulation of "perfect" laboratory tests.

Anticipated Objections

People usually respond to this demonstration in one of two ways. The first is to say that the model only presents a quantification of what has long been obvious to all good clinicians. (I agree.) The second response is one of disbelief, based on objections to the ("additional") assumptions made in calculating the results of the last diagnostic strategy:

Disbeliever: You have assumed that the diseases within a cell are equiprevalent. This is not very likely, and it ignores the value of "clinical experience" in estimating the actual prevalence.

Answer: True. But clinical experience won't help the "perfect" data strategies, which do not use clinical information, and clinical experience can only help, not hinder, the last strategy. For example, let's say that for the cell comprising symptom 3 and sign 3, the clinician has learned that the prevalence of the disease is such that G>F>E. If he switches his testing sequence from

E,F,G to G,F,E, he would decrease the average number of laboratory tests needed to achieve a diagnosis within that cell.

Disbeliever: But you have also assumed that all presentations of the disease are equiprevalent. Yet you couldn't know this without knowing the natural history of each disease. Furthermore, this assumption contradicts the previous one, that the diseases are equiprevalent, because disease A appears in only one cell, while disease E appears in many cells. If you corrected for true prevalence, wouldn't it change the result and the conclusion?

Answer: It would change the numerical value of the result, but not the conclusion. The mean values for each of the individual cells in Table 27-3 range from 0 to 3.3 tests per cell. Therefore, no matter how the individual cells were weighted for prevalence, the mean value for the universe will still be between 0 and 3.3. Thus, the highest possible value is still lower than the 5.4, which was the best result of the strategies using only "perfect" laboratory data, and the conclusion would not change.

Developing a More Sophisticated Model

One could refine this model by finding the actual values for sensitivity, specificity, and prevalence of disease, preferably performing the calculations by means of a high speed computer with an elevated threshold for boredom.

Diagnosis by Exclusion: the Importance of a Negative Test

The utility of refuting diagnoses so as to achieve other diagnoses is now little appreciated due to the loss of the differential diagnosis and the multiplication of subspecialists, each of whom can make a handful of diagnoses, but not the same handful.

Consider a situation in which the diagnostic possibilities comprise three diseases of equal prevalence. There are two readily available tests. The first is an inexpensive, noninvasive test such as a blood chemistry, with sensitivity as given in Table 27-4. The second is a relatively expensive, but still benign imaging procedure, with sensitivity and predictive value of a positive test as given in Table 27-4. Patients who are without a definitive diagnosis may be subjected to a third test, which is perfectly sensitive and pathognomonic, but is risky and requires hospitalization. Which test should be ordered first?

Many persons vote for ordering test 2 because test 1 is not useful in making a positive diagnosis of disease B. But actually, test 1 is very useful for making that diagnosis, within this context, because if it is negative, it would immediately rule out the other two possibilities, disease A or C. (In other contexts, the test might not be helpful; therefore, in many textbooks it might not be described because, being universally negative, the test would not seem helpful.)

Let's calculate some probabilities. If we order test 2, there is a 90% chance of getting an abnormal result in each disease, and a 90% chance that the abnormal result will be diagnostic. Thus, for each disease, there is only an 81% chance of a correct diagnosis. Since the diseases are equiprevalent, the likelihood of reaching a

Table 27-2. Part of Table 27-1 from Clinician's Viewpoint

Symptoms	None	1	2	3	1&2	2&3
1	A,B,C,D,E,F					E
2	B,C,D,E,F					E
3	E,F,G,H,I,J	—	E	E,F,G	—	E
1&2	B,C,D,E,F					E
1&3	E,F					E
2&3	E,F,G					E
1,2,&3	E,F					E

Source: *Sapira (1981).*

Table 27-3. Diagnostic Matrix Derived from Table 27-2

Symptoms	0	1	2	3	1&2	2&3
1	3.3	1.7	1.7	1.0	1.0	0
2	3.3	1.7	1.7	1.7	1.0	0
3	3.3	—	0	1.7	—	0
1&2	2.8	1.7	1.7	1.0	1.0	0
1&3	1.0	—	0	1.0	—	0
2&3	1.7	—	0	1.7	—	0
1,2&3	1.0	—	0	1.0	—	0

Source: *Sapira (1981).*

Table 27-4.

Disease	Test 1 Sensitivity	Test 2 Sensitivity	Predictive Value of a Positive Test
A	100%	90%	90%
B	0%!	90%	90%
C	100%	90%	90%

diagnosis on the basis of test 2 alone is 81%. Now applying test 1 to the remaining 19%, we can diagnose disease B if the test is negative, leaving two thirds of the 19% (12.7%) to undergo the invasive test.

If we start with test 1, we immediately diagnose the one third of the cases due to disease B. Performing test 2 on the remainder, 81% will again be correctly diagnosed. The diagnosis has been made now in (.33) + (.67)(.81), or 87.3%, leaving 12.7% to undergo the invasive test.

Although the same number of patients have to undergo the invasive test if we use the second strategy, a third of all the patients have been spared the cost, inconvenience, risk, and delay of test 2.

Some people who pick test 2 first give the reason that a single test will make the diagnosis in 81%, rather than only 33%. But this is meaningless, since eventually all the cases must be diagnosed.

A second reason given for picking the wrong strategy (doing test 2 first) is based upon the assumption that the differential diagnosis is incomplete. If this is true, the problem has been misstated, and no best strategy can be calculated.

If this strategy seems difficult to understand, consider a simpler version, in which there are only two diagnoses in the differential, diseases A and B. (This was actually the situation in the clinical circumstance that prompted this analysis.) Simply go back to Table 27-1 and cover up the line representing disease C. Now, it is easy to see that ordering test 1 gives a certain and correct answer *all the time*. This section shows the power of refuting hypotheses, although some clinicians, accustomed to making "positive diagnoses," have a very difficult time understanding it in the actual clinical situation. Note that the use of this method *requires the construction of an accurate differential diagnosis*.

Very advanced. For a larger number of diseases, there is no decrement to the superiority of the strategy of using test 1 first. Prove this to yourself by composing a differential of four diseases by adding disease D. Let the sensitivities and the positive predictive values be the same as for disease C. Once again, the two strategies will have the same number of patients who have to go on to the dreaded third, invasive test to achieve the diagnosis. Since strategy 1 (test 1 first) alone completes some of its diagnoses in the first round ("takes its cut off the top"), it will always be superior.

Similarly, note that the result is also independent of the actual sensitivities and predictive value of test 2, assuming that the latter does not become 100%. Try changing them to 80%; the superior strategy is still the same.

But if the "bad" test 1 is changed, the whole set of solutions changes. It does not matter that the test cannot distinguish between diseases A and C; its virtue is that it is completely insensitive to disease B, making it in a negative sense completely diagnostic within the context of the problem. Yes, it is a trick. So were the Chamberlin obstetrical forceps.

An example of such a test 1 might be an elevated T4 test, which is always negative in hypothyroidism, or cyanosis, which is always absent in patients with congenital heart disease who do not have a right-to-left shunt. (This type of test is analogous to the "barking dog" clue explicated by Sherlock Holmes, see Ch. 26, p. 458.)

The other reason why the test 1 first strategy is superior is that test 1 is cheap and safe. If this were not so, and if test 2 had those characteristics, the strategy of doing test 1 first would no longer be preferred since it would just "save" one third of the patients from a cheap test, while the strategy of doing test 2 first would now save 81% of patients from the more costly or dangerous test 1. Similarly, test 3 must be relatively inaccessible and more noxious within the physician's and patient's value hierarchy. This set of relationships between the tests is crucial for determining the preferred strategy.

In the real world, test 1 might be something simple like auscultating the heart or looking at the patient's blood smear. Test 2 might be a liver spleen scan or a cerebral angiogram. Test 3 might be a blind biopsy or exploratory surgery.

In general, the components of the history and physical examination tend to have the characteristics of test 1. Thus, this model can be used to demonstrate the utility of the clinical examination in a general way.

Increasing the Level of Complexity as a Problem Solving Device

Let us say that a physician has examined a patient and determined that the patient is disoriented to time. By considering the differential diagnosis of "disorientation to time" and performing the rest of the mental status examination, one can make a specific diagnosis, perhaps "organic brain syndrome."

Next, one could review the past medical records and determine that the patient has been disoriented either acutely or for some time. If the former, one does the differential diagnosis of "acute organic brain syndrome"; if the latter, the differential diagnosis of the "chronic organic brain syndrome."

Next, one could perform a neurologic examination and determine whether or not focal findings are present. Let us say that they are not. The level of complexity now changes to "acute organic brain syndrome, no focal findings" or "chronic organic brain syndrome, no focal findings."

At this point, the differential diagnosis of the former would be given by the outline in Table 27-5.

It is worth noting that the same table outlines the differential diagnosis of the chronic organic brain syndromes, as well as for stupor, coma, and syncope. Of course, the emphasis changes: for example, with syncope the mechanisms subsumed under part I, C (such as bradycardias, tachyarrhythmias, and vagal syncopes) increase in importance, while the metabolic causes are less prevalent.

Let us assume for the sake of argument that your patient has the "chronic organic mental syndrome—no focal signs," and using the outline given in Table 27-5 above you have gone to the library to look up all the possibilities. The final list for this differential diagnosis is mind boggling. You become discouraged because you have been taught that only 10% to 20% of the chronic organic brain syndromes are due to reversible etiologies. What should you do?

First, you might go down the list and eliminate all the irreversible etiologies. You will then have advanced one more level of complexity (all this with the same patient and problem) to the differential diagnosis of "chronic organic brain syndrome—no focal neurologic findings—no reversible causes."

Since the differential diagnosis is nothing but a list of testable hypotheses, you could then match each item on the list with a *specific* laboratory test that would detect the disease in question were it present. In this way, your differential diagnosis would write the *orders* for working up the patient.

The orders would look like the items in Table 26-14. (Notice that the history and physical examination for both the acute and the chronic brain syndromes would already point you to a number of diagnoses.)

Let us suppose that the thyroid function studies come back with a low thyroxine level, low T3 resin uptake (and just to be unambiguous) a low free thyroxine index, a low triiodothyronine, a low free triiodothyronine, a low reverse triiodothyronine, and normal serum proteins. (You may also fantasize that the patient has a low

Table 27-5. Outline of Causes for Organic Brain
Syndromes (as Well as Other Conditions of Central Neuropenia)

I. Inadequate metabolic supply
   A. Hypoxia (e.g., decreased arterial pO_2, CO, or cyanide poisoning, methemoglobinemia, or sulfhemoglobinemia)
   B. Decreased glucose (hypoglycemia)
   C. Decreased delivery of substrates to the brain (decreased cerebral perfusion due to vascular obstruction, decreased cardiac output as in shock, etc.)

II. Inadequate metabolic milieu
   A. Systemic alterations in metabolism reflected in the brain (hypothyroidism, nutritional deficiencies such as B-12 deficiency, thiamine, niacin, etc.)
   B. Alterations of pH (acidosis or alkalosis, respiratory or metabolic)
   C. Alterations in ionic composition (e.g., as in uremia, especially acute; poisonings, etc.)

III. Inadequate physical milieu
   A. Mechanical disease of the central nervous system
      1. Trauma
      2. Tumors and other space-occupying lesions
   B. Inflammation (bacterial, fungal, etc.)
   C. Central nervous system syphilis
   D. Alterations in osmolality (hyperosmolar and hypoosmolar syndromes)
   E. Alterations in CSF pressure
   F. Etc.

basal oxygen consumption, a low thyroid 131I uptake at 6 and 24 hours, and a low butanol extractable iodine, although just a fraction of these available tests would be required.) Such a patient has unequivocal hypothyroidism. Let us further assume that all of the other tests are negative and that following treatment, the organic brain syndrome resolved.

You are finished with the case analysis, right? Wrong. You now should do the differential diagnosis of hypothyroidism, which is primarily the distinction between primary and secondary hypothyroidism. Let us assume that the thyroid-stimulating hormone is low. Now you have diagnosed secondary hypothyroidism.

Are you finished? No. Now you must do the differential diagnosis of secondary hypothyroidism (pituitary versus hypothalamic). Let us assume that it turns out to be pituitary. Are you finished yet?

No. You might want to determine whether the cause is pituitary apoplexy, hypophysitis, sarcoid infiltration of the pituitary, or any of the other items on that particular differential diagnosis.

Eventually, you may come to a point at which further progress is impractical, and here you might stop. But the point is that you can constantly improve your diagnostic acumen by forcing yourself always to progress to the next level of complexity.

An additional example is the analysis of edema (see Ch. 25, p. 446).

A Nonstrategy of Nondiagnosis

The word "diagnosis" comes from the Greek *gnosis* meaning to know or understand, and the Greek *dia* meaning through or thorough, as in diameter. Thus, when you make the diagnosis, it means that you know the thing thoroughly. "The diagnosis" is not an imperfect or inaccurate impression, although "my diagnosis" might be.

Sometimes residents say that they do not need a diagnosis because they can "manage" the patient. When I observe the results of their "management" of such undiagnosed patients, I am often reminded of how one of my patients once used that term. She was a prostitute, who referred to herself as a dancer, and to her procurer as her manager.

Diagnosis by Observing the Natural History

The term "diagnosis by observing the natural history" needs to be distinguished from "not making a diagnosis." The former was often used in earlier centuries when most patients were finally diagnosed at autopsy, and few diseases had effective treatments. Back then, following the patient until the disease "revealed itself" seldom did any harm.

Today, the main application of this strategy is in the outpatient evaluation of patients with poorly discerned findings, not suggestive of the need for immediate further diagnostic activities. For example, a patient with aches and pains alone might be followed with "undifferentiated rheumatic disorder" until such time as it became clear that he had rheumatoid arthritis, ankylosing spondylitis, palindromic rheumatism, or some other recognized entity, of which the first manifestations had been truly nondiagnostic. Similarly, for physicians who believe in the distinction between Raynaud's phenomenon (secondary to another disorder) as opposed to Raynaud's disease (unassociated with another disorder), it is obvious that the patient must be followed for several years to determine whether another disease, such as lupus erythematosus or progressive systemic sclerosis, will manifest itself or not.

To call a strategy "diagnosis by observing the natural history of the disease" (as opposed to "waiting for the diagnosis to fall out of the sky") one must be able, at the initiation of the process of observation, to list almost every single disease that the patient might eventually turn out to have, as well as the ways in which it will become clear that he has or does not have each of them.

A Personal Memoir

Between 1959 and 1970, when I was learning to think under the diligent examples and vigorous expectations of the Pittsburgh faculty, I was always perplexed by how quickly they made "the" diagnosis, usually correctly. The weekly performance at Clinicopathologic Conferences, the like of which I have not seen nor read before, during, or since, was so astounding, that I carried a set of Pittsburgh CPC protocols with me for over a decade after I was a full professor myself, trying to recapitulate their thinking from the notes I had made of their diagnostic explication. Someday, I told myself, I too would become a Great Rounder, but I would slow things up for my students and explain *how* the thing is done, not only that it *can* be done.

The present chapter is an admittedly feeble attempt, which falls short of the goal, not only by reason of the author's limitations, but also because there is something inherently unteachable in all this. I have noticed that as one progresses and gains *experience*,* there is some sort of automatic selfregulating internal system that reprograms one's thinking and improves one's diagnostic ability, provided that one was initially well educated and continues to read and see patients.

That said, the present chapter is a best attempt at recapitulating those ideas and techniques that have seemed at least to facilitate discussion of these issues, and so possibly to shorten the student's own apprentice time.

Appendix 27-1. Analysis for the Problem on Page 533

Let X = hypokalemia with hyperkaliuria. Etiology 1 = nonrenal causes; etiology 2 = renal tubular acidosis (RTA) (2a =

---

*The key word is *experience*. Remember the internist's rebuttal to the surgeon who had claimed, "*I* have never seen *that*": "Excuse me, Doctor you've *seen* it. You just haven't *recognized* it." Dr. Andy Lonigro of Missouri has a similar story whose punch line is, "No, Doctor, you have *not* had 20 years of experience. You've had 1 year of experience repeated 20 times." The point is the same.

RTA type 1; 2b = RTA type 2). It would be a fallacy to conclude that the patient under discussion must have mineralocorticoid excess because he could alternately have renal tubular acidosis type 2.

Appendix 27-2. A Method for Solving the Problem on Page 536

First take any six balls, and compare them with any other six balls. If the pans balance, the lighter ball is obviously the one excluded. If the pans do not balance, the lighter ball is one of the six in the pan that has risen. Take these six and weigh three against three for the second trial. Obviously, the lighter ball is in the pan that rises. For the third and final trial, take any two of the three balls remaining under suspicion and compare them. If one pan rises, it contains the lighter ball. If the pans balance, the lighter ball is the one that was excluded from this final trial.

References

Bernard C: *An Introduction to the Study of Experimental Medicine.* Green HC (trans.). Dover Publications, New York, 1957.

Blacklow RS: *MacBryde's Signs and Symptoms,* ed 6. JP Lippincott, Philadelphia, 1983.

Feinstein AR: *Clinical Judgment.* Williams & Wilkins, Baltimore, 1967.

Sapira JD: Logical handling of clinical data. *South Med J* 73:1437–1438, 1980.

Sapira JD: Diagnostic strategies. *South Med J* 74:582–584, 1981.

Stead EA: *What This Patient Needs Is a Doctor.* Wagner GS, Cebe B, Rozear MP (eds). Carolina Academic Press, Durham, NC, 1978.

Wittgenstein L: *Philosophical Remarks.* Rhees R (ed), Hargreaves R, White R (trans.). University of Chicago Press, Chicago, 1975.

28
Some Bedside Laboratory Tricks

"As Ponocrates grew familiar with Gargantua's vicious manner of studying, he began to plan a different course of education for the lad; but at first he let him go on as before knowing that nature does not endure abrupt changes without great violence."

The Old Education and the New, Gargantua, *Book 1, Rabelais*

Although not traditionally considered part of the clinical examination, laboratory diagnosis is simply an extension of the physical examination, albeit one that is now usually performed by persons unseen and not by the physician. Formerly, much of the laboratory examination was performed by the personal physician with the same advantages accruing as with the interview and the physical examination. Because some of these procedures are so simple and also because both they and their disappearance from recent textbooks are so instructive, a *selection* is provided for the entertainment and enlightenment of young Gargantuas. The selection is based on matters that came up in the course of teaching at the bedside. Many procedures that are well known and widely practiced are omitted for those very reasons.

BLOOD

Whole Blood

Erythrocyte Sedimentation Rate

The rate at which erythrocytes in anticoagulated whole blood sediment is an indirect measure of fibrinogen and globulin. Thus, it is a poor man's interleukin-1 assay. It is elevated in a wide variety of conditions of infection, inflammation, tissue necrosis, and neoplasia. Because of its nondiagnosticity for single diseases, it has lost favor, since it is now possible to distinguish, for example, angina pectoris from infarction or rheumatoid arthritis from osteoarthritis on other grounds. Still, the test has utility for screening large numbers of patients and for following therapy in inflammatory conditions, such as rheumatoid arthritis. I also use it on a yearly basis when following hypochondriacal patients.

A method:

1. Place blood, anticoagulated with EDTA or oxalate, in a Wintrobe tube, which is placed in a rack or taped to the wall behind the patient's bed. Be sure the tube is perfectly vertical.

2. One hour later, note how many millimeters of settling has taken place. (Measure from the top of the plasma to the top of the red cell column.)

3. Correct the sedimentation rate according to the hematocrit (Fig. 28-1). If the hematocrit is not already known, it can be determined on the same sample in the Wintrobe tube.

Interpretation. False-positive elevations in the sedimentation rate occur in old age and pregnancy.* False negatives (normal sedimentation rates) occur in typhoid fever, brucellosis, and 2% of cavitary tuberculosis cases. Some viral infections do not increase the sedimentation rate, while some mild viral infections may do so (Ham et al., 1957; Wintrobe, 1967).

Lee-White Clotting Time

Current usefulness. Although replaced in most laboratories by the various partial thromboplastin times, this test is still useful for diagnosing decreased amounts of procoagulants and for monitoring heparin therapy, if the partial thromboplastin time is not available. It can also be used in the "50/50" mixing test (vide infra), even if a partial thromboplastin time is not available, simply as a matter of convenience.

A method:

1. Draw fasting blood from a vein and place 2 ml in a Pyrex tube 8 × 15 × 100 mm. (Wider tubes yield longer clotting times, and smaller volumes yield shorter clotting times.) Note "zero time," defined as the moment that blood first appears in the syringe.

Caveats: The blood should be allowed to run down the side of the tube, and specifically should not be "jet-sprayed" into the tube or handled in any way that will produce bubbles (Waldron & Duncan, 1954).

2. After 5 minutes have elapsed, begin tilting the tube to a 45-degree angle at 1-minute intervals.

3. The clotting time is the interval at which the tube can be inverted without displacing the clot. The normal time is 5 to 8 minutes (Todd & Sanford, 1948).

---

*For the *Westergren* sedimentation rate, an age-correction formula has been derived (Miller et al., 1983) from a population of patients aged 20 to 65. For men, the upper limit of normal is obtained by dividing the age in years by 2. For women, add 10 to the age and divide the sum by 2.

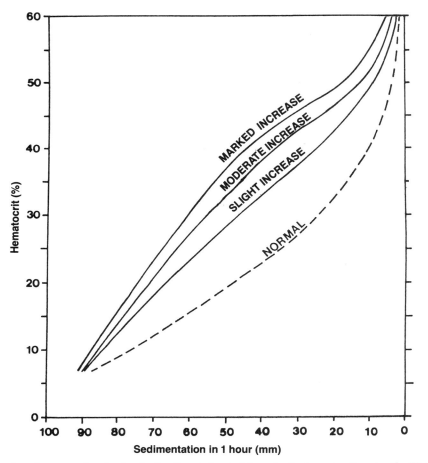

Figure 28-1. *Reference chart for correcting the depth of sedimentation in 1 hour for the hematocrit, using the Wintrobe-Landsberg method (after Hynes & Whitby, 1938). The sedimentation rate is to be corrected from the observed hematocrit to a sedimentation that corresponds to a hematocrit of 45%. The normal range for the corrected sedimentation rate is 0 to 10 mm.*

Plot the point corresponding to the observed hematocrit and the observed sedimentation rate. This will fall in one of the zones indicating the approximate degree of increase in the rate. (Follow the nearest curve to the point where it intersects the line corresponding to a hematocrit of 45%. Read the corrected sedimentation rate. For example, if the observed sedimentation is 50 mm and the observed hematocrit is 25%, then the sedimentation in 1 hour corrected to a hematocrit of 45% is approximately 11 mm. If the observed sedimentation is 8 mm and the observed hematocrit is 56%, then the sedimentation in 1 hour corrected to a hematocrit of 45% is approximately 30 mm.)

Variations.   This test has been modified to use two, three, and even four tubes. One begins the stopwatch immediately after filling the tubes and starts tilting the first tube. When that one has clotted, proceed to the next one in turn. The intertilting interval may be shortened to 30 seconds, but increased handling shortens the clotting time.

In some versions of the test, the tubes are placed in a 37° C water bath. In others, the tubes are prechilled by rinsing in iced saline. Under warmer conditions, the clotting time is slightly shorter.

Interpretation.   When two tubes are used, the clotting time is the average, unless the tubes vary by more than 5 minutes, in which case only the clotting time of the second tube is reported. The normal value is 4 to 12 minutes (Frommeyer & Epstein, 1957).

For three or four tubes, the clotting time is taken to be the time at which the last tube can be inverted. The normal is 5 to 15 minutes for three tubes, and less than 17 minutes for four tubes (Wintrobe, 1967).

○   The most important issue in interpreting results is that the test be performed under the same conditions each time.

History.   The importance of drawing blood from the vein so as to avoid contact with tissue thromboplastin was already known to Howell in 1905. The test had been performed using a coagulometer by Pratt in 1903, and Morawitz and Bierch performed it using a glass tube in 1907. Addis had added the step of inverting the test tube for determining the end point at least by 1910. And other workers had performed essentially the same test, as noted by Lee and White, who wrote, "the method described is not completely new. . . ." (Lee & White, 1913).

"50/50" Mixing Test for Circulating Anticoagulants

A patient with a prolonged clotting time may have a circulating anticoagulant instead of a simple deficiency of a clotting factor. To make this distinction, the clotting time (or other test of impaired coagulation, such as the automated PTT) is repeated, using a mixture of equal parts of the patient's blood and that of a normal person. The abnormal clotting test will become normal if the patient has insufficient clotting factors, but not if a circulating anticoagulant is present. Preincubation at 37°C will increase the positive yield (Clyne & White 1988).

The rationale for this test is as follows: If one views the clotting factors as operating in an enzymatic cascade, an improvement from near zero to 50% of normal will provide sufficient material to run the reaction. However, if there is an anticoagulant sufficient to impair normal levels of enzymes, the clotting test will still be abnormal if the anticoagulant is only diluted out by one half.

Blood Clot Tests

Observe a perfectly vertical tube of blood that has been taped to the wall next to the patient's bed.

1. If no clot ever forms, the fibrinogen content of the blood is thought to be very low, less than 60 mg/dl.

2. If the clot dissolves within 20 or 30 minutes, the patient has hypofibrinogenemia or accelerated fibrinolysis.

3. Clot retraction begins at about 1 hour and reaches a maximum in less than a day. With normal clot retraction, the clot becomes progressively smaller, leaving a space of completely clear serum behind it. Impaired clot retraction occurs more slowly than normal. Also, the red cells are not trapped effectively, so that they leak out of the clot, fall through the serum, and coat the floor of the test tube.

Clot retraction depends upon normal platelet number and function. If the platelets are decreased in number, there will be a decrease in clot retraction. Impaired clot retraction in the presence of a normal platelet count makes the diagnosis of "thrombasthenia" (weak platelets), or what we would now refer to as the family of numerically-adequate-but-functionally-inferior platelet syndromes. In fact, this is the only bedside test that distinguishes "thrombasthenia" from vascular defects (such as those found in scurvy or amyloidosis).

False negatives (falsely normal-appearing clot retraction despite impaired platelet function): With hypofibrinogenemia, fibrinolysis, or severe anemia, the abnormally small clot may mimic a normal clot that has retracted.

False positives: Polycythemia may cause the clot to appear "too big" despite normal retraction.

(For more on platelets, see "Rumpel-Leede test," Ch. 7, p. 109, and "platelets," p. 545.)

4. Leave the tube of blood up for more than a day to check for normal fibrinolysis.

Test for Heparin-Induced "White Clot" Syndrome

Occasionally, heparin induces immune-mediated platelet aggregation, causing thrombocytopenia and paradoxic thromboemboli. The emboli are ghostly white, and consist of platelet aggregates and fibrin.

A method. Mix platelet-rich plasma from a control subject with platelet-poor plasma from a patient. If the patient has white clot syndrome, his plasma will sensitize the platelets of the control subject. With the addition of 1 unit of heparin per cubic centimeter of plasma, plus adenosine diphosphate solution, a platelet aggregate will form. This may be obvious to inspection, or can be quantitated with a platelet aggregometer (Stanton et al., 1988).

Formed Elements of the Blood

First, clinical microscopy was purged from the curriculum because there was no National Board Examination in it. Then, manual differential counts were automated, to the further detriment of patients, as certain kinds of findings were lost. This section is concerned with what was lost (and can be regained) rather

than with cost effectiveness. It is intended to show neophytes and those who instruct them that there is both utility and pleasure in finding things for one's self in the laboratory, in exact analogy to interviewing and examining one's own patient.

How to Make a Blood Smear

1. Place a thick glass slide on a solid surface, frosted side up. Write the patient's name and the date in pencil on the frosted area.

2. Place a drop of blood very near one end of the slide. Hold the other end with the fingers of your nondominant hand.

3. With your dominant hand, pick up a second glass slide to be used as a spreading device. Hold it at a 45-degree angle to the first slide, and place its edge near the drop of blood, between the drop and your nondominant hand. (The drop will now be in the 45-degree angle formed by the two slides.) (See Fig. 28-2.)

4. Bring the second slide back toward the drop of blood. When it touches the drop, surface tension will cause the drop suddenly to spread out all along the length of the touching slides. (See Fig. 28-2.)

5. Quickly move the second slide toward your nondominant hand. This will pull the blood behind it and spread the blood over the glass without pressing on the blood corpuscles. (See Fig. 28-2.)

6. A perfect blood film will have a feathery edge. Usually, it takes two or three practice runs under supervision to produce such an edge, but once you learn the skill you will never lose it.

7. Allow the slide to dry (fix). Stain it according to the local ground rules, or the following procedure.

Staining a Peripheral Blood Smear

1. Place the smear on a support such as a cork nailed to a board or two rods hung over a sink.

2. When it is completely air-dried (fixed), pour Wright's stain on it so as to cover the entire slide. Wait 3 to 5 minutes.

3. Add the prepared buffer. Use enough to make the surface of the stain appear iridescent, but not so much that the overlying fluid becomes transparent enough to see the smear beneath it. Mix in the traditional manner by gently blowing on the slide, not

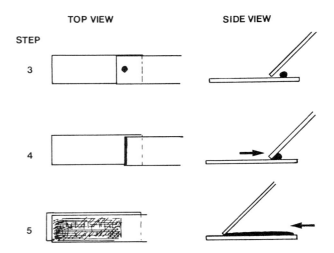

Figure 28-2. Preparing a blood smear (see text).

with a dowel rod or wooden applicator, lest the smear be disturbed.

4. After a few minutes, rinse with a wash bottle or under the tap and shake dry. Remaining topside bubbles may be blown off.

5. Blot with absorbent paper from the side. (Try not to touch the smear itself.)

6. The order of examination is: 1) red cells, 2) white cells, and 3) platelets.

Red Cells

The red cell number has already been implicitly measured by estimating the hematocrit from the nail beds and conjunctiva. Keep in mind such estimates of anemia and polycythemia when attempting to estimate the white count and platelet count from the relative numbers of cells on the smear (vide infra).

The diameter of the normal red cell is approximately the same as the nucleus of a small lymphocyte.

Information about red cell size can also be obtained from the mean corpuscular volume (MCV), which the electronic cell counter determines by displacement of an electrolyte solution, provided that there is no elliptocytosis, rouleaux formation (vide infra), or cold agglutinins (Rappaport et al., 1988). (In fact, the electronic cell counter's measurement of MCV is more accurate than the hematocrit; the latter is not measured but rather calculated from the MCV and the red cell count, giving an error of 3% to 5% compared with the spun hematocrit.)

Considerable variation in the shape of the red cells (poikilocytosis) is a significant finding not available from an inspection of the electronic hemogram. Abnormal cells include drepanocytes (also called banana cells and sickle cells), spherocytes, microspherocytes, stomatocytes, elliptocytes, burr cells, spur cells, helmet cells, bite cells, tear-drop cells, basophilic cells, and schistocytes. Cabot rings, Howell-Jolly bodies, malarial parasites, nucleated red cells, and so forth are examples of red cell inclusions that cannot be detected without inspection of the smear.

Rouleaux formation is the appearance of the red cells as rolls or "stacks of coins." A normal phenomenon in the thick portion of the smear, rouleaux formation is "called" only in the thin part of the smear and therefore requires much experience. It results from changes in the surface charge of the red cells, due to coating with increased amounts of globulin. Dr. Eugene Robin once diagnosed a case of multiple myeloma from noting the rouleaux formation, and so can you.

Cold agglutinins can also cause rouleaux formation on slides prepared in the customary manner. This can be diagnosed with confidence if such rouleaux are not seen on a second slide made from blood kept warm through the smearing and fixing stages, as with an incandescent lamp.

Anisocytosis is an abnormal variation in the size distribution of the red cells.

Unless your electronic counter has an accurate measure of the size distribution of the red cells (RDW or red cell distribution width), one would not know whether the patient had a dimorphic population of red cells without examining the smear. If the electronic counter does provide both these measures (MCV and RDW), there is no need to make size estimates from the smear, except to learn how to do it against the day when such a device might not be available. (The same principle applies, though unstated, to the other tests in this section.)

White Cells

With practice, one can estimate the *white blood cell count* (WBC) from the peripheral smear, if one has estimated the hematocrit.

An Arneth *lobe count,* looking for hypersegmented polymorphonuclear leukocytes, is performed by counting only those lobes that are seen to be connected by a thin thread of chromatin, not those that are simply overlapped. In counting 100 to 200 cells, one only need see 5% five-lobed polymorphonuclear leukocytes to know that an abnormality is present. If you find a single six-lobed polymorphonuclear leukocyte, you can stop counting instantly.

The causes of hypersegmented polymorphonuclear leukocytes are well known and are found in standard texts, with two important exceptions. 1) The most common cause of hypersegmented polymorphonuclear leukocytes in the present hospital population is the uremic syndrome. This is immediately reversed by the administration of supplemental folate, even though pretreatment serum folate levels may have been borderline or even normal (Siddiqui et al., 1970). 2) Patients with severe iron deficiency may have hypersegmented neutrophils that disappear with iron therapy. It is likely that iron deficiency inhibits formininotransferase, thus producing a functional folate deficiency despite normal levels of folate in both the serum and red blood cells (Beard & Weintraub, 1969).

A *Barr body* is a tiny projection from the nucleus, which is thought to represent the "extra" X chromosome in female cells. Males may appear to have Barr bodies on up to 5% of their neutrophils. Over 10% of leukocytes from females (genotype XX) will have Barr bodies. Although the Barr body has been likened to a drumstick (with the thick part distal to the nucleus proper), many XY nuclei will have drumsticks. A true Barr body looks more like a lollipop or a balloon on a stick.

The payoff for examining blood smears is to find the 1 out of 600 phenotypically male patients whose hypogonadism is suddenly explicable based upon the XXY chromosomes of Klinefelter's syndrome.

Döhle bodies are pale-blue inclusions seen in Wright-stained polymorphonuclear leukocytes. By histochemical analysis, they are composed of ribonucleoprotein and/or ribonucleic acid. Once thought to be diagnostic of scarlet fever, they appear in the blood of 7% of hospitalized patients, specifically in the conditions listed in Table 28-1. They are not seen in healthy student nurses (Abernathy, 1964, 1966) or patients with urticaria or serum sickness (Granger & Pole, 1913).

Döhle bodies with red granules within them are called Amato bodies. These have the same significance as Döhle bodies, although they too were once thought to be diagnostic of scarlet fever (Toomey & Gammel, 1927).

Structures identical to Döhle bodies in light microscopic appearance have also been seen in various congenital syndromes, including the May-Heggelin anomaly, Chediak-Higashi syndrome, the pseudo-Pelger-Huet syndrome, the Fechtner syndrome, and so forth (Peterson et al., 1985).

Auer rods are pink (by Wright's stain) intracytoplasmic rods or clumps that come from the azure granules that in turn come from lysosomes. They are most frequent in inmature cells. They were discovered by Auer, who reported seeing them in lymphocytic leukemia (Auer, 1906) and this continues to be reported (Juneja et al., 1987). Both reported them in tuberculosis in 1913 (Freeman, 1960)

Table 28-1. Döhle Bodies: Associations

Infections
  Scarlet fever (100% in first 2 days) (Granger & Pole, 1913)
  Tuberculosis (11% to "practically all") (Bachman & Lucke, 1918)
  Lobar pneumonia (67%–100% (Granger & Pole, 1913)
  Empyema
  Bronchitis
  Viral upper respiratory infection
  Pertussis (rare) (Bachman & Lucke, 1918)
  Amebiasis
  Purulent infections
  Erysipelas (64%) (Granger & Pole, 1913)
  German measles (rare) (Bachman & Lucke, 1918)
  Chickenpox (rare) (Bachman & Lucke, 1918)
  Measles (45% in the first 5 days) (Granger & Pole, 1913)
  Diphtheria (68% in the first 5 days) (Granger & Pole, 1913)
  Tonsillitis (58%) (Granger & Pole, 1913)
  Typhus

Neoplastic
  Carcinoma
  Myelogenous leukemia
  Lipoma
  Myoma

Neurologic
  Concussion
  "Anxiety neurosis"

Other
  Diabetes
  Uremia
  Anemia
  Severe burns
  Pregnancy (Abernathy, 1966)

Iatrogenic
  After the infusion of diphtheria toxin
  After blood transfusion
  After cyclophosphamide treatment

Source: Abernathy (1964, 1966).

and this too has been replicated (Leavell & Twomey, 1964). They are seen in 21% of acute myelogenous leukemia, or 66% to 75% if peroxidase staining is used (Jain et al., 1987).

The *eosinophil* count obtained by multiplying the white count by the percentage of eosinophils is only accurate when the percentage of eosinophils is at least 5% to 6%, even if the white count is very high. Accuracy can be improved by counting 200 white cells instead of the usual 100.

Eosinophilia is called when there are more than 310 eosinophils per mm³. The differential diagnosis of eosinophilia (which includes parasites, allergic conditions, some infectious conditions such as tuberculosis, malignant conditions, and a number of other causes, all diagnosable on other grounds) is out of fashion in most medical centers. Thus, there is little awareness of a frequent new cause of eosinophilia in the modern medical center—therapeutic radiation-induced eosinophilia (Ghossein et al., 1975).

Any degree of eosinophilia rules out the diagnosis of Cushing's syndrome, and the absence of eosinophils rules out the diagnosis of chronic adrenocortical insufficiency.

Platelets

An estimation of platelet number should routinely be made from the smear, and the examiner's skill augmented by feedback from the electronic platelet count. Begin by estimating 25,000 platelets per mm³ for every platelet seen in a high-power field.

Electronic cell counters may produce a spurious thrombocytopenia in three circumstances (Kjeldsberg & Hershgold, 1974): 1) Platelet satellitism occurs in blood collected in EDTA. Platelets adhere to polymorphonuclear leukocytes, which are excluded by size from the count. 2) Platelet agglutinins can cause the platelets to clump together; the clump is also optically excluded by the counter due to its size. 3) Giant platelets are excluded for the same reason.

Spurious thrombocytosis may be produced by the electronic cell counter in three circumstances (Rappaport et al., 1988), all of which can be recognized on the smear: 1) fragmented white cells (smudge cells), as in leukemia or sepsis; 2) fragmented red cells, as in thrombotic thrombocytopenic purpura, disseminated intravascular coagulation, microangiopathic hemolytic anemia, or cardiopulmonary bypass; 3) marked microcytosis of the red cells as in microspherocytosis.

(Also see "Rumpel-Leede Test" in Ch. 7, p. 109, and "Blood Clot Tests," p. 543.)

Earlobe Histiocytes (Low Power)

In the *first* drop of blood (Smith, 1964) taken from the lanced earlobe of a patient with subacute bacterial endocarditis, it is often, but not always, possible to find large histiocytes, which are at least one and a half times as large as monocytes (Daland et al., 1956; Van Nuys, 1907). (This is an example of empiric but not scientific fact since we do not know why this should be true, only that it is.)

Sensitivity. In various large series, the sensitivity for subacute bacterial endocarditis has been reported as 21% to 33% (Hill & Bayrd, 1960; Smith, 1964).

False positives. Earlobe histiocytes are not pathognomonic for bacterial endocarditis. If one uses strict criteria and requires at least 10% of the differential count to be these unusual cells, the differential diagnosis also includes malaria and trypanosomiasis.

Other cutoffs. Large histiocytes may constitute 2% of the differential count in septicemia, rheumatic fever with active carditis, tuberculosis, Hodgkin's disease, chronic sinusitis, subsiding hepatitis, mediastinal tumor, agranulocytosis, localized bacterial infection (Smith, 1964), and systemic lupus erythematosus.

If one accepts 1% histiocytosis as evidence of a positive sign, one will start to include perinephric abscess, infectious mononucleosis, mastoiditis, ulcerative colitis, subsiding acute appendicitis, trichinosis, acute and chronic myelocytic leukemia, typhoid fever, paroxysmal nocturnal hemoglobinuria, cholera, severe hemolysis, transfusion reactions, chronic meningococcemia, sickle-cell anemia (Greenberg, 1964), and anemia of the newborn (erythroblastosis fetalis?) (Hill & Bayrd, 1960; Smith, 1964).

Large histiocytes may be found in normal persons, but never constitute more than 1% of the differential count (Hill & Bayrd, 1960; Smith, 1964).

Leukocytes Containing Bacteria

In patients with septicemia, a low-power scan of a thin blood film prepared from the *first* drop of earlobe blood and stained with Gram's stain (or Jenner-Giemsa, Leishman, or May-Grünwald-Giemsa) may reveal intracellular organisms. The ear that the patient has *not* been lying on gives better results. The feathered edge of the smear is the best place to find the infected leukocytes.

Gram Stain of the Buffy Coat

This incredibly simple technique (see p. 553 for the Gram stain) permits the identification of bacteria in the blood about 24 to 48 hours before the laboratory reports a positive culture, and rarely in cases with negative culture results (Humphrey, 1944). See Table 28-2 for the diagnostic value of this technique (which has also been applied to the peripheral blood film and blood aspirated from skin lesions) in various studies. No studies have yet been reported giving a comparison of buffy coat staining with the earlobe histiocyte test performed in the same patients.

In contaminated blood transfusion reactions, one should also Gram stain the *plasma* of blood centrifuged briefly (for 2 to 3 minutes). (Also see "Ascitic Fluid," p. 553.)

Serum and Plasma

Distinguishing Hemoglobinuria from Myoglobinuria

Most urine tests for hemoglobin are also positive for myoglobin. Thus, given a positive dipstick test, how can one distinguish between prior hemoglobinemia and prior myoglobinemia?

Hemoglobin in the blood binds to haptoglobin. The molecular size of the hemoglobin-haptoglobin complex is too large to pass the glomerulus and appear in the urine, and only when the binding capacity of haptoglobin is exceeded will hemoglobin appear in the urine. Thus, any time that plasma hemoglobin spills into the urine, a simultaneous serum (plasma) sample will be mahogany in appearance and positive for hemoglobin by benzidine or other dipstick. (The hemoglobin can react with the dipstick even when bound to haptoglobin.)

Because myoglobin does not bind to haptoglobin to any significant extent, myoglobinuria can be distinguished from hemoglobinuria secondary to hemoglobinemia by the fact that the myoglobinuria will *not* be accompanied by pigmented, dipstick-positive serum (or plasma).

Schumm's Test

$$ This is a test for methemalbumin, which appears acutely in the plasma following any episode of hemoglobinemia. The test re-quires a decent student laboratory, a hand spectroscope, and a sunny day (the light source for the spectroscope).

Method. Cover nine volumes of plasma with a one-volume layer of ether. Add one volume of concentrated ammonium sulfide to the plasma layer (*beneath* the ether) with a pipette. Stir all the components together, and examine for a sharply defined band at 558 micra.

Salicylate Intoxication

A rapid approximation of serum salicylate levels may be obtained with Phenistix (see p. 550). The dipstick turns brown at concentrations up to 40 mg/dl, and purple at concentrations over 90 mg/dl (Clarkson, 1978).

Viscosity

A viscometer for studying a patient suspected to have the hyperviscosity syndrome may be made from a red cell or white cell diluting pipette, or even from the barrel of a tuberculin syringe (sans plunger).

Fill the container with the serum to be tested, and determine the time it takes to drip out. Compare the number of elapsed seconds with a control. In hyperviscosity syndrome, the value is usually twice normal.

Cryoglobulins

Cryoglobulins are globulins precipitable by cold. They occur in: 1) multiple myeloma, 2) a variety of "collagen-vascular" diseases and other entities characterized by circulating antigen-antibody complexes, and 3) polyclonal hypergammaglobulinemia such as that caused by cirrhosis of the liver. They are sometimes found accidentally by the clinical laboratory when a serum sample stored in the refrigerator for later analysis is found to have "coagulated."

Cryofibrinogen is fibrinogen that is precipitable by cold. Cryofibrinogens are found as accompaniments to many inflammatory diseases and some tumors, and rarely as a primary disease. They are rarely found accidentally by the clinical laboratory since they are not present in serum, and most refrigerator-stored samples are not plasma.

Table 28-2.   Results of Studies Examining Blood Film or Buffy Coat for Bacteria

Reference	Method	Sensitivity	Predictive Value of a Negative Test	False Positives
Brooks et al., 1973	Buffy coat examined on 135 specimens sent for blood culture	5/14 (36%)	135/144 (94%)	0
Powers & Mandell, 1974	Buffy coat examined in 16 patients suspected of having endocarditis (6 of whom did not) and 6 normal controls	6/10 (60%)	12/16 (75%)	0
Smith, 1966	Earlobe blood of septicemic patients	17/57 (30%)		
Thomas, 1943	Examination of peripheral blood film in rapidly fatal cases of meningococcemia	6/12 (50%)		
Hoefs & Runyon, 1985	Ascitic buffy coat in spontaneous bacterial peritonitis	(55%)		
Bush & Bailey, 1944	Examination of peripheral blood film in rapidly fatal cases of meningococcemia[a]	3/6 (50%)		
McLean & Caffey, 1931	Examination of blood film obtained from hemorrhagic purpuric lesion in meningococcemia	15/18 (83%)		

[a]*The patients with organisms seen on peripheral smear all had negative blood cultures. The cells containing the Gram-negative diplococci superficially resembled basophils.*

Because the test is so simple (and because many laboratories will respond to a request for cryoproteins by performing the tests for cold agglutinins or cold hemolysins, which are unrelated), the method is presented here:

1. Put a plasma sample and a serum sample in the refrigerator.
2. Look at the two tubes the next morning. Tilt them. Is there a solid gel at the bottom?

If there is a gel in both tubes, one is dealing with a cryoglobulin. If there is a gel only in the bottom of the plasma tube, one is dealing with a cryofibrinogen.

Sia Water Test

This test for abnormal quantities or types of globulins is now performed by adding one drop of serum to a 30-cm cylinder of distilled water. Normally, when the serum hits the water, there is no change in the water's appearance. But when the test is positive, there will be an opacity in the shape of a tear or upside down parachute as the serum falls through the water.

This test was invented in China for diagnosing the hyperglobulinemia of kala azar. Originally, 20 ml of blood were shaken with 0.6 ml of distilled water, and turbidity read at 5, 15, 30, and 60 minutes (Sia, 1924).

Some persons perform the test by putting a drop of distilled water into the serum, and some put a drop of serum into a short test tube full of distilled water.

According to the loose criterion, *any* degree of turbidity is a positive test. Using this criterion, the test is 12% to 20% sensitive for myeloma protein (Laurell & Waldenstrom, 1961; Pruzanski & Watt, 1972) and 57% sensitive for macroglobulin (Laurell & Waldenstrom, 1961). Proteins migrating in the alpha and ß range almost always give a negative test. False positives occur in some normal persons.

According to the strict criterion, flocculation must occur as soon as the serum falls into the water. This is called a "3 + test." It requires that the M-component be 2.4 g/dl or higher, but eliminates the false positives occurring in normal persons. However, this result is generally seen only in about 25% of patients with macroglobulinemia (Laurell & Waldenstrom, 1961).

Lipids

To make a quick determination of the type of hyperlipoproteinemia (if any) that a patient has, allow a serum sample to sit overnight in the refrigerator.

In the rare type I hyperlipoproteinemia, there will be a creamy supernatant over a clear infranatant. (Such blood may look like cream of tomato soup as it is drawn.)

Type II hyperlipoproteinemia is the only type in which the serum may look perfectly normal. However, some type IIB sera will develop a cloudy or turbid infranatant.

The rare type III will have a creamy supernatant and a cloudy or turbid infranatant. Sometimes, these separate poorly by the next morning, and simply appear cloudy throughout.

The common type IV will have a clear supernatant and a turbid infranatant, or sometimes will be cloudy throughout if separation has been poor.

Since type V is a combination of types I and IV, it not unexpectedly will have a creamy supernatant over a turbid infranatant.

Further analysis can be done by electrophoresis or cholesterol and triglyceride ratios, but these are beyond the scope of this work.

While the above is not foolproof, it offers an excellent chance of making a very quick diagnosis after very little effort, especially if one correlates the findings with the xanthomas discussed in Chapter 7 (p. 117).

Ketoacidosis and Hydroxyacidosis

The ubiquity of the Autoanalyzer has made it possible for ketoacidosis (due to acetoacetate) and hydroxyacidosis (due to hydroxybutyrate and/or lactate) to be diagnosed in the aggregate along with the other causes of anion gap acidosis.

At the same time, there has been less interest in measuring serum acetone (expressed in terms of the weakest dilution—1:2n—that gives a positive reaction with Acetest tablets). This test also measures acetoacetate, but not the hydroxyacids.

Since each 1:1 dilution of serum that is required to reach a negative test for acetone represents about 4 mEq per liter of acid (3 of hydroxybutyrate and 1 of acetoacetate), it would seem that one could determine whether all of the anion gap had been accounted for. Alas, the redox pair (acetoacetate/hydroxybutyrate) shifts toward the latter (unmeasured) hydroxyacids in situations of greater acidosis. Thus, an improvement in patients with diabetic ketoacidosis, for instance, may be accompanied by an improvement in all biochemical parameters except for serum acetone, which becomes positive in even stronger dilution although the total amount of the redox pair is reduced.

A bedside test for ß-hydroxybutyrate would be extremely helpful in this regard because one could determine the exact ratio at any given moment in any given sample and know whether the anion gap had been adequately explained or whether it would be necessary to measure lactate or even whether there was a simultaneous but masked decreased anion gap.*

It has been stated that the addition of a drop of hydrogen peroxide to a serum sample containing ß-hydroxybutyrate would convert the latter to acetoacetate. Then the difference between the acetoacetate titration with and without added hydrogen peroxide would be due to hydroxybutyrate. (This seems to be based upon the decades-old Hart's test for ß-hydroxybutyrate in the urine, which involved studying a diluted sample that had also been treated with heat and glacial acetic acid.)

Unfortunately, the test does not work in the suggested form on serum since the addition of the hydrogen peroxide interferes with (i.e., "bleaches") the color development of both the tablet and dipstick currently used to assay for "acetone."

Osmolal Gaps

The osmolal gap† is the difference between the measured osmolality and the following quantity:

$$2(Na^+ + Cl^-) + BUN/2.8 + blood\ glucose/18.$$

Osmolal gaps greater than 10 mOsm/kg are found in cases in which the following substances have appeared in the serum: methanol, ethanol (divide the osmolal gap by 4.24 to obtain mg/dl of ethanol), isopropyl alcohol, acetone, ether, trichloroethane, glycerin, isoniazid, diatrizoate, mannitol, sorbitol, and

---

*A decreased anion gap occurs with: 1) elevation of an unmeasured (or unconsidered) cation (potassium, calcium, lithium, or magnesium), or 2) decreased albumin, or 3) increased abnormal globulins.

†Dr. Al Shapiro of Pennsylvania asked technician applicants to distinguish between osmolality and osmolarity. There is no practical difference with the usual biologic fluids because the density of water is 1 g/cc under customary conditions. Purists who like challenges are invited to reconcile the definitions given in the 24th edition of *Dorland's Illustrated Medical Dictionary* with those of Homer Smith (1956).

some solutions infused for the treatment of shock (Smithline & Gardner, 1976).

Urine

Color

Unusual colors in the urine may result from the metabolism of both endogenous and exogenous substances (Table 28-3). A detailed history is most important, but measuring the urine pH, observing for color change on standing, and certain other tests may be useful (Raymond & Yarger, 1988). (See the tests for hemoglobinuria [p. 548] and porphyrins [p. 549] and the ferric chloride test [p. 550].)

Specific Gravity

The osmolality of the urine can be estimated from the specific gravity. Given a standard diet, every increase of .003 in the specific gravity is about 100 mOsm of solutes. To correct for glucosuria, subtract .004 from the specific gravity for 1% sugar (which is 270 mg/dl, or 2 + to 3 + depending upon the brand of dipstick). To correct for 3 + proteinuria (which represents about 1 g/dl), subtract .003. The remaining specific gravity is that due to solutes. These conversions work *only* for urine.

In studies done by Dr. Holly Sata of California, the dipstick specific gravity varied from the hydrometer value by an average of .005 unit, and was not good enough to rely upon in individual cases. (Using the conversion formula given above, the hydrometer gave a better estimate of measured osmolality than did the dipstick.)

The dipstick specific gravity was found to respond correctly to monovalent salts but not to glucose or urea; protein was overestimated. A pH change from 5 to 7 further decreased the specific gravity reading by as much as 0.10 unit (Kirschbaum, 1983).

While it is clearly optimal to measure the osmolality, if the measurement is not available, the specific gravity should be measured with a hydrometer or refractometer.

Chemistry

Hemoglobin and Myoglobin

As previously noted (p. 546), hemoglobinuria secondary to hemoglobinemia is characterized by benzidine-positive material, usually of a mahogany color, in both plasma and urine. Hemoglobinuria secondary to bleeding into the urinary tract with no prior intravascular hemolysis (hemoglobinemia) is characterized by clear serum and residual unhemolyzed red cells seen on microscopic examination of the urine. Myoglobinuria from myoglobinemia is characterized by clear serum and benzidine-positive pigment in the urine with few or no red cells seen on microscopic examination.

Porphyrins

Bedside porphyrin metabolism.   All diseases that may be accompanied by the excess production of porphyrins can be divided into two classes: the porphyrinurias and the true porphyrias. The former include diseases such as lead poisoning, hepatic cirrhosis, malignancies, hemolytic anemias, and a variety of other conditions. However, one does not screen these patients

Table 28-3. Urine Color

Color of Urine	Substance
Pink	Hemoglobin, myoglobin
Pink to red	Beets, oxyhemoglobin, doxorubicin, ibuprofen, phenytoin, phensuximide
Pink to red in large concentrations	Porphyrins
Pink to red in alkaline urine	Phenolphthalein, phenolsulfonephthalein, bromsulfalein, santonin
Pink to red in acid urine	Urorosein
Pink to red on contact with hypochlorite bleach	Aminosalicylic acid
Deep red after large doses	Antipyrine
Red if excreted in large amounts	Congo red
Red	Pyridium, indirubin from malabsorption (Sapira et al., 1971)
Red-orange	Rifampin
Red-brown	Porphobilin, chloroquin, ibuprofen, phenothiazines, phensuximide, phenytoin
Red-brown in alkaline urine	Levodopa, methyldopa
Red-violet in acid urine, yellow-brown in acid urine	Chrysophonic acid formed from anthracine (aloe, cascara segrada, rhubarb, senna)
Blue or green (the latter possibly owing to mixture with yellow of urine)	Methylene blue, chlorophyll breath mints, magnesium salicylate, Doan's pills, iodochlorohydroxyquin, pyocyanin from *Pseudomonas*
Blue	Indigotin ("blue diaper disease") (Sapira et al., 1971)
Blue or blue-green	Mitoxantrone (Anonymous, 1988)
Purple	Chlorzoxazone
Purple in alkaline urine	Phenolphthalein
Greenish tint	Thymol
Olive green to black on exposure to air	Phenol
Deep yellow in acid urine	Santonin
Yellow to brown	Bilirubin, sulfamethoxazole, nitrofurantoin, primaquin
Yellow-orange	Carrots, vitamin A, aminopyrine, warfarin
Yellow-orange in alkaline urine	Sulfasalazine
Yellow to amber	Urobilin
Light brown to dark brown	Methemoglobin
Brown, black (or pink)	Myoglobin
Black on standing	Homogentisic acid
Brown to black on standing	Melanin pigment or precursors

Source: *Ham et al. (1957) and Raymond and Yarger (1988).*

for urinary porphyrins for two reasons: First, the production of measurable quantities of porphyrins in the urine of these patients is so inconstant (with the possible exception of lead poisoning) that the test is not useful as a diagnostic screen. Second, there are other easier ways to screen for these diseases. They are mentioned here only because they may give false positives in the tests to be described.

The true porphyrias, on the other hand, are not so easily diagnosed, and here the determination of urinary porphyrins (for porphyria cutanea tarda), as well as red cell porphyrins and fecal porphyrins (for some of the very rare inherited porphyrias) becomes useful. (Acute intermittent porphyria, one of the most common causes of undiagnosed recurrent abdominal pain, is best diagnosed by testing for porphobilinogen, vide infra.)

Screening for urinary porphyrins
(after Snapper & Kahn, 1967):

1. Add 25 ml of 10% NaOH to 75 ml of hemoglobin-free urine in a glass cylinder, and let it stand overnight.

2. If the precipitate is white the next morning, the test is negative. But if it is brown, porphyrins are present, or the patient has taken cascara. (Shining a Wood's light on the precipitate will produce a red fluorescence in either case.)

3. Redissolve the precipitate in 10% HCl and examine under the Wood's light. If the red fluorescence is present, porphyrins of some type are in the sample, and further study is mandatory. (The red fluorescence of cascara disappears in 10% HCl.)

Other fluorescent tests for porphyrins:

1. A reagent for extracting porphyrins from urine or stool may be made from 4 parts of ethyl acetate (or amyl alcohol) and 1 part glacial acetic acid. Add one volume of this mixture to two volumes of the substance to be studied. Shake. Examine the tube with a Wood's light for red fluorescence.

(This reagent may be improved and adapted to blood testing by adding some ether. But the latter is so hard to find at present, that alternatives are suggested below. Additionally, if you are thinking about erythropoietic porphyrias, you are beyond the screening stage.)

2. For fecal porphyrins, just smear the feces from the rectal examination onto a piece of filter paper, cover with acetic acid, and search for red fluorescence with the Wood's light.

3. For red cell fluorescence, use the fluorescent microscope in the pathology department to examine an *unstained* blood smear, as well as a control smear, for fluorescence, being sure that the excitation and emission filters are set correctly. *Under no circumstances should you attempt to improvise a fluorescent microscope* by shining a Wood's light through the microscope as this could damage your eyes.

Urine porphobilinogen tests. The purpose of these tests is to detect porphobilinogen in the urine of patients suffering from acute intermittent porphyria. They are not used to detect any other porphyrias or porphyrinurias.

The Watson-Schwartz test is performed as follows:

1. Shake about 5 ml of urine with the same volume of Ehrlich's urobilinogen reagent. (This can be found in most clinical laboratories, which purchase it premixed from commercial suppliers. If you have to make your own, add 600 to 700 mg of *p*-dimethylaminobenzaldehyde to 150 ml of concentrated HCl and top it off with distilled water to make a total volume of 250 ml.)

2. If a red or pink color occurs, you have detected something, possibly only urobilinogen. Add an equal volume of saturated sodium acetate solution.

3. Add some chloroform and shake. Eventually two layers will emerge. (This may take some time if you shake too violently. But you must shake vigorously enough to allow the red pigment to partition between the two phases. If in a hurry, simply centrifuge for a minute in the urinalysis centrifuge.)

4. If the pigment is predominantly in the chloroform layer (the one on the bottom), the test is positive for urobilinogen, not porphobilinogen. But if the pink color remains in the aqueous (upper) phase, you should do one more extraction to remove interfering substances. Pour some of the upper phase into another tube, and extract against toluene or butanol. If the pigment still remains in the aqueous phase, you may make a provisional diagnosis of acute intermittent porphyria.

Significance: A single false-negative Watson-Schwartz test was found in an asymptomatic member of a large kindred (Mahood & Killough, 1966). The false-positive rate was 0.0% in a series of 1,000 consecutive urines if the butanol extraction step was used. Without this step, the false-positive rate was 5.9% (Townsend, 1964). Purple false positives (due to indoles) may be obtained in the carcinoid syndrome and from compliant patients receiving at least 750 mg per day of methyldopa.

The Watson-Schwartz test was superior to the Hoesch test (vide infra) when performed in Dr. Watson's laboratory (Pierach et al., 1977), but in all fairness the Hoesch test has its champions.

The Hoesch test is an alternate that circumvents the problem of false positives due to urobilinogen, pyridium therapy, and (one hopes) all the other contaminants to which urine is heir. No extraction need be done. However, one cannot appropriate the clinical laboratory's urobilinogen reagent, but must make up some of Ehrlich's original reagent, by dissolving 2 g of *p*-dimethylaminobenzaldehyde in 100 ml of 6 *N* HCl. Place a few milliliters of fresh urine in a test tube and add about 2 drops of the reagent. A red color is porphobilinogen (Lamon et al., 1974).

Bence Jones Protein

A method:

1. Check the pH of the urine with a pH meter or pH paper. If it is above pH 5, add acetic acid or acetate buffer to bring the pH to 5.

2. Place the urine in a water bath at 400°C and raise the temperature of the water bath. When the temperature of the *urine* is between 40° and 60°C, a precipitate or flocculence or murkiness will develop if Bence Jones protein is present. (But the precipitate may not immediately collect at the bottom of the tube.)

3. Snapper adds an equal volume of 4% sulfosalicylic acid at this point, bringing the pH to 3. This precipitates not only all the Bence Jones protein, but also any albumin that is present. (You already know whether albumin is present because it will show as protein on the dipstick, but Bence Jones protein will *not*.)

4. Now boil the urine. Bence Jones protein will dissolve, but albumin will not. If you are uncertain about the results, pour the boiling urine through filter paper, which will retain the denatured albumin, but not the dissolved Bence Jones protein. Put the filtrate into an ice bath, and when it cools down to about 50°, you will be able to see the Bence Jones protein precipitate again.

Historical note. Some famous places do not even have a student or house staff laboratory. Those that do have a laboratory may not have a water bath or even a thermometer. Accordingly, the following quick and dirty method has been invented. It requires no reagents or equipment, although the astute will be able to improve it to the degree that such are available to them.

An alternate method:

1. Place the patient's fresh (and hence acidic) urine into a test tube. (If urine is allowed to stand, bacteria will grow and may make the urine alkaline.) If the urine contains albumin, it must first be removed by precipitation and filtration as above.

2. Place the test tube in a beaker about half the height of the test tube, so that some of the urine can be seen above the level of the beaker.

3. Place a piece of a telephone directory page or newspaper into the beaker so that part of it may be read *through* the urine in the test tube, unobscured by the additional glass wall of the beaker.

4. Place the whole thing in a microwave oven, turn it on, and wait for the urine to boil, as you observe through the door of the microwave. If Bence Jones protein is present, one can often observe a turbidity in the tube before the urine boils. By the time the urine boils, the turbidity will have cleared, although not always completely. (The degree of turbidity is judged by the ease of reading the printing through the urine.)

Urinary Catalase

A method. The following method (Gagnon et al., 1959) is recommended by simplicity.

1. Soak a disc of Schleicher and Schell 507-GH filter paper in 1 or 2 drops of urine, then place it in a 16-mm test tube to which 5 ml of 3% hydrogen peroxide are added. (Obviously, the disc has to be smaller than the diameter of the test tube.)

2. Observe whether the disc floats to the top. Allow 45 minutes before calling the test negative.

Interpretation. Normally, the disc does not float. However, if catalase appears in the urine, it will catalyze the formation of water and oxygen from the hydrogen peroxide solution. The oxygen bubbles attach to the paper disc and cause it to float. Obviously, the speed of flotation is proportional to the catalase concentration of the urine.

Catalase can appear in the urine when renal parenchymal cells are destroyed, when red or white cells appear in the urine, and when there is proliferation of the 90% of bacteria that cause pyelonephritis and also produce catalase. (The 10% that do not produce catalase, such as Enterococci, may still produce a positive catalase test because of leukocyturia.) The catalase test may even be positive when routine urine cultures are negative, as during protoplast formation (Braude & Berkowitz, 1961; Sapira & Shapiro, 1967), or when the microscopic examination is negative because of lysis of the red and white blood cells.

Ferric Chloride Test and Phenistix

A 10% solution of ferric chloride shaken with an equal volume of urine will react slowly with a wide range of phenols and related materials. It takes about 2 minutes for a maximum color change to occur (Cassidei et al., 1978). Salicylates produce a brown color at a concentration of 25 to 50 mg/dl, and a purple color at concentrations greater than 150 mg/dl. In the presence of 5-hydroxyindoleacetic acid from carcinoid syndrome (Yamaguchi &

Hayashi, 1978) or desferrioxamine (Finlay, 1978), a deep red-brown color develops. Acetoacetate gives a purple color, and phenylpyruvic acid a grey-blue color when it occurs in the quantities seen in phenylketonuria (Broder, 1987).

Phenistix, which are reagent strips impregnated with ferric chloride, were once used in screening for phenylketonuria, but have been replaced because of false negatives (Medical Research Council Steering Committee, 1981). However, the sticks (if available) can still be used in lieu of the ferric chloride solution for the purposes mentioned above.

Very high doses of phenothiazines may mimic the reaction given by salicylates, but can be differentiated by adding a drop of concentrated sulfuric acid to the reagent strip. This strong acid bleaches out the color due to salicylates, but intensifies that due to phenothiazines (Clarkson, 1978).

Forrest Reagents for Psychoactive Drug Overdose

In the early 1960s, psychoactive drug compliance was a major question facing psychopharmacologists. A series of papers by Forrest and Forrest in *Clinical Chemistry* and *The American Journal of Psychiatry* gave formulas for solutions that turned color when shaken with an equal volume of urine containing various psychoactive drugs, the intensity of the color being proportional to the concentration of the substance. While these solutions became obsolete for this purpose in the 1970s, they still have great potential for diagnosing drug overdose in the emergency room. Two that I have found useful are as follows:

1. Universal reagent for the detection of high-dose phenothiazines:
5 parts	5% ferric chloride
40 parts	20% perchloric acid
50 parts	50% nitric acid
    Shake with urine, and check immediately for a purple color.
2. Imipramine reagent:
    Equal amounts of:
    0.2% potassium dichromate
    30% sulfuric acid
    20% perchloric acid
    50% nitric acid
    Shake with urine, and read the green color.

False negatives are found with the simultaneous ingestion of ascorbic acid (James et al., 1980).

The pharmaceutical manufacturing association having outstripped "shake" chemistry, it is not known what other current psychoactive drugs will react with those reagents. Could you think up a good senior research project?

Microscopy

Preserving Wet Mounts of Urine and Other Fluids

From time to time, an attending physician will wish to review a joint fluid, a urinalysis, or some other wet mount the morning after it was examined.

A method. If the histology department is not open, and glass sealant cannot be obtained, simply place a cover slip over the fluid and seal the edges with fingernail polish.

If a specific finding has been noticed, but its position cannot be noted because the microscope has no coordinates, simply take a wax crayon and mark the *bottom* of the slide, in the beam of the light, so that the interesting field can be quickly relocated.

Never mark the top of the slide, especially if it is a Gram or acid-fast stain.

A Field Finder slide can be purchased from Lovins Engineering Company in Silver Spring, Maryland. This is simply a glass slide, the same size as the standard microscope slide, with an imprinted grid. This can be placed on top of the examined slide. Each square of the grid has an identifying number visible under the microscope but not interfering with the view. (If the specimen slide does not have a frosted labeling surface, be sure to mark an end for orientation.)

Three-Glass Test

In males, the microscopic examination of the urine for pus can be made more diagnostic by collecting the specimen in three glasses or containers. The stream is started in the first container, then moved to the second container, then completed in the third container, all without stopping the stream.

In urethritis, the pus is predominantly or exclusively in the first glass; in prostatitis, in the first and third glasses; and in bladder and kidney infections, in all three glasses.

Crystals

Calcium oxalate dihydrate crystals (Fig. 28-3) occur in normal urine. These resemble little diamonds, and in three dimensions are actually octahedrons (double pyramids, placed base to base). They *may* also be seen in the urine of patients with ethylene glycol intoxication.

If the oxalate is excreted in the form of calcium oxalate monohydrate, it may appear in the form of urate-like needles and other thin crystal forms as shown on the left in Figure 28-3. These have in the past been called "hippurate crystals." In ethylene glycol poisoning, they may occur in huge numbers, alone or mixed with the calcium oxalate dihydrate octahedrons (Terlinsky et al., 1981).

Urate crystals (in acid urine) and phosphate crystals (in alkaline urine) are not helpful. They can even be predicted from the urine pH.

Red Blood Cell Casts

In an unstained urine, red cell casts appear as orange translucent casts, the same size and shape as the more frequently seen types of casts. They are not red, like red cells, but clearly orange. Once seen, they will never be confused with anything else.

The presence of red cell casts signifies glomerulitis (glomerulonephritis, antigen-antibody complex disease as in infectious endocarditis, etc.) until proven otherwise. They may also be

seen in bleeding into the lumen of the nephron as in polycystic kidney disease. They are *never* normal.

Fat Embolization

Fat embolization is often accompanied by fat droplets in the urine, which may be detected with any supravital fat stain, such as Sudan III (see also p. 554).

Oval Fat Bodies

Oval fat bodies are degenerative tubular cells that have sloughed into the urine. In some, but not all, patients with nephrotic syndrome there is a hyperlipoproteinemia causing the tubular cell, through incompletely understood mechanisms, to undergo fatty degeneration. When this fat crystallizes inside the sloughed cell, an oval fat body is created. This can be identified with a fat stain such as the Sudan III stain (discussed under stool fat stains on p. 554), or more simply with a pair of polarizing lenses (which can be carried in one's wallet).

A method (polarized light):

1. Obtain two polarizing lenses. These are simply two squares of polarizing paper, two pieces of polarizing glass, or two glass polarizing lenses (obtainable from American Optical). In dire straits, the two lenses from a pair of polaroid sunglasses can be used.

2. Check that these are in fact polarizing by looking through them en face at a light source. As you rotate one upon the other through 90 degrees, there will be a change from complete transmittance of light to total black.

3. Place one of these lenses on top of the light source of the microscope, below the condenser. This one is called the "polarizer."

4. The other lens, called the "analyzer," can be placed anywhere between your eye and the stage containing the slide with the sample. In some microscopes, it is possible to disassemble the eyepieces and place the analyzer into the barrel of the scope. (This has the advantage of leaving your hands free, and of polarizing both eyepieces of a binocular microscope.) However, if this is not possible, you can always simply hold the analyzer between your eye and one of the eyepieces, and rotate it to see the light intensity change as before. (The change will not be complete because the light coming to your other eye through the other eyepiece is not passing through the analyzer.)

5. Turn the analyzer so that the field is very dark and the outline of cells can just barely be seen. Now scan the slide rapidly. Oval fat bodies, if present, will appear as bright lights, as will a lot of other refractile material that can be found in the urine.

If you think you have an oval fat body, rotate the analyzer. As the field becomes lighter, the oval fat body (or other refractile material) will be less bright; but as the field becomes darker, the oval fat body becomes lighter and brighter.

6. Focus on the suspected oval fat body. If it truly is an oval fat body, you will see four bright bands radiating out from the center, in alternation with four dark bands. The bright bands will emerge from the center at right angles to each other, forming what is called a "Maltese Cross" in medicine. (In heraldry, it is actually a formée cross (Webster, 1976), since the true Maltese Cross has notched ends, and the oval fat body does not.)

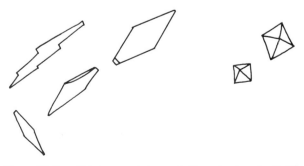

Figure 28-3. *Calcium oxalate crystal in urine (see text). The monohydrate of ethylene glycol poisoning is at the left, and the dihydrate is shown on the right.*

7. Any other small round crystal can give a false positive. Starch granules from surgical gloves are such good false positives that they can be used for teaching polarizing microscopy. Simply put some on a glass slide, and follow the steps above.*

8. This technique can also be used for crystals (see joint fluid, vide infra).

"Telescoped Urine"

This term has nothing to do with the optics of the telescope or a "far away" appearance to the urine, but rather to the mechanics of the old collapsible telescope or spyglass. It refers to urine in which the acute, subacute (if there is such), and chronic stages of a renal disease are all collapsed in time into the same urine sample. For example, the red cells and red cell casts of acute glomerulitis may accompany the broad, wide casts of chronic renal disease. "Telescoped urine" means that the patient has both acute and chronic renal failure.

Urinary Eosinophilia

Urinary eosinophilia was first advanced as a test for allergic interstitial nephritis, but has been faulted on two grounds: the absence of perfect diagnosticity and the relative inefficiency of Wright's stain as compared with Hansel's stain (Nolan et al., 1986).

Using the latter stain and accepting even 1% eosinophils as a positive test for eosinophilia, the differential diagnosis includes allergic interstitial nephritis, other acute interstitial nephritides, chronic interstitial nephritis, transplant rejection, rapidly progressive glomerulonephritis, eosinophilic cystitis, and (rarely) prostatitis. The test has been negative to date in acute bacterial pyelonephritis and acute tubular necrosis.

Other Body Fluids and Secretions

Joint Fluid Crystals

A Method

1. Place the joint fluid on a clean glass slide and cover it with a cover glass. (If it is to be saved, it should also be sealed as described on p. 550.)

2. Next search for crystals using polarized light (as described on p. 551).

3. If crystals are found, it will next be necessary to determine whether they are positively or negatively birefringent. This requires a first-order red compensator, which may be made quickly and cheaply as follows: Take a clean glass slide and put two layers of *good*-quality transparent tape in sequence on top of the slide. From below to above, you now have: glass slide, first layer of tape, second layer of tape.

---

*With the increasing use of starched gloves during procedures, this false positive has become a real problem (Kirkpatrick & Sirmon, 1989). The real oval fat bodies, however, occur in renal tubular epithelial cells, while the starch granules do not. Second, the starch granules, but not the oval fat bodies, will turn grey in unpolarized light if exposed to a drop of iodine solution (e.g., from the Gram stain kit). Finally, if one focuses up and down on the four arms of the cross, they will go in and out of focus simultaneously in the case of an oval fat body, but will focus asynchronously with this maneuver in the case of most starch granules.

This incredibly simple device has created a lot of difficulty for a large number of otherwise intelligent persons. First, you cannot use "frosty" or other nontransparent tapes. Second, one should use a clean glass slide and clean (nonoily) fingers. Accept no creases or bubbles. One is building a crystal; grease, dirt, poor-quality materials, and other optical aberrances will destroy the device. Finally, be sure to use *broad* tape for best results. (If light can go around the edge of the crystal, the optical result will be impure.)

4. Place the first-order red compensator on top of the polarizer in the same orientation as the crystal that you are inspecting in the fluid (e.g., if the crystal goes from right to left [east to west], the first-order red compensator must be placed with its ends pointing in that same axis). Look at the *background* color of the field. The goal is a color that is variously described as magenta, pink, red, or even rust. If the background is blue or green, you can change it by lifting up the first-order red compensator, and rotating the polarizer beneath it about 90 degrees. After doing this, replace the first-order red compensator in the same axis as the crystal being inspected, and recheck the background color. (You may also have to rotate the analyzer to some degree.) Repeat this adjustment in decreasing degrees of rotation until you have the strongest red (or pink or magenta) that you can obtain.

5. Now look at the crystal. If it is yellow (negatively birefringent), it is a monosodium urate monohydrate crystal, and the diagnosis is gout. If it is blue (positively birefringent), it is a calcium pyrophosphate dihydrate crystal, and the diagnosis is pseudogout.

False Positives

Joint fluid stored in Becton-Dickinson lithium heparin tubes may contain crystals of lithium heparin, which will also be positively birefringent (blue in step 5). Triamcinolone acetate crystals in the joint fluid, either from prior therapeutic injections or from withdrawing the joint fluid through a needle or syringe that is potentially contaminated with triamcinolone acetate, will also appear blue. Cholesterol crystals from joints afflicted with rheumatoid arthritis ("gold paint" effusion) may appear blue, but these are almost never needle-shaped crystals, but rather broad notched rhomboid plates. Rarely, hydroxyapatite crystals may be seen in monocytes of synovial fluid from patients experiencing acute arthritis or exacerbations of osteoarthritis (although usually hydroxyapatite appears in chunks). These could be confused with either urate or calcium pyrophosphate, as hydroxyapatite crystals are both positively and negatively birefringent (Schumacher et al., 1977).

6. As a double check, you can rotate the compensator slide or the polarizer to give a blue-green background (i.e., by 90 degrees). Gout crystals that were yellow will now appear blue, and previously blue crystals will now appear yellow (Gatter, 1977).

Unstained Sputum

Gross Findings

Three-layered sputum (lipid foam, water, and cellular debris, from top to bottom) is diagnostic of retained lung secretions and purulent exudate where clearance is impaired (e.g., lung abscess or, rarely, saccular bronchiectasis).

Actinomycosis produces sulfur granules and "cayenne pepper seeds."

Of all the causes of hemoptysis, pulmonary infarction alone produces (rarely) "currant jelly."

Microscopic Findings

1. Under *low power*, one can identify macrophages (about 30 μm) and Curschmann spirals. Macrophages guarantee that the sputum is alveolar. Curschmann spirals, which are mucous plug casts of bronchioles, probably make the diagnosis of bronchial asthma.

2. Under *high dry*, one can better identify macrophages, which are usually filled with ingested debris. In smokers, the debris is often the color of a fine maduro wrapper.

One can also see Charcot-Leyden crystals (which are diagnostic of bronchial asthma) and not be concerned that one is looking at precipitated dye.

Finally, one can identify polymorphonuclear neutrophils (which indicate infection) by their multilobed nuclei. These may be distinguished from other cells with two-lobed nuclei and very large granules. The latter are eosinophils and suggest the presence of allergic diseases such as bronchial asthma.

3. Other interesting findings include the lipid-laden macrophages of lipoid pneumonia and the ciliated bronchial epithelium. The latter is seen with severe coughing from asthma or viral upper respiratory infection (Epstein, 1972).

Quellung Reaction

1. Pneumococci may be diagnosed on an unstained sputum smear by means of the Quellung reaction, provided that one has put away a supply of polyvalent antipneumococcal antiserum. Such slides may even be carried around dry (M. Mufson, personal communication, 1976).

2. Place 1 drop of the serum on the slide. Pneumococci only and always will exhibit the characteristic swelling.

Gram Stain

Invented by Henry Christian Gram to improve the visibility of bacteria in tissue sections, this stain has been adapted to the bacteriologic examination of a variety of body fluids, exudates, and even the buffy coat. Gram actually used aniline gentian violet instead of crystal violet, and he used no counter stain. So, the answer to the question, "Who invented the Gram stain (as we presently do it)?" is—not Gram!

A Method (after Kolmer, 1944; Todd & Sanford 1948)

1. Smear a generous amount of the material on a clean glass slide with the labeled side up.

2. Allow the material to air dry, and then fix it by passing it through a flame a few times. It is not necessary or desirable to charbroil the material.

3. Apply the crystal violet stain for 1 minute if you are using a 1.4% solution in a 1:4 mixture of 95% ethanol and 1% aqueous ammonium oxalate. If you use a 2% solution of crystal violet in methanol, you only have to stain for 30 seconds. (With stronger staining solutions, only 10 seconds may be necessary for each step.)

4. Wash off *gently* with tap water. If you are having trouble with understaining (as when using weak solutions), you may wish to just pour off the stain and omit the rinsing with tap wa-

ter. If your stains are coming out with pale blue or red pneumococci, be sure to leave the stain on for a full minute.

5. Add Gram's iodine (made by dissolving 1 g of iodine and 2 g of a potassium iodide in 300 ml of distilled water) for at least 30 seconds (or at least until the smear appears black.)

6. Decolorize the Gram-negative bacteria by applying the decolorizer (acetone, ethanol, or a 1:1 mixture of the two) until no further blue stain floats off the slide. This can take from 15 seconds to 2 minutes. (Overdecolorizing* is usually not the result of leaving the decolorizer on too long, but to the deterioration of the iodine solution in step 5 due to light exposure. It may be rejuvenated with a pinch of baking soda.)

7. Wash with tap water and counterstain with 1% safranin (10 ml of saturated alcoholic safranin solution in 90 ml of water) for at least 30 seconds and preferably for 1 minute if you wish to see the hemophilus coccobacillus lying in the proteinaceous background. (Actually, you can use almost anything for the counterstain, even the carbol-fuchsin from the acid-fast stain kit.)

8. Wash with tap water, dry, and observe. The nuclei of leukocytes should be red, not blue as with the Wright's stain. If they are blue, you left the crystal violet on for too long or the decolorizer not enough. The stain may be variable in different regions of the slide, and the same coccus may be negative in one area and positive in another, so use the leukocyte nucleus color as a local control.

Pleural Fluid: Selected Topics

1. The diagnosis of tuberculous pleural effusion is often missed because the few antigenic tubercle bacilli that set off the allergic effusion are usually not found. To overcome this problem, let the fluid sit for a time, and a pellicle will form at the top of the fluid. This coagulum may actually contain the tubercle bacilli.

2. It is said that the pleural effusion of tuberculosis is *never* accompanied by mesothelial cells; however, exceptions have been seen (Light et al., 1973).

3. To determine whether anatomically deformed lymphatics are contributing to the formation of body fluids, such as a rapidly reaccumulating pleural effusion, have the patient eat a few ice cream cones before the next thoracentesis, and see whether the fluid becomes lactescent. Opalescence due to a chylous effusion (as opposed to debris) can be extracted into ether. (Don't forget that ether is flammable or explosive.) The same trick works with ascitic fluid.

Ascitic Fluid

Gram stain of the buffy coat of ascitic fluid is invaluable in the diagnosis of a disease notoriously difficult to diagnose: spontaneous bacterial peritonitis. Here, the sensitivity is 55% (Hoefs & Runyon, 1985). For comparison, only 24% of such patients are culture positive on admission!

The advantage of the test is not only that it makes the diagnosis, but it also provides instantaneous morphologic information useful in providing guidance for immediate therapy.

---

*Manifested by all red organisms—even the pneumococcus!

Cerebrospinal Fluid

Subarachnoid Hemorrhage Versus Traumatic Taps

Subarachnoid hemorrhage is characterized by blood in the cerebrospiral fluid (CSF), but so is a traumatic tap. If the blood clears by the time the third or fourth tube is collected, traumatic tap is the diagnosis, while if the supernatant is xanthochromic, the blood has been in the CSF for at least 12 hours, or is present in large quantities.

There are equivocal cases, in which the measurement of a CSF bilirubin will be helpful since in a traumatic tap the blood will not have had time to be metabolized by the reticuloendothelial cells into bilirubin (the source of the xanthochromia of the crude test above). *Caveats*: 1) This test does not work in jaundiced patients, who have bilirubin in the CSF on that account. 2) You must determine some normal CSF bilirubins to get the baseline normal "ceiling" for each laboratory. This value is about 0.40 mg/dl, but varies from automated laboratory to laboratory, and even between machines and methods in those laboratories that have more than one machine or method for the automated determination of bilirubin.

A Weekend Method for Concentrating CSF Cells

This method is useful if the cytospin is not available on the weekend when the patient has his lumbar puncture.

1. Take a glass slide and mark a target area about 1 cm in diameter (the inner diameter of the rubber washer to be used in step 3) on the *bottom* of the slide with a wax pencil.

2. Take a piece of bibulous paper and cut a hole that matches the size of the target. Cover the slide with the paper, with the hole over the target area (Fig. 28-4).

3. Place a rubber washer on top of the hole in the paper.

4. Place the fluid in a 3-ml syringe from which the plunger has been removed.

5. Place the syringe over the rubber washer. (You may want

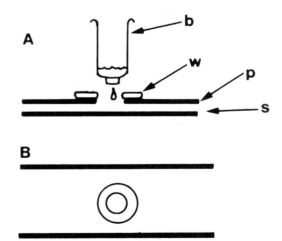

Figure 28-4. *Apparatus required for concentrating CSF cells. A, Side view: b = barrel of the syringe; w = washer, with a section taken through the center; p = paper; and s = glass slide. The paper appears not to be touching the slide, but in practice lies right on top of it. B, Top view with the syringe removed. The "doughnut" is the washer. The center of the doughnut would be glass, and all the area peripheral to it would be paper over glass.*

to clamp this all together, on a ring stand, for instance.) Allow the fluid to drip down into the well made by the rubber washer. The liquid will freely diffuse laterally through the bibulous paper, leaving the cells in the well, just over the spot marked by the crayon. The protein in the CSF will fix the cells to the glass. If the fluid is not to be stained immediately, it can be refrigerated and stained by the technician on Monday morning.

Plasma cells are seen in the CSF in myeloma, brain abscess, cerebral metastases, and after and during aseptic meningitis (Bosch & Oehmichen, 1976; Glasser et al., 1977; Manconi et al., 1978; Sato et al., 1986).

Eosinophilia of the CSF, an unusual finding, may be due to parasitic infections. Other less common causes include fungal meningitis (*Coccidiodes immitis*); meningitis due to mycobacteria, *Treponema pallidum*, or rickettsia; malignancy (lymphoma); allergic reaction to foreign bodies; and the hypereosinophilic syndrome. Recently it has been described in neurosarcoidosis (Scott, 1988).

Fat Staining

Fat staining of the CSF is a good way to diagnose fat embolism (Cross, 1965). (Also see urine, p. 551; however, fat staining of the sputum gives a large number of false positives.)

The use of glucose detection tape for diagnosing cerebrospinal fluid rhinorrhea is discussed in Chapter 12 (p. 218).

Stool Examination for Pancreatic and Small-Bowel Malabsorption

A Method

1. Smear a smidgen of stool (e.g., from the rectal examination) on a glass slide.

2. Mix 1 drop of glacial acetic acid into it.

3. Add 1 drop of a fat stain. (Sudan III, Sudan IV, or scarlet red have all been used; I use the first.)

4. Place a cover slip on top of the mixture and *gently* heat over a flame (or in the microwave oven) so that any fatty acids present will melt. If using a flame, take care not to smoke the slide, or boil it, or ignite the alcohol in the stain. The student handling the slide should resemble Koch more than the Statue of Liberty.

5. Allow the slide to cool for about 10 minutes. This will let any (unstained) fatty acids crystallize out as thin needles, usually in bunches. (On the other hand, the triglycerides will be stained with Sudan III as round orange globules, provided you did not burn the slide.)

Interpretation

1. If one sees *only* fatty acid crystals, the diarrhea is due to intestinal insufficiency, since the pancreatic enzymes have digested the triglycerides into fatty acids, but the fatty acids have not been absorbed.

2. If there are large numbers (more than 12 per high power field at high-dry) of orange globules, one is dealing with pancreatic insufficiency. (In this situation, colonic bacteria may metabolize *some* of the triglycerides into fatty acids, which are not absorbed by the colon. However, the predominant form is still the orange globule.)

With pancreatic insufficiency, two double checks are available. First, in addition to insufficient lipase, there is undoubtedly insufficient luminal carboxypeptidase. In that case, dietary meat fibers (muscle fibers) may be seen in the stool.

Muscle fibers may also be seen in the stool of patients who masticate poorly, but these fibers will have rounded ends (where the pancreatic carboxypeptidase has attempted to compensate for insufficient maceration), whereas with pancreatic insufficiency the meat fibers will have sharp ragged edges (indicating that mastication was good but not much further happened in the lumen of the gut.)

If the muscle fibers are only of the skeletal type (nonbranching), the patient has been eating the better cuts of meat. But if the muscle fibers are branched (as in smooth muscle and heart muscle), the patient has been eating the cheaper cuts of meat, such as chitlings, sausages, and salamis other than andouille. It is amazing how many people will bet that you cannot "guess" what kind of meat the patient had the day before he entered the hospital.

The second check for pancreatic insufficiency is that microscopic octahedral starch crystals (which can possibly be confused with sardine scales) will appear in the stool. When in doubt, add a drop of Lugol's solution or Gram's iodine to a smidgen of stool. Only starch crystals will appear grey-black (Todd & Sanford, 1948).

False Negatives

While some persons have such minimal disease that it may not be detected by this method, others have been taught in the school of experience that certain foods produce symptoms, and so have altered their dietary intake to avoid the offending materials, often unconsciously. Obviously, if nothing has gone into the top of the tube, you won't be able to detect anything at the bottom of the tube. Accordingly, one should arrange for a hasty food emporium to provide a few preparatory meals consisting of a burger (for meat fibers), an order of fries (for the starch granules), and a shake (for the triglycerides).

Similarly, this screening test should be performed before the barium enema. The latter does not alter the physiology, but so adulterates and displaces the native stool that nothing can be seen under the microscope but the bland and boring lunar terrain of barium salts.

Another type of false negative occurs in protein-losing enteropathy, in which the tests, including the one for meat fibers, will be completely negative. In these diseases (such as Menetrier's disease), the gut is losing only protein molecules, which cannot be seen microscopically. The pancreatic hydrolytic function and the absorptive function are both intact, but the absorptive function is overwhelmed by the outpouring of fluid.

False Positives

The use of suppositories, mineral oil, and dietetic salad dressing may all cause false positives for triglycerides.

A caveat. Until one gains some experience with this test it may be necessary to compare results with a quantitative stool fat determination. The correlation is excellent (Drummey et al., 1961). Alternately, one could learn at the elbow of one who has done the test, but since the paper heralding the rediscovery of this technique is already older than most residents, such instruction is rarely available.

Vaginal Secretions

The examination of vaginal secretions for infection is discussed in Chapter 22 (see Table 22-1, p. 403).

Ice Water Test for Pericardial Disease

Following the ingestion of 750 ml of ice water, normal subjects and patients with heart disease (regardless of cardiac enlargement) show (at 3 to 5 minutes) a decrease in the T-wave amplitude in leads 2, 3, and aVF, and an increase of T-wave amplitude in aVL, aVR, V-1, V-2, and V-4. This normal effect of cold stimulation on the T-wave vector is minimal or absent in subjects in whom the heart muscle is thermally insulated by fluid, inflammation, or pericardial thickening (Friedman & McClure, 1962).

References

Abernathy MR: Incidence of Döhle bodies in physiologic and pathologic conditions. *Lab Digest* 28:3–5, 1964.

Abernathy MR: Döhle bodies associated with uncomplicated pregnancy. *Blood* 27:380–385, 1966.

Anonymous: Mitoxantrone. *Med Lett Drugs Ther* 30:67–68, 1988.

Auer J: Some hitherto undescribed structures found in large lymphocytes of an acute leukemia. *Am J Med Sci* 131:1002–1015, 1906.

Bachman RW, Lucke BH: The differential blood count, the Arneth formula, and Doehle's inclusion bodies in pulmonary tuberculosis. *NY Med J* 107:492–495, 1918.

Beard MEJ, Weintraub LW: Hypersegmented neutrophil granulocytes in iron deficiency anemia. *Br J Haematol* 16:161–163, 1969.

Bosch I, Oehmichen M: [Diagnostic significance of plasma cells in the cerebrospinal fluid, special reference to their demonstration in brain abscess]. *Nervenarzt* 47:618–622, 1976.

Braude AI, Berkowitz H: Detection of urinary catalase by disk flotation. *J Lab Clin Med* 57:490–494, 1961.

Broder JN: The ferric chloride screening test. *Ann Emerg Med* 16:1188, 1987.

Brooks GF, Pribble AH, Beaty HN: Early diagnosis of bacteremia by buffy coat examinations. *Arch Intern Med* 132:673–675, 1973.

Bush FW, Bailey FR: The treatment of meningococcus infections with especial reference to the Waterhouse-Friderichsen [*sic.*] syndrome. *Ann Intern Med* 20:619–631, 1944.

Cassidei L, Dell'Atti A, Sciacovelli O: Improvement of the FeCl₃ test for phenylpyruvic acid. *Clin Chim Acta* 90:121–127, 1978.

Clarkson AR: Phenistix in screening. *Aust Fam Physician* 7:1324–1328, 1978.

Clyne LP, White PF: Time dependency of lupuslike anticoagulants. *Arch Intern Med* 148:1060–1063, 1988.

Cross HE: Examination of CSF in fat embolism. *Arch Intern Med* 115:470–474, 1965.

Daland GA, Gottlieb L, Wallerstein RO, Castle WB: Hematologic observations in bacterial endocarditis. *J Lab Clin Med* 48:827–845, 1956.

Drummey GD, Benson JA, Jones CM: Microscopic examination of the stool for steatorrhea. *N Engl J Med* 264:85–87, 1961.

Epstein RL: Constituents of sputum: A simple method. *Ann Intern Med* 77:259–265, 1972.

Finlay HVL: Phenistix urine test strip and desferrioxamine. *Br Med J* 2:356, 1978.

Freeman JA: The ultrastructure and genesis of Auer bodies. *Blood* 15:449–465, 1960.

xxxx xxxx

Friedman B, McClure HH: A simple bloodless and painless presumptive test for pericardial fluid and thickening. *Am J Med Sci* 244:321–333, 1962.

Frommeyer WB, Epstein RD: Hemorrhagic diseases. In: Ham TH (ed),

A Syllabus of laboratory Examinations in Clinical Diagnosis. Harvard University Press, Cambridge, 1957.

Gagnon M, Hunting WM, Esselen WB: New method for catalase determination. *Anal Chem* 31:144, 1959

Gatter RA: Use of the compensated polarizing microscope. *Clin Rheum Dis* 3:91-103, 1977. [This is the best single source on all facets of this subject.]

Ghossein NA, Bosworth JL, Stacey P, Muggia FM, Krishnaswamy V: Radiation-related eosinophilia. *Radiology* 117:413-417, 1975.

Glasser, L, Payne, C, and Corrigan, JJ, Jr: The in vivo development of plasma cells: A morphologic study of human cerebrospinal fluiud. *Neurology* 27:448-459, 1977.

Granger J, Pole CK: The inclusion bodies in scarlet fever. *Bri J Child Dis* 10:9-16, 1913.

Greenberg MS: Earlobe histiocytosis as a clue to the diagnosis of subacute bacterial endocarditis. *Ann Intern Med* 61:124-127, 1964.

Ham TH, Shwachman H, Hills AG: Proteins of plasma and serum—sedimentation rate of red cells. In: Ham (ed), *A Syllabus of Laboratory Examinations in Clinical Diagnosis.* Harvard University Press, Cambridge, 1957.

Hill RW, Bayrd ED: Phagocytic reticuloendothelial cells in subacute bacterial endocarditis with negative cultures. *Ann Intern Med* 52:310-319, 1960.

Hoefs JC, Runyon BA: Spontaneous bacterial peritonitis. *DM* 31(9):1-48, 1985.

Humphrey AA: Use of the buffy layer in the rapid diagnosis of septicemia. *Am J Clin Pathol* 14:358-362, 1944.

Hynes M, Whitby EH: Correction of the sedimentation rate for anemia. *Lancet* 2:249-251, 1938.

Jain NC, Cox C, Bennett JM: Auer rods in the acute myeloid leukemias: Frequency and methods of demonstration. *Hematol Oncol* 5:197-202, 1987.

James GP, DJang MH, Hamilton HH: False-negative results for urinary phenothiazines and imipramine in Forrest's qualitative assays. *Clin Chem* 26:345-347, 1980.

Juneja HS, Rajaraman S, Alperin JB, Bainton DF: Auer rod-like inclusions in prolymphocytic leukemia. *Acta Haematol* 77:115-119, 1987.

Kirkpatrick WG, Sirmon MD: Pseudocrystalluria and pseudolipiduria. *Am J Med* 87:242, 1989.

Kirschbaum BB: Evaluation of a colorimetric reagent strip assay for urine specific gravity. *Am J Clin Pathol* 79:722-725, 1983.

Kjeldsberg CR, Hershgold EJ: Spurious thrombocytopenia. *JAMA* 227:628-630, 1974.

Kolmer JA: *Clinical Diagnosis by Laboratory Examinations* (ed 1, revised). Appleton-Century, New York, 1944.

Lamon J, With TK, Redeker AG: The Hoesch test: Bedside screening for urinary porphobilinogen in patients with suspected porphyria. *Clin Chem* 20:1438-1440, 1974.

Laurell C-B, Waldenstrom J: Sera with exceptional appearance and the euglobulin reaction as screen test. *Acta Med Scand* [Suppl] 367:97-100, 1961.

Leavell BS, Twomey J: Possible leukemoid reaction in disseminated tuberculosis: Report of a case with auer rods. *Trans Am Clin Climatol Assoc* 75:166-174, 1964.

Lee RI, White PD: A clinical study of the coagulation time of the blood. *Am J Med Sci* 165:495-503, 1913.

Light RW, Erozan YS, Ball WC Jr: Cells in pleural fluid: Their value in differential diagnosis. *Arch Intern Med* 132:854-860, 1973.

Mahood WH, Killough JH: Acute intermittent porphyria: A clinical and laboratory study of a large family. *Ann Intern Med* 64:259-267, 1966.

Manconi PE, Marrosu MG, Spissu A, Todde PF, Ferelli A: Plasma cell reaction in cerebrospinal fluid: an additional case report. *Neurology* 28:856-857, 1978.

McLean S, Caffey J: Endemic purpuric meningococcus bacteremia in early life. *Am J Dis Child* 42:1053-1074, 1931.

Medical Research Council Steering Committee for the MRC/DHSS Phenylketonuria Register: Routine neonatal screening for phenylketonuria in the United Kingdom 1964-1978. *Br Med J* 282:1680-1684, 1981.

Miller A, Green G, Robinson D: Simple rule for calculating normal erythrocyte sedimentation rate. *Br Med J* 286:266, 1983.

Nolan CR, Anger MS, Kelleher SP: Eosinophiluria: A new method of detection and definition of the clinical spectrum. *N Engl J Med* 315:1516-1519, 1986.

Peterson LC, Rao KV, Crosson JT, White JG: Fechtner syndrome—a variant of Alport's syndrome with leukocyte inclusions and acanthocytosis. *Blood* 65:397-406, 1985.

Pierach CA, Cardinal R, Bossenmaier I, Watson CJ: Comparison of the Hoesch and the Watson-Schwartz tests for urinary porphobilinogen. *Clin Chem* 23:1666-1668, 1977.

Powers DL, Mandell GL: Intraleukocytic bacteria in endocarditis patients. *JAMA* 227:312-313, 1974.

Pruzanski W, Watt JG: Serum viscosity and hyperviscosity syndrome in IgG multiple myeloma. *Ann Intern Med* 77:553-560, 1972.

Rappaport ES, Helbert B, Beissner RS, Trowbridge A: Automated hematology: Where we stand. *South Med J* 81:365370, 1988.

Raymond JR, Yarger WE: Abnormal urine color: Differential diagnosis. *South Med J* 81:837-841, 1988.

Sapira JD, Shapiro AP: Beta-glucuronidase excretion in hypertensive patients. *Am J Med Sci* 253:174-179, 1967.

Sapira JD, Somani S, Shapiro AP, Scheib ET, Reihl W: Some observations concerning mammalian indoxyl metabolism and its relationship to the formation of urinary indigo pigments. *Metabolism* 20:474-486, 1971.

Sato Y, Mizoguchi K, Ohta Y: [Abnormal cerebrospinal fluid plasma cells in a case of myeloma]. *No To Shinkei* 38:399-403, 1986.

Schumacher PR, Smolyo AP, Tse RL, Maurer K: Arthritis associated with apatite crystals. *Ann Intern Med* 87:411-416, 1977.

Scott TF: A new cause of cerebrospinal fluid eosinophilia: Neurosarcoidosis. *Am J Med* 84:973-974, 1988.

Sia RHP: A simple method for estimating quantitative differences in the globulin precipitation test in kala-azar. *China Med J* 38:34-43, 1924.

Siddiqui J, Freeburger R, Freeman RM: Folic acid, hypersegmented polymorphonuclear leukocytes and the uremic syndrome. *Am J Clin Nutr* 23:11-16, 1970.

Smith H: *Principles of Renal Physiology.* Oxford University Press, New York, 1956.

Smith H: The prevalence and diagnostic significance of "histiocytes" and phagocytic mononuclear cells in peripheral blood films. *Med J Aust* 2:205-210, 1964.

Smith H: Leucocytes containing bacteria in plain blood films from patients with septicemia. *Australas Ann Med* 15:210-221, 1966.

Smithline N, Gardner KD Jr: Gaps—anionic and osmolal. *JAMA* 236:1594-1597, 1976.

Snapper I, Kahn AI: *Bedside Medicine*, ed 2. Grune & Stratton, New York, 1967.

Stanton PE Jr, Evans JR, Lefemine AA, Vo NM, Rannick GA, Morgan CV Jr, Hinton PJ, Read M: White clot syndrome. *South Med J* 81:616-620, 1988.

Terlinsky AS, Grochowski J, Geoly KL, Stauch BS, Hefter L: Identification of atypical calcium oxalate crystalluria following ethylene glycol ingestion. *Am J Clin Pathol* 76:223-226, 1981.

Thomas HM: Meningococcic meningitis and septicemia. *JAMA* 123:265-272, 1943.

Todd JC, Sanford AH: *Clinical Diagnosis by Laboratory Methods*, ed 11. WB Saunders, Philadelphia, 1948.

Toomey JA, Gammel JA: Scarlet fever: V. Amato bodies in scarlet fever. *Am J Dis Child* 34:841-844, 1927.

Townsend JD: An evaluation of a recent modification of the Watson-Schwartz test for porphobilinogen. *Ann Intern Med* 60:306-307, 1964.

Van Nuys F: An extraordinary blood: The presence of atypical phagocytic cells. *Boston Med Surg J* 156:390, 1907.

Waldron JM, Duncan GG: Variability of the rate of coagulation of whole blood. *Am J Med* 17:365-373, 1954.

Webster's Third New International Dictionary. G & C Merriam Co, Springfield, MA, 1976.

Wintrobe MM: *Clinical Hematology*, ed 6. Lea & Febiger, Philadelphia, 1967.

Yamaguchi Y, Hayashi C: Simple determination of high urinary excretion of 5-hydroxyindole-3-acetic acid with ferric chloride. *Clin Chem* 24:149–150, 1978.

29
General References

"You go back to the classics of a subject for the practical purpose of saving yourself a lot of work. You get an accumulation of observation, method, and technique that subsequent experience has confirmed, and you can take it at second-hand and don't have to work it all out afresh for yourself. Maybe you can improve on it, here and there, and that is all right, but if you don't know the classics of your subject, you often find that you have been wasting a lot of time over something that somebody went all through, clear back in the Middle Ages . . .

. . . When I was at Ems a couple of years ago, one of their experimenters had just discovered that the Ems salts helped out a little in cases of pyorrhea. That was known four hundred years ago. It is mentioned in a report on the springs, written in the sixteenth century. Then it was forgotten, and discovered again only the other day."

Albert Jay Nock, *Pantagruelism*,
a speech to the faculty of medicine at Johns Hopkins
October 28, 1932, the 400th anniversary
of the publication of *Pantagruel*

"The work of M. Laennec is a book eminently practical, but we fear that its length can only be a great obstacle to its utility."

A French review by L. Rouzet, January 1820
cited in *Thorax* 36:487–492, 1981

Most of the following textbooks have been referred to throughout this work. They may be recommended, provided that the reader understands that each is faulted by undocumented statements, elision, or in many cases simply the passage of time. Nevertheless, each has its virtues.

Adams FD: *Physical Diagnosis*, ed 14. Williams & Wilkins, Baltimore, 1958, reprinted 1961, 962 pp. (This was the last version of the text originally written by Cabot [vide infra], until it was resurrected in 1974 by Burnside. The current incarnation of Cabot's original work can be read much more quickly than that available a quarter century ago, having only 223 pages versus 926 in the 1958 edition. But the pagination sequences indicate the decrepitude of American medical education regarding clinical examination.)

Alexander L: The neurologic examination. In: *Pullen's Medical Diagnosis*, last published in 1950. (This book is difficult to find. The present work makes use of some of the illustrations.)

"Bailey": Clain A (ed): *Hamilton Bailey's Demonstrations of Physical Signs in Clinical Surgery*, ed 15. Williams & Wilkins, Baltimore, 1973, 572 pp. (This is an example of a masterpiece that has outlived its author, and is still called "Bailey" even though Clain is now the editor. It is a benchmark work both in the quality of its illustrations and in the number of editions and sales. It is a true chrestomathy—it does not really teach a systematic approach, and the picture of examining equipment used within its pages does not even include a stethoscope [although this instrument is mentioned in the 16th edition], let alone an ophthalmoscope!)

Baker AB, Joynt RJ: *Clinical Neurology*, revised ed. Harper & Row, New York, 1986. ("Baker" remains a clearly written, authoritative description of neurologic diseases.)

Bauer J: *Differential Diagnosis of Internal Diseases*. Grune & Stratton, New York, 1967. (Another single-authored refutation of the notion that there is "too much knowledge" for one person to be broadly competent.)

Cabot RC: *Physical Diagnosis*, ed 11. William Wood & Co, Baltimore, 1934, 540 pp. (Cabot was a Harvard medical student rooming with a law student, who was rehearsing for mock trials. Cabot transferred the mock trial to medicine and thus concocted the CPC, the clinicopathologic conference. One of the best teaching devices ever invented, it is currently in eclipse because of its antinarcissistic effects and the intellectual demands it makes upon the participants.)

The first edition of this work came out in 1900. The last edition that Cabot wrote by himself was the 11th. I used this work well into the 1980s, until one day it grew legs and walked out of my office. In 1938, Cabot took a partner, FD Adams, who wrote the 13th edition by himself, *vide supra*.)

Cassell EJ: *Talking with Patients: Volume 2 Clinical Technique*. MIT Press, Cambridge, 1985. (An illustrative passage:

It is sad that even during the period when this crucial technique (interviewing) is being learned, most instructors never listen to their students taking an entire history. The reason usually given for this lapse in teaching is, of course, that the process takes so long. Can you imagine a surgeon saying that surgeons in training are not supervised for a whole operation because it takes too long?)

"Cope": Silen W (ed): *Cope's Early Diagnosis of the Acute Abdomen*, ed 15. Oxford University Press, New York, 1979, 280 pp. (The first edition by Sir Zachary Cope appeared in 1921; the book, like "Bailey," is happily outliving the author, who died in 1974. Although the posthumous edition has been revised by an American surgeon, William Silen, it is still known as "Cope." If American medical students were forced to use this book, it would probably modify their behavior as practitioners to the extent that millions of dollars could be saved annually in unnecessary presurgical studies. Acknowledged to be a classic by the medical literate, it reminds me of the wag's definition of a classic—something everybody should read, but no one does.)

DeGowin EL: *Bedside Diagnostic Examination*. Macmillan, New York, 1965, 687 pp. (DeGowin was the spiritual successor to Adams, but had the misfortune to appear just a few years before that revolution in American medical education (1968), which the present author views with such dismay. Due to the educational times, DeGowin never had the sales that it deserved. The most recent edition by Richard DeGowin (the father, Elmer, having died), has a slightly different format, which can make it hard to find things, but DeGowin was for two decades the benchmark for physical diagnosis texts.)

DeJong RN: *The Neurologic Examination*, ed 4. Harper & Row, New York 1979. (In less than 800 pages of clearly written text, here is everything you need to know.)

Dorland's Illustrated Medical Dictionary, ed 23. WB Saunders, Philadelphia, 1957.

Flexner A: *Medical Education in the United States and Canada*. A report to the Carnegie Foundation for the Advancement of Teaching, New York, 1910, 346 pp. (This is the famous Flexner report, which was reissued by the Carnegie Foundation in 1960. The Arno Press has a reprint edition issued in 1972 (ISBN 0-405-03952-2). The principles enunciated in part I still hold, although society has evolved sufficiently to make the special chapters on the medical education of women and "the Negro" obsolete. Conversely, the state-by-state descriptions of the medical schools, given in part II, that seemed quite laughable just 20 years ago, are in many instances now frighteningly accurate.)

Forgacs P: The functional basis of pulmonary sounds. *Chest* 73:399–405, 1978. (Forgacs cites his own classic studies.)

"French's": Hart FD (ed): *French's Index of Differential Diagnosis*, ed 12, 1,032 pp. John Wright and Sons, Bristol, 1985. (Affectionately known as "French's," this is a rather complete listing of the diagnostic possibilities for certain leading signs and symptoms. First published in 1912, its continued existence should serve as a refutation to those troglodytes who think medicine can be reduced to protocols.)

Friedberg CK: *Diseases of the Heart*, ed 2. WB Saunders, Philadelphia, 1956, 1,161 pp. (After all these years, this is still a better sourcebook for much clinical cardiology than the popular multiauthored texts which have succeeded it in time, but not in heuristic worth.)

Hillman RS, Goodell BW, Grundy SM, McArthur JR, Moller JH: *Clinical Skills: Interviewing, History Taking, and Physical Diagnosis*. McGraw-Hill, New York, 1981, 399 pp. (This book is strong on the interview, although the physical examination, in spots, is treated in a somewhat cavalier manner.)

Judge RD, Zuidema GD (eds): *Physical Diagnosis: A Physiologic Approach to the Clinical Examination* (ed 2). Little, Brown, Boston, 1963, 495 pp. (More recent editions, which include Dr. Faith Fitzgerald's contributions, represent a great improvement.)

Leopold SS: *The Principles and Methods of Physical Diagnosis*. WB Saunders, Philadelphia, 1952, 430 pp. (A great deal of Norris and Landis [vide infra] went into this much shorter work.)

"Major": Delp MH, Manning RT (eds): *Major's Physical Diagnosis*. WB Saunders, Philadelphia, 1975, 759 pp. (Anything with Major's name on it is well written. The decline in this work's popularity is more a reflection on the changing audience than on the new editors.)

Morgan WL Jr, Engel GL: *The Clinical Approach to the Patient*. WB Saunders, Philadelphia, 1969. (Although this is not much of a physical diagnosis book—nor does it claim to be—for explication and emphasis of those clinical and interpersonal skills needed by the junior clerk, this book still has no peer.)

Norris G, Landis HRM: *Diseases of the Chest*, ed 6. WB Saunders, Philadelphia, 1938, 1,019 pp. (This is actually a textbook of physical diagnosis confined to the lungs and heart. The authors produced over 1,000 referenced, well-written, well-organized, practical pages on the physical examination of those two organs. This work was highly scientific for its time, and when compared with contemporary physical

diagnosis texts, is still rather scholarly. Note that the date of publication preceded the phonocardiogram, so all of the cardiac auscultation graphics consist of what the authors heard and taught.)

Perloff JK: *Physical Examination of the Heart and Circulation*. WB Saunders, Philadelphia, 1982, 278 pp. (This work is so good that it makes other medical writers jealous. Its strength is that the author has actually done that which he writes about and is not merely repeating what others have written. Further, he has the perspective required to deal effectively yet gracefully with some of the silliness of physical examination pedantry, and the writing skill to do so briefly. There are also excellent references to the works of others, but not so many as to make the style tedious.)

Pinel P: *The Clinical Training of Doctors: An Essay of 1793*, edited and translated with an introductory essay by DB Weiner. Johns Hopkins University Press, Baltimore, 1980, 102 pp. (An essay of 1793, lost for decades because of a series of historic accidents. Its timeliness is uncanny. This is the same Pinel who is better known, though erroneously, for taking the chains off patients in the Bicetre asylum.)

Prior JA, Silberstein JS: *Physical Diagnosis*. CV Mosby, St. Louis, 1959, 388 pp. (Recent editions have been much improved by Havener's chapter on ophthalmoscopy.)

Roberts HJ: *Difficult Diagnosis: A Guide to the Interpretation of Obscure Illness*. WB Saunders, Philadelphia, 1958, 913 pp. (This one-author tour de force is an example of the outstanding thinking available to medical students of my generation. The author never published a second edition. A present multiauthored volume of the same name is less useful except to illustrate that whereas formerly there was not "too much knowledge" for one person to master, presently there may be too many "experts" to permit breadth and perspective in a medical work.)

Sapira JD, Cherubin CE: *Drug Abuse*. American Elsevier, New York, 1975. (A useful guide to medical diseases of the drug abuser.)

Snapper I, Kahn AI: *Bedside Medicine*, ed 2. Grune & Stratton, New York, 1967. (This text is referred to as "Snapper" because he was the famous sole author of the first edition of this work. Kahn was the silent junior author acknowledged at the time of the second edition. This text is a masterpiece of clinical detective work utilizing the disease concept, with emphasis on knowing the natural history of the disease, the history of the patient, and the physical findings.)

Stern TN: *Clinical Examination*. Yearbook Medical Publishers, Chicago, 1964. (Since one may now be a diplomate of both the National Board of Medical Examiners and the American Board of Internal Medicine with no external evaluation of one's clinical examination skills, pleasant single-author books like this one, once so plentiful, have disappeared, there being so little audience for them. The professors of my medical school were apparently right when they predicted that the disease would replace the patient as the focal point of university medicine. See also Altschule MD: *Essays on the Rise and Decline of Bedside Medicine*. Lea & Febiger for Tots Gap Medical Research Laboratories, Inc., Philadelphia, 1989.)

Stevenson I: *The Diagnostic Interview*, ed 2. Harper & Row, New York, 1971, 273 pp. (A single volume that effectively instructs in both interviewing and history taking. Highly recommended for the person who wishes to be a physician rather than a "health care provider.")

Wiener SL, Nathanson M. (This refers to a series of articles that appeared in the journal *Medical Times* during the winter-spring of 1976–1977. This series was abstracted from a full-length manuscript about frequently observed errors in the history and physical. While a very brief version of this work also appeared in *JAMA*, as far as I can determine, the complete manuscript was never published.)

Wood P: *Diseases of the Heart and Circulation*, ed 2. JB Lippincott, Philadelphia, 1956, or ed 3, 1968, 1,161 pp. (The third edition was actually produced as a labor of love by his former students and colleagues, but the second edition was written only by Wood.)

And so here, O Reader, has the time come for us two to part. Toilsome was our journey together; not without offence; but it is done. To me thou wert as a beloved shade, the disembodied or not yet embodied spirit of a Brother. To thee I was but as a Voice. Yet was our relation a kind of sacred one; doubt not that! For whatsoever once sacred things become hollow jargons, yet while the Voice of Man speaks with Man, hast thou not there the living fountain out of which all sacredness sprang and will yet spring? Man, by the nature of him, is definable as "an incarnated Word." Ill stands it with me if I have spoken falsely; thine also it was to hear truly. Farewell. (Carlyle, *The French Revolution*, Finis)

Good night, gentlemen. *Perdonatemi*, and don't be thinking too much about my faults, since you are not in the habit of giving any too much thought to your own. (Rabelais, *First Book of the Pantagruel*)

Index